51.99

369 0276928

51.99

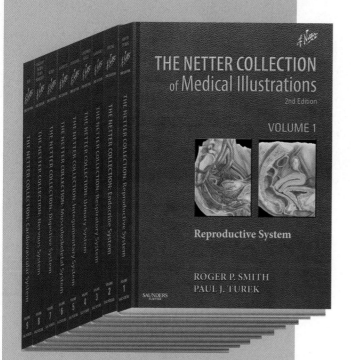

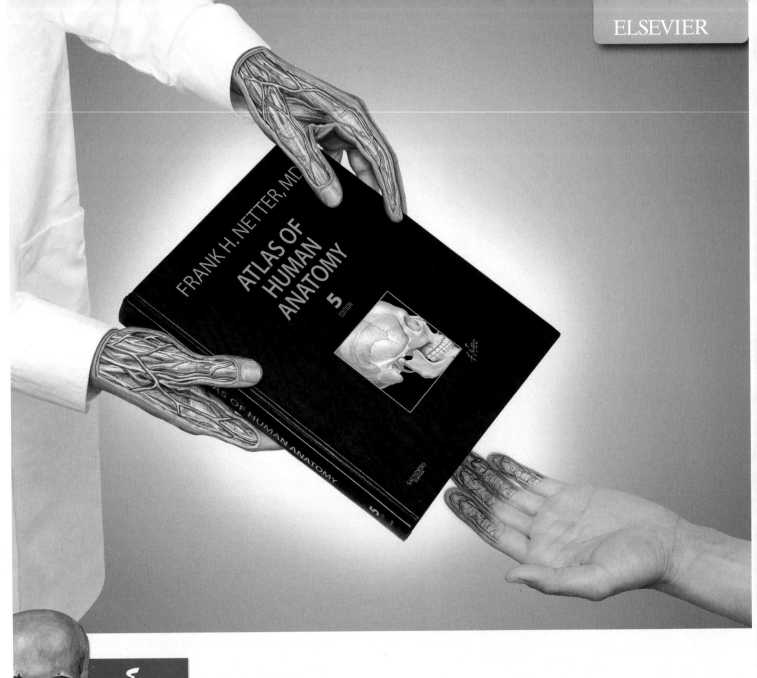

Netter's
Pediatrics

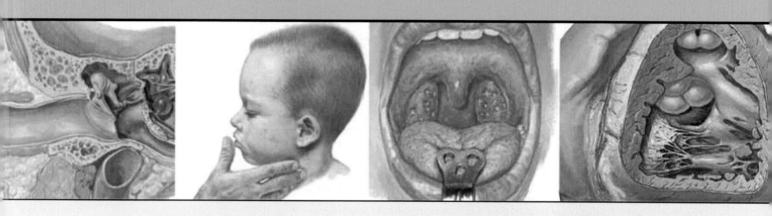

EDITORS

TODD A. FLORIN, MD
Fellow, Division of Pediatric Emergency
  Medicine
The Children's Hospital of Philadelphia
Instructor, Department of Pediatrics
The University of Pennsylvania School
  of Medicine
Philadelphia, Pennsylvania

STEPHEN LUDWIG, MD
Senior Advisor for Medical Education
John H. and Hortense Cassell Jensen Endowed
  Chair
The Children's Hospital of Philadelphia
Professor of Pediatrics and Emergency Medicine
The University of Pennsylvania School
  of Medicine
Philadelphia, Pennsylvania

ASSOCIATE EDITORS

PAUL L. ARONSON, MD
Fellow, Division of Pediatric Emergency
  Medicine
The Children's Hospital of Philadelphia
Instructor, Department of Pediatrics
The University of Pennsylvania School
  of Medicine
Philadelphia, Pennsylvania

HEIDI C. WERNER, MD
Fellow, Division of Emergency Medicine
Children's Hospital Boston
Instructor of Pediatrics
Harvard Medical School
Boston, Massachusetts

Illustrations by Frank H. Netter, MD

CONTRIBUTING ILLUSTRATORS

Carlos A. G. Machado, MD

John A. Craig, MD

James A. Perkins, MS, MFA

Tiffany S. DaVanzo, MA, CMI

Anita Impagliazzo, MA, CMI

ELSEVIER
SAUNDERS

ELSEVIER
SAUNDERS

1600 John F. Kennedy Blvd.
Ste 1800
Philadelphia, PA 19103-2899

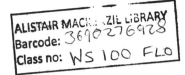
NETTER'S PEDIATRICS   ISBN: 978-1-4377-1155-4

ISBN: 978-1-4377-1155-4

Acquisitions Editor: Elyse O'Grady
Developmental Editor: Marybeth Thiel
Editorial Assistant: Chris Hazle-Cary
Publishing Services Manager: Patricia Tannian
Senior Project Manager: John Casey
Designer: Steven Stave

Printed in United States of America

Last digit is the print number: 9 8 7 6 5 4 3 2 1

About the Editors

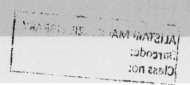

Stephen Ludwig, MD, is Senior Advisor for Medical Education and Senior Attending Physician at The Children's Hospital of Philadelphia, Department of Pediatrics. He is the Chairman of the Graduate Medical Education Committee and Designated Institutional Official. Dr. Ludwig holds the John H. and Hortense Cassell Jensen Endowed Chair. In addition, he is a Professor of Pediatrics and Emergency Medicine at The University of Pennsylvania School of Medicine.

Dr. Ludwig is a past president of the Academic Pediatric Association (APA) and a member of the Board of Directors, as well as a founding member of the Pediatric Emergency Medicine Special Interest Group. He is a member of the International Society of Child Abuse and Neglect. Dr. Ludwig is a founding member of the Ray Helfer Society. Currently, he serves as Chairman of the Residency Review Committee (RRC) for Pediatrics of the Accreditation Council for Graduate Medical Education (ACGME). He has been a member of the Board of Directors of the American Board of Pediatrics and was Chair of the Program Directors Committee until 2009. He has received many awards from The University of Pennsylvania, Association of Pediatric Program Directors (APPD), and APA. He was elected to the Institute of Medicine in 1998. Recently, Dr. Ludwig has been selected by the Board of Directors of the Federation of Pediatric Organizations as the recipient of the 2010 Joseph W. St. Geme, Jr. Leadership Award.

Dr. Ludwig has over 150 publications to his credit and serves on several editorial boards. He is Co-Editor in Chief of *Pediatric Emergency Care*. He is the Editor of the *Textbook of Pediatric Emergency Medicine*, now in its sixth edition.

Dr. Ludwig received his medical degree from Temple University School of Medicine and completed his pediatric internship and residency at the Children's Hospital National Medical Center in Washington, DC. He holds board certification in General Pediatrics and certificate 001 in Pediatric Emergency Medicine from the American Board of Pediatrics.

Todd A. Florin, MD, is currently a senior fellow in Pediatric Emergency Medicine at The Children's Hospital of Philadelphia. Dr. Florin graduated from the University of Rochester with a bachelor of arts in music with a vocal performance and conducting focus and received his medical degree from the University of Rochester School of Medicine and Dentistry.

He was a resident in Pediatrics from 2005-2008 and Chief Resident from 2008-2009 at The Children's Hospital of Philadelphia. In addition to his fellowship training, he is currently pursuing his masters of science in clinical epidemiology at the Center for Clinical Epidemiology and Biostatistics at The University of Pennsylvania School of Medicine. Dr. Florin is the recipient of a Young Investigator Award from the Academic Pediatric Association and a grant from the Loan Repayment Program of the National Institutes of Health. After completing fellowship, Dr. Florin intends to pursue an academic career combining clinical pediatric emergency medicine, medical education, and research in pediatric acute care epidemiology. He continues to be an active singer and conductor and has just completed his eighth summer season as a principal conductor with the College Light Opera Company in Falmouth, Massachusetts.

Paul L. Aronson, MD, received his bachelor of arts in drama from Duke University and his medical degree from New York University. He completed his residency and chief residency in pediatrics at The Children's Hospital of Philadelphia, at which he is currently a fellow in pediatric emergency medicine. His main academic interest is in medical education with a particular focus on evidence-based medicine. He is the recipient of the senior resident and fellow teaching awards from the residency program at The Children's Hospital of Philadelphia. He lives in Philadelphia with his wonderful wife, Jenny (a fifth grade teacher), and their two loving cats, Emma and Duke. He would especially like to thank his parents for their support and for teaching him that true success is measured by character and a happy family.

Heidi C. Werner, MD, is currently a senior fellow in Pediatric Emergency Medicine at The Children's Hospital Boston. Dr. Werner graduated from Princeton University with a bachelor of arts in molecular biology and received her medical degree from Columbia College of Physicians and Surgeons. She was a resident in pediatrics from 2005-2008 and Chief Resident from 2008-2009 at The Children's Hospital of Philadelphia. After fellowship training, Dr. Werner intends to pursue an academic career combining clinical pediatric emergency medicine, medical education ,and research in pediatric bedside emergency ultrasound.

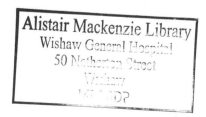

About the Artists

Frank H. Netter, MD

Frank Netter was born in 1906, in New York City. He studied art at the Art Student's League and the National Academy of Design before entering medical school at New York University, where he received his MD degree in 1931. During his student years, Dr. Netter's notebook sketches attracted the attention of the medical faculty and other physicians, allowing him to augment his income by illustrating articles and textbooks. He continued illustrating as a sideline after establishing a surgical practice in 1933, but he ultimately opted to give up his practice in favor of a full-time commitment to art. After service in the United States Army during World War II, Dr. Netter began his long collaboration with the CIBA Pharmaceutical Company (now Novartis Pharmaceuticals). This 45-year partnership resulted in the production of the extraordinary collection of medical art so familiar to physicians and other medical professionals worldwide.

In 2005, Elsevier, Inc., purchased the Netter Collection and all publications from Icon Learning Systems. There are now over 50 publications featuring the art of Dr. Netter available through Elsevier, Inc. (in the US: www.us.elsevierhealth.com/Netter and outside the US: www.elsevierhealth.com).

Dr. Netter's works are among the finest examples of the use of illustration in the teaching of medical concepts. The 13-book *Netter Collection of Medical Illustrations*, which includes the greater part of the more than 20,000 paintings created by Dr. Netter, became and remains one of the most famous medical works ever published. *The Netter Atlas of Human Anatomy*, first published in 1989, presents the anatomical paintings from the Netter Collection. Now translated into 16 languages, it is the anatomy atlas of choice among medical and health professions students the world over.

The Netter illustrations are appreciated not only for their aesthetic qualities, but, more important, for their intellectual content. As Dr. Netter wrote in 1949, "... clarification of a subject is the aim and goal of illustration. No matter how beautifully painted, how delicately and subtly rendered a subject may be, it is of little value as a *medical illustration* if it does not serve to make clear some medical point." Dr. Netter's planning, conception, point of view, and approach are what inform his paintings and what makes them so intellectually valuable.

Frank H. Netter, MD, physician and artist, died in 1991.

Learn more about the physician-artist whose work has inspired the Netter Reference collection: http://www.netterimages.com/artist/netter.htm.

Carlos A. G. Machado, MD

Carlos Machado was chosen by Novartis to be Dr. Netter's successor. He continues to be the main artist who contributes to the Netter collection of medical illustrations.

Self-taught in medical illustration, cardiologist Carlos Machado has contributed meticulous updates to some of Dr. Netter's original plates and has created many paintings of his own in the style of Netter as an extension of the Netter collection. Dr. Machado's photorealistic expertise and his keen insight into the physician/patient relationship informs his vivid and unforgettable visual style. His dedication to researching each topic and subject he paints places him among the premier medical illustrators at work today.

Learn more about his background and see more of his art at: http://www.netterimages.com/artist/machado.htm.

Preface

This book serves as a tribute to medical education and mentoring in all its forms. It spans a cycle of mentoring that began for me more than 40 years ago. It underscores the value of the mentoring process from that time to today.

More than 40 years ago, as a medical student, I relied on the masterful work of Frank Netter. In every sense he seemed like a helpful sage mentor. Learning from other standard textbooks was certainly possible, but the Netter drawings took me by the hand, opened my mind to anatomy, physiology, pathogenesis, and clinical signs and symptoms in a very personal way. *Gray's Anatomy Textbook* had all the detail, but studying it felt almost austere, untouchable. Frank Netter was warm and welcoming the way any good mentor establishes a positive learning environment. Dr. Netter and those who followed him taught entire generations of physicians through the 1960s, 1970s, and 1980s. The old adage that a picture is worth a thousand words was multiplied many times over by a Netter illustration. When offered the opportunity to co-edit this book, which might help to recirculate the Netter illustrations, it was my immediate reaction to sign on. Our hope was that these illustrations would be available to touch the lives of the next generations of pediatric trainees.

However, this volume had other mentoring dimensions as well. First was the opportunity to work with three outstanding chief residents, Todd Florin, MD, the co-editor, and Paul Aronson, MD, and Heidi Werner, MD, the two associate editors. Having worked with them over three years of pediatric residency at The Children's Hospital of Philadelphia and during one additional year as chief residents, the choice to continue our collaboration was a mentor's dream. It was a chance to produce something of enduring value as a team. Although all of our careers have moved forward in new directions, this was a chance to hold on to a certain chemistry we shared. This is the first major textbook that will bear their names, but you will hear their names often in the future, as I am certain they will be leaders in pediatrics. This may be their first book, but I assure you it will not be their last.

When formulating our concepts of the book, we decided to make it a mentoring project in itself. All of the chapters were written by more-junior faculty, fellows, and residents. Each was supervised by a section editor who helped these young but talented authors get their chapters written, edited, and into print. For some authors this represents their first major publication. For many there were lessons learned along the way. For all there was a chance to build a relationship with a more senior section editor. To these section editors we owe a great debt of gratitude.

With all the technologic advances in medicine and our deepening understanding of the basis of diseases and therapeutics, we are all still benefiting from the time-worn traditions of medicine. *Netter's Pediatrics* showed us the way. Senior faculty working one on one with more-junior people. Mentoring — the apprenticeship model — still at the heart of our academic process.

Our hope is that this volume will aid you in the care of children. We hope these words and drawings will bring the subject matter alive and help you derive as much practice knowledge and pleasure from using *Netter's Pediatrics* as we experienced in bringing it to you.

Stephen Ludwig, MD
Philadelphia, 2011

Dedication

To my families—
The one at home and the one at work.
I am ever grateful to both.
SL

To
My patients, you are my greatest educators
My teachers, you are my inspiration
My parents, you are my foundation
My wife, Kemper, you are my rock
TAF

To my beautiful and very patient best friend and wife, Jenny.
You make me a better person, and everything I do is possible
because of your love and support.
To my family and family-in-law, I am truly grateful for your love
and generosity.
To my many teachers, mentors, and colleagues at The
Children's Hospital of Philadelphia, from whom I have
learned so much.
To my patients, who have ultimately taught me everything I
know in pediatrics. It is a true privilege to be a pediatrician.
PLA

To my husband, my parents, and my children for their loving
support.
HCW

Acknowledgments

This is a book of "firsts." The first time that Frank Netter's drawings of pediatric illness have been brought together in a single volume. The first time that many of the young residents and fellows represented in this book have written a book chapter. For Dr. Ludwig, the first time that he has collaborated on such a large project with three of his chief residents. For Drs. Florin, Aronson, and Werner, the first time they are editing a textbook. "Firsts" are exciting—they create an atmosphere of adventure, passion, cautious anticipation. They also require significant effort and time, often beyond the hours and days of the typical workweek. As a result, many people not directly listed in the pages that follow had a tremendous impact on the successful production of this book.

We would first like to thank all of the contributing authors and section editors from The Children's Hospital of Philadelphia and The University of Pennsylvania School of Medicine. All of the first authors are residents and fellows at the early stages of their pediatric careers whose passion, intellect, and dedication shine through in the pages that follow. Without their hard work, *Netter's Pediatrics* could not exist. We would also like to especially thank the faculty members at our institution that served as section editors for this book. These physicians have shown a clear and dedicated commitment to mentorship through their contributions and hard work in guiding these young authors through the process of writing this book.

Our patients and their parents provide continuous inspiration and motivation. We thank you all for the privilege to care for you and your children and for being our most valued teachers. It is primarily our patients that motivate us to produce a volume to teach the current and next generation of pediatric health care providers.

Many of the beautiful images in this book were drawn by Frank Netter. However, many images needed to be edited, and some new images were drawn from scratch. We would like to thank all of the artists that contributed to this book: Jim Perkins, Tiffany DaVanzo, Anita Impagliazzo, and the DragonFly Media Group. "A picture is worth a thousand words," and these talented artists were incredible in their ability to bring concepts to life through their beautiful artwork.

Special thanks go to our editorial team at Elsevier—Anne Lenehan Woodcock, Elyse O'Grady, and especially Marybeth Thiel—who were instrumental in guiding us through the production of this first edition of *Netter's Pediatrics*. Their encouragement and guidance were critical in the process of writing and editing the book.

Special recognition goes to Ms. Carolyn Trojan, whose extraordinary organizational skills and commitment were vital in producing a new multi-authored textbook.

Finally, we would like to extend our most emphatic thanks to our families, without whom a project of this scope would not be possible. Without their tremendous love and support, our work would lack meaning. First, we would like to acknowledge our spouses—Kemper Florin, Zella Ludwig, Jenny Shieh, and Howard Horn—whose patience, encouragement, support, and love make everything possible. Second, thanks to our children and grandchildren—Susannah Ludwig and Mike Poppleton, Elisa Ludwig and Jesse Pires, Aubrey Ludwig and Jared Ellman, Jack Ellis Poppleton, and Archer and Ella Horn—who challenge us and inspire us to remember the truly important things in life. Finally, thanks to our parents who gave us the foundation to become who we are today.

Editors

Todd A. Florin, MD
Fellow, Division of Pediatric Emergency Medicine
The Children's Hospital of Philadelphia
Instructor, Department of Pediatrics
The University of Pennsylvania School of Medicine
Philadelphia, Pennsylvania

Stephen Ludwig, MD
Senior Advisor for Medical Education
John H. and Hortense Cassell Jensen Endowed Chair
The Children's Hospital of Philadelphia
Professor of Pediatrics and Emergency Medicine
The University of Pennsylvania School of Medicine
Philadelphia, Pennsylvania

Paul L. Aronson, MD
Fellow, Division of Pediatric Emergency Medicine
The Children's Hospital of Philadelphia
Instructor, Department of Pediatrics
The University of Pennsylvania School of Medicine
Philadelphia, Pennsylvania

Heidi C. Werner, MD
Fellow, Division of Emergency Medicine
Children's Hospital Boston
Instructor of Pediatrics
Harvard Medical School
Boston, Massachusetts

Section Editors

Louis M. Bell, MD
Associate Chair for Clinical Activities
Department of Pediatrics
The Patrick S. Pasquariello, Jr, MD Endowed Chair in
   Pediatrics
Chief, Division of General Pediatrics
The Children's Hospital of Philadelphia
Professor of Pediatrics
The University of Pennsylvania School of Medicine
Philadelphia, Pennsylvania

Mercedes M. Blackstone, MD
Attending Physician
Division of Emergency Medicine
The Children's Hospital of Philadelphia
Assistant Professor of Clinical Pediatrics
The University of Pennsylvania School of Medicine
Philadelphia, Pennsylvania

Terri Brown-Whitehorn, MD
Attending Physician
Division of Allergy and Immunology
The Children's Hospital of Philadelphia
Assistant Professor of Clinical Pediatrics
The University of Pennsylvania School of Medicine
Philadelphia, Pennsylvania

James M. Callahan, MD
Director, Medical Education
Division of Emergency Medicine
The Children's Hospital of Philadelphia
Associate Professor of Clinical Pediatrics
The University of Pennsylvania School of Medicine
Philadelphia, Pennsylvania

Matthew A. Deardorff, MD, PhD
Attending Physician
The Children's Hospital of Philadelphia
Assistant Professor of Pediatrics
The University of Pennsylvania School of Medicine
Philadelphia, Pennsylvania

Richard S. Finkel, MD
Director, Neuromuscular Program
Division of Neurology
The Children's Hospital of Philadelphia
Clinical Professor in Neurology and Pediatrics
The University of Pennsylvania School of Medicine
Philadelphia, Pennsylvania

Joshua R. Friedman, MD, PhD
Attending Physician
Division of Gastroenterology, Hepatology, and Nutrition
The Children's Hospital of Philadelphia
Assistant Professor of Pediatrics
The University of Pennsylvania School of Medicine
Philadelphia, Pennsylvania

Rose C. Graham, MD, MSCE
Attending Physician
Mission Children's Specialists
Pediatric Gastroenterology
Asheville, North Carolina

Fred Henretig, MD
Attending Physician
Division of Pediatric Emergency Medicine
The Children's Hospital of Philadelphia
Professor of Pediatrics
The University of Pennsylvania School of Medicine
Philadelphia, Pennsylvania

Leslie S. Kersun, MD
Attending Physician
Division of Oncology
The Children's Hospital of Philadelphia
Assistant Professor of Clinical Pediatrics
The University of Pennsylvania School of Medicine
Philadelphia, Pennsylvania

Jason Y. Kim, MD, MSCE
Attending Physician
Division of Infectious Diseases
The Children's Hospital of Philadelphia
Assistant Professor of Clinical Pediatrics
The University of Pennsylvania School of Medicine
Philadelphia, Pennsylvania

Sara B. Kinsman, MD, PhD
Attending Physician
Division of Adolescent Medicine
The Children's Hospital of Philadelphia
Assistant Professor of Clinical Pediatrics
The University of Pennsylvania School of Medicine
Philadelphia, Pennsylvania

Michael A. Levine, MD, FAAP, FACP
Division Chief
Division of Endocrinology and Diabetes
The Children's Hospital of Philadelphia
Professor of Pediatrics
The University of Pennsylvania School of Medicine
Philadelphia, Pennsylvania

Christina L. Master, MD
Associate Pediatric Residency Program Director
The Children's Hospital of Philadelphia
Associate Professor of Clinical Pediatrics
The University of Pennsylvania School of Medicine
Philadelphia, Pennsylvania

Kevin E. C. Meyers, MB BCh
Attending Physician
Division of Nephrology
The Children's Hospital of Philadelphia
Associate Professor of Pediatrics
The University of Pennsylvania School of Medicine
Philadelphia, Pennsylvania

David A. Munson, MD
Attending Physician
Division of Neonatology
The Children's Hospital of Philadelphia
Assistant Professor of Clinical Pediatrics
The University of Pennsylvania School of Medicine
Philadelphia, Pennsylvania

Howard B. Panitch, MD
Director of Clinical Programs
Division of Pulmonary Medicine
The Children's Hospital of Philadelphia
Professor of Pediatrics
The University of Pennsylvania School of Medicine
Philadelphia, Pennsylvania

Beth Rezet, MD
Attending Physician
Division of General Pediatrics
The Children's Hospital of Philadelphia
Clinical Associate Professor of Pediatrics
The University of Pennsylvania School of Medicine
Philadelphia, Pennsylvania

James R. Treat, MD
Attending Physician, Dermatology
Division of General Pediatrics
The Children's Hospital of Philadelphia
Assistant Professor of Clinical Pediatrics
The University of Pennsylvania School of Medicine
Philadelphia, Pennsylvania

Paul M. Weinberg, MD
Senior Cardiologist
Director, Fellowship Training Program in Pediatric
    Cardiology
The Children's Hospital of Philadelphia
Professor of Pediatrics and Pediatric Pathology and
    Laboratory Medicine
The University of Pennsylvania School of Medicine
Philadelphia, Pennsylvania

Pamela F. Weiss, MD, MSCE
Attending Physician
Division of Rheumatology
The Children's Hospital of Philadelphia
Assistant Professor of Clinical Pediatrics
The University of Pennsylvania School of Medicine
Philadelphia, Pennsylvania

Char M. Witmer, MD
Attending Physician
Division of Hematology
The Children's Hospital of Philadelphia
Assistant Professor of Pediatrics
The University of Pennsylvania School of Medicine
Philadelphia, Pennsylvania

Contributors

Saba Ahmad, MD
Fellow, Division of Neurology
The Children's Hospital of Philadelphia
Philadelphia, Pennsylvania

Craig A. Alter, MD
Attending Physician
Division of Endocrinology
The Children's Hospital of Philadelphia
Associate Professor of Pediatrics
The University of Pennsylvania School of Medicine
Philadelphia, Pennsylvania

Brett R. Anderson, MD, MBA
Pediatric Resident
Department of Pediatrics
The Children's Hospital of Philadelphia
Philadelphia, Pennsylvania

Marsha Ayzen, MD
Pediatric Resident
Department of Pediatrics
The Children's Hospital of Philadelphia
Philadelphia, Pennsylvania

Rochelle Bagatell, MD
Attending Physician
Division of Oncology
The Children's Hospital of Philadelphia
Associate Professor of Pediatrics
The University of Pennsylvania School of Medicine
Philadelphia, Pennsylvania

H. Jorge Baluarte, MD
Medical Director, Renal Transplant Program
Division of Nephrology
The Children's Hospital of Philadelphia
Professor of Pediatrics
The University of Pennsylvania School of Medicine
Philadelphia, Pennsylvania

Vaneeta Bamba, MD
Attending Physician
Division of Endocrinology
The Children's Hospital of Philadelphia
Assistant Professor of Clinical Pediatrics
The University of Pennsylvania School of Medicine
Philadelphia, Pennsylvania

David R. Bearden, MD
Child Neurology Fellow, Division of Neurology
The Children's Hospital of Philadelphia
Philadelphia, Pennsylvania

Ulf H. Beier, MD
Fellow, Division of Nephrology
The Children's Hospital of Philadelphia
Philadelphia, Pennsylvania

Lauren A. Beslow, MD
Fellow, Division of Neurology
The Children's Hospital of Philadelphia
Philadelphia, Pennsylvania

Shazia Bhat, MD
Pediatric Resident
Department of Pediatrics
The Children's Hospital of Philadelphia
Philadelphia, Pennsylvania

Christopher P. Bonafide, MD
Fellow, Division of General Pediatrics
The Children's Hospital of Philadelphia
Philadelphia, Pennsylvania

Jill L. Brodsky, MD
Fellow, Division of Endocrinology and Diabetes
The Children's Hospital of Philadelphia
Philadelphia, Pennsylvania

Naomi Brown, MD
Pediatric Resident
Department of Pediatrics
The Children's Hospital of Philadelphia
Philadelphia, Pennsylvania

Jason B. Caboot, MD
Fellow, Division of Pulmonary Medicine
The Children's Hospital of Philadelphia
Philadelphia, Pennsylvania

Andrew C. Calabria, MD
Fellow, Division of Endocrinology & Diabetes
The Children's Hospital of Philadelphia
Philadelphia, Pennsylvania

Leslie Castelo-Soccio, MD, PhD
Fellow, Dermatology
Division of General Pediatrics
The Children's Hospital of Philadelphia
Philadelphia, Pennsylvania

Ann Chahroudi, MD, PhD
Division of Infectious Diseases
Department of Pediatrics
Emory University School of Medicine
Atlanta, Georgia

David Chao, MD
Fellow, Pediatric Emergency Medicine
The Children's Hospital of Philadelphia
Philadelphia, Pennsylvania

Kathryn Chatfield, MD, PhD
Fellow, Division of Genetics
The Children's Hospital of Philadelphia
Philadelphia, Pennsylvania

Lori A. Christ, MD
Pediatric Resident
Department of Pediatrics
The Children's Hospital of Philadelphia
Philadelphia, Pennsylvania

Andrew Chu, MD
Fellow, Division of Gastroenterology, Hepatology, and
  Nutrition
The Children's Hospital of Philadelphia
Philadelphia, Pennsylvania

R. Thomas Collins II, MD
Fellow, Division of Cardiology
The Children's Hospital of Philadelphia
Philadelphia, Pennsylvania

Lawrence Copelovitch, MD
Attending Physician
Division of Nephrology
The Children's Hospital of Philadelphia
Assistant Professor of Clinical Pediatrics
The University of Pennsylvania School of Medicine
Philadelphia, Pennsylvania

Jennifer A. Danzig, MD
Fellow, Division of Endocrinology
The Children's Hospital of Philadelphia
Philadelphia, Pennsylvania

Carrie Daymont, MD
Fellow, Division of General Pediatrics
The Children's Hospital of Philadelphia
Philadelphia, Pennsylvania

Diva D. DeLeón, MD
Attending Physician
Division of Endocrinology and Diabetes
The Children's Hospital of Philadelphia
Assistant Professor of Pediatrics
The University of Pennsylvania School of Medicine
Philadelphia, Pennsylvania

Michelle Denburg, MD
Fellow, Division of Nephrology
The Children's Hospital of Philadelphia
Philadelphia, Pennsylvania

Melissa Desai, MD, MPH
Pediatric Resident
Department of Pediatrics
The Children's Hospital of Philadelphia
Instructor in Pediatrics
The University of Pennsylvania School of Medicine
Philadelphia, Pennsylvania

Erin Pete Devon, MD
Pediatric Resident
Department of Pediatrics
The Children's Hospital of Philadelphia
Philadelphia, Pennsylvania

Aaron Donoghue, MD, MSCE
Attending Physician
Divisions of Emergency Medicine and Critical Care
Assistant Professor of Pediatrics
The Children's Hospital of Philadelphia
The University of Pennsylvania School of Medicine
Philadelphia, Pennsylvania

Nicholas Evageliou, MD
Attending Physician
Division of Hematology and Oncology
The Children's Hospital of Philadelphia
Assistant Professor of Clinical Pediatrics
The University of Pennsylvania School of Medicine
Philadelphia, Pennsylvania

Mirna M. Farah, MD
Attending Physician
Division of Pediatric Emergency Medicine
The Children's Hospital of Philadelphia
Associate Professor of Clinical Pediatrics
The University of Pennsylvania School of Medicine
Philadelphia, Pennsylvania

Kristen A. Feemster, MD, MPH, MSHP
Fellow, Division of Infectious Diseases
The Children's Hospital of Philadelphia
Philadelphia, Pennsylvania

James Aaron Feinstein, MD
Pediatric Resident
Department of Pediatrics
The Children's Hospital of Philadelphia
Philadelphia, Pennsylvania

Amy Feldman, MD
Chief Pediatric Resident
Department of Pediatrics
The Children's Hospital of Philadelphia
Philadelphia, Pennsylvania

Ryan J. Felling, MD, PhD
Pediatric Neurology Resident
The Johns Hopkins Hospital
Baltimore, Maryland

John J. Flibotte, MD
Pediatric Resident
Department of Pediatrics
The Children's Hospital of Philadelphia
Philadelphia, Pennsylvania

Stephen G. Flynn, MD
Pediatric Resident
Department of Pediatrics
The Children's Hospital of Philadelphia
Instructor in Pediatrics
The University of Pennsylvania School of Medicine
Philadelphia, Pennsylvania

Elizabeth E. Foglia, MD
Attending Physician
Division of General Pediatrics
The Children's Hospital of Philadelphia
Philadelphia, Pennsylvania

Lisa Forbes, MD
Fellow, Division of Allergy and Immunology
The Children's Hospital of Philadelphia
Philadelphia, Pennsylvania

Jackie P. D. Garrett, MD
Pediatric Resident
Department of Pediatrics
The Children's Hospital of Philadelphia
Philadelphia, Pennsylvania

Laura Gober, MD
Fellow, Division of Allergy and Immunology
The Children's Hospital of Philadelphia
Philadelphia, Pennsylvania

Michael D. Gober, MD, PhD
Resident Physician, Department of Dermatology
Hospital of The University of Pennsylvania
Philadelphia, Pennsylvania

Kelly C. Goldsmith, MD
Aflac Cancer Center and Blood Disorders Service
Children's Healthcare of Atlanta
Assistant Professor
Emory University
Atlanta, Georgia

Monika Goyal, MD
Fellow, Division of Emergency Medicine
The Children's Hospital of Philadelphia
Instructor, Department of Pediatrics
The University of Pennsylvania School of Medicine
Philadelphia, Pennsylvania

Abby Green, MD
Pediatric Resident
Department of Pediatrics
The Children's Hospital of Philadelphia
Philadelphia, Pennsylvania

Adda Grimberg, MD
Scientific Director, Diagnostic and Research Growth Center
Division of Endocrinology and Diabetes
The Children's Hospital of Philadelphia
Associate Professor of Pediatrics
The University of Pennsylvania School of Medicine
Philadelphia, Pennsylvania

Chad R. Haldeman-Englert, MD
Assistant Professor
Department of Pediatrics, Section of Medical Genetics
Wake Forest University School of Medicine
Winston-Salem, North Carolina

E. Kevin Hall, MD
Fellow, Heart Failure and Transplantation
Children's Hospital Boston
Boston, Massachusetts

Fiona Healy, MD
Pulmonary Fellow, Division of Pulmonary Medicine
The Children's Hospital of Philadelphia
Philadelphia, Pennsylvania

Jessica L. Hills, MD
Attending Physician
Division of General Pediatrics
The Children's Hospital of Philadelphia
Clinical Assistant Professor of Pediatrics
The University of Pennsylvania School of Medicine
Philadelphia, Pennsylvania

Melissa A. Hofmann, MD
Pediatric Resident
Department of Pediatrics
The Children's Hospital of Philadelphia
Philadelphia, Pennsylvania

Daniel B. Horton, MD
Pediatric Resident
Department of Pediatrics
The Children's Hospital of Philadelphia
Philadelphia, Pennsylvania

Anna Hunter, MD
Fellow, Division of Gastroenterology, Hepatology, and
    Nutrition
The Children's Hospital of Philadelphia
Philadelphia, Pennsylvania

Elif E. Ince, MD
Fellow, Division of Neonatology
The Children's Hospital of Philadelphia
Philadelphia, Pennsylvania

Reena Jethva, MD, MBA
Attending Physician
St. Christopher's Hospital for Children
Assistant Professor
Drexel University College School of Medicine
Philadelphia, Pennsylvania

Anitha S. John, MD, PhD
Fellow, Adult Congenital Heart Disease
The Mayo Clinic
Rochester, Minnesota

Amanda Jones, MD
Pediatric Resident
Department of Pediatrics
The Children's Hospital of Philadelphia
Philadelphia, Pennsylvania

Eden Kahle, MD
Pediatric Resident
Department of Pediatrics
The Children's Hospital of Philadelphia
Instructor of Pediatrics
The University of Pennsylvania School of Medicine
Philadelphia, Pennsylvania

Jennifer M. Kalish, MD, PhD
Fellow, Division of Human Genetics
The Children's Hospital of Philadelphia
Philadelphia, Pennsylvania

Melissa Kennedy, MD
Fellow, Division of Gastroenterology, Hepatology, and
  Nutrition
The Children's Hospital of Philadelphia
Philadelphia, Pennsylvania

Soorena Khojasteh, MD
Pediatric Resident
Department of Pediatrics
The Children's Hospital of Philadelphia
Instructor of Pediatrics
The University of Pennsylvania School of Medicine
Philadelphia, Pennsylvania

Roy J. Kim, MD, MPH
Assistant Professor of Pediatrics
Department of Pediatrics
Division of Endocrinology
University of Texas Southwestern Medical Center
Dallas, Texas

Dorit Koren, MD
Attending Physician
Division of Endocrinology and Diabetes
The Children's Hospital of Philadelphia
Clinical Associate
The University of Pennsylvania School of Medicine
Philadelphia, Pennsylvania

Matthew P. Kronman, MD
Divisions of Infectious Diseases and General Pediatrics
The Children's Hospital of Philadelphia
Departments of Pediatrics and Epidemiology
The University of Pennsylvania School of Medicine
Philadelphia, Pennsylvania

David R. Langdon, MD
Clinical Director, Division of Endocrinology and Diabetes
The Children's Hospital of Philadelphia
Clinical Associate Professor of Pediatrics
The University of Pennsylvania School of Medicine
Philadelphia, Pennsylvania

Christopher LaRosa, MD
Fellow, Division of Nephrology
The Children's Hospital of Philadelphia
Philadelphia, Pennsylvania

Javier J. Lasa, MD
Fellow, Division of Cardiology
The Children's Hospital of Philadelphia
Philadelphia, Pennsylvania

Lara Wine Lee, MD, PhD
Pediatric Resident
Department of Pediatrics
The Children's Hospital of Philadelphia
Philadelphia, Pennsylvania

Melissa Leyva-Vega, MD
Fellow, Division of Gastroenterology, Hepatology, and
  Nutrition
The Children's Hospital of Philadelphia
Philadelphia, Pennsylvania

Scott M. Lieberman, MD, PhD
Fellow, Division of Rheumatology
The Children's Hospital of Philadelphia
Philadelphia, Pennsylvania

Jessica Sparks Lilley, MD
Fellow, Pediatric Endocrinology
Vanderbilt University School of Medicine
Nashville, Tennessee

Julie M. Linton, MD
Pediatric Resident
Department of Pediatrics
The Children's Hospital of Philadelphia
Philadelphia, Pennsylvania

Elizabeth Lowenthal, MD
Fellow, Division of General Pediatrics
The Children's Hospital of Philadelphia
Philadelphia, Pennsylvania

Sheela N. Magge, MD, MSCE
Attending Physician
Division of Endocrinology and Diabetes
The Children's Hospital of Philadelphia
Assistant Professor of Pediatrics
The University of Pennsylvania School of Medine
Philadelphia, Pennsylvania

Jennifer Mangino, MD
Fellow, Divisions of Hematology and Oncology
The Children's Hospital of Philadelphia
Philadelphia, Pennsylvania

Olivera Marsenic, MD
Pediatric Nephrologist
Assistant Professor of Pediatrics
Oklahoma University Health Sciences Center
Oklahoma City, Oklahoma

Pamela A. Mazzeo, MD
Pediatric Resident
Department of Pediatrics
The Children's Hospital of Philadelphia
Instructor of Pediatrics
The University of Pennsylvania School of Medicine
Philadelphia, Pennsylvania

Jennifer L. McGuire, MD
Fellow, Division of Neurology
The Children's Hospital of Philadelphia
Philadelphia, Pennsylvania

Paul McNally, MB, MRCPI
Consultant Respiratory Physician
Our Lady's Children's Hospital, Crumlin
Dublin, Ireland

Jane E. Minturn, MD, PhD
Attending Physician
Division of Oncology
The Children's Hospital of Philadelphia
Assistant Professor of Pediatrics
The University of Pennsylvania School of Medicine
Philadelphia, Pennsylvania

Manoj K. Mittal, MD, MRCP (UK), FAAP
Attending Physician
Division of Emergency Medicine
Assistant Professor of Clinical Pediatrics
The University of Pennsylvania School of Medicine
Philadelphia, Pennsylvania

Melissa Mondello, MD
Pediatric Resident
Department of Pediatrics
The Children's Hospital of Philadelphia
Philadelphia, Pennsylvania

Kathryn M. Murphy, RN, PhD
Associate Director, Diabetes Center for Children
Division of Endocrinology and Diabetes
The Children's Hospital of Philadelphia
Philadelphia, Pennsylvania

Sage Myers, MD
Fellow, Division of Pediatric Emergency Medicine
The Children's Hospital of Philadelphia
Philadelphia, Pennsylvania

Frances Nadel, MD, MSCE
Attending Physician
Division of Pediatric Emergency Medicine
The Children's Hospital of Philadelphia
Associate Professor of Clinical Pediatrics
The University of Pennsylvania School of Medicine
Philadelphia, Pennsylvania

Kyle Nelson, MD, MPH
Attending Physician
Division of Pediatric Emergency Medicine
The Children's Hospital of Philadelphia
Assistant Professor of Pediatrics
The University of Pennsylvania School of Medicine
Philadelphia, Pennsylvania

Gustavo Nino, MD
Fellow, Division of Pulmonary Medicine
The Children's Hospital of Philadelphia
Philadelphia, Pennsylvania

Bettina Mucha-Le Ny, MD
Fellow, Division of Human Genetics
The Children's Hospital of Philadelphia
Philadelphia, Pennsylvania

Michael L. O'Byrne, MD
Pediatric Resident
Department of Pediatrics
The Children's Hospital of Philadelphia
Philadelphia, Pennsylvania

Vikash S. Oza, MD
Pediatric Resident
Department of Pediatrics
The Children's Hospital of Philadelphia
Philadelphia, Pennsylvania

Andrew A. Palladino, MD
Attending Physician
Division of Endocrinology and Diabetes
The Children's Hospital of Philadelphia
Assistant Professor of Pediatrics
The University of Pennsylvania School of Medicine
Philadelphia, Pennsylvania

Shefali Parikh, MD
Fellow, Division of Hematology and Oncology
The Children's Hospital of Philadelphia
Philadelphia, Pennsylvania

Tara Petersen, MD
Chief Pediatric Resident
Department of Pediatrics
The Children's Hospital of Philadelphia
Philadelphia, Pennsylvania

Amy L. Peterson, MD
Fellow, Division of Cardiology
The Children's Hospital of Philadelphia
Philadelphia, Pennsylvania

Connie M. Piccone, MD
Fellow, Division of Hematology and Oncology
The Children's Hospital of Philadelphia
Philadelphia, Pennsylvania

Sara E. Pinney, MD
Attending Physician
Division of Endocrinology
The Children's Hospital of Philadelphia
Assistant Professor of Pediatrics
The University of Pennsylvania School of Medicine
Philadelphia, Pennsylvania

Jill Posner, MD, MSCE
Attending Physician Pediatric Emergency Medicine
The Children's Hospital of Philadelphia
Associate Professor of Clinical Pediatrics
The University of Pennsylvania School of Medicine
Philadelphia, Pennsylvania

Kari R. Posner, MD
Fellow, Pediatric Emergency Medicine
The Children's Hospital of Philadelphia
Philadelphia, Pennsylvania

Madhura Pradhan, MD
Attending Physician
Division of Nephrology
The Children's Hospital of Philadelphia
Assistant Professor of Clinical Pediatrics
The University of Pennsylvania School of Medicine
Philadelphia, Pennsylvania

Ryan M. Raffaelli, MD
Fellow, Division of Nephrology
The Children's Hospital of Philadelphia
Philadelphia, Pennsylvania

Homaira Rahimi, MD
Fellow, Division of Rheumatology
The Children's Hospital of Philadelphia
Philadelphia, Pennsylvania

Kristin N. Ray, MD
Pediatric Resident
Department of Pediatrics
The Children's Hospital of Philadelphia
Philadelphia, Pennsylvania

Susan R. Rheingold, MD
Attending Physician
Division of Oncology
The Children's Hospital of Philadelphia
Assistant Professor of Pediatrics
The University of Pennsylvania School of Medicine
Philadelphia, Pennsylvania

Nicole Ryan, MD
Fellow, Division of Neurology
The Children's Hospital of Philadelphia
Philadelphia, Pennsylvania

Benjamin A. Sahn, MD, MS
Pediatric Resident
Department of Pediatrics
The Children's Hospital of Philadelphia
Philadelphia, Pennsylvania

Esther Maria Sampayo, MD, MPH
Attending Physician
Division of Pediatric Emergency Medicine
The Children's Hospital of Philadelphia
Assistant Professor of Pediatrics
The University of Pennsylvania School of Medicine
Philadelphia, Pennsylvania

Matthew G. Sampson, MD
Fellow, Division of Nephrology
The Children's Hospital of Philadelphia
Clinical Instructor in Pediatrics
The University of Pennsylvania School of Medicine
Philadelphia, Pennsylvania

Alisa B. Schiffman, DO
Fellow, Division of Endocrinology and Diabetes
The Children's Hospital of Philadelphia
Philadelphia, Pennsylvania

Dana Aronson Schinasi, MD
Fellow, Division of Pediatric Emergency Medicine
The Children's Hospital of Philadelphia
Philadelphia, Pennsylvania

Sandra Schwab, MD
Attending Physician
Division of Pediatric Emergency Medicine
The Children's Hospital of Philadelphia
Assistant Professor of Clinical Pediatrics
The University of Pennsylvaina School of Medicine
Philadelphia, Pennsylvania

Halden F. Scott, MD
Fellow, Division of Pediatric Emergency Medicine
The Children's Hospital of Philadelphia
Instructor in Pediatrics
The University of Pennsylvania School of Medicine
Philadelphia, Pennsylvania

Jeffrey A. Seiden, MD
Attending Physician
Division of Pediatric Emergency Medicine
The Children's Hospital of Philadelphia
Assistant Professor of Clinical Pediatrics
The University of Pennsylvania School of Medicine
Philadelphia, Pennsylvania

Dana Sepe, MD
Fellow, Division of Oncology
The Children's Hospital of Philadelphia
Philadelphia, Pennsylvania

Nilika B. Shah, MD
Pediatric Resident
Department of Pediatrics
The Children's Hospital of Philadelphia
Philadelphia, Pennsylvania

Rachana Shah, MD
Fellow, Division of Endocrinology and Diabetes
The Children's Hospital of Philadelphia
Instructor of Pediatrics
The University of Pennsylvania School of Medicine
Philadelphia, Pennsylvania

Samir S. Shah, MD, MSCE
Attending Physician
Divisions of Infectious Diseases and General Pediatrics
The Children's Hospital of Philadelphia
Assistant Professor of Pediatrics
The University of Pennsylvania School of Medicine
Philadelphia, Pennsylvania

Eric D. Shelov, MD
Pediatric Hospitalist
Division of General Pediatrics
The Children's Hospital of Philadelphia
Clinical Associate
The University of Pennsylvania School of Medicine
Philadelphia, Pennsylvania

Angela J. Sievert, MD, MPH
Fellow, Division of Hematology and Oncology
The Children's Hospital of Philadelphia
Instructor in Pediatrics
The University of Pennsylvania School of Medicine
Philadelphia, Pennsylvania

Sanjeev K. Swami, MD
Fellow, Division of Infectious Diseases
The Children's Hospital of Philadelphia
Philadelphia, Pennsylvania

Christina Lynch Szperka, MD
Fellow, Division of Neurology
The Children's Hospital of Philadelphia
Philadelphia, Pennsylvania

Kathryn S. Taub, MD
Fellow, Division of Neurology
The Children's Hospital of Philadelphia
Philadelphia, Pennsylvania

Alexis Teplick, MD
Fellow, Division of Hematology and Oncology
The Children's Hospital of Philadelphia
Philadelphia, Pennsylvania

Deepika Thacker, MD
Fellow, Division of Cardiology
The Children's Hospital of Philadelphia
Philadelphia, Pennsylvania

Oana Tomescu, MD, PhD
Attending Physician
Craig Dalsimer Division of Adolescent Medicine
The Children's Hospital of Philadelphia
Philadelphia, Pennsylvania

Howard Topol, MD
Pediatrics Resident
Department of Pediatrics
The Children's Hospital of Philadelphia
Philadelphia, Pennsylvania

Shamir Tuchman, MD, MPH
Attending Physician
Division of Nephrology
The Children's Hospital of Philadelphia
Philadelphia, Pennsylvania

Levon H. Utidjian, MD
Pediatric Resident
Department of Pediatrics
The Children's Hospital of Philadelphia
Philadelphia, Pennsylvania

Carly R. Varela, MD
Fellow, Division of Oncology
The Children's Hospital of Philadelphia
Philadelphia, Pennsylvania

Shirley D. Viteri, MD
Fellow, Department of Anesthesiology and Critical Care
  Medicine
The Children's Hospital of Philadelphia
Clinical Instructor
The University of Pennsylvania School of Medicine
Philadelphia, Pennsylvania

Amy T. Waldman, MD
Attending Physician
Division of Child Neurology
The Children's Hospital of Philadelphia
Assistant Professor of Pediatrics
The University of Pennsylvania School of Medicine
Philadelphia, Pennsylvania

Elizabeth M. Wallis, MD
Pediatric Resident
Department of Pediatrics
The Children's Hospital of Philadelphia
Instructor in Pediatrics
The University of Pennsylvania School of Medicine
Philadelphia, Pennsylvania

Daniel A. Weiser, MD
Fellow, Division of Hematology and Oncology
The Children's Hospital of Philadelphia
Philadelphia, Pennsylvania

Jessica Wen, MD
Fellow, Division of Gastroenterology, Hepatology, and
  Nutrition
The Children's Hospital of Philadelphia
Philadelphia, Pennsylvania

Deborah Whitney, MD
Attending Physician
Division of General Pediatrics
The Children's Hospital of Philadelphia
Clinical Assistant Professor of Pediatrics
The University of Pennsylvania School of Medicine
Philadelphia, Pennsylvania

Jennifer J. Wilkes, MD
Pediatric Resident
Department of Pediatrics
The Children's Hospital of Philadelphia
Philadelphia, Pennsylvania

Kamillah Wood, MD
Pediatric Chief Resident
Department of Pediatrics
The Children's Hospital of Philadelphia
Philadelphia, Pennsylvania

Courtney J. Wusthoff, MD
Clinical Neurophysiology Fellow
Division of Neurology
The Children's Hospital of Philadelphia
Philadelphia, Pennsylvania

Joyce Yang, MD
Pediatric Resident
Department of Pediatrics
The Children's Hospital of Philadelphia
Philadelphia, Pennsylvania

Mark R. Zonfrillo, MD
Fellow, Division of Pediatric Emergency Medicine
The Children's Hospital of Philadelphia
Philadelphia, Pennsylvania

Contents

Fred Henretig and James M. Callahan

Care of the Acutely Ill Child

Resuscitation

David Chao and Frances Nadel

Cardiopulmonary resuscitation (CPR) is the series of emergency interventions provided to a person who appears dead or in respiratory *extremis*, with the goal of restoring vital functions through optimization of cardiac output and tissue oxygen delivery. The two main components are external cardiac massage (chest compressions) and assisted respirations.

Most children who require CPR do not survive. Those who do survive often have significant neurologic deficits from the hypoxia and ischemia associated with the cardiopulmonary arrest. However, some children do return to their premorbid function. This may be related to recognition and treatment of impending cardiorespiratory failure, early bystander CPR, or rapid correction of the life-threatening event. It is difficult to predict which patients will have a return of spontaneous circulation and ultimately survive. Therefore, high-quality CPR should be begun immediately while more information is gathered to guide therapy.

The incidence of out-of-hospital cardiopulmonary arrest is difficult to ascertain from the current literature. However, data from multicenter registries support many widely held beliefs about pediatric out-of-hospital arrests. The incidence of nontraumatic, out-of-hospital cardiac arrest is highest for infants (children younger than 1 year of age). The most common cause in this age group is sudden infant death syndrome (SIDS). The presenting rhythm is usually asystole, and survival to discharge is rare ($\approx3\%$). For all other pediatric age groups, trauma is the leading cause of death. Although asystole is the most common arrest rhythm, ventricular tachycardia (VT) and ventricular fibrillation (VF) do occur and are more common in older children, especially adolescents. Survival in patients with ventricular dysrhythmias is higher than in patients with cardiopulmonary arrest associated with rhythms that are not responsive to cardioversion or defibrillation, such as asystole and pulseless electrical activity (PEA). For nontraumatic arrests, survival even for older children remains low, about 9% in those older than 1 year of age.

ETIOLOGY AND PATHOGENESIS

Cardiopulmonary arrest may result from many causes. Sepsis, respiratory infection, pulmonary conditions, drowning, SIDS, and injuries can lead to respiratory failure or shock. Without effective intervention, cardiopulmonary failure (inadequate perfusion and ineffective or absent respiration) ensues. Most pediatric arrests occur after an initial respiratory arrest (rather than circulatory failure) and if prolonged result in terminal rhythms of bradycardia; PEA; and, finally, asystole. Patients in asystole likely have experienced a significant hypoxic–ischemic insult.

CLINICAL PRESENTATION

The signs and symptoms of children requiring immediate resuscitation are typically the result of failure of the delivery of two vital substrates—oxygen and glucose—to end organs (Table 1-1). Recognition of these manifestations through a physical examination that focuses on airway, gas exchange, and cardiovascular stability allows for rapid resuscitation of those who have failure of substrate delivery and identification of those at risk for failure.

INITIAL ASSESSMENT

Evaluation of a critically ill or injured child should begin with a *general assessment*. Physical examination clues help the provider determine the extent of illness or injury (i.e., whether the condition is life threatening or not) and identify systems that require closer attention during the remainder of the assessment. The Pediatric Assessment Triangle of the Pediatric Advanced Life Support (PALS) course outlines the following components of the general assessment:

Appearance: muscle tone, interaction, consolability, look or gaze, speech or cry
Work of breathing: increased work of breathing, decreased or absent respiratory effort, or abnormal sounds
Circulation: abnormal skin color or bleeding

The initial assessment can be done without laying hands on the patient and should take no more than several seconds. If the patient's condition is life threatening, additional support should be recruited immediately. After these rapid initial impressions, the clinician should aim to perform a swift yet careful primary assessment.

PRIMARY ASSESSEMENT

The primary assessment evaluates and addresses vital functions in a systematic way with priority to systems that are most crucial for sustaining life. Conveniently, the components of the primary assessment can be remembered as the "ABCDEs"—*airway, breathing, circulation, disability,* and *exposure and environment*. If a life-threatening abnormality is identified at any point, the aberration should be addressed before moving on in the assessment.

With the publication of new guidelines for cardiopulmonary resuscitation in 2010, it has been recommended that the standard sequence of "ABC" be switched to "CAB" for patients who need cardiopulmonary resuscitation. This recommendation is based on the recognition that most cardiopulmonary arrests occur in adults and that even in children and adolescents sudden arrest is more likely to be due to a cardiac arrhythmia. Prompt institution of cardiac compressions to provide artificial circulation is important to ensure the best possible outcome for individual patients. This is especially important in out-of-hospital settings where early initiation of bystander CPR has been shown to be one of the strongest predictors of survival and good neurologic outcome. In medical settings the approach to resuscitation may be individualized based on the clinical scenario.

Table 1-1 Signs of a Life-Threatening Condition	
Airway	Complete or severe airway obstruction
Breathing	Apnea, significant work of breathing, bradypnea
Circulation	Absence of detectable pulses, poor perfusion, hypotension, bradycardia
Disability	Unresponsiveness, depressed consciousness
Exposure	Significant hypothermia, significant bleeding, petechiae or purpura consistent with septic shock, abdominal distension consistent with acute abdomen

Adapted from American Academy of Pediatrics and American Heart Association: Pediatric Advanced Life Support. Dallas, TX, American Heart Association Publication, 2006.

Close attention to securing the airway and providing artificial ventilation remain important but in the setting of cardiopulmonary arrest chest compressions should not be delayed.

Airway

The patient's airway is the first priority. There are fundamental differences between the airway of a child and that of an adult. The pediatric airway (Figure 1-1) is more anterior than the adult airway, requiring less manipulation to bring the oral, pharyngeal, and tracheal axes into alignment. In addition, the head-to-body proportion is larger in infants than in adults, and thus extreme hyperextension of the neck may exacerbate airway obstruction in younger children. The pediatric airway is narrower, and the tongue is relatively large compared with the jaw, increasing the risk of airway obstruction. The pediatric larynx is located more anteriorly and cephalad than the adult larynx.

The provider should assess airway patency using the "look, listen, and feel" approach. The provider should *look* at the chest wall and *listen* to the mouth and nose to detect whether there is evidence of air movement. Findings suggesting airway obstruction include increased respiratory effort with retractions, abnormal inspiratory sounds, or episodes during which no airway or breath sounds are produced despite respiratory effort. If a child is speaking, crying, or otherwise verbalizing, the airway is intact. Attention should be paid to the quality of the sounds. A hoarse or high-pitched cry should alert the provider to the possibility of airway compromise without complete obstruction. Finally, the provider should *feel* for air movement using a hand or cheek close to the patient's mouth.

The most effective maneuvers for opening an obstructed pediatric airway are the *head tilt–chin lift* or *jaw thrust* techniques (Figure 1-2). In the head tilt–chin lift maneuver, the head is tilted back slightly (without overextending), and the chin is lifted gently with one finger on the bony prominence to avoid placing pressure on the soft tissues of the neck. A roll or towel may be placed under the shoulders to maintain the position.

If there is a risk of a neck injury, it is critical to stabilize the cervical spine during evaluation of the airway and avoid extending the neck. Manual cervical spine stabilization is accomplished by holding the head in the midline position while applying gentle cephalad traction. A cervical collar may be applied, taking care to size the collar appropriately. It is important to remember that neither manual nor collared stabilization provides true immobilization.

The jaw thrust maneuver should be attempted in these cases by lifting the jaw forward with the provider's third or fourth fingers (or both) "hooked" under the angles of the mandible while avoiding compression of the soft tissues. The goal is to pull the mandibular block of tissue forward so that the lower central incisors are anterior to the upper central incisors.

At any point, if it is determined that the patient is unable to independently maintain the patency of his or her airway, the provider should open the airway to maintain adequate ventilation and protection from the aspiration of stomach contents. Simple suctioning should be attempted first because it may relieve an airway obstructed by secretions or foreign materials.

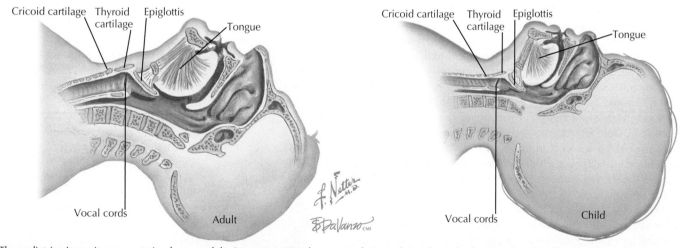

The pediatric airway is more anterior than an adult airway, requiring less manipulation to bring the oral, pharyngeal, and tracheal axes into alignment. The infant has a relatively large occiput, predisposing the neck to flexion and thus an increased propensity for airway obstruction when supine. Furthermore, extreme hyperextension may also result in airway obstruction in younger children as a result of the increased flexibility of the young airway. A child's airway is narrower and the tongue is relatively large compared to the jaw, increasing the risk of airway obstruction. The larynx is located more anteriorly and cephalad than the adult larynx, making the angle of entry into the trachea more acute.

Figure 1-1 *Pediatric and adult airway anatomy.*

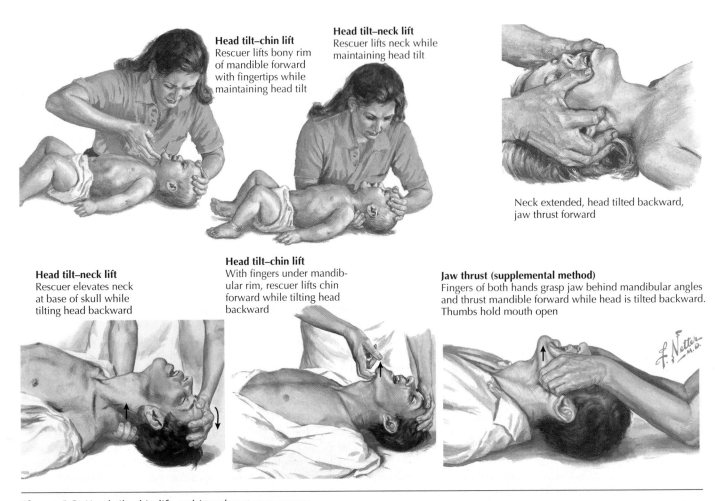

Head tilt–chin lift
Rescuer lifts bony rim of mandible forward with fingertips while maintaining head tilt

Head tilt–neck lift
Rescuer lifts neck while maintaining head tilt

Neck extended, head tilted backward, jaw thrust forward

Head tilt–neck lift
Rescuer elevates neck at base of skull while tilting head backward

Head tilt–chin lift
With fingers under mandibular rim, rescuer lifts chin forward while tilting head backward

Jaw thrust (supplemental method)
Fingers of both hands grasp jaw behind mandibular angles and thrust mandible forward while head is tilted backward. Thumbs hold mouth open

Figure 1-2 *Head tilt–chin lift and jaw thrust maneuvers.*

Bag–valve–mask (BVM) ventilation (see below) may provide an open airway if a good mask seal is achieved and airway positioning is maintained.

In an unconscious patient, an oropharyngeal airway can be used to help stent the mandibular block of tissue away from the posterior hypopharynx (Figure 1-3). A nasopharyngeal (NP) airway is another option. NP airways are well tolerated in unconscious and semiconscious patients and may even be used in conscious individuals with upper airway obstruction. NP airways should be used with caution when midface trauma is suspected because of the risk of inserting the airway through fractured bone into intracranial structures. Laryngeal mask airways (LMAs) are supraglottic airway devices that are being increasingly used in resuscitation settings to help bypass the soft tissues of the anterior oropharynx and to deliver oxygen directly to the proximal trachea.

When the patency of the airway cannot be maintained by other means, endotracheal intubation offers a relatively stable artificial airway. The following formula is used to determine the appropriate size (inner diameter) for an uncuffed endotracheal tube (ETT): (Age in years/4) + 4. Cuffed ETTs are being used with increasing frequency in children. The appropriate size can be determined using the above formula and then subtracting 0.5 (mm) from the result. One should have tubes one size larger and smaller at the ready in case this estimate is not quite

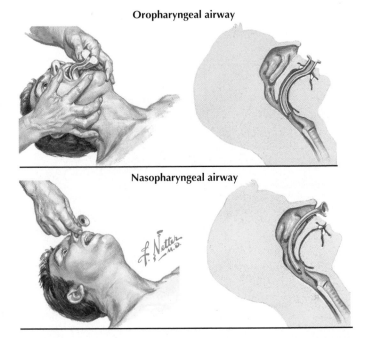

Oropharyngeal airway

Nasopharyngeal airway

Figure 1-3 *Oral and nasopharyngeal airways.*

appropriate for the individual patient. An appropriately sized laryngoscope blade should be chosen; the two most common types are Miller (straight) and Macintosh (curved) blades.

Pharmacologic agents (premedications such as atropine and lidocaine, sedatives, and paralytics) may be used to increase patient comfort, improve patient safety, and increase the chances of successful intubation. These are not necessary when the patient presents in cardiopulmonary arrest. In other settings, premedications should be selected based on the clinical scenario and prepared to be given. All equipment should be checked before sedative or neuromuscular blocking agents are administered to the patient. A useful mnemonic for preparing materials for intubation is "SOAP ME" for suction, oxygen, airway equipment, pharmacy or personnel, and monitoring equipment. After medications have been given, it is important to preoxygenate the patient using 100% oxygen via facemask.

Direct laryngoscopy can be accomplished by positioning the patient's head and then using the right thumb and index finger to "scissor" open the mouth. The laryngoscope blade is inserted under direct vision toward the right corner of the mouth over the tongue and over the epiglottis (if using a straight blade) or into the vallecula (if using a curved blade). The tongue should be "swept" toward the left side the mouth while the laryngoscope handle is pulled upward at a 45-degree angle, taking care not to damage the teeth or gums (Figure 1-4). Suctioning may

be needed to clear secretions to visualize the vocal cords, which should fall into the direct line of sight. The provider should maintain his or her view of the larynx and insert the ETT while watching it pass through the vocal cords. The tube should be placed so that the second of the distal vocal cord markers is at the level of the vocal cords. A projection for how deep to place the tube (centimeter mark at the teeth) can be calculated using the following formulas: [(Age in years/2) + 12] or [3 × (External diameter of the ETT)].

Confirmation of proper insertion of the ETT can be accomplished in several ways. Primary confirmation should always be confirmed by the detection of exhaled carbon dioxide (CO_2) through the use of a colorimetric CO_2 detector or use of inline capnography. Capnography has the added advantage of showing exhaled levels of CO_2. In patients in cardiopulmonary arrest, exhaled CO_2 may not be present even with proper tube placement. Listening for symmetric breath sounds in bilateral lung fields, observing symmetric chest wall rise, and maintaining a good oxygen saturation are all secondary signs of good tube placement. Visualizing mist in the ETT with expiration is helpful but may occur with misplacement of the tube into the esophagus as well. When time permits, a chest radiograph should be obtained to confirm placement, including depth of the ETT. The tip of the tube should be approximately 1 cm above the carina.

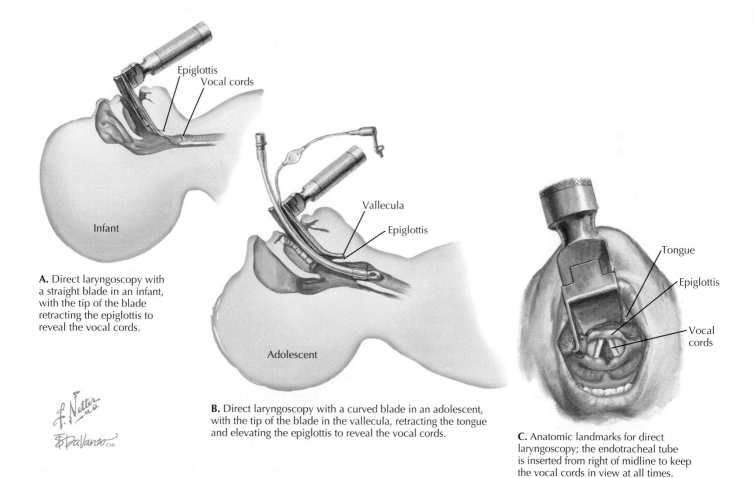

Epiglottis
Vocal cords

Infant

A. Direct laryngoscopy with a straight blade in an infant, with the tip of the blade retracting the epiglottis to reveal the vocal cords.

Vallecula
Epiglottis

Adolescent

B. Direct laryngoscopy with a curved blade in an adolescent, with the tip of the blade in the vallecula, retracting the tongue and elevating the epiglottis to reveal the vocal cords.

Tongue
Epiglottis
Vocal cords

C. Anatomic landmarks for direct laryngoscopy; the endotracheal tube is inserted from right of midline to keep the vocal cords in view at all times.

Figure 1-4 *Endotracheal intubation.*

Breathing

After the airway has been stabilized, assessment of ventilation and gas exchange should be initiated. Observation of chest wall movement can provide clues regarding adequacy of respiratory effort. In infants, adequate chest wall movement is characterized by uniform expansion of the lower chest and upper abdomen. In older children and adolescents, observation should focus on upper chest expansion. Auscultation over the trachea assesses central airway patency. Breath sounds should then be auscultated over the upper lung fields while focusing on adequacy of air movement and symmetry of breath sounds. Adequate gas exchange can be assessed using pulse oximetry, capnography, and blood gases. Because hypoxia is the major means of pediatric cardiac arrest, supplemental oxygen should be given to all critically ill patients to maximize oxygen delivery.

If the patient's efforts at ventilation or oxygenation are compromised, assisted ventilation should be initiated. BVM ventilation (Figure 1-5) is a skill at which all physicians working in acute-care settings should become adept. Masks of various sizes should be available, and the smallest mask that completely covers the mouth and nose should be selected. Airway patency is maximized when the patient's head is placed in the "sniffing position," with the neck slightly flexed while the head is rotated into extension.

When using the chin lift maneuver, the provider's nondominant hand should be used to hold the mask in place by forming a "C" around the connector with the thumb and index fingers while the remaining fingers maintain the chin lift along the angle of the mandible. If the jaw thrust is used, the mask should be secured with the thumb and index fingers of both hands with the remaining third or fourth fingers maintaining the jaw thrust at the angles of the mandible. Downward pressure on the mask should be used to provide countertraction against the upward force generated by the jaw maneuver, maintaining an adequate seal of the mask against the face. The provider should concentrate on trying to "lift" the jaw up to the mask. With either maneuver, the mask should fit snugly on the face, and the provider should assess for an adequate seal (attempting to minimize air leaks), which is the most important aspect of effective BVM ventilation.

After an adequate seal has been achieved, ventilation can be accomplished by administering positive pressure via the resuscitation bag. A two-person technique is preferred, with one person holding the mask in place and the other providing breaths. The amount of positive pressure generated should be dictated by the adequacy of chest wall excursion—the patient's chest wall movements should be similar to normal deep respirations. The recommended number of respirations depends on age—infants and children should receive 15 to 20 breaths/min (≈1 breath every 3-5 seconds), and adolescents should receive 10 to 12 breaths/min (≈1 breath every 5-6 seconds).

Although BVM ventilation is a safe procedure, there are potential complications. Equipment failure is a common and avoidable complication that may lead to inadequate oxygenation and ventilation. Oxygen sources and the patency of connections should be checked routinely as well as when problems arise. Other complications of BVM ventilation include cervical cord damage in cases of traumatic injury, hyperventilation,

Two-handed technique

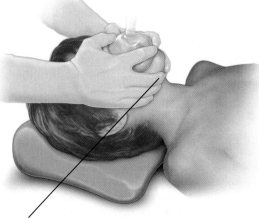

Three fingers are used to gently pull the mandible up into the mask using a gentle jaw thrust rather than pushing the mask down into the face.

One-handed technique

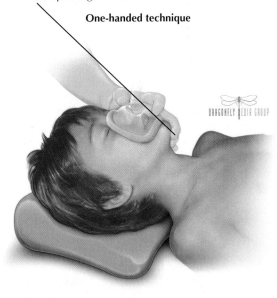

Figure 1-5 *Maintaining airway patency and securing the mask in bag–valve–mask ventilation.*

pneumonitis associated with reflux and aspiration of stomach contents, pneumothorax, and gastrointestinal tract distension.

Circulation

The goals of the circulatory assessment are to evaluate cardiovascular function and end-organ perfusion. Cardiovascular dysfunction can be reflected by changes in skin color, temperature, heart rate, heart rhythm, blood pressure, pulses, and capillary refill time. End-organ dysfunction can be reflected by changes in brain perfusion (manifesting as altered mental status), skin perfusion, and renal perfusion (manifesting as decreased urine output).

Heart rate should be appropriate for the child's age (Table 1-2) but may be affected by clinical conditions other than poor circulation (e.g., fever, dehydration, pain). Normal blood

Table 1-2 Normal Heart Rates by Age

Age	Awake Rate (beats/min)	Mean (beats/min)	Sleeping Rate (beats/min)
Newborn to 3 months	85-205	140	80-160
3 months to 2 years	100-190	130	75-160
2 years to 10 years	60-140	80	60-90
>10 years	60-100	75	50-90

Adapted from American Academy of Pediatrics and American Heart Association: Pediatric Advanced Life Support. *Dallas, TX, American Heart Association Publication, 2006.*

pressure is also age dependent (Table 1-3) and can also be affected by associated clinical conditions. In children, compensatory mechanisms (tachycardia, increased stroke volume, and vasoconstriction) may cause blood pressure to be preserved even though there is inadequate tissue perfusion. This is termed *compensated shock* (see Chapter 2). However, hypotension should be treated as shock until proven otherwise in critically ill or injured children because it represents a state in which compensatory mechanisms have failed (uncompensated shock). It is important to measure blood pressure using a properly sized cuff.

Assessment of perfusion should include palpation of both central (most commonly femoral) and peripheral (radial and dorsalis pedis) pulses. In infants, the brachial pulse is checked. Weak central pulses portend impending circulatory failure. A discrepancy between central and peripheral pulses may suggest worsening shock but may be caused by appropriate vasoconstriction in a cold environment. Prolonged capillary refill times may also be seen during times of inadequate perfusion. However, both ambient temperature and the patient's body temperature may cause prolonged capillary refill to be a nonspecific finding.

Compromised circulation may be the result of a number of different factors, including blood loss, dehydration, neurologic injury, and infection. Ideally, during the primary assessment, providers obtain vascular access. Large-bore intravenous (IV) lines are preferable; however, it may be difficult to establish venous access in a critically ill child who has compromised perfusion. The intraosseous (IO) route is a quick and reliable technique. Newer IO devices have been developed (including spring-loaded needles and battery-powered handheld drills),

Table 1-3 Definition of Hypotension by Systolic Blood Pressure and Age

Age	Systolic Blood Pressure (mm Hg)
Term neonates (0-28 days)	<60
Infants (1-12 months)	<70
Children (1-10 years)	<70 + (Age in years × 2)
Children (>10 years)	<90

BP, blood pressure
Adapted from American Academy of Pediatrics and American Heart Association: Pediatric Advanced Life Support. *Dallas, TX, American Heart Association Publication, 2006.*

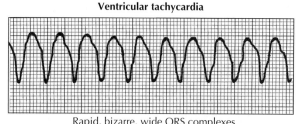
Ventricular tachycardia

Rapid, bizarre, wide QRS complexes

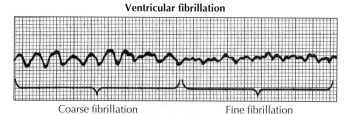
Ventricular fibrillation

Coarse fibrillation   Fine fibrillation

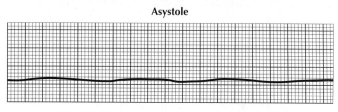
Asystole

Figure 1-6 *Arrest rhythms.*

which may be easier to use, especially in larger children. Fluid resuscitation is indicated in states of circulatory compromise. The goal is to prevent cardiopulmonary arrest, which is the cessation of blood circulation resulting from ineffective or absent cardiac activity.

Cardiac arrest is associated with the following arrest rhythms (Figure 1-6): asystole, PEA, VF, and pulseless VT. Asystole is characterized by the absence of discernible electrical activity ("flatline"). PEA is a condition in which the patient has no palpable pulse despite showing electrical activity on cardiac monitoring (but excludes VF, VT, and asystole). VT is characterized by organized, wide QRS (>0.08 sec) complexes. Pulseless VT must be distinguished from VT with a pulse because they are treated differently. VF is a form of pulseless arrest that is characterized by chaotic, disorganized electrical activity on cardiac monitoring with an absence of coordinated contractions. For all of these rhythms, it is important to provide supplemental oxygen (100%) and to initiate CPR immediately.

CPR (Figure 1-7) is indicated for the management of cardiopulmonary arrest. Studies have consistently shown that CPR, when performed correctly, saves lives. The mantra "push hard, push fast, minimize interruptions, allow full chest recoil, and do not overventilate" should guide the provider's efforts.

Recommendations for compression to breath ratios are summarized. In newborns, a ratio of 3:1 is recommended. In infants and children, the compression to ventilation ratio is different depending on whether there is a single rescuer or two rescuers performing CPR. A single rescuer should give 30 compressions for every 2 breaths, whereas 2 rescuers should perform CPR using the ratio of 15 compressions for every 2 breaths. In both scenarios, the goal is to provide at least 100 compressions per minute. After an artificial airway has been placed, continuous

Chest compressions: adult and child*

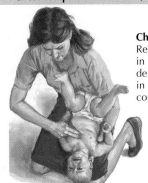

Central point of pressure area

Xiphoid

Liver

Posterior movement of xiphoid may lacerate liver. Lowest point of pressure on sternum must be at xiphisternal junction or slightly above

Patient horizontal on rigid surface

Rescuer palpates rib margin and follows medially to xiphisternal junction

With middle finger in xiphisternal junction, rescuer places index finger on lower end of sternum

Heel of other hand is placed on sternum next to index finger of palpating hand

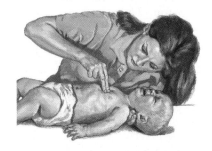

Heel of palpating hand is now placed on top of hand on sternum, and compression initiated. Fingers do not touch chest wall during compression

*Compression method for adult is 2 hands (heel of 1 hand, other hand on top); for child 2 hands (heel of 1 hand with second hand on top) OR 1 hand (heel of 1 hand); for infant 2 fingers.

Chest compressions: infant (children younger than 12 months, excluding the newly born [see Chapter 106])

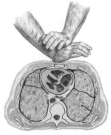

Chest thrusts
Rescuer holds infant on thigh in head-down position and delivers up to 4 chest thrusts in same manner as chest compressions (see next)

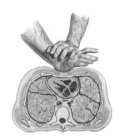

Compression and ventilation
Tips of index and middle fingers are used for compression over midsternum. Compression rate in infants is 100 per minute. A single rescuer gives 2 ventilations after 30 compressions, while two rescuers should give 2 ventilations after every 15 compressions, observing closely for rise and fall of chest

Compression depth

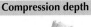

Compression depth is at least 2 inches in an adult and at least 1/3 the depth of the chest in the infant and child (about 1 1/2 inches [4 cm] in infants and 2 inches [5 cm] in most children)

Figure 1-7 *External chest compressions.*

compressions at a rate of at least 100 compressions/min with ventilations at a rate of about 8 to 10 breaths/min (1 breath every 6-8 sec) should be performed. Resuscitation of the newly born infant is discussed in Chapter 106.

Synchronized cardioversion is indicated for VT accompanied by a pulse. The initial dose is 0.5 to 1 J/kg. If ineffective, an additional dose of 2 J/kg should be administered. Defibrillation is indicated for VT without a pulse and VF. If using a manual defibrillator, the initial dose is 2 J/kg, and an automated external defibrillator (AED) may be used for patients older than 1 year of age.

Although a full discussion of resuscitation medications is beyond the scope of this chapter, it is important to be familiar with the most important pharmacologic agents used during resuscitation. Epinephrine, an adrenergic agent with both α- and β-agonist properties, is used to promote vasoconstriction, which is important in increasing aortic diastolic pressure and coronary perfusion pressure. It also increases automaticity of cardiac muscle and makes cardiac muscle more susceptible to the effects of cardioversion and defibrillation. It is used as a first-line agent in pulseless arrest with nonshockable rhythms (i.e., asystole and PEA) and symptomatic bradycardia (heart rate <60 beats/min with poor perfusion despite CPR). It is also used for VF and pulseless VT that do not respond to defibrillation. Although the dose and concentration used are route dependent (0.01 mg/kg of 1:10000 IV or IO and 0.1mg/kg of 1:1000 via ETT), the appropriate volume to give is easily remembered as 0.1 mL/kg. CPR should be continued for at least one full cycle (2 minutes) of compressions after any intervention and until medications for the treatment of cardiorespiratory arrest have taken effect.

After the return of spontaneous circulation, it is important that meticulous attention be paid to post-resuscitation care including glucose monitoring and control, fluid resuscitation, and support of cardiovascular stability through vasoactive medications.

Disability

Disability assessment focuses on evaluation of the two main components of the central nervous system, the cerebral cortex and the brainstem. A number of scales are used to assess neurologic function. The AVPU Pediatric Response Scale is quick and simple to apply in critical situations. Level of consciousness is described as:

A: alert (child is awake, active, and appropriately responsive)
V: voice (child responds to voice)
P: pain (child responds only to painful stimulus)
U: unresponsive (child does not respond to any stimulus)

A more detailed assessment for older children and adolescents, the Glasgow Coma Scale, is the most widely used method (Figure 1-8). The patient's *best* responses in each of the categories (eye opening, verbal response, motor response) are added to produce a score out of 15. A change of 2 points reflects a clinically significant change in neurologic status. This scale is modified when used in infants and younger children.

The pupils should also be examined during this part of the assessment to help assess brainstem function. Normally, the pupils constrict in response to light and dilate in dark environments. An abnormal size of pupils, failure of pupils to react to light, and asymmetry of pupil size are all abnormalities that should be noted during the primary assessment.

An additional "D" that is included for a noninjured, critical patient is a "D-stick" (fingerstick glucose measurement) because many medical conditions leading to critical illness are characterized or accompanied by disturbances in blood sugar. For the treatment of hypoglycemia, the appropriate dose of dextrose to administer as an IV bolus is 0.5 to 1 g/kg, which is equivalent to 5 to 10 mL/kg of D10W (dextrose 10% in water).

Exposure

Complete exposure by undressing an injured or ill child should ideally be accomplished simultaneously by ancillary staff while the other components of the primary survey are addressed. Complete exposure is important to facilitate a comprehensive physical examination as part of the secondary survey. Another important "E" is "environment." The provider should take care to institute warming measures for the exposed child if clinically indicated, and the environment should be free of contaminants that may exacerbate the child's clinical condition (e.g., a child

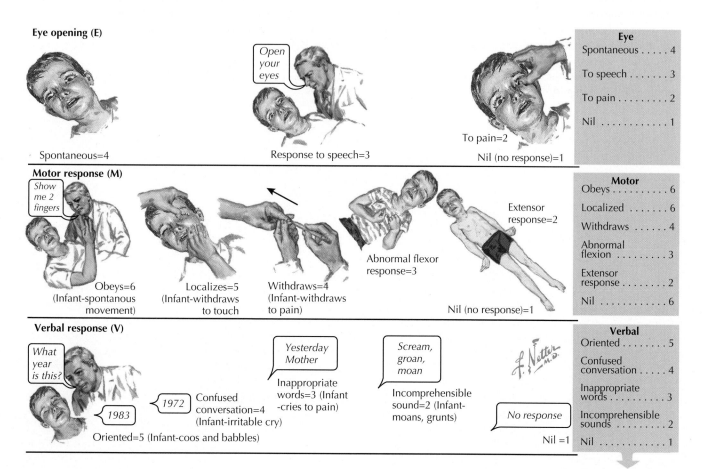

Figure 1-8 *Glasgow Coma Scale.*

who experienced inhalation injury should be taken out of the smoky environment).

SECONDARY ASSESSMENT

After completion of the primary assessment, including addressing any abnormalities discovered during the course of evaluation, the provider should initiate the *secondary survey*, which includes a focused history and physical examination. The SAMPLE mnemonic is helpful in addressing the important parts of the focused history: *signs and symptoms*, *allergies*, *medications*, *past medical history*, *last meal*, and *events* leading to current condition. Questions should be directed toward attempting to determine factors that may help to explain impaired respiratory, circulatory, or neurologic function. A focused physical examination is best approached in a head-to-toe fashion.

FUTURE DIRECTIONS

Outcomes from pediatric resuscitation have improved incrementally over the past several decades. Research has brought about advances in our understanding of the pathophysiology and management of cardiopulmonary arrest and its consequences. Current areas of research include therapeutic hypothermia, oxygen toxicity and reperfusion injury, the molecular genetics behind causes of cardiopulmonary arrest, and genetic polymorphisms and their implications in response to therapy. Pre- and postconditioning of the myocardium and brain epithelium, emergency preservation and resuscitation (EPR), postresuscitation myocardial support, mechanical circulatory support, quality CPR, and the epidemiology of CPR are also subjects of significant inquiry. The once dismal prognosis of critically ill and injured children continues to improve as discoveries of promising therapeutic advances are made in pre- and postresuscitation care.

SUGGESTED READINGS

American Academy of Pediatrics and American Heart Association: *Pediatric Advanced Life Support*, Dallas, TX, 2006, American Heart Association Publication.

Atkins DL, Everson-Stewart S, Sears GK, et al: Resuscitation Outcomes Consortium Investigators. Epidemiology and outcomes from out-of-hospital cardiac arrest in children: The Resuscitation Outcomes Consortium Epistry-Cardiac Arrest, *Circulation* 119(11):1484-1491, 2009.

Berg MD, Schexnayder SM, Chameides L, et al: Pediatric Basic Life Support: 2010 American Heart Association guidelines for cardiopulmonary resuscitation and emergency cardiovascular care: part 13, *Circulation* 122:S862-S875, 2010.

King C, editor: Cardiopulmonary life support procedures. In Henretig FM, King C, editors: *Textbook of Pediatric Emergency Procedures*, Philadelphia, 1997, Lippincott Williams & Wilkins.

Kleinman ME, Chameides L, Schexnayder SM, et al: Pediatric Advanced Life Support: 2010 American Heart Association guidelines for cardiopulmonary resuscitation and emergency cardiovascular care: part 14, *Circulation* 122:S876-S908, 2010.

Ludwig SL, Lavelle JM: Resuscitation—pediatric basic and advanced life support. In Fleisher G, Ludwig S, Henretig FM, editors: *Pediatric Emergency Medicine*, ed 5, Philadelphia, 2006, Lippincott Williams & Wilkins.

Schexnayder SM, Zaritsky AL, editors: Pediatric Resuscitation, *Pediatr Clin North Am* 55(4), 2008.

Topjian AA, Berg RA, Nadkarni VM: Pediatric cardiopulmonary resuscitation: advances in science, techniques, and outcomes, *Pediatrics* 122(5):1086-1098, 2008.

Shock

Kari R. Posner and Aaron Donoghue

2

Shock is an acute clinical syndrome of circulatory dysfunction in which there is failure to deliver sufficient oxygen and substrate to meet metabolic demand. All practitioners who care for children must understand and identify shock promptly to initiate an effective treatment plan. This, in turn, can help prevent the progression and poor outcomes that characterize the natural clinical course of shock. The goal is to prevent end-organ damage; failure of multiple organ systems; and, ultimately, death.

ETIOLOGY AND PATHOGENESIS

Normal circulatory function is maintained by the interplay between the heart and blood flow with the purpose of delivering oxygen and nutrients to the tissues. Cardiac output is calculated by multiplying the stroke volume (volume of blood ejected by the left ventricle in a single beat) by the heart rate (ejection cycles per minute). Stroke volume is dependent on the filling volume of the ventricle (preload), resistance against which the heart is pumping blood (afterload), and myocardial contractility. During childhood, the heart rate is faster, and the stroke volume is smaller than during adulthood. In children, increasing the heart rate is the primary means to increase the cardiac output.

Shock develops as the result of conditions that cause decreased intravascular volume, abnormal distribution of intravascular volume, or impaired cardiovascular function. Children effectively compensate for circulatory insufficiency by increasing their heart rate, systemic vascular resistance (SVR), and venous tone. Children can therefore maintain normal blood pressures despite significantly compromised tissue perfusion. Thus, in pediatric patients, it is especially important to recognize that hypotension is not part of the definition of shock.

The clinical manifestations of shock can be directly related to the abnormalities seen on the tissue, cellular, and biochemical levels. Microcirculatory dysfunction; tissue ischemia; and release of biochemical, vasoactive, and inflammatory mediators are all part of the spectrum of pathophysiologic aberrations seen in shock. Poor perfusion of vital organs results in impaired function. For example, inadequate perfusion of the brain and kidneys results in depressed mental status and decreased urine output, respectively. As poorly perfused cells switch to anaerobic metabolism to generate energy, lactic acid accumulates resulting in a metabolic acidosis that further interferes with cell function. Hypoperfusion also initiates inflammatory events, such as the activation of neutrophils and release of cytokines, that cause cell damage and microischemia.

The prevalence of causes of shock varies by patient age, as well as region of the world. Hypovolemic shock from diarrheal illness is the leading cause of pediatric mortality worldwide, but is very rare in the United States. Congenital lesions (including heart disease) and complications of prematurity are most common in neonates and infants. Malignant neoplasms (for whom infectious complications are prevalent), infectious causes, and unintentional injuries are more common in older children and young adolescents. Injury, homicide, and suicide become more prevalent in older adolescents.

Compensated (Early) Shock

In compensated shock, homeostatic mechanisms have temporarily balanced metabolic supply and demand. In this state, the systolic blood pressure is normal in the presence of inadequate tissue perfusion. The earliest symptoms of shock result from an effort to maintain cardiac output and perfusion of vital organs (heart, brain, and kidneys). The body's initial mechanism to maintain cardiac output and compensate for low stroke volume is to increase heart rate (tachycardia). Other compensatory mechanisms include increasing SVR, cardiac contractility, and venous tone. As shock continues, the early compensatory mechanisms fail to meet the metabolic demands of the tissues, and uncompensated shock ensues. Here, as the microcirculation is affected, the child shows signs of brain, kidney, and cardiovascular compromise.

Uncompensated (Late) Shock

Uncompensated shock occurs when attempts to maintain blood pressure and perfusion are no longer successful, resulting in hypotension. When hypotension develops, the child's condition may deteriorate rapidly to cardiovascular collapse and subsequent cardiac arrest. Eventually, the child in uncompensated shock develops multiple organ dysfunction syndrome (MODS) secondary to ongoing shock and exaggerated inflammatory responses. Irreversible shock implies irreversible damage to vital organs resulting in death, regardless of therapy.

CLASSIFICATION OF SHOCK

Hypovolemic Shock

The most common type of shock in children is hypovolemic shock. Hypovolemia is defined as a decrease in circulating blood volume. The most common cause of hypovolemic shock is fluid loss associated with diarrhea and vomiting. Other causes include blood losses (e.g., trauma and gastrointestinal disorders), plasma losses (peritonitis, hypoproteinemia, burns), and water losses (osmotic diuresis, heatstroke). In hypovolemic shock, preload is decreased, SVR may be increased as a compensatory mechanism, and cardiac contractility is typically normal or may be increased.

Distributive Shock

Distributive shock is the result of abnormal distribution of blood volume (i.e., poor flow to the splanchnic circulation with excessive flow to the skin) caused by vasodilatation from changes in vasomotor tone and peripheral pooling of blood, resulting in inadequate tissue perfusion. SVR can be low, producing increased blood flow to the skin that keeps the extremities warm (warm shock), as well as a widened pulse pressure and bounding peripheral pulses. Conversely, SVR may be increased, resulting in decreased blood flow to the skin, resulting in cool extremities, with a narrowed pulse pressure and weak pulses (cold shock). Generally, cardiac output is normal or increased. Distributive shock commonly occurs in anaphylaxis; central nervous system or spinal injuries; drug ingestions; and most commonly in children, sepsis.

Cardiogenic Shock

Cardiogenic shock results from myocardial dysfunction and can usually be distinguished from other forms of shock because of associated signs of congestive heart failure (i.e., rales, gallop rhythm, hepatomegaly, jugular venous distension). Pump failure, arrhythmias, and congenital heart disease may all contribute to the inadequate perfusion seen in cardiogenic shock. A patient may exhibit tachycardia, increased SVR, and signs of decreased cardiac output as a result of a decrease in myocardial contractility. Causes of cardiogenic shock in children include viral myocarditis, arrhythmias, drug ingestions, complications of cardiac surgery, trauma, metabolic derangements, and congenital heart disease. Cardiogenic shock can also occur with obstruction of blood flow, as seen with a tension pneumothorax, massive pulmonary embolism, or critical coarctation of the aorta or other obstructive vascular lesions. A patient may also show evidence of both intrinsic cardiac disease and obstruction of blood flow with a cardiac tamponade or ductal-dependent congenital abnormality. It is important to recognize that infants that present with shock caused by a ductal-dependent cardiac lesion require blood flow through the ductus arteriosus to maintain adequate oxygen delivery.

Neurogenic Shock

Neurogenic shock may occur in the setting of pediatric trauma. Spinal cord injury may produce hypotension caused by a loss of sympathetic tone. The classic picture of neurogenic shock is hypotension without tachycardia or cutaneous vasoconstriction. The pulse pressure is usually widened. Patients sustaining spinal injuries often have concurrent torso trauma. Therefore, patients with known or suspected neurogenic shock should be treated initially for hypovolemia.

Septic Shock

Sepsis is defined as the presence of the systemic inflammatory response syndrome (SIRS) caused by a presumed or confirmed infection (Box 2-1). Sepsis may occur because of bacterial, viral, fungal, or parasitic infections. Septic shock is defined as sepsis and cardiovascular dysfunction. Classifying septic shock may be difficult because of the developmental variability in physiologic response to sepsis. A clinical picture consistent with hypovolemic, distributive, or cardiogenic shock may be present in a child with sepsis. Additionally, studies have demonstrated that the cardiovascular pathophysiology of children with sepsis can

Box 2-1 Systemic Inflammatory Response Syndrome Criteria

Must have two of the following criteria, one of which must be abnormal temperature or leukocyte count:
   Core **temperature** of >38.5°C or <36°C
   Tachycardia (mean HR >2 standard deviations above normal for age) in absence of external stimuli, chronic drugs or pain, or otherwise unexplained persistent elevation over a 0.5- to 4-hour time period *or* **bradycardia** for children younger than 12 months of age (mean HR <10th percentile for age) in the absence of external vagal stimuli, β-adrenergic blocker drugs, congenital heart disease, or otherwise unexplained persistent depression over a 0.5-hour period
   Mean **respiratory rate** >2 standard deviations above normal for age
   Leukocyte count elevated or depressed for age or >10% immature neutrophils

HR, heart rate.
Adapted from American Academy of Pediatrics and American Heart Association. *Pediatric Advanced Life Support.* Dallas, 2006, AHA.

evolve over time, and the adjustment of hemodynamic therapy is commonly necessary.

CLINICAL MANIFESTATIONS AND EVALUATION

Shock remains a clinical diagnosis (Figure 2-1). Early recognition of the clinical signs of shock (including familiarity with normal ranges for vital signs by age; see Chapter 1) should lead to directed management. An accurate history should be obtained from the family and, if possible, the child, simultaneously with treatment initiation.

A history of fluid loss, as with a gastrointestinal bleed, gastroenteritis, or diabetic ketoacidosis, is consistent with hypovolemic shock. A detailed trauma history is useful because an injured child may have hypovolemic shock from hemorrhage (i.e., with blunt abdominal trauma), neurogenic shock with spinal cord injury, or obstructive shock from tension pneumothorax. A child who has had fever or is immunocompromised may have features consistent with septic shock. Exposure to an allergen, such as a food or an insect bite, could suggest distributive shock caused by anaphylaxis. A history of ingestion or medications should always be included when speaking to the family because shock may be attributable to toxin exposure. Patients with underlying heart disease may present in cardiogenic shock. Patients with a history of adrenal insufficiency (i.e., chronic steroid therapy, congenital adrenal hyperplasia, or hypopituitarism) can present with adrenal crisis and shock.

A complete physical examination should be performed, including vital signs and pulse oximetry. When a child presents in shock, it is sometimes difficult to obtain an accurate weight, which can be essential for determining fluid requirements and medication doses. If the patient's weight cannot be measured, one may be estimated using a length-based tape system (e.g., the Broselow tape) or the child's age.

Children in shock tend to be tachypneic, as well as tachycardic. Blood pressure should be monitored closely. Remember,

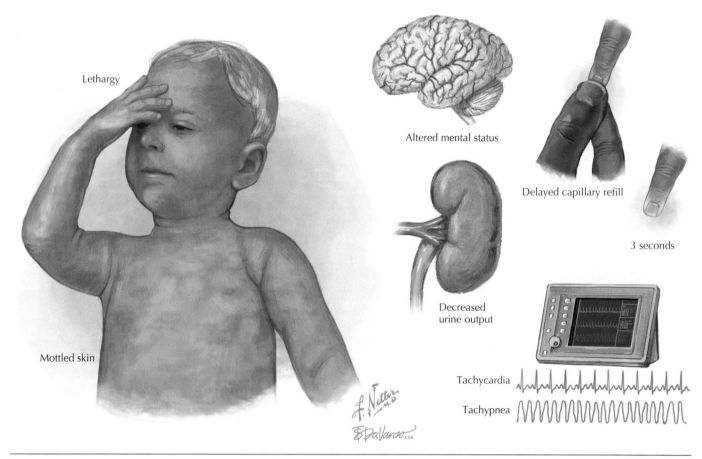

Lethargy

Altered mental status

Delayed capillary refill

3 seconds

Decreased urine output

Mottled skin

Tachycardia

Tachypnea

Figure 2-1 *Clinical manifestations of shock.*

children with shock may have normal blood pressures. Narrow pulse pressure may occur as a result of a compensatory increase in SVR, as in hypovolemic or cardiogenic shock. Widening of the pulse pressure can be seen as the result of decreased SVR, as can occur with distributive shock. The child's temperature should also be measured because fever—or in young infants, hypothermia—may suggest septic shock.

When first examining an ill child, one should do a rapid assessment of mental status. Change in the level of consciousness of a child may indicate decreased cerebral oxygenation or perfusion. Signs of diminished perfusion to the brain include confusion, irritability, lethargy, and agitation.

Examining the child's skin is another way to assess perfusion and the degree of shock. A child with normal cardiorespiratory function should have warm and pink nailbeds, mucous membranes, palms, and soles. As shock progresses and poor perfusion develops, the skin may become cool, pale, or mottled. Capillary refill, although limited by clinician variability as well as ambient temperature and the child's body temperature, can help to evaluate children in shock. Light pressure is applied to blanch the fingernail bed. The pressure is released, and the amount of time until color returns is measured. Normal is less than 2 seconds; volume depletion or poor perfusion can increase this time to greater than 3 seconds.

The evaluation of a child with poor perfusion and shock should always include an assessment of pulses. This includes the rate, strength, and regularity of the central and peripheral pulses. In healthy children, the carotid, brachial, radial, femoral, dorsalis pedis, and posterior tibial pulses are readily palpable. A rapid pulse is a nonspecific clinical sign of distress. An irregular pulse is a warning of cardiac dysrhythmia. A weak pulse raises the concern for shock and a severe hypovolemic state. An absence of central pulses indicates ineffective or absent cardiac contractions and signifies the need for immediate resuscitative action.

After the initial evaluation of airway, breathing, and circulation (the ABCs), a complete physical examination can help elucidate the type of shock. For example, central cyanosis, a gallop rhythm, crackles on lung examination, hepatomegaly, or heart murmur may indicate an underlying cardiac condition. Children with stridor, wheeze, urticaria, or edema may have anaphylactic shock. Purpura or petechiae can be seen in children with septic shock. Bruises and abrasions can be seen with traumatic injury and may give a clue to underlying hemorrhagic shock.

MANAGEMENT

General Principles

Early recognition of compensated shock is critical to ensuring appropriate and expedient therapy. Initial therapy of shock is universal, regardless of the cause of the shock state, with the goals of optimizing blood oxygen content, improving cardiac output, reducing oxygen demand, and correcting metabolic abnormalities

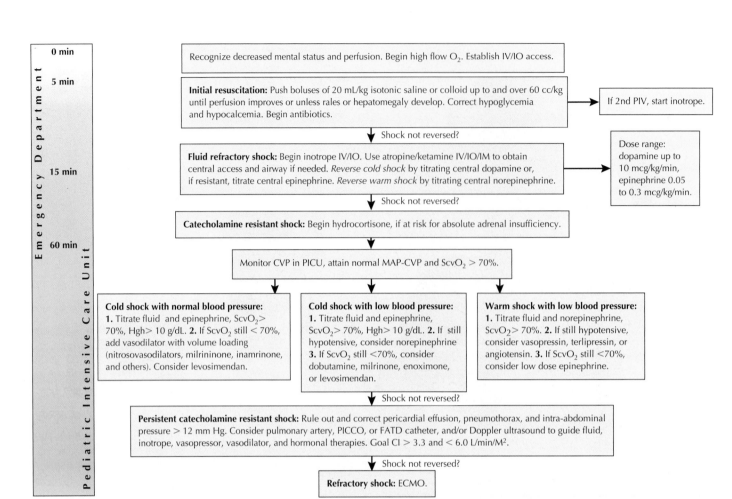

Figure 2-2 *Algorithm for management of pediatric septic shock.* From Brierley J, Carcillo J, Choong K, et al: 2007 American College of Critical Care Medicine clinical practice parameters for hemodynamic support of pediatric and neonatal septic shock. Crit Care Med 37(2):666-688, 2009.

(Figure 2-2). General principles of resuscitation should be applied immediately on presentation to medical care (see Chapter 1). Ultimately, after initial management has commenced, correction of the underlying cause is essential (e.g., stopping blood loss in hemorrhagic shock, antibiotics for shock caused by bacterial infection).

Immediate attention to the ABCs is mandatory. Maintenance of a patent airway with positioning or endotracheal intubation should be performed immediately if airway compromise is present. Hypoxemia should be corrected without delay; all patients with compromised perfusion should receive supplemental oxygen at 100% FiO₂ (fraction of inspired oxygen). Insufficient respiratory effort should be addressed with positive-pressure ventilation.

Imminently life-threatening causes of shock should be identified and corrected. For example, a child with upper airway obstruction from anaphylaxis should receive epinephrine. If a child has severe respiratory distress, asymmetric breath sounds, and poor perfusion, a tension pneumothorax might need to be decompressed.

Vascular access is indicated in all cases. If possible, large-bore intravenous (IV) catheters should be inserted in peripheral veins. If an IV line is unable to be placed promptly, intraosseous (IO) cannulation should be performed. IV fluid boluses of

20 mL/kg of isotonic saline should be given rapidly and repeated as needed with reassessment occurring simultaneously. Rapid fluid administration should be actively performed using either a pressure bag or a push–pull system rather than using passive gravity flow for administration. IV fluids should be given with care in cardiogenic shock, so as to not worsen associated pulmonary edema.

Adequate hemoglobin is essential for optimal oxygen carrying capacity. Thus, in cases of hemorrhagic shock, O-negative packed red blood cells should be rapidly administered early in the resuscitation. Even in cases of nontraumatic shock, children who have cyanotic heart disease or neonates may require less fluid and higher hematocrit percentages to ensure adequate oxygen carrying capacity. Life-threatening metabolic abnormalities should be identified and corrected early. Hypoglycemia should be treated with 0.5 to 1 g/kg of IV dextrose. Hypocalcemia (especially decreased ionized calcium) is common in septic shock and can occur as acidosis resolves; it should be corrected with either calcium gluconate or calcium chloride.

Circulatory Support

Depending on the cause, patients in shock may require large volumes of fluid as well as vasoactive medications. Clinical

Table 2-1 Vasoactive Medications

Agent	α-1 Receptor Activity	β-1 Receptor Activity	β-2 Receptor Activity	Dopaminergic Receptor Activity	Predominant Clinical Effects
Dopamine	Minimal; increases with dose	+	0	++	CO ↑ SVR ↑
Epinephrine	+++	+++	++	0	CO ↑ SVR ↓ (low dose) SVR ↑ (higher dose)
Dobutamine	0	+++	++	0	CO ↑ SVR ↓
Norepinephrine	+++	++	0	0	SVR ↑ CO ↔ or ↑
Phenylephrine	+++	0	0	0	SVR ↑
Milrinone*	0	0	0	0	CO ↑ SVR ↓

CO, cardiac output; SVR, systemic vascular resistance.
*Milrinone is a phosphodiesterase inhibitor which acts in a separate receptor pathway than catecholamines.

studies of septic shock in children have demonstrated an association between higher volumes of fluid administration and survival. Current guidelines for septic shock recommend up to and over 60 mL/kg in the first 15 to 60 minutes. Every hour that goes by without implementation of this therapy is associated with a 1.5-fold increase in mortality. A retrospective chart review of 90 children with septic shock showed that those who received less than 20 mL/kg of fluid within the first hour had a mortality rate of 73%. Early fluid resuscitation was associated with a threefold reduction in the odds of death.

Vasoactive agents help improve cardiac output through their effects on myocardial contractility, heart rate, and vascular tone. These drugs target at least three types of receptors. The β_1-receptors mediate inotropic (contractility), chronotropic (rate), and dromotropic (increased conduction velocity) activity. The β_2-receptors mediate vasodilatation and smooth muscle relaxation in blood vessels and bronchial tree. The α-receptors mediate arteriole constriction systemically and bronchial muscle constriction. The dopaminergic receptors mediate smooth muscle relaxation and increase renal blood flow and sodium excretion.

Table 2-1 outlines commonly used vasoactive agents, their targeted receptors, and their hemodynamic effects. Data are varied on the choice of initial agent; current recommendations from the American College of Critical Care Medicine state that dopamine, epinephrine, or norepinephrine may be appropriate first-line therapy for septic shock, provided they are administered through a central venous catheter. Dopamine or low-dose epinephrine may be given via a peripheral vein while central venous access is obtained.

Special Circumstances: Shock in Neonates

Neonatal physiology poses specific challenges regarding the management of shock. As mentioned previously, optimal oxygen-carrying capacity may demand a higher hematocrit in a newborn. Hypoxemia may occur more readily because of the presence of smaller and fewer alveoli, absent collateral channels of ventilation, and poor chest wall compliance; uncorrected hypoxemia may result in bradycardia in neonates. Additionally, myocardial performance is more drastically affected by acidosis

and hypocalcemia in neonates. Prompt correction of hypoxemia, acidosis, and hypocalcemia is essential. Neonates are also more prone to hypoglycemia, which should be looked for and treated appropriately.

When faced with a neonate with shock, early consideration should be given to ductal-dependent congenital heart disease. Lesions marked by ductal-dependent systemic blood flow, such as aortic stenosis, hypoplastic left heart syndrome, coarctation of the aorta, and interrupted aortic arch, may present as shock in the neonatal period (see Chapter 44). Infants with these lesions depend on blood flow from the pulmonary artery across the ductus arteriosus into the aorta for perfusion of all or part of the systemic circulation. Although this is deoxygenated blood, the oxygen content is sufficient to meet the metabolic demands of the tissues. Therefore, when the ductus arteriosus closes, circulatory failure and tissue hypoxia occur.

Prostaglandin E1 (PGE_1 or alprostadil) is the definitive initial therapy for neonates with ductal-dependent congenital heart disease who have not yet undergone surgical palliation or correction. An infusion at 0.1 μg/kg/min is required to reopen a closing ductus arteriosus. Side effects of prostaglandin include flushing, hypotension, pyrexia, bradycardia, seizures, and apnea. Emergent evaluation by a pediatric cardiologist should be pursued, but initiation of PGE_1 therapy should not be delayed pending the evaluation.

FUTURE DIRECTIONS

Current research in shock in children is predominantly in the realm of septic shock. Goal-directed therapy of septic shock, an established concept in adults, is less well investigated in children and will continue to be an important topic in future investigations. Diagnostic laboratory studies, such as serum lactate and B-type natriuretic peptide levels, may hold promise in early detection and ongoing monitoring of children with shock. Newer noninvasive techniques for cardiac output measurement (e.g., pulse contour waveform analysis, partial carbon dioxide rebreathing) have begun to be used successfully in children and may be applied more broadly in the years to come. Massive transfusion therapy in children with hemorrhagic shock is

another area in which advances in therapy for adults are beginning to be investigated in pediatric patients. Additional advanced
critical care therapies, such as steroid or thyroid hormone
replacement, renal replacement therapy, newer hemodynamic
agents (e.g., levosimendan), and extracorporeal circulatory
support, have been studied in pediatric patients, but their exact
role remains unclear.

SUGGESTED READINGS

American College of Surgeons Committee on Trauma: *Advanced Trauma Life Support for Doctors (ATLS)*, 8th ed. Chicago, 2008, American College of Surgeons.

American Heart Association: *Pediatric Advanced Life Support (PALS) Provider Manual*, Dallas, 2006, American Heart Association Publications.

Bell L: Shock. In Fleisher G, Ludwig S, editors: *Textbook of Pediatric Emergency Medicine*, ed 6, Philadelphia, 2010, Lippincott Williams & Wilkins, pp 46-57.

Brierley J, Carcillo JA, Choong K, et al: Clinical practice parameters for hemodynamic support of pediatric and neonatal septic shock: 2007 update from the American, *Crit Care Med* 37(2):666-688, 2009.

Ceneviva G, Paschall JA, Maffei F, Carcillo JA: Hemodynamic support in fluid-refractory pediatric septic shock, *Pediatrics* 102(2):e19, 1998.

Goldstein B, Giroir B, Randolph A: Pediatric sepsis consensus conference: definitions of sepsis and organ dysfunction in pediatrics, *Pediatr Crit Care Med* 6(1):2-8, 2005.

McKiernan C, Lieberman S: Circulatory shock in children: an overview, *Pediatr Rev* 26:451-460, 2005.

Rivers E, Nguyen B, Havstad S, Ressler J, et al: Early goal-directed therapy in the treatment of severe sepsis and septic shock, *N Engl J Med* 345:1368-1377, 2001.

Respiratory Distress

Shirley D. Viteri and Esther Maria Sampayo

3

Respiratory distress is defined as an alteration in the normal biomechanical and physiologic mechanisms of respiration. Respiratory distress is manifested by complaints of difficulty breathing and a variety of findings on physical examination showing increased respiratory effort. The degree of these findings can vary from mild to severe. Respiratory distress is one of the most common conditions for which children present for acute care. In contrast to adults, children experience significant morbidity and mortality as a result of respiratory conditions because of their different anatomy and physiology as well as decreased pulmonary reserve. Rapid assessment and appropriate management of children with respiratory distress is imperative, given that patients who cannot be adequately managed in the acute setting may progress to acute cardiopulmonary failure and ultimately death.

ETIOLOGY AND PATHOGENESIS

The main function of the respiratory system is to supply sufficient oxygen to meet metabolic demands and to remove carbon dioxide. A variety of processes, including ventilation (gas delivery to and from the lungs), perfusion (amount of venous blood brought to the pulmonary bed), and diffusion (the movement of gases across the alveolar membrane), are involved in tissue oxygenation and carbon dioxide removal. Abnormalities in any one of these mechanisms, including hypoventilation, diffusion impairment, intrapulmonary shunt (when alveoli are perfused but not ventilated), and ventilation/perfusion mismatch (a disparity between gas delivery and pulmonary venous blood delivery), can lead to respiratory failure.

Respiratory distress can either be a manifestation of a primary respiratory problem or a secondary effect resulting from the disruption of another organ system. The pathogenesis and resultant signs and symptoms are directly linked to the underlying cause. In general, causes of respiratory distress may be classified as involving (1) the airway; (2) the lungs, chest wall, or both; (3) the central nervous system (CNS) respiratory drive or control; or (4) the neuromuscular system. Alternatively, the respiratory system may be compromised by dysfunction in other organ systems (i.e., cardiovascular, gastrointestinal, endocrine, hematologic) that affect respiratory function or trigger respiratory compensatory mechanisms.

Observed manifestations of distress reflect attempts by the patient to address the underlying inadequacies of their current respiratory status. Several core principles can explain these manifestations depending on the underlying cause:

1. Inadequate minute ventilation: Hypoxemia or hypercarbia can lead to increased minute ventilation by increasing tidal volume, respiratory rate, or both, as is seen in pneumonia with hypoxemia and resultant tachypnea.
2. Disordered regulatory system: Interference with the normal signal pathways of respiration by either depression (e.g., narcotic overdose) or stimulation of the drive to breathe (e.g., metabolic acidosis).
3. Disorders of mechanical structures: Disruption of the normal physical mechanisms of breathing, as in airway obstruction or muscular disorders.

CLINICAL PRESENTATION

Initial Assessment

The evaluation of a child with acute respiratory distress includes determining the severity as well as the underlying cause. Given that respiratory distress may range in severity from mild to severe, the clinical presentation can be quite varied. In all cases, the first key to the assessment is to ensure the patency of the airway, adequate breathing, and intact circulation (see Chapter 1). After these basic life support principles have been addressed, the physical examination may proceed.

History

A thorough history, including existing medical problems and recent events leading to the current presentation, provides important clues to the underlying cause (Table 3-1). For example, a patient with a foreign body obstruction or anaphylaxis may have an acute presentation of severe respiratory distress compared with a child with an infectious cause in whom the presentation may be more gradual.

Physical Examination

VITAL SIGNS

Vital signs, including temperature, heart rate, blood pressure, respiratory rate, and pain score, should be promptly obtained in all patients with respiratory distress. Pulse oximetry, although not classically part of the vital signs, should also be noted to detect hypoxia. Tachypnea (rapid breathing) is one of the most consistent findings among children with respiratory distress and may be caused by fever, hypoxemia, hypercarbia, metabolic acidosis, pain, or anxiety (Table 3-2). However, many children with significant respiratory disease may have normal respiratory rates. Bradypnea may also occur in response to hypoxia in younger infants or from respiratory fatigue, CNS depression, or increased intracranial pressure. Pulsus paradoxus, an exaggeration of the normal decrease in blood pressure during inspiration, of greater than 10 mm Hg correlates well with the degree of airway obstruction but is very difficult to assess in children and therefore not routinely measured.

RESPIRATORY EXAMINATION

The respiratory examination can give many clues as to the cause of respiratory distress because the clinical manifestations may be indicative of the location of the disease process within the

Table 3-1 Focused History for a Patient with Respiratory Distress

Component	Comments and Examples
Onset, duration, and chronicity	• Abrupt onset: suggests upper airway conditions such as foreign body, allergy, or irritant exposure • Gradual onset: more consistent with process such as infection or heart failure
Alleviating and provoking factors	• A child with respiratory distress caused by upper airway obstruction may have some degree of relief by assuming the "sniffing position" to maximize airway patency
Treatment attempted	• A child with wheezing secondary to asthma may respond readily to inhaled bronchodilators, but a child with wheezing caused by foreign body aspiration may continue to show symptoms after treatment
Respiratory symptoms	• Cold symptoms: may indicate viral upper respiratory infection • Cough: "seal-like" or "barky" cough is commonly heard in patients with croup • Eliciting descriptions of the difficulty breathing may provide clues to the underlying cause (e.g., supraclavicular or suprasternal retractions point to upper airway obstruction) • Color change: pallor may indicate anemia; cyanosis is indicative of decreased oxygen content in the blood, as seen in some forms of congenital heart disease and in methemoglobinemia • Respiratory effort: poor effort may be seen in patients with underlying muscular dystrophies • Change in voice: whereas muffled or hoarse voice points to upper airway pathology, lower airway disease does not typically change the character of the voice
Systemic or associated symptoms	• Fever: presence suggests an infectious cause • Hydration status, including intake and output (urine, emesis, diarrhea, excessive perspiration, or high respiratory rate) • Weight loss or failure to gain weight: may indicate systemic process (e.g., inborn error of metabolism) or the severity of respiratory distress is impairing growth (as seen in congestive heart failure) • Abdominal pain: may suggest abdominal pathology such as obstruction or appendicitis or may represent referred pain from diaphragmatic irritation (as in basilar pneumonia)
Past medical history	• Underlying disorders may predispose patients to certain conditions: for example, a patient with sickle cell disease and respiratory distress may be exhibiting signs of acute chest syndrome; a patient with known gastroesophageal reflux and coarse lung findings on examination could have an aspiration pneumonia
Exposures or environmental factors	• For example, a patient involved in a fire may not only be affected by thermal injury to the airways but also systemic toxins such as carbon monoxide and cyanide • A patient with allergy and a potential exposure to the allergen could be showing signs of anaphylaxis
Trauma	• History of trauma suggests diagnoses such as pneumothorax, flail chest, cardiac tamponade, or abdominal injury
Immunization status	• Children with incomplete or lack of immunization against *Haemophilus influenzae* type B are at increased risk for this form of epiglottitis
Last oral intake	• If advanced airway management becomes necessary (e.g., positive-pressure ventilation), the presence of stomach contents may increase the risk of pulmonary aspiration

upper or lower respiratory tract (or both) (Figure 3-1). Initially, observe the general appearance of the patient, specifically for depth, rhythm, and symmetry of respirations; color; increased work of breathing; perfusion; and mental status. Patients with complete upper airway obstruction have aphonia, which is no audible speech, cry, or cough secondary to lack of effective air movement caused by a foreign body, angioedema, or epiglottitis. The presence of nasal flaring indicates dyspnea or upper airway obstruction. Facial edema and urticaria may signify anaphylaxis. The patient may show signs of acute or chronic hypoxemia in the form of cyanosis or clubbing, respectively (Figure 3-2).

Cyanosis is not evident until more than 5 g/dL of hemoglobin is desaturated, which correlates with an oxygen saturation of less than 70% to 75%. Cyanosis is a late finding in children with hypoxemia and is seen in children with low cardiac output as well as low arterial oxygen saturation. Cyanosis in the presence of normal oxygen saturation may be indicative of methemoglobinemia.

Sounds noted on auscultation are useful in localizing the source of respiratory distress. Stertor, a sound from the upper airways resembling snoring, may indicate a degree of adenotonsillar hypertrophy, nasal congestion, or neuromuscular weakness. Hoarseness points to laryngeal or vocal cord dysfunction. A barky cough results from subglottic or tracheal obstruction. Stridor indicates abnormal turbulent air flow through a partially obstructed extrathoracic airway and can occur in both phases of respiration; if occurring during inspiration, the obstruction is most likely in the glottic or subglottic region; if in the expiratory phase, the sound is generated from the carina or below; if present in both phases (biphasic), the trachea may be involved (see Chapter 36). Grunting is a means by which patients

Table 3-2 Definition of Tachypnea by Age

Age	Breaths per Minute
Younger than 2 months	>60
2-12 months	>50
1-5 years	>40
Older than 5 years	>20

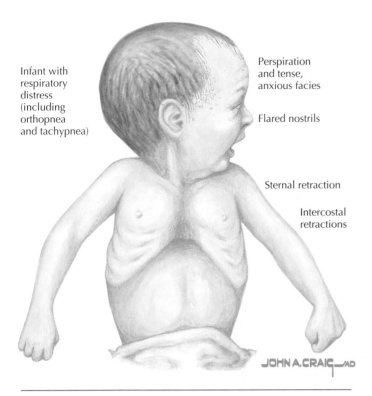

Infant with respiratory distress (including orthopnea and tachypnea)

Perspiration and tense, anxious facies

Flared nostrils

Sternal retraction

Intercostal retractions

Figure 3-1 *Physical examination findings in respiratory distress.*

generate intrinsic end-expiratory pressure against a closed glottis; in children, this is a sign of hypoxia that may indicate lower airway disease such as pneumonia. Grunting may also be associated with pain or an intraabdominal process. Retractions, the inward collapse of the chest wall, are caused by high negative intrathoracic pressure with increased respiratory effort and are more obvious in children because of the high compliance of the chest wall. Supraclavicular and suprasternal retractions occur in patients with upper airway obstruction; intercostal retractions signify lower tract disease or obstruction. Subcostal retractions may be seen with either upper or lower airway obstruction.

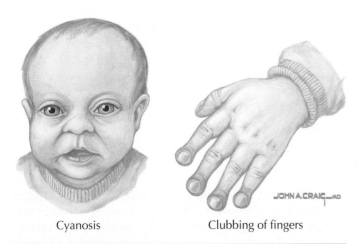

Cyanosis

Clubbing of fingers

Figure 3-2 *Physical examination findings demonstrating hypoxemia.*

Thoracoabdominal dissociation, or paradoxical breathing in which the chest collapses on inspiration while the abdomen is protruding, is a sign of respiratory failure from weakness or fatigue. Wheezing is classically a sign of lower airway obstruction and usually occurs during expiration (see Chapter 37). It may be associated with underlying medical conditions such as asthma, bronchiolitis, congestive heart failure, and congenital malformations. Inspiratory wheezing may indicate upper airway extrathoracic obstruction secondary to a foreign body, edema, or a fixed intrathoracic obstruction. Crackles (or rales) indicate fluid in the small- to medium-sized airways and may be heard in pneumonia, bronchiolitis, or myocarditis with heart failure. Rhonchi (coarse rales) involve secretions in the larger bronchi. A friction rub is heard when the pleura are inflamed and may be heard in patients with pneumonia or lung abscess and with pleural effusions or empyema. Bronchophony, egophony, and whispered pectoriloquy, which may be difficult to elicit in pediatric patients, occur because of consolidations in or around the lung, as seen in patients with pneumonia or pleural effusion.

Palpation and percussion of the neck or chest may also reveal crepitus suggestive of subcutaneous emphysema secondary to an air leak, such as in a pneumothorax. Whereas hyperresonance on percussion suggests air trapping, dullness suggests consolidation, a mass, or pleural fluid.

Differential Diagnosis

The differential diagnosis of respiratory distress can be summarized by organ system (Box 3-1).

EVALUATION AND MANAGEMENT

Algorithm

An algorithmic approach that merges history and physical examination findings is helpful in eliciting the underlying cause of respiratory distress while also providing guidance for further testing (Figures 3-3 and 3-4).

Initial Management

The emergent evaluation of children with respiratory distress must first identify the respiratory status of the patient by ensuring the patency of the airway, breathing, and circulation (see Chapter 1) before proceeding. Patients in severe respiratory distress and impending respiratory failure should be evaluated immediately for the life-threatening causes of respiratory distress, which include complete or rapidly progressing partial airway obstruction, as in foreign body or epiglottitis, tension pneumothorax, and cardiac tamponade (Table 3-2 and Figure 3-4). Children with respiratory failure secondary to inadequate oxygenation or ventilation may exhibit pallor or central cyanosis; altered mental status; decreased chest wall movement; or marked tachypnea, bradypnea, or apnea.

Abnormal vital signs should also be noted given that several simple interventions can promptly lessen the degree of the patient's distress. For example, for a patient with a fever that may be contributing to respiratory distress, antipyretics are

---

Box 3-1 Differential Diagnosis of Respiratory Distress*

Respiratory System
Upper airway (nasopharynx, oropharynx, larynx, trachea, bronchi)
- Anatomic: craniofacial abnormalities, choanal atresia, tonsillar hypertrophy, macroglossia, midface hypoplasia, micrognathia, laryngomalacia, tracheomalacia, hemangioma, webs, cysts, laryngoceles, laryngotracheal cleft, papilloma, subglottic stenosis, vocal cord paralysis, tracheal stenosis, fistula, bronchomalacia, bronchogenic cyst
- Infectious: *nasal congestion*, Ludwig's angina, *peritonsillar abscess*, tonsillitis, *croup*, **epiglottitis**, retropharyngeal abscess, *tracheitis*, bronchitis
- Environmental or traumatic: chemical or thermal burn, **aspiration of foreign body**
- Mass, including malignancy
- Inflammatory: angioneurotic edema, anaphylaxis
Lower airway (bronchioles, acini, interstitium)
- Inflammatory: *asthma, allergy*, angioneurotic edema, *meconium aspiration*, near drowning, submersion, gastroesophageal reflux, aspiration
- Infectious: *bronchiolitis, pneumonia* (bacterial, viral, atypical bacterial, Chlamydia, pertussis, fungal, *Pneumocystis* spp.), abscess
- Congenital malformation: congenital emphysema; cystic adenomatoid malformation; sequestration; pulmonary agenesis, aplasia, or hypoplasia; pulmonary cyst
- Environmental or traumatic: chemical or thermal burn, smoke, carbon monoxide, cyanide, hydrocarbon, near drowning, drug-induced pulmonary fibrosis, bronchopulmonary traumatic disruption, pulmonary contusion, high-altitude pulmonary edema
- Other: persistent fetal circulation, *transient tachypnea of the newborn, respiratory distress syndrome*, bronchiectasis, interstitial lung disease, bronchopulmonary dysplasia, cystic fibrosis, pulmonary edema, hemorrhage, embolism, atelectasis, mass
Chest wall and intrathoracic
- Pneumothorax, tension pneumothorax
- Pneumomediastinum
- Pleural effusion
- Empyema
- Chylothorax
- Hemothorax
- Diaphragmatic hernia
- Cyst, mass
- Spinal deformity (kyphoscoliosis)
- Pectus excavatum or carinatum
- Rib fracture, flail chest
Central Nervous System
- Structural abnormality: agenesis, hydrocephalus, mass, arteriovenous malformation
- Infectious: meningitis, encephalitis, abscess, poliomyelitis

- Dysfunction or immaturity: apnea, hypoventilation, hyperventilation
- Inherited degenerative disease: spinal muscular atrophy
- Intoxication or toxins: alcohol, barbiturates, benzodiazepines, opiates, tetanus
- Seizure
- Trauma: hemorrhage, birth asphyxia, spinal cord injury, anoxic encephalopathy
- Other: transverse myelitis, acute paralysis, myopathy
Peripheral Nervous System
- Phrenic nerve injury
- Environmental or toxins: tick paralysis, heavy metal poisoning, organophosphates, botulism, snakebite
- Metabolic: inborn errors of metabolism, carnitine deficiency, porphyria
- Inflammatory: dermatomyositis, polymyositis
- Other: Guillain-Barré syndrome, multiple sclerosis, myasthenia gravis, muscular or myotonic dystrophy, muscle fatigue
Cardiovascular System
- Structural: *congenital heart disease*, pericardial effusion, **pericardial tamponade**, aortic dissection or rupture, mass, coronary artery dilation or aneurysm, pneumopericardium, great vessel anomalies
- Other: arrhythmia, myocarditis, myocardial ischemia or infarction, congestive heart failure
Gastrointestinal System
- Appendicitis
- Necrotizing enterocolitis
- Mass (including hepatomegaly, splenomegaly)
- Ascites
- Obstruction
- Perforation, laceration
- Hematoma
- Contusion
- Esophageal foreign body
Hematologic System
- Acute chest syndrome
- Anemia
- Polycythemia
- Methemoglobinemia
Metabolic and Endocrine
- Acidosis: exercise, *fever*, hypothermia, *dehydration*, sepsis, shock, inborn errors of metabolism, liver *disease*, renal disease, *diabetic* ketoacidosis, salicylates
- Electrolyte disturbances: hypo- or hyperkalemia, hypo- or hypercalcemia, hypophosphatemia, hypo- or hypermagnesemia
- Hypo- or hyperglycemia
- Mitochondrial disorders leading to disruption of oxygen metabolism

*Common causes are *italicized;* life-threatening causes are in bold.
Reprinted with permission from Weiner DL: Synopsis of Pediatric Emergency Medicine, ed 4. Philadelphia, Lippincott Williams & Wilkins, 2002, pp 221-227.

---

indicated. For a patient who has tachycardia caused by dehydration that is contributing to respiratory distress, an intravenous bolus of isotonic fluid can provide intravascular volume repletion and normalization of the tachycardia. Increased respiratory rate and hypoxia on pulse oximetry may indicate a need for supplemental oxygen.

A patient with respiratory distress of any degree may have an obstruction in the airway that should be managed with measures such as repositioning to maximize the patency of the airway, suctioning of excessive secretions, and inspection for a foreign body. Physical examination findings such as drooling, stridor, change in cry or voice, and dysphagia likely signify an upper

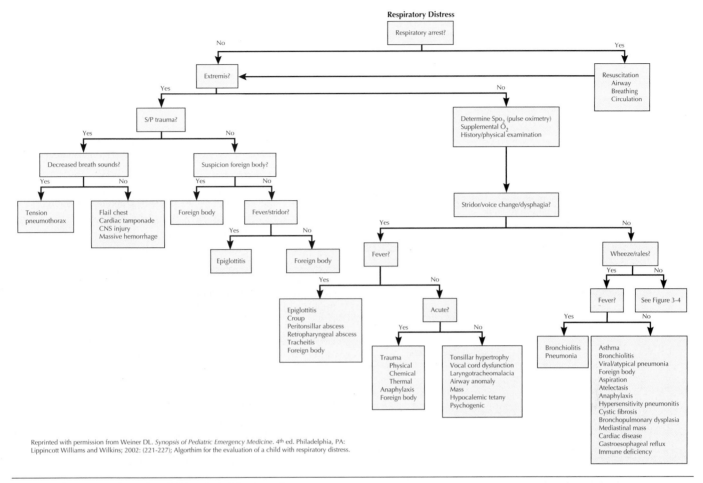

Figure 3-3 *Approach to the child with respiratory distress.*

airway condition. The presence of fever in these children indicates an infectious cause such as epiglottitis, croup, tracheitis, retropharyngeal abscess, or peritonsillar abscess. Absence of fever favors alternate diagnoses, such as vocal cord dysfunction or angioedema secondary to anaphylaxis.

If signs such as crackles or wheezing are present by auscultation, respiratory distress is likely attributable to a process located in the lung parenchyma (e.g., pneumonia) or larger lower airways (e.g., asthma). As with upper airway disease, the presence of fever favors infectious causes.

Simple tachypnea without other lung findings may still indicate infectious causes (i.e., pneumonia, empyema, or sepsis), anatomic abnormalities (i.e., pneumothorax or congenital heart disease), or even underlying metabolic and CNS causes that interfere with the normal mechanisms of respiration.

Diagnostic Studies

RADIOGRAPHS

In the younger age groups, the physical examination, including the respiratory examination, may not clearly elucidate the underlying disease process. Radiographs may be helpful in these cases and in other instances to corroborate physical examination findings. A child who exhibits a barking cough suspicious for laryngotracheobronchitis (more commonly known as croup)

may have the pathognomonic "steeple sign," the radiographic projection of the narrowing of the subglottic trachea on a neck radiograph. Croup is usually a diagnosis made only on clinical grounds, but radiographs may be helpful when the diagnosis is in question or the presentation is unusual. In a child who exhibits fever, drooling, and is sitting upright in the "sniffing position" (neck flexed and head mildly extended), a lateral neck radiograph may show prevertebral widening classically seen in retropharyngeal abscess. Chest radiographs, both anteroposterior and lateral projections, are also helpful in evaluating for heart size, which may signify an underlying cardiac anomaly; consolidations in the lung fields, which may represent infection, atelectasis, or effusion; and inadequate lung expansion, which may be present with pneumothorax, foreign body, or poor external muscle strength.

If the history and physical examination indicate an obstructive component, neck radiographs or lateral decubitus chest radiographs can aid in the diagnosis. Lateral and anteroposterior radiographs of the neck are useful for the diagnosis of retropharyngeal abscess, epiglottitis, foreign body aspiration, or tracheitis in stable children. Abdominal radiographs may reveal intestinal obstruction or perforation causing respiratory distress from abdominal competition. Other advanced imaging studies to consider based on the clinical situation include barium swallow, airway fluoroscopy, computed tomography, and

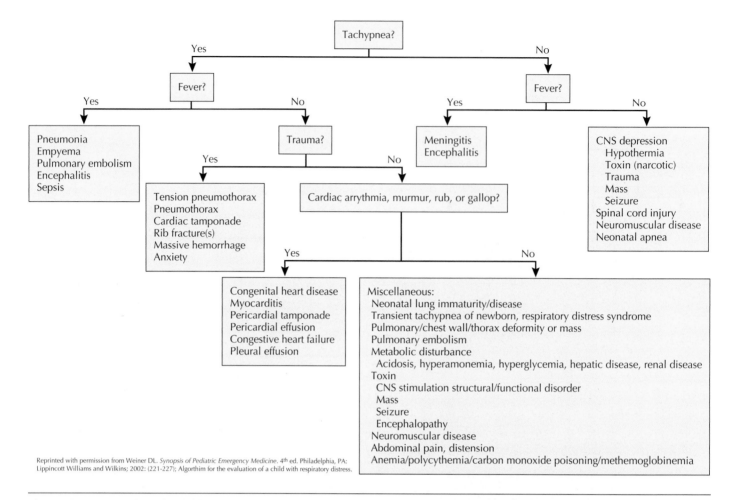

Reprinted with permission from Weiner DL. *Synopsis of Pediatric Emergency Medicine*. 4th ed. Philadelphia, PA: Lippincott Williams and Wilkins; 2002: (221-227); Algorthim for the evaluation of a child with respiratory distress.

Figure 3-4 *Approach to the child with respiratory distress (continued).*

magnetic resonance imaging. A ventilation-perfusion scan or pulmonary angiography of the chest may also be helpful in the diagnosis of entities such as pulmonary embolus.

BLOOD TESTS

Blood tests may also be useful to guide further therapy. A blood gas analysis, ideally an arterial sample, will reflect oxygenation, ventilation, and acid–base status, all of which may be amenable to immediate treatment (Figure 3-5). A venous blood gas analysis can provide some information about ventilation but is less useful in assessing oxygenation. Blood chemistry analysis that includes electrolytes and total carbon dioxide may provide evidence of a metabolic acidosis that could be contributing to the patient's respiratory distress. Other tests such as carboxyhemoglobin or methemoglobin levels may be useful if the clinical history and physical examination raise suspicion. A complete blood count can indicate an elevated white blood cell count that may support a diagnosis of infection or may show anemia or polycythemia, both of which may lead to tachypnea. A toxicology screen may be useful in a child with altered mental status, respiratory depression (opiate overdose), or unexplained tachypnea (metabolic acidosis). Specimens should be sent for microbiologic culture as deemed necessary.

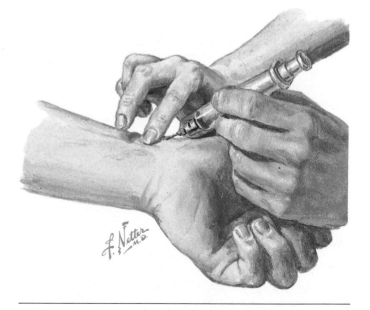

Figure 3-5 *Arterial puncture for blood gas analysis.*

SUGGESTED READINGS

Lipps-Kim J: Respiratory distress. In Zaoutis LB, Chiang VW, editors: *Comprehensive Pediatric Hospital Medicine*, Philadelphia, 2007, Mosby Elsevier, pp 218-222.

Perez Fontan JJ, Haddad GG: Respiratory pathophysiology. In Behrman RE, Kliegman RM, Jenson HB, editors: *Nelson Textbook of Pediatrics*, Philadelphia, 2004, WB Saunders, pp 1376-1379.

Weiner DL: Respiratory distress. In Fleisher GR, Ludwig S, editors: *Textbook of Pediatric Emergency Medicine*, Philadelphia, 2000, Lippincott Williams & Wilkins, pp 553-564.

Weiner DL: *Synopsis of Pediatric Emergency Medicine*, ed 4, Philadelphia, 2002, Lippincott Williams & Wilkins, pp 221-227.

Weiner DL, Fleisher GR: Emergent evaluation of acute respiratory distress in children. In Wiley JF, editor: UpToDate Online 18.3. www.uptodate.com/contents/emergent-evaluation-of-acute-respiratory-distress-in-children.

Diabetic Ketoacidosis

Jennifer A. Danzig and Mirna M. Farah

4

Diabetes is a chronic disease defined by hyperglycemia caused by insulin deficiency. (Chapter 71 provides a detailed discussion of diabetes mellitus.). This may be the result of a lack of insulin production, as in type 1 diabetes mellitus (T1DM) or the body's ineffective use of the insulin it produces, as in type 2 diabetes mellitus. The most common form of diabetes in children is T1DM.

The World Health Organization and International Diabetes Foundation have established the diagnosis of diabetes as meeting any of the following criteria: (1) fasting (≥8 hours) plasma glucose above 126 mg/dL; (2) plasma glucose above 200 mg/dL 2 hours after a glucose load as given by an oral glucose tolerance test; (3) any random plasma glucose above 200 mg/dL along with the presence of symptoms of diabetes, including increased thirst and urination or unexplained weight loss, or (4) a hemoglobin A1C ≥6.5%.

Diabetes is one of the most common chronic diseases in the United States. Approximately 8.0% of the U.S. population meets criteria for diabetes. It is estimated that about 150,000 people in the United States younger than 20 years of age have diabetes; about one in every 500 children and adolescents has T1DM. There is a bimodal distribution of age at onset, with a peak age at presentation around age 5 years and another at early puberty.

This chapter focuses on the care of acutely ill children with T1DM presenting with diabetic ketoacidosis (DKA), a complication of T1DM in which hyperglycemia, dehydration, electrolyte derangement, ketonemia, and acidemia result from absolute insulin deficiency. DKA can be the presenting manifestation of T1DM in up to 25% of children; it is also seen in children with known T1DM secondary to failure of or noncompliance with insulin therapy.

ETIOLOGY AND PATHOGENESIS

T1DM is the result of an inflammatory process within the pancreas. It is thought that children inherit a susceptibility to the disease through specific genes. There is then a triggering event, such as a viral infection, that is either directly toxic to pancreatic β-cells or triggers a widespread generalized immune response. Affected individuals tend to become symptomatic when 90% of β-cell mass is destroyed and carbohydrate intolerance occurs.

DKA is a result of insulin deficiency. Insulin is a hormone that responds to an increase in serum glucose via receptor-mediated utilization. This includes stimulation of glucose uptake from the blood by peripheral tissues; glycogen synthesis in the liver; and inhibition of processes that increase serum glucose, such as gluconeogenesis and glycogenolysis (Figure 4-1). In the absence of insulin, blood glucose levels increase. There is inability to store glucose that is absorbed through the gut, and because of the absence of insulin's suppression of these pathways, production of new glucose via gluconeogenesis continues. This process is perpetuated by increased production of hormones that increase blood glucose, including glucagon, cortisol, and catecholamines. As blood glucose increases, osmotic diuresis occurs, resulting in urinary losses of electrolytes. Because the body cannot use the glucose that has been supplied, it responds as if in the fasting state. Fat is then broken down into free fatty acids to be used as fuel. Free fatty acids are converted to keto-acids, including β-hydroxybutyrate and acetoacetate, leading to metabolic acidosis (Figure 4-2).

The presenting signs and symptoms of DKA reflect this progression. Initially, hyperglycemia and hyperosmolarity cause osmotic diuresis leading to polyuria and compensatory polydipsia. Progressive insulin deficiency leads to catabolism of protein and fat stores, resulting in weight loss and fatigue. As production of counterregulatory hormones increases, ketosis worsens, leading to acute symptoms of nausea, vomiting, and abdominal pain. Progressive dehydration can lead to lethargy and confusion. Ongoing metabolic acidosis stimulates respiratory compensation via hyperpnea, leading to deep, sighing breaths known as Kussmaul respirations.

CLINICAL PRESENTATION

Patients with DKA typically present with acute symptoms of nausea and vomiting. In patients presenting with T1DM for the first time, there may be a history of polyuria, polydipsia, enuresis, or weight loss. As ketosis progresses, patients may become obtunded and unable to provide a history. Therefore, a glucose measurement should be obtained quickly in any patient who presents with altered mental status. (Hypoglycemia may also be manifested as altered mental status.) Ketosis may also result in presence of a fruity breath, which can help direct the diagnosis. On physical examination, patients generally show signs related to the degree of dehydration from chronic hyperglycemia and osmotic diuresis. This may include tachycardia, presence of dry mucous membranes, and delayed capillary refill. DKA should be suspected in patients with signs of dehydration who maintain a high urine output. Abdominal examination often reveals diffuse tenderness. It is important to document a detailed neurologic examination at presentation because patients who present with normal mental status may have an acute change in status with therapy. DKA leads to physical examination findings affecting many systems (Table 4-1).

Differential Diagnosis

The diagnosis of DKA can be difficult because of the presenting signs and symptoms, which are similar to those of other acute illnesses. The history of polyuria and polydipsia are also signs of urinary tract infection or diabetes insipidus. The weight loss and abdominal pain may be indicative of anorexia or inflammatory bowel disease. Abdominal pain can also be a symptom of appendicitis or other acute surgical problems in the abdomen. Vomiting may be a symptom of gastroenteritis. The presence of hyperpnea may be concerning for pneumonia or an asthma

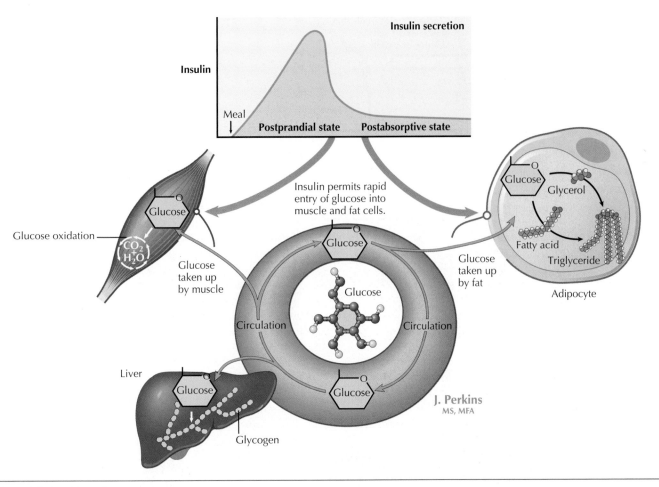

Figure 4-1 *Insulin action.*

exacerbation. In patients who are obtunded, DKA may be confused with head trauma or central nervous system infection. Laboratory testing can be both misleading and helpful in terms of narrowing the differential diagnosis. Elevation of stress hormones, including epinephrine and cortisol, in DKA may lead to leukocytosis, suggestive of infection. In addition, infection may be a precipitating factor in development of DKA, and patients may manifest with a chief complaint related to the underlying infectious process. The best way to narrow the differential diagnosis is by rapidly obtaining serum glucose, electrolytes, blood

Table 4-1 Physical Exam Findings in Diabetic Ketoacidosis

Physical Examination Component	Findings	Interpretation
General	Can range from alert and interactive to obtunded based on the degree of dehydration and acidosis	Obtain a glucose measurement immediately on any patient presenting with altered mental status
HEENT	Dry mucous membranes, blurred vision, presence of fruity odor to breath	Ketosis tends to result in fruity odor to breath
Cardiovascular	Tachycardia	Indicative of dehydration
Lungs	Kussmaul respirations	Deep, sighing breaths used as respiratory compensation for metabolic acidosis
		Lungs are clear to auscultation, indicating the absence of an underlying lung pathology
Abdomen	Diffuse abdominal tenderness	Ileus may result from ketosis and can mislead the diagnosis toward an acute abdominal process
Extremities	Delayed capillary refill, decreased skin turgor	Indicative of dehydration
Intake and output	Increased	Indicative of thirst and increased fluid intake caused by osmotic diuresis

HEENT, head, ears, eyes, nose, and throat.

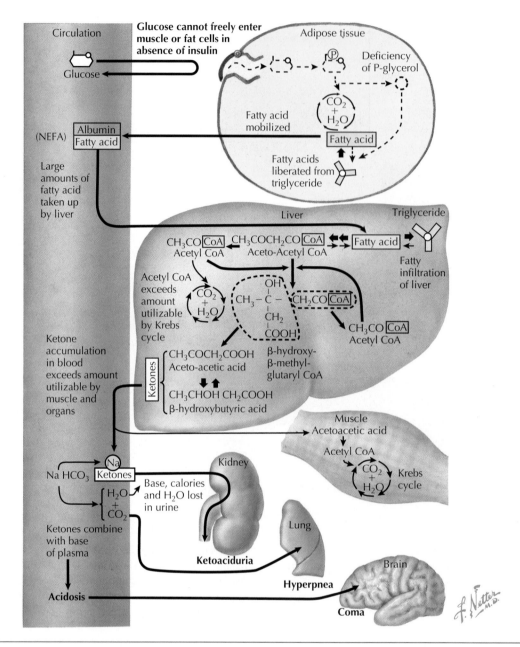

Figure 4-2 *Ketoacidosis.*

pH, and urinalysis. DKA is defined as blood glucose above 240 mg/dL with the presence of ketones in the urine or blood and pH below 7.3.

EVALUATION AND MANAGEMENT

The management of patients with DKA focuses on correction of the dehydration, electrolyte loss, acidosis, and hyperglycemia. This requires frequent monitoring and admission to the hospital.

Dehydration

Management begins with an initial bolus of *isotonic* crystalloid fluid (hypotonic fluids should be avoided), usually 10 to 20 mL/kg of normal saline given over 1 hour. Initial fluid therapy is aimed at correcting the cardiovascular compensation for the degree of dehydration. Patients who present in shock may need more rapid fluid resuscitation. However, care must be taken not to administer too much fluid initially because of the risk of potentially fatal cerebral edema (see Complications). In general, the vital signs and clinical status should be reassessed between boluses of 10 mL/kg to avoid fluid overload. The goal is to gradually replace the fluid deficit over 36 to 48 hours.

Electrolyte Loss

DKA results in electrolyte loss, specifically related to sodium, potassium, and phosphate. Sodium deficit at presentation is attributable to hyperosmolarity resulting from hyperglycemia and osmotic shift of water into the intravascular space, resulting in dilutional hyponatremia. Serum sodium is reduced by 1.6 mEq/L for each 100-mg/dL increase in glucose; thus, it is important to calculate the sodium concentration corrected for hyperglycemia with the formula:

$$\text{Corrected sodium} = \text{Measured sodium} + ([\text{Serum glucose} - 100]/100) \times 1.6$$

It is important to follow the serum sodium as treatment continues; an increase in sodium does *not* indicate a worsening of the hypertonic state. In contrast, a failure of the sodium value to increase may indicate overly rapid rehydration and increase the risk for complications, namely cerebral edema. All children with DKA are total body potassium depleted but the initial serum potassium concentration may be low, normal, or elevated. Treatment of hyperglycemia with insulin and acidosis correction will move potassium intracellularly, resulting in hypokalemia. Therefore, except in cases of extreme elevation of serum potassium concentration (e.g., >5mEq/dL) or when patients are anuric, potassium should be added to rehydration fluids regardless of the initial serum potassium concentration. The initial concentration of potassium added to intravenous (IV) fluids should be 40 mmol/L if the initial serum potassium is in the "normal" range. The concentration of potassium should then be adjusted based on frequent reassessments of serum potassium. Generally, half of the potassium is given as potassium chloride, and half is given as potassium phosphate. The phosphate loss in DKA results in reduction in 2,3-diphosphoglycerate, which is important in the affinity of hemoglobin for oxygen. As a result, less oxygen is available to the tissues, resulting in increased anaerobic metabolism, production of lactic acid, and worsening metabolic acidosis. It is important to recognize that phosphate administration may result in hypocalcemia, so serum calcium concentration should be monitored simultaneously. It is recommended to follow electrolyte values every 2 hours during initial treatment for DKA.

Acidosis

In DKA, production of ketoacids and bicarbonate loss results in acidosis. With correction of DKA, there is replacement of intravascular fluids and improvement in peripheral perfusion, which help to improve acidosis. In addition, with the administration of insulin (see below), ketoacids are metabolized to produce bicarbonate and replace bicarbonate losses. The administration of bicarbonate has been shown to worsen cerebral edema and may cause exacerbation of hypokalemia; thus, it is not recommended in the acute management of DKA. If it is believed that bicarbonate is necessary (e.g., in cases of extreme acidosis, i.e., blood pH <7.0), it should be given in small doses and over a slow infusion. Even with pH below 7.0, bicarbonate is not recommended in most cases.

Hyperglycemia

Because DKA results from insulin deficiency, insulin administration is critical to correction. Insulin treatment generally begins after the first hour of therapy, when the fluid bolus is complete. Insulin is generally given as a continuous infusion at a rate of 0.1 U/kg/h. Hyperglycemia will be corrected by insulin faster than the acidosis, and ketosis will resolve. Therefore, as the serum glucose decreases, it is necessary to administer some dextrose along with the insulin infusion until the acidosis resolves and the ketones begin to clear. Generally, addition of dextrose-containing solutions begins when the glucose has reached 300 mg/dL. Some institutions have adopted the use of a "two-bag system" in which fluids of identical electrolyte content and the presence or absence of dextrose are infused simultaneously (i.e., one bag of normal saline without dextrose and one bag with 10% dextrose in normal saline). With this method, the amount of dextrose provided can be gently titrated based on hourly assessment of serum glucose, with the target blood glucose range between 100 and 200 mg/dL. This helps to ensure a gradual decline in serum glucose, with a goal of decreasing by 50 to 100 mg/dL/h.

Monitoring

Patients with DKA should be followed closely to avoid and detect complications. Patients should not be allowed to eat or drink by mouth until the acidosis has resolved. Serum glucose should be tested every hour. Blood pH (via venous blood gas) and electrolytes need to be followed at least every 2 hours until major abnormalities are corrected. Urinalysis is also checked with each void to monitor for clearance of urine ketones. Continuous electrocardiographic monitoring is recommended for patients receiving high concentrations of potassium.

Complications

Cerebral edema is the complication most associated with morbidity and mortality in DKA, occurring in approximately 1% of patients. The cause is not clearly identified, but current hypotheses include cerebral hypoperfusion during DKA treatment and rapid fluid shifts caused by rapid changes in osmolarity. Risk factors at presentation include pH below 7.0, age younger than 3 years, low pCO_2, high blood urea nitrogen, treatment with bicarbonate, lack of increase in serum sodium during treatment, corrected serum sodium above 155 mEq/L, and glucose above 1000 mg/dL. The symptoms include headache, new findings on neurologic examination (abnormal response to pain, posturing, cranial nerve palsy), a sudden decline in mental status, and hypertension. Cerebral edema is a clinical diagnosis, and if it is suspected, treatment should begin rapidly with infusion of IV mannitol at 0.25 to 1.0 g/kg, elevation of the head of the bed, and reduction in the rate of IV fluids by one-third. When stabilized, an emergent cranial computed tomography should be performed.

Resolution

When pH and bicarbonate have normalized, ketones have decreased, and the patient feels well enough to begin to maintain hydration by mouth, treatment can be switched to a regimen of subcutaneous insulin. Because the half-life of IV insulin is several minutes, a subcutaneous insulin injection should be given before the insulin infusion is stopped. Management after DKA resolves is discussed in Chapter 71.

When the patient is beyond the acute stage of illness, it is important to determine what caused the patient to develop DKA. Some patients present with diabetes for the first time and have families that are unfamiliar with the signs and symptoms of DKA. For these patients, it important to provide education about diabetes management and to develop a good relationship with an endocrinologist for follow-up. For some patients, acute illnesses can increase the need for insulin that is not met by the current maintenance regimen. In these instances, identification and treatment of the underlying illness is necessary.

In patients with known T1DM, it is important to determine if DKA is the result of noncompliance with the demanding insulin regimen of several injections per day or with failure of insulin pump therapy (see Figure 71-2). Insulin pump therapy is designed to deliver subcutaneous insulin continuously with bolus dosing on demand. In these patients, it is important to emphasize compliance and education with current equipment.

FUTURE DIRECTIONS

Although efforts to prevent or reverse T1DM have not met good results thus far, there have been significant developments in the management of patients with diabetes. Advances in glucose monitoring and ease of insulin delivery have made living with T1DM easier and less painful than in the past. While awaiting the next development in diabetes management, patients should be empowered to optimize control while living with a chronic disease.

SUGGESTED READINGS

American Diabetes Association. Available at http://www.diabetes.org.

Cooke DW, Plotnick L: Management of diabetic ketoacidosis in children and adolescents, *Pediatr Rev* 29:431-436, 2008.

Glaser N, Barnett P, McCaslin I, et al: Risk factors for cerebral edema in children with diabetic ketoacidosis, *N Engl J Med* 344:264-269, 2001.

Sherry NA, Levitsky LL: Management of diabetic ketoacidosis in children and adolescents, *Paediatr Drugs* 10(4):209-215, 2008.

Vanelli M, Chiarelli F: Treatment of diabetic ketoacidosis in children and adolescents, *Acta Bio Medica* 74:59-68, 2003.

Weinzimer SA, Magge S. Type 1 diabetes mellitus in children. In Moshang T, Jr, ed, Bell LM, series ed. *Pediatric Endocrinology: The Requisites in Pediatrics*, ed 1, Philadelphia, 2005, Elsevier Mosby, pp 3-18.

The Acute Abdomen

Dana Aronson Schinasi and Sandra Schwab

5

Abdominal pain is a chief complaint frequently encountered in the pediatric office, urgent care, and emergency department settings. Although typically minor and self-limited, acute abdominal pain may also signify a medical or surgical process requiring immediate treatment. The clinician's role is to identify patients who have serious or potentially life-threatening conditions, such as acute appendicitis, bowel obstruction, or peritonitis. The most difficult challenge lies in making a timely diagnosis so treatment can be initiated and potential morbidity prevented.

In this chapter, a clinical guideline is presented for the evaluation and management of children with acute abdominal pain. Appendicitis is the most common surgical emergency in children and adolescents and deserves special mention. Key features of its pathophysiology, clinical presentation, evaluation, and management are highlighted throughout this chapter.

ETIOLOGY AND PATHOGENESIS

Abdominal pain falls into three clinical categories: visceral, parietal (somatic), and referred pain. A general understanding of these is helpful in determining the cause of abdominal pain.

Visceral pain is poorly localized and is often described as dull and aching. It is caused by stretching, distension, or ischemia of the viscera. *Parietal (somatic) pain* is well localized, discrete, and often described as sharp and intense in character. Pain is stimulated by stretching, inflammation, or ischemia of the parietal peritoneum. The pattern of pain in appendicitis has features of both visceral and parietal pain. Initially, the pain is visceral in nature: vague, poorly localized, and periumbilical. As the peritoneum becomes inflamed over the ensuing 12 to 48 hours, the pain migrates to and localizes in the right lower quadrant (RLQ).

Referred pain is often perceived at sites distant from the affected organ and may be described either as sharp and localized or as a vague aching sensation (Figure 5-1). Examples include irritation of the parietal pleura of the lung perceived as abdominal wall pain and inflammation of the gallbladder perceived as scapular pain.

It is helpful to classify the cause of acute abdominal pain by age (Table 5-1). There are many potential causes of abdominal pain, including infectious, anatomic, traumatic, inflammatory, functional, and oncologic.

CLINICAL PRESENTATION

Differential Diagnosis

The differential diagnosis for abdominal pain in children is very broad, and it can be approached in different ways (Figure 5-2). Certain conditions occur more commonly at specific ages and therefore it may be useful to classify causes of acute abdominal pain based on age. Pain may also be classified as surgical or medical (Table 5-1).

Across all ages, gastroenteritis and appendicitis are the most common medical and surgical causes of acute abdominal pain, respectively. Malrotation with midgut volvulus is the single most devastating abdominal surgical emergency of childhood (see Chapter 109).

Life-threatening causes of abdominal pain include those related to trauma, intestinal obstruction, and peritoneal irritation. Examples of processes that present with intestinal obstruction are intussusception, midgut volvulus, and extrinsic obstruction caused by adhesions from prior surgery. Peritoneal irritation may be secondary to inflammation or perforated viscus; examples include necrotizing enterocolitis in a neonate, acute appendicitis, and ruptured ectopic pregnancy.

Abdominal pain can also be classified based on the location of the pain. A classic approach is by dividing the abdomen into four quadrants (Figure 5-3). This can help the practitioner direct the workup to rule in or out the most common diagnoses based on the location of symptoms. For example, hepatic and gallbladder disease usually present with right upper quadrant pain (see Chapter 115). Appendicitis classically presents with migration of pain to the RLQ. Gastritis or peptic ulcer disease may present with left upper quadrant pain (see Chapter 108).

History

The initial evaluation of acute abdominal pain is particularly challenging in pediatrics because children often cannot describe, articulate, or localize their symptoms. This is often exacerbated by anxiety, making it harder for the clinician to examine and identify positive findings.

Pain Character

Acute abdominal pain caused by a medical or surgical emergency typically increases in intensity over time, may awaken the child at night, and likely interferes with activity. In addition to the age of patient and the location of the pain, other important features of the history include the onset, frequency and duration, pattern, associated symptoms, and pertinent medical history.

Infants and young children can seldom localize their pain, and parents often describe an inconsolable child who lies with his or her legs drawn up to the chest. Asking the parents if they think the child is in pain can be helpful to distinguish pain from fussiness or irritability. Pain that is intermittent, with paroxysms of cramping inconsolable pain alternating with return to normal state, is characteristic of intussusception (Figure 5-4). Peritoneal irritation is suggested by pain that is worse with movements that change the tension of the abdominal wall, such as a bumpy car ride or walking. Pain that improves after vomiting or a bowel movement reflects a small bowel or large bowel cause, respectively.

The pain of acute appendicitis is progressive in character without intermittent relief. The initial pain of early evolving appendicitis is classically periumbilical. As the inflammatory

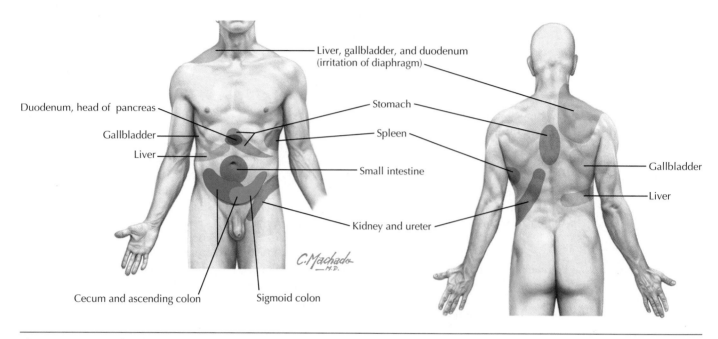

Figure 5-1 *Visceral referred pain.*

process progresses to affect the surrounding abdominal wall structures, the pain shifts to the RLQ (Figure 5-5). This progression is very helpful if obtained on history. Patients may describe a sudden temporary decrease in pain, which often coincides with perforation and temporary relief of intraluminal pressure.

Associated Symptoms

Certain infectious processes are associated with abdominal pain: fever, headache, and sore throat suggest streptococcal pharyngitis (see Chapter 35); dysuria and vomiting may be attributable to a urinary tract infection (see Chapter 93); tachypnea and cough point to a lower lobar pneumonia (see Chapter 91). An associated rash may suggest a vasculitis such as Henoch-Schönlein purpura as the cause of the abdominal pain (see Chapter 28). Whereas nonbloody diarrhea suggests gastroenteritis, bloody diarrhea could also signal hemolytic uremic syndrome, inflammatory bowel disease, or bacterial enteritis. Abdominal pain that is accompanied by vomiting but without diarrhea should prompt a more careful evaluation for potentially life-threatening conditions such as intussusception, midgut volvulus, adhesive small bowel obstruction, or pancreatitis.

Table 5-1 Medical and Surgical Causes of Acute Abdominal Pain*

	Infant	Child	Adolescent
Surgical	**Intussusception**	**Appendicitis**	**Trauma**
	Incarcerated hernia	**Intussusception**	**Appendicitis**
	Volvulus	**Incarcerated hernia**	**Ectopic pregnancy**
	Appendicitis	**Trauma**	Testicular or ovarian torsion
		Testicular torsion	
Medical	Colic	Renal stones	Renal stones
	GERD	Acute gastroenteritis	Cholecystitis
	Acute gastroenteritis	Urinary tract infection	Acute gastroenteritis
	Viral syndromes	Lobar pneumonia	Urinary tract infection
	Milk-protein allergy	Functional abdominal pain	Pelvic inflammatory disease
	Neoplasm	Viral syndromes	Dysmenorrhea
		Streptococcal pharyngitis	Inflammatory bowel disease
		Constipation	**Diabetic ketoacidosis**
		Hemolytic uremic syndrome	**Pancreatitis**
		Inflammatory bowel disease	
		Diabetic ketoacidosis	
		Sickle cell crisis	

*Classified based on age: infant, younger than 2 years old; child, 2 to 11 years old; adolescent, 12 years and older. Acute life-threatening conditions are listed in **bold**.
  GERD, gastroesophageal reflux disease.
Adapted from Fleischer GR, Ludwig S, Henretig F: Textbook of Pediatric Emergency Medicine, ed 4. Philadelphia, Lippincott Williams & Wilkins, 2000.

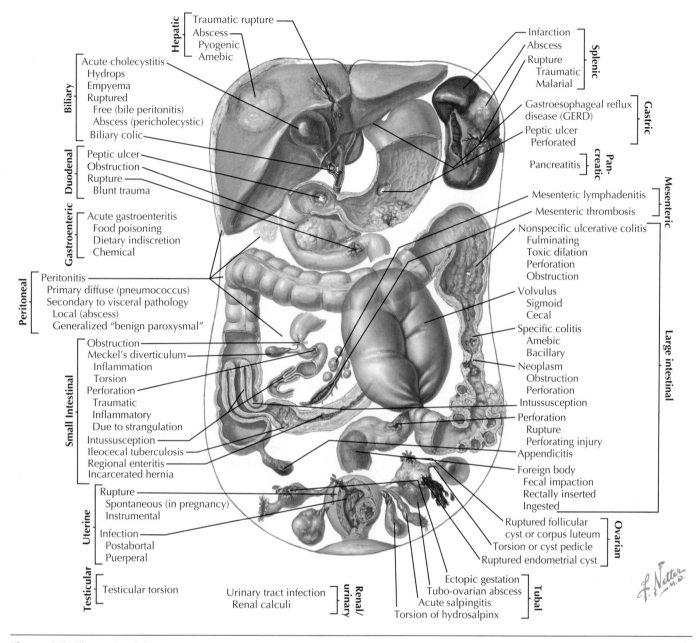

Figure 5-2 *The acute abdomen.*

Appendicitis is classically accompanied by anorexia before the onset of pain, although this is not always the case. Fever is variable, and vomiting usually occurs after the pain has migrated to the RLQ. Diarrhea is occasionally seen with appendicitis, often caused by pelvic irritation after perforation. The diagnosis of appendicitis can be difficult in children because classic symptoms are often not present, especially in infants and very young children.

Pertinent Medical History

Certain chronic medical conditions are associated with abdominal complications. Patients with sickle cell disease are predisposed to cholecystitis, splenic sequestration, and abdominal vaso-occlusive crises (see Chapter 53). Patients with diabetic ketoacidosis often present with accompanying abdominal pain (see Chapter 4). Patients with Hirschsprung's disease are at risk for enterocolitis and toxic megacolon, and those with nephrotic syndrome may develop primary bacterial peritonitis. Patients with a history of abdominal surgery are predisposed to adhesions, which may cause obstruction.

Physical Examination

Clinicians can gain considerable information from the patient's general appearance even as observed from afar. A child in severe pain may prefer to be curled up in a position that shortens the rectus muscles and protects the abdomen. Patients with peritonitis often appear acutely ill and prefer to lie still. Intussusception should always be considered in a young child with altered

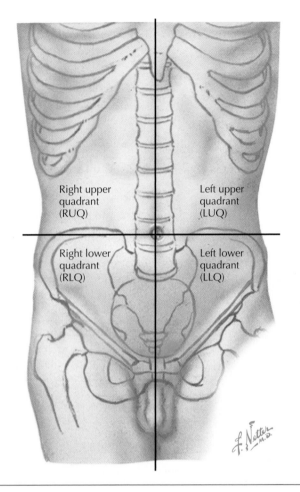

Figure 5-3 *Quadrants of the abdomen.*

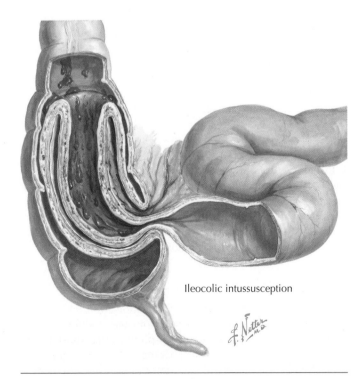

Ileocolic intussusception

Figure 5-4 *Intussusception.*

mental status. Clinicians should pay attention to vital signs, specifically for the presence of fever, tachycardia, or hypotension. Signs of poor perfusion may be seen with peritonitis or hypovolemia.

The abdominal examination is optimally performed when the child is quiet, calm, and cooperative. Clinician should consider examining young patients in the parent's lap, if possible. Start in the area away from reported pain. Evaluate for distension and the presence or absence of bowel sounds. Palpate while paying close attention to presence of masses or focal tenderness. A mass may be indicative of neoplasm, intussusception, or stool. Reproducible focal tenderness points to an intraabdominal inflammatory process. Patients with peritoneal irritation present with percussion pain, involuntary guarding, or rebound tenderness. Rebound is elicited by deep palpation followed by a sudden release. Pay attention to the child's face when attempting these maneuvers because they may not always be able to express localization. The rectal examination is sometimes useful in helping to narrow the differential diagnosis: note the presence of hard stool in the rectal vault (constipation), blood (intussusception, inflammatory bowel disease, infection, milk-protein allergy), or an inflamed retrocecal appendix.

Signs on examination that suggest an acute surgical cause include marked abdominal distension, severe tenderness, rigidity, involuntary guarding, and rebound tenderness. Classic presentations of acute surgical conditions include a neonate with bilious vomiting (midgut volvulus), colicky abdominal pain (intussusception), and RLQ pain (appendicitis). Surgical subspecialists should be alerted early when a surgical cause is suspected. A delay in the diagnosis of appendicitis is associated with rupture and associated complications, especially in young children younger the age of 2 years. A delay in diagnosis increases risk of perforation and postoperative complications to as high as 39%.

Overall, the cause is less likely to be serious in an otherwise healthy child who has a nonfocal examination, is without obvious discomfort to deep palpation, and is without constitutional or extraabdominal findings.

EVALUATION AND MANAGEMENT

The clinician's first priority is to stabilize patients who are critically ill, focusing on identifying and addressing abnormalities in airway, breathing, and circulation. Next, the clinician must identify potential acutely life-threatening processes requiring emergent surgical intervention (Table 5-1). Typically, these are distinguished based on the patient's history and physical examination, as discussed previously. Laboratory testing and imaging studies may be useful adjuncts in identifying the diagnosis.

Laboratory Testing

Testing should be tailored to the pertinent findings during the history and physical exam in order to come to a timely diagnosis. In most children older than 5 years of age with abdominal pain, tests are needed only to confirm a diagnosis that is suspected clinically. Radiographic studies can be useful and diagnostic in many instances.

In the presence of clinical evidence of obstruction, peritonitis, or a mass, a complete blood count (CBC) with differential

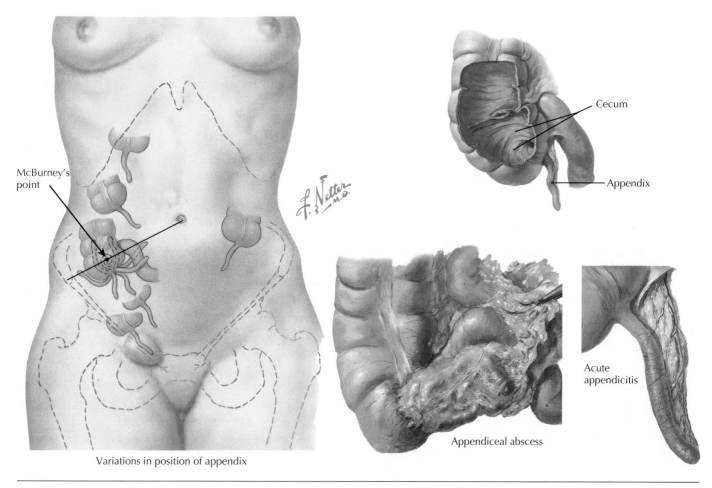

McBurney's point

Variations in position of appendix

Cecum

Appendix

Acute appendicitis

Appendiceal abscess

Figure 5-5 *Acute appendicitis.*

is indicated to evaluate for anemia or thrombocytopenia. When the diagnosis is uncertain, a CBC can help point towards or away from an inflammatory process. Note that in acute appendicitis before rupture, white blood cell count may only be minimally elevated or even normal. C-reactive protein (CRP) has gained favor as an early inflammatory marker, and many investigators are exploring its clinical utility in the pediatric emergency department.

A urinalysis to evaluate hydration status and the presence of infection is useful. Serum electrolytes should also be obtained in ill patients to assess fluid and electrolyte balance, as well as acidosis. However, checking routine serum electrolytes is not necessary in the face of acute gastroenteritis. Additional laboratory tests that may be helpful are hepatic function panel, amylase, lipase, and inflammatory markers.

A qualitative urine pregnancy test must always be sent in any postpubertal female patient with abdominal pain.

Imaging Studies

Imaging studies should be performed when the history and physical examination reveal focal findings or suggest concerning diagnoses.

Abdominal plain films are useful in evaluating for obstruction (air-fluid levels, distended bowel), mass, or perforation (free air). An optimal radiographic study requires supine and upright views to evaluate the bowel gas pattern and movement of intestinal loops. Although the results are most often normal, radiographic signs of appendicitis include a sentinel loop (localized bowel obstruction), an appendicolith, or obliteration of the psoas shadow.

Any child with suspected midgut volvulus (i.e., report of bilious vomiting in an infant) needs an emergent contrast study to clarify the rotational status of his or her small intestine. Failure to diagnose and surgically correct midgut volvulus in a timely manner can lead to infarction of the entire small intestine. Infarction is a preventable catastrophe that may result in long-term total parenteral nutrition dependence and potentially death.

Ultrasonography (US) is the imaging modality of choice for evaluation of the biliary tree and suspected urolithiasis and in the diagnosis of ovarian or testicular pathology, such as torsion or tubo-ovarian abscess. Additionally, US aids in diagnosis of intussusception, pyloric stenosis and appendicitis. Advantages are that it is safe, noninvasive, and does not use radiation; however, the ability to obtain results often depends on the skill of the technician. The sensitivity and specificity of US for diagnosing appendicitis are greater than 90%. Signs of appendicitis on US include a noncompressible tubular structure in RLQ, wall thickness larger than 2 mm, overall diameter larger than 6 mm, free fluid in the RLQ, thickening of the mesentery, and localized tenderness with compression.

Because of the risks of radiation, especially in children, computed tomography (CT) should be reserved to rule in or out significant pathology. CT with contrast is most useful when considering a wide variety of diagnoses, such as intraabdominal mass, pancreatitis, intraabdominal abscess, and appendicitis. Noncontrast CT is indicated in the evaluation of urolithiasis when US is inconclusive. The sensitivity and specificity of CT for diagnosing appendicitis are greater than 90% and 85% to 90%, respectively. The signs of appendicitis on CT include wall thickness larger than 2 mm, appendicolith, abscess or phlegmon, free fluid greater than expected for age, thickening of the mesentery, and fat stranding.

Management

In a critically ill patient with acute abdominal pain or when a potentially life-threatening process is identified, the clinician's role is to simultaneously stabilize the patient, perform the necessary diagnostic steps to identify the underlying cause, and initiate a treatment plan. Supportive care, such as monitoring and intravenous fluids, should be provided. Patients with severe pain should receive effective analgesia. The classic teaching of withholding opiates from patients with abdominal pain for fear of complicating the diagnostic process has fallen out of favor and is not supported by recent studies. Antibiotics should be administered when indicated because they have been shown to delay progression of certain disease processes.

Patients who are stable, do not appear acutely ill, and for whom a definitive diagnosis is not reached upon initial evaluation may benefit from hospitalization for continued monitoring and serial abdominal examinations. Repeat examination may identify evolving clinical features.

Patients who are well appearing with a reassuring history and examination may be discharged with appropriate follow-up.

FUTURE DIRECTIONS

Improvements in timely diagnosis and decreased complications have been made in patients presenting with abdominal pain. One area of ongoing research and development is the use of advanced radiologic imaging. Investigation of reliable modalities that do not use radiation, such as US and magnetic resonance imaging, are especially appealing to practitioners dealing with pediatric patients. Other areas of investigation include use of laboratory markers, such as CRP or lactate, to identify patients with acute abdominal pathology.

SUGGESTED READINGS

Ashcraft KW: Consultation with the specialist: acute abdominal pain, *Pediatr Rev* 21:363-366, 2000.

Behrman RE, Kliegman RM, Jenson HB: *Nelson Textbook of Pediatrics*, ed 18, Philadelphia, 2007, WB Saunders.

Fleischer GR, Ludwig S: *Textbook of Pediatric Emergency Medicine*, ed 6, Philadelphia, 2010, Lippincott Williams & Wilkins.

Leung A, Sigalet D: Acute abdominal pain in children, *Am Fam Phys* 67(11):2321-2326, 2003.

Drowning

Halden F. Scott and Kyle Nelson

6

*D*rowning is defined as a process of respiratory impairment from submersion or immersion in a liquid. Although complicated terminology to define drowning has been used in the past, the 2002 World Congress on Drowning established this universal definition, and recommends against the use of other terms, including "near drowning" and "dry drowning."

Pediatric drowning is the second leading cause of accidental childhood death in the United States, surpassed only by motor vehicle collisions. It is most common in young toddlers and adolescents, and boys are more likely to drown in all age groups. Toddlers are most likely to drown in small, household water sources such as bathtubs and buckets. Inadequate adult supervision is often responsible, although children have usually been out of sight for less than 5 minutes. Toddlers have large heads relative to their bodies, making them more likely to fall forward into buckets or tubs and less able to right themselves (Figure 6-1). Adolescents are more likely to drown during recreational activities such as boating and in natural bodies of water. Alcohol use contributes to up to 50% of teenage drownings. Pediatric drownings carry high morbidity and mortality; 30% to 50% of drowning victims die, and 10% survive with severe neurologic impairment.

ETIOLOGY AND PATHOGENESIS

Hypoxemia is the driving force of the process of drowning, initially caused by apnea and then caused by aspiration. After submersion, drowning victims typically hold their breath and struggle. Small amounts of water are aspirated, and involuntary laryngospasm and hypoxia ensue. With continued hypoxia, the vocal cords relax, and larger amounts of water are aspirated. Even greater amounts of water are swallowed than aspirated, and vomiting is common. The cascade of pulmonary damage from drowning can occur with aspiration of as little as 1 to 3 mL/kg of water.

The effects of aspiration and continued submersion are many (Figure 6-2). Within the alveoli, water prevents diffusion of oxygen across the capillary/alveolar membrane. The capillary endothelium becomes increasingly permeable, resulting in pulmonary edema. Aspiration of gastric contents contributes to lung injury. As pulmonary edema and intrapulmonary shunt progress, hypoxia, hypercarbia, and acidosis ensue. These metabolic disturbances decrease myocardial contractility, increase systemic vascular resistance, and contribute to arrhythmias. If submersion continues long enough, drowning will progress to cardiac arrest. Clinically, there is little difference between fresh and salt-water drownings; however, there are some putative pathophysiologic differences. Whereas fresh water is particularly destructive to surfactant, salt water causes osmotic forces to draw additional fluid into the alveoli. Electrolyte disturbances are rare; however, ingestion of large amounts of fresh water can cause hyponatremia, and salt water ingestion can cause hypernatremia. Ingestion of large quantities of fresh water in the setting of hypoxemia may lead to hemolysis, although this is also a rare event.

Hypothermia is often present and causes peripheral vasoconstriction, which preserves blood flow to the central organs. Increased core blood flow triggers central volume receptors to perceive greater blood volume and thus produce less antidiuretic hormone, resulting in diuresis and volume depletion.

CLINICAL PRESENTATION

The duration of submersion and hypoxia will determine the clinical presentation and outcome in drowning victims. Submersions less than 5 minutes are associated with intact survival, but submersions more than 25 minutes have almost universally poor outcomes. Many victims are rescued from the water in cardiac arrest, and immediate, effective cardiopulmonary resuscitation (CPR) can improve survival rates and neurologic outcome. After pulses are restored, signs of shock may be present, including hypotension, diminished peripheral pulses, altered level of consciousness, acidosis, and decreased urine output. Patients may appear cold, cyanotic, and unresponsive. More mildly affected patients may have isolated pulmonary findings such as wheezes, crackles, cough, or hypoxia. Neurologic findings range from an alert child to any amount of central nervous system compromise, including coma with flexor or extensor posturing.

Many studies have evaluated factors associated with good outcomes, and better prediction is possible with parameters measured later in the hospital course than at initial presentation or in the field. There have been reports of pediatric survivors with good outcomes despite ominous predictors such as submersion over 1 hour. Thus, all patients should receive aggressive initial resuscitation in the field and emergency department (ED), regardless of circumstances surrounding the drowning. After initial resuscitation, failure to exhibit reflexes or response to external stimuli within the first 24 hours of care predicts a poor neurologic outcome.

Unusually good outcomes have occurred in cold-water drownings in children. It is believed that sudden exposure of the face to icy water triggers a protective "diving reflex" that causes apnea, bradycardia, and vasoconstriction. The resultant decreased metabolic demands seem to improve the chances of neurologic recovery compared with warm-water drownings of similar duration. An alternative theory is that rapid cerebral cooling leads to decreased cerebral metabolic demand and is responsible for these outcomes. Ultimately, these good outcomes are relatively rare, and the reasons for them remain unclear.

It is important to consider potential coexistent injuries and risk factors for drowning. Drowning may be associated with other trauma, including head injury, blunt abdominal trauma, and spinal injury (Figure 6-3). Seizures, cardiac arrhythmias, hypoglycemia, and intoxication can all contribute to a drowning event.

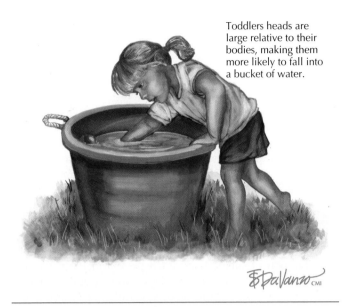

Toddlers heads are large relative to their bodies, making them more likely to fall into a bucket of water.

Figure 6-1 *Toddlers have high centers of gravity.*

EVALUATION AND MANAGEMENT

Unresponsive patients should be evaluated according to Basic Life Support guidelines and receive CPR as indicated at the scene (see Chapter 1). The Heimlich maneuver and attempts to drain water from the lungs should be avoided. Further cooling of the patient should be prevented by removing wet clothing and insulating the patient with dry blankets. Prehospital care and ED providers should evaluate the patient's airway and ventilatory efforts, provide oxygen, and consider intubation. Unresponsive and hypoxic patients most likely require intubation because vomiting is common, and lung injury will probably continue to worsen. If cervical spine (c-spine) injury is a possibility, resuscitation should occur with c-spine immobilization throughout. Gastric decompression is an important step in early resuscitation. Use of a nasogastric or orogastric tube to remove stomach contents decreases vomiting and aids in ventilation by allowing easier distension of the lungs.

Initial laboratory studies should include an arterial blood gas analysis, chest radiograph, complete blood count, electrolytes, and urinalysis. Attention should be paid to reversing hypoxemia and metabolic acidosis. Shock is common after initial resuscitation of drowning victims. Myocardial dysfunction caused by hypoxia, acidosis, hypothermia, and volume loss contribute to decreased perfusion. Both volume resuscitation and inotropic support may be required. Dobutamine is an inotrope recommended for drowning patients if cardiovascular support is required.

Hypothermia was once universally treated with active rewarming; however, emerging evidence suggests that maintaining cooler temperatures may be protective. Ice water drownings have better outcomes than expected, and hypothermia after cardiac arrest in adults may improve neurologic outcome. Thus, the decision to aggressively rewarm should be made carefully. All patients with a core temperature below 28°C with coagulopathy, hypotension, or arrhythmia should be actively rewarmed. A target temperature of 32° to 34°C is recommended

for comatose drowning patients. Active rewarming may use external heating blankets and lamps, and internal rewarming may include warm intravenous fluids, warm bladder irrigation, and even cardiac bypass or extracorporeal membranous oxygenation (ECMO) for the most unstable patients. Passive rewarming should be used to keep all patients from becoming cooler. Hyperthermia is detrimental for all patients and should be avoided in patients who are being actively rewarmed. Continuous temperature monitoring with special hypothermia thermometers (which can read lower temperatures than routine thermometers) is recommended.

Lung injury rapidly evolves in the initial hours after drowning, and the patient may require prolonged mechanical ventilation and possibly nonconventional ventilatory modalities or ECMO. Decreased lung compliance, edema, surfactant deficiency, and alveolar damage can progress to acute respiratory distress syndrome (ARDS). Although ARDS is commonly managed with permissive hypercapnia, in a drowning patient with suspected brain injury, normocapnia preserves cerebral perfusion, making ventilatory strategies more challenging. Diuretics have not been shown to be helpful in treating pulmonary edema from drowning and may even be harmful in patients who are volume depleted. Fluid status and renal function should be carefully monitored. Pneumonia can occur and should be treated if clinically apparent; however, prophylactic antibiotics are not recommended except for drowning in grossly contaminated water such as sewage. *Aeromonas* is an organism that has been associated with severe pneumonia after drowning.

Although primary hypoxic injury to the brain cannot be reversed, prevention of secondary neurologic injury is a goal of acute postresuscitative care. This involves careful monitoring of all body systems to maintain normotension, normoglycemia, and normocapnia and to prevent hypoxia. Seizures are common and should be promptly controlled with anticonvulsants. Monitoring of intracranial pressure or placement of a ventriculostomy drain has not been shown to improve outcomes in drowning victims. Long-term sequelae of hypoxic-ischemic brain injury from drowning may range from mild cognitive difficulties to seizures to persistent vegetative states. Some children may develop reactive airway disease as well.

After acute resuscitation and management of airway, breathing, and circulation, evaluation for concomitant injury and the underlying cause of drowning should occur. Circumstances surrounding the event help guide this workup, and evaluation of a patient with a suspected traumatic mechanism should follow the approach to the trauma patient (see Chapter 8). A history of high-impact trauma such as diving, striking an object, or being in a motorized boat increases the likelihood of requiring computed tomography scans to evaluate for c-spine, intraabdominal, or head injuries. The serum glucose level should be checked both to detect causative hypoglycemia and to preserve normoglycemia. Hypoxic-ischemic injury to the liver and kidneys may present as coagulation abnormalities and acute tubular necrosis.

Seizures are the most common underlying medical cause of drowning. Arrhythmias should also be considered. An electrocardiogram should be evaluated in an otherwise healthy person who drowns without a traumatic mechanism or apparent cause. A congenitally prolonged QT interval can lead to arrhythmia

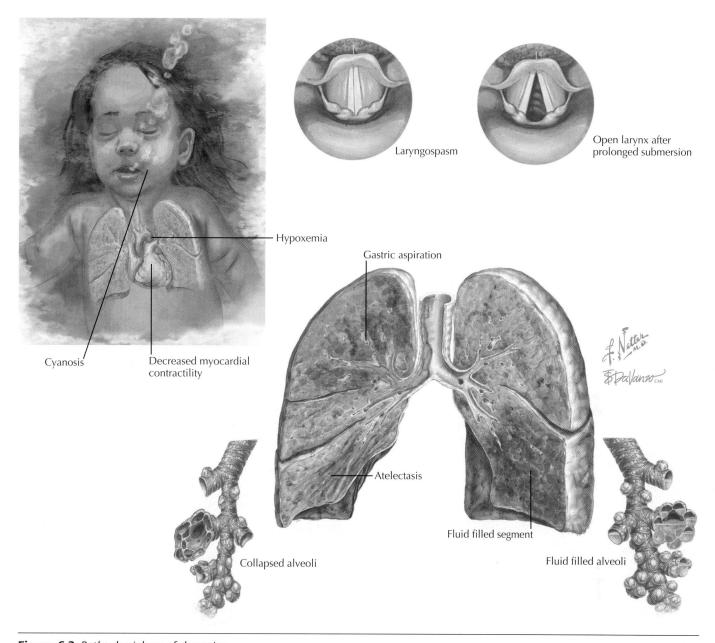

Laryngospasm

Open larynx after
prolonged submersion

Hypoxemia

Gastric aspiration

Cyanosis

Decreased myocardial
contractility

Atelectasis

Fluid filled segment

Collapsed alveoli

Fluid filled alveoli

Figure 6-2 *Pathophysiology of drowning.*

and loss of consciousness with subsequent drowning in the water. Cold-water exposure, exercise, and breath holding appear to trigger arrhythmia in patients with congenital long QT syndrome. If it is suspected, family members should also be evaluated. Urine and blood testing for drugs of abuse may be considered in adolescents. Child abuse sometimes leads to drowning, and a careful history and physical examination should be performed to evaluate for other signs that this might be a possibility.

Many drowning victims have no symptoms. Patients with Glasgow Coma Scale scores greater than 13 who remain asymptomatic for 6 to 8 hours may be considered for discharge. Some advocate routine chest radiography in such patients before discharge. Even mild symptoms during the first 6 hours should

prompt hospitalization because lung disease can continue to progress. Any patient with a submersion lasting more than 1 minute with apnea or cyanosis should be admitted for observation.

Prevention

Although U.S. drowning rates have declined over the past 20 years, more than 80% of drownings are thought to be preventable. Improved prevention efforts, particularly fencing laws for home pools, are credited with the declining drowning rate. Close adult supervision of toddlers can protect against drowning in young children. Adults should be within touching distance of young children who are near any form of water. Pools should

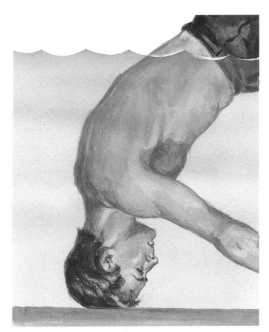

Mechanism. Vertical blow on head as in diving or surfing accident.

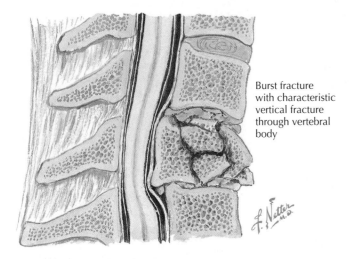

Burst fracture with characteristic vertical fracture through vertebral body

Figure 6-3 *Injury to the cervical spine during drowning.*

be enclosed with fencing on all sides, isolating pools from the house with a self-closing, latching gate. Fencing legislation has decreased drowning deaths by 50% to 70%. Because most children drown in their home pools, parents who own pools should be educated in CPR. Continued attention to public instruction

in CPR is critical. Effective bystander CPR can improve outcomes in drowning victims.

Adolescents should be educated about water safety and the increased dangers of intoxication during water recreation. Use of personal flotation devices reduces drowning deaths during water-based recreation. Swimming lessons have not been shown to reduce the risk of drowning on a population-based level, and overestimation of one's swimming ability can contribute to drownings, particularly in adolescents.

Certain medical conditions warrant specific precautions. Children and adults with seizure disorders should take showers, not baths, because of the risk of drowning if they have a seizure while bathing. All children with neurologic impairments should be supervised closely while swimming.

FUTURE DIRECTIONS

Data on the use of therapeutic hypothermia continue to be gathered, with trials beginning in pediatric patients. This information may guide the resuscitation of comatose pediatric drowning patients in the future and improve our understanding of the optimal target temperature for rewarming. Neuromonitoring techniques such as near-infrared spectroscopy are being refined and may also aid in improved postresuscitative care and prognostication. Surfactant therapy has not been proven beneficial in ARDS; however, several case reports exist on its use in pediatric drowning, and it may be an area of future investigation.

SUGGESTED READINGS

Bierens JJ, editor: *Handbook on Drowning*, The Netherlands, 2004, Springer, Available at http://www.drowning.nl.

Bierens JJ, Knape JT, Gelissen HP: Drowning, *Curr Opin Crit Care* 8:578-586, 2002.

Layon AJ, Modell JH: Drowning: update 2009, *Anesthesiology* 110:1390-1401, 2009.

Meyer RJ, Theodorou AA, Berg RA: Childhood drowning, *Pediatr Rev* 27:163-169, 2006.

Moon RE, Long RJ: Drowning and near-drowning, *Emerg Med* 14:377-386, 2002.

Thompson DO, Rivara F: Pool fencing for preventing drowning in children. The Cochrane Collection Web Site Available at http://www2.cochrane.org/reviews/en/ab001047.html. Accessed March 9, 2011.

Watson RS, Cummings P, Quan L, et al: Cervical spine injuries among submersion victims, *J Trauma* 51:658-662, 2001.

Zuckerbraun NS, Saladino RA: Pediatric drowning: current management strategies for immediate care, *Clin Pediatr Emerg Med* 6:49-56, 2008.

7

Burns

Todd A. Florin and Jill Posner

*B*urns and fire-related injuries account for significant morbidity and mortality in the pediatric population. In children
younger than 18 years of age, fires and burns are the third
leading cause of death from unintentional injury in the United
States. Approximately one-third of all burns occur in children
and adolescents younger than 20 years of age. Boys and children
younger than 5 years of age are at highest risk of burn injuries.
Burns may be thermal (resulting from flame, scald, steam, or
contact), electrical, or chemical in cause (Figure 7-1). In children younger than 5 years of age, scalds resulting from bathing
injuries or hot liquid spills account for the majority of burns.
Fire and flames are the leading causes of burns in children older
than 5 years of age. Electrical burns are seen primarily in adolescents. Child abuse accounts for up to 20% of burns in children and thus needs to be considered in all cases of pediatric
burns, particularly in those with inconsistent mechanisms or
specific patterns of injury (see Chapter 12). Carbon monoxide
poisoning can occur with smoke inhalation and is responsible
for many early deaths related to fire.

Significant advances in burn treatment have occurred over
the past 50 years. Of those children younger than 16 years of
age with burns of more than 80% of body surface area (BSA),
mortality rate has declined to just below 25%. This is largely a
result of aggressive prehospital, emergency, and inpatient hospital care in addition to the development of specialized burn
centers. Many burn injuries are preventable using relatively
simple measures. Lowering the temperature of water heaters
from 130° to 120°F increases the time to causing a full-thickness
burn from less than 30 seconds to 10 minutes. Smoke detectors
in homes can alert occupants to potential thermal dangers in the
home. Flame-retardant children's sleepwear has decreased the
incidence of full-thickness burns caused by flames or fire.

ETIOLOGY AND PATHOGENESIS

The clinical effects of burn injuries result from the loss of integrity of the skin and its vital functions. The skin serves to protect
the body from infection, controls heat loss, and plays a vital role
in fluid regulation. The epidermis prevents water loss and has a
protective fatty acid layer that kills many infectious organisms.
The deeper dermis contains sweat glands and vessels that
regulate evaporative and radiant heat loss. Therefore, burns
may result in infection, extensive fluid loss and disorders of
thermoregulation.

Three zones of injury typically occur with a burn: hyperemia,
stasis, and coagulation necrosis. Hyperemia is the result of vasodilatation secondary to inflammatory mediators without direct
cell injury. Stasis occurs in the dermis and is characterized by
vasoconstriction and thrombosis that results in reversible cell
injury. Coagulation necrosis results in an irreversible surface
injury known as an eschar.

Larger burns may produce systemic effects (Figure 7-2). Bacterial colonization of burned tissue may result in infection

caused by disruption of the protective epidermal barrier and the
inability of immune system elements and antibiotic agents to
penetrate burned tissue. Capillary permeability is increased by
the release of osmotically active substances into the interstitial
space and the release of vasoactive mediators into the systemic
circulation. Edema with resulting intravascular hypovolemia
results in both injured and noninjured tissues. Circulating
factors reduce myocardial function, thus decreasing cardiac
output. Direct heat damage and a microangiopathic hemolytic
process result in acute hemolysis of erythrocytes. All of these
acute processes may result in renal failure, liver dysfunction,
mental status changes, and hypoxia. After the initial injury, a
hypermetabolic and immunosuppressive state may ensue, resulting in malnutrition, infection, and multisystem organ failure.

CLINICAL PRESENTATION

The diagnosis of a burn injury is typically evident from the
patient's history and clinical presentation. The differential diagnosis includes erythroderma, toxic epidermal necrolysis, and
staphylococcal scalded skin syndrome; however, these are
quickly distinguished from burns based on history and presentation. Certain patterns of injury are classic for an intentional burn
as a result of child abuse (Figure 7-3). Scald injuries of the buttocks and thighs accompanied by perineal or foot injury that
spares the flexion creases is classic for intentional injury with
defensive posturing. Symmetric burns of the hands or feet with
clear lines of immersion are classic for forced submersion injuries. Small, round, deep burns are suggestive of intentional cigarette burns. Any deep wound with some geometric pattern may
suggest a contact burn, such as an iron. Suspicion should be
raised for abuse in any case with a nonspecific history, a mechanism that is inconsistent with the clinical presentation, delayed
presentation, or a classic injury pattern.

Burns are traditionally classified by the depth of skin injury
(Figure 7-4). Superficial burns, formerly known as first-degree
burns, involve the epidermis only and present with pain and
redness over the affected areas without significant edema or
blistering. These burns resolve in 3 to 5 days without residual
scarring. Of note, superficial burns are not included in burn
surface area (BSA) calculations.

Partial-thickness burns, formerly known as second-degree
burns, are divided into superficial and deep based on the depth
of extension through the dermis. Superficial partial-thickness
burns extend through the epidermis and the top half of the
dermis. Blistering and weeping is usually present along with
pink-red color because of the extensive dermal capillary network,
edema caused by increased capillary permeability, and severe
pain caused by the exposed sensory nerve receptors in the
dermis. These burns typically heal in 2 to 3 weeks without scarring because epithelial regenerative cells are intact. Deep
partial-thickness burns extend deep into the dermis. These are
typically less tender than superficial burns as a result of fewer

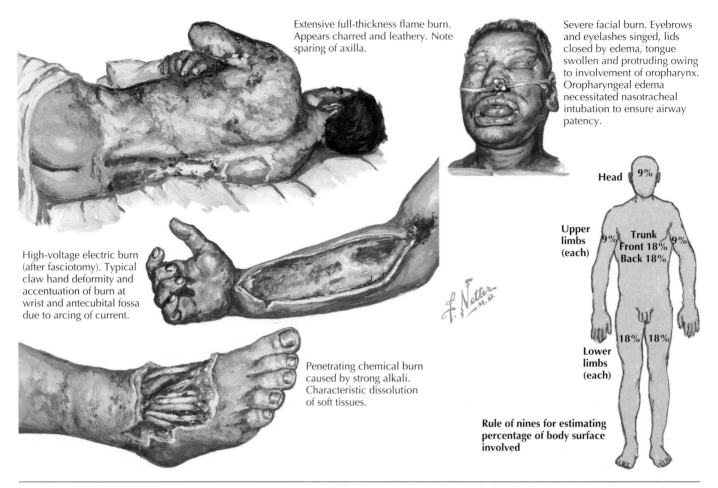

Extensive full-thickness flame burn. Appears charred and leathery. Note sparing of axilla.

Severe facial burn. Eyebrows and eyelashes singed, lids closed by edema, tongue swollen and protruding owing to involvement of oropharynx. Oropharyngeal edema necessitated nasotracheal intubation to ensure airway patency.

High-voltage electric burn (after fasciotomy). Typical claw hand deformity and accentuation of burn at wrist and antecubital fossa due to arcing of current.

Penetrating chemical burn caused by strong alkali. Characteristic dissolution of soft tissues.

Head 9%
Upper limbs (each) 9%
Trunk Front 18% Back 18% 9%
18% 18%
Lower limbs (each)

Rule of nines for estimating percentage of body surface involved

Figure 7-1 *Causes and clinical types of burns.*

exposed viable sensory nerve receptors. Deep partial-thickness burns are also paler and dryer compared with superficial injuries and may have a speckled appearance resulting from thrombosed vessels. Blisters may be present. These burns may take several weeks to heal, often with scar formation, necessitating skin grafting.

Full-thickness, or third-degree, burns involve total destruction of the epidermis and dermis revealing the subcutaneous fat. These wounds are insensate because the dermal cutaneous nerves are destroyed. Pain is typically caused by surrounding partial-thickness burns. These wounds appear white, leathery, charred, or translucent, with vessels showing through the wound. These burns cannot reepithelialize and only heal from the periphery. As a result, most full-thickness burns require skin grafting.

To adequately determine the extent of burn injury, the surface area and burn depth must be assessed. This is essential for guiding therapy, disposition, and prognosis. In adults and children older than age 15 years, the "rule of nines" is used to assess BSA—9% for the head and neck and each upper extremity and 18% for the trunk, back, and each lower extremity (Figure 7-1). The rule of nines cannot be used for children younger than age 15 years because of their proportionally larger head and different body proportions. Specialized charts that estimate burn area based on age can be used to estimate BSA for younger children.

A rough estimate may be provided using the child's palm, which represents approximately 1% of BSA.

Electrical burns result from electrical current passing through the body and generating thermal energy that damages tissues. Most injuries in younger children are low voltage (<120 V) as a result of toddlers chewing on plugs or electrical cords. These may result in deep burns with eschar formation at the corners of the mouth. These may scar and contract, and delayed labial artery bleeding may occur weeks after the injury when the eschar separates. High-voltage injuries (>500 V) may occur in adolescent boys because of risk-taking behaviors. These injuries may appear insignificant on the surface; however, deep and internal injuries may be extensive. Patients are at risk for cardiac arrhythmia, muscle destruction, renal failure, and compartment syndrome. Typically, BSA calculations are inadequate in severe electrical burns because much of the damage is internal.

Chemical burns may occur from skin contact with acidic or alkaline substances. Acids, such as household toilet cleaners, cause tissue protein coagulation necrosis, thus limiting the depth of injury. Alkaline agents, such as lye, bleach, and detergents, may result in a deep liquefaction necrotic injury. Edema resulting from these burns may cause full-thickness injuries to appear more superficial. Ingestion of acid or alkaline agents may result in esophageal injury, and splash injuries to the eye may result in blindness.

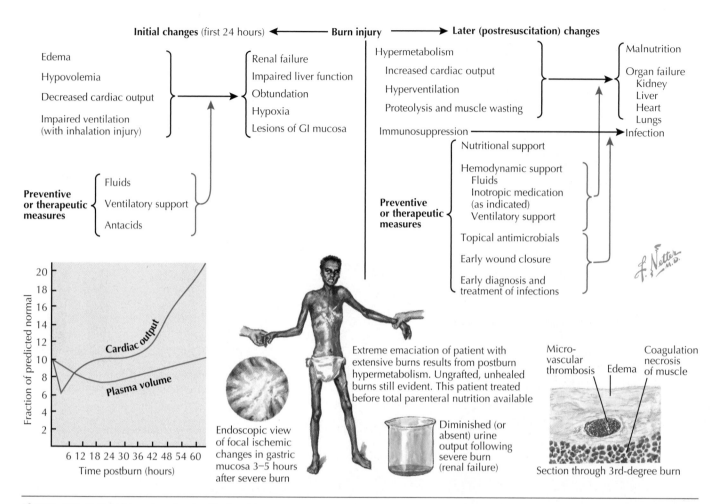

Initial changes (first 24 hours) ◄——— Burn injury ———► Later (postresuscitation) changes

Edema

Hypovolemia

Decreased cardiac output

Impaired ventilation
(with inhalation injury)

Renal failure

Impaired liver function

Obtundation

Hypoxia

Lesions of GI mucosa

Hypermetabolism

Increased cardiac output

Hyperventilation

Proteolysis and muscle wasting

Immunosuppression ————————► Infection

Malnutrition

Organ failure
Kidney
Liver
Heart
Lungs

**Preventive
or therapeutic
measures**

Fluids

Ventilatory support

Antacids

**Preventive
or therapeutic
measures**

Nutritional support

Hemodynamic support
Fluids
Inotropic medication
(as indicated)
Ventilatory support

Topical antimicrobials

Early wound closure

Early diagnosis and
treatment of infections

Endoscopic view
of focal ischemic
changes in gastric
mucosa 3–5 hours
after severe burn

Extreme emaciation of patient with
extensive burns results from postburn
hypermetabolism. Ungrafted, unhealed
burns still evident. This patient treated
before total parenteral nutrition available

Diminished (or
absent) urine
output following
severe burn
(renal failure)

Micro-
vascular
thrombosis

Edema

Coagulation
necrosis
of muscle

Section through 3rd-degree burn

Figure 7-2 *Metabolic and systemic effects of burns.*

EVALUATION AND MANAGEMENT

As with any trauma patient, airway, breathing, and circulation should be assessed first in all patients with burns. If these are all stable; the burn is minor (superficial or superficial partial thickness); and the burn does not involve the face, hands, feet, or perineum, the burn may be handled with basic first aid measures. Early cooling of the wound is accomplished by running cool water over the area within the first 30 minutes to stop thermal damage and prevent edema. Ice, grease, butter, and ointments should be avoided. The approach to intact blisters is controversial because blister fluid is thought to have both protective and damaging properties. If a blister is large, likely to rupture, or painful, clinicians generally rupture the blister. A clean bandage and topical antibiotics should be used to cover these minor burns.

If burns are significant (i.e., involve extensive BSA, deep partial-thickness or full-thickness burns involving face, hands, feet, or perineum), a physician should promptly evaluate them. As already noted, the physician should first assess the patient's airway, breathing, and circulation. Inhalation of hot gases as a result of house fires may lead to airway edema, which may obstruct the airway. Therefore, early intubation should be considered in patients with facial burns, singed facial hairs, hoarseness, or any other signs or symptoms consistent with potential

airway damage. All severely burned children should receive 100% oxygen. There should be a low threshold for considering lower airway injury if the mechanism is consistent with smoke or steam inhalation. Rapid assessment of circulation is paramount because burn shock may occur in patients with burns over 20% of BSA. The patient should receive appropriate vascular access, and fluid resuscitation should be initiated early. Evidence has suggested that adequate initial fluid resuscitation improves outcomes for these patients. Because of the extravasation of water and sodium through abnormally permeable capillaries in the first 24 hours after injury, initial fluid resuscitation should occur with isotonic crystalloid solutions, such as lactated Ringer's solution. The Parkland formula (4 mL/kg per percent of total affected BSA) can be used to estimate fluid requirements. Half of the required fluid is given in the first 8 hours after the burn, and the remaining fluid is given over the next 16 hours. Careful monitoring of perfusion, blood pressure, and urine output is important in detecting the development of shock.

In all serious burns, the physician must be aware of the risk of burn sepsis. Antiseptic techniques should be scrupulous to diminish pathogen colonization of burned areas. Topical antibiotics should also be used to reduce bacterial colonization. In general, prophylactic broad-spectrum antibiotics should be avoided because they do not significantly reduce the risk of infection and do increase the likelihood of developing resistant organisms.

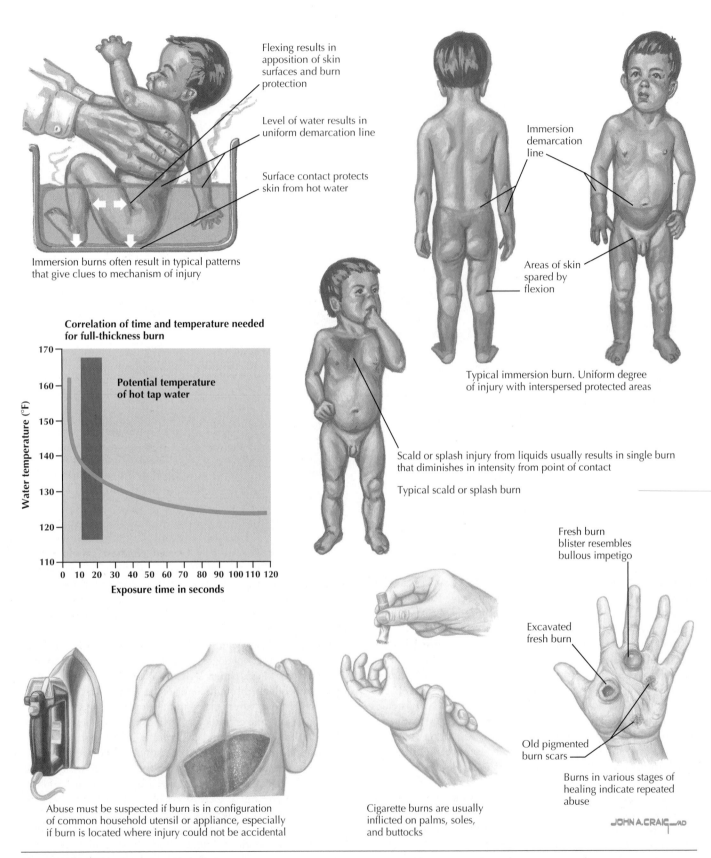

Flexing results in apposition of skin surfaces and burn protection

Level of water results in uniform demarcation line

Surface contact protects skin from hot water

Immersion burns often result in typical patterns that give clues to mechanism of injury

Immersion demarcation line

Areas of skin spared by flexion

Typical immersion burn. Uniform degree of injury with interspersed protected areas

Correlation of time and temperature needed for full-thickness burn

Water temperature (°F)

Potential temperature of hot tap water

Exposure time in seconds

Scald or splash injury from liquids usually results in single burn that diminishes in intensity from point of contact

Typical scald or splash burn

Fresh burn blister resembles bullous impetigo

Excavated fresh burn

Old pigmented burn scars

Burns in various stages of healing indicate repeated abuse

Abuse must be suspected if burn is in configuration of common household utensil or appliance, especially if burn is located where injury could not be accidental

Cigarette burns are usually inflicted on palms, soles, and buttocks

JOHN A. CRAIG—AD

Figure 7-3 *Child abuse: burn injuries.*

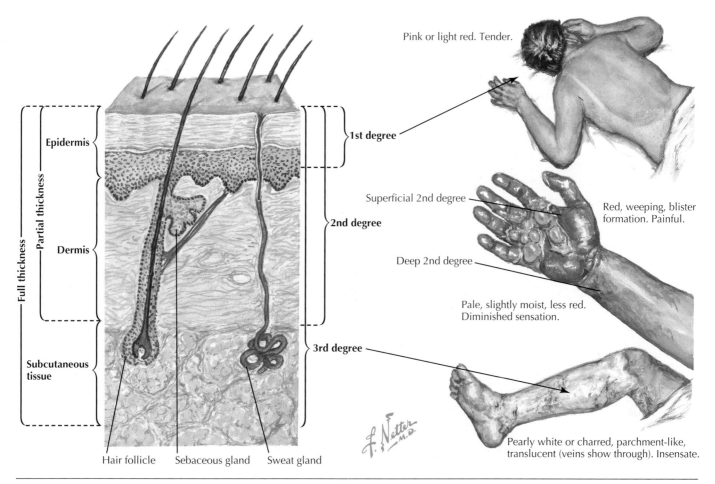

Figure 7-4 *Classification of burns.*

The burn wounds should be covered loosely with clean sheets until they are ready to be assessed and treated to protect the wounds and minimize pain. The wounds should be cleaned with large volumes of sterile warm saline, and loose tissue should be debrided gently with sterile gauze. Temporary skin substitutes, such as Biobrane, may help to reduce pain, facilitate healing, and decrease the length of hospitalization. These dressings consist of a silicone outer layer that acts as a protective epidermal barrier and an inner surface consisting of collagen peptides that bind to wound surface fibrin and facilitate reepithelialization. Topical antibiotics, such as silver sulfadiazine, bacitracin, or mafenide acetate, should be used for larger and more contaminated burns. Escharotomy should be considered in all full-thickness burns that have the potential to threaten circulation to an extremity. Surgical excision and skin grafting should be considered in deep partial-thickness and full-thickness burns (Figure 7-5). Pain control should be attended to promptly in patients with partial-thickness burns, with morphine being the drug of choice for severe burns and acetaminophen or ibuprofen for use with minor burns.

Appropriate disposition of these patients is essential to optimize treatment outcome. Specialized burn centers have been developed that have the resources to provide aggressive medical, psychological, and rehabilitative care to children with significant burns. The American Burn Association has developed criteria for referral of patients to burn centers (Box 7-1). Appropriate

---

Box 7-1 American Burn Association Criteria for Referral to a Burn Center

1. Partial-thickness burns of >10% of the total body surface area
2. Burns that involve the face, hands, feet, genitalia, perineum, or major joints
3. Third-degree burns in any age group
4. Electrical burns, including lightning injury
5. Chemical burns
6. Inhalation injury
7. Burn injury in patients with preexisting medical disorders that could complicate management, prolong recovery, or affect mortality
8. Any patients with burns and concomitant trauma (e.g., fractures) in which the burn injury poses the greatest risk of morbidity or mortality
9. Burned children in hospitals without qualified personnel or equipment for the care of children
10. Burn injury in patients who will require special social, emotional, or rehabilitative intervention

Excerpted from Committee on Trauma, American College of Surgeons: *Guidelines for the Operation of Burn Centers, Resources for Optimal Care of the Injured Patient*, 2006, pp 79-86.

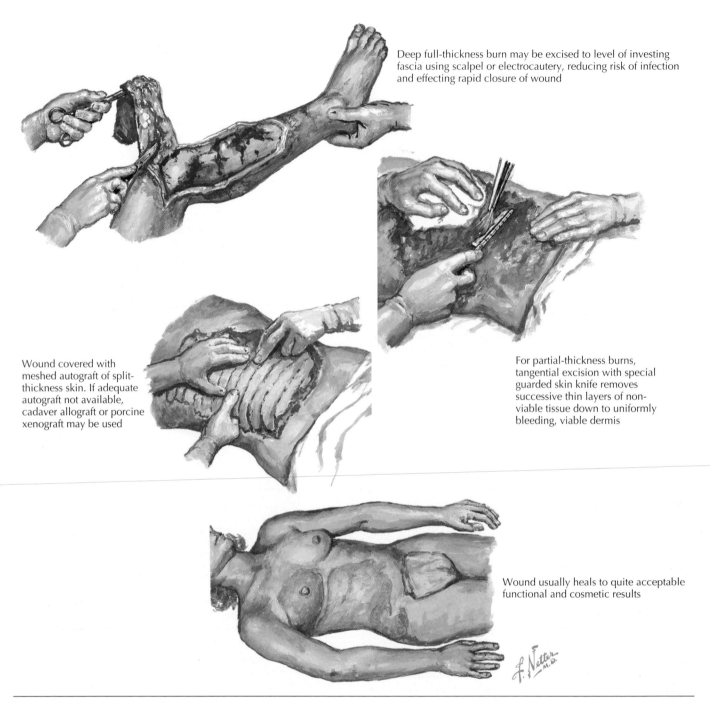

Deep full-thickness burn may be excised to level of investing fascia using scalpel or electrocautery, reducing risk of infection and effecting rapid closure of wound

Wound covered with meshed autograft of split-thickness skin. If adequate autograft not available, cadaver allograft or porcine xenograft may be used

For partial-thickness burns, tangential excision with special guarded skin knife removes successive thin layers of non-viable tissue down to uniformly bleeding, viable dermis

Wound usually heals to quite acceptable functional and cosmetic results

Figure 7-5 *Excision and grafting for burns.*

and timely treatment and disposition can potentially improve the outcomes and quality of life of children with burn injuries.

SUGGESTED READINGS

American Burn Association. Available at http://www.ameriburn.org.

Church D, Elsayed S, Reid O, et al: Burn wound infections, *Clin Microbiol Rev* 19(2):403-434, 2006.

Holland AJA: Pediatric burns: the forgotten trauma of childhood, *Can J Surg* 49(4):272-277, 2006.

Patel PP, Vasquez SA, Granick MS, Rhee ST: Topical antimicrobials in pediatric burn wound management, *J Craniofacial Surg* 19(4):913-922, 2008.

Palmieri TL, Greenhalgh DG: Topical treatment of pediatric patients with burns: a practical guide, *Am J Clin Dermatol* 3(8):529-534, 2002.

Schulman CI, Ivascu FA: Nutritional and metabolic consequences in the pediatric burn patient, *J Craniofacial Surg* 19(4):891-894, 2008.

Whitaker IS, Cantab MA, Prowse S, Potokar TS: A critical evaluation of the use of Biobrane as a biologic skin substitute, *Ann Plastic Surg* 60(3):333-337, 2008.

Injury and Trauma

8

Sage Myers and James M. Callahan

*I*njury is one of the most important public health threats to children in the United States. Trauma causes more deaths in children and adolescents than all other causes combined. The care of injured children is a vitally important and specialized skill. Differences between child and adult anatomy and physiology make injury patterns and responses to injury unique to the pediatric age group.

Effective trauma resuscitation and treatment require the rapid acquisition and communication of large amounts of information about patients' respiratory and cardiovascular stability as well as the extent of their injuries. It is common practice to follow a structured examination technique and management strategy during the evaluation of trauma patients, such as that taught in Advanced Trauma Life Support (ATLS) courses. Use of these principles helps to minimize secondary injury in pediatric trauma victims and ensures the best possible outcomes in these patients.

ETIOLOGY AND PATHOGENESIS

Injury is the leading cause of death from ages 1 to 19 years in the United States. In addition, injury causes 30% of all deaths in children younger than 1 year of age. Eighty percent of all deaths related to trauma occur at the scene of the injury or in the emergency department (ED). This highlights the need for effective prevention strategies and the importance of appropriate prehospital and ED care for pediatric trauma victims.

The most common causes of injuries and resultant injury patterns are age specific. In infants (younger than 1 year of age), a high percentage of injuries are nonaccidental in nature, and it is important to maintain a high index of suspicion for possible inflicted injuries (see Chapter 12). Falls are the most common cause of injury in children from 1 to 14 years of age. Motor vehicle collisions and motor vehicle–pedestrian incidents are the most common causes of fatal injuries in children ages 1 to 18 years. Drowning (see Chapter 6) is the second most common cause of fatalities in younger children, and firearm-related deaths are the next most common cause in adolescents ages 15 to 18 years.

In children and adolescents presenting to trauma centers because of injury, a head injury is part of the presenting findings in 60% of patients. Different patterns of injury are evident in children of various ages and can often be predicted by the mechanism of injury and the size and age of the patient. For example, when struck by motor vehicles, younger and smaller children may primarily sustain head injuries. Older toddlers and young school-aged children may sustain injuries consistent with Waddell triad's (closed head injury, intraabdominal injury, midshaft femur fracture), and adolescents may sustain primarily extremity injuries. The clinical presentation of pediatric trauma victims varies depending on the mechanism and severity of their injuries. Evaluation and management are aimed at assessing the nature and severity of the patient's injuries while beginning stabilization and deciding on the needed course of therapy.

EVALUATION AND MANAGEMENT

Primary Survey (see Chapter 1)

The primary survey is structured to generate information vital to the immediate treatment of life-threatening issues. It is often referred to as the ABCs (airway, breathing, and circulation) but is better thought of as ABCDE (airway, breathing, circulation, disability, and exposure and environment), which is delineated below. Children who have sustained injuries are at risk of secondary injuries caused by hypoxia, hypercarbia, and poor perfusion. Recognition and correction of these conditions are the goals of this rapid portion of their assessment.

AIRWAY

Initial evaluation of the airway is of utmost importance. A child who can phonate normally has a patent airway. In an unconscious patient, inspection for foreign body in the pharynx and for midface or mandibular injuries, which could compromise airway patency, should occur, as well as observation of obvious stridor or stertor with respiratory effort. Hoarseness or crepitus over the tracheal cartilage should raise concern for laryngeal fracture. After these areas have been examined, the physician should quickly move to secure an airway if necessary or move on to the assessment of ventilatory efficacy.

Readers are directed to Chapter 1 for complete information about airway evaluation and management. However, it is important to reiterate here the need for inline stabilization of the cervical spine (c-spine) during this assessment and treatment, especially if intubation is attempted. The collar should be opened or removed before direct laryngoscopy because it can impede successful visualization of the larynx. *An assistant should hold the patient in the midclavicular line with the ears firmly between the lower arms to eliminate movement of the c-spine during intubation.*

BREATHING

Evaluation of effective ventilatory effort occurs after the airway evaluation. The chest wall excursion should be observed for symmetric chest rise. Visual inspection, including of the axillae and back, should identify open wounds. The clinicians should evaluate for symmetry and adequacy of breath sounds by auscultating the chest. Asymmetric chest rise or asymmetric breath sounds suggest the possibility of pneumothorax, hemothorax, flail chest, or an open chest wound.

Asymmetry in breath sounds may signify pneumothorax or hemothorax. This is important to note on the initial examination even when it appears clinically insignificant because a

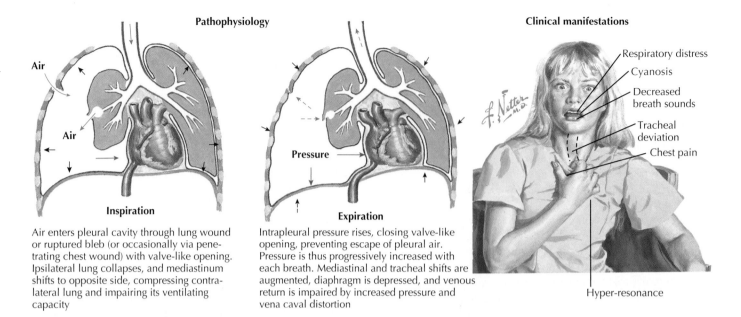

Pathophysiology

Clinical manifestations

Air

Air

Inspiration

Air enters pleural cavity through lung wound or ruptured bleb (or occasionally via pene-trating chest wound) with valve-like opening. Ipsilateral lung collapses, and mediastinum shifts to opposite side, compressing contra-lateral lung and impairing its ventilating capacity

Pressure

Expiration

Intrapleural pressure rises, closing valve-like opening, preventing escape of pleural air. Pressure is thus progressively increased with each breath. Mediastinal and tracheal shifts are augmented, diaphragm is depressed, and venous return is impaired by increased pressure and vena caval distortion

Respiratory distress

Cyanosis

Decreased breath sounds

Tracheal deviation

Chest pain

Hyper-resonance

Figure 8-1 *Tension pneumothorax.*

simple pneumothorax can be quickly converted to a tension pneumothorax when a patient is ventilated with positive pressure by bag–valve–mask (BVM) or endotracheal ventilation. Also, children are especially sensitive to the development of tension pneumothorax because of their relatively compliant and mobile mediastinum. Radiographs can be used to determine the presence and amount of air or blood in the pleural space. In a more clinically stable patient, a small simple pneumothorax may be treated noninvasively with inpatient monitoring, oxygen therapy, and serial chest radiography. Larger pneumothoraces or hemothoraces should be managed with chest tube drainage.

An absence of breath sounds, especially in conjunction with hypotension, should alert the clinician to possible tension pneumothorax. Tracheal deviation to the opposite side and hyper-resonance of the chest to percussion may be less obvious in pediatric patients, and the more mobile mediastinum in this age group may produce vascular collapse in a more rapid fashion. Needle decompression can be immediately undertaken in such circumstances, with the introduction of a large-bore over-the-needle catheter (e.g., a 14-gauge intravenous [IV] catheter) into the second intercostal space in the midclavicular line. Needle decompression necessitates the subsequent placement of a chest tube. Massive hemothorax can present in a similar fashion, although the chest should be dull to percussion, and severe hypotension often predominates because of the significant blood loss (Figure 8-1).

Open chest wounds create loss of the usual negative pressure upon inspiration that is needed to inflate the lung. If the chest wall defect is large compared with the airway, air will preferentially be brought into the defect as opposed to the airway, significantly impairing effective ventilation. An occlusive dressing should be placed over sucking chest wounds, closed on three sides, to allow for air to escape during exhalation but preventing air from entering during inspiration.

CIRCULATION

After the respiratory assessment, hemodynamic status should be evaluated by auscultation of heart sounds; palpation of central pulses (femoral or brachial), paying attention to both the rate and quality; and rapid evaluation of skin color, capillary refill, and level of consciousness. Any obvious area of external hemorrhage should be identified and addressed with pressure dressings; whip stitching; or in the case of massive scalp wounds, stapling to control bleeding.

Complete details on hypoperfusion and shock may be found in Chapter 2. In patients who have sustained significant traumatic injuries, IV access should be secured as quickly as possible with two large-bore IV catheters placed in large peripheral veins. If peripheral access attempts are unsuccessful in a patient showing signs of shock, clinicians should proceed quickly to obtain interosseous (IO) access. IO lines should not be placed distal to any obvious fractures.

Shock in a trauma patient should be presumed to be attributable to hypovolemia secondary to hemorrhage. Because most pediatric trauma victims have sustained blunt trauma, hemorrhage may be attributable to internal injuries such as splenic or hepatic lacerations and not readily visualized. However, other causes of traumatic shock must be considered, especially in patients with shock unresponsive to fluid resuscitation or with hemodynamic collapse. Chief among these causes are tension pneumothorax, tension hemothorax, and cardiac tamponade.

Cardiac tamponade is more common with penetrating chest wounds but can be caused by rupture of the myocardium with blunt traumatic force. As with tension pneumothorax, patients with cardiac tamponade present with tachycardia, hypotension, and distended jugular veins. However, with tamponade, there is no tracheal deviation. Pulsus paradoxus, which is exaggeration of the normal decrease in blood pressure with spontaneous inspiration, may be present in association with tamponade.

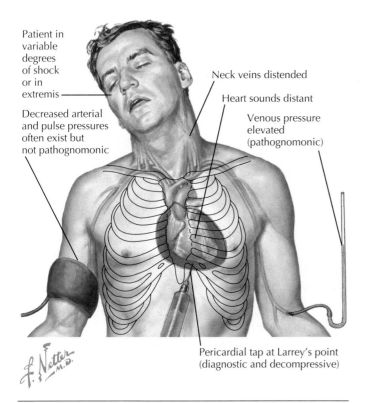

Patient in variable degrees of shock or in extremis

Decreased arterial and pulse pressures often exist but not pathognomonic

Neck veins distended

Heart sounds distant

Venous pressure elevated (pathognomonic)

Pericardial tap at Larrey's point (diagnostic and decompressive)

Figure 8-2 *Cardiac tamponade and pericardiocentesis.*

Rapid bedside ultrasonography can help make the diagnosis, but if unavailable or if the patient is hemodynamically unstable, pericardiocentesis can be used to diagnose and treat tamponade (Figure 8-2).

Finally, hypotension in the pediatric trauma patient can, rarely, be caused by spinal cord injury. This should be suspected in a patient with an appropriate injury mechanism who is observed to have bradycardia, or a lack of appropriate tachycardia, in the face of hypotension.

The rapid installation of IV fluids is standard first-line therapy for shock. Boluses of 20 mL/kg of 0.9% saline solution or lactated Ringer's solution should be given rapidly. If there is no response after 40 mL/kg is administered, then blood products should be given. In a child with decompensated shock caused by trauma, O-negative packed red blood cells (PRBCs) should be pushed rapidly until type-specific or cross-matched blood is available. In patients who require massive transfusion, fresh whole blood or fresh-frozen plasma and platelets in addition to PRBCs should be considered. If shock is not rapidly reversed with transfusion therapy, identification of the source of hemorrhage must be achieved, and operative management to halt the hemorrhage must be immediately undertaken.

DISABILITY

After the patient's hemodynamic status has been stabilized, the neurologic status is evaluated. The symmetry, size, and briskness of pupillary response should be documented along with the level of responsiveness. Numerical scales, such as the Glasgow Coma

Scale (GCS, see Figure 1-8), are used to generate structured assessments of the level of responsiveness. This allows for comparisons in mental status evaluations over time, comparisons of assessments performed by different clinicians, and improved communication among providers. The GCS has been adapted for use in preverbal patients as well. A more straightforward, although somewhat less nuanced, system for rapid neurologic evaluation is the AVPU (awake, verbal, pain, unresponsive) system. Abnormalities in the pupillary response or level of consciousness should increase concern for intracranial injuries and alert the team to prepare for possible interventions such as intubation for airway protection or to improve ventilation, mannitol, or hypertonic saline administration for increased intracranial pressure (ICP) or emergent neurosurgical intervention.

In patients who are alert and can cooperate with the examination, the patient's strength and sensation should be assessed in all four extremities. Tenderness and deformities of the cervical, thoracic, and lumbar spine should also be assessed. In preverbal children, this assessment can be challenging. Observation of spontaneous movement, watching how the patient reaches for objects, and the patient's response to touch or painful stimulus should be assessed. The spine should be palpated, but it is difficult to ascertain tenderness in these children.

EXPOSURE AND ENVIRONMENT

The final step in the primary survey is to ensure that all clothing has been removed from the patient so that all areas of the body can be visually inspected for injury. In this step, the patient's core temperature should be evaluated with the understanding that trauma patients are often cold because of the environment and significant blood loss. Rewarming should be undertaken, as well as the prevention of heat loss now that the patient is fully exposed. Children, especially, lose a significant amount of heat through their skin because of their relatively large body surface area. The ambient temperature of the resuscitation area should be kept warm, and when inspection for injury is completed, warm blankets should be used to cover the patient to prevent heat loss.

Some sources have suggested adding "Family" as the final part of the primary survey in the care of injured children to prompt providers to remember to inform family members quickly about the child's status and injuries as well as to consider allowing family members to be present for the resuscitation. Family presence at resuscitation has not been shown to hinder care and has been shown to increase family satisfaction. When family members are present for resuscitation efforts, a trained health care associate (nurse, social worker, or chaplain) must be assigned to be with and communicate to the family members to help them understand the efforts that are being undertaken.

Secondary Survey

The goal of the secondary survey is to detail all likely injuries with a head-to-toe evaluation of the patient. It is best if this is done in an ordered way to avoid inadvertently leaving out body areas.

Temporal fossa hematoma

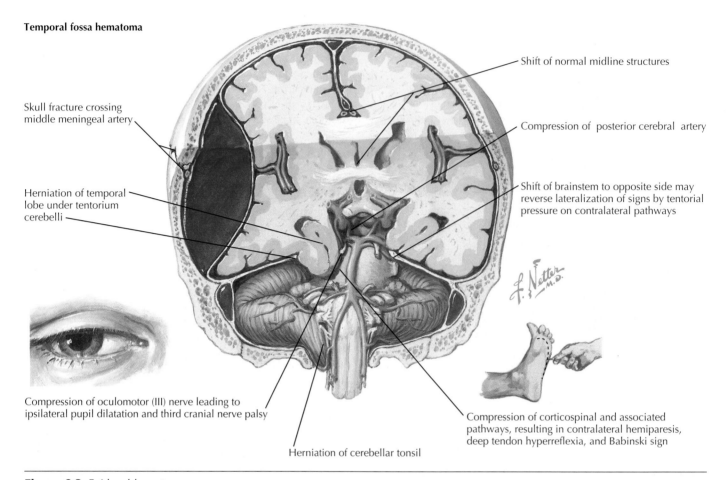

Shift of normal midline structures

Compression of posterior cerebral artery

Shift of brainstem to opposite side may reverse lateralization of signs by tentorial pressure on contralateral pathways

Skull fracture crossing middle meningeal artery

Herniation of temporal lobe under tentorium cerebelli

Compression of oculomotor (III) nerve leading to ipsilateral pupil dilatation and third cranial nerve palsy

Herniation of cerebellar tonsil

Compression of corticospinal and associated pathways, resulting in contralateral hemiparesis, deep tendon hyperreflexia, and Babinski sign

Figure 8-3 *Epidural hematoma.*

HEAD

The initial evaluation of the head involves inspection for evidence of injury to the skull, as well as assessment of level of consciousness and neurologic status, which may indicate underlying brain injuries. Locations of all hematomas, lacerations, abrasions, depressions, and areas of tenderness should be documented. Because the middle meningeal artery runs through the temporal bone, hematomas or other signs of injury in the temporal region raise concerns for the possibility of an underlying epidural hematoma as a result of tearing of this artery. Epidural hematomas (Figure 8-3) are often described as presenting with a lucid interval followed by a rapid deterioration in mental status when the volume of blood filling the epidural space reaches the threshold to cause significant mass effect. On computed tomography (CT), epidural hematomas are seen as a convex fluid collection between the skull and brain. Significant epidural hematomas represent a neurosurgical emergency because evacuation of the growing hematoma before herniation can be lifesaving.

Subdural hematomas are a second, more common intracranial hemorrhage. They may be seen without significant external signs of trauma. Subdural hematomas (Figure 8-4) are usually caused by tearing of small bridging veins from the surface of the cortex to the inner layer of the dura mater. These injuries are often caused by high-force, rapid flexion and extension of the

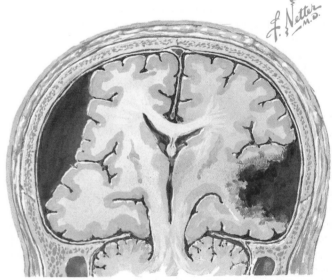

Section showing acute subdural hematoma on right side and subdural hematoma associated with temporal lobe intracerebral hematoma ("burst" temporal lobe) on left

Figure 8-4 *Subdural hematoma.*

head. CT will show concave fluid collections between the skull and brain. Although subdural hematomas are less likely to lead to the rapid onset of significant symptoms than are epidural hematomas, they are more often associated with significant underlying brain damage because of the mechanism of injury. In infants and toddlers, it is important to remember that subdural hematomas can be associated with nonaccidental injury from shaking the child or as part of the shake and impact syndrome (see Chapter 12).

Both epidural hematomas and subdural hematomas can become large enough to lead to significant increases in ICP (see Chapter 10). When ICP increases, herniation of brain tissue across the tentorium or downward through the foramen magnum may occur. Bradycardia, hypertension, and irregular respirations (Cushing's triad) indicate impeding herniation. Transtentorial herniation is heralded by a decreased level of consciousness and asymmetric pupillary responses. Rapid therapy, including brief periods of hyperventilation and IV administration of 0.25 to 1.0 g/kg of mannitol or 5 mL/kg of 3% sodium chloride solution may temporize the situation until more definitive therapy, such as surgical evacuation of a hematoma or drainage of cerebrospinal fluid (CSF) through an intraventricular catheter, can occur.

Most children with significant head injuries caused by blunt trauma do not have surgically correctable lesions (e.g., epidural or subdural hematomas). Instead, diffuse axonal injury, which is characterized by diffuse edema and small, punctate hemorrhages on CT, is more common. All children with a decreased level of consciousness or other neurologic abnormalities after head injury should undergo CT to define their injuries and help to plan their immediate and subsequent care.

The care of children and adolescents with severe head injuries requires meticulous attention to the ABCs. Hypoxia, hypercarbia, and poor perfusion (shock) can all lead to secondary injuries in children who have sustained significant neurologic injury. In the face of increased ICP, cerebral perfusion pressure (CPP = Mean arterial pressure – Intracranial pressure) will be further compromised in patients who are allowed to remain in shock.

If mean arterial pressure (MAP) decreases, perfusion to areas of injury decreases, and injuries may be worsened. Therefore, attempts to manage ICP may be counterproductive unless CPP is preserved through the maintenance of MAP with appropriate volume resuscitation.

Most children who sustain head injuries have seemingly mild injuries and look well on initial presentation. In these children, the relatively low risk of underlying significant intracranial injuries must be weighed against the radiation involved in imaging the brain and the possible risk of malignancies in the future associated with this imaging. A decision rule based on a large, multicenter, prospective study has identified historical and physical findings associated with intracranial injuries on CT scans in children (Box 8-1). CT scans are rarely indicated in the absence of any of these findings in children.

Linear, nondisplaced skull fractures are the most common type of skull fracture in children, rarely require intervention, and are associated with a relatively good prognosis. Skull fractures that are diastatic or which extend into preexisting suture lines are more likely to require correction to prevent future

---

Box 8-1 Factors Associated with Positive Findings on Computed Tomography Scans in Children with Seemingly Mild Head Injuries

Children younger than 2 years old
- Altered mental status
- Occipital, parietal, or temporal scalp hematomas
- Loss of consciousness >5 sec
- Severe mechanism of injury
- Palpable or possible skull fracture
- Not acting normally per parent

Children 2 years old or older
- Altered mental status
- Level of consciousness
- History of vomiting
- Severe mechanism of injury
- Signs of basilar skull fracture
- Severe headache

Adapted from Kuppermann N, Holmes JF, Dayan PS, et al: Identification of children at very low risk of clinically-important brain injuries after head trauma: a prospective cohort study. Lancet 374:1160-1170, 2009.

---

development of leptomeningeal cysts at these sites. Skull fractures with significant depression causing risk to underlying brain tissue may also require surgical correction.

Basilar skull fractures require special evaluation and treatment because they raise concern for other injuries associated with the significant forces needed to produce them, as well as their unique location, which may lead to significant complications, including late intracranial hemorrhages, carotid artery dissections, and intracranial infections. Basilar skull fractures should be suspected when any of the following are present: "raccoon eyes" caused by periorbital ecchymoses; Battle sign or postauricular ecchymoses; hemotympanum; clear rhinorrhea or clear otorrhea caused by CSF leakage from the nose or ear, respectively; or cranial nerve VII or VIII dysfunction (Figure 8-5). Neurosurgical input should be obtained early in management.

Children with concussion after head trauma can have significant symptoms and prolonged recovery despite normal head imaging. Concussion—or more accurately, mild traumatic brain injury—is defined as a brief alteration in brain function with or without loss of consciousness caused by a blow or jolt to the head. Children and adolescents with concussions may have significant and long-lasting symptomatology, including headaches, dizziness, amnesia, confusion, difficulty concentrating, nausea, and vomiting. Older grading systems based on the *initial* signs and symptoms of injury are not predictive of subsequent outcomes and are no longer used by most experts.

The International Conference on Concussion in Sport has suggested that measures of recovery must be included in the determination of injury severity as well as in determining when someone who has sustained a concussion is ready to resume activities such as work and school attendance and return to sports participation. To limit the duration of symptoms in children after concussions, rest (including the concept of cognitive rest) should be encouraged and strict return-to-activity guidelines should be followed. This involves a gradual increase in both physical and mental activities.

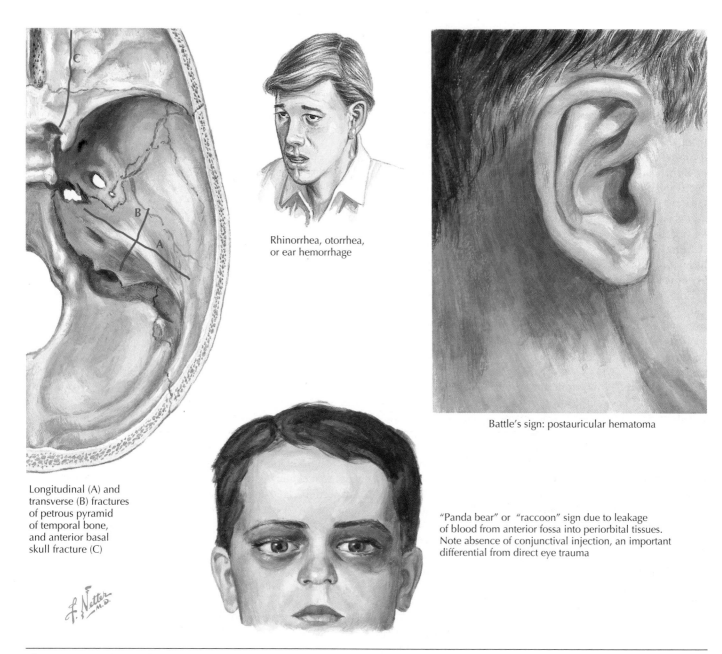

Longitudinal (A) and transverse (B) fractures of petrous pyramid of temporal bone, and anterior basal skull fracture (C)

Rhinorrhea, otorrhea, or ear hemorrhage

Battle's sign: postauricular hematoma

"Panda bear" or "raccoon" sign due to leakage of blood from anterior fossa into periorbital tissues. Note absence of conjunctival injection, an important differential from direct eye trauma

Figure 8-5 *Basilar skull fracture: physical findings.*

Facial and eye injuries should be considered in all children with head injury. A thorough examination, including assessment of the stability of the facial bones and oral structures and a thorough examination of the eye and extraocular movements, must be completed. Injuries to the facial bones, including the maxilla and mandible, may lead to airway compromise, secondary infections, and cosmetic deformities if not recognized promptly and treated appropriately.

In alert patients, examination of the eye must include the assessment of the patient's visual acuity and inspection of the globe, including the cornea, anterior chamber, and fundus, for signs of injury. Any concern for penetrating trauma to the globe or a hyphema or other serious injuries necessitates emergent evaluation by an ophthalmologist. In children in whom the extraocular movements are decreased, facial CT scans should be performed to assess for orbital fractures and possible entrapment of the extraocular muscles or other processes affecting the ophthalmic nerve.

NECK AND SPINE

Any child who has sustained a severe head injury should be assumed to have a c-spine injury and remain in spinal immobilization until there is clear clinical or radiologic evidence that there is no spinal injury. Plain radiographs and CT scans may aid in this evaluation, but in patients with a decreased level of consciousness, magnetic resonance imaging may be required. As long as immobilization is maintained, this can be delayed until the child has been stabilized and other major traumatic injuries have been addressed. In awake patients, clinical signs of spine injuries include posterior midline tenderness and limitation of motion. Even in patients with a normal level of consciousness, clinical clearance of the c-spine is especially difficult in patients who are preverbal and young children who are uncooperative because of fear, anxiety, or pain associated with other injuries. It is important to remember that children are at risk of spinal cord injury without radiologic abnormalities (SCIWORA) because of the relative ligamentous laxity found in their c-spines. Therefore, normal radiographs may not completely rule out injury to the spinal cord itself, and MRI may be necessary for complete diagnosis. Detailed discussion of spinal injuries can be found in Chapter 24.

Evaluation of the anterior neck should involve palpation to ensure that the trachea is in a midline position. Deviation should raise concern for tension pneumothorax or hemothorax. Blunt trauma to the anterior neck, hyperextension of the neck, or blunt trauma to the chest with forced exhalation against a possible closed glottis may cause laryngeal injury. Signs of laryngeal injury include a change in voice, dysphagia, odynophagia, hemoptysis, stridor, crepitus along the anterior neck, and obscuration of the cartilaginous landmarks.

In a patient with suspected laryngeal injury who requires intubation, consideration must be given to the possible complication of converting a partial tracheal laceration to a complete transaction or the creation of a false track when performing direct laryngoscopic intubation. As with prolonged BVM ventilation, laryngeal mask airways can also carry the risk of expanding subcutaneous and mediastinal free air. Preparation for possible surgical airway placement and the use of flexible fiberoptics for intubation may decrease these risks.

Evaluation of the neck should also involve inspection for signs of penetrating injury. The neck is often divided into three zones (Figure 8-6) according to the collection of structures at risk of injury, with zone I covering the area between the thoracic inlet and the cricoid cartilage, zone II covering the cricoid cartilage to the angle of the mandible, and zone III above the angle of the mandible. Injuries to zones I and II may be associated with pneumothorax or hemothorax. Injuries in zone II are the easiest to explore surgically but also the most likely to involve major vascular structures and therefore are often brought directly to the operating room for exploration if they extend through the platysma. If clinically stable, zone I and III injuries are often evaluated with diagnostic imaging to determine appropriate management before surgical exploration.

Finally, although not always apparent in the initial evaluation, clinicians must have a high index of suspicion for injuries to the carotid artery, including carotid artery dissection, pseudoaneurysm, and thrombosis. Symptom onset, including stroke, may be delayed from the time of trauma. Ultrasonography, CT angiography, magnetic resonance angiography, and conventional angiography have all been used for diagnosis.

CHEST

The evaluation of the chest should involve the familiar initial steps of *inspection* for external signs of trauma; *palpation* for deformities, crepitus, and tenderness; and *auscultation* of breath sounds. Children may sustain significant lung injury, including pulmonary contusions and pneumothorax (see above) without rib fractures because of their compliant rib cages. Therefore, external signs of trauma may be limited despite significant internal injuries.

Injuries to the chest wall, including the ribs, may occur. Flail chest should be suspected in any child with asymmetric chest rise, significant tenderness and crepitus on palpation of the ribs, and a high-velocity mechanism. Flail chest occurs when a segment of the chest wall becomes discontinuous with the rest of the thorax, usually requiring two or more ribs to be broken in two or more places to create this "floating" chest segment. Splinting because of pain from this injury can cause significant impairment of appropriate respiration, and the injury to the underlying lung tissue can further impair oxygenation and ventilation. Pain control and close monitoring for respiratory decompensation are required.

Simple rib fractures create significant pain and require appropriate analgesia but should heal completely without other intervention. However, splinting from inadequately controlled pain may lead to atelectasis and worsen any coexisting

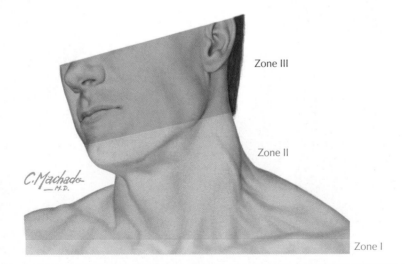

Figure 8-6 *Zones of the neck.*

pulmonary issues. Fractures of ribs 1 to 3 require significant force and should alert the clinician to be aware of the possibility of other high-impact injuries.

Injuries to the chest may also involve mediastinal structures. Blunt cardiac injury may result in myocardial contusion, myocardial rupture, or chordae rupture with valvular insufficiency. Patients with myocardial rupture should present with cardiac tamponade. Patients with myocardial contusion will likely present with chest pain and tachycardia. Cardiac arrhythmias, evaluated with a 12-lead electrocardiogram, may also occur.

Although rare, aortic disruption may occur in blunt injuries, especially those associated with a rapid deceleration. Patients with aortic injuries who survive to the hospital tend to have incomplete lacerations, often located near the ligamentum arteriosum. Although initially hemodynamically stable, these incomplete lacerations carry a high risk of further acute deterioration if there is rupture of the contained hematoma. Such injuries should be considered when an appropriate mechanism exists; widened mediastinum, obliteration of the aortic knob, or deviation of the trachea or deviation of the nasogastric tube to the right (without other cause) may be present on plain radiographs of the chest. The presence of an apical cap, fractures of the first or second rib, and left-sided hemothorax are also concerning for aortic injuries. Transesophageal echocardiography and CT angiography are commonly used for diagnosis.

Esophageal injury is rare, with injury from penetrating trauma being more common than with blunt mechanisms. The presence of subcutaneous air or mediastinal air on a chest radiograph should increase suspicion for an esophageal injury, and its presence should be confirmed with contrast esophagography.

Finally, consideration should be given to the possibility of diaphragmatic rupture, especially in patients with sudden compressive forces to the abdomen such as may be seen with a lap belt in a motor vehicle collision. Protrusion of abdominal contents into the chest may lead to progressive respiratory distress. However, many traumatic diaphragmatic hernias remain asymptomatic, and diagnosis can be difficult. Placement of a nasogastric tube can assist with diagnosis before imaging. Chest radiographs and chest CT scans can be used for diagnosis, but sensitivity is not perfect. Therefore, diagnosis often occurs at a time remote from the injury. Indications on chest radiographs that should increase suspicion include elevation or blurring of the hemidiaphragm, a gastric tube in the chest, and obscuration of the hemidiaphragm by an abnormal gas shadow.

ABDOMEN

Abdominal injury is relatively common in children as a result of the large size of their abdomens relative to the rest of their bodies. In addition, their abdominal organs are less protected by their rib cages and abdominal musculature. The abdomen should be examined for tenderness, rigidity, and distension. CT scan is the initial imaging modality of choice in evaluating abdominal injuries in children. The sensitivity of focused assessment sonography in trauma (FAST) examination is operator dependent. To date, there have been mixed results in studies of efficacy in pediatric trauma victims; therefore, FAST is not routinely recommended for children. Direct peritoneal lavage is rarely used in the pediatric population.

The spleen is the most commonly injured abdominal organ (Figure 8-7). Patients with splenic lacerations may present with left upper quadrant pain that radiates to the left shoulder with or without signs of peritoneal irritation. The liver is also commonly injured in children sustaining trauma (Figure 8-8). Liver lacerations may present with right upper quadrant tenderness that may radiate to the right shoulder after blunt trauma. Hemodynamically stable children with spleen or liver lacerations can be conservatively managed with bed rest and close monitoring of vital signs and hematocrit levels. Children with unstable vital signs that do not improve with aggressive volume resuscitation may require operative intervention or embolization of bleeding vessels by an interventional radiologist experienced in the

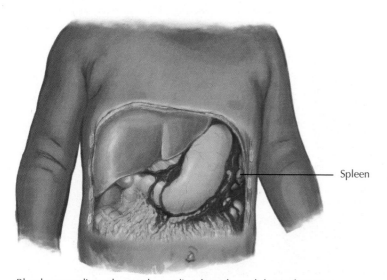

Blood surrounding spleen and spreading throughout abdominal cavity

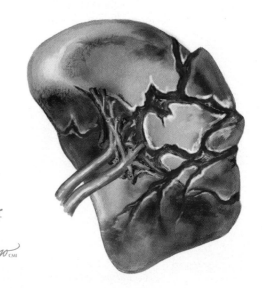

Multiple lacerations in spleen

Figure 8-7 *Splenic laceration.*

treatment of children with significant injuries. Children who have sustained significant splenic injuries, especially those who undergo splenectomy, are at increased risk of overwhelming sepsis with encapsulated bacteria (e.g., *Streptococcus pneumoniae*). Pneumococcal vaccination and consideration of long-term antibiotic prophylaxis (e.g., daily oral penicillin) should be considered based on the child's age and clinical situation.

Although the kidneys are more protected than other abdominal organs, renal injury should be suspected in children with injury to the flank or back, significant back pain, or gross hematuria (Figure 8-9). Urinalysis can be used as screening for more subtle injury, and CT or renal ultrasonography can be used to confirm and detail injuries.

Injury to the bowel is difficult to diagnosis, requiring a high degree of suspicion. Possible injuries to the intestines include perforation, hematomas, and mesenteric injuries. The initial CT scan may show pneumoperitoneum or extravasation of contrast, but often it is normal or shows nondescript bowel wall edema. Persistent abdominal pain, tenderness, or vomiting may be the only symptoms. Injuries to the abdomen by handlebars have been shown to lead to a significant risk of bowel and pancreas injury. Also, motor vehicle collisions during which children are restrained with inappropriately positioned seatbelts riding above the pelvis can lead to the significant abdominal injury triad of the "seatbelt sign" (abdominal wall contusion caused by the seatbelt), bowel injury, and Chance fracture (compression or flexion-distraction fracture of the lumbar spine). Bowel injuries often require surgical intervention to fully evaluate the extent of the injury and to allow for repair. Late diagnosis of bowel injuries may be associated with the development of peritonitis.

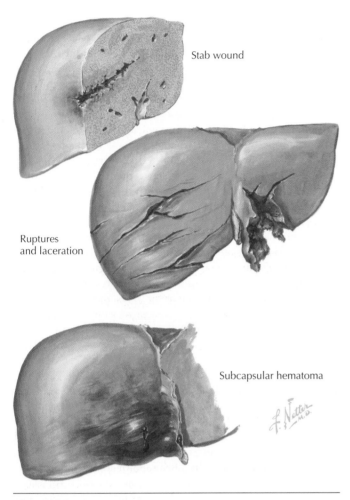

Stab wound

Ruptures and laceration

Subcapsular hematoma

Figure 8-8 *Liver trauma.*

Nonpenetrating trauma of kidney

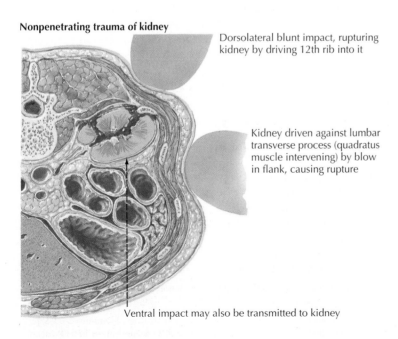

Dorsolateral blunt impact, rupturing kidney by driving 12th rib into it

Kidney driven against lumbar transverse process (quadratus muscle intervening) by blow in flank, causing rupture

Ventral impact may also be transmitted to kidney

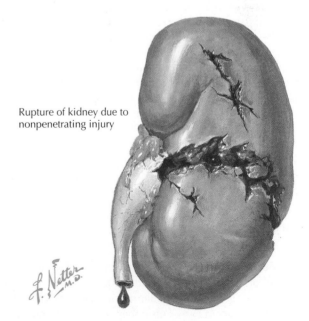

Rupture of kidney due to nonpenetrating injury

Figure 8-9 *Renal trauma.*

PELVIS

The pelvis should be evaluated for tenderness to palpation and stability. Determination that the pelvis is unstable on clinical examination correlates with open-book fractures of the pelvis. These injuries should be treated with placement of a pelvic splint to decrease the volume of the pelvis and the likelihood of severe hemorrhage. Lateral compression pelvic fractures, in contrast, are less often associated with significant blood loss and more frequently associated with injury to the bladder and urethra. Importantly, pelvic fractures are associated with other high-impact abdominal and retroperitoneal injuries that should be considered in the full evaluation of such patients.

EXTREMITIES AND NEUROLOGIC STATUS

The final steps in the secondary survey include a rapid but complete evaluation of the extremities and evaluation for focal neurologic deficits. This is usually accomplished by palpation of the full extent of each extremity noting tenderness, lacerations, and deformity. Tenderness to palpation or observed deformity should prompt radiologic evaluation. Further discussion of common pediatric fractures can be found in Chapter 22. Neurologic evaluation is often accomplished in conjunction with the extremity evaluation, briefly testing strength and sensation of each extremity, with cooperation acting as a quick evaluation of mental status. Focal deficits raise concern for intracranial or spinal cord injury depending on the location and extent. Appropriate imaging of the head and spine should follow from the clinical examination, as appropriate.

RADIATION

Many of the injuries discussed are definitively diagnosed using radiographs or CT scans. These imaging modalities are often necessary for the appropriate treatment of injured children. However, the use of ionizing radiation must be balanced with the risk of possible long-term iatrogenic injury caused by radiation exposure. Children, especially infants and toddlers, are particularly at risk for the development of secondary cancers caused by radiation because of the increased years of life after radiation and the increased susceptibility to the carcinogenicity of ionizing radiation. Therefore, ionizing radiation for diagnosis should be limited to instances in which there is either a significant clinical suspicion or the possibility of high-morbidity injuries. When imaging is necessary, pediatric radiation dose protocols that abide by the ALARA (as low as reasonably achievable) principles should be used.

PREVENTION

The majority of pediatric injuries occur in or around motor vehicles, in organized sports, and at home. Significant prevention efforts should be targeted at these locations. In the car, children should be restrained in a rear-facing car safety seat until they are 2 years of age or until they reach the highest weight or height specified by the manufacturer of their carseat. Children should remain in rear-facing seats until they can no longer fit in them. Children who are 2 years of age or older, or those younger than 2 years who have outgrown the rear-facing weight and height limits of their carseat should be restrained forward facing in an appropriate five-point restraint safety seat up to the highest weight or height specified by the manufacturer of the carseat. All children whose weight or height is above the forward-facing limit for their car safety seat should use a belt-positioning booster seat until the vehicle lap-and-shoulder seat belt fits properly, typically when they have reached 4 feet 9 inches in height and are between 8 and 12 years of age. The lap portion of the belt should fit low across the hips and pelvis, and the shoulder portion should fit across the middle of the shoulder and chest.

In sports, specific safety equipment should be provided and appropriately used to protect areas of likely injury for a given sport. For bicycle, skateboard, and scooter use, helmets should be worn at all times, and the use of wrist guards should be encouraged. In organized sports, appropriate supervision and the enactment and enforcement of rules that promote safe play should be mandatory. Safe areas to ride bicycles, fields for playing sports, and places for pedestrians to walk are all important.

At home, specific safety-proofing for a child's given developmental stage should be encouraged. For example, cabinet-locking devices should be placed on any cabinets holding potential toxins, including cleaning products and medications. Safety gates should be placed on all stairs and doorways to potentially harmful areas of the house. Increased vigilance of children around streets and training of older children in street safety may also decrease the likelihood of injury. Appropriate fences on all four sides with locking gates should isolate swimming pools and hot tubs. Children should never swim alone, and toddlers should always wear life preservers when in or around water even if they have taken swimming lessons.

Injury prevention strategies such as these have led to a greater than 30% reduction in "accidental" deaths in children in the United States in the past 30 years. Times when parents seek medical care for their children for minor injuries can be thought of as "teachable moments" when injury prevention techniques can be discussed with families in the hopes of increasing or maintaining compliance in the future.

SUGGESTED READINGS

AAP Joint Statement: Management of pediatric trauma, *Pediatrics* 121:849-854, 2008.

Abujamra L, Joseph MM: Penetrating neck injuries in children: a retrospective review, *Pediatr Emerg Care* 19(5):308-313, 2003.

American College of Surgeons Committee on Trauma: *Advanced Trauma Life Support for Doctors (ATLS) Student Course Manual*, ed 7, Chicago, 2004, ACS.

Avarello JT, Cantor RM: Pediatric major trauma: an approach to evaluation and management, *Emerg Med Clin of North Am* 25:803-836, 2007.

DeRoss AL, Vane DW: Early evaluation and resuscitation of the pediatric trauma patient, *Semin Pediatr Surg* 13(2):74-79, 2004.

Durbin DR and American Academy of Pediatrics, Committee on Injury, Violence, and Poison Prevention: Policy Statement—Child Passenger Safety, *Pediatrics* 127:788-793, 2011.

Gaines BA, Ford HR: Abdominal and pelvic trauma in children, *Crit Care Med* 30(suppl):S416-S423, 2002.

Garcia VF, Brown RL: Pediatric trauma beyond the brain, *Crit Care Clin* 19:551-561, 2003.

Kirkwood MW, Yeates KO, Wilson PE: Pediatric sport-related concussion: a review of the clinical management of an oft-neglected population, *Pediatrics* 117:1359-1371, 2006.

Kleinerman RA: Cancer risks following diagnostic and therapeutic radiation exposure in children, *Pediatr Radiol* 36(suppl 2):121S-125S, 2006.

Kuppermann N, Holmes JF, Dayan PS, et al: Identification of children at very low risk of clinically-important brain injuries after head trauma: a prospective cohort study, *Lancet* 374:1160-1170, 2009.

Mami AG, Nance ML: Management of mild head injury in the pediatric patient, *Adv Pediatr* 55:385-394, 2008.

Meehan WP III, Bachur RG: Sport-related concussion, *Pediatrics* 123:114-123, 2009.

McCrory P, Meeuwisse W, Johnston K, et al: Consensus statement on concussion in sport: the 3rd International Conference on Concussion in Sport, Zurich, Nov 2008, *Br J Sports Med* 43:76-84, 2009.

O'Connell KJ, Farah MM, Spandorfer P, Zorc JJ: Family presence during pediatric trauma team activation: an assessment of a structured program, *Pediatrics* 120(3):e565-e574, 2007.

Wegner S, Colletti JE, Wie DV: Pediatric blunt abdominal trauma, *Pediatr Clin North Am* 53:243-256, 2006.

Poisoning

Melissa Desai and Fred Henretig

9

Poisoning is one of the most common medical emergencies in young children and adolescents. Children are exposed to toxic substances more than any other age group. According to the American Association of Poison Control Centers (AAPCC), there were almost 2.5 million total human exposures in 2007, of which 65% were in children younger than 21 years old. Of these exposures, approximately 10% to 15% were intentional and include suicide attempts, and 80% to 85% of them were unintentional and occurred through exploratory behavior, environmental exposure, or neonatal exposure.

ETIOLOGY AND PATHOGENESIS

The cause of childhood poisoning can vary dramatically from one case to another, but the most frequent causes are ingestions of readily accessible household products such as cosmetics, hair products, cleaning substances, and analgesics. The most lethal or potentially lethal poisonings, however, are most commonly related to pharmaceuticals, including antimalarials, β-blockers, calcium channel blockers, camphor, antidiarrheals, salicylates, opioids, and tricyclic antidepressants (TCAs).

The mechanism of toxicity varies from one agent to another, yet there are some classic presentations that can be seen with particular ingestions (Table 9-1). Ingestions that can be lethal in small doses are reviewed in more depth here.

Tricyclic Antidepressants

According to the 2007 AAPCC report, antidepressants were the third most common cause of fatalities secondary to poisoning. TCAs, in particular, have a potent anticholinergic effect that can present as mydriasis, urinary retention, and gastroparesis. Death most often occurs from cardiotoxicity, in particular arrhythmias and hypotension. TCAs have a dose-dependent response in that ingestions less than 5 mg/kg are often asymptomatic, but fatalities can be seen with doses of 15 mg/kg and most often with doses greater than 30 mg/kg.

Antimalarials

Although these medications are rarely used in the United States as antiparasitic agents, they are becoming more common in households because some (e.g., hydroxychloroquine) act as second-line antiinflammatory therapy for rheumatoid arthritis and lupus. The toxic effects of antimalarials result from blockage of sodium and potassium channels, which causes subsequent cardiotoxicity, arrhythmia, and hypotension. Respiratory alterations (tachypnea, dyspnea, pulmonary edema, and respiratory failure) as well as central nervous system (CNS) side effects (seizures and coma) are also observed. Chloroquine doses of 5 to 10 mg/kg are therapeutic, but ingestions of 30 to 50 mg/kg can be lethal. Given the dangers of even moderate dose exposures, patients ingesting more than 10 mg/kg should be observed for cardiac dysfunction.

Calcium Channel Blockers and Beta-Adrenergic Blockers

Calcium channel blockers are most often used to treat hypertension, angina, migraines, and glaucoma, and they work by antagonizing L-type voltage-gated calcium channels in vascular smooth muscle and cardiac tissue. By preventing calcium influx into these cells, calcium antagonists cause vasodilatation as well as depression of both myocardial conduction and contractility. In large doses, this can lead to life-threatening bradycardia, heart block, and hypotension. Beta-adrenergic blockers can have similar cardiotoxicity in overdose (Table 9-1).

Camphor

Camphor is a component found in many nasal decongestants and topical anesthetic ointments. It can be toxic by oral ingestion, inhalation, or inappropriate dermal use. If ingested, camphor can cause oropharyngeal irritation, a burning sensation, nausea, and vomiting. It can also have CNS effects of apnea, coma, agitation, anxiety, hallucinations, hyperreflexia, myoclonic jerks, and seizures. Death can occur from doses of greater than 500 mg of camphor and usually results from intractable seizures or respiratory failure.

Salicylates

Aspirin, oil of wintergreen, and Pepto-Bismol all contain various quantities of salicylates. Symptoms of salicylate poisoning include nausea, vomiting, and altered mental status. Additionally there is often a classic laboratory finding of an elevated anion gap metabolic acidosis with a respiratory alkalosis. In severe cases, usually involving doses greater than 150 mg/kg, patients may manifest with agitation, delirium, seizures, pulmonary edema, coma, cardiovascular collapse, or death.

Sulfonylureas

Oral hypoglycemic agents are dangerous because patients may present with a delayed clinical onset of hypoglycemia accompanied with behavior changes, irritability, seizures, weakness, and eventually coma. Toxicity can occur from ingestions of even one or two sulfonylurea pills, and therefore overnight (fasting) observation and glucose monitoring is recommended after ingestion of most sulfonylureas.

Opioids

Opioids are found in analgesics, cough suppressants, and antidiarrheal medications. Ingestions present with a classic triad of respiratory depression, miosis, and CNS depression; death may result from respiratory depression. Children are most commonly exposed to codeine and oxycodone, and medical attention is important for those who ingest codeine in doses greater than

Table 9-1 Clinical Manifestations of Selected Toxic Ingestions

Ingestion	Clinical Findings
Acetaminophen	Nausea, vomiting, anorexia early in course; late findings of jaundice and liver failure
Antihistamines	Initially CNS depression but stimulation in higher doses (hyperactivity, tremors, hallucinations, seizures)
Aspirin	Tachypnea, respiratory alkalosis, metabolic acidosis, tinnitus, coagulopathy, slurred speech, seizures
β-Blockers	Bradycardia, hypotension, coma or convulsions, hypoglycemia, bronchospasm
Calcium channel blockers	Bradycardia, hypotension, junctional arrhythmias, hyperglycemia, metabolic acidosis
Caustics	Coagulation necrosis (acid) or liquefaction necrosis (alkali), scarring, strictures, burning, dysphagia, glottic edema
Digoxin	Nausea, vomiting, visual disturbances, lethargy, electrolyte disturbances, hyperkalemia, prolonged AV dissociation and heart block, arrhythmias
Disc batteries	Corrosive when in contact mucosal surfaces
Ethanol	Nausea, vomiting, stupor, anorexia; late toxicity: triad of coma, hypothermia, hypoglycemia Lethal (cardiorespiratory depression) if >400-500 mg/dL (life-threatening hypoglycemia may occur at much lower levels in young children)
Ethylene glycol	CNS depression, metabolic acidosis, convulsions and coma, hypocalcemia, renal failure Laboratory findings: anion gap metabolic acidosis, osmolal gap, urine oxalate crystals
Hypoglycemic agents	Hypoglycemia, coma, seizures
Iron	Hemorrhagic necrosis of GI mucosa, hypotension, hepatotoxicity, metabolic acidosis, coma, seizure, shock
Isopropyl alcohol	Altered mental status, gastritis, hypotension Laboratory findings: elevated osmolal gap, ketonuria (no metabolic acidosis or hypoglycemia)
Lead	Abdominal pain, constipation, anorexia, listlessness, encephalopathy (peripheral neuropathy; rare in children), microcytic anemia
Methanol	CNS depression, delayed metabolic acidosis, optic disturbances Laboratory findings: anion gap metabolic acidosis, osmolal gap
Tricyclic antidepressants	Lethargy, disorientation, ataxia, urinary retention, decreased GI motility, coma, seizures Cardiovascular alterations: sinus tachycardia, widened QRS complex; may progress to hypotension, ventricular dysrhythmias, cardiovascular collapse

AV, atrioventricular; CNS, central nervous systeml; GI, gastrointestinal.
Compiled from Eldridge DL, Van Eyk J, Kornegay C: Pediatric toxicology. Emerg Med Clin North AM 15:283-308, 2007 and Osterhoudt K, Shannon M, Burns Ewald M, Henretig F: Toxicologic emergencies. In Fleisher GR, Ludwig S (eds): Textbook of Pediatric Emergency Medicine, ed 6. Philadelphia, Lippincott Williams & Wilkins, 2010, pp 1171-1223.

5 mg/kg. Methadone, however, is a longer acting medication and can be toxic in doses as low as 5 mg. Therefore, the AAPCC recommends close observation for opioid-naïve children ingesting more than 5 mg of methadone or any dose of extended-release opioids.

Antidiarrheals

Antidiarrheals often contain opioids (e.g., Lomotil, a combination of diphenoxylate and atropine). The diphenoxylate inhibits gastrointestinal (GI) motility, as can the atropine. The anticholinergic effects of atropine may also cause agitation, tachycardia, dry mucous membranes, facial flushing, and hyperthermia. The expected anticholinergic effect of mydriasis may not be present; rather, miosis may be present from the opioid component. Monitoring for 24 hours after any Lomotil ingestion is recommended because of the risk of delayed or recurrent CNS and respiratory depression (as long as 12-24 hours after ingestion).

CLINICAL PRESENTATION

Patients with poisonings may present with a wide array of clinical signs and symptoms. Most often, children present with nonspecific signs, including nausea and vomiting, as well as altered mental status. Depending on the exposure, patients may also have burns or rashes, alterations in their respiration, and

metabolic changes that are not typically seen in a more common illness. Nevertheless, there are characteristic clinical features, representing in particular altered central and autonomic nervous system findings, which have been termed "toxidromes" (Table 9-2).

EVALUATION AND MANAGEMENT

As with the management of any patient, the initial focus of a patient with a possible poisoning must begin with the ABCs (airway, breathing, and circulation). The first step is to assess airway patency and reflexes, then breathing (both respiration and ventilation), and finally circulation. For patients with altered mental status, the next step is to determine their disability (e.g., neurologic status using the Glasgow Coma Score) and blood glucose. It is also imperative to place patients on cardiorespiratory monitors so their cardiac and respiratory status can be continually reassessed, as well as obtain frequent vital signs so changes can be detected as early as possible.

After initial stabilization, attention can be turned to discerning what the ingestion may have been; the most fruitful place to turn is a brief and focused history. Some patients may not present with a clear history of poisoning, but rather with an acute illness that does not quite fit with the history. The concern for ingestion should be raised in any child who presents with a suspicious clinical picture, particularly if they are toddlers or

Table 9-2 Toxidromes

	Mental Status	Heart Rate	Blood Pressure	RR	Pupils	Laboratory and Electrocardiographic Findings
Acetaminophen	Early: nausea, vomiting Late: Confusion, stupor, somnolence, coma					Elevated AST, ALT, bilirubin after 24 hours
Salicylates	Disorientation, lethargy, coma, seizures	Increased		Increased		Respiratory alkalosis, progressive anion gap metabolic acidosis, hyper- or hypoglycemia, electrolyte imbalances
Anticholinergics	Delirium, psychosis, coma, convulsions	Increased	Increased		Large, sluggish	Sinus tachycardia (TCAs will have increased QRS interval)
Benzodiazepines	Drowsy, lethargic, coma	Decreased (effects slight unless co-ingestants)		Decreased (effects slight unless co-ingestants		
Calcium channel blockers	Drowsy, confusion	Decreased	Decreased			Heart block, metabolic acidosis, hyperglycemia
Stimulants	Agitation, delirium, psychosis, convulsions	Increased	Increased	Increased	Large, reactive	
Narcotics	Drowsy, coma	Decreased	Decreased	Decreased	Pinpoint	Respiratory acidosis
Organophosphates	Confusion, coma	Decreased or increased	Decreased or increased	Increased	Small	
Sedative/hypnotics	Somnolence, coma	Decreased	Decreased	Decreased	Variable	

ALT, alanine aminotranferease; AST, aspartate aminotransferase; TCA, trycyclic antidepressant.
Compiled and adapted from Larsen LC, Cummings DM: Oral poisonings: guidelines for initial evaluation and treatment. Am Fam Phys 57(1):85-92, 1998 and Osterhoudt K, Shannon M, Burns Ewald M, Henretig F: Toxicologic emergencies. In Fleisher GR, Ludwig S (eds): Textbook of Pediatric Emergency Medicine, ed 6. Philadelphia, Lippincott Williams & Wilkins, 2010, pp 1171-1223.

adolescents. For observed or highly suspected poisonings, gathering information on the patient with respect to who, what, where, and when the incident or illness onset occurred may lead to uncovering the cause of the poisoning. It is also important to determine a patient's weight; what medications or chemicals are in the house; the timing of the incident; how much of the toxin was potentially ingested; and where the exposure took place, both in terms of where the patient was at the time and what body part(s) were exposed. Attention must also be paid to a patient's coexisting medical conditions so they can be appropriately managed as well.

In addition to the history, the physical examination of a patient with a poisoning can be extremely revealing. Close attention to heart rate, respiratory pattern, pupillary response, mental status, abdominal examination, and reflexes can be clues to particular exposures. For example, patients poisoned with stimulants, including cocaine, amphetamines, caffeine, and theophylline, present with mydriasis, tremors, tachycardia, hypertension, tachypnea, hyperthermia, diaphoresis, mania, convulsions, and tachyarrhythmias (Figure 9-1). Poisoning with depressants, on the other hand, including opioids, alcohol, benzodiazepines, and muscle relaxants, can lead to lethargy, decreased responsiveness to verbal and physical stimulation, miosis (especially opioids,

barbiturates, and alcohol), bradycardia, hypotension, bradypnea, hypothermia, and coma (see Figure 9-1). Other signs and symptoms characteristic of a particular substance can be characterized as a toxidrome (Table 9-2).

The laboratory workup should begin with a bedside test for blood glucose, complete blood count, electrolytes, liver function testing, and urinalysis. Studies have shown that urine and serum toxicologic studies are less important emergently but are still often part of a patient's initial evaluation. Additionally, if agents such as salicylates, acetaminophen, ethanol, methanol, ethylene glycol, digoxin, iron, lithium, or anticonvulsants are suspected, serum drug levels can be helpful for instituting the appropriate therapeutic management of the ingestion. Electrocardiography is essential for patients with arrhythmias or cardiotoxic drug ingestion, and chest radiography may be helpful in patients who have or are at risk of developing aspiration or pulmonary edema.

Treatment of a poisoning is fourfold: patient stabilization, minimizing toxin exposure and absorption, enhancing elimination (when possible), and managing the sequelae of the exposure. There are several methods of minimizing topical and inhaled toxin exposure, including irrigation of exposed eyes, removal of soiled clothing followed by washing of the skin and hair, and movement of the patient to fresh air, as appropriate.

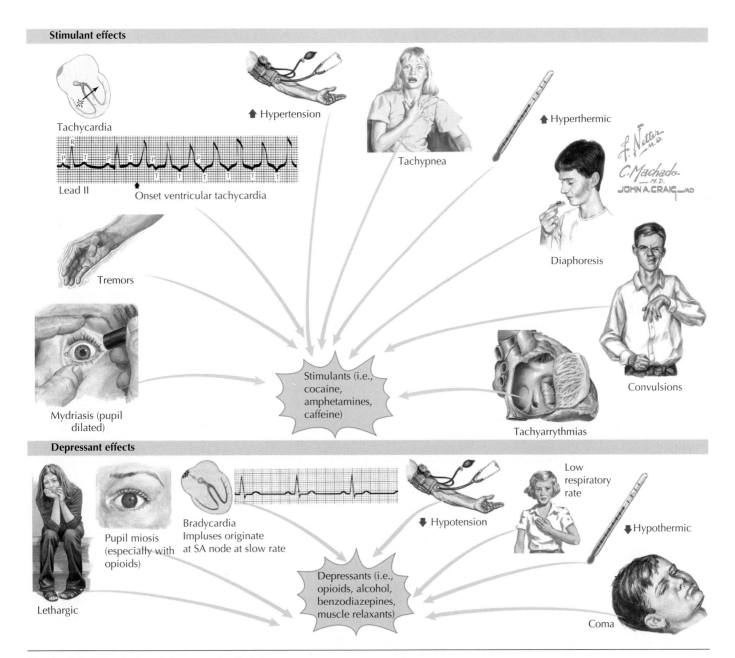

Figure 9-1 *Stimulant and depressant effects.*

Ingested poison absorption may be mitigated by gastric decontamination, but this has raised many controversies with respect to the efficacy and safety of the various decontamination methods. The current recommendations are outlined below.

Activated Charcoal

When necessary, activated charcoal has been shown to be the most effective method of gastric decontamination if administered in a timely manner. A single dose of activated charcoal has its greatest benefit if administered within 1 hour of an ingestion, but it can be useful even several hours later in some situations (e.g., anticholinergic, salicylate, or opioid ingestion with delayed gastric emptying or intestinal motility or significant overdoses of delayed-release medications). Charcoal decontamination should be considered if the toxin is known to adsorb to charcoal,

if the patient is at risk for significant toxicity, and if the patient has an intact GI tract. The complications are negligible compared with the other methods of gastric emptying, but aspiration has occurred rarely and can be fatal. Charcoal is not useful for iron, other heavy metals, lithium, alcohols, and cyanide ingestions because these compounds do not bind to charcoal.

Gastric Lavage

Lavage is not routinely used for decontamination because of variable results, lack of evidence with respect to improved outcomes, and significant adverse effects associated with its use. It should be considered when a life-threatening amount of poison has been ingested and if activated charcoal would not provide for sufficient decontamination, as might be the case with large iron or lithium ingestions. To do a lavage, a patient is placed on his or her left side, and a large orogastric tube is placed into the stomach. Fluid is aspirated back, and small aliquots of approximately 15 mL/kg (maximum, 250 mL) of water are administered and then aspirated back until the aspirate is clear. The most likely complications are aspiration, oxygen desaturation, esophageal irritation, and dysrhythmia.

Whole-Bowel Irrigation

This method of decontamination is not routinely recommended, but it is indicated for toxic ingestions of sustained-release or enteric-coated drugs, metals such as iron and lithium, and drug packets that may have a long absorption time or are not bound by charcoal. The intent of whole-bowel irrigation is to prevent absorption of ingested materials by provoking a liquid stool through administration of a large volume (≥1 L) of a polyethylene glycol electrolyte solution at a fast rate, typically via nasogastric tube. It may be effective if used within 4 hours of enteric-coated aspirin ingestion or even up to 12 to 16 hours after the ingestion of some sustained-release medications.

Dilution

The method of using water or milk to dilute a toxin is useful in situations in which local irritation or corrosion can be life threatening, but not for medication ingestions in which dilution may increase dissolution of the toxin and thereby increase absorption. It is only recommended if it can be initiated within the first few minutes after such exposures and only if there is no evidence of airway compromise.

Ipecac

The American Academy of Pediatrics issued a policy statement in 2004 recommending that ipecac no longer be used for home or health care facility decontamination because of the potential harmful side effects and the fact that positive results are so variable. The findings of various studies have ranged between a 0% to 40% decrease in drug absorption if ipecac is used within 1 hour of an ingestion, but the likelihood of administering ipecac in such a short period of time, especially outside of the home, is unlikely. Even if it can be done, the rare side effects of lethargy, diarrhea, persistent emesis, aspiration, and a delay in additional oral therapies are deemed too risky by most authorities to justify the potential positive results.

Cathartics

Neither saccharide (sorbitol) nor saline (magnesium citrate) cathartics have been proven effective in GI decontamination.

Table 9-3 Antidotes and Management of Selected Toxic Exposures

Ingestion	Potential Antidote / Other management
Acetaminophen	N-acetylcysteine, activated charcoal within 4 hours
Antihistamines	Activated charcoal or WBI for extended-release formulations, anticonvulsants, physostigmine
Benzodiazepine	Flumazenil
β-adrenergic blockers	Glucagon, activated charcoal if early after ingestion, WBI for delayed-release formulations, atropine, IVF, pressors
Calcium channel blockers	Calcium, activated charcoal if early after ingestion, WBI for delayed-release formulations, atropine, IVF, pressors, insulin/glucose
Carbon monoxide	100% oxygen, hyperbaric oxygen
Caustic agents	ABCs, steroids for esophageal burns (controversial); in-hospital monitoring for mediastinitis, pneumonitis, and peritonitis
Cholinesterase inhibitors	Atropine, pralidoxime
Cyanide	ABCs, 100% oxygen, sodium nitrite/sodium thiosulfate or hydroxocobalamin
Digoxin	Digoxin immune FAb, activated charcoal, electrolyte management
Disc batteries	Removal if in esophagus; if below esophagus, watch for 3 days, and if not out, then consult regarding potential removal
Ethanol	Respiratory management, correction of hypoglycemia, temperature control, thiamine (in chronic alcoholism)
Ethylene glycol and methanol	Ethanol or 4-methylpyrazole if level >20 mg/dL, sodium bicarbonate, calcium, pyridoxine, thiamine, folate, hemodialysis
Iron	Deferoxamine, WBI, hemodynamic support for possible GI bleed, management of acidosis, hypoglycemia, and hypotension
Isoniazid	Pyridoxine
Lead	Chelation with edetate calcium disodium, 2,4-dimercaptopropanol, succimer, and anticonvulsants as needed
Methemoglobinemic agents	Methylene blue
Opioids	Naloxone
Salicylates	Correct electrolytes, fluid resuscitation, urine alkalinization, hemodialysis
Sulfonylurea	Dextrose, octreotide
TCAs	Sodium bicarbonate to reduce cardiotoxicity, pressor support prn, activated charcoal

ABCs, airway, breathing, and circulation; GI, gastrointestinal; IVF, intravenous fluids; TCA, tricyclic antidepressant; WBI, whole-bowel irrigation.
Compiled and adapted from Larsen LC, Cummings DM: Oral poisonings: guidelines for initial evaluation and treatment. Am Fam Phys 57(1):85-92, 1998 and Osterhoudt K, Shannon M, Burns Ewald M, Henretig F: Toxicologic emergencies. In Fleisher GR, Ludwig S, Henretig FM (eds): Textbook of Pediatric Emergency Medicine, ed 5. Philadelphia, Lippincott Williams & Wilkins, 2006, pp 951-1007.

Some clinicians use cathartics for decontamination as a single dose in conjunction with activated charcoal, but repeat doses may increase diarrhea, cramping, and hypernatremic dehydration. Nevertheless, its efficacy remains equivocal.

Enhancement of toxin elimination is infrequently effective, but it may be lifesaving in select cases. Urine alkalinization is effective in increasing salicylate excretion. Additionally, hemodialysis is used for life-threatening toxicity caused by salicylates, toxic alcohols, lithium, and theophylline.

Some poisonings are amenable to specific antidotal therapy, which may counter the toxin itself or its dangerous metabolites (Table 9-3). Three treatments in particular—oxygen (for any patient with hypoxia, carbon monoxide exposure, or cyanide toxicity), glucose (for hypoglycemia caused by insulin, oral hypoglycemics, ethanol, and so on), and naloxone (for opioid-induced respiratory depression)—are important and safe enough to consider for emergent use as empiric therapy for altered mental status in suspect cases. The local poison control center is another valuable resource to help ensure adequate patient management regardless of the exposure. All poisonings or suspected poisonings should be reported to the local poison control center (800-222-1222) so they can assist with appropriate treatment and monitoring on a case-by-case basis.

FUTURE DIRECTIONS

Childhood poisonings lead to significant morbidity and mortality each year. If each exposure or possible exposure is called into the local poison control center, public health measures can be focused on the areas that currently lead to the most morbidity and mortality with respect to pediatric poisonings. Efforts can then be aimed at reducing such exposures by instituting safety mechanisms on potentially dangerous substances. One such effective innovation was the creation of child-resistant pill bottle caps, which are difficult for young children to open. Additional interventions need to be made to further reduce exposure to the more common household products, including cosmetics, household cleaners, and personal care products, because these currently make up the majority of pediatric poisonings. Furthermore, there exists quite a bit of gray area around issues such as optimal gastric decontamination or antidote therapy. Additional basic and clinical research, tied in with public health efforts, can work to help minimize the morbidity and mortality that currently surround pediatric poisonings.

SUGGESTED READINGS

Bronstein AC, Spyker DA, Cantilena LR, et al: 2007 Annual Report of the American Association of Poison Control Centers' National Poison Data System (NPDS): 25th annual report, *Clin Toxicol* 46(10):927-1057, 2008.

Eldridge DL, Van Eyk J, Kornegay C: Pediatric toxicology, *Emerg Med Clin North Am* 15:283-308, 2007.

Erickson TB, Ahrens WR, Aks SE, et al: *Pediatric Toxicology: Diagnosis and Management of the Poisoned Child*, New York, 2004, McGraw-Hill Professional.

Larsen LC, Cummings DM: Oral poisonings: guidelines for initial evaluation and treatment, *Am Fam Phys* 57(1):85-92, 1998.

Osterhoudt K, Shannon M, Burns Ewald M, Henretig F: Toxicologic emergencies. In Fleisher GR, Ludwig S, editors: *Textbook of Pediatric Emergency Medicine*, ed 6, Philadelphia, 2010, Lippincott Williams & Wilkins, pp 1171-1223.

Tenenbein M: Recent advances in pediatric toxicology, *Pediatr Clin North Am* 46(6):1179-1188, 1999.

Neurologic Emergencies

Stephen G. Flynn and Jeffrey A. Seiden

10

*P*ediatricians may encounter neurologic emergencies caused by both primary nervous system dysfunction and secondary systemic illness in children with and without underlying neurologic diseases. True neurologic emergencies include acute seizures, altered level of consciousness (ALOC), increased intracranial pressure (ICP), spinal cord compression, and stroke. This chapter focuses on acute seizures (specifically status epilepticus [SE]), ALOC, and the emergent aspects of increased ICP. A detailed discussion of other neurologic disorders is presented in Section XIII.

STATUS EPILEPTICUS

A seizure is defined as a transient, involuntary alteration of consciousness, behavior, motor activity, sensation, or autonomic function as a result of hypersynchrony and increased rate of cerebral neural discharges (Figure 10-1). Between 3% and 6% of children have at least one seizure in the first 16 years of life. Many seizures are associated with fever. Seizures can occur in individuals with underlying tendencies to seize (i.e., epilepsy) or secondary to other processes that primarily or secondarily affect the central nervous system. Seizures are discussed in detail in Chapter 74.

SE is the most common medical neurologic emergency of childhood and is defined as a group of seizures in rapid succession without remittance or a continuous prolonged episode. Historically, SE had been defined as a seizure that lasted more than 30 minutes. However, in a recent study, first- and second-line medications were effective in terminating seizures in 86% of cases when the duration was less than 20 minutes at presentation and only 15% of cases when it exceeded 30 minutes. As a result, most experts now define SE as a seizure lasting more than 5 minutes in recognition of the importance of rapid recognition and treatment.

Etiology and Pathogenesis

Common to the pathophysiology of all seizures is the hypersynchrony of neuronal discharges. The inciting cause varies and may include metabolic, anatomic, infectious, and primary neurologic processes (see Chapter 74). Uncovering the cause of SE is essential because it guides subsequent evaluation and management of a patient in SE.

Clinical Presentation

HISTORY

A brief, focused history should be obtained in the initial evaluation of a seizing patient with the goal of uncovering the precipitating event(s). Important historical features to obtain include recent head trauma, illnesses, fever, exposure to toxins, and current medications. It is important to know if the patient has epilepsy or has seized before, and if so, what antiseizure

medications are prescribed, adherence to this regimen, and recent changes to the treatment regimen. Finally, it is important to know what medications, if any, have been given to stop the current seizure. It is important to know whether the seizure is associated with fever because febrile seizures are unique to children 6 months to 6 years of age and may be evaluated and treated differently than seizures not associated with fever (see Chapter 74).

PHYSICAL EXAMINATION

Clinically, seizures are divided into those with generalized onset and those with partial (focal or localization related) onset. Generalized seizures usually involve the entire cerebral cortex, and consciousness is lost. In generalized tonic-clonic seizures, the child falls to the ground unresponsive, the eyes deviate, the muscles contract, and there may be incontinence of urine or stool. The body then begins to shake rhythmically in the clonic phase. After the seizure, there is a postictal period of decreased responsiveness; occasionally, there may be weakness or paralysis of an area of the body (Todd's paralysis). Absence seizures are a type of generalized seizure characterized by brief loss of consciousness, typically without loss of posture or tone and no postictal period. Simple partial seizures typically present with focal motor signs, although sensory, autonomic, and psychic phenomena are possible. Unlike generalized seizures, consciousness is typically not impaired in partial seizures.

Other than seizure type, the physical examination in a child in SE should focus on eliciting the cause of the seizure. Fever may be a sign of infection. Meningismus and a toxic appearance can be suggestive of meningitis. A toxidrome may lead the clinician to look for potential toxic ingestions (see Chapter 9). Significant hypertension implies hypertensive encephalopathy. Although a complete neurologic examination is difficult in a seizing patient, focal neurologic signs can suggest intracranial or spinal lesions. The entire body should be examined for signs of trauma. Dysmorphic features may be associated with nervous system abnormalities.

Differential Diagnosis

There are other paroxysmal events that can mimic seizures in children that must be considered in the differential diagnosis. Breath-holding spells occur in children 6 months to 4 years of age and consist of a period of crying resulting from an inciting event, such as trauma, followed by breath holding and ensuing pallor or cyanosis. The child becomes rigid and may have twitching movements but quickly returns to a full level of alertness. Syncope, a brief loss of consciousness and muscle tone, can be differentiated from seizure by history and physical examination (see Chapter 48). Sleep disorders, such as night terrors, benign myoclonus, and sleep paralysis, can mimic seizures.

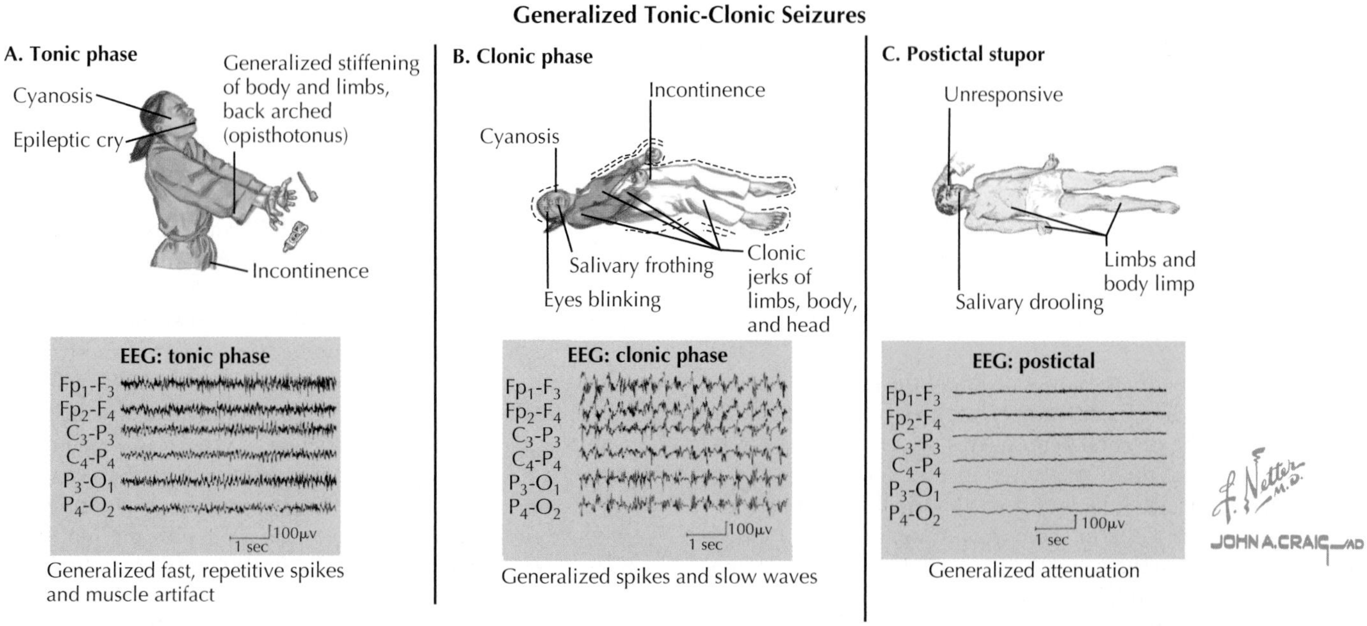

Generalized Tonic-Clonic Seizures

A. Tonic phase

Cyanosis

Epileptic cry

Generalized stiffening of body and limbs, back arched (opisthotonus)

Incontinence

EEG: tonic phase

Fp₁-F₃
Fp₂-F₄
C₃-P₃
C₄-P₄
P₃-O₁
P₄-O₂

$]100\mu v$
1 sec

Generalized fast, repetitive spikes and muscle artifact

B. Clonic phase

Incontinence

Cyanosis

Salivary frothing

Eyes blinking

Clonic jerks of limbs, body, and head

EEG: clonic phase

Fp₁-F₃
Fp₂-F₄
C₃-P₃
C₄-P₄
P₃-O₁
P₄-O₂

$]100\mu v$
1 sec

Generalized spikes and slow waves

C. Postictal stupor

Unresponsive

Limbs and body limp

Salivary drooling

EEG: postictal

Fp₁-F₃
Fp₂-F₄
C₃-P₃
C₄-P₄
P₃-O₁
P₄-O₂

$]100\mu v$
1 sec

Generalized attenuation

Figure 10-1 *Seizures.*

Evaluation and Management

The initial management of a child with SE includes assessment and support of the patient's airway, breathing, and circulation (ABCs). The administration of supplemental oxygen is recommended, and intravenous (IV) access should be established. Initial laboratory testing should include basic electrolytes and a bedside glucose test. Children in SE should be protected from trauma, although objects should not be placed in the patient's mouth to prevent tongue biting.

Children who arrive in the emergency department actively convulsing should be assumed to be in SE and given pharmacologic agents to stop the seizure. If hypoglycemia is present, 0.5 g/kg of IV dextrose should be given using the "rule of 50s" (multiply the volume of fluid in mL/kg by the concentration of dextrose to equal 50, e.g., 2 mL/kg of 25% dextrose in water, 5 mL/kg of 10% dextrose in water). Other electrolyte abnormalities should be addressed as well. Hyponatremia, hypocalcemia, and hypomagnesemia can all result in seizure. Patients with hyponatremia (usually <125 mEq/L) are treated with 3 to 5 mL/kg of 3% saline IV, hypocalcemia with 0.3 mL/kg of 10% calcium gluconate IV, and hypomagnesemia with 50 mg/kg of magnesium sulfate IV.

Benzodiazepines are the first-line anticonvulsant medications for treating children with SE (Table 10-1). IV lorazepam is usually preferred, but if IV access is not available, midazolam can be given via the buccal or intramuscular route or diazepam can be administered rectally. Although these agents have similarly rapid onsets of action, lorazepam lasts much longer than other benzodiazepines (≤12-24 hours). As a result, one must be mindful to administer another agent for long-term seizure control when using other benzodiazepines as a first-line agent. If the patient does not have seizure remittance after benzodiazepine administration, phenytoin (or fosphenytoin) is widely considered the next anticonvulsant agents to use. Although

phenobarbital has been used as a second-line agent in SE, phenytoin is preferred because by acting on voltage-gated sodium channels, its mechanism of action is different than lorazepam. Lorazepam and phenobarbital, on the other hand, are both GABA (γ-aminobutyric acid) receptor agonists. Phenobarbital and some newer anticonvulsant medications, such as levetiracetam, are considered third-line agents for SE. Consultation with a pediatric neurologist and/or pediatric intensivist are warranted when treatment beyond benzodiazepines is used.

ALTERED LEVEL OF CONSCIOUSNESS

Consciousness is the state of being awake and aware of one's self and surroundings. Alteration of this state may signify severe, life-threatening pathology. The most extreme form of ALOC is

Table 10-1 Suggested Treatment Algorithm for Status Epilepticus

Immediately	Benzodiazepine:
	    IV lorazepam (0.1 mg/kg up to 4 mg)
	or
	    PR diazepam (0.5 mg/kg up to 10 mg)
	or
	    IM midazolam (0.2 mg/kg up to 5 mg)
	or
	    Buccal midazolam (0.5 mg/kg up to 10 mg)

5 minutes	Repeat benzodiazepine dose
10 minutes	IV phenytoin or fosphenytoin (20-30 mg/kg)

20 minutes	Consult neurology or PICU
	Consider third-line agents:
	    Phenobarbital
	    Valproate
	    Levetiracetam

IM, Intramuscular; IV, intravenous; PICU, pediatric intensive care unit; PR, per rectum.

coma, in which one has a complete lack of awareness and responsiveness. Lethargy is a depressed state of consciousness resembling deep sleep; the patient can be aroused but quickly returns to this state without stimulation. Obtundation refers to a profoundly decreased response to external stimuli. These terms are somewhat subjective, and several schemas to quantify level of consciousness are used clinically, including the AVPU (awake, verbal, pain, unresponsive) scale (see below under Management) and the Glasgow Coma Score (see Chapter 8).

Etiology and Pathogenesis

ALOC occurs when there is dysfunction of the reticular activating system in the brainstem and pons, which is responsible for wakefulness, or the cerebral hemispheres, which are responsible for awareness. For these structures to function properly, the nervous system needs to be free from abnormal irritation, body temperature needs to be in the normal range, adequate blood flow needs to exist to these areas to bring vital energy-producing substrates, and the body needs to be free of metabolic waste products or toxins. Whenever there is an alteration in one of these factors, ALOC ensues. There are myriad causes for the aforementioned alterations in consciousness. The mnemonic VITAMINS outlines the most prevalent causes (Table 10-2).

Evaluation and Management

The initial management of ALOC includes assessment and support of the patient's ABCs. This is followed by a detailed history that may help narrow the differential diagnosis. Questions should focus on the patient's past medical history (e.g., diabetes mellitus, epilepsy) as well as the circumstances surrounding the onset of symptoms (e.g., head trauma, possible toxin ingestion, presence of fever). Specific questions about physical signs and symptoms such as headache, irritability, vomiting, gait disturbances, and behavioral abnormalities should also be asked.

Subsequent examination of the patient begins with a global neurologic assessment using the AVPU scale or the Glasgow Coma Scale and an evaluation of vital signs, including core temperature. Pupillary response can provide important clues to the underlying cause of ALOC. A unilateral dilated pupil can indicate mass effect and increased ICP, and bilateral enlarged pupils might represent severe global intracranial dysfunction or an ingestion of sympathomimetic or anticholinergic substances. Pinpoint bilateral pupils may result from ingestion of opiates. The patient should next be examined for signs of head trauma such as scalp hematoma, retinal hemorrhage, hemotympanum, cerebrospinal fluid (CSF) otorrhea or rhinorrhea, postauricular hematoma, periorbital hematoma, and other visible signs of head injury. Evaluation for infection, especially in the setting of fever, should include testing for meningeal irritation using Kernig's (resistance to bent knee extension with the hip in 90 degrees flexion) and Brudzinski's (involuntary knee and hip flexion with passive neck flexion) signs (Figure 10-2). Other stigmata of infectious causes for ALOC include petechiae or purpura found in patients with meningococcal sepsis.

Laboratory evaluation of patients with ALOC should be determined based on the most likely causes. A bedside glucose test along with basic electrolytes, blood urea nitrogen, and creatinine can uncover correctable metabolic derangements. Blood gas analysis, complete blood count with differential, and toxicologic screening of blood and urine may also be helpful. An empiric trial of the opioid antagonist naloxone should be considered in patients with unexplained ALOC, especially with associated respiratory depression and miosis, and in toddler or adolescent patients because of their higher risk of poisoning (see Chapter 9). Brain imaging is helpful in revealing possible hemorrhage, malignancy, abscess, hematoma, cerebral edema, and

Table 10-2 Causes of Altered Level of Consciousness ("VITAMINS")	
Vascular	Stroke, AVM, venous thrombosis
Infection	Meningitis, encephalitis, brain abscess, sepsis
Trauma	Subdural hematoma, epidural hematoma, concussion, cerebral edema, cerebral contusion
A lot of toxins	Opioids, anticholinergics, TCAs, salicylates, anticonvulsants, sedatives
Metabolic derangements	Hypoglycemia, DKA, hyperammonemia, uremia, hypo- or hypernatremia, hypo- or hypercalcemia, hypo- or hypermagnesemia, metabolic acidosis, liver failure
Intussusception	ALOC may predominate early in some cases
Neoplasm	Increased ICP, direct effect of brainstem tumors
Seizure	Status epilepticus, postictal phase

ALOC, altered level of consciousness; AVM, arteriovenous malformation; DKA, diabetic ketoacidosis; ICP, intracranial pressure; TCA, tricyclic antidepressant.

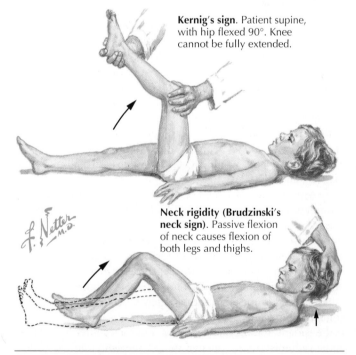

Kernig's sign. Patient supine, with hip flexed 90°. Knee cannot be fully extended.

Neck rigidity (Brudzinski's neck sign). Passive flexion of neck causes flexion of both legs and thighs.

Figure 10-2 *Kernig's and Brudzinski's signs.*

hydrocephalus. A high index of suspicion for nonaccidental trauma must be maintained, especially in infants with ALOC, even in the absence of physical signs of injury. If fever or other signs of CNS infection are present, lumbar puncture is warranted, and empiric antibiotic therapy with a third-generation cephalosporin (e.g., cefotaxime) should be started, with other antibiotics, such as ampicillin or vancomycin, added if indicated by age and clinical situation. Electroencephalography (EEG) may also be necessary to evaluate for nonconvulsive seizures in patients with ALOC. Ultimately, definitive treatment depends on the results of the diagnostic evaluation.

INCREASED INTRACRANIAL PRESSURE

Etiology and Pathogenesis

Elevated ICP in children is most often a complication of traumatic brain injury. Other common causes include hydrocephalus, brain tumors, and intracranial infections. Prompt recognition and treatment of increased ICP is vital to avoid morbidity and mortality. The intracranial compartment is a fixed internal volume composed of brain parenchyma (80%), CSF (10%), and blood (10%) protected by the skull. ICP is a function of the volume and compliance of each component. The Monro-Kellie doctrine states that because the intracranial compartment is a fixed space, an increase in volume of one compartment requires displacement of other structures, an increase in ICP, or both. Cerebral blood flow must be maintained to provide oxygen and nutrients for metabolic activity. Cerebral perfusion pressure (CPP) is used clinically to define the adequacy of cerebral perfusion. It is defined as:

$$CPP = MAP - ICP$$

Normal CPP in children can be estimated to be around 50 to 60 mm Hg based on normal ICP of less than 20 mm Hg and mean arterial pressure (MAP) greater than 70 to 80 mm Hg. Inadequate CPP caused by systemic hypotension or elevated ICP may result in ischemic brain injury. Therefore, management of increased ICP must take into account the ultimate goal of maintaining CPP.

Clinical Manifestations

Children with increased ICP may present with headache, decreased consciousness secondary to increased pressure in the midbrain reticular formation, or vomiting. Headache is an early symptom and is typically characterized by a progressive increase in frequency and severity, nocturnal awakening, and worsening with Valsalva maneuvers (cough, defecation, micturition). Infants may present with a bulging fontanelle, poor feeding, lethargy, and flat affect. Funduscopic examination may reveal papilledema, but the absence of this finding does not rule out increased ICP, especially if it has developed acutely (Figure 10-3). The presence of retinal hemorrhages should raise suspicion for nonaccidental head trauma (e.g., shaken baby syndrome; see Chapter 12). Infants may have a "sun-setting" appearance of their eyes, split sutures, or a bulging fontanelle. Dilated pupils (unilateral or bilateral) may be present along with cranial nerve

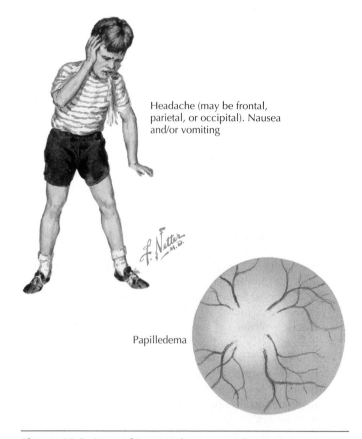

Headache (may be frontal, parietal, or occipital). Nausea and/or vomiting

Papilledema

Figure 10-3 *Signs of increased intracranial pressure.*

palsies (most commonly the third and sixth nerves). Such cranial nerve palsies can cause double vision and head tilt as the patient tries to correct for the visual discrepancy. Hemiparesis, hyperreflexia, and hypertonia are late signs of increased ICP. Development of Cushing's triad (bradycardia, systemic hypertension, and irregular respirations) is a late indication of impending cerebral herniation, with bradycardia being the earliest feature.

Evaluation and Management

The initial management of a child with suspected increased ICP includes assessment and support of the patient's ABCs. Endotracheal intubation should be considered if there is concern for loss of airway protective reflexes, severe hypoxia or hypoventilation, or acute cerebral herniation. Hyperventilation (goal $PaCO_2$ of 30-35 mm Hg), which leads to cerebral vasoconstriction and decreased cerebral blood flow, should be performed to acutely decrease ICP in the case of acute herniation. However, overly aggressive hyperventilation may lead to ischemic injury. Especially in cases of head injury and multisystem trauma, MAP must be supported to preserve CPP. After initial hemodynamic stabilization has been achieved, the patient should undergo computed tomography (CT) of the brain, which may reveal an underlying cause for the increased ICP. It is important to remember that ICP can be elevated in the setting of a normal initial CT. In one study, 33% of patients with initially normal head CTs developed CT scan abnormalities within the first few days after closed head injury. Thus, close monitoring in an intensive care unit is necessary for patients with suspected increased ICP.

Pharmacologic therapy may be warranted in the management of suspected increased ICP. Recalling the goal of preserving CPP, one must address both ICP and MAP when deciding on appropriate management strategies. Early neurosurgical consultation is mandatory. Medical management might include the following:

1. *Medications that decrease ICP:*
   a. **Mannitol:** Mannitol establishes an osmotic gradient between plasma and brain parenchyma, leading to a net reduction in brain water content. Because mannitol is an osmotic diuretic, one must be careful to avoid hypovolemia with resultant hypotension, which may lead to an overall decrease in CPP despite improving ICP.
   b. **Hypertonic saline:** IV hypertonic saline establishes an osmotic gradient that reduces brain water content, thus decreasing ICP. Hypertonic saline is not a diuretic, so it does not carry the same risk of hypovolemia and hypotension. As a result, many prefer its use over mannitol in cases of traumatic injury.
   c. **Corticosteroids:** Corticosteroids may be helpful in decreasing vasogenic edema secondary to their antiinflammatory effects. However, their effects are delayed and have not been proven to be useful in the setting of acute traumatic brain injury. Corticosteroids may be helpful in the initial management of increased ICP resulting from a mass lesion.
   d. **Barbiturate coma:** Pentobarbital is used when other drug modalities have failed in ICP reduction. It decreases metabolic rate and demand for CBF, thus lowering ICP. However, cardiac suppression may result and cause hypotension, which needs to be addressed with isotonic fluids and inotropic agents.
2. *Rapid correction of hypoxia, hypercarbia, and hypotension:* Supplemental oxygen should be administered to increase tissue oxygenation and prevent ischemic injury. Normal saline should be administered to maintain adequate MAP; pressor support may be necessary if IV fluids are not sufficient.
3. *Elevation of the head of the bed to 30 degrees:* This maneuver lowers ICP by encouraging venous drainage. However, greater degrees of elevation may result in a decrease in CPP.
4. *Antipyretics and cooling blankets:* Fever increases cerebral metabolism, thereby increasing CBF and increasing ICP.
5. *Administration of prophylactic anticonvulsants for patients at high risk of seizure* (severe traumatic brain injury, depressed skull fracture, or parenchymal abnormality). Some of these agents, such as IV phenytoin, may result in systemic hypotension, so blood pressure should be carefully monitored during and after their administration.
6. *Maintenance of analgesia to blunt response to pain stimuli.*
7. *Tight control of blood sugar levels:* Hyperglycemia has been shown to lead to poorer outcomes in children with increased ICP. Hypoglycemia in infants and children may also result in poorer outcomes as less substrate for metabolic demand is delivered to brain parenchyma already at risk for ischemic injury.

SUGGESTED READINGS

Abend NS, Huh JW, Helfaer MA, Dlugos DJ: Anticonvulsant medications in the pediatric emergency room and intensive care unit, *Pediatr Emerg Care* 24(10):705-721, 2008.

Chiang VW: Seizures. In Fleisher GR, Ludwig S, Henretig FM, editors: *Textbook of Pediatric Emergency Medicine*, Philadelphia, 2006, Lippincott Williams & Wilkins, pp 629-636.

Lewena S, Young S: When benzodiazepines fail: how effective is second line therapy for status epilepticus in children? *Emerg Med Australas* 18:45-50, 2006.

Lobato RD, Sarabia R, Rivas JJ, et al: Normal computerized tomography scans in severe head injury. Prognostic and clinical management implications, *J Neurosurg* 65(6):784-789, 1986.

Apparent Life-Threatening Event and Sudden Infant Death Syndrome

11

Tara Petersen and Manoj K. Mittal

APPARENT LIFE-THREATENING EVENT

Apparent life-threatening events are frightening events often of sudden onset, affecting predominantly young infants. A National Institutes of Health (NIH) consensus conference in September 1986 defined an apparent life-threatening event (ALTE) as "an episode that is frightening to the observer and that is characterized by some combination of apnea (central or occasionally obstructive), color change (usually cyanotic or pallid but occasionally erythematous or plethoric), marked change in muscle tone (usually marked limpness), choking, or gagging. In some cases, the observer fears that the infant has died."

The community incidence of ALTE has been reported as 2.4 to 9.4 per 1000 live births. It accounts for 0.6% to 1% of emergency department (ED) visits by infants. The median age of infants with ALTE is about 50 days. The incidence is similar in boys and girls.

Etiology and Pathogenesis

The most frequently identified problems associated with an ALTE are digestive (≈50%, most commonly gastroesophageal reflux [GER]), neurologic (30%), respiratory (20%), cardiovascular (5%), metabolic and endocrine (<5%), and diverse other problems (including child abuse). However, up to 50% of cases remain unexplained. The presence of a condition capable of causing ALTE does not equal causation in an individual case. This is particularly true of GER. A study of a cohort of infants with both apnea and GER found that episodes of apnea were seldom associated with GER. However, in instances where they were associated, the predominant sequence of events was obstructive or mixed apnea followed by reflux.

Clinical Presentation

ALTE is a presenting complaint and not a diagnosis. It represents a heterogeneous group of potential underlying disorders. As the NIH definition indicates, it encompasses a broad range of conditions, varying from choking or gagging to obstructive apnea to central apnea.

Because ALTE is a diagnosis based on symptomatology rather than pathophysiology, the differential diagnosis and recommended medical evaluation can be broad. A careful history is often the most helpful part of the evaluation. Determination of whether the infant has been chronically ill or previously well is of utmost importance because a history of previous similar episodes, failure to thrive, poor feeding, and prematurity may provide important clues as to an identifiable cause for the observed symptoms.

A clear description of the event from the caregiver who witnessed the event often contains valuable insight into an underlying cause. Normal infant behaviors such as irregular breathing during REM (rapid eye movement) sleep, periodic breathing, respiratory pauses (5–15 sec), and transient coughing or gagging during feeding may be misinterpreted as abnormal behavior. It is important to carefully use the history and physical examination to distinguish these normal behaviors from underlying pathology.

Infection, gastrointestinal pathology, toxic ingestion, metabolic decompensation, and trauma (both accidental and nonaccidental) are among some of the serious conditions that may initially be identified as an ALTE. Chronic conditions may also present initially as an ALTE (Box 11-1).

Evaluation and Management

Diagnostic evaluation and the need for laboratory or radiographic studies should be directed by a thorough history and physical examination. The importance of a detailed history and examination was highlighted in a 2005 study that found the diagnosis of ALTE was suggested or made by historical or physical examination findings in approximately 70% of cases.

Both the caretaker who witnessed the episode and any emergency personnel or first responders involved in the case should be interviewed. Key historical elements include:

- **State** immediately preceding the event: Was the child asleep, awake or crying?
- **Position**: Was the infant prone, supine, in a car seat, or being held by the caregiver?
- **Relationship to feeding**: How many hours or minutes had elapsed since the last feeding? Is there any history of emesis, gagging or choking?
- **Respiratory effort**: Did the infant seem to be struggling to breathe or choking? Was there an increased or decreased respiratory effort? Was there complete cessation of breathing, and if so, for how long?
- **Color**: Did the child appear cyanotic, pallid, grey, red, or purple?
- **Tone**: Did the infant appear limp, rigid, or demonstrate tonic or clonic movements?
- **Noise**: Did the infant cough or have stridor? Was there crying or gasping? Did the infant make any sound at all?
- **Eyes:** Were the infant's eyes open or closed? Did they appear to be dazed, staring, rolling, or bulging?
- **How long did the event last:** Seconds versus minutes? Witnessing an ALTE is frightening to the observer because

---

Box 11-1 Conditions That May Present Initially as Apparent Life-Threatening Event

- Infections: sepsis, meningitis, encephalitis, urinary tract infection, respiratory tract infections (most notably RSV and pertussis)
- Gastrointestinal: volvulus, intussusception, gastroesophageal reflux, swallowing incoordination
- Toxic exposure: unintentional or intentional ingestion, carbon monoxide poisoning
- Metabolic decompensation: inborn errors of metabolism, endocrinopathies or electrolyte imbalances
- Trauma (accidental or nonaccidental): suffocation, aspiration, inflicted injury
- Cardiac: arrhythmias, cardiomyopathies
- Respiratory: abnormalities of respiratory control, upper airway obstruction, vocal cord dysfunction, laryngotracheomalacia, vascular ring
- Neurologic: central hypoventilation syndrome, seizure or apnea associated with Chiari or other hindbrain malformation
- Genetic: congenital anomalies

RSV, respiratory syncytial virus.

---

the infant's life may be perceived to be in danger. Thus, seconds may seem like minutes. It is often helpful to count out the seconds or minutes to provide a reference point for comparison.

- **Did the event require intervention:** Did the infant spontaneously return to his or her behavioral baseline? Was gentle or vigorous physical stimulation required? Were rescue breaths given? Did the infant receive cardiopulmonary resuscitation (CPR) by the caregiver or medical personnel?

A careful physical examination should pay particular attention to any abnormalities identified when obtaining the history. Growth parameters, including height, weight, and head circumference should be obtained and compared with age- and gender-appropriate standards. A comprehensive set of vital signs, including body temperature, heart rate, respiratory rate, and pulse oximetry should be obtained. During both the history and physical examination, it is also important to observe the interaction between the caregiver and the infant, as nonaccidental trauma is part of the differential diagnosis.

There is no consensus statement on what laboratory or radiographic studies to obtain for infants presenting with ALTE. Thus, further diagnostic testing should be based on the information obtained during the initial history and physical examination. A retrospective study of ED evaluation of infants presenting with ALTE showed that of the 81% of the patients who underwent some diagnostic test in the ED, fewer than 3% had a positive result. Infants presenting with ALTE do not routinely require evaluation for serious bacterial infections. In well-appearing infants, blood culture and cerebrospinal fluid studies may not be needed. This evaluation may, however, be considered if there are clear signs of infection and should include viral studies.

Multichannel polysomnography may be helpful in infants with recurring ALTEs or infants who experience a particularly

severe episode without an identifiable cause or explanation. This test typically spans the course of 12 to 24 hours and includes:

1. Measurement of thoracic and abdominal wall movement to evaluate for the presence of obstructive apnea
2. Electrocardiography to evaluate for the presence of arrhythmia and heart rate (especially bradycardia) in the presence of apneic events
3. Pulse oximetry
4. Airflow sensors (thermistors that sense alterations in heat exchange and end-tidal CO_2 monitoring)
5. When indicated by history:
   a. Esophageal pH monitoring to evaluate for GER
   b. EEG to evaluate the sleep–wake state of the infant and for underlying signs of seizure activity

Polysomnography may assist in identifying the underlying cause of an ALTE; however, it cannot predict the risk of future ALTE episodes or of sudden infant death syndrome (SIDS).

Infants with an ALTE have historically been considered a high-risk group for sudden subsequent death with most reports recommending a mandatory period of inpatient observation. More recent studies have, however, found the natural history of an ALTE to be more benign and have questioned its association with SIDS. In a recent prospective study that enrolled 300 infants with ALTE, no infant died during hospital stay or within 72 hours of discharge. None was diagnosed with serious bacterial infection (bacterial meningitis, bacteremia, or urinary tract infection). Only 12% of infants in this cohort had a significant intervention warranting hospital admission, thus questioning the need for mandatory admission for all infants presenting to EDs with ALTE. Criteria predicting an admission that was truly warranted were prematurity, absence of history of choking, color change to blue, and abnormal examination findings in the ED. Inpatient observation with cardiorespiratory monitoring should also be considered in cases in which concern for continued physiologic compromise exists or if the event is so distressing to the caregiver that a brief period of observation in the ED is not sufficient to alleviate his or her fears. Specific medical or surgical treatment should be reserved for infants with an identifiable cause. In all cases of ALTE episodes requiring hospital admission, the caregivers should receive appropriate training in infant CPR.

HOME APNEA MONITORING

According to the 2007 American Academy of Pediatrics (AAP) Policy Statement on Home Apnea Monitoring, home cardiorespiratory monitoring should not be prescribed to prevent SIDS in healthy term infants with or without a history of ALTE. However, cardiorespiratory monitoring may be warranted for premature infants who are at high risk of recurrent episodes of apnea, bradycardia, and hypoxemia after hospital discharge. The current recommendation is to limit the use of home monitoring in this population to approximately 43 weeks postmenstrual age or after the cessation of extreme episodes, whichever comes last. Additionally, home monitoring may be warranted for infants who are technology dependent, have unstable airways, or have chronic lung disease. In all of these cases, parents should be advised that home cardiorespiratory monitoring has not been proven to prevent sudden unexpected deaths in infants.

Future Directions

More research is needed to define the pathophysiology of ALTE. Larger, multicenter, prospective studies are needed to better define the characteristics of the very small subgroup of infants with ALTEs who may have an associated serious bacterial or viral infection (such as enteroviral meningitis), so that invasive testing can be better targeted. In addition, larger studies are needed to validate history and examination findings that predict significant intervention during hospital stay, and thus warrant admission to the hospital.

SUDDEN INFANT DEATH SYNDROME

SIDS is defined as the sudden death of an infant younger than 1 year of age during sleep whose cause remains unexplained despite a complete investigation, including history, examination, autopsy, and death scene investigation. Babies with SIDS appear to be healthy before death. Because most SIDS deaths occur while the infants are sleeping, the disorder is also referred to as "crib death" or "cot death."

SIDS is the leading cause of infant mortality between 1 month and 1 year of age in the United States. In a study by the National Institute of Child Health and Development, the median age for SIDS deaths was 11 weeks; the peak incidence was between 2 and 4 months, and 90% occurred before 6 months of age. The SIDS rate in industrialized countries varies from 0.1 to 0.8 per 1000 infants. Preterm infants are at a higher risk for SIDS than term infants, with the postmenstrual age of peak vulnerability for SIDS occurring 4 to 6 weeks earlier among preterm than term infants. The risk of SIDS is also higher among African American and American Indian babies, in infants born to women who smoked during pregnancy, infants born to very young women, and in male infants.

Etiology and Pathogenesis

The most recent research suggests that SIDS is a polygenic, multifactorial condition inclusive of genetic, environmental, behavioral, and sociocultural factors. Well-established extrinsic risk factors for SIDS include prone sleep positioning; use of pillows, soft mattresses, or blankets in cribs; sleeping on sofas or other soft furniture in which the infant could become wedged; bed sharing; high ambient temperature in the sleeping environment; and prenatal and postnatal exposure to tobacco (Figure 11-1).

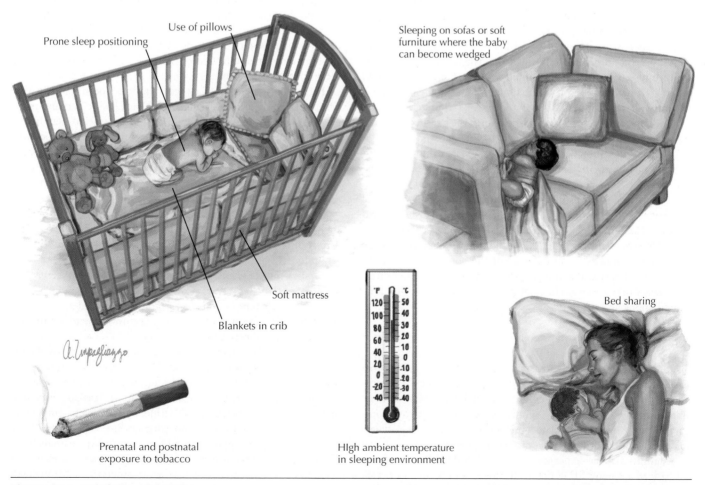

Figure 11-1 *Risk factors for SIDS.*

For many years, an ATLE was believed to be the predecessor of SIDS. This led to the widespread use of home apnea monitors in an attempt to prevent SIDS. However, studies such as the Collaborative Home Infant Monitoring Evaluation (CHIME) have demonstrated that ALTE neither precedes nor predicts SIDS. This has led to a change in focus from home apnea monitoring to the proven efficacy of the prevention methods outlined below.

Several factors argue against a causal relationship between ALTE and SIDS. Most notably, the timing of ALTE events versus SIDS deaths is distinctly different. Eighty percent of SIDS deaths occur between midnight and 6 AM, 82 percent of ALTE episodes occur between 8 AM and 8 PM. Upon review of effective preventive measures, interventions proven to reduce the incidence of SIDS (most notably supine sleep position) have not resulted in a decreased incidence of ALTE. In fact, the vast majority of SIDS victims do not experience ALTE before death. Further statistical analysis reveals that prior ALTE episodes were reported in only 5% of SIDS victims.

Because neither ALTE nor SIDS appears to exist beyond infancy, emerging evidence suggests that underlying brain immaturity may play a role in the pathogenesis. As noted above, the highest incidence of SIDS occurs between the second and fourth months of life, a period of intensive developmental changes in ventilatory, cardiac, and sleep–wake patterns in normal infants. The coincidence of timing suggests that infants are vulnerable to sudden death during a critical period of autonomic maturation. Additionally, classic studies on the infant nervous system show profound cardiovascular compromise in infants upon stimulation of the immature autonomic nervous system in the presence of apnea or hypoxia during sleep. This compromise was not noted in adult models. Currently, abnormalities in neurologic serotonin signaling and brainstem functioning as well as genetic polymorphisms interacting with specific environmental risk factors remain at the heart of ongoing research.

The final common pathway that seems to explain most cases of SIDS involves (1) a life-threatening event that causes asphyxia and brain hypoperfusion (e.g., rebreathing exhaled gases in prone position, gastroesophageal regurgitation causing obstructive apnea or activation of laryngeal receptors causing reflex apnea); (2) failure of arousal in response to asphyxia so that the infant does not turn his or her head and recover from the apnea; (3) hypoxic coma as a consequence of the continued asphyxia; (4) extreme bradycardia and gasping, and (5) failure of autoresuscitation because of ineffectual gasping, resulting in uninterrupted apnea and death.

Clinical Presentation

SIDS is a diagnosis of exclusion. Diagnoses that should be considered in suspected SIDS cases include accidental or nonaccidental trauma, congenital adrenal hyperplasia, cardiac arrhythmia, prolonged QT syndrome, cardiomyopathy, congenital heart defects, inherited metabolic disorders (e.g., fatty acid oxidation disorders), pneumonia, and sepsis.

A family that has experienced one SIDS death has a 2% to 6% risk of a second SIDS death. In the case of recurrent SIDS deaths, inherited disorders must be ruled out. Additionally,

although nonaccidental trauma and homicide are rare, they are important considerations when evaluating the cause of infant death, particularly with a subsequent sudden unexpected death in a family or with a single caregiver (see Chapter 12).

Evaluation and Management

An infant coming to the ED in cardiopulmonary arrest should be managed as per the principles of Pediatric Advanced Life Support (PALS) with a brief period of well-executed CPR. CPR is a series of interventions aimed at restoring and supporting vital functions after apparent death (see Chapter 1). This involves cardiorespiratory monitoring, careful management of airway and breathing (including definitive airway management with artificial ventilation), vigorous monitored chest compressions, intraosseous and/or intraventricular access, and two to three doses of epinephrine. During this period, the patient's history should be reviewed with the parent, if available, and with the emergency medical services personnel, and the infant should be examined thoroughly with a primary and secondary survey. The examination should include evaluation for signs of prolonged death such as rigor mortis, corneal clouding, and dependent lividity. The infant should be transferred to the pediatric intensive care unit if resuscitative efforts achieve cardiorespiratory stability. Infants who arrive in the ED in asystolic arrest have a poor prognosis. Prolonged resuscitation efforts past 20 minutes, without return of spontaneous circulation, are usually futile in the absence of treatable problems such as hypothermia, drug overdose, or ventricular tachycardia or fibrillation. The team leader should make the diagnosis of death and decide about discontinuation of resuscitative efforts based on the foregoing.

Family presence in the resuscitation room is gradually becoming the norm in pediatric EDs. This is because many parents want to be with their children during what may be the last moments of life. They also want to be sure that they and the ED staff have done all that is possible to resuscitate the child. If parents want to be in the resuscitation area, a nurse or social worker who can serve as a support person and interpret the ongoing resuscitative efforts should accompany them.

A well-prepared ED should have a plan in place for issues such as bereavement measures and postmortem care and notification of medicolegal authorities, the infant's pediatrician, and any referring physicians and consultants.

First-response teams should be trained to make observations at the scene, including the position of the infant, any marks on the body, body temperature and rigor, type of bed and position of clothing and bedding, room temperature, type of ventilation and heating, and reactions of caretakers.

The loss of an infant is devastating for all concerned. Families who suffer such a loss from SIDS may encounter a police investigation, a waiting period for autopsy results, and a lack of emotional closure. It is important for the professional response teams to remain supportive, empathic, and nonaccusatory while obtaining essential information surrounding the death of the infant. Emotional support should be offered to the caregivers in the ED by both the medical staff and by a social worker or a grief counselor. The parents may be informed that a SIDS death happens quickly and silently without causing any pain and suffering to the infant. Additionally, information obtained in the acute care setting should be relayed to the family's pediatrician or family practice physician so that appropriate follow-up can be arranged, including age-appropriate support for surviving siblings.

Prevention and Future Directions

Because of the lack of evidence available to support the use of home monitoring, the current and future management of SIDS focuses on risk reduction strategies. Infants should be placed in the supine position every time they are laid down for sleep. The prone sleeping position is associated with an increased risk of SIDS in a number of observational studies. Similarly, the AAP recommends against placing infants on their side for sleep because of the instability of this position. As a result of the national Back to Sleep campaign launched in 1994, the SIDS rate in United States has fallen by more than 50%.

In addition to sleep position, the sleep environment (inclusive of sleep surface, sleepwear, bedding and the incidence of co-sleeping) appears to affect the risk of SIDS. It is recommended that infants sleep on a firm surface, such as on a safety-approved crib mattress covered with a fitted sheet without blankets, pillows, wedges, rolls, or toys in their bassinet or crib, since these objects increase the risk of suffocation. Infants should sleep in a shared room but in a separate bed. Bed sharing has benefits such as bonding and promoting breast feeding, but has been linked to higher rates of SIDS, especially for infants younger than 4 months of age, if either parent smokes, drinks alcohol before bedtime, or is abusing prescription or illicit drugs. Additionally, there is a consistent association between increased risk of SIDS and sharing a sofa or couch with parents.

Studies have suggested that pacifier use may help reduce the risk of SIDS. The mechanism is unknown, but it is hypothesized that it may lower the arousal threshold in sleeping infants. Overheating the room should be avoided because it increases the SIDS risk. A recent study suggested that having a fan in the room may reduce the risk of SIDS by 70%. Mothers should avoid smoking during pregnancy and around the infants.

Home cardiorespiratory monitoring of apnea and bradycardia has not been shown to prevent SIDS and is therefore not recommended.

About 20% of SIDS deaths occur while the infant is under the care of a nonparent caregiver. Accordingly, it is important that all childcare providers be apprised of the above precautions and safe practices to further lower the SIDS rate.

SUGGESTED READINGS

APPARENT LIFE-THREATENING EVENT

Brand DA, Altman RL, et al: Yield of diagnostic testing in infants who have had an apparent life-threatening event, *Pediatrics* 115:885, 2005.

Claudius I, Keens T: Do all infants with apparent life-threatening events need to be admitted? *Pediatrics* 119:679-683, 2007.

DeWolfe CC: Apparent life-threatening event: a review, *Pediatr Clin North Am* 52(4):1127-1146, 2005.

Fu LY, Moon RY: Apparent life-threatening events (ALTEs) and the role of home monitors, *Pediatr Rev* 28:203-208, 2007.

Kiechl-Kohlendorfer U, Hof D, Peglow UP, et al: Epidemiology of apparent life threatening events, *Arch Dis Child* 90:297-300, 2005.

Mittal MK, Shofer FS, Baren JM: Serious bacterial infections in infants who have experienced an apparent life threatening event, *Ann Emerg Med* 54(4):523-527, 2009.

SUDDEN INFANT DEATH SYNDROME

American Academy of Pediatrics: Policy Statement: Apnea, Sudden infant death syndrome, and home monitoring, *Pediatrics* 111:914-917, 2003.

Collaborative Home Infant Monitoring Evaluation (CHIME): National Institute of Health. Available at http://www.nichd.nih.gov/research/supported/chime.cfm.

Kinney HC, Thach BT: The sudden infant death syndrome, *N Eng J Med* 361(8):795-805, 2009.

Moon RY, Fu FY: Sudden infant death syndrome, *Pediatr Rev* 28:209-214, 2007.

Ramanathan R, Corwin MJ, Hunt CE, et al: Cardiorespiratory events recorded on home monitors: comparison of healthy infants with those at increased risk for SIDS, *JAMA* 285:2199-2207, 2001.

Child Abuse and Neglect

Stephen Ludwig

12

PHYSICAL ABUSE

Physical abuse is defined as nonaccidental physical injury to a child by parental acts or omissions. There has been an alarming increase in reported cases of child abuse throughout the United States in the past 3 decades. In all states, health professionals are now legally required to report their suspicions of abuse to their state's child protection services (CPS) or police.

Clinical Presentation

Determination of suspected abuse is based on compilation of information from five data sources: (1) history, (2) physical examination, (3) laboratory and radiographic information, (4) observation of parental–child interaction, and (5) a detailed family social history.

When examining any child with an injury, the clinician should be suspicious of abuse if the history reveals an unusual delay in seeking medical care, the parents' explanation of the injury is not compatible with the physical findings, the cause of the injury is unknown or "magical," or there is a history of similar or repeated episodes. Parents may be reluctant to give information or their reaction may be inappropriate to the seriousness of the injuries. Other worrisome signs are a lack of primary care (no immunizations, no source of health care), a history of parental mental illness or substance abuse, and high levels of family stress.

While examining the child, maintain a high index of suspicion for abuse or neglect if the child's weight is below the third percentile for age and there is poor personal hygiene, lack of adequate clothing, behavioral disturbance (especially undue compliance with the examiner), or an abnormal interaction between the parent and child (unwarranted roughness or extreme aloofness). But realize that abuse may occur by parents of any socioeconomic or educational level.

Remove all of the child's clothing and examine the skin carefully for contusions, abrasions, burns, and lacerations in various stages of resolution. Any bruise on a child who is not yet cruising or walking is unusual. Certain skin lesions are typical for specific types of abuse; such as circular cigarette burns; human bite marks; J-shaped curvilinear or loop-shaped marks from a wire, cord, or belt; circumferential rope burns; "grid" marks from an electric heater; and symmetrical scald burns on the buttocks or extremities (Figure 12-1). Other dermatologic manifestations include cutaneous signs of malnutrition (decreased subcutaneous fat, increased creases), scalp hematomas, signs of trauma to the genital area, and signs of injuries at different stages of healing (Figure 12-2).

Fractures are suggested by refusal to bear weight or move an extremity, gross deformity, or soft tissue swelling and point tenderness over an extremity. However, most metaphyseal chip fractures are not associated with deformity (Figure 12-3). Neurologic manifestations may include retinal hemorrhages, unexplainable irritability, coma, or convulsions (see Figure 12-3). Finally, an acute abdomen, poisoning, or any traumatic injury that cannot be explained may in fact represent forms of child abuse.

The differential diagnosis of the abused child includes conditions with skeletal involvement: accidental trauma, osteogenesis imperfecta, Caffey's disease, scurvy, rickets, birth trauma, and congenital infection. Diseases with dermatologic manifestations include bleeding disorders (idiopathic thrombocytopenic purpura, leukemia, hemophilia, von Willebrand's disease), recurrent pyodermas, and scalded skin syndrome. Sudden infant death syndrome and accidental poisonings may be mistaken for child abuse. The most common clinical problem is the differentiation between accidental and nonaccidental trauma.

Evaluation and Management

If there is any fracture or other suggestion of any form of abuse in a child younger than 2 years of age, obtain a complete skeletal survey for trauma. For older patients, if the physical examination suggests a fracture, obtain specific radiographs. Order other radiologic studies, such as a head computed tomography or magnetic resonance imaging scan, as indicated by the nature of the injuries. Ophthalmologic consultation may be needed to identify retinal hemorrhage.

If the parents deny any knowledge of the cause of skin bruises, obtain a complete blood count with differential, platelet count, prothrombin time, partial thromboplastin time, and a bleeding time. The differential diagnosis and other possible laboratory studies are shown in Table 12-1.

Physicians and other health care workers are required to report the *suspicion* of abuse. Use the information gathered in the assessment phase to determine the level of suspicion. Depending on local laws, notify the CPS or police by telephone if abuse or neglect is suspected. Generally, the CPS is required to investigate all cases reported and may not refuse to accept a referral made in good faith by a competent reporter. Usually, a physician, nurse, or social worker must complete a written report within 48 hours. However, do not delay reporting if there are other children at home because in some cases, siblings will have also been abused.

The CPS worker must evaluate the case and decide whether the child can safely return home or must go to a temporary shelter or foster placement. The physician may need to hospitalize the child for medical care or if that is the only option to provide safety. Arrange appropriate follow-up for patients who do not require hospitalization. Notify the parents about your intention to report or hospitalize the child. If the parents refuse to allow hospitalization, it may be necessary to have security or law enforcement officials intervene. In most states, hospital personnel may place a child under temporary protective custody without either parental consent or a family court order, although it is the responsibility of the CPS worker to decide whether the child can be placed in the custody of a relative or guardian.

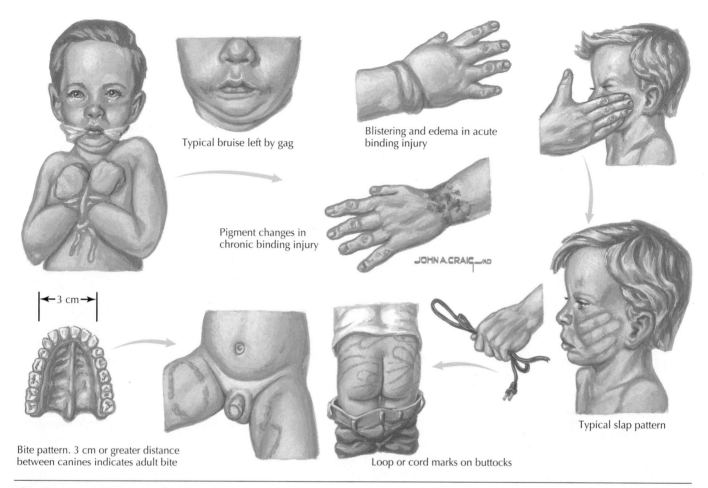

Typical bruise left by gag

Blistering and edema in acute binding injury

Pigment changes in chronic binding injury

JOHN A. CRAIG—MD

|← 3 cm →|

Bite pattern. 3 cm or greater distance between canines indicates adult bite

Loop or cord marks on buttocks

Typical slap pattern

Figure 12-1 *Child abuse injury patterns.*

Working with the families of abused children can be a difficult experience. Avoid an accusatory attitude because most of these parents love their children and deserve a supportive approach. Keep the parents informed and involved and emphasize that the goal of all concerned is to keep the child safe and, when possible, the family together. Explain the role of the social worker and supportive services and assure confidentially. Careful documentation is critical; the record will be needed for legal reference.

SEXUAL ABUSE

Sexual abuse is the exposure of a child to sexual stimulation inappropriate for his or her age, cognitive development, or position in the relationship. The legal definition is nonconsensual sexual contact. Incest is legally defined as marriage or intercourse (oral, anal, genital) with a person known to be related as an ancestor, descendant, brother, sister, uncle, aunt, nephew, or niece. Rape is legally defined as nonconsensual sexual intercourse; a person having legitimate access to the child is the typical perpetrator.

Clinical Presentation

A number of signs, symptoms, and behavioral changes may signal the possibility of sexual abuse, including difficulties in school, sudden change in behavior, fears, unwillingness to go to certain places, enuresis and encopresis, sleep disturbances, running away, and attempted suicide. Sexual abuse victims may exhibit seductive or regressive behavior. More specific complaints include difficulty walking or sitting and genital trauma, discharge, pain, or itching. Sexually transmitted disease (STD) in a child younger the age of 12 years is sexual abuse until proven otherwise. Consider sexual abuse in girls who become pregnant.

Evaluation and Management

Maintain a high index of suspicion in order to identify sexual abuse promptly. Ensure privacy for the patient and whoever accompanies the child and keep the number of staff members involved to a minimum. Because sexual abuse usually evokes intense feelings, maintaining objectivity requires effort.

The key to establishing the diagnosis in these cases is careful history taking. Use language that is appropriate for the child's age and ask specifically about all types of sexual contact. It may be useful to use anatomically correct dolls or pictures to encourage the child to describe the sexual contact in as much detail as possible. Try to ascertain when the last sexual activity occurred and what the child has done since the assault (changed clothes, bathed, urinated, defecated). Assure the child that he or she was right to reveal information about the sexual abuse.

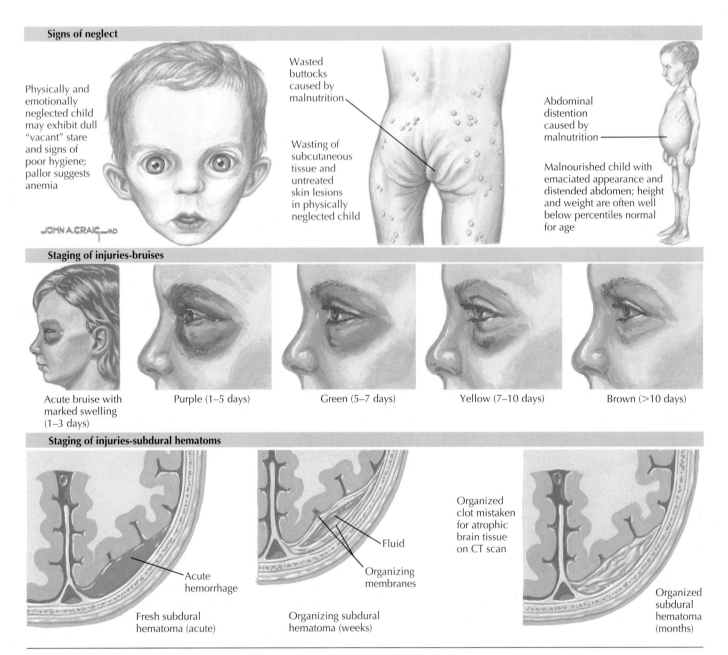

Signs of neglect

Physically and emotionally neglected child may exhibit dull "vacant" stare and signs of poor hygiene; pallor suggests anemia

JOHN A. CRAIG—AD

Wasted buttocks caused by malnutrition

Wasting of subcutaneous tissue and untreated skin lesions in physically neglected child

Abdominal distention caused by malnutrition

Malnourished child with emaciated appearance and distended abdomen; height and weight are often well below percentiles normal for age

Staging of injuries-bruises

Acute bruise with marked swelling (1–3 days)

Purple (1–5 days)

Green (5–7 days)

Yellow (7–10 days)

Brown (>10 days)

Staging of injuries-subdural hematoms

Acute hemorrhage

Fresh subdural hematoma (acute)

Fluid

Organizing membranes

Organizing subdural hematoma (weeks)

Organized clot mistaken for atrophic brain tissue on CT scan

Organized subdural hematoma (months)

Figure 12-2 *Signs of neglect and staging of injuries.*

Consent for physical examination is often an issue. However, consent from the minor (regardless of age) is all that is required because the examination also serves to rule out STDs. Do not force the patient if the examination is refused.

If the abuse has occurred within the past 72 hours, be thorough in terms of evidence collection. If the patient has not changed clothes since the sexual activity, have him or her undress on a sheet and save all clothing for legal evidence. If the child has changed but not bathed, collect only the underwear. If the child has pubic hair, comb it onto a paper towel and seal the towel, combings, one plucked pubic hair, and the comb in a labeled envelope. These samples may be used for DNA evidence. Perform a complete and careful physical examination looking for marks, bruises, or other signs of physical injury or illness and note the child's Tanner stage of pubertal development.

In most cases, the revelation of sexual abuse occurs long after the actual contact. If sexual contact has not occurred within 72 hours and there are no physical complaints (e.g., bleeding), refer the patient to a specialized sexual abuse center. Also refer the child if the emergency department (ED) does not have the personnel or time to do a proper in-depth evaluation.

With either prompt or delayed revelation, a careful genital examination is necessary. Perform a perineal-genital examination in young children in the frog-leg, supine, or knee-chest prone position (Figure 12-4). Using a saline-moistened cotton Q-Tip, swab any areas of possible seminal fluid deposition, and placed it on a labeled slide to air dry. In girls, spread the labia with two fingers to examine the hymenal ring, the introitus, and the area between the labia majora and minora. In prepubertal girls, if there are no acute signs of pelvic injury, a speculum

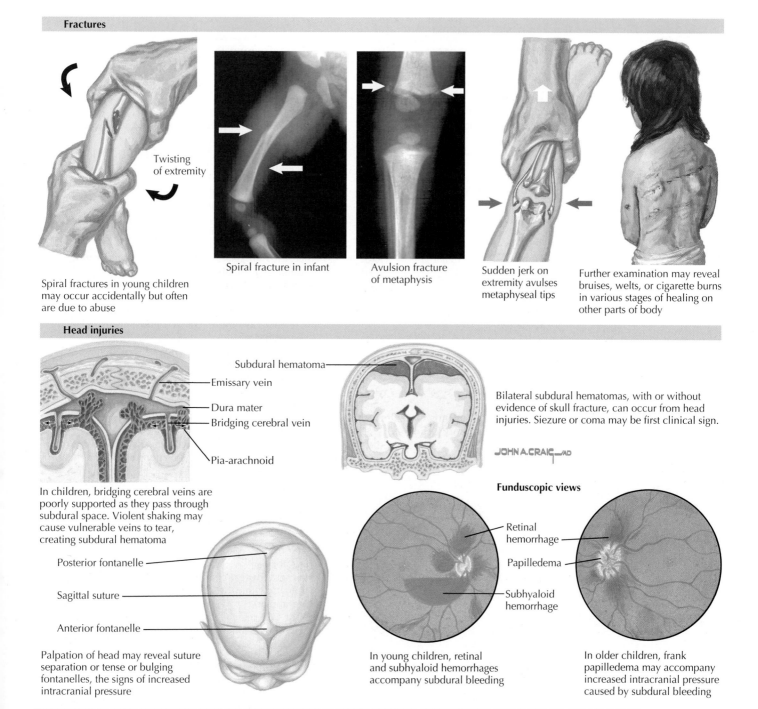

Fractures

Twisting of extremity

Spiral fractures in young children may occur accidentally but often are due to abuse

Spiral fracture in infant

Avulsion fracture of metaphysis

Sudden jerk on extremity avulses metaphyseal tips

Further examination may reveal bruises, welts, or cigarette burns in various stages of healing on other parts of body

Head injuries

Subdural hematoma
Emissary vein
Dura mater
Bridging cerebral vein
Pia-arachnoid

Bilateral subdural hematomas, with or without evidence of skull fracture, can occur from head injuries. Siezure or coma may be first clinical sign.

JOHN A. CRAIG—AD

In children, bridging cerebral veins are poorly supported as they pass through subdural space. Violent shaking may cause vulnerable veins to tear, creating subdural hematoma

Posterior fontanelle
Sagittal suture
Anterior fontanelle

Palpation of head may reveal suture separation or tense or bulging fontanelles, the signs of increased intracranial pressure

Funduscopic views

Retinal hemorrhage
Subhyaloid hemorrhage

Papilledema

In young children, retinal and subhyaloid hemorrhages accompany subdural bleeding

In older children, frank papilledema may accompany increased intracranial pressure caused by subdural bleeding

Figure 12-3 *Fractures and head injuries in child abuse.*

examination is not necessary. If there are obvious signs of physical injury (bleeding, lacerations) (Figure 12-5), consult with a pediatric gynecologist or pediatric surgeon on the need for pelvic examination under anesthesia.

In boys, examine the penis and scrotum for bruises, swelling, teeth marks, erythema, and other signs of trauma (see Figure 12-5). In both boys and girls, spread the buttocks with both hands to examine the anus and perineal area. If there are obvious signs of physical injury or severe pain, anoscopy or sigmoidoscopy is indicated under anesthesia if necessary.

Box 12-1 lists the specific laboratory evaluation of a sexually abused child. Obtain gonorrhea and chlamydial cultures from the cervix (postmenarchal), vagina (premenarchal), urethra, rectum, and pharynx if the symptoms of an STD are present. Examine vaginal specimens for the presence of *Trichomonas* spp. Obtain wet preps from all affected areas to look for sperm up to 6 hours after assault from the mouth and up to 24 hours from the rectum or vagina. If a speculum exam is performed, obtain a Pap smear and ask the hospital laboratory to specifically note the presence of sperm. Immotile sperm are present up to

Table 12-1 Differential Diagnosis and Abnormal Laboratory Studies to Support a Non-abuse Diagnosis

Findings	Differential Diagnosis	Distinguishing Features and Tests
Bruising (extensive or deep)	Trauma	Physical examination
	ITP	Decreased platelets
	Hemophilia	Increased PT, PTT
	Von Willebrand's disease	Increased bleeding time
	Henoch-Schönlein purpura	Rash on lower extremities; rule out sepsis; normal platelet count
	Purpura fulminans	Clinical appearance (findings of sepsis); decreased platelet count
	Ehlers-Danlos syndrome	Joint hyperextensibility
Dehydration	Renal or prerenal	Increased BUN, creatinine, urine specific gravity Prerenal: BUN/creatinine >20:1
Failure to thrive	Organic or nonorganic	History, physical examination; abnormal studies based on symptoms
Abdominal pain	Trauma	Hematuria; increased liver enzymes
	Tumor	Increased amylase; abdominal ultrasonography; abnormal urinalysis
	Infection	Increased WBC, ESR; abdominal ultrasonography
Fractures (multiple or in stages of healing)	Various trauma	
	Osteogenesis imperfecta	Blue sclerae; radiography: decreased bone density
	Rickets	Increased calcium; decreased phosphorus, alkaline phosphatase Radiography: cupping at ends of long bones, widened metaphysic
	Hypophosphatasia	Decreased calcium, alkaline phosphatase; increased phosphorus
	Leukemia	Abnormal peripheral smear, bone marrow, biopsy
	Previous osteomyelitis or septic arthritis	Increased WBC, ESR, CRP; positive culture
	Neurogenic sensory deficit	Detailed neurologic examination
Metaphyseal or epiphyseal lesions	Trauma	Radiographs consistent with mechanism of injury
	Scurvy	Radiographs: periosteal elevation; nutritional history
	Rickets	(See above)
	Menkes syndrome	Decreased copper, ceruloplasmin; hair analysis
	Syphilis	Abnormal serology
	Little League elbow	History of use
	Birth trauma	Neonatal history
Subperiosteal ossification	Trauma	
	Osteogenic malignancy	Radiographs; biopsy
	Syphilis	(See above)
	Infantile cortical hyperostosis	No metaphyseal changes
	Osteoid osteoma	Dramatic clinical response to aspirin
	Scurvy	(See above)
CNS injury	Trauma	CT or MRI scan
	Aneurysm	CT or MRI scan
	Tumor	MRI scan

BUN, blood urea nitrogen; CNS, central nervous system; CT, computed tomography; ESR, erythrocyte sedimentation rate; MRI, magnetic resonance imaging; PT, prothrombin time; PTT, partial thromboplastin time; WBC, white blood cell.

2.5 weeks after intercourse. Obtain a pregnancy test on all pubertal girls but do not obtain a Venereal Disease Research Laboratory (VDRL) test; a positive result can be used as damaging evidence during subsequent court proceedings. HIV testing may be indicated (at 1 month, 6 months, and 1 year after contact) in areas of high incidences or if the perpetrator has any risk factors for HIV infection.

If the alleged perpetrator is a family member or someone with family-like contact with the child, report the suspected sexual abuse to the CPS. It is not the responsibility of the ED staff to determine whether or not the abuse actually occurred. In many jurisdictions, child sexual abuse is also reported to the police. Make careful documentation in writing of all findings on the physical examination; diagrams and drawings are very useful. Take photographs of any bruises or other evidence of physical injury. Label all specimens taken for evidence and place them in evidence envelopes to be logged and secured by the security department of the hospital or given directly to the police. Ensure that the chain of legal evidence is unbroken.

Give treatment for gonorrhea and chlamydial infections as outlined in Table 12-2 if there is a high suspicion of infection or if the patient is not likely to return (emancipated minor).

Offer a postcoital contraceptive to the postmenarchal adolescent girl who is seen within 72 hours. Lo-Ovral (0.3 mg

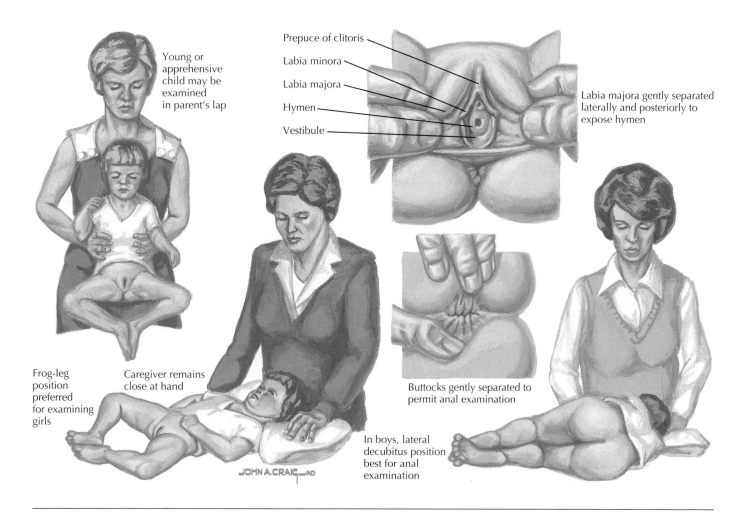

Young or apprehensive child may be examined in parent's lap

Prepuce of clitoris

Labia minora

Labia majora

Hymen

Vestibule

Labia majora gently separated laterally and posteriorly to expose hymen

Frog-leg position preferred for examining girls

Caregiver remains close at hand

Buttocks gently separated to permit anal examination

In boys, lateral decubitus position best for anal examination

JOHN A. CRAIG—AD

Figure 12-4 *Pediatric genital examination.*

norgestrel, 0.03 mg ethinyl estradiol), four tablets at once and three tablets 12 hours later, is one efficacious regimen that has few side effects (nausea and vomiting).

Reassure the child that his or her body is not harmed, that he or she was not responsible for the sexual assault, and that you believe the patient and will do everything to protect him or her

from further assault. Some victims and parents may need reassurance that the encounter will not alter the child's sexual preference in the future.

PHYSICAL ABANDONMENT AND NEGLECT

The most common form of physical neglect is nutritional neglect that results in failure to thrive. Failure to thrive may have causes that are rooted in physical conditions such as malabsorption; HIV infection and immunologic defects; or psychosocial causes such as neglect, maternal depression, and drug addiction. There are also mixed medical/psychosocial causes, such as when a relatively minor medical condition throws an already stressed family into chaos and results in the loss of ability to provide the child with adequate caloric intake. Beyond failure to thrive, some families are neglectful in providing adequate medical care, housing, clothing, hygiene, and educational support.

Abandonment of infants and small children is the most extreme form of parental neglect. Abandoned children may suffer physical and psychological harm unless there is immediate, appropriate intervention. Other forms of neglect may be less pervasive as parents fail to meet a child's need for food,

---

Box 12-1 Possible Laboratory Studies in Sexual Abuse

- *Neisseria gonorrhoeae* cultures: oropharynx, vagina or urethra, rectum
- *Chlamydia trachomatis* cultures: vagina or urethra, rectum
- Clothing, hair fingernail scrapings, and other physical evidence
- Serum pregnancy test (if appropriate)
- HIV testing (depending on the locale and nature of the abuse)
- Stool fecal occult blood test (in cases of anal penetration)
- If contact occurred within the past 72 hours:
  - Detection of sperm: obtain specimens from the mouth, vagina, and rectum; place the swaps in saline; then dry mount on slide
  - Determination of blood group: saliva

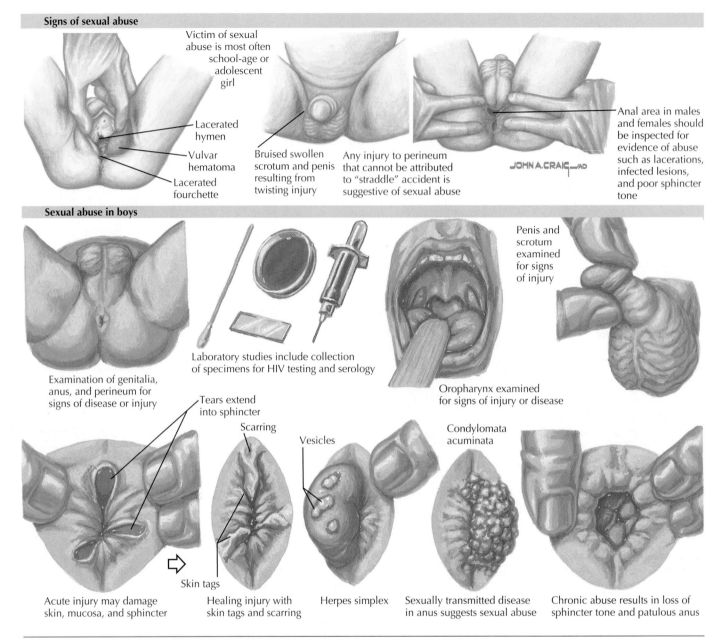

Signs of sexual abuse

Victim of sexual abuse is most often school-age or adolescent girl

Lacerated hymen

Vulvar hematoma

Lacerated fourchette

Bruised swollen scrotum and penis resulting from twisting injury

Any injury to perineum that cannot be attributed to "straddle" accident is suggestive of sexual abuse

JOHN A. CRAIG—AD

Anal area in males and females should be inspected for evidence of abuse such as lacerations, infected lesions, and poor sphincter tone

Sexual abuse in boys

Examination of genitalia, anus, and perineum for signs of disease or injury

Laboratory studies include collection of specimens for HIV testing and serology

Oropharynx examined for signs of injury or disease

Penis and scrotum examined for signs of injury

Tears extend into sphincter

Scarring

Vesicles

Condylomata acuminata

Skin tags

Acute injury may damage skin, mucosa, and sphincter

Healing injury with skin tags and scarring

Herpes simplex

Sexually transmitted disease in anus suggests sexual abuse

Chronic abuse results in loss of sphincter tone and patulous anus

Figure 12-5 *Pediatric sexual abuse.*

clothing, shelter, medical care, education, or supervision. The long-term effects of neglect may be more injurious than those of abuse because the indolent nature of neglect causes it to be underreported and uncorrected.

Clinical Presentation

The evaluation of failure to thrive is largely based on the history and physical examination findings. These findings should guide a laboratory evaluation. In extreme cases or when the child is of a vulnerable age, hospitalization for feeding observation and calorie counts may be warranted.

Every abandoned child must undergo a thorough physical examination, with particular attention to a general assessment of the state of hydration, nutrition, body temperature, and hygiene. Undress and examine the child thoroughly for physical stigmata of abuse or neglect.

Evaluation and Management

The first priority is to try to locate the parent or another family member known to the child. Then perform the physical examination and obtain appropriate laboratory studies to document any harm resulting from abandonment and to find any treatable conditions.

The next step is to report this form of child neglect to the local CPS or police, depending on local child abuse reporting laws and protocols.

Disposition options in the management of an abandoned child include transfer to the custody of a relative who is judged

Table 12-2 Treatment of Sexually Transmitted Infections in Children

Infection	Recommended Treatment
Chlamydia trachomatis (vulvovaginitis and urethritis)	**Children < 45 kg:** Erythromycin base or ethylsuccinate 50 mg/kg/d orally divided into 4 doses daily (maximum, 2 g/d) for 14 days **Children > 45 kg but < 8 years old:** Azithromycin 1 g orally in single dose **Children > 8 years old:** Azithromycin 1 g orally in single dose *or* Doxycycline 100 mg orally twice a day for 7 days
Neisseria gonorrhoeae (vulvovaginitis, urethritis, cervicitis, pharyngitis, and proctitis)	**Children < 45 kg:** Ceftriaxone, 125 mg, in a single dose
Treponema vaginalis	**Children < 45 kg:** Metronidazole, 15 mg/kg /d orally in three divided doses (maximum 2 g/day) for 7 days
Bacterial vaginosis	**Children < 45 kg:** Metronidazole, 15 mg/kg /d orally in two divided doses (maximum, 1 g/d) for 7 days
HSV–primary infection	**Children < 45 kg:** Acyclovir, 80 mg/kg/d, orally, in three or four divided doses (maximum, 1.2 g/d) for 7-10 days
Treponema pallidum	Treatment regimen depends on syphilis stage
Human papillomavirus (external anogenital warts)	**Children < 45 kg:** Patient applied: Podofilox 0.5% solution or gel* *or* Imiquimod 5% cream* Provider administered: Cryotherapy *or* Podophyllin resin 10%-25%* *or* Trichloroacetic acid *or* Bichloroacetic acid *or* Surgical removal

*Contraindicated in pregnancy.
Based on data from the following sources: Centers for Disease Control and Prevention. Sexually Transmitted Diseases Treatment Guidelines—2006. MMWR Morbid Mortal Wkly Rep 55(No. RR-11):1-94, 2006.
   Pickering LK (ed): Prophylaxis after sexual victimization of preadolescent children. sexual victimization and STIs. Red Book: 2006 Report of the Committee on Infectious Diseases, ed 26. Elk Grove Village, IL, American Academy of Pediatrics, 2006, pp 172-177.

suitable by the CPS worker or placement in temporary shelter or foster care. However, if medical care is necessary or community-based resources do not exist, admit the child to the hospital. In most states, abandoned children who are referred to the local CPS may be legally placed, on a temporary basis, in another home without a court order. Proper court proceedings must follow to justify and continue an emergency placement.

In the hospital, a parent who has abandoned his or her child may be extremely defensive and at times hostile to the staff. Do not induce further hostility by raising the levels of parental guilt or fear. Instead, focus on the mutual concern for the child.

For children with neglect short of abandonment, meticulously document the aspects and findings of neglect and refer the family to their primary care provider.

SUGGESTED READINGS

American Academy of Pediatrics Committee on Child Abuse and Neglect: Guidelines for the evaluation of sexual abuse of children: subject review, *Pediatrics* 103:186-191, 1999.

American Academy of Pediatrics Section on Radiology: Diagnostic imaging of child abuse, *Pediatrics* 105:1345-1348, 2000.

Atabaki S, Paradise JE: The medical evaluation of the sexually abused child: lessons from a decade of research, *Pediatrics* 104:178-186, 1999.

Christian CW, Lavelle JM, DeJong AR, et al: Forensic evidence findings in prepubertal victims of sexual assault, *Pediatrics* 106:100-104, 2000.

Reece RM, Ludwig S: *Child Abuse: Medical Diagnosis and Management*, Philadelphia, 2001, Lippincott Williams & Wilkins.

Swanston HY, Tebbutt JS, O'Toole BI, et al: Sexually abused children 5 years after presentation: a case-control study, *Pediatrics* 100:600-608, 1997.

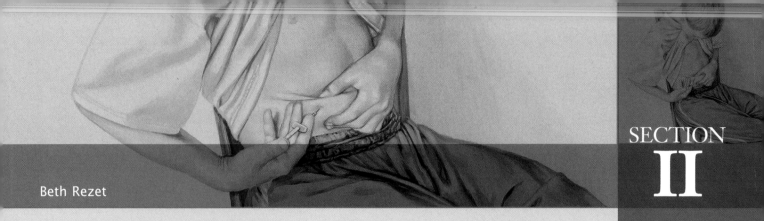

Beth Rezet

Nutrition

Nutritional Requirements and Growth

13

Carrie Daymont and Beth Rezet

Adequate nutrition is essential for good health at all ages. However, because of rapid growth and development, nutritional requirements vary throughout infancy and childhood. Assessment of a child's growth is a crucial part of any evaluation of a child, whether the child is well or ill. Assessment of growth depends on an understanding of the wide variation in the normal range of growth. This chapter provides an introduction to nutritional requirements and growth throughout childhood.

NUTRITIONAL REQUIREMENTS

Fluids and Electrolytes

Weight-based recommendations for adequate fluids in children have been made based on metabolic rates. The Holliday-Segar method recommends 100 mL/kg/d for the first 10 kg of weight, 50 mL/kg/d for the next 10 kg of weight, and then 25 mL/kg/d for each kilogram above 20 kg. This estimate does not take excess losses into account; children with diarrhea, vomiting, severe burns, and other sources of fluid loss could require even more fluids. This may provide an overestimate of fluid requirements because these estimates have not been tested in children.

In general, infants who are voiding six times in 24 hours are getting adequate fluids. Infants' immature kidneys are not capable of producing either very concentrated or very dilute urine; therefore, it is essential that the fluid and electrolytes consumed be balanced. Breast milk and properly prepared commercial infant formula contain appropriate amounts of electrolytes for infants. Free water should not be given to infants younger than 6 months of age, and intake should be limited until 1 year of age. The electrolyte composition of cow's milk is not appropriate for infants.

Healthy children are generally able to regulate their own fluid intake when it is provided, and many children get a substantial amount of fluid through the high water content of most foods. Urine output and signs and symptoms of dehydration can be used to assess fluid status in older children.

Calories

Neonates need approximately 110 to 120 kcal/kg/d for appropriate growth. Calorie requirements steadily decrease to approximately 90 kcal/kg/d in toddlers. After 3 years of age, calorie requirements vary by gender, age, weight, and activity. Children with very low levels of activity, such as children with profound mental or motor disability who receive tube feedings, usually have significantly lower energy requirements than healthy children. When offered but not forced to take food, most infants and children are able to self-regulate their calorie, or energy,

intake to optimal levels over time. Children are generally able to increase their calorie intake when needed, such as during brief periods of rapid weight gain in infancy and pubertal growth spurt and then decrease their intake back to appropriate levels for typical growth. If a toddler is gaining weight well, parents of picky eaters should provide healthy food options and can be reassured that the child is appropriately regulating his or her calorie intake (Figure 13-1).

Macronutrients

PROTEIN

Protein should make up approximately 10% to 35% of a child's diet. In infancy, protein requirements are based on the protein consumed by "on-demand" feeding of breastfed infants (≈1.5 g/kg/d for infants up to 6 months of age). Commercial infant formulas provide somewhat higher values of protein; there is no evidence that this increase in protein is either beneficial or harmful. Protein requirements decrease to a recommended daily allowance of 0.85 g/kg/d in adolescents.

Human milk and animal protein generally provide adequate levels of all essential amino acids. However, plant sources of protein, such as beans, nuts, and grains, do not provide adequate levels of all essential amino acids. Children who consume their protein from plant sources primarily need to receive a balance of legumes and grains to ensure adequate essential amino acid intake. Parents may need to consult with a nutritionist regarding alternative diets to ensure the provision of adequate sources of all essential amino acids and vitamins.

FAT

Fat is an important nutrient, particularly for children younger than 2 years of age who have high energy needs and require fatty acids for nervous system myelination. Children younger than 2 years of age should get approximately 25% to 40% of their calories from fat. From age 1 to 2 years of age, children of normal weight should drink whole milk to ensure adequate fat intake. Children who are overweight can drink 2% milk to reduce fat and caloric intake, but they should not be placed on a low-fat diet at this age. Older children should get 10% to 35% of their calories from fat. Children who are overweight or obese in particular should aim for a fat intake that does not exceed this range.

CARBOHYDRATES

Carbohydrates make up approximately 45% to 65% of total caloric intake. Most carbohydrate intake should come from complex carbohydrates rather than simple sugars, which contribute to dental caries as well as obesity. Fruits have significant

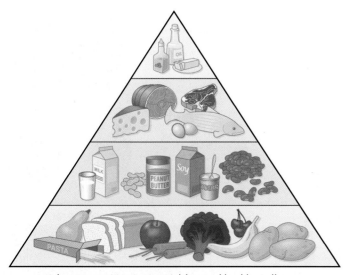

Adequate nutrition is essential for good health at all ages.

J. Perkins
MS, MFA, CMI

Figure 13-1 *Diet.*

amounts of sugar but also supply vitamins and fiber and are part of a healthy diet for children. Most other sources of sugar, such as soda, candy, and many juices, do not contain other significant sources of nutrients and should be limited. One hundred percent fruit juice contains vitamins but lacks fiber and provides more concentrated sugar than whole fruit. Therefore, the American Academy of Pediatrics (AAP) recommends no more than 4 to 6 oz per day of 100% fruit juice between 6 months and 6 years of age and no more than 8 to 12 oz per day of 100% fruit juice after 6 years of age. Excess juice intake contributes to obesity by increasing caloric intake and can contribute to failure to thrive in children who drink juice in place of eating more nutritious food. Low-carbohydrate diets are not generally recommended for children and should never be followed without supervision by a nutritionist or physician.

Micronutrients

This section briefly discusses three of the most important micronutrients and the problems that can arise when they are deficient. Chapter 16 addresses these and other deficiencies in more detail.

CALCIUM

Adequate calcium intake during childhood is important for long-term bone health. Recommendations for calcium intake have been published by the Food and Nutrition Board of the National Academy of Sciences and affirmed by the AAP. Breast milk and infant formula provide adequate calcium intake for infants (210-270 mg/d). Preterm infants who are formula fed should receive preterm formula with increased calcium. Children who are 1 to 3 years of age should receive 500 mg/d of calcium, which can be supplied in two or three servings of dairy products per day. Children between 4 and 8 years of age need

800 mg/d of calcium, and children older than 9 years of age need 1300 mg/d of calcium achieved by consuming, respectively, three and four servings of dairy a day.

Children who do not consume adequate dairy products can get calcium through calcium-fortified orange juice, other naturally occurring sources such as tofu or leafy green vegetables, or oral supplements. Soy milk does not naturally contain calcium and vitamin D, so it should be fortified with calcium and vitamin D.

VITAMIN D

Adequate vitamin D intake is also important for long-term bone health, and recent research has shown its importance in a wide variety of other functions (Figure 13-2). Vitamin D can be ingested or synthesized when the skin is exposed to ultraviolet light. Vitamin D deficiency in infants causes rickets and when very severe can lead to hypocalcemic seizures. Vitamin D deficiency is relatively common in the United States. Risk factors include breastfeeding, darker skin, little sun exposure, and fat malabsorption. Infant formula is supplemented with vitamin D, but breastfed infants are at risk for rickets without vitamin D supplementation. Infants who are breastfed should receive a vitamin D supplement with 400 IU of vitamin D per day to prevent rickets. Children who do not receive at least 400 IU of vitamin D in their diets should also receive a supplement. Future research may show that the current recommendations for vitamin D are too low and should be revised.

IRON

Prevention of iron deficiency in infants and young children is crucial because it can lead to neurologic deficits in developing children that may not be reversible. The iron in breast milk is highly bioavailable and provides adequate levels of iron for infants of mothers who maintain an adequate source of their own dietary or supplemental iron. After 6 months of age breastfed infants should also be given iron-rich foods, such as proteins or iron-fortified rice cereal, to provide adequate iron intake. Commercial infant formulas that are fortified with iron also provide adequate iron. Studies have shown that iron-fortified formulas do not lead to gastrointestinal symptoms, and formulas with low iron should not be used. Preterm infants require additional iron, which can be given as a multivitamin with iron. The iron in cow's milk is not very bioavailable and should not be given to infants. Meat and egg yolk are good sources of iron that is readily bioavailable. Many cereals are fortified with significant amounts of iron, although their shelf life may make the iron less bioavailable. Iron is also found in many fruits and vegetables, but consideration should be given to giving a daily iron supplement of 10 mg of elemental iron to children who do not eat meat.

OTHER MICRONUTRIENTS

Deficiencies of other micronutrients are rare in the United States, but children with metabolic diseases or very restricted diets can have deficiencies in other micronutrients, such as zinc or vitamin C.

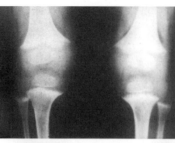

Impaired growth
Craniotabes
Frontal bossing
Dental defects
Chronic cough
Pigeon breast (tunnel chest)
Kyphosis
Rachitic rosary
Harrison groove
Flaring of ribs
Enlarged ends of long bones
Enlarged abdomen
Coxa vara
Bowleg (genu varum)

Clinical findings
(all or some present in variable degree)

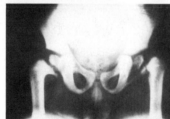

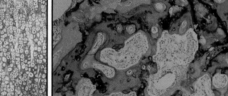

▲ Coxa vara and slipped capital femoral epiphysis. Mottled areas of lucency and density in pelvic bones

◀ Flaring of metaphyseal ends of tibia and femur. Growth plates thickened, irregular, cupped, and axially widened. Zones of provisional calcification fuzzy and indistinct. Bone cortices thinned and medullae rarefied

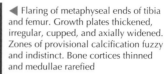

▶ Radiograph of rachitic hand shows decreased bone density, irregular trabeculation, and thin cortices of metacarpals and proximal phalanges. Note increased axial width of epiphyseal line, especially in radius and ulna

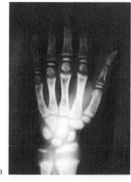

Radiographic findings

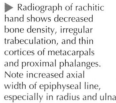

◀ Section of rachitic bone shows sparse, thin trabeculae surrounded by much uncalcified osteoid (osteoid seams) and cavities caused by increased resorption

▲ Radiograph shows variegated rarefaction of pelvic bones, coxa vara, deepened acetabula, and subtrochanteric pseudofracture of right femur

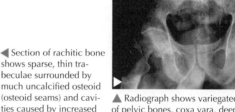

◀ (Left) Cartilage of epiphyseal plate in immature normal rat. Cells of middle (maturation) zone in orderly columns, with calcified cartilage between columns
◀ (Right) After 6 weeks of vitamin D–and phosphate-deficient diet. Large increase in axial height of maturation zone, with cells closely packed and irregularly arranged

Figure 13-2 *Bone health.*

COUNSELING

Infants

The AAP recommends breastfeeding for at least the first year of life, with exclusive breastfeeding for the first 6 months (Figure 13-3). Solid foods should be introduced at age 6 months, including iron-rich high protein foods and iron-fortified cereals and pureed fruits, vegetables, and meats. Infants diets can be slowly expanded to more complex textures as tolerated, always avoiding foods that could cause choking. When breastfeeding is not an option, infants should be given properly prepared commercial iron-fortified infant formula with introduction of solid foods between 4 and 6 months of age. Juice, with its high sugar content, should be avoided or limited to no more than 4 oz/d.

Parents of infants should also be counseled on distinguishing the signs of hunger and satiety in infants to allow children to self-regulate their energy intake. Moving lips, sucking on hands, and rooting are some signs of hunger that precede fussing or crying. Releasing the nipple, biting the nipple, pulling head away, and shaking the head are some signs of satiety. Healthier eating habits will result if parents are encouraged to respond to their baby's cues rather than adhering to a feeding schedule or to measured amounts of foods. Parents may find the normal erratic eating patterns of babies and toddlers to be confusing and frustrating. Confirming that the baby is satisfied and is adequately gaining weight can be very assuring.

Children

Parents should provide children with a variety of healthy foods. Telling children to "clean their plates" or overly restricting the type or amount of food inhibits their ability to respond to their own feelings of satiety.

BEVERAGES

Fluids can be a good source of nutrients or a large source of empty calories. Recommended beverages change with age (Table 13-1). Parents should choose nutrient-rich liquids or water and avoid empty-calorie options such as soda.

GROWTH

During well-child visits, assessment of growth serves as a screening tool for a wide variety of medical problems that may need further evaluation. In children presenting with an illness, assessment of growth can provide clues about the nature and time course of the illness. Because there is such wide variation in the distribution of normal growth, the challenge for clinicians is to as the chapter on disorders of growth in the endocrinology section (Chapter 73), and disease-specific chapters.

Types of Measurements

Weight is the most important and most commonly used measure of growth in children. Length (in children younger than 2 years), height (in children older 2 years), and head circumference are also useful. From these measures, weight-for-length percentiles or body mass index (BMI) can be calculated. Methods that can indicate body fat percentage, such as subscapular skin-fold thickness and arm circumference, are used less often but can be helpful when assessing children with suspected malnutrition.

Measurement Methods

It is crucial that all measurements are accurately assessed. Infants should be weighed without clothing or a diaper, and older children should be weighed with very light clothing because apparent weight loss or weight gain may be an artifact of differences in clothing. All staff taking measurements should be properly trained, and equipment should be calibrated to ensure proper measurements. A stadiometer should be used for measuring length and height.

Use of Growth Curves

Growth in children is typically assessed by plotting a child's measurement and age on a gender-specific growth curve (Figure 13-4). Growth curves allow clinicians to compare a child's measurements with those of other children of the same age and to evaluate patterns in an individual child's growth if measurements from multiple points in time are plotted on the same curve. On weight and BMI charts, the upper lines are not true percentiles; they have been adjusted so that the increasing prevalence of obesity does not lead to the classification of overweight children as having a healthy weight.

There are two standard forms commonly used in the United States: the Centers for Disease Control and Prevention (CDC) charts published in 2000 based on data from multiple national cross-sectional studies including both healthy children and those with medical problems and the World Health Organization (WHO) charts published in 2006 based on a prospective longitudinal study of healthy, breastfed children on six continents. The CDC and WHO's length curves are similar. The WHO curves classify more children as being overweight and fewer children as underweight than the CDC curves. The WHO curves also classify more children as being macrocephalic than the CDC curves.

Assessing a Child's Growth

Growth is usually assessed in two ways: (1) current, attained growth relative to same-age peers and (2) growth velocity relative to peers. Using the 5th and 95th percentile parameters as cutoffs for normal growth is sensitive but not specific. It is important to remember that in using these cutoffs, approximately 10% of all children will be labeled as outside the normal

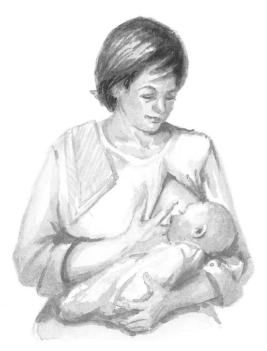

The AAP recommends breastfeeding for at least the first year of life, with exclusive breastfeeding for the first six months.

JOHN A. CRAIG—AD

Figure 13-3 *Breastfeeding.*

determine whether children with unusual growth patterns are unhealthy or if they are healthy patients with a less common growth pattern. This segment focuses on how to assess growth and growth patterns seen in healthy patients. Further information on disorders of growth can be found in this section, as well

Table 13-1	Recommended Fluids by Age for Healthy, Typically Growing Children
Age	**Fluid Recommendations**
0-6 months	• Breast milk • Properly prepared commercial infant formula
6-12 months	• Breast milk • Properly prepared commercial infant formula • Water: no more than 8 oz/d • 0-4 oz/d of 100% fruit juice
12-24 months	• Breast milk • Whole milk: 16-24 oz/d (2% milk if child is overweight or obese) • Water • 0-4 oz/d of 100% fruit juice
2-6 years	• Water • Low-fat milk (skim or 1% milk) • 0-4 oz/d of 100% fruit juice
6-18 years	• Water • Low-fat milk (skim or 1% milk) • 0-8 oz/d of 100% fruit juice

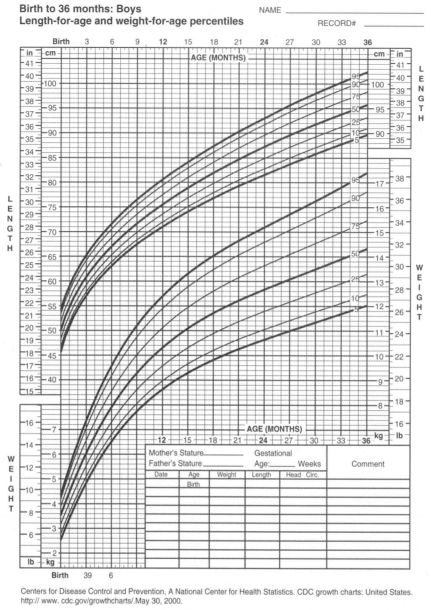

Birth to 36 months: Boys
Length-for-age and weight-for-age percentiles

NAME _____

RECORD# _____

Centers for Disease Control and Prevention, A National Center for Health Statistics. CDC growth charts: United States.
http:// www. cdc.gov/growthcharts/.May 30, 2000.

Figure 13-4 *Weight and height growth curves for boys ages 0 to 36 months.*

range, including many healthy children. A child's growth veloc- ity can be estimated by determining if a child is following a certain percentile line or is crossing percentile lines. Crossing two or more major percentile lines can be indicative of a problem. However, a shift in percentiles in the first year of life may merely reflect a child's transition to his or her genetic potential.

WEIGHT

Neonates can lose up to 10% of their birth weight and should be at or above their birthweight by 10 to 14 days after birth. Expected weight gain early in infancy is approximately 26 to 31 g/d decreasing to 7 to 9 g/d at 12 months of age. Breastfed infants typically gain weight more quickly than formula-fed

infants between 4 and 6 months but then gain weight more slowly and are ultimately slightly leaner, on average, than formula-fed infants. Children do not always gain weight steadily and may have periods of relatively little weight gain followed by periods of more rapid weight gain. If an infant or child loses weight or has not been gaining adequate weight, a careful history and physical examination should be used to determine possible causes, and the child should be reevaluated.

HEIGHT AND LENGTH

As with weight, periods of slower gain in height may be followed by more rapid gains in height. A significant change in height percentile is less common than for weight percentile, particu- larly after the first year of life. Children grow at a slightly decreasing velocity from infancy until puberty. The average gain in length is 4 cm/mo in the neonatal period, decreasing to 0.8 cm/mo at 2 years of age. At puberty, children have a growth spurt, gaining several inches in height, and have minimal gain in height after puberty. The pubertal growth spurt starts later and lasts longer in boys, which accounts for much of their increased average height.

WEIGHT FOR HEIGHT AND BODY MASS INDEX

For infants and young children, weight relative to length can be evaluated with weight-for-length percentiles on the CDC 2000 or WHO growth curves or with the WHO curves for BMI. For older children, weight relative to height should be evaluated using BMI percentile. These charts are helpful when evaluating children who have familial short or tall stature. If these children are out of the normal range on the weight growth curve but have a normal weight for height, one can be reassured that their abnormal weight is likely proportional to their height. Overweight and obesity are discussed further in the Chapter 15.

HEAD CIRCUMFERENCE

Head circumference should be measured by placing a tape measure around the head parallel to the floor with the tape just above the eyebrows in front and around the most prominent part of the occiput. In infants, a head circumference that is rapidly crossing increasing percentiles is concerning for hydrocephalus. A head circumference that is not increasing or is crossing decreasing percentile lines is concerning for a failure of brain growth.

FUTURE DIRECTIONS

In many parts of the world, children are hungry, and research continues to focus on high-energy, nutrient-rich, compact, portable foods to combat starvation. Obesity treatment and prevention is a focus of many current investigations. Research is also ongoing in the timing of introduction of solid foods, particularly in relation to food allergies. Research is continuing on recommendations for vitamin D requirements and prevention of deficiencies.

SUGGESTED READINGS

Barlow SE: Expert committee recommendations regarding the prevention, assessment, and treatment of child and adolescent overweight and obesity: summary report, *Pediatrics* 120(suppl 4):S164-S192, 2007.

Kleinman R, editor: *Pediatric Nutrition Handbook*, ed 6, Elk Grove, IL, 2009, American Academy of Pediatrics.

Kramer MS, Kakuma R: The optimal duration of exclusive breastfeeding: a systematic review, *Adv Exp Med Biol* 554:63-77, 2004.

Roche A: *Human Growth*. New York, 2003, Cambridge University Press.

Summerbell CD, Waters E, Edmunds L, et al: Interventions for preventing obesity in children. *Cochrane Database Syst Rev* (3):CD001871, 2005.

U.S. Preventive Services Task Force: *Screening for Iron Deficiency Anemia— Including Iron Supplementation for Children and Pregnant Women: Recommendation Statement*, Rockville, MD, 2006, Agency for Healthcare Research and Quality.

Malnutrition

Elizabeth Lowenthal and Beth Rezet

14

Malnutrition is an impairment of physical or mental health (or both) resulting from failure to meet nutritional requirements characterized by inadequate or excess availability of calories, protein, and micronutrients. Despite the increasing problem of obesity in many parts of the world, nutritional deficiency remains the most prevalent form of malnutrition worldwide. Inadequate consumption of food, lack of essential dietary nutrients, and impaired absorption because of disease are the most common contributors to malnutrition in children. Worldwide, malnutrition is estimated to be a contributing factor in more than half of all childhood deaths. Children in low-income countries are most susceptible to malnutrition around the time of weaning.

Acute malnutrition is characterized by low weight for height, small mid-upper arm circumference (MUAC), or nutritional edema. A chronically malnourished child is stunted and has a low weight for age. The severity of malnutrition is typically defined as mild, moderate, or severe. Severe malnutrition has the highest case fatality rate, but mild malnutrition is responsible for the largest overall burden of nutritionally preventable illnesses. This chapter focuses on the manifestations and management of patients with severe acute malnutrition. Identification and management of mild and moderate malnutrition are also reviewed.

CLINICAL PRESENTATION

Chronic malnutrition is identified by low height for age, also known as stunting. Chronically malnourished children are shorter than other children their age and may fail to meet their long-term growth potential. Acute malnutrition is characterized by low weight for height and low MUAC with or without symmetric edema. Severe acute malnutrition is defined as severe wasting, nutritional edema, or both. An acutely malnourished child has low body fat reserves and may also have limited protein stores. Children with severely low levels of serum protein often develop symmetric edema. Table 14-1 displays criteria used to define moderate and severe malnutrition. This chapter uses the World Health Organization (WHO) definitions to classify the severity of malnutrition. It is common for stunting and wasting to occur concomitantly. Children with combined chronic and acute malnutrition are both short for age and thin for height.

Scales for assessing weight, stadiometers for measuring height, and tape measures for evaluating MUAC are all essential tools in settings where severe malnutrition is diagnosed and managed. Growth charts (discussed in Chapter 13) are also necessary to allow for the quantification of the degree of malnutrition. In very low-resource settings when scales are not available, MUAC tapes alone may be used to screen for and follow up severe acute malnutrition (Figure 14-1).

The three common forms of protein-energy malnutrition are marasmus, kwashiorkor, and a mixed form called marasmic kwashiorkor. Whereas marasmus is typically considered to be a reflection of caloric deficiency, kwashiorkor is thought to be reflective primarily of a deficiency of protein. Marasmus can be recognized visually by decreased subcutaneous fat leading to prominent bones and the appearance of "loose skin," especially around the buttocks. Kwashiorkor is characterized by bilateral pitting edema and a protuberant belly (Figure 14-2). Malnutrition is commonly associated with visible hair and skin changes. The hair is commonly thin, scanty, straight, and lightly pigmented. Skin changes are varied and commonly include xerosis, itchy rashes, and poor wound healing.

Other physical examination findings that are commonly seen with severe malnutrition are outlined in Table 14-2.

DIFFERENTIAL DIAGNOSIS

When diagnosing malnutrition, underlying causes should be investigated. Infections with HIV, tuberculosis, malaria, and parasites commonly cause or exacerbate malnutrition. Failure to identify and treat these underlying conditions would prohibit appropriate recovery. Other common causes of severe malnutrition can be found in Chapter 17, specifically Table 17-1.

PHYSIOLOGIC CHANGES ACCOMPANYING MALNUTRITION

Profound physiologic changes occur in children with severe acute malnutrition. All body systems undergo significant functional changes with severe malnutrition. Table 14-3 outlines some of the most significant physiologic changes that occur with severe acute malnutrition and the treatment approaches that are necessary to avoid complications related to these physiologic abnormalities.

Micronutrient deficiencies are also common among children with severe malnutrition. Vitamin A deficiency should be assumed to be present, and high-dose vitamin A should be provided on day 1 of treatment. For infants younger than 6 months of age, a high-dose vitamin A is 50,000 IU; 100,000 IU should be given to infants between 6 and 12 months, and 200,000 IU should be given to children over 12 months of age. When clinical signs of vitamin A deficiency are present, an additional large dose of vitamin A should be given on day 2 of rehabilitation and a third dose about 2 weeks later. Ocular signs of vitamin A deficiency are often easily recognizable and include night blindness, conjunctival xerosis with foamy white Bitot's spots, keratomalacia, and corneal ulceration (Figure 14-3).

DIAGNOSTIC EVALUATIONS

In many settings where severe acute malnutrition is endemic, resource limitations prevent any evaluation beyond physical examination and history taking. When available, laboratory evaluation would include tests for suspected causes such as infection, stool for ova and parasites, cultures, serology, complete

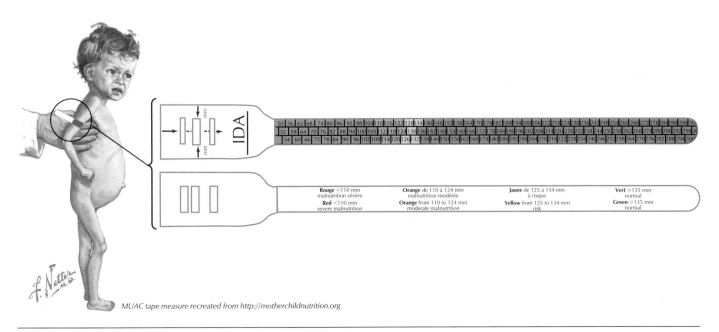

Figure 14-1 *Measurement of mid-upper arm circumference.*

blood count, and serum electrolytes, as well as any indicated radiographic imaging.

MANAGEMENT

A severely malnourished child is also often severely ill, and management must progress through stages of recovery. The first week of treatment for severe malnutrition is referred to as the stabilization phase because appropriate management during this period makes the child less vulnerable to malnutrition-related death and is critical for survival. There are physiologic differences between a healthy child and a severely malnourished child that must be taken into account in devising management plans during at least the first 6 weeks of rehabilitation. Close follow-up of a malnourished child should continue for at least 6 months after presentation with severe malnutrition. Figure 14-4 outlines the main goals of each phase of management of a severely malnourished child.

Inappropriate stabilization and rehabilitation of a severely malnourished child can have fatal consequences. Severely

malnourished children cannot tolerate typical amounts of protein, sodium, or fat found in routine infant formulas, and they require frequent feeds with simple carbohydrates. During stabilization, breast milk and F-75 milk formula (75 kcal and 0.9 g protein per 100 mL) are recommended by the WHO for feeding. For infants with severe malnutrition who are acutely and severely ill, exclusive breastfeeding is often unsuccessful; therefore, supplementation with F-75 should be attempted. Deaths related to an excessive renal solute load during malnutrition recovery can be avoided by using F-75 formula. Between

Table 14-1 World Health Organization Criteria for Defining Moderate and Severe Malnutrition		
	Moderate Malnutrition	**Severe Malnutrition**
Height for age	−3 to −2 SD below the mean (85th to 89th percentile)	<−3 SD below the mean (<85th percentile)
Weight for height	−3 to −2 SD below the mean (70th to 79th percentile)	<−3 SD below the mean (<70th percentile)
Symmetric edema	No	Yes

SD, standard deviation.

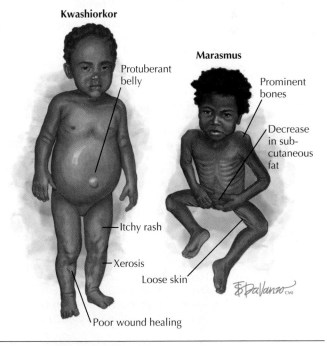

Figure 14-2 *Kwashiorkor and marasmus.*

Table 14-2 Common Physical Examination Findings in Severe Acute Malnutrition

Physical Finding	Significance
Low height for age	• Indicates stunting
Low weight-for-height and low MUAC	• Indicates wasting
Edema	• Indicates protein deficiency
Extreme pallor	• Anemia present
Sunken eyes	• May indicate decreased subcutaneous fat around eyes
	• Rapid change is more likely indicative of dehydration
Corneal and conjunctival lesions	• Suggestive of vitamin A deficiency
Weak pulses	• Weak or absent radial, carotid, femoral, or brachial pulses suggest the presence of shock
Hypothermia	• Commonly associated with serious infection in malnourished children
Cold hands and feet without central hypothermia	• May signify dehydration or sepsis
Mental status changes	• Severely malnourished children are commonly apathetic when left alone and irritable when handled
	• Sudden changes in mental status may indicate a serious complication of illness
Dry mouth and absent tears	• Common in malnutrition because of atrophy of salivary and lacrimal glands
	• Not a reliable indicator of dehydration in malnourished children
Shedding and ulceration of skin, particularly of the perineum, groin, limbs and armpits	• Commonly seen with kwashiorkor
	• Prone to infectious complications

MUAC, mid-upper arm circumference.

80 and 100 kcal/kg of F-75 should be given daily during the stabilization phase by way of small feedings every 2 to 3 hours.

After stabilization with F-75, advancement to F-100 (100 kcal and 2.9 g protein per 100) is recommended as a "catch-up" formula to help rebuild wasted tissues. In some areas of the world, easily transportable, ready-to-use therapeutic foods (RUTFs) such as "plumpy nut" bars are used in addition to or instead of F-100.

In addition to high-dose vitamin A supplementation (discussed above), micronutrient supplementation in the form of a vitamin mix containing riboflavin; pyridoxine; thiamine; and vitamins C, D, E, and K should be provided daily. Folate should also be supplemented giving 5 mg on day 1 and then 1 mg/d throughout rehabilitation and follow-up. Iron can have toxic effects during acute severe malnutrition and should not be given during the first week of treatment.

Table 14-3 Major Physiologic Changes with Severe Acute Malnutrition

Body System	Major Physiologic Changes	Treatment Approaches
Cardiovascular	• Decreased cardiovascular output and stroke volume • Low blood pressure • Increase in blood volume may rapidly lead to heart failure • Decrease in blood volume may compromise tissue perfusion	• Do not give IV fluids unless child is in shock • Restrict blood transfusions to 10 mL/kg and give diuretics • Monitor perfusion and cardiac status closely
Dermatologic	• Loss of subcutaneous fat and atrophied glands make typical signs of dehydration less reliable	• Rehydrate with ReSoMal and F-75 diet
Gastrointestinal	• Decreased intestinal motility • Decreased production of gastric acids and pancreatic enzymes • Decreased nutrient absorption	• Provide frequent small meals
Hepatic	• Decreased gluconeogenesis and increased risk of hypoglycemia • Decreased protein synthesis • Decreased capacity to metabolize and excrete toxins	• Provide frequent small carbohydrate-rich meals • Limit protein intake to 1-2 g/d during stabilization • Decrease use of or decrease dose of hepatotoxic and hepatically metabolized drugs
Immunologic	• All aspects of immunity are impaired • Typical signs of infection are absent	• Provide broad-spectrum antibiotics during stabilization • Avoid sick contacts
Renal and electrolytes	• Increased intracellular sodium • Decreased intracellular potassium and magnesium • Decreased glomerular filtration rate • Decreased excretion of sodium, phosphorus, acids, and water	• Avoid excess sodium and water intake • Do not give more protein than needed to maintain tissues • Supplement potassium and magnesium

IV, intravenous.

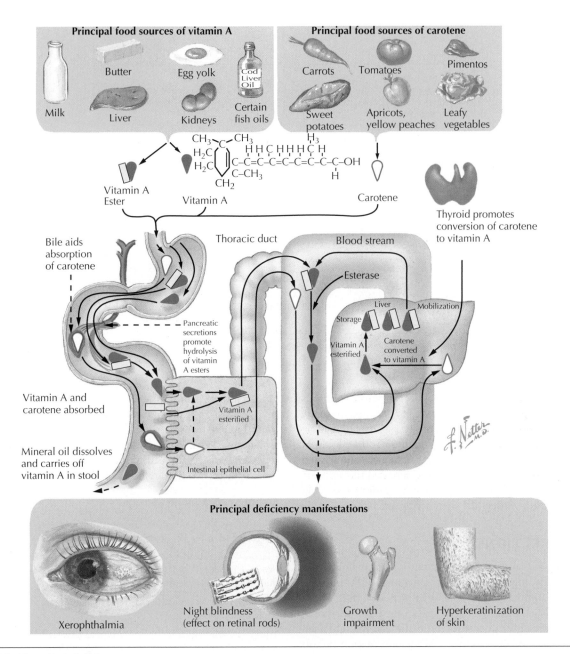

Figure 14-3 *Vitamin A deficiency.*

Studies have shown that a high percentage of severely malnourished children have bacterial infections when first admitted to hospitals. Empiric antibiotic treatment of presumed infection in a severely malnourished child has been shown to improve nutritional recovery, lower the incidence of septic shock, and reduce mortality. Clotrimoxazole (25 mg sulfamethoxazole + 5 mg trimethoprim/kg) given twice a day for 5 days is one recommended regimen for severely malnourished children without specific signs of infection.

Children with mild and moderate malnutrition can be treated starting at the rehabilitation phase. Non-edematous children should gain a minimum of 5 g/kg/d of body weight. During rehabilitation, careful attention should be given to assessing the family's food access, feeding strategies, and food choices. Attention must also be paid to malnourished children's psychological

and intellectual development; emotional and physical stimulation are essential. Successful management of malnourished children requires that both medical and psychosocial problems be recognized and corrected. Without correction of food access issues and behavioral problems, relapse is likely.

MANAGEMENT OF DEHYDRATION IN SEVERELY MALNOURISHED CHILDREN

Dehydration occurs commonly in severely malnourished children, and inappropriate management can be rapidly fatal. Intravenous fluids should be avoided except in cases of shock because of the increased risk of overhydration and heart failure in malnourished children. Children with severe malnutrition require low-sodium rehydration solutions with higher levels of

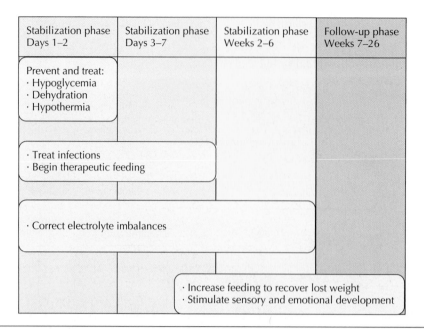

Figure 14-4 *Phases in management of acute severely malnourished children.*

potassium than typically found in oral rehydration solutions (ORS) used for well-nourished children. Use of a ready-made solution (ReSoMal) should be given orally (or via nasogastric tube) at a decreased rate for severely malnourished children. This rate is slower than what would be given to a well-nourished child because of the malnourished child's increased risk of heart failure from rapid fluid shifts. During rehydration, the child should be monitored closely for signs of cardiac failure.

FUTURE DIRECTIONS

Children younger than the age of 6 months with malnutrition are at particularly high risk of poor outcomes. HIV-infected children with malnutrition are likewise at increased risk. There is a lack of published information related to the best nutritional rehabilitation strategies for severely malnourished children younger than the age of 6 months. More information is also needed on the optimal treatment of severe malnutrition in HIV-infected children, including changes in antiretroviral drug dosing that may be prudent in severely malnourished children. Experts have hypothesized that severely malnourished children

younger than 6 months of age and those with HIV infection may have significant physiologic differences that would make them benefit from care that differs from that offered to older and non–HIV-infected children. Further research in the next few years is likely to lead to different recommendations for the care of these two particularly vulnerable groups.

SUGGESTED READINGS

Ashworth A: Efficacy and effectiveness of community-based treatment of severe malnutrition, *Food Nutr Bull* 27(3 suppl):S24-S48, 2006.

Chagan M, Berkley JA, Rollins N, et al; Blantyre Working Group: Case management of HIV-infected severely malnourished children: challenges in the area of highest prevalence, *Lancet* 371(9620):1305-1307, 2008.

Collins S, Dent N, Binns P, et al: Management of severe acute malnutrition in children, *Lancet* 368(9551):1992-2000, 2006.

World Health Organization: *Community-Based Management of Severe Acute Malnutrition*. Available at www.who.int/nutrition/publications/severemalnutrition/en/.

World Health Organization: Management of Severe Malnutrition: A manual for Physicians and Other Senior Health Workers, Geneva, 2009, WHO Library.

Obesity

Amanda Jones and Beth Rezet

15

Obesity is currently one of the most significant health problems in the United States, and the prevalence of this disease is increasing worldwide. A combination of metabolic, genetic, environmental, behavioral, and social factors affects a person's risk for developing obesity. As the epidemic of obesity increases, there is a concomitant increase in the comorbid diseases associated with obesity, such as diabetes, hypertension, dyslipidemia, nonalcoholic fatty liver disease, sleep apnea, and orthopedic problems.

It is estimated that approximately 15% of children in the United States meet the criteria for being obese. The prevalence of obesity is greatest in children of African-American, Native American, and Mexican American descent. Preventing and treating obesity involve balancing caloric intake with energy expenditure. This basic concept is increasingly difficult in our society given the availability of inexpensive, high-calorie foods and the relatively sedentary lifestyle of most children.

ETIOLOGY AND PATHOGENESIS

The causes of obesity are multifactorial, with both genetic and environmental influences playing roles in the balance between caloric intake and energy expenditure. Patients with at least one obese biologic parent have a threefold increased risk of developing obesity in their lifetime; having two obese biologic parents is associated with a 10-fold increased risk for developing obesity. Rarely, a genetic syndrome or endocrine disease contributes to the cause of a patient's obesity. Examples of these disorders include Prader-Willi syndrome, Cushing's disease, and hypothyroidism. Evaluation for these causes should be based on physical examination findings and history.

Clinical Presentation

The standardized measurement of weight appropriateness is the body mass index (BMI), which is validated in children older than 2 years of age. Before age 2 years, it is often useful to rely on a patient's weight-to-height measurement. In adults (age 18 years and older), the term *overweight* corresponds to a BMI of 25 to 30, and a BMI of 30 or greater correlates with obesity. Throughout childhood, there is an increase in both weight and height, and it is therefore necessary to refer to BMI percentiles, which are adjusted for age and gender:

- Healthy weight: 5% to 85% BMI for age and gender
- Overweight: 85% to 95% BMI for age and gender
- Obesity: >95% BMI for age and gender

BMI is calculated using a formula (weight (kg) ÷ [height (m)]^2) or by using a BMI calculator, such as that provided by the Centers for Disease Control and Prevention (http://www.cdc.gov/healthyweight/assessing/bmi/index.html.) BMI should be calculated and plotted on the appropriate standardized graph to ascertain the BMI percentile at every well-child visit.

The history and physical examination of an obese patient should focus on identifying the problem, treatment options, and comorbidities. To assess for a patient's risk for or diagnosis of obesity, one inquires about a patient's lifestyle, including a general assessment of the patient's dietary and eating habits, with particular attention placed on consumption of fruits and vegetables as well as high-calorie foods that are low in nutritional value, such as sweetened drinks, and an assessment of the patient's daily screen time (both television and video games) and physical activity. Family history should include any first-degree relatives with obesity or common comorbidities of obesity, such as hypertension, cardiovascular disease, diabetes, and liver disease.

Laboratory evaluation such as fasting glucose, liver enzymes (alanine aminotransferase [ALT], aspartate aminotransferase [AST]), and fasting lipids are used to screen patients for the common comorbidities associated with obesity. Additional tests should be ordered based on the history and physical examination (Table 15-1).

MANAGEMENT

Prevention

Pediatric prevention of obesity starts at birth, encouraging the current recommendation that infants be breastfed for at least the first 6 months of life. Helping parents to respond to satiety cues will encourage healthy eating habits. Early emphasis on healthy habits relating to food and physical activity allows parental control over some environmental factors. Establishing these habits early can lead to a lifelong preventive approach.

Treatment Options

BEHAVIORAL

The management of obesity requires a multidisciplinary approach and should involve the patient's family in all aspects of treatment planning. Research provides evidence that behavior modification is the most useful modality in the treatment of pediatric obesity. It is essential to use motivational interviewing and consider the readiness of the patient and his or her family in adopting the lifestyle changes necessary for management of obesity. Lifestyle interventions can focus on any or all areas of a child's life: home, school, and childcare settings (Figure 15-1).

Excessive television viewing has been linked with obesity. This is most likely to be a combination of the sedentary nature of passive viewing as well as the commercial advertising of high-calorie foods. Reducing the number of hours of screen time,

Table 15-1 Evaluation for Comorbidities Associated with Obesity

Comorbidity	Relevant History	Physical Examination Findings	Laboratory Findings
Prediabetes (laboratory screen, age 9 y)	Family history	Acanthosis nigricans	Fasting glucose, 100-125 mg/dL or random glucose, 140-199 mg/dL
Diabetes (laboratory screen, age 9 y)	Family history, polyuria, polydipsia	Acanthosis nigricans	Fasting glucose >126 mg/dL or random glucose >200 mg/dL
Hypertension	Family history		SBP or DBP >95% on three separate encounters
Dyslipidemia (laboratory screen age 9 y)	Family history (laboratory screen at age 2 y if positive)	Central fat distribution	Fasting LDL >110 mg/dL or fasting triglycerides >150 mg/dL or fasting HDL <40 mg/dL
NFLD (laboratory screen age 9 y)	May be asymptomatic or may have nonspecific complaints	RUQ pain, hepatomegaly	Elevated AST, ALT (twice normal)
Cholelithiasis	Abdominal pain, nausea, vomiting, fatty food intolerance	Epigastric or RUQ pain, jaundice	+Ultrasonography
Metabolic syndrome		Abdominal obesity (waist-to-hip ratio >0.9*)	See criteria for diabetes, hypertension and dyslipidemia
PCOS	Anovulation or irregular menstrual cycles	Hyperandrogenism (hirsutism, acne), acanthosis nigricans	Ultrasound demonstrating polycystic ovaries, elevated free testosterone level
Pseudotumor cerebri	Headache, vision loss	Papilledema	+MRI
Sleep apnea	Snoring, difficulty breathing during sleep, frequent awakenings, daytime sleepiness (may be manifested by behavioral problems)	Enlarged tonsils or adenoids	+Sleep study
SCFE	Pain in hips, knees, or both; limp	Limp, leg length discrepancy, bowing of the knees	+Radiography
Blount disease	Pain in hips, knees, or both; limp	Limp, leg length discrepancy, bowing of the knees	+Radiography
Depression	Social history (specifically inquire about teasing and bullying)		

*Adult data.

ALT, alanine aminotransferase; AST, aspartate aminotransferase; DBP, diastolic blood pressure; HDL, high-density lipoprotein; LDL, low-density lipoprotein; MRI, magnetic resonance imaging; NFLD, nonalcoholic fatty liver disease; PCOS, polycystic ovarian syndrome; RUQ, right upper quadrant; SCFE, slipped capital femoral epiphysis; SBP, systolic blood pressure.

including television, video games, texting and computers, may have a significant effect on lowering a child's risk of obesity.

The American Heart Association has published recommendations for diet and exercise for children age 2 years and older. These include a diet rich in fruits, vegetables, whole-grain breads, and cereals with only a limited amount of juices, sugar-sweetened beverages, and processed foods. Children can easily consume excess calories in the form of beverages, and it is therefore important to follow current recommendations that include limiting juice intake to 4 to 6 oz/d, to include three servings of milk (whole milk until 2 years of age and then skim or 1% thereafter), and to frequently offer water (after age 6 months). Additionally, it is suggested that parents concentrate on limiting portion sizes and refer to nutritional labels when serving and preparing meals (see Figure 15-1).

Many children eat at least one meal daily that is provided by school. Meals that are available through government-subsidized programs are subject to nutritional standards based on adequate daily caloric content and not necessarily on low sugar, low fat, or high fiber. Additionally, there are many other foods offered "a la carte" and through vending machines and snack bars in schools that are not as well controlled for nutritional content. Efforts have been made in recent years to enact nutritionally sound policies for both government subsidized meals and other foods offered during the school day.

For a number of reasons, over the past 30 to 40 years, schools have dramatically decreased their curriculum involving physical activity. Recent recommendations have included the addition of 60 minutes of vigorous physical activity in an average school day (see Figure 15-1).

PHARMACOLOGIC

Pharmacologic treatment of obesity could be considered as an adjunct to dietary and behavioral modifications in older children and youth. The medications approved for use in the pediatric population are orlistat and metformin, the latter of which is not specifically approved for the treatment of obesity.

Orlistat (Xenical) inhibits the absorption of fats by reversibly inhibiting gastric and pancreatic lipases. Adverse effects of Orlistat include abdominal discomfort and diarrhea. Metformin (Glucophage) is approved for use in type II diabetes, decreasing

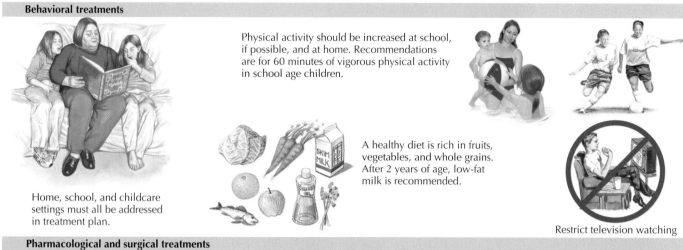

Behavioral treatments

Physical activity should be increased at school, if possible, and at home. Recommendations are for 60 minutes of vigorous physical activity in school age children.

Home, school, and childcare settings must all be addressed in treatment plan.

A healthy diet is rich in fruits, vegetables, and whole grains. After 2 years of age, low-fat milk is recommended.

Restrict television watching

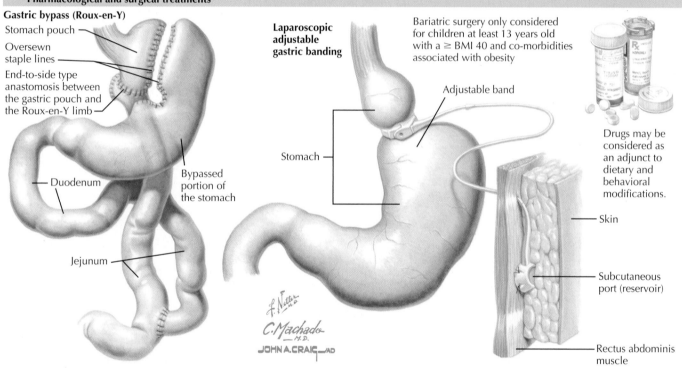

Pharmacological and surgical treatments

Gastric bypass (Roux-en-Y)

Stomach pouch

Oversewn staple lines

End-to-side type anastomosis between the gastric pouch and the Roux-en-Y limb

Duodenum

Bypassed portion of the stomach

Jejunum

Laparoscopic adjustable gastric banding

Bariatric surgery only considered for children at least 13 years old with a ≥ BMI 40 and co-morbidities associated with obesity

Adjustable band

Stomach

Drugs may be considered as an adjunct to dietary and behavioral modifications.

Skin

Subcutaneous port (reservoir)

Rectus abdominis muscle

Figure 15-1 *Treating obesity.*

endogenous glucose production and inducing peripheral insulin sensitivity. It may also be prescribed for the treatment of women with polycystic ovarian syndrome. Appetite suppressants such as amphetamines and antidepressants associated with appetite suppression are not currently approved for pediatric use.

SURGERY

The term *bariatric surgery* refers to various procedures that have been shown to produce long-term weight loss results and reduction in obesity-related comorbidities. It is an established treatment option for adults with morbid obesity, defined as BMI of 40 or greater. These procedures include those that induce a state of malabsorption and those that restrict a patient's intake by

decreasing stomach size. Currently, the two procedures offered in the pediatric population are gastric bypass with roux-en-Y anastomosis and gastric banding. Bariatric surgery is only considered for children at least 13 years old with BMIs of 40 or greater and comorbidities associated with obesity and for whom other treatment options have failed. It is also important that patients undergoing this form of treatment be committed to following strict nutritional guidelines and medical follow-up required after surgery.

FUTURE DIRECTIONS

There is a need for strong evidence-based recommendations in the prevention and treatment of pediatric obesity. It is clear that this will be multifactorial involving dietary, physical activity, environmental, and policy interventions with individual and community support for patients and families.

SUGGESTED READINGS

Baranowski T, Berkowitz R, et al. Working Group Report on Future Research Directions in Childhood Obesity Prevention and Treatment: Available at http://www.nhlbi.nih.gov/meetings/workshops/child-obesity/. Accessed National Heart, Lung and Blood Institute, National Institutes of Health, 2007.

Barlow SE, the Expert Committee: Expert Committee recommendations regarding the prevention, assessment, and treatment of child and adolescent overweight and obesity: summary report, *Pediatrics* 120(suppl):S164-S192, 2007.

Woodrow Wilson School of Public and International Affairs at Princeton University and the Brookings Institute: *Childhood Obesity, The Future of Children* 16(1), 2006. Princeton, NJ: Princeton University Press.

Nutritional Deficiencies

Amanda Jones and Beth Rezet

16

Assessment of a pediatric patient's nutritional status includes evaluation of the child's current and past medical problems, dietary intake, growth parameters, physical examination, and often laboratory tests. Establishing normal growth and development, prevention, and early identification of nutritional deficiencies is the goal in assessing a patient's nutritional status. When evaluating a patient for specific nutritional deficiencies, clinical findings as well as laboratory data may be helpful. Children with mild nutritional deficiencies often present with non-specific signs and symptoms that are discussed in Chapter 17. However, when severe deficiencies are present, the presentation will be more pronounced, as described in this chapter. Serum albumin can be used to determine long-term nutritional status, and serum prealbumin provides assessment of the adequacy of short-term dietary intake (see section on malnutrition for further information). A complete blood count (CBC) with red blood cell (RBC) indices can be used to identify deficiencies of iron, folate, vitamin B_{12}, and anemia of chronic disease. Laboratory assessment of fat-soluble vitamins (A, E, and D) is more easily measured than are water-soluble vitamins.

DEFICIENCIES

Iron

There has been a significant decrease in iron-deficiency anemia in the past 30 years as a direct result of universal screening guidelines as well as iron fortification of formulas and cereals. It is important for pediatricians to monitor their patients' iron intake because primary prevention is necessary to prevent irreversible mental, motor, and behavioral effects.

The greatest risk factor for the development of iron-deficiency anemia is the early introduction of cow's milk (before age 1 year) because of its low iron content and poor bioavailability. Nursing mothers should maintain an adequate source of their own dietary or supplemental iron. Breast milk has low iron content, but it is highly bioavailable. After 6 months of age, breastfed infants require iron-rich foods such as egg yolk, leafy green vegetables, proteins, or iron-fortified cereals. After the introduction of cow's milk at age 1 year it is important to limit intake to no more than 16 to 24 oz/d to prevent iron deficiency.

All infants can be screened for iron-deficiency anemia between 9 and 12 months of age by assessing dietary iron intake and with laboratory data. Although a hemoglobin value determines anemia, a CBC with RBC indices helps to delineate iron-deficiency from other anemias. One may choose to use an empiric treatment of iron-fortified vitamins when mild iron-deficiency anemia is suspected. Determining serum iron levels and total iron binding capacity will support the use of elemental iron treatment.

Iodine

Iodine is an essential component of thyroid hormone that is crucial for growth and development. Iodine is absorbed through the intestines in the form of iodide and is then taken up by the thyroid gland for incorporation into thyroxin (T4) and triiodothyronine (T3). Before the iodization of salt in 1920, iodine deficiency was endemic in the United States, and it is still the most common preventable cause of mental retardation worldwide. A deficiency of iodine is the most common cause of goiter, an enlargement of the thyroid gland, which, if large enough, may produce symptoms such as hoarseness or dysphagia as a result of local compression. Iodine deficiency and subsequent thyroid hormone deficiency can manifest with symptoms of hypothyroidism, such as weight gain, fatigue, and constipation. The most severe consequence of iodine deficiency is congenital hypothyroidism (mental retardation, deaf-mutism, gait abnormalities, and short stature), which can be prevented by adequate iodine intake both during pregnancy and early infancy (Figure 16-1).

Zinc

Zinc, an essential cofactor necessary for growth and development, is often available in adequate levels for full-term infants fed formula or who are breastfed by mothers who themselves have adequate zinc levels. Zinc deficiency is usually caused by intestinal loss from diarrhea or malabsorptive states but can also be caused by renal disease, malignancy, and skin conditions such as acrodermatitis enteropathica. The clinical diagnosis is supported by findings that include growth failure, dermatitis (an erythematous, scaly rash found on the face and perineal region), and impaired wound healing. Laboratory measurements of zinc are often unreliable because of fluctuations seen in various disease states.

Vitamin A

Vitamin A includes retinols, β-carotenes, and carotenoids. Retinols are the most bioactive form and are found in animal proteins. β-carotenes are derived from plants, such as spinach and other leafy greens. More than half of the vitamin A in the body is stored in the liver in a form bound to retinol-binding protein (RBP); the remaining vitamin A can be found in the kidneys, lungs, and adipose tissue and circulating in the blood. Vitamin A deficiency, although uncommon in the United States, may be caused by increased requirements; decreased intake (associated with poverty); or decreased intestinal absorption, including any process that decreases fat absorption such as bowel disease or cholestasis. Clinical findings associated with vitamin A deficiency most often involve the eyes and the skin. Ophthalmologic consequences include retinal pathology leading to blindness, Bitot spots caused by excessive keratin deposition in the superficial conjunctiva, xerophthalmia, and keratomalacia. Dermatologic manifestations include dry skin; pruritus; dry hair; dry, cracked fingernails; and follicular hyperkeratosis. Deficiency is also associated with anemia, impaired osteoclast activity, and immune dysfunction.

Types of congenital hypothyroidism

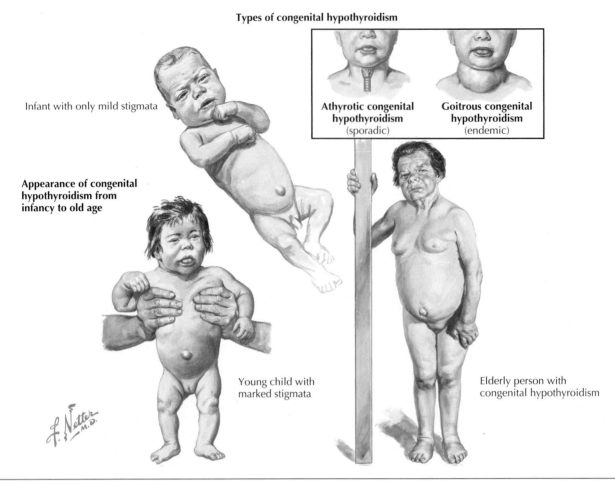

Infant with only mild stigmata

Appearance of congenital hypothyroidism from infancy to old age

Athyrotic congenital hypothyroidism (sporadic)

Goitrous congenital hypothyroidism (endemic)

Young child with marked stigmata

Elderly person with congenital hypothyroidism

Figure 16-1 *Congenital hypothyroidism.*

Vitamin B

The vitamin B complex includes eight water-soluble vitamins with distinct roles in cellular metabolism. Deficiency often arises from poor nutritional intake because there are minimal stores of vitamin B in the body. Nutritional sources of vitamin B include most animal products such as beef, poultry, fish, and eggs. It is important to note that vitamin B_{12} is not available through consumption of plants, and this should be considered when caring for patients on vegetarian and vegan diets.

The role of the vitamin B complex is varied but primarily affects the skin and muscle systems. Deficiency of vitamin B_1 (thiamine) causes beriberi, the symptoms of which include weight loss, extremity pain and weakness, emotional disturbances, and cardiac abnormalities (Figure 16-2). Korsakoff's syndrome, which is characterized by an irreversible psychosis, is a consequence of chronic thiamine deficiency. Lack of vitamin B_2 (riboflavin) is associated with dermatologic findings such as cheilosis, angular cheilitis, glossitis, and seborrheic dermatitis and with congenital abnormalities such as cleft lip and transverse limb deficiency. Vitamin B_3 (niacin) is a key component in required coenzymes in the body, and its deficiency may lead to pellagra, diarrhea, dermatitis, and dementia. The symptoms of vitamin B_5 (pantothenic acid) and vitamin B_6 (pyridoxine)

deficiencies include paresthesias, depression, and fatigue, although lack of these vitamins is uncommon. In infants, deficiency of pyridoxine may cause seizures that are refractory to antiepileptic drugs. Deficiency of vitamin B_7 (biotin) is rare and has been linked to growth impairment in infants.

Vitamin B_9 (folic acid) deficiency in pregnancy may lead to neural tube defects; deficiency in children and adults may lead to a macrocytic anemia. Humans do not produce folic acid and are therefore dependent on dietary sources, such as leafy greens and fortified breads, flours, and cereals. Folate deficiency may occur with chronic diarrhea, congenital malabsorptive states, and drug interactions. Diagnosis of deficiency can be determined by a serum folate level or a peripheral blood smear demonstrating hypersegmented neutrophils and macrocytes. Treatment for folic acid deficiency includes supplementation with 0.5 to 1 mg/d. Vitamin B_{12} (cobalamin) deficiency, which may be seen with gastrointestinal disorders, may lead to a megaloblastic anemia as well as cognitive difficulties. Deficiency is rare in infants because of large vitamin B_{12} stores but can be found in some inherited disorders of metabolism as well as in infants breastfed by mothers with vitamin B_{12} deficiencies. Diagnosis of deficiency is evident by a low vitamin B_{12} level. Treatment of vitamin B_{12} deficiency includes administration of doses of 50 to 100 mg via intramuscular injection.

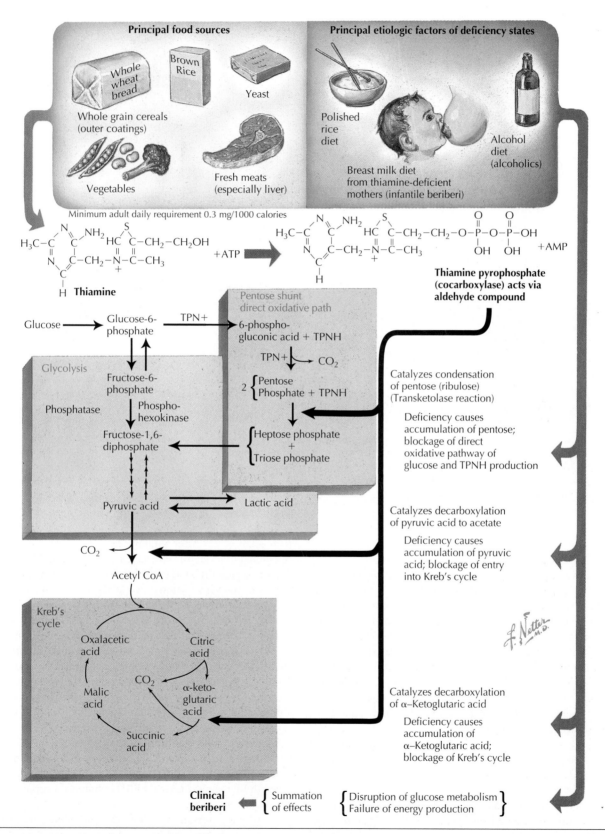

Figure 16-2 *Vitamin B (thiamine) deficiency (beriberi).*

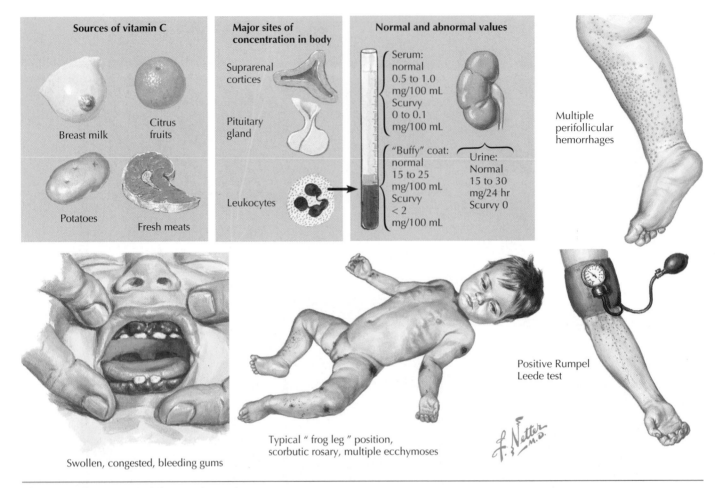

Figure 16-3 *Vitamin C deficiency (scurvy).*

Vitamin C

Vitamin C (ascorbic acid) is not synthesized by humans and therefore must be obtained through the diet in the form of fruits and vegetables. Vitamin C deficiency manifests as scurvy with symptoms such as gingival hemorrhages, petechial rash, and ecchymosis caused by defective collagen synthesis of blood vessel walls. Children with vitamin C deficiency may also present with bony tenderness, pseudoparalysis, and poor wound healing. Diagnosis of vitamin C deficiency can be made clinically by assessing physical signs and symptoms as well as characteristic radiologic findings, such as costochondral beading known as scorbutic rosary (Figure 16-3).

Vitamin D

Vitamin D plays a major role in bone mineralization by regulating the levels of calcium and phosphorus in the body through absorption in the intestines and reabsorption in the kidney. Whereas vitamin D_2 (ergocalciferol) is provided in the diet, vitamin D_3 (cholecalciferol) is produced in the skin when 7-dehydrocholesterol reacts with ultraviolet B (UVB) light. Foods naturally rich in vitamin D include eggs and fatty fishes, although foods such as milk, cereal, and bread are often fortified

with vitamin D. After vitamin D is produced in the skin or consumed in food, it is converted in the liver and kidney to 1,25 dihydroxyvitamin D $(1,25(OH)_2D)$, the physiologically active form of vitamin D known as calcitriol. Vitamin D deficiency may result from a lack of exposure to UVB radiation; inadequate intake; fat malabsorption; liver or kidney disease, which can impair its conversion to active metabolites; and rarely, genetic disorders. Deficiency is most commonly seen in breastfed infants with inadequate vitamin D supplementation. Dark-skinned children are at increased risk of vitamin D deficiency because increased amounts of melanin in the skin reduce the body's ability to produce endogenous vitamin D in response to sunlight exposure. American Academy of Pediatrics (AAP) guidelines published in 2008 recommend supplementation of 400 IU/day vitamin D for all infants. The AAP also recommends that older children and adolescents who do not obtain 400 IU/d through diet should take a 400-IU vitamin D supplement daily (Figure 16-4).

Deficiency results in disorders of bone mineralization, leading to rickets in children and osteomalacia in adults, as well as inadequate serum calcium and phosphorus concentrations. Clinical presentation of rickets may include bone abnormalities such as genu valgus and varus, craniotabes, and costochondral deformities (which produce the classic "rachitic rosary" on chest radiography).

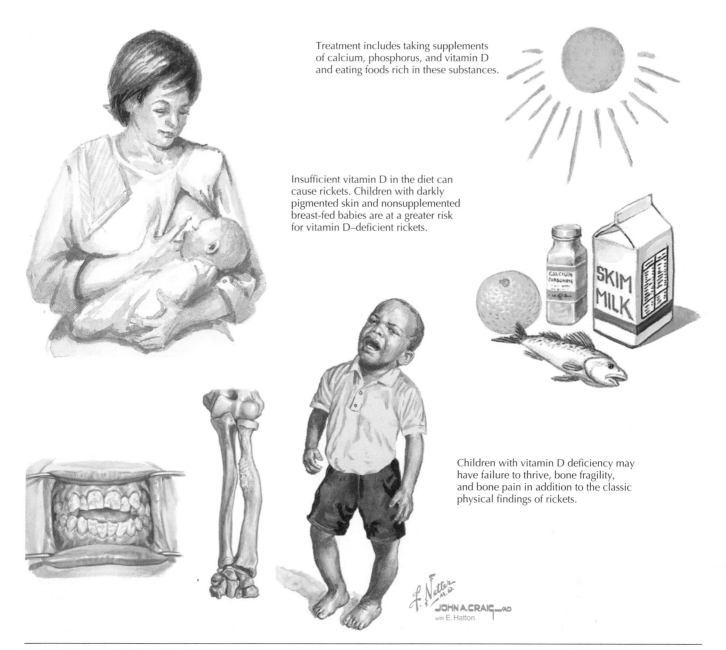

Treatment includes taking supplements of calcium, phosphorus, and vitamin D and eating foods rich in these substances.

Insufficient vitamin D in the diet can cause rickets. Children with darkly pigmented skin and nonsupplemented breast-fed babies are at a greater risk for vitamin D–deficient rickets.

Children with vitamin D deficiency may have failure to thrive, bone fragility, and bone pain in addition to the classic physical findings of rickets.

Figure 16-4 *Vitamin D deficiency.*

FUTURE DIRECTIONS

Research is continuing on the various roles of vitamin D, recommendations for vitamin D and calcium requirements, and prevention of deficiencies.

SUGGESTED READINGS

Black RE, Allen LH, Bhutta ZA, et al: Maternal and child undernutrition: global and regional exposures and health consequences, *Lancet* 371(9608):243-260, 2008.

Kleinman RE: *Pediatric Nutrition Handbook.* American Academy of Pediatrics Committee on Nutrition, 2004, Elk Grove Village, IL.

Misra M, Pacaud D, Petryk A, et al: Vitamin D deficiency in children and its management: review of current knowledge and recommendations, *Pediatrics* 122(2):398-417, 2008.

Failure to Thrive

17

Carrie Daymont and Beth Rezet

DEFINITION

Failure to thrive (FTT) is a growth deficit in infancy and early childhood. FTT is usually defined as both poor weight gain and low weight for age defined as falling below the 3rd or 5th percentile on a growth curve representative of the population. Poor weight gain can be defined as crossing two decreasing major percentile lines or a rate of weight gain that is less than 2 standard deviations below the mean for age (assessed using weight velocity curves). Weight is affected earlier and more severely than length in FTT.

ETIOLOGY AND PATHOGENESIS

FTT can arise from organic disease or nonorganic (psychosocial) factors and is very often multifactorial. The underlying cause of FTT in almost all cases is undernutrition.

Nonorganic Factors

Various psychosocial factors can lead to FTT. Child characteristics such as low appetite, food aversion, and oral-motor dysfunction make children susceptible to FTT and may interact with caregiver and social factors that exacerbate the problems. Many of the same psychosocial conditions that lead to FTT are also risk factors for obesity, suggesting that individual children respond to the same factors differently.

Although FTT can occur in children of all social classes, children living in poverty are disproportionately affected by FTT. Many children in the United States and other developed countries are "food insecure" and do not consistently have access to a minimally nutritious diet. This is particularly a problem in families that depend on the federal Women Infants and Children (WIC) program, which provides formula and food to supplement what a family is able to provide. Families may attempt to extend the supplement to supply all of an infant's nutritional needs not realizing the dangers of using a diluted baby formula that is prepared with additional water. Supplemental coupons from WIC or food stamps are not intended to supply all of a family's nutritional needs.

Even if a family is food secure, stressors associated with poverty can cause attachment problems, leading to difficulty in feeding for susceptible children. Families living in shelters or with many family members may have little control over when and where children are fed. Children whose temperaments and appetites require more routine or more frequent meals sometimes fail to thrive in these settings. Domestic violence can be associated with FTT through its detrimental effects on the caregiver, child, or both. Caregiver mental or physical illness, including postpartum depression (Figure 17-1), can also lead to disturbances of attachment. Children who are failing to thrive are at increased risk for abuse and neglect compared with the general population, but most experts believe that the majority of children with FTT are not abused or neglected (Figure 17-2). Some children in stressful living environments appear to have problems absorbing and using calories for growth because they grow poorly despite apparently adequate caloric intake and lack of organic causes for growth failure.

Cognitively impaired caregivers may prepare formula improperly or lack knowledge of an appropriate toddler diet. Some children prefer fruit juice or another single food over more nutrient-dense choices, and caregivers may not recognize this as a problem or be effective in encouraging children to eat a more balanced diet.

Caregiver health beliefs may also contribute to FTT. The influence of cultural expectations and norms, a parent's relationship with the medical system, and individual beliefs may result in a family's resistance to recognition of the problem or acceptance of intervention. Some caregivers may be so vigilant and concerned about nutrition and obesity that they may choose a restricted diet that is not appropriate for their child's age.

Organic Factors

Organic factors can cause FTT by decreasing intake, decreasing absorption, or increasing metabolic demands. For example, poor motor coordination can cause decreased intake; celiac disease can cause malabsorption, and heart failure can increase metabolic demands.

CLINICAL PRESENTATION

Patients may present throughout infancy and early childhood, although most cases of FTT start in the first year of life. Weight is generally affected earlier and more severely than length. Psychosocial dwarfism is a distinct problem that occurs in patients older than 3 years of age and primarily affects height. Waterlow's categorization of FTT as mild, moderate, and severe is determined by comparing a child's growth parameters with the median values for the child's age and height. Growth patterns demonstrating each of the three classes of FTT are shown in Figure 17-3.

Children who were born prematurely or with intrauterine growth retardation (IUGR) should be evaluated in the context of their gestational age and birth weight. Many children with prematurity and IUGR will catch up to their peers; however, if these children have not started to show significant catch-up growth in the first 6 months of life, they are unlikely to reach normal size. Children of short parents may be of low height and weight because of their genetic potential; however, the parents may have not reached their full genetic potential secondary to their own malnourishment as children.

Children with FTT generally have decreased height and weight in middle childhood compared with children who grew adequately during infancy. Long-term cognitive delays had been a concern for these children in the past, but recent

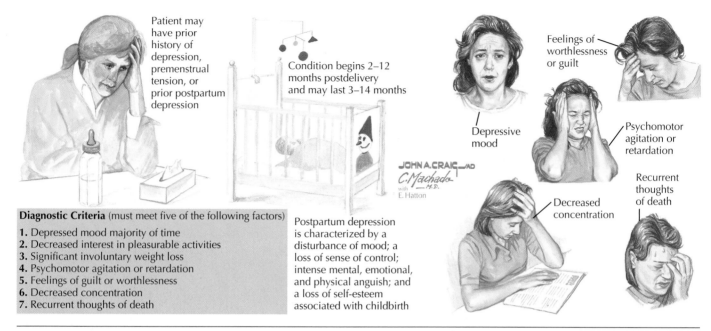

Patient may have prior history of depression, premenstrual tension, or prior postpartum depression

Condition begins 2–12 months postdelivery and may last 3–14 months

Feelings of worthlessness or guilt

Depressive mood

Psychomotor agitation or retardation

Recurrent thoughts of death

Decreased concentration

Diagnostic Criteria (must meet five of the following factors)
1. Depressed mood majority of time
2. Decreased interest in pleasurable activities
3. Significant involuntary weight loss
4. Psychomotor agitation or retardation
5. Feelings of guilt or worthlessness
6. Decreased concentration
7. Recurrent thoughts of death

Postpartum depression is characterized by a disturbance of mood; a loss of sense of control; intense mental, emotional, and physical anguish; and a loss of self-esteem associated with childbirth

Figure 17-1 *Postpartum depression.*

research using community-based, rather than hospital-based patient samples, shows no significant difference in IQ between children with a history of FTT and children with adequate growth.

DIFFERENTIAL DIAGNOSIS

The differential diagnosis for FTT is broad and often multifactorial. As already noted, many psychosocial stressors and many chronic medical conditions could contribute to FTT. A list of some conditions to consider in the differential diagnosis is presented in Box 17-1.

EVALUATION AND MANAGEMENT

Evaluation

DIET AND FEEDING

A 3-day diet history detailing the quantity and frequency of specific liquids and solids should be obtained. In infancy, evaluation of breast feeding includes observation of the nursing dyad, attention to proper latching and positioning, the duration and frequency of feeds, and assessment of maternal diet and medical history. For formula-fed infants, correct formula preparation in addition to the frequency and quantity of feeds should be addressed. Many foods, such as juice and typical snack foods, are calorie rich but not nutrient dense and can displace more nutritious food, leading to poor weight gain.

Assessing the feeding environment, including the child's behavior during feeding and the parents' response to the child as well as the location, timing, and consistency of feedings can provide insight in evaluating the cause of FTT. Discussing a child's response to food transitions and assessing differences in a child's food intake outside the home (e.g., at daycare) may provide direction for intervention.

PSYCHOSOCIAL FACTORS CONTRIBUTING TO FAILURE TO THRIVE

A culturally sensitive approach should be used when assessing issues such as food insecurity, domestic violence, caregiver physical and mental health, and family health beliefs. By first framing the relationship between possible stressors in the home environment and FTT, the provider allows for a more open and honest discussion of these issues. The provider can use tools from the validated assessment of household food insecurity and hunger

---

Box 17-1 Differential Diagnosis of Failure to Thrive: Conditions to Consider

Nonorganic or Psychosocial
- Child abuse
- Domestic abuse of caregiver
- Food insecurity
- Disturbed attachment
- Caregiver mental or physical illness
- Neglect of child
- Chaotic living situation (e.g., shelter)
- Caregiver health beliefs

Allergic
- Food allergy

Cardiovascular
- Congenital heart disease
- Cardiomyopathy

Endocrine
- Hypothyroidism

Gastrointestinal
- Celiac disease*
- Chronic diarrhea
- Gastroesophageal reflux

Genetic
- Prader-Willi syndrome (in infancy)
- Silver-Russell syndrome

Hematologic
- Schwachman-Diamond syndrome

Immunologic
- HIV*

Infectious Disease
- *Giardia**
- Urinary tract infection*

Metabolic
- Galactosemia

Neurologic
- Spinal muscular atrophy

Renal
- Renal tubular acidosis*

Respiratory
- Cystic fibrosis*
- Obstructive sleep apnea

*In persistent FTT, these conditions should be considered even in the absence of signs or symptoms.

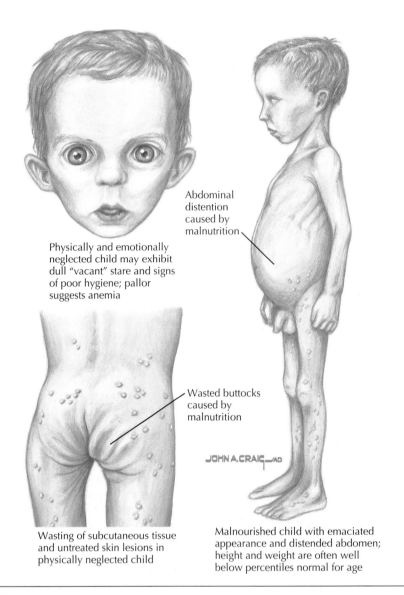

Physically and emotionally neglected child may exhibit dull "vacant" stare and signs of poor hygiene; pallor suggests anemia

Abdominal distention caused by malnutrition

Wasted buttocks caused by malnutrition

JOHN A. CRAIG—MD

Wasting of subcutaneous tissue and untreated skin lesions in physically neglected child

Malnourished child with emaciated appearance and distended abdomen; height and weight are often well below percentiles normal for age

Figure 17-2 *Signs of neglect.*

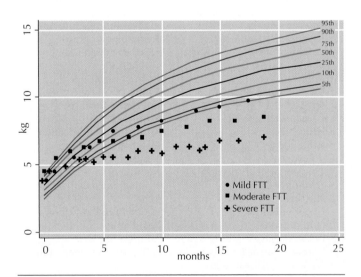

Figure 17-3 *Growth chart with points depicting growth patterns of mild, moderate, and severe failure to thrive.*

developed by Radimer by assessing responses to statements such as: "I wonder if my food is going to run out ?"

Psychosocial factors may be best assessed through observation of the adult–child interaction demonstrating possible attachment disturbances of a parent not responding to the cues of the child. Observation during a home visit by a clinician or health educator of both food preparation and feeding may be an effective method of ascertaining appropriate preparation, food refusal, and caregiver response. Food insecurity and other aspects of the home environment are also generally best assessed through a home visit.

ORGANIC CAUSES OF FAILURE TO THRIVE

Most organic causes of FTT can be detected through thorough histories and physical examinations without laboratory evaluation. The history should include a birth history and birth growth parameters as well as family history, including parental height. Symptoms such as diarrhea, vomiting, respiratory problems, or abnormalities on physical examination should prompt further evaluation. Subtle signs such as atopy may suggest possible food allergies and snoring or mouth breathing may be associated with obstructive sleep apnea. Recurrent infections may be a sign of an immune deficiency and should be evaluated further, but they may also be a sign of the decreased effectiveness of the immune system in a malnourished child. Some conditions can cause or contribute to FTT without apparent signs or symptoms, and if children have no apparent cause for FTT and are not adequately responding to treatment, consideration should be given to testing for those conditions listed in Box 17-1: HIV infection, cystic fibrosis, celiac disease, *Giardia* and urinary tract infections, and renal tubular acidosis, all of which may cause FTT without other symptoms.

In addition to performing a complete physical examination, a clinician should observe feeding to evaluate for problems with motor coordination leading to difficulty feeding.

ASSOCIATED CONDITIONS

Children with FTT are at increased risk for developmental problems from iron-deficiency anemia, rickets, and lead poisoning. Children with FTT should have an evaluation of a complete blood count and serum lead level and should be evaluated for rickets.

Management

Children with FTT require frequent follow-up to assess adequacy of weight gain and to assess for new signs or symptoms suggesting organic disease. FTT is often managed in a multidisciplinary outpatient setting that can address the complex factors leading to FTT. The staff may include a pediatrician, speech therapist, nutritionist, and social worker.

TREATMENT OF UNDERLYING CAUSE

When a specific underlying cause can be identified, treatment of that condition may be the only intervention necessary. There often is impressive catch-up growth after tonsillectomy and adenoidectomy for sleep apnea. Nonorganic causes can be more difficult to treat. However, advocating for children with FTT can lead to weight gain in certain circumstances. Children in families experiencing domestic violence can show dramatic catch-up growth when they are no longer living with the perpetrator or those living in a shelter may gain weight once in their own home.

TREATMENT OF FEEDING DIFFICULTIES

Caregivers should be counseled to provide food at consistent times, to sit and eat with their children, and to minimize distractions during mealtimes. For toddlers especially, caregivers must make sure that nutritious snacks are offered between meals because toddlers generally consume smaller meals more frequently than older children. Food refusal behaviors such as spitting and throwing food should be ignored. Children benefit from receiving lots of positive attention for accepting food.

Caregivers should be counseled to avoid providing juice and nutritionally deficient food because they can decrease children's appetite for nutritious food. Marketing, social norms, and individual beliefs can make it difficult for caregivers to appreciate the connection between excess juice intake and poor food intake. The intake of nutritionally dense foods, such as cheese and peanut butter, should be promoted. Foods can be made more nutritionally dense by adding protein powders or fats such as butter, cream, or mayonnaise.

SUPPLEMENTAL FEEDS

In early, mild FTT, providing high-calorie foods along with feeding guidance may be sufficient to increase caloric intake to the amount needed for catch-up growth. However, some children do not respond well to feeding interventions. Children may be able to increase intake to levels that are within the normal range for age but are not sufficient for catch-up growth. In these cases, supplemental feedings are needed so children can return to the normal weight range for their age. The benefits of supplemental feedings must be balanced with the risk that they may cause children to decrease their intake of foods and ultimately make it more difficult for them to eat a sufficient amount of typical foods. During infancy, increasing the caloric density of formula above 20 kcal/kg is an effective way of increasing calories without increasing volume. Precision and return demonstration of formula preparation are essential. When caloric density is increased above 24 kcal/kg in young infants, providers and caregivers should watch for signs of diarrhea or dehydration, which can occur with solute overload.

The use of prepared supplemental formulas with caloric densities of 30 kcal/kg can be helpful to increase daily calorie consumption in older children. In children with moderate or severe FTT who are not achieving catch-up growth with oral feeds, placement of a nasogastric tube and ultimately a gastrostomy tube may be necessary. For some children, tube feedings can interfere with oral feeding and cause significant stress for the family. Alternatively, providing calories through tube feedings may be positive for the family by decreasing the stress centered around feeding times.

HOSPITALIZATION

Most children with FTT, even those started on tube feedings, can be managed as outpatients. Children with severe FTT require hospitalization for initiation of supplemental feeds to ensure adequate weight gain and monitor for refeeding syndrome. Observation in the hospital may help identify problematic feeding behaviors, although demonstration of adequate weight gain in the hospital does not distinguish between organic and nonorganic causes of FTT.

SOCIAL SERVICES

There are several reasons to consider contacting social services in children with FTT. Evaluation for FTT may lead a clinician to suspect child abuse or neglect. Social services intervention may also be required when a child has persistent growth failure and caregivers have not followed through with recommendations for treatment or evaluation despite outreach from clinicians. Finally, in some communities, services such as home visits may only be available if social services are involved.

FUTURE DIRECTIONS

More research is needed to effectively treat and, ideally, prevent FTT. The effects of food insecurity on children and families is an active area of research. Longitudinal studies would help to determine the long-term outcomes in children with FTT. More research is also needed to demonstrate therapies that significantly improve long-term growth. Research and advocacy related to reducing the effects of poverty on children and the number of children living in poverty could prevent many cases of FTT.

SUGGESTED READINGS

Black MM, Dubowitz H, Krishnakumar A, et al: Early intervention and recovery among children with failure to thrive: follow-up at age 8, *Pediatrics* 120(1):59-69, 2007.

Kleinman R, editor: Failure to thrive. In *Pediatric Nutrition Handbook*, ed 6, Elk Grove, IL, 2009, American Academy of Pediatrics, pp 601-636.

Radimer KL, Olson CM, Green JC, et al: Understanding hunger and developing indicators to assess it in women and children, *J Nutr Educ* 24(suppl):36S-45S, 1992.

Zenel JA Jr: Failure to thrive: a general pediatrician's perspective, *Pediatr Rev* 18(11):371-378, 1997.

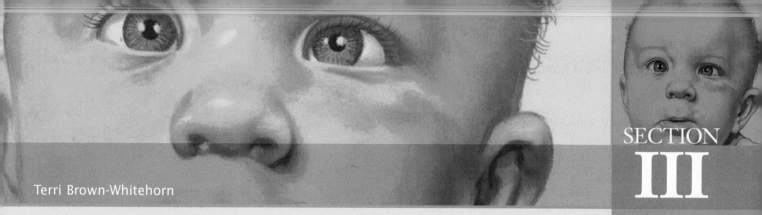

Terri Brown-Whitehorn

Allergy and Immunology

SECTION
III

Anaphylaxis

Jackie P. D. Garrett and Terri Brown-Whitehorn

18

Anaphylaxis is an acute, rapidly progressive, potentially life-threatening systemic allergic reaction. Traditionally, anaphylactic reactions were caused by an immunoglobulin E– (IgE-) mediated mechanism, and "anaphylactoid" reactions were caused by non-IgE mediated mechanisms. More recently, definitions have changed. Anaphylactic reactions are caused by *any* immune-mediated mechanism (IgE, IgG, or immune complex), and nonallergic anaphylaxis refers to nonimmune-mediated reactions. Regardless of the mechanism, the reactions are indistinguishable. Clinically, patients typically present with varying degrees of dermatologic (e.g., hives), respiratory (e.g., wheezing), gastrointestinal (e.g., vomiting), and circulatory (e.g., hypotension) manifestations. Reactions can range from mild to severe and may be fatal. The most common causes of anaphylaxis in the pediatric population include foods, drugs, venom, and latex. The true incidence of anaphylactic reactions is unknown because of underdiagnosis and underreporting. In the United States, the potential risk of anaphylaxis approximates 1% of the general population. Currently, it is approximated that the death rate of anaphylaxis is 1 to 3 per million people per year.

ETIOLOGY AND PATHOGENESIS

IgE-mediated anaphylaxis, a type I hypersensitivity reaction, is the most understood form of anaphylaxis (Figure 18-1). A person is exposed to an antigen, and upon reexposure, cross-linkage of IgE occurs followed by an immediate release of potent mediators from tissue mast cells and peripheral basophils. These mediators include histamine, leukotrienes, nitric oxide, and neutral proteases, which all lead to vasodilatation, increased vascular permeability, bronchoconstriction, and additional inflammation. At times, the reaction occurs with the first known exposure.

Other mechanisms include direct stimulation of mast cells and basophils, as is observed with morphine and exercise- and cold-induced anaphylaxis. Blood products and radiocontrast media may lead to activation of complement and subsequent reactions. Anaphylaxis to aspirin and nonsteroidal antiinflammatory drugs (NSAIDs) may result from the interference of the arachidonic acid pathway. Other agents may act through one or more of the above mechanisms.

The most common IgE-mediated reactions occur with food, drugs, venom, and latex. The leading cause of anaphylaxis in children is food. In the United States, the most common foods implicated in anaphylactic reactions include milk, eggs, soy, wheat, peanuts, tree nuts, and fish (although almost any food can cause a reaction). Children often develop tolerance and outgrow reactions to milk, egg, soy, and wheat; this is less likely to occur with peanuts, tree nuts, and fish. Drug allergy is another common cause of IgE-mediated anaphylaxis, with penicillin and other β-lactam antibiotics being the most commonly implicated agents. Other medications, such as aspirin and NSAIDs, may also lead to reactions. Fire ants and hymenoptera (e.g., honey

bees, yellow jackets, hornets, and wasps) are common causes of anaphylaxis in both children and adults. Children with spina bifida and health care workers are at higher risk for latex allergy. Although latex allergy had been on the rise, current use of latex precautions, latex-free gloves, and health care provider awareness have stabilized the incidence of latex reactions. There is also an entity known as exercise-induced anaphylaxis. Three groups of patients present with anaphylaxis after exercising: some of whom have known specific food triggers, others in whom any food ingestion may lead to symptoms, and a third group in which there is no known food trigger. Those with a food trigger have symptoms when they exercise within 4 hours of a meal. Other causes of anaphylaxis include immunizations, radio contrast material, blood products, allergy immunotherapy, and those that remain unknown (idiopathic).

CLINICAL PRESENTATION

Patients with anaphylaxis may have different clinical manifestations (Table 18-1). Anaphylaxis is often underdiagnosed or misdiagnosed because of clinicians' failure to recognize symptoms. There has been a recent attempt to standardize the diagnostic criteria to help clinicians to better recognize anaphylaxis (Box 18-1 and Figure 18-2). Approximately 90% of children with allergic reactions have skin manifestations, which include hives, angioedema (see Chapter 20, Figures 20-1 and 20-2), pruritus, or flushing. Although the remainder may not have skin involvement, they are still having a reaction, and that reaction may be more severe than those that occur with skin findings present. Tongue and throat swelling, dysphagia, and choking are manifestations of upper airway edema. Lower respiratory tract symptoms, such as coughing and wheezing, are the next most common symptoms. Vomiting, diarrhea, and abdominal pain are often seen, especially in food-induced anaphylaxis. Cardiovascular manifestations include tachycardia, hypotension, shock, and (rarely) bradycardia. Children may also be lethargic, and some have described a "feeling of impending doom."

Symptoms can develop within minutes of exposure, although most occur within 30 minutes to 1 hour. Most anaphylactic reactions are uniphasic in which the patient has a reaction, is treated, and improves. A biphasic response may also occur in which a patient becomes asymptomatic after the initial reaction and then develops a second reaction that may be the same or more severe than the initial reaction. Protracted anaphylaxis has also been described in which patients have symptoms that persist for days. Both biphasic and protracted reactions seem to occur less frequently in the pediatric population.

Differential Diagnosis

Given the involvement of multiple organ systems in anaphylaxis, many other life-threatening diagnoses can present similarly (Table 18-2). Vocal cord dysfunction presents with inspiratory

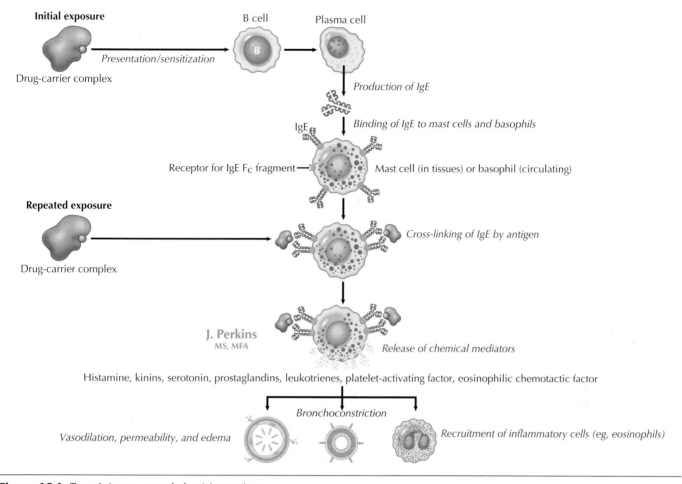

Initial exposure

Drug-carrier complex

Presentation/sensitization

B cell

Plasma cell

Production of IgE

IgE

Binding of IgE to mast cells and basophils

Receptor for IgE F$_C$ fragment —

Mast cell (in tissues) or basophil (circulating)

Repeated exposure

Drug-carrier complex

Cross-linking of IgE by antigen

J. Perkins
MS, MFA

Release of chemical mediators

Histamine, kinins, serotonin, prostaglandins, leukotrienes, platelet-activating factor, eosinophilic chemotactic factor

Bronchoconstriction

Vasodilation, permeability, and edema

Recruitment of inflammatory cells (eg, eosinophils)

Figure 18-1 *Type 1 (acute, anaphylactic) reactions.*

stridor and coughing. Wheezing and stridor are also signs of an airway foreign body, croup, bronchiolitis, or an asthma exacerbation. Patients complaining of oral pruritus after food ingestion may have an oral allergy. This is typically self-limited and does not progress to anaphylaxis. Circulatory failure in the form of hypotension, tachycardia, and poor peripheral perfusion may be indicative of a systemic inflammatory response or shock (see Chapter 2). Vasovagal reactions usually present with history of syncope (see Chapter 48). Although urticaria can be an early sign of anaphylaxis, it also is an isolated local cutaneous reaction or may be associated with underlying infection (see Chapter 20). Flushing may occur after ingestion of particular food products, including additives such as monosodium glutamate (MSG) and sulfites, which are found in smoked foods and preservatives. "Red man syndrome" occurs with the use of vancomycin, presents with flushing, and typically resolves with termination of the infusion. Other diagnoses that present with multisystemic involvement include panic attacks, capillary leak syndrome, hereditary angioedema, and systemic mastocytosis. A good history will help distinguish these diagnoses from anaphylactic reactions.

EVALUATION AND MANAGEMENT

The diagnosis and treatment of anaphylaxis are based on history of event, clinical manifestations, and examination. No diagnostic tests are available that will help to guide management in the immediate setting. However, some diagnostic tests such as serum histamine, urinary histamine, and serum tryptase can be helpful after the acute event (Table 18-3). If performed judiciously and expeditiously, these values can prove useful in supporting the clinical diagnosis of anaphylaxis. Serum histamine levels can be drawn if a patient presents within 1 hour of reaction. β-Tryptase levels are often recommended because they peak 60 to 90 minutes after an anaphylactic reaction and may remain elevated for 6 hours. Positive results are helpful, but a patient may still have had an anaphylactic reaction if results are negative.

After someone has a reaction, the cause is then pursued. Often, referral to a specialist is recommended. Knowledge of positive and negative predictive values and sensitivity and specificity of various tests is important. False-positive and false-negative testing can occur; therefore, *specific* skin prick testing and cap radioallergosorbent testing (RAST) is often useful to confirm one's suspicion (Figure 18-3). Of note, intradermal testing should *never* be used for food allergy testing. Intradermal tests are performed for allergies to pollens. The authors do not recommend broad panels of testing; however, if there is a suspicion for a specific food, then the clinician should test accordingly.

Management

For patients who have already had an anaphylactic reaction, prevention of future reactions is of highest priority. Ideally,

Table 18-1 Signs and Symptoms of Anaphylactic Reactions

Systems	Signs and Symptoms
Cutaneous	Angioedema
	Conjunctival erythema
	Edema or pruritus of mouth
	Flushing
	Periorbital edema and erythema
	Periorbital pruritus
	Urticaria
Respiratory	***Upper Respiratory***
	Dysphagia
	Dysphonia
	Hoarseness
	Nasal congestion
	Pruritus of nose, throat, or both
	Pruritus of external auditory canals
	Rhinorrhea
	Sneezing
	Stridor
	Throat tightness
	Lower Respiratory
	Bronchospasm
	Coughing
	Chest tightness
	Dyspnea
	Shortness of breath
	Wheezing
Cardiovascular	Arrhythmia
	Chest pain
	Hypotension
	Syncope
	Tachycardia
Gastrointestinal	Abdominal pain
	Diarrhea
	Nausea
	Vomiting
Neurologic	Altered mental status
	Headache
	Hypotonia
	Sense of impending doom

Box 18-1 Proposed Diagnostic Criteria for Classic Anaphylaxis

Need Any One of Three Criteria to Qualify As Anaphylaxis

1. Acute onset of an illness (minutes to hours) with involvement of
   Skin mucosal tissue (e.g., hives; generalized itch or flush; swollen lips, tongue, or uvula)
   and
   Airway compromise (e.g., dyspnea, wheeze or bronchospasm, stridor, reduced PEF)
   or
   Hypotension or associated symptoms (e.g., hypotonia, syncope)
2. Two or more of the following after exposure to known allergen for that patient (minutes to hours)
   a. History of severe allergic reaction
   b. Skin or mucosal tissue involvement
   c. Airway compromise
   d. Hypotension or associated symptoms
   e. In suspected food allergy: gastrointestinal symptoms (e.g., abdominal pain, vomiting)
3. Hypotension after exposure to known allergen for that patient (minutes to hours)
   Infants and children: low SBP (age specific) or >30% decrease in SBP*
   Adults: SBP ,100 mm Hg or >30% decrease from baseline

*Low systolic BP for children is defined as <70 mm Hg from 1 month to 1 year; <70 mm Hg + (2× age) from 1 to 10 years; and <90 mm Hg from age 11 to 17 years.
BP, blood pressure; PEF, peak expiratory flow.
From Sampson HA, Munoz-Furlong A, Bock SA, et al: Symposium of the definition and management of anaphylaxis: summary report. J Allergy Clin Immunol 115:584-591, 2005.

EMERGENCY MANAGEMENT

Managing an anaphylactic reaction begins like any other emergent clinical scenario, with the assessment of airway, breathing, and circulation. Supplemental oxygen should be administered as needed, and the Trendelenburg position is recommended when possible. The treatment of choice in a patient with anaphylaxis is epinephrine (1:1000 solution) given in a dose of 0.01 mL/kg up to a maximum of 0.3 mL/dose for children and 0.5 mL/dose for adults. The dose should be given intramuscularly (IM) because absorption of epinephrine is faster if given IM compared with the subcutaneous route. Epinephrine can be readministered every 5 minutes with a maximum of three doses. Epinephrine infusions, along with other vasopressors such as dopamine, have been used in severe cases. An intravenous (IV) line must also be placed as soon as possible to aid with fluid replacement because patients with severe reactions, such as anaphylactic shock, may need rapid administration of large volumes of fluids.

Antihistamines, including H1 and H2 blockers, have been used for the treatment of anaphylaxis. Medications such as diphenhydramine (1-2 mg/kg; maximum, 50 mg) can be given orally or IV depending on the severity of the reaction. H2 blockers, such as ranitidine (1 mg/kg; max IV, 50 mg/dose; max PO, 150 mg/dose), have been used in combination with H1 blockers in the most severe cases. For those with history of asthma or who

avoidance of the inciting agent is the best prevention. However, accidental exposures may occur, so knowledge of appropriate management of allergic reactions is essential. An anaphylaxis management plan should be developed for each patient with a known anaphylactic history and should contain the following: name of patient, known allergen, type of reaction, corresponding dose and type of medication for each clinical scenario, and when to seek additional medical care. For example, a child who has a known milk allergy accidentally drinks some milk and develops facial hives. Per his anaphylaxis management plan, he is given a proper dose of diphenhydramine for his weight with resolution. He may not need to seek immediate medical attention if the reaction does not progress. Another child who has the same allergy and same exposure may develop an immediate wheeze and angioedema. Because the reaction is more severe, this child would be given epinephrine, and emergency services (911) would be called. In all cases, the family would have access to the plan to help guide their decisions during an anaphylactic reaction.

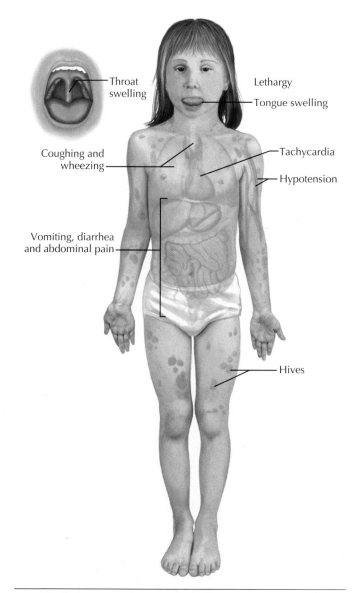

Figure 18-2 *Anaphylaxis.*

Table 18-2 Differential Diagnosis by Symptoms

System	Diagnosis
Circulatory	Shock
	SIRS
Cutaneous	Vasovagal reaction
	Carcinoid syndrome
	Monosodium glutamate ingestion
	Red man syndrome
	Scombroid fish poisoning
	Sulfite ingestion
Respiratory	Airway foreign body
	Asthma exacerbation
	Oral allergy
	Vocal cord dysfunction
Other/Mixed	Capillary leak syndrome
	Hereditary angioedema
	Munchausen syndrome
	Panic attack
	Systemic mastocytosis

SIRS, systemic inflammatory response syndrome.

radiograph contrast media, premedicating with corticosteroid and diphenhydramine is recommended. If one has a known reaction to a drug and there are no other alternatives, then a consultation with an allergist is warranted. Antibiotic desensitization protocols have been established and successful in many patients with IgE-mediated reactions. Of note, during the desensitization protocol, the patient remains at risk for anaphylaxis, and after a patient is desensitized to the antibiotic, he or she must stay on protocol. If that patient misses a dose, he or she may need to repeat the protocol again. Also, if the antibiotic is needed in the future, the protocol must be repeated again.

Patients taking β-blocker therapy present a special challenge to treatment of anaphylaxis. These patients may have reactions that are resistant to standard therapy for anaphylaxis. Hypotension and bradycardia are often difficult to treat. Glucagon is the drug of choice in these patients because it has both inotropic

have persistent wheezing despite epinephrine, β-2 adrenergic agents, such as albuterol, should be used. The exact role of corticosteroids in the management of anaphylaxis is unclear, but they may prevent or ameliorate the late phase reaction by acting on inflammatory mediators. There is also no recommended dose or drug of choice, but agents such as prednisone or prednisolone can be given orally (1-2 mg/kg; maximum 60 mg/day) or methylprednisolone can be given IV (1-2 mg/kg; maximum 125 mg).

HOSPITAL MANAGEMENT

Anaphylaxis in a hospitalized patient is treated the same way. The offending agent, if known and applicable (e.g., an antibiotic infusion), should be stopped. If the antigen has been injected, as with allergy immunotherapy, use of a tourniquet proximal to injection site is recommended. Care should be taken to release the tourniquet every 5 minutes, and it should be left no longer than 30 minutes. For patients with previous reaction to IV

Table 18-3 Laboratory Evaluation

Tests	Marker	Time
Histamine	Released by mast cells	Serum: within 1 hour of event
		Urine: methylhistamine can be collected up to 24 hours after event
Tryptase (although prefer beta tryptase)	Released by mast cells	Serum: within 6 hours of event (earlier the better)
Skin prick testing	IgE-mediated skin response to specific allergen (only test to a specific allergen)	After exposure (may need to perform 4 weeks after event)
Cap RAST	Measures IgE levels in patient's blood (only test to a specific allergen)	After exposure (may need to perform 4 weeks after event)

IgE, immunoglobulin E; RAST, radioallergosorbent test.

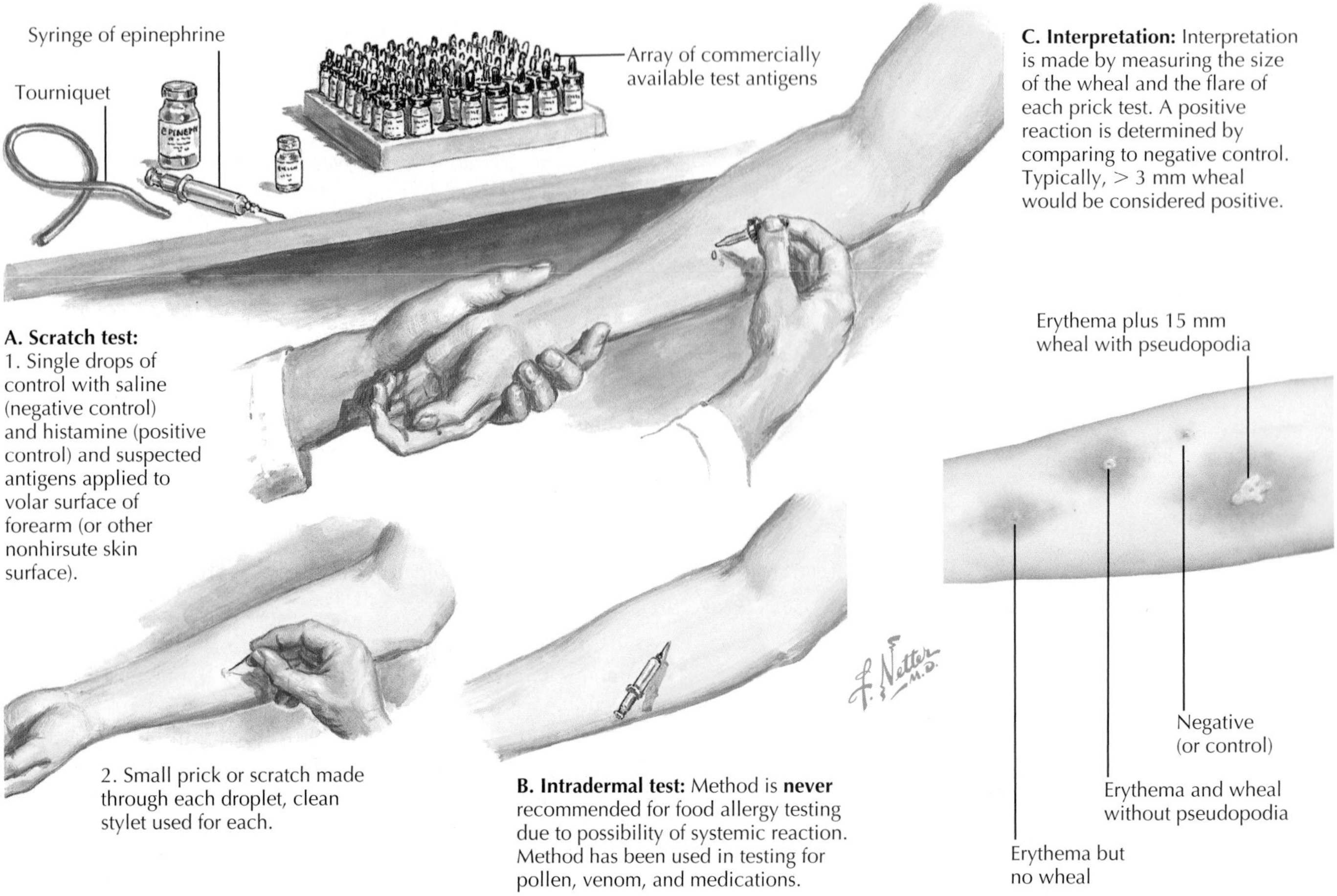

Syringe of epinephrine

Tourniquet

Array of commercially available test antigens

C. Interpretation: Interpretation is made by measuring the size of the wheal and the flare of each prick test. A positive reaction is determined by comparing to negative control. Typically, > 3 mm wheal would be considered positive.

Erythema plus 15 mm wheal with pseudopodia

A. Scratch test:
1. Single drops of control with saline (negative control) and histamine (positive control) and suspected antigens applied to volar surface of forearm (or other nonhirsute skin surface).

Negative (or control)

Erythema and wheal without pseudopodia

2. Small prick or scratch made through each droplet, clean stylet used for each.

B. Intradermal test: Method is **never** recommended for food allergy testing due to possibility of systemic reaction. Method has been used in testing for pollen, venom, and medications.

Erythema but no wheal

Figure 18-3 *Skin testing for allergy.*

and chronotropic effects on the heart. Atropine is useful only for patients with bradycardia.

DISPOSITION

There is no standardized observation period after an anaphylactic reaction. Not all patients with anaphylactic reactions require hospitalization. For more mild reactions, 8 hours of observation may be appropriate. Indications for inpatient care include patients with a moderate to severe reaction, such as respiratory or circulatory compromise at time of presentation, or wheezing with concomitant asthma.

OUTPATIENT MANAGEMENT

Avoidance, education, and an anaphylaxis plan are important aspects of management. Patients must understand their risk of future reactions. A referral to an allergist is recommended. In cases of venom allergy, immunotherapy is often beneficial. In cases of food allergy, label reading and avoidance are important. And finally, in cases of drug allergy, desensitization protocols may be helpful.

Upon discharge from an emergency department or inpatient unit, patients must be prescribed an epinephrine auto injector

(e.g., EpiPen). They must be trained in how and when to use their epinephrine auto injector. Patients and families should be instructed that after an epinephrine auto injector is used, they should proceed immediately to the hospital. The twin pack may be used to readminister epinephrine for the same exposure as they proceed to hospital. An anaphylaxis management plan is useful for the family and can be given to other family members, babysitters, and school nurses. A MedicAlert bracelet for certain types of anaphylaxis is helpful as well. When a history of anaphylaxis is elicited, it is important that a clinician ensure that patients have their epinephrine auto injector prescription renewed at appropriate times and with them at all times along with diphenhydramine.

FUTURE DIRECTIONS

Anaphylaxis is a medical emergency with a whole host of potential causes. We do not know why patients develop anaphylaxis, why some outgrow their allergies and others do not, or why some develop new reactions to things they once tolerated. This poses many questions and research opportunities for now and the future. Although the treatment of anaphylaxis is often successful, patients still die from anaphylaxis. Ways to improve awareness, prevention, and treatment are also of great importance.

SUGGESTED READINGS

Ellis AK, Day JH: Diagnosis and management of anaphylaxis, *Can Med Assoc J* 169(4):307-312, 2003.

Lieberman PL: Anaphylaxis. In Adkinson NF, Bocher BS, Busse WW, et al, editors: *Middleton's Allergy: Principles & Practice*, ed 7, 2009, pp 1027-1049.

Martelli A, Ghiglioni D, Sarratud T, et al: Anaphylaxis in the emergency department: a paediatric perspective, *Curr Opin Allergy Clin Immunol* 8(4):321-329, 2008.

Moneret-Vautrin DA, Morisset M, et al: Epidemiology of life-threatening and lethal anaphylaxis: a review, *Allergy* 60(4):443-451, 2005.

Neugut AI, Ghatak AT, Miller RL: Anaphylaxis in the United States: an investigation into its epidemiology, *Arch Intern Med.* 161(1):15-21, 2001.

Sampson HA, Munoz-Furlong A, Bock SA, et al: Symposium of the definition and management of anaphylaxis: summary report, *J Allergy Clin Immunol* 115:584-591, 2005.

Tang AW: A practical guide to anaphylaxis, *Am Fam Phys* 68:1325-1332, 1339-1340, 2003.

Atopic Dermatitis

19

Christopher P. Bonafide and Terri Brown-Whitehorn

Atopic dermatitis (AD) is a chronic inflammatory skin disease affecting 10% to 20% of children and accounting for approximately 1 million outpatient visits per year. More than half of patients affected present before 12 months of age with an itchy rash on the face and extremities. AD is often associated with asthma, allergic rhinitis, and food allergy. The natural history of atopic disease, progressing from AD to asthma and allergic rhinitis, is often referred to as the atopic march.

ETIOLOGY AND PATHOGENESIS

The chronic skin lesions of AD result from a complex interplay of genetic, immune, infectious, and environmental factors. In combination, these factors produce areas of persistently pruritic, inflamed skin that significantly impact the quality of life of patients. Immunologically, the systems affected most are the *epidermal barrier*, the first line of defense for the immune system, and the *humoral immune system*, which modulates the immune response to antigenic challenges by regulating antibody production.

The epidermis provides a critical barrier to keep infectious organisms, irritants, and allergens from entering the body. Genes encoding epithelial structural proteins have been strongly implicated in the pathogenesis of AD. Filaggrin is a key protein involved in keratinization that is encoded by a gene within the epidermal differentiation complex on chromosome 1q21. Defects in the gene encoding Filaggrin have been named as major causes of AD. Spink 5 is a protease inhibitor involved in intercellular attachment, which is also important in maintaining an intact epidermal barrier. It is deficient in Netherton's syndrome, a disorder that includes severe AD.

In addition to the genes encoding epidermal barrier components, genes encoding cytokines produced by type 1 and type 2 helper T cells have also been implicated in AD. These cytokines, including interleukins (ILs) 4, 5, 12, and 13 and granulocyte-macrophage colony-stimulating factor, are important in the regulation of immunoglobulin E (IgE) synthesis. IL-18, also implicated in AD, is involved in the switching between type 1 and type 2 helper T cell responses. Children with AD have an imbalance toward a type 2 helper T cell response, resulting in a switch in B cell antibody production toward an IgE response, contributing to the development of atopic disease.

A number of other factors are important in the pathogenesis of AD. Reduced levels of ceramide, lipid molecules that make up an important component of the epidermal barrier, contribute to the compromised epidermal barrier function. The barrier is further compromised by increased proteolytic enzyme activity via increased production and a decrease in endogenous protease inhibitors. External factors, including mechanical injury from scratching affected skin, proteases from bacteria and dust mites, and the use of pH-altering soaps also contribute to a weakened skin barrier, facilitating bacterial colonization and penetration of allergens. The combination of defects in the immune system, compromised skin barrier integrity, and external pathogens and irritants sets up the cycle of chronic inflammation characteristic of AD.

CLINICAL PRESENTATION

Most children with AD initially present at a very young age, with more than half presenting in the first year of life and more than two-thirds presenting before age 5 years.

History

The chief complaint of a "red, itchy rash" is common for children with AD. The child may have a pattern of similar episodes of skin eruption in a similar distribution in the past. Certain foods, clothing, soaps, lotions, or allergenic exposures (pollen, pets) exacerbate the rash of AD. There may be a history of other atopic diseases such as food allergy, asthma, or allergic rhinitis in the child or in the immediate family.

Physical Examination

Physical examination of acute AD lesions reveals red papules and plaques that may also feature scaling, oozing, and crusting. In addition to acute lesions, children and adolescents with chronic AD may also have areas of thickened, dark skin (lichenification) at sites of prior acute lesions. The distribution of the rash is characteristic and varies by age. In infants, the cheeks, scalp, wrists, and extensor surfaces of the arms and legs are most affected (Figure 19-1). The diaper area is typically spared. The perioral and perinasal areas are rarely involved, leading to the characteristic "headlight sign" of pallor in these areas. In children and adolescents, the neck, hands, and flexor surfaces of the upper and lower extremities are more commonly affected (Figure 19-2).

Complications

The defects in the epithelial barrier leave the skin susceptible to invasion by viruses and bacteria. Two common secondary infections include superinfection with *Staphylococcus aureus* and eczema herpeticum.

STAPHYLOCOCCUS AUREUS SUPERINFECTION

The skin of most individuals with AD is colonized with *S. aureus*. Regions of the skin affected by AD are susceptible to bacterial invasion of the skin and subcutaneous soft tissues, resulting in superinfection. A local inflammatory response results with subsequent pain, erythema, edema, and warmth at the site. Serous drainage, crusting, and lymphadenopathy may be present. Fever and an elevated white blood cell count may occur if the lesions are extensive or if the bacteria have invaded the bloodstream. Surface cultures with antibiotic sensitivities should be considered to help guide appropriate therapy.

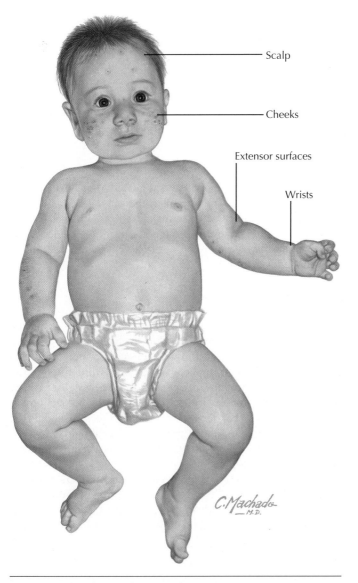

Figure 19-1 *Infant with atopic dermatitis.*

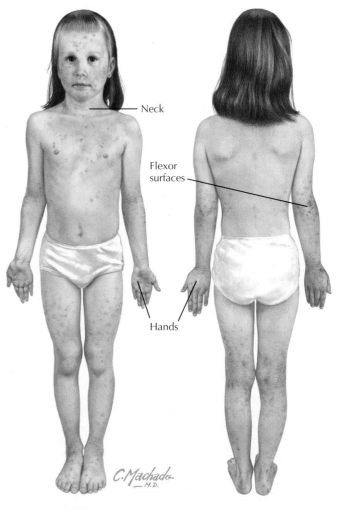

Figure 19-2 *Child with atopic dermatitis.*

ECZEMA HERPETICUM

Secondary infection with herpes simplex virus (HSV) is a potentially life-threatening complication that may affect children with AD of all ages. Vesicular lesions typically appear in groups superimposed on areas of skin affected by AD between 2 days and 2 weeks after exposure to HSV-1 or HSV-2. The lesions evolve to appear as "punched-out" hemorrhagic lesions with crusting (Figure 19-3). Associated symptoms may include fever, fatigue, and lymphadenopathy. Diagnosis may be made by Tzanck prep, direct fluorescent antibody, polymerase chain reaction, or viral culture from swabs of the affected area.

EVALUATION AND MANAGEMENT

Laboratory Testing

There are no laboratory studies essential in the diagnosis of AD. If checked for other reasons, a white blood cell count with differential may reveal an eosinophilia; a serum IgE may be

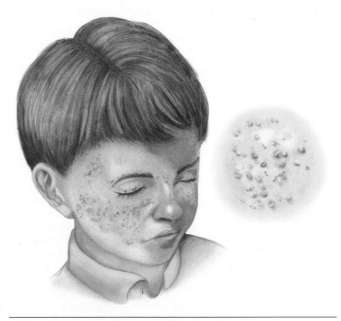

Figure 19-3 *Eczema herpeticum.*

Box 19-1 Hanifin and Rajka Diagnostic Criteria for Atopic Dermatitis

Major Criteria (At Least Three):
1. Pruritus
2. Dermatitis in a distribution characteristic for age
   a. Infants: face and extensor surfaces
   b. Older children and adolescents: flexor surfaces
3. Chronic or relapsing course of dermatitis
4. Personal or family history of asthma, allergic rhinitis, or AD

Minor Criteria (At Least Three):
1. Early age of onset
2. Xerosis
3. Cheilitis
4. Perifollicular accentuation
5. Facial pallor or erythema
6. Ichthyosis, keratosis pilaris, or palmar hyperlinearity
7. Hand and foot dermatitis
8. Nipple dermatitis
9. Pityriasis alba
10. Accentuated infraorbital folds (Dennie-Morgan lines)
11. Infraorbital darkening
12. Cataracts (anterior subcapsular)
13. Recurrent conjunctivitis
14. Keratoconus
15. White dermographism
16. Anterior neck folds
17. Susceptibility to skin Infections (*Staphylococcus aureus*, herpes simplex virus)
18. Sensitivity to emotional factors
19. Intolerance to certain foods
20. Exacerbation of pruritus or dermatitis with sweating
21. Exacerbation of pruritus or dermatitis when wearing wool
22. Immediate (type 1) skin test reactivity
23. Elevated IgE level

From Hanifen JM, Rajka G: Diagnostic features of atopic dermatitis, Acta Derm Venerol (Stockh) 92(suppl 92):44-47, 1980.
AD, atopic dermatitis; IgE, immunoglobulin E.

elevated. In severe or refractory cases of AD, an evaluation by a pediatric allergist with skin testing (see Figure 18-3) or IgE assays for specific allergens (also known as radioallergosorbent testing [RAST]) may aid in identifying triggers that should be avoided. RAST results should be interpreted with caution because the assays often have high false-positive rates, and in the case of food allergens, subsequent elimination of foods, such as milk or eggs, poses nutritional risks.

Diagnosis

Hanifin and Rajka developed and validated a set of diagnostic criteria for AD in 1980 that remain the standard. Diagnosis is based on the presence of three major and three minor criteria (Box 19-1). The differential diagnosis of AD includes other primarily dermatologic diseases as well as systemic disease and immunodeficiency (Table 19-1).

Approach to Therapy

The foundation of AD management includes moisturizing the skin and reducing inflammation. Moisturizing is best achieved using topical emollients with low alcohol and water content to reduce stinging when applied and drying with evaporation. Applying an effective moisturizer such as Aquaphor, Eucerin, or petroleum jelly at least twice per day helps to reduce the xerosis and heal the skin barrier. After bathing, the skin should be patted dry rather than rubbed, and moisturizer should be applied to seal in moisture. Emollients should be applied 30 minutes after any topical medications.

The first-line therapy for reducing the inflammation associated with AD is topical corticosteroids. Ointments contain less alcohol than creams and are generally preferred because of better skin penetration, although older children and adolescents may prefer creams because of their less greasy feeling. These

Table 19-1 Differential Diagnosis of Atopic Dermatitis

Diagnosis	Differentiating features
Contact dermatitis	History of contact with an allergen
	Distribution of eruption (exposed extremities for poison ivy, site of contact with button of pants for nickel)
Seborrheic dermatitis	Nonpruritic
	Salmon colored, "greasy" appearance
Nummular eczema	Discrete round areas of erythema, scaling, and lichenification
Keratosis pilaris	Appearance of "goosebumps"
	Noninflammatory follicular papules
Psoriasis	Discrete plaques with well-defined irregular borders
	Thick scaling
	Nail involvement
Acrodermatitis enteropathica	U-shaped perioral rash with extremity and perineal involvement
	History of failed treatment for presumed fungal diaper dermatitis
	Associated with chronic diarrhea, growth delay, hair loss
Wiskott-Aldrich syndrome	T-cell immunodeficiency with severe AD, thrombocytopenia, and recurrent infections
Severe combined immunodeficiency	Combined (B and T cell) immunodeficiency with severe AD, diarrhea, failure to thrive, and life-threatening infections
Netherton syndrome	Disorder characterized by ichthyosis in the first 10 days of life, hair shaft abnormalities leading to easy breakage, and AD and other allergic disease
	Mental retardation may also be present

AD, atopic dermatitis.

Box 19-2 Consider Referral to a Pediatric Dermatologist or Allergist for Children Who:

- Are refractory to topical therapy
- Experience frequent flares
- Experience recurrent infections
- Require hospitalization for atopic dermatitis treatment
- Have associated symptoms that suggest systemic disease

agents are available in a wide range of potencies. Maintenance therapy is typically initiated using a low-potency corticosteroid with a low likelihood of side effects, such as hydrocortisone 1% or 2.5%. Use of medium-potency agents such as fluocinolone 0.025% or triamcinolone 0.1%, or high-potency agents such as fluocinonide 0.05% may be used for short periods of time to treat severe flares but should not be used on the face or groin. Higher-potency agents are more commonly associated with side effects, including skin atrophy, striae, telangiectasias, hypopigmentation, and hypothalamic–pituitary–adrenal axis suppression. Side effects are more likely to occur when these agents are applied to thin skin such as on the face, neck, or groin. For severe flares not controlled by topical therapy, a short course of systemic corticosteroids may be effective. Referral to an AD expert should be considered for children whose AD management is challenging (Box 19-2).

TOPICAL CALCINEURIN INHIBITORS

Topical calcineurin inhibitors (TCIs) are nonsteroidal agents that are considered second-line therapy to reduce the inflammation associated with AD. Examples include tacrolimus ointment and pimecrolimus cream. They can be applied to any body surface and do not have the same side-effect profile as the topical corticosteroids. The Food and Drug Administration issued a black box warning for these medications in 2006 because of concerns that the long-term safety of TCIs had not been established, and very limited data showed an increased incidence of lymphoma and skin cancers with high doses of TCIs. Despite the warning, TCIs remain a valuable treatment option for short-term use in children older than 2 years old.

ADDITIONAL PHARMACOLOGIC THERAPIES

Symptomatic therapy for nighttime pruritus can provide significant improvements in sleep and quality of life for children with AD. Sedating antihistamines, such as diphenhydramine and hydroxyzine, can be helpful for children with acute flares. Nonsedating antihistamines, such as cetirizine, loratadine, and fexofenadine, are often used to help manage the pruritus the children experience day to day. Children with severe AD and pruritus may benefit from the nighttime use of the tricyclic antidepressant doxepin, which has antihistamine activity in addition to its anxiolytic and sedative properties.

NONPHARMACOLOGIC INTERVENTIONS

Educating the patient and family about AD management is essential in the care of children with this chronic disease.

Patients with AD and their families should be encouraged to avoid known triggers for their AD flares. These triggers may include personal hygiene products, such as bath soaps, baby wash, and deodorant; certain fabrics such as wool; and food allergens, such as milk, eggs, peanuts, and shellfish. Environmental allergens, such as dust, pets, and pollens, often play a role in AD. In cases of AD in which allergies are suspected to be contributing to the illness, an evaluation by a pediatric allergist can be very helpful in identifying specific triggers to avoid. Probiotics and herbal supplements have been studied in the treatment of AD and are currently not considered effective treatment options.

Prevention of Atopic Dermatitis in Infants

In infants, exclusive breastfeeding for the first 4 months of life has been shown to decrease the cumulative incidence of AD at 2 years of age compared with feeding with cow's milk formula. There is no substantial evidence that supports delaying solid food introduction (including potential allergens such as cow's milk, fish, and eggs unless the child has a suspected allergy) beyond 4 to 6 months of age as a means of preventing the development of AD.

Treatment of Complications

Treatment of *S. aureus* superinfection can usually be successful on an outpatient basis using oral antibiotics active against *S. aureus*, with consideration of antibiotics active against methicillin-resistant *S. aureus* (MRSA) as first-line therapy based on local resistance patterns. Small areas may respond to topical mupirocin alone. Hospitalization should be considered in young infants, those with severe disease, and children with signs of systemic illness. Ongoing therapy of the AD with moisturizers and topical steroids should be continued in children with bacterial superinfections.

Children with eczema herpeticum should be treated with acyclovir. Topical corticosteroids and TCIs should be discontinued during the acute phase of illness. Hospitalization and intravenous administration of acyclovir may be necessary in severe or disseminated cases. Ophthalmologic consultation should be considered to evaluate for herpetic keratoconjunctivitis.

TREATMENT OF *STAPHYLOCOCCUS AUREUS* SKIN COLONIZATION

Patients with AD have a high prevalence of *S. aureus* skin colonization compared with the general population. As previously discussed, this colonization can lead to secondary infection. In addition, it has been suggested that *S. aureus* eradication may improve AD disease severity independent of secondary infections, but the data are conflicting on this topic. One approach to reducing the skin burden of *S. aureus* has been with topical therapy with mupirocin. Adjunctive therapy using dilute bleach baths (one-half of a cup of bleach in a bathtub filled with water is an example of one regimen) and intranasal administration of mupirocin ointment has the potential to reduce the skin burden of *S. aureus*, decreasing the likelihood of secondary infection and reducing AD severity. A regimen of long-term bleach bath therapy and mupirocin has been shown to reduce the severity of AD in children with active signs of secondary infection.

FUTURE DIRECTIONS

Our understanding of the pathogenesis of AD is improving rapidly. The Filaggrin and Spink 5 genes, critical in the development of an intact epithelial barrier, and the proteins they encode are examples of potential targets for AD therapy. In addition, our understanding of the altered immune response in AD may provide additional opportunities for novel therapies to reduce the burden of this disease.

SUGGESTED READINGS

Bieber T: Atopic dermatitis, *N Engl J Med* 358(14):1483-1494, 2008.

Hanifen JM, Rajka G: Diagnostic features of atopic dermatitis, *Acta Derm Venerol (Stockh)* 92(suppl 92):44-47, 1980.

Krakowski AC, Eichenfield LF, Dohil MA: Management of atopic dermatitis in the pediatric population, *Pediatrics* 122(4):812-824, 2008.

Palmer CNA, Irvine AD, Terron-Kwiatkowski A, et al: Common loss-of-function variants of the epidermal barrier protein filaggrin are a major predisposing factor for atopic dermatitis, *Nat Genet* 38(4):441-446, 2006.

Zutavern A, Brockow I, Schaaf B, et al: Timing of solid food introduction in relation to atopic dermatitis and atopic sensitization: results from a prospective birth cohort study, *Pediatrics* 117(2):401-411, 2006.

Urticaria and Angioedema

Laura Gober and Terri Brown-Whitehorn

20

Urticaria, or hives, is a pruritic and episodic rash that most commonly occurs without an identifiable trigger. It occurs in approximately 25% of the population. The occurrence of urticaria increases to 50% in those affected by allergic disorders, such as asthma, allergic rhinitis, or atopic dermatitis. Acute urticaria, defined as symptoms lasting less than 6 weeks, accounts for two-thirds of all urticaria. Chronic urticaria, which can be subdivided into chronic idiopathic urticaria (CIU) and physical urticaria, is classified by symptom duration of greater than 6 weeks with symptoms on at least 2 days per week. CIU occurs in approximately 0.1% to 3% of the population and is more prevalent in females. Features of physical urticarias can be common, especially dermatographism, which occurs in almost half of the general population, including those with no history of chronic urticaria.

Chronic urticaria can have a significant social and financial impact. The hallmark of urticaria is pruritus, which contributes to difficulty sleeping and in activities of daily life. Urticaria can be a frustrating disease for patients because typically there is no identifiable trigger for exacerbations, leading to an unpredictable course. The effect on quality of life is comparable to that of coronary heart disease and atopic dermatitis. Patients with chronic urticaria also have multiple medications, medical visits, work and school absences, and use of the emergency department, all of which contribute to the economic burden of the disease.

ETIOLOGY AND PATHOGENESIS

Urticaria is characterized by the waxing and waning appearance of pruritic, erythematous papules or plaques with superficial swelling of the dermis (Figure 20-1). The swelling observed with urticaria and angioedema results from the movement of plasma from small blood vessels into adjacent connective tissue. Unlike atopic dermatitis, the pruritus of urticaria is driven by histamine. Histologically, urticarial lesions consist of a lymphocyte-predominant perivascular infiltrate. In CIU, the cellular infiltrate is similar to that seen in allergen-induced late phase skin response, and the cytokine profile is both T_H1 and T_H2.

Acute Urticaria

There is no identifiable trigger in more than 50% of cases of acute urticaria. Viral infections are the most common cause in children. Hives typically occur a few days after the start of viral symptoms. In regards to other potential triggers, urticaria should be classified as allergic or nonallergic. Allergic, or IgE-mediated, urticaria can be attributed to food, drug, or insect allergies. Unlike in adults, in whom less than 1% of acute urticaria is thought to be caused by food allergy, food allergy needs to be considered in children because it is a more common cause of acute urticaria. Nonallergic, or non–IgE-mediated, urticaria may be attributed to an immune response, such as in serum sickness, or to pseudoallergens, such as aspirin and other

salicylates. Vasoactive amines found in cheeses, beer, and wine can also elicit urticaria. In general, IgE-mediated food allergies, specifically to milk, wheat, egg, soy, and nuts, are more common than non–IgE-mediated food-induced hives.

Chronic Idiopathic Urticaria

CIU, as the name implies, typically lacks an identifiable, consistent trigger. The episodic onset of disease is more commonly observed in adults than children. The disease duration is on average 3 to 5 years, with greater duration if severe disease, angioedema, or autoimmune features are present. The pathogenesis of CIU is still unknown, although autoantibodies and cells typically involved in IgE-mediated reactions, such as mast cells and basophils, have been implicated. About 30% to 40% of patients with CIU are classified as having autoimmune urticaria, a subgroup of CIU defined by the presence of histamine-releasing autoantibodies. The majority of these autoantibodies are directed against the α subunit of the high-affinity receptor, FcεRI; the remainder target IgE. These autoantibodies have been hypothesized to be pathogenic, although this remains controversial because they can also be found in healthy individuals, in addition to those with other autoimmune diseases, such as systemic lupus and dermatomyositis. Injection of autologous serum, also known as the autologous serum skin test (ASST), leads to a wheal-and-flare response in CIU patients, suggesting that the causative agent is in the serum. Patients with CIU have a higher prevalence of other autoantibodies such as antimicrosomal and antithyroglobulin thyroid autoantibodies and a higher frequency of certain HLA class II alleles (DR4, DQ8) associated with autoimmunity.

More recently, the role of mast cells and basophils has been investigated. Skin biopsies of patients with CIU demonstrate mast cell degranulation accompanied by increased mast cell releasibility that reverses with disease remission. Basophils, which typically are not present in the skin, are observed in both lesional and nonlesional CIU skin biopsies. Basopenia has been described in CIU and is a marker of more severe disease. More recently, basophil activation markers have been shown to be enhanced in CIU patients along with defects in basophil signaling through the IgE receptor.

Physical Urticaria

Physical urticarias have a specific trigger that directly induces hives within minutes, with hives lasting minutes to a few hours. Physical urticarias are further classified into multiple subtypes (Table 20-1), each having a different physical trigger; thus, an individual can have more than one subtype. Mast cell degranulation is included in the pathogenesis of most subtypes of physical urticaria, including dermatographic, cholinergic, cold, and solar urticaria, but serum immunoglobulin may also be involved as demonstrated by passive transfer experiments.

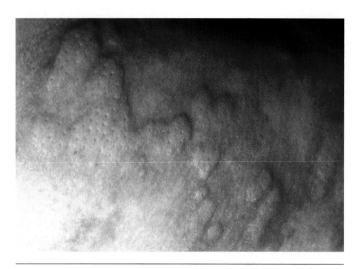

Figure 20-1 *Urticaria.*

ANGIOEDEMA

Angioedema, which is a swelling of the dermis, subcutaneous, and submucosal tissues, often coexists with urticaria but typically persists past 24 hours (Figure 20-2). Angioedema is described as painful or burning in quality. The lack of pruritus in angioedema may be caused by fewer mast cells in the lower dermis and subcutis. Idiopathic angioedema coexists with urticaria, occurring in up to 50% of those with CIU. Angiotensin-converting enzyme (ACE) inhibitors can also trigger angioedema via the bradykinin pathway.

CLINICAL PRESENTATION

Urticarial lesions are intensely pruritic and can affect any location on the body. They are typically transient, lasting less than 24 hours. Unlike atopic dermatitis, excoriation is not a typical finding in urticaria, regardless of the degree of pruritus experienced. Lesions can vary in size and can be confluent. Similar to urticaria, angioedema can occur anywhere on the body, although it frequently involves face, lips, tongue, throat, and extremities, but unlike urticaria, it commonly involves mucous membranes. Cold urticaria is the exception because it may involve swelling of the tongue or palate. Urticarial lesions usually demonstrate complete resolution without skin pigment changes.

Patients with long-lasting lesions or the presence of other systemic symptoms should be evaluated for other diseases (see Box 20-1). *Urticarial vasculitis* is classified by painful or pruritic lesions lasting longer than 48 hours and may leave residual skin changes unrelated to excoriation. Concurrent systemic

Table 20-1 Physical Urticarias with Relative Triggers and Provocation			
Type	**Features**	**Reaction Times**	**Provocation Test**
Dermatographic	Mechanical shearing forces lead to lesions	1. Immediate: within 2–5 min; lasts 30 min 2. Intermediate: within 30 min–2 h; lasts 3–9 h 3. Late onset (rare): within 4–5 h; lasts 24–48 h	Stroke forearm or back with tongue blade
Delayed pressure	Constant application of pressure to skin results in erythema and superficial and deep swelling	Within 3–12 h; lasts ≤48 h	Application of weight to one area for a minimum of 10 min
Vibratory	Occurs after vibratory stimuli (e.g., lawn mowing)	Within minutes; lasts ≤24 h	Challenge with vibratory stimuli (e.g., vortex mixer) for 5 min
Familial cold	Immediate type characterized by burning papules or macules and systemic symptoms such as arthralgias and fever; delayed type occurs after cold exposure	Delayed type occurs within 9–18 h of cold exposure; lasts 2–3 days	
Cold contact	Occurs with skin cold exposure; may have angioedema and rare cases of anaphylaxis after total-body exposure to cold	Within 2–5 min as skin rewarms	Ice cube placement to area for 10–20 min
Heat contact	Occurs at sites of heat application; divided into immediate and nonfamilial and delayed familial	1. Immediate: within 5 min; lasts ≤1 h 2. Delayed: within 6–8 h; lasts 12–24 h	Local contact with hot water or object
Solar	Induced by sunlight or indoor lighting exposure (wavelengths 280–760 nm)	Within 2–3 min; lasts 3–4 h	Expose to UV light
Cholinergic	Caused by an increase in core body temperature	Within minutes; lasts <1 h	Physical activity (e.g., running in place for 5 min)
Aquagenic	Contact with water induces small hives similar to those seen in cholinergic urticaria	Within 2 min; lasts ≤1 h	Apply water compress for 30 min
Contact	Inciting triggers are plants, foods, drugs, and chemicals	Within minutes; lasts <a few hours	
Adrenergic	Pin-sized wheals elicited by stress	Within minutes; lasts <1 h	

From Koutou-Fili K, Borici-Mazi R, Kapp A. et al. Physical urticaria: classification and diagnostic guidelines. An EAACI position paper. Allergy 1997;52(5):504-513.
UV, ultraviolet.

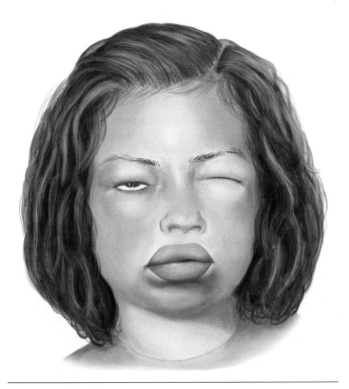

Figure 20-2 *Angioedema.*

complaints or abnormal laboratory findings indicative of an inflammatory process, such as an elevated erythrocyte sedimentation rate (ESR) or C-reactive protein (CRP) or low complement levels, are seen. A skin biopsy is required to rule out urticarial vasculitis. *Urticaria pigmentosa*, a subset of mastocytosis, may mimic urticaria, although these lesions are typically pigmented and last longer than urticaria. The presence of fever

---

Box 20-1 Differential Diagnosis of Urticaria and Angioedema

Acute Urticaria
• IgE mediated
  • Food allergy
  • Drug allergy
  • Stinging insect allergy
• Non–IgE mediated
  • Papular urticaria secondary to insect bite
  • Urticaria multiforme
  • Transfusion reaction
  • Infections
Chronic Urticaria or Angioedema
• With urticaria
  • Idiopathic urticaria
  • Physical urticarias
  • Urticarial vasculitis
  • Urticaria pigmentosa
  • Serum sickness
  • Infection
  • Muckle-Wells syndrome
  • Schnitzler's syndrome
• Without urticaria
  • Idiopathic angioedema
  • Hereditary angioedema
  • Malignancy

---

with urticaria can occur in Schnitzler's syndrome and Muckle-Wells syndrome. *Schnitzler's syndrome* is described as recurrent urticaria with arthralgia, fever, and elevation in inflammatory markers in association with an elevation in IgM. *Muckle-Wells syndrome* is a periodic fever syndrome with urticaria associated with periodic, unexplained fevers.

History

In diagnosing either acute or chronic urticaria, a thorough history is the most important element along with a detailed physical examination. The history should elicit the time of onset of hives (because some patients may experience diurnal variation) and the specific days that the patient is affected because there may be an association with certain environmental exposures or stressors. A description of the lesions, including their shape, size, distribution, color, pigmentation, and the quality of pain or itch, is important in confirming the diagnosis of urticaria. To identify acute triggers, the history should elicit recent use of medications, including antibiotics, nonsteroidal antiinflammatory drugs (NSAIDs), and aspirin; food ingested shortly before symptom occurrence (especially within 2 hours of lesion appearance); implanted surgical devices; insect stings; and changes in environment. Questions regarding recent infections or to evaluate for symptoms of thyroid disease are important (see Chapter 68). For female patients, it is important to investigate if there is a variation of hives in relation to hormonal changes observed with menses or pregnancy. Physical triggers are important for defining physical urticarias. Further evaluation of life stressors may assist in understanding the timing of lesions. It is also important to evaluate how the patient is coping and what therapeutics, including nonprescription medications or dietary changes, are being used and if they are providing any relief. Some patients with chronic urticaria are on restricted diets, which are unnecessary and may lead to nutritional deficits. Medication side effects should also be evaluated.

For patients with angioedema without a history of urticaria, it is important to ask about family history of angioedema. Hereditary angioedema (HAE), an autosomal dominant disease involving a defect in C1 esterase inhibitor function, presents with isolated angioedema that can sometimes be disfiguring and life threatening if the airway is involved. It is important to question about episodic abdominal pain and abdominal surgeries in these patients because many times their sole presenting symptoms are abdominal pain and vomiting.

Physical Examination

The physical examination is important in solidifying the diagnosis of urticaria, but it cannot distinguish between acute and chronic urticaria. The examination should focus on the size, distribution, and color of the lesions. Whereas wheals are characteristically pink or red because of histamine-induced dilatation of vessels in the skin and are easily blanched, vasculitic lesions have a darker red or purple appearance resulting from vascular damage and leakage. Cholinergic urticaria has a characteristic "fried egg" appearance with a small wheal and surrounding large flare (Figure 20-3). The physical examination should include testing for dermatographism, which can be elicited by applying

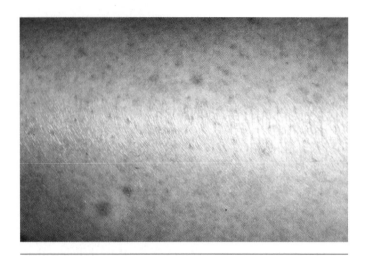

Figure 20-3 *Cholinergic urticaria.*

linear pressure to skin using a blunt object, such as a tongue depressor. In some types of physical urticaria, eliciting urticaria with additional maneuvers is diagnostic, as in the ice-cube test for cold urticaria. The physical examination should include thyroid palpation to assess for thyroid gland abnormalities.

EVALUATION AND MANAGEMENT

Laboratory Testing

No routine laboratory testing is indicated in urticaria unless the clinician is attempting to identify the trigger or if the patient has an atypical clinical presentation. For patients with acute urticaria suspected of having a food allergy, specific skin testing and specific IgE measurements may be helpful, although the latter should only be done if skin test results are positive or if it is contraindicated. There is a high percentage of false-positive test results in skin testing to foods, so testing should occur only to foods of concern. Skin testing is difficult to perform in patients with chronic urticaria because of the high prevalence of dermatographism and delayed pressure features in this group, as well as their dependence on antihistamines. Patients with physical urticaria do not need laboratory testing. In CIU, laboratory testing acts as an adjunct to history and examination, especially in patients who fail to respond to conventional therapies or who have uncharacteristic lesions. If there are concerns for vasculitis or autoimmune disorders, an ESR and antinuclear antibody (ANA) are good screening tests. Complement levels, specifically C3 and C4, should be considered. Other laboratory screening tests, such as a complete blood count with differential, complete metabolic panel, and urinalysis, should be obtained if there are concerns for systemic disease. Patients with significant angioedema without urticaria should also have complement levels, specifically C4, and C1 inhibitor function testing; C4 levels are typically low in patients with HAE during acute episodes. Symptoms consistent with thyroid disease warrant thyroid screening with a thyroid-stimulating hormone and thyroid autoantibody testing. If there are signs, symptoms, or laboratory tests concerning for malignancy, a chest radiograph is recommended.

Even though viral infections, especially viral upper respiratory infections, are common causes of acute urticaria, testing for viruses does not change therapy or outcomes. Other infectious agents have been implicated in urticaria, and testing for these should be guided by the history and examination. Hepatitis, especially hepatitis C, has been reported to manifest as chronic urticaria; thus, screening studies for hepatitis B and C should be considered in patients with risk factors. In patients with symptoms of gastroesophageal reflux or gastritis, it may be indicated to obtain *Helicobacter pylori* serology because this organism is thought to trigger autoantibody production in some patients with CIU. If there is peripheral eosinophilia, the stool should be tested for ova and parasites. Bacterial and fungal cultures do not need to be ordered for urticaria because these are unusual triggers of hives.

Management

The treatment of CIU is a greater challenge than that of acute and physical urticarias. Patients may be less frustrated if they are educated on the natural history of CIU. For all types of urticaria, if there is a clear avoidable trigger, such as in confirmed food allergy or physical urticaria, it should be eliminated. In chronic urticaria, it is unlikely that foods are contributing in a significant manner, and there are no conclusive data supporting diets with avoidance of foods high in salicylates. For all patients, avoidance of aspirin and salicylate-containing medications, as well as NSAIDs, is advisable. Both aspirin and NSAIDs can aggravate urticaria and angioedema via inhibition of prostaglandin synthesis; thus, patients should switch to selective cyclooxygenase-2 inhibitors if a chronic analgesic agent is needed. For patients with angioedema, ACE inhibitors should be avoided. All patients should avoid morphine and codeine-containing products that can directly stimulate skin mast cells.

The mainstay of treatment for urticaria is symptom alleviation using antihistamines. Because of the soporific side effect of antihistamines, less sedating H1-blockers, such as loratadine and cetirizine, are preferred for more regular use, with the classic sedating H1-blockers, such as diphenhydramine and hydroxyzine, reserved for use on an as-needed basis. Different H1-blockers may be tried because one may work better per individual; for select patients with CIU, the simultaneous use of multiple H1-blockers may be necessary. H2-blockers can provide an added benefit in combination with H1-blockade and may even increase serum concentration of the H1-blocker. Doxepin is a tricyclic antidepressant with some H1- and H2-receptor antagonist properties, and it can be used for nighttime itch, with the added benefit of assisting with disease-associated depression. It should be used with caution because it is very sedating; can decrease the effectiveness of other drugs, such as cimetidine and macrolides; and is contraindicated if a patient is taking monoamine oxidase inhibitors because of the risk for developing prolonged QT syndrome.

Evidence for leukotriene receptor antagonist (LTRA) use in chronic urticaria is conflicting. Some benefit has been observed in CIU and physical urticaria (specifically cold-induced and delayed pressure subtypes), as well as acute urticaria caused by aspirin or food. The Food and Drug Administration has placed a warning indicating that LTRA drugs may alter children's moods; thus, these medications should only be used in children without underlying mood disorders and in conjunction with other therapies, such as antihistamines, with discontinuation of the LTRA if no added benefit is observed.

For severe cases of acute urticaria, a short course of systemic corticosteroids can lead to rapid symptom alleviation. Systemic corticosteroids also have a role in severe, antihistamine-resistant CIU when rapid control is warranted, as with episodes of significant angioedema. The use of systemic corticosteroids should be judicious because of the side effect profile with prolonged use, including greater risk for osteoporosis, peptic ulcer disease, diabetes, and hypertension, to name a few. Also, it is important that the patients and their families are aware that hives may recur after the corticosteroid effect has worn off because corticosteroids do not alter the disease process. Topical corticosteroids play no role in the treatment of patients with urticaria, with the exception of perhaps some minimal benefit in localized delayed pressure urticaria.

Unlike HAE, angioedema associated with acute or chronic urticaria is rarely life threatening, but it may respond to epinephrine. Thus, an epinephrine autoinjector may provide that subset of patients with relief. There is no role for epinephrine, steroids, or antihistamines in patients with HAE.

More recently, immunomodulators have been used for the treatment of patients with severe, steroid-dependent chronic urticaria. Cyclosporine, sulfasalazine, and dapsone have demonstrated some benefit in a subset of patients. Dapsone, which inhibits neutrophil function, may be beneficial for patients with neutrophil-predominant infiltrates on skin biopsy. Isolated reports of cyclophosphamide and methotrexate use in CIU appear to demonstrate some benefit. Colchicine and hydroxychloroquine have also been suggested as therapeutics. For patients with suspected autoimmune CIU, plasmapheresis has been used to remove autoantibodies with temporary amelioration of disease. Intravenous immunoglobulin infusions have also been studied in patients with functional autoantibodies with a transient beneficial effect. Overall, these therapeutics should be used with caution and only when the patient has failed all other therapies. Most of these therapies also require frequent side effect monitoring, including laboratory testing.

Patients with CIU have a higher incidence of thyroid disease and thyroid autoantibodies compared with the general population, so only patients with underlying thyroid disease should be treated for underlying process. Euthyroid patients with thyroid autoantibodies should not be treated with thyroid hormone replacement.

FUTURE DIRECTIONS

Even with the various medications available, patients with severe disease still may not reach symptomatic control; thus, novel therapies are needed. Rituximab, a monoclonal anti-CD20 antibody, may decrease autoantibodies, thus making it a potential therapeutic for CIU patients with an autoimmune profile. Other biologics, such as the TNF-α antagonists, which have known antiinflammatory properties and are used for other autoimmune and skin inflammatory diseases, such as psoriasis, may be a potential therapeutic for CIU. Of all the biologics available, omalizumab, a monoclonal anti-IgE antibody, has been most studied and demonstrated to improve disease activity in CIU and cold-induced urticaria. Omalizumab alters both mast cell and basophil anti-IgE–induced histamine release, decreases free IgE serum levels, and reduces FcεRI expression on mast cells and basophils, all mechanisms that may lead to fewer targets for autoantibodies.

Overall, the current available treatments for urticaria are inadequate, increasing patient frustration and morbidity of disease. A better understanding of underlying disease mechanisms is essential to guide new, targeted therapeutics.

SUGGESTED READINGS

Brodell LA, Beck LA: Differential diagnosis of chronic urticaria, *Ann Allergy Asthma Immunol* 100:181-188, 2008.

Dibbern DA, Dreskin SC: Urticaria and angioedema: an overview, *Immunol Allergy Clin North Am* 24:141-162, 2004.

Greaves MW: Chronic urticaria in childhood, *Allergy* 55:309-320, 2000.

Kaplan AP: Clinical practice. Chronic urticaria and angioedema, *N Engl J Med* 346:175-179, 2002.

Kaplan AP: Urticaria and angioedema. In Adkinson NF, Bochner BS, Busse WW, et al, editors: *Middleton's Allergy: Principles and Practice*, ed 7, Philadelphia, 2008, Mosby, pp 1063-1075.

Kaplan AP, Greaves M: Pathogenesis of chronic urticaria, *Clin Exp Allergy* 39:777-787, 2009.

Zuberbier T: Urticaria, *Allergy* 58:1224-1234, 2003.

Approach to the Child with Primary Immunodeficiency

Lisa Forbes and Terri Brown-Whitehorn

Primary immunodeficiencies are a diverse group of inherited disorders with defects in one or more components of the immune system. Persistent, recurrent, or hard to treat infections are hallmark features of primary immunodeficiency diseases (PIDs). Early diagnosis and referral to a pediatric allergist/immunologist is essential. Treatments such as prophylactic antibiotics or antifungals; immunoglobulin replacement; early recognition of infection; and at times, hematopoietic stem cell transplant can save lives, help prevent infections and end organ damage, and improve long-term outcomes and quality of life.

Primary immunodeficiency disorders are rare, with the exception of IgA deficiency (prevalence of 1:500–700 whites). Overall, the incidence of primary immunodeficiency is one in 10,000, with a range of one in 10,000 to one in 200,000. The prevalence differs among ethnic groups and countries of origin. There are approximately 400 new cases of primary immunodeficiency diagnosed in the United States each year. Approximately 80% are diagnosed before 5 years of age. The male-to-female ratio is roughly 2:1. According to recent registry data, antibody defects account for 65% of primary immune deficiency, combined defects account for 15%, phagocyte defects account for 10%, complement defects account for 5%, and cellular defects without antibody dysfunction account for 5%. Although immunodeficiency may be secondary to many disease processes, including infection, metabolic disorders, protein-losing states, medications, and oncologic and rheumatologic disorders, this chapter focuses on the approach to the PIDs.

ETIOLOGY AND PATHOGENESIS

The pathogenesis of primary immune defects is related to the underlying cellular defect, which may be further divided into problems with the innate and adaptive immune system. Immune defects are distinguished by the cellular mechanism involved, including B cells and humoral or antibody defects, T cells and cell-mediated defects, combined B and T cell defects, phagocytic defects, complement defects, and newly described defects in pattern recognition molecules (Toll-like receptors [TLRs] and signaling molecules). The innate immune system is composed of phagocytes (dendritic cells, macrophages, and neutrophils), complement components, natural killer (NK) cells, TLRs, and signaling molecules. These cells are the first line of defense and respond to pathogens in a nonspecific manner. The adaptive immune system includes B cells, T cells, and combined defects. These cells recognize and respond to pathogens in a specific manner, leading to long-lasting immunity. There are also genetic disorders of immune regulation that cross both arms of the immune system. Specific disorders are often associated with particular infectious organisms (Table 21-1).

Disorders of the Innate Immune System

PHAGOCYTES

Phagocytes are responsible for detecting and migrating to the site of intruder by recognition of microbial products, antibody-mediated detection, or complement. In turn, these cells produce cytokines and signal the adaptive immune system to fight an infection or react to the danger signal. Abnormalities lead to severe and unusual infections. Representative disorders include congenital neutropenia, chronic granulomatous disease, and hyper immunoglobulin E (IgE) syndrome. Four specific genetic defects in phagocyte NADPH oxidase have been described in chronic granulomatous disease. A neutrophil defect should be considered in children who have recurrent abscesses, *Staphylococcus* infections, granulomas, and an unusual sensitivity to *Aspergillus* or atypical mycobacterium.

NATURAL KILLER CELLS

NK cells confer immunity against viruses, intracellular bacteria, and parasites and provide cytotoxicity against tumor cells. The three disorders that affect NK cells and related interferon gamma (INF-γ)/interleukin-12 (IL-12) pathway are NK cell deficiency (e.g., CD16 deficiency), IFN-γ receptor 1 and 2 defects, and Griscelli syndrome (albinism with immunodeficiency). Patients with defects in the IFN-γ/IL-12 pathway typically present with atypical mycobacterium infection. Patients with isolated NK cell defects are susceptible to herpes viral infections.

COMPLEMENT

The complement system shares responsibility in host defense, induction of the adaptive immune system, inflammation, and clearance of apoptotic cells and immune complexes. The clinical manifestations of deficiencies early in the complement cascade are susceptibility to infections with *Streptococcus pneumoniae* and *Haemophilus influenzae* and rheumatologic abnormalities, such as systemic lupus erythematosus (see Chapter 29). *Neisseria* infections are more common with defects in later components of the complement cascade. Hereditary angioedema results from a defect in C1 esterase inhibitor enzyme function.

TOLL-LIKE RECEPTORS

TLRs are a recently discovered component of the innate immune system. They are a family of pattern recognition receptors whose sole job is immunologic surveillance. TLRs recognize microbial products and danger signals and activate pathways that produce cytokines to recruit the appropriate immune response. Most defects in the TLRs or signaling molecules downstream affect children early in life until the adaptive immune system can mature

Table 21-1 Infectious Organisms Associated with Immunodeficiency

Organism	B Cell Defects	T Cell Defects	Combined B and T Cell Defects	Phagocyte Defects	Other
Streptococcus pneumoniae or *Haemophilus influenzae*	XLA, CVID, selective antibody deficiency, selective IgA deficiency		Hyper IgM (CD-40L deficiency), MHC class I deficiency		IRAK-4 deficiency, NEMO defects, early complement deficiency
Staphylococcus aureus	XLA			CGD, LAD, neutropenia, Chediak-Higashi syndrome	IPEX syndrome, IRAK-4 deficiency, hyper IgE syndrome
Mycobacterial infections		Idiopathic CD4 deficiency	SCID	CGD	IL-12 and IL-23 receptor defects, IFN-gR1 and IFN-gR2 defects, NEMO defects
Candida spp.		Idiopathic CD4 deficiency	SCID, MHC class II deficiency	Myeloperoxidase deficiency, WAS	APECED, NEMO defects, CMCC, hyper IgE
Aspergillus fumigatus		Idiopathic CD4 deficiency	SCID	CGD, LAD	Hyper IgE
Cryptococcus neoformans		Idiopathic CD4 deficiency			Hyper IgE
Histoplasma capsulatum		Idiopathic CD4 deficiency	Hyper IgM (CD-40L deficiency)		AD IFN-gR1 deficiency, hyper IgE
Pneumocystis carinii	XLA, CVID	Idiopathic CD4 deficiency	SCID, Zap70, hyper IgM (CD-40L and CD40 deficiency)	WAS	NEMO defects
Neisseria meningitidis					Terminal complement deficiency
Viral infections	XLA, CVID (enterovirus)	Idiopathic CD4 deficiency	SCID, MHC class II deficiency		NK cell deficiency (Herpesviral family), NEMO defects (enterovirus), WHIM (human papillomavirus), XLP (EBV)

AD IFN-gR1, autosomal dominant interferon gamma receptor 1; APECED, autoimmune polyendocrinopathy candidiasis ectodermal dystrophy; CGD, chronic granulomatous disease; CMCC, chronic mucocutaneous candidiasis; CVID, common variable immunodeficiency; EBV, Epstein Barr virus; IFN, interferon; IPEX, immune dysregulation enteropathy X-linked; IRAK, interleukin-1 receptor-associated kinase; LAD, leukocyte adhesion disorder; MHC, major histocompatibility complex; NEMO, NF-κB essential modulator defect; NK, natural killer; SCID, severe combined immune deficiency; XLA, X-linked agammaglobulinemia; XLP, X-linked lymphoproliferative syndrome; WAS = Wiskott-Aldrich syndrome; WHIM, warts hypogammaglobulinemia infection myelokathexis syndrome.

and contribute to immune regulation. IRAK-4 (interleukin-1 receptor-associated kinase 4) deficiency is an example of a specific defect of the TLR pathway.

Disorders of the Adaptive Immune System

HUMORAL IMMUNE SYSTEM

The humoral immune system defects, including B cell and antibody defects, make up the most common PIDs. These defects include selective IgA deficiency, transient hypogammaglobulinemia of infancy, X-linked agammaglobulinemia (XLA, or Bruton agammaglobulinemia), hyper IgM syndrome (CD40 ligand deficiency), IgG subclass deficiency, selective antibody deficiency, and common variable immune deficiency (CVID). Patients with humoral defects are typically older than 6 months; they may be diagnosed in the toddler or school-age group. Although CVID can be diagnosed at an earlier age, it is typically diagnosed in adolescents and adults. Children with transient hypogammaglobulinemia of infancy have low quantitative IgG levels with normal IgG function, as noted by protective titers to immunization. Over time, the quantity of IgG normalizes. Children with other humoral

defects are unable to respond normally to bacterial infections. Specific defects have been described for some disorders. In XLA, the absence of the *Btk* gene leads to impairment in B cell development, maturation, function, and receptor signaling. Diagnosis is made by absence of mature B cells. Patients with hyper IgM most commonly have a defect in CD40 ligand (on T cells). Without CD40 ligand binding to CD40 on B cells, the normal switch from IgM to IgG or IgA does not occur. In CVID, patients may have normal mature B cells. However, they have defects in differentiation to immunoglobulin-secreting plasma cells. Characteristic infections seen in humoral defects include severe enteroviral infections in patients with XLA, *Pneumocystis carinii* pneumonia or *Cryptosporidium parvum* (associated with sclerosing cholangitis) in patients with hyper IgM, and *Giardia* infections in patients with XLA or CVID. In addition to infection, some of these patients are more at risk for autoimmune disease and malignancy.

CELL-MEDIATED IMMUNE SYSTEM

Defects in the cell-mediated immune system are often quite severe. T cell disorders often begin in early infancy and childhood. These defects affect T cell development or function with varying degrees of defects in the other lymphocytes (i.e., B cells and NK cells). Severe combined immunodeficiency (SCID) is the most serious immune defect and is considered a "medical emergency." These patients present in infancy with severe viral infections, opportunistic infections, bronchiolitis, and failure to thrive. They typically have absolute lymphocyte counts of less than 2800 cells/microliter and nonfunctioning lymphocytes. Without a bone marrow transplant, these children generally die by 2 years of age. Prompt diagnosis and treatment with transplant increases the survival rate to upward of 90%. One must also consider complete DiGeorge syndrome or secondary immune defects (e.g., HIV) in these very ill infants. Patients with SCID may have a single gene defect or may be a part of an immunodeficiency syndrome such as 22q11.2 deletion syndrome, cartilage hair hypoplasia, or CHARGE (coloboma of the eye, heart defects, atresia of the nasal choanae, retardation of growth or development, genital or urinary abnormalities, and ear abnormalities and deafness) syndrome.

Other T cell immunodeficiencies include chronic mucocutaneous candidiasis, CD4 lymphopenia, and OKT4 epitope deficiency. People with Wiskott-Aldrich syndrome (WAS) present with eczema, thrombocytopenia (small platelets), and T cell defects. Children with ataxia telangiectasia also have T cell defects presenting with ataxia and recurrent infections. These children are also at increased risk for lymphoma.

OTHER DEFECTS OF THE ADAPTIVE IMMUNE SYSTEM

Many other immune defects have been described. If a child presents with insulin-dependent diabetes mellitus, autoimmune disease, noninfectious diarrhea, lymphadenopathy, food allergy and recurrent infections, and a defect in the *FoxP3* gene, a diagnosis of IPEX syndrome (immune dysregulation, polyendocrinopathy, enteropathy, X linked) is likely.

CLINICAL PRESENTATION

History

Children with primary immune deficiencies can present in a variety of ways (Table 21-2). Classically, the most severe defects occur early on with recurrent or persistent viral illnesses, failure to thrive, or chronic diarrhea. Older toddlers and school-aged children may present with recurrent ear infections, sinus infections, pneumonias, or poor growth. When obtaining the history, one must pay particular attention to patient's age at time of infection, type(s) of infection, site of infection, and ability to treat infection with oral or intravenous (IV) antimicrobials, as well as the number of hospitalizations. The overall health, growth, and development of the patient are important. The birth history and maternal prenatal history must be obtained. Prior miscarriages may be an indication of a genetic problem. The presence of maternal infection during pregnancy may lead to an immunodeficiency in a newborn. The immunization history is crucial when evaluating for an antibody defect or a T cell abnormality. The child's response to immunizations is a way to look at the function of the immune system. Also, it is important to recognize that children with suspected or known severe immune defects should not receive live viral vaccines. Included in the history should be

a comprehensive family history. Many of the primary immunodeficiencies are X-linked or associated with known genetic mutations. At times, there is a family history of autoimmune disease. A list of medications should be obtained, including any that may have been given in the past such as chemotherapeutics or antiepileptics. Finally, a detailed review of systems may be helpful detailing concomitant medical or development concerns and phenotypes leading to the diagnosis of a genetic syndrome.

Physical Exam

The physical examination can sometimes give clues as to the possible immune defect and guide laboratory evaluation. Assessing the child's growth and evaluating the growth curves are important. Some children have failure to thrive or they "fall off the growth chart." Characteristic facial abnormalities have been seen in some of the genetic and syndromic deficiencies, such as hyper IgE syndrome. The absence of tonsils and palpable lymph nodes may indicate a B or T cell abnormality, such as XLA or SCID. Lymphadenopathy and splenomegaly may be associated with autoimmune lymphoproliferative disorder (ALPS). Erythroderma and lymphopenia in the newborn period can be indicative of a form of SCID called Ommen syndrome. Nail and hair abnormalities can be seen in some of the rare immune defects. Telangiectasias and photosensitivity, along with ataxia, are associated with ataxia telangiectasia. Patients with cartilage hair hypoplasia classically present with short limb dwarfism. Patients with X-linked anhydrotic ectodermal dysplasia with immunodeficiency (also known as NEMO or NF-κB essential modulator defect) have conical teeth with delayed eruption and osteopetrosis. Developmental delays have also been described in some of the immune defects.

Differential Diagnosis

When a child presents with recurrent infections, one must keep in mind that there are other causes that should be considered. The differential diagnosis includes cystic fibrosis; ciliary dyskinesia; and secondary immune defects from treatment of malignancies or underlying infections, such as HIV or cytomegalovirus (CMV).

EVALUATION AND MANAGEMENT

Laboratory Studies

If one is concerned about an underlying immunodeficiency, screening blood tests are necessary. For most patients, this includes obtaining a complete blood count (CBC) with differential, quantitative immunoglobulins (IgG, IgA, IgM, and IgE), and antibody titers to immunizations (diphtheria, tetanus, pneumococcal serotypes, and H. influenzae B) or naturally occurring antibodies (isohemagglutinin titers). When obtaining a CBC with differential, calculating the absolute lymphocyte count and the absolute neutrophil count is important. "Normal" lymphocyte values change with the age of the child, and thus appropriate references should be consulted for normal values when obtaining these tests. If there are further concerns or abnormalities in this screening laboratory evaluation, additional testing can be performed, and referral to a specialist is warranted

Table 21-2 Clinical Presentation of the Primary Immunodeficiencies

Clinical Presentation	B Cell Defect	T Cell Defect	Natural Killer Defect	Neutrophil Defect	Other
Recurrent pneumonia	X	X		X	X (make sure CF is considered)
Recurrent sinusitis	X	X			
Recurrent otitis	X				
Enteroviral infection	X (XLA)	X			
Recurrent abscesses				X	
Failure to thrive		X	X		
Recurrent diarrhea		X			
Fungal infections		X		X	
Recurrent viral infections		X			

Primary Immune Defect	Clinical Presentation
B cell defect	Recurrent bacterial infections Recurrent otitis Recurrent sinusitis Recurrent pneumonia Enteroviral infection Absence of tonsils and lymph nodes on examination
T cell defects	Recurrent viral infections Severe viral infections Thrush Fungal infections Bacterial infections (similar to B cell defects) Mycobacterial infections Diarrhea Failure to thrive
Neutrophil defects	Recurrent abscesses Granulomatous disease Catalase positive organisms *Aspergillus* infection or pneumonia
Natural killer cell defects	Recurrent viruses Atypical mycobacterium Herpes viral infection
Complement defects	Recurrent *Neisseria* infections Severe *Streptococcus* and Hib infections Autoimmune disease

CF, cystic fibrosis; Hib, *Haemophilus influenzae* type B; XLA, X-linked agammaglobulinemia.

(Table 21-3). For T cell defects, lymphocyte subsets along with functional assays, including mitogens or antigens, are important. In children where a neutrophil defect is suspected, absolute neutrophil number, morphology, and functional assays should be performed. A dihydrorodamine reduction (DHR) assay or nitrotetrazolium blue (NBT) assay is available to assess oxidative burst, the abnormality in chronic granulomatous disease (CGD). Complement deficiencies can be screened with a CH50 and C4 levels. Some assays look at absolute numbers and function of NK cells. DNA mutation analysis is available for some of the immune deficiencies with known genetic mutations. If a child has an abnormal immune evaluation or if there is a suspected defect or concern, immediate referral to an immunologist may be necessary.

Radiographic Studies

Although radiographic studies have minimal role in specific diagnosis, they can be useful in detecting clinical manifestations of the immunodeficiency. Chest radiographs are often obtained in infants and children with suspected pneumonia. In infants, an absence of the thymus may indicate SCID. Patients with adenosine deaminase (ADA) deficiency (a type of SCID) may also present with anterior cupping of the ribs. To evaluate for abscesses and granulomatous disease of the gastrointestinal tract, imaging studies are useful.

Management

Genetic counseling is essential for families of patients with primary immunodeficiency. Some infants can be diagnosed in utero. There has even been a reported case of an in utero bone marrow transplant for SCID. Otherwise, in the neonatal period, newborns with known or suspected combined defects should be placed in protective isolation. All blood products must be irradiated and CMV negative. Some of these children are placed on antibiotic and/or antifungal prophylaxis pending laboratory results and diagnosis.

Table 21-3 Laboratory Evaluation of Immunodeficiencies

Laboratory Test	Abnormality Seen	Possible Immune Defect
CBC		
Absolute lymphocyte count	Changes as patient ages; <2800 cells/ microliter in an infant is concerning	SCID
Absolute neutrophil count	Decreased	Congenital neutropenia
Platelet count	Decreased	WAS (small platelets, eczema, and T cell immunodeficiency)
DHR assay	Assesses neutrophil oxidative burst; absent burst is diagnostic	Chronic granulomatous disease
CH50 assay	If negative	Complement deficiency
T cell markers (CD3, CD4, CD8)	Low	Multiple immunodeficiencies, including SCID, CVID, selective deficiency
B cell markers (CD19, CD20)	Absent mature B cells only	XLA
	Absent mature B cells with decreased or absent T cells or NK cells	SCID
IgG	Low or absent	XLA
		Hyper Ig M
		CVID
		SCID
		Transient hypogammaglobulinemia of infancy
IgA	Absent	Selective IgA deficiency
		CVID
IgM	Elevated IgM in the absence of IgG, IgA, and IgE	Hyper IgM
IgE	Elevation	Hyper IgE syndrome (Job's syndrome)
		Severe atopy
Antibody titer assessment: diphtheria, tetanus, pneumococcal	Normal response with protective titers; less likely to be primary immune defect	Less likely to be primary immune defect
		IgA deficiency
		Transient hypogammaglobulinemia of infancy
Antibody titer assessment: diphtheria, tetanus, pneumococcal	Nonprotective titers	May need booster and reassess titers 4 weeks later
		Abnormalities seen in all B cell abnormalities, selective pneumococcal deficiency, and common variable immune defect
Lymphocyte stimulation by mitogens (PHA, PWM, and Con A)	Absent	SCID
		Complete DiGeorge syndrome

CBC, complete blood count; Con A, concanavalin A; CVID, common variable immune deficiency; DHR, dihydrorodamine reduction; Ig, immunoglobulin; NK, natural killer; PHA, phytohaemagglutinin; PWM, Pokweed mitogen; SCID, severe combined immunodeficiency; WAS, Wiskott-Aldrich syndrome; XLA, X-linked agammaglobulinemia.

In children with SCID, stem cell transplants are lifesaving. Human leukocyte antigen– (HLA-) matched siblings are preferred and have a lower incidence of graft-versus-host disease. When an HLA-matched sibling is not available for a patient with SCID, haploidentical or matched urelated donor transplants are performed. Bone marrow transplantation has been performed in patients with other immune defects, WAS, chronic granulomatous disease, leukocyte adhesion defects, and complete DiGeorge syndrome.

For children with more severe humoral immune defects, replacement IV immunoglobulin is standard of care administered either intravenously or subcutaneously. These patients do not need immunizations except for the yearly influenza vaccine because they have passive immunity through the infusion. Live virus vaccines should be avoided in children with primary immunodeficiency, especially in patients with severe T cell defects or severe agammaglobulinemia.

Antimicrobial prophylaxis is recommended for patients with CGD and WAS. Prophylactic antibiotics have been used in patients with humoral immunodeficiencies as an adjuvant to IV immunoglobulin. Antifungal prophylaxis is also recommended for patients with CGD.

Patients with underlying immune defects remain at risk for infections. Unnecessary exposure to individuals with infection must be avoided. These children can become quite sick very quickly. Aggressive management of any infection is imperative. Up-to-date knowledge of these disorders is important. Often, these children present with a fever, and the cause needs to be elucidated. In the event of infection, identification of the organism is helpful and strongly recommended. Some of these children may also be at risk for autoimmune disease or cancer.

FUTURE DIRECTIONS

As described in this chapter, early diagnosis of underlying primary immune disorders will help save lives, prevent infections, treat infections, and improve long-term outcome and quality of life. With specific genetic mutations known and others being pursued, gene therapy may become the therapy of choice in the future. At this time, improvements and strides in awareness, diagnosis, and overall care of these patients are of great importance.

SUGGESTED READINGS

Ballow M: Approach to the patient with recurrent infections, *Clin Rev Allergy Immunol* 34:129-140, 2008.

Bonilla FA, Bernstein IL, Khan DA, et al: Practice parameter for the diagnosis and management of primary immunodeficiency, *Ann Allergy Asthma Immunol* 94(suppl):S1-S63, 2005.

Carneiro-Sampaio M, Coutnho, A: Immunity to microbes: lessons from primary immunodeficiencies, *Infect Immun* 75(4):1545-1555, 2007.

Slatter MA, Gennery AR: Recurrent infections in childhood, *Clin Exp Immunol* 152:389-396, 2008.

Stiehm ER, Ochs HD, Winkelstein JA: Immunodeficiency Disorders in Infants and Children, ed 5, Philadelphia, 2004, Elsevier Saunders.

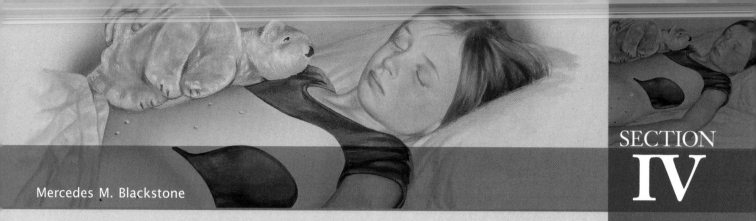

Mercedes M. Blackstone

SECTION

IV

Bone and Joint Disorders

Common Fractures

Monika Goyal

22

*P*ediatric orthopedic trauma comprises approximately 10% to 15% of all childhood injuries, and almost half of all children will sustain a childhood fracture. Because of the dynamic nature of skeletal growth and immaturity of the bony architecture, fractures in children differ from those in adults in regard to patterns of occurrence, diagnosis, and treatment. Injuries in children more frequently result in fractures than ligamentous injuries or sprains because the increased porosity and pliability of bones in children makes them more susceptible to fracture. Moreover, children are susceptible to growth plate injuries, which may be difficult to diagnose but can result in long-term growth abnormalities or growth arrest. Therefore, careful attention is required in the evaluation and management of pediatric patients presenting with orthopedic injuries.

Each age group has typical mechanisms of injury and common fractures. When evaluating newborns and infants with injuries, one should maintain a high index of suspicion for nonaccidental trauma because this is a leading cause of fracture in this age group (see Chapter 12). Injuries in toddlers and school-aged children most often result from falls. During adolescence, injuries become similar to those of adults and are often sustained in sports or through high-energy mechanisms, such as motor vehicle collisions.

The evaluation of a patient with a possible fracture begins with a thorough history and physical examination. Important information to gather on history includes mechanism of injury and the presence of any numbness or tingling. Physical examination should begin with visual inspection for obvious deformity; palpation for point(s) of maximal tenderness; and a thorough neurovascular examination, including comparison of pulses, capillary refill, sensation, and motor function between affected and unaffected regions. Radiographic evaluation should follow history and physical examination if suspicion for fracture remains and almost always begins with plain films. It is important to obtain multiple views, which include the joint above and below the area of injury.

FRACTURE DESCRIPTION

After a fracture has been identified, to effectively communicate with orthopedic consultants and other health care providers, it is important to use fracture nomenclature so that appropriate decisions can be made regarding management and treatment. Consultants should always be made aware of the patient's neurovascular status. Radiographic interpretation of the fracture should include the type of image; anatomic location (Figure 22-1); whether it is complete or incomplete, open or closed, and intra- or extraarticular; and the presence of physeal (growth plate) disruption, displacement, angulation, shortening, or comminution (Figure 22-2).

Fractures that extend across the width of a bone are complete fractures, and those that do not extend all the way across are incomplete fractures. Incomplete fractures are more common in children than adults and are described in more detail below.

Complete fractures can be further characterized according to their orientation as transverse fractures (those running at right angles to the long axis of the affected bone), oblique fractures (those that cross the shaft at an angle), and spiral fractures (fractures in which the break is helical). Any fracture that divides the bone into more than two separate segments is said to be comminuted (see Figure 22-2).

When describing the relationships of the fragments to each other, it can be helpful to describe *position* and *alignment*. The position of the bone refers to the relationship to the normal anatomy of the bone; the fracture is *displaced* when there is a loss of apposition or when the bony fragments are overriding or rotated. *Alignment* refers to the bone fragment's relationship to the longitudinal axis of the bone. Fractures that are not in good alignment are described as *angulated*. Often, the degree of displacement and angulation of the fracture are also described.

Perhaps the most important feature of a fracture is the distinction between an open and closed fracture (see Figure 22-2). In open fractures, the overlying skin is disrupted, and the fracture communicates with the outside environment, thus leading to increased risk of infection. Open fractures are an orthopedic emergency and necessitate operative repair.

COMMON FRACTURE TYPES IN CHILDREN

Physeal Fractures

Fractures involving the physis occur frequently in children and account for up to 20% of all pediatric fractures. Although several classification systems for the description of physeal fractures exist, the Salter-Harris classification system is the most widely used. This classification system, based on the radiographic appearance of the fracture, describes the degree of involvement of the physis, epiphysis, metaphysis, and joint and has both prognostic and therapeutic implications (Figure 22-3).

SALTER-HARRIS TYPE I FRACTURE

A Salter-Harris type I fracture involves separation of the epiphysis and most of the physis from the metaphysis. Diagnosis can be difficult if displacement is minimal because radiographs often appear normal. Therefore, this type of fracture is diagnosed clinically when there is swelling and tenderness over a growth plate. Management consists of immobilization and orthopedic follow-up because healing usually occurs within 3 to 4 weeks, and complications are rare. These fractures rarely result in growth disturbance.

SALTER-HARRIS TYPE II FRACTURE

Salter-Harris type II fractures are the most common type of pediatric physeal fractures. These fractures extend through the

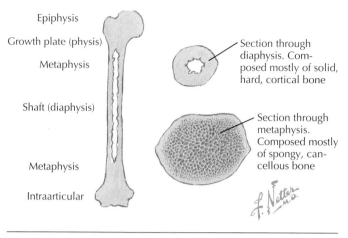

Figure 22-1 *Basic science of bone.*

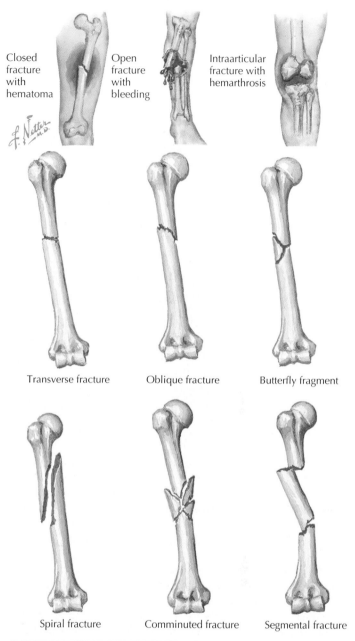

Figure 22-2 *Fracture patterns.*

physis into the metaphysis. Similar to Salter-Harris type I fractures, these fractures rarely result in growth disturbance, and management consists of immobilization and orthopedic follow-up.

SALTER-HARRIS TYPE III FRACTURE

Salter-Harris type III fractures extend through the physis and then propagate through the epiphysis into the intraarticular space. Growth disturbance may occur if anatomic position is not reestablished. Therefore, these fractures require emergent orthopedic consultation and may need surgical reduction.

SALTER-HARRIS TYPE IV FRACTURE

Salter-Harris type IV fractures involve the metaphysis, physis, articular surface, and epiphysis. Similar to Salter-Harris type III fractures, these fractures may result in growth arrest and deformity if anatomic position is not reestablished, often through surgical repair. As such, emergency orthopedic consultation is required.

SALTER-HARRIS TYPE V FRACTURE

Salter-Harris type V fractures result from a compression or crush injury with resultant disruption of the growth plate. Similar to Salter-Harris type I fractures, these fractures can be difficult to diagnose because radiographs may be normal, and the diagnosis is often made in hindsight. Because these fractures disrupt the germinal matrix, they can cause severe injury with growth arrest and can have a poor prognosis. When recognized, these fractures again merit emergent orthopedic consultation.

Greenstick Fractures

Greenstick fractures are the most common fracture pattern in children. They describe an incomplete fracture of cortex in which the fracture line does not extend completely through the width of the bone. Depending on the degree of

angulation, reduction by an orthopedic surgeon may be necessary (Figure 22-4).

Torus Fractures

Torus, or buckle, fractures are common fractures in young children. They result from a compressive load resulting in metaphyseal compaction of trabecular bone and buckling of cortical bone. These fractures are often seen in the distal radius after a fall onto an outstretched hand. As the child matures, the stiffness of the metaphyseal region increases, and the incidence of torus fractures decreases. These fractures are stable and can be managed with simple immobilization for 3 to 4 weeks and orthopedic follow-up (see Figure 22-4).

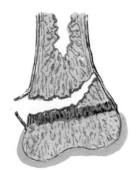

Periosteum

Metaphysis

Fracture

Growth plate (physis)

Epiphysis

Articular cartilage

Type I. Complete separation of epiphysis from shaft through calcified cartilage (growth zone) of growth plate. No bone actually fractured; periosteum may remain intact. Most common in newborns and young children

Type II. Most common. Line of separation extends partially across deep layer of growth plate and extends through metaphysis, leaving triangular portion of metaphysis attached to epiphyseal fragment

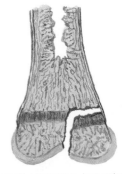

Type III. Uncommon. Intra-articular fracture through epiphysis, across deep zone of growth plate to periphery. Open reduction and fixation often necessary

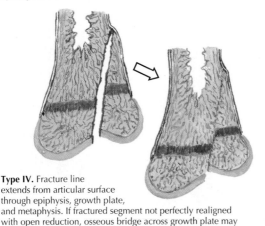

Type IV. Fracture line extends from articular surface through epiphysis, growth plate, and metaphysis. If fractured segment not perfectly realigned with open reduction, osseous bridge across growth plate may occur resulting in partial growth arrest and joint angulation

Type V. Severe crushing force transmitted across epiphysis to portion of growth plate by abduction or adduction stress or axial load. Minimal or no displacement makes radiographic diagnosis difficult; growth plate may nevertheless be damaged, resulting in partial growth arrest or shortening and angular deformity

Figure 22-3 *Injury to growth plate (Salter-Harris classification).*

Bowing Fractures

Bowing fractures represent a plastic deformity of the bone and are unique to children. These fractures occur when a longitudinal force exceeds the bone's ability to recoil to its normal position and results in a bend in the bone without a fracture. These fractures most commonly involve the radius and ulna. Bowing fractures can sometimes be subtle, and comparison views of the contralateral arm may be necessary. If the deformity occurs in a child younger than 4 years or if the deformation is less than 20 degrees, the angulation usually corrects with growth. However, open reduction may be required for these fractures if they have bowing greater than 20 degrees and the patient is older than 6 years old (see Figure 22-4).

Apophyseal Avulsion Fractures

Avulsion fractures are quite common in children. Tendons and ligaments attach to secondary ossification centers known as apophyses in the developing skeleton, and avulsion fractures occur when a fragment of bone is pulled off during muscle contraction. Common sites of injury occur in the pelvis, tibial tubercle, and phalanges. Apophyseal injuries do not interfere with growth and usually heal with conservative management.

FRACTURES OF THE UPPER EXTREMITY

Clavicle Fractures

The clavicle is the most commonly fractured bone in childhood. In neonates, these fractures can occur during the birthing process secondary to shoulder compression and can present with pseudoparalysis. Clavicle fractures in older children may be caused by a direct blow to the clavicle or indirect forces transmitted to the clavicle from a fall onto an outstretched hand. Most fractures involve the lateral two-thirds of the clavicle. Diagnosis can often be made on physical examination because patients typically have swelling, tenderness, and occasionally crepitus at the fracture site. Although neurovascular injury is rare, it is important to conduct a neurovascular examination to assess for any associated brachial plexus injury.

Most clavicle fractures heal well without complication, and management consists of immobilization in a figure-of-8 clavicle strap or sling and swathe. Patients with open fractures, neurovascular or respiratory compromise, significantly displaced midshaft fractures, or grossly unstable distal injuries need orthopedic consultation because closed reduction may be indicated. The vast majority of clavicle fractures heal quickly, usually within 3 to 6 weeks. A bony callus appears during the healing process but disappears with bone remodeling (Figure 22-5).

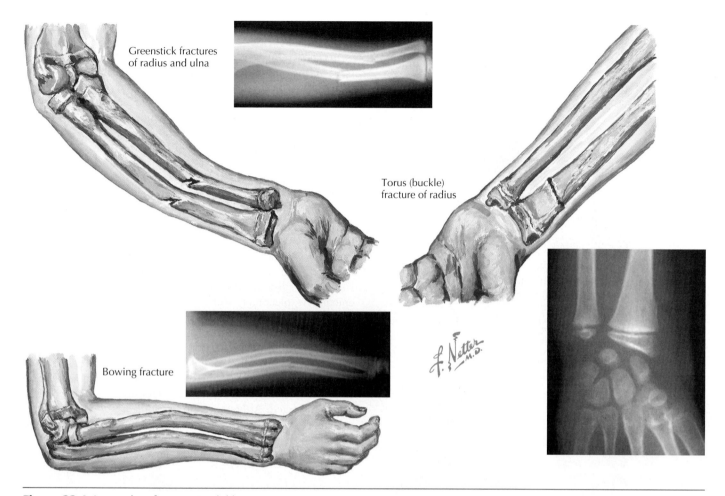

Greenstick fractures of radius and ulna

Torus (buckle) fracture of radius

Bowing fracture

Figure 22-4 *Incomplete fracture in children.*

Fractures of the Humerus

Fractures of the humerus include supracondylar fractures (discussed in the Elbow Fractures section below), proximal humerus fractures, and midshaft fractures. The latter two fractures are relatively rare. Child abuse should be considered when a child younger than 3 years of age presents with a spiral fracture of the humerus.

Humeral fractures have a remarkable ability to remodel and thus rarely result in nonunion. Most of these fractures can be managed with a shoulder immobilizer or sling and swathe with orthopedic referral.

Elbow Fractures

ANATOMY OF THE ELBOW

When evaluating elbow injuries, it is important to understand the ossification centers of the elbow and the average ages at which they appear because it is easy to mistake an ossification center for a fracture on radiography. A mnemonic aid for remembering the order in which these ossification centers appear is CRITOE (capitellum, age 1 year; radial head, age 3 years; internal [medial] condyle, age 5 years; trochlea, age 7 years; olecranon, age 9 years; external [lateral] condyle, age 11 years).

An adequate radiographic evaluation of the elbow consists of an anteroposterior view of the joint in extension and a lateral view

with the elbow flexed at 90 degrees (Figure 22-6). When evaluating elbow radiography, it is important to look for abnormalities of the fat pads, the anterior humeral line, and the radiocapitellar line on lateral views of the elbow. There are two elbow fat pads that overly the joint capsule along the distal humerus, one anterior and another posterior. Of the two, only the anterior fat pad is normally visible on a lateral radiograph as a small lucency just anterior to the coronoid fossa. When there is fluid in the joint space, as with a hemarthrosis from a fracture, the fat pads are displaced upward and outward thereby accentuating the anterior fat pad and making the posterior fat pad visible. The posterior fat pad sits deep in the olecranon fossa and is not visible under normal circumstances (see Figure 22-6). The anterior humeral line is also used to identify occult elbow injury. It is drawn along the anterior cortex of the distal humerus on a true lateral view of the elbow and should normally intersect the middle third of the capitellum; displacement may be consistent with a supracondylar fracture. The radiocapitellar line is drawn down the radius and should bisect the capitellum. Failure to do so may suggest an occult radial neck fracture or radial head dislocation.

SUPRACONDYLAR FRACTURES

Supracondylar fractures account for more than half of all elbow fractures in children and often occur from a fall onto an outstretched hand with hyperextension of the elbow. Most

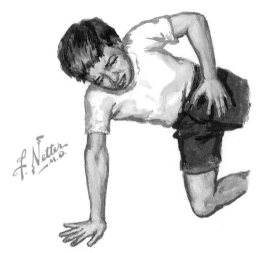

Commonly caused by fall on outstretched hand with force transmitted via shoulder to clavicle

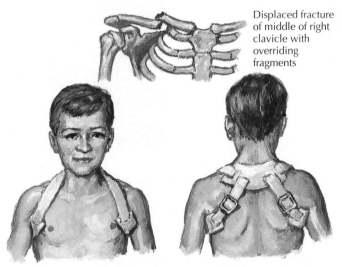

Displaced fracture of middle of right clavicle with overriding fragments

Fracture immobilized with snug, commercially available shoulder harness or figure-of-8 bandage for 3–4 weeks

Figure 22-5 *Fracture of clavicle in children.*

supracondylar fractures require open or closed reduction. Only minimally displaced or nondisplaced supracondylar fractures may be immobilized with orthopedic referral.

Neurovascular injury is a common complication of supracondylar fractures. Although actual laceration of the brachial artery is rare, the vessel may be compressed or contused or undergo vasospasm at the fracture site, leading to distal ischemia. Patients are also at risk for developing a forearm compartment syndrome, which can lead to Volkmann's ischemic contracture and a nonfunctional hand and wrist. Neurologic deficits, usually transient, are also common, and radial, medial, and ulnar nerve palsies have all been associated with supracondylar fractures (see Figure 22-6).

Forearm Fractures

After the clavicle, the radius and ulna are the most frequently broken bones in children. The most common mechanism of

injury is a fall onto an outstretched hand. Most of these fractures involve the distal forearm, with the majority of them being torus or greenstick fractures. Although an isolated fracture of one of the bones can occur, there is often concomitant injury to the paired bone. Additionally, a fracture or dislocation at one end may be associated with a similar abnormality at the opposite end; therefore, it is important to include the wrist and elbow when ordering radiographs of the forearm.

In general, isolated fractures of the ulna are rare. A fracture of the proximal ulna may be associated with concomitant dislocation of the radial head, know as a Monteggia fracture. A fracture at the distal third of the radius in association with distal radioulnar joint dislocation is called a Galeazzi fracture (Figure 22-7). These fractures require closed reduction. Most proximal radius fractures in young children involve the radial neck, usually resulting in Salter-Harris type I and type II radial neck fractures. Proximal radius fractures can occur in conjunction with elbow dislocations and are often associated with medial epicondyle, olecranon, and coronoid process fractures. Nondisplaced or minimally displaced fractures of radial head and neck can often be treated with splinting and orthopedic follow-up. Fractures with a high degree of angulation or displacement may need reduction or surgical repair.

Most fractures of the radius and ulna heal without significant complications. However, rotational abnormalities must be accurately corrected. Although complications are uncommon, vascular compromise or compartment syndrome can develop with any forearm fracture; therefore, a thorough neurovascular examination is imperative when evaluating forearm injuries.

Fractures of the Hand and Wrist

FRACTURES OF THE WRIST

Wrist fractures are common in children and mostly involve the distal radius. These are often caused by a fall on an outstretched hand. Most often, these fractures are Salter-Harris type I and II fractures. Most are conservatively managed with immobilization and orthopedic referral.

Although the carpal bones are rarely fractured in childhood, scaphoid fractures are the most common carpal fracture. These typically occur in adolescence from falling onto an outstretched hand. Examination may elicit tenderness along the anatomic snuffbox, pain with wrist extension and flexion, pain with forced supination, and pain with longitudinal compression of the thumb. Plain radiographs often do not reveal an acute fracture; therefore, if a scaphoid fracture is clinically suspected, the wrist should be immobilized with orthopedic referral. Radiographs can then be repeated 7 to 14 days after injury or a magnetic resonance imaging (MRI) or computed tomography (CT) scan can be obtained to better elucidate the fracture. Because the rate of nonunion for scaphoid fractures in pediatric patients is low, many can be managed nonoperatively.

METACARPAL FRACTURES

The most commonly encountered metacarpal fracture in children is a fractured distal fifth metacarpal, which often results from striking something with a closed fist (the so-called boxer's fracture). These require closed reduction if angulation is more

Bones of the elbow

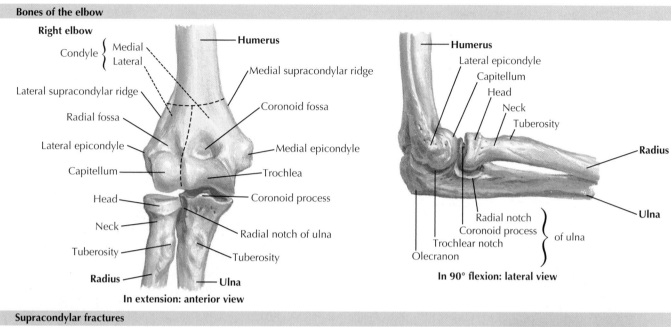

Supracondylar fractures

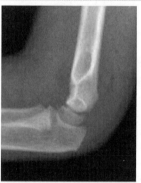

Extension type Posterior displacement of distal fragment (most common)

Humerus
Posterior fat pad
Anterior fat pad
Elevated posterior fat pad
Ulna

Flexion type Anterior displacement of distal fragment (uncommon)

Lateral radiograph of elbow in a 5-year-old female who fell from monkey bars sustaining injury to left elbow. Radiograph shows elevation of anterior and posterior fat pads. No apparent fracture on this view, but subsequent radiographs confirmed presence of a nondisplaced supracondylar humerus fracture.

Figure 22-6 *Bones and fractures of the elbow.*

than 30 to 40 degrees but can usually be managed with immobilization and orthopedic follow-up. Most other metacarpal fractures are nondisplaced or minimally displaced and are treated by immobilization for 2 to 4 weeks.

FRACTURES OF THE PHALANGES

The different phalangeal fracture patterns in children include physeal, diaphyseal, and tuft fractures. Evaluation of the fractured digit should include assessment of the skin integrity, the nail bed, any gross deformity, tendon function, and rotational alignment. The most common fractures of the hand in pediatrics are distal phalanx fractures, or tuft fractures. These are usually crush injuries complicated by lacerations. These injuries are treated with wound care, nailbed repair, and finger splinting.

Middle and proximal phalangeal fractures commonly occur at the physis and are usually Salter-Harris type II fractures. When evaluating patients with these fractures, it is important to assess for rotational deformity with the fingers flexed because any malrotation or angular deformity requires closed reduction to preserve hand function (Figure 22-8).

FRACTURES OF THE PELVIS AND LOWER EXTREMITIES

Fractures of the Pelvis

Pelvic fractures in children include pelvic ring fractures, avulsion fractures, and acetabular fractures. Pelvic ring fractures are rare in children and involve high-energy accidents. These are

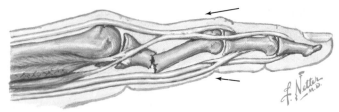

Fractures of proximal ulna often characterized by anterior angulation of ulna and anterior dislocation of radial head (Monteggia fracture)

In less common type of Monteggia fracture, ulna angulated posteriorly and radial head dislocated posteriorly

Galeazzi fracture

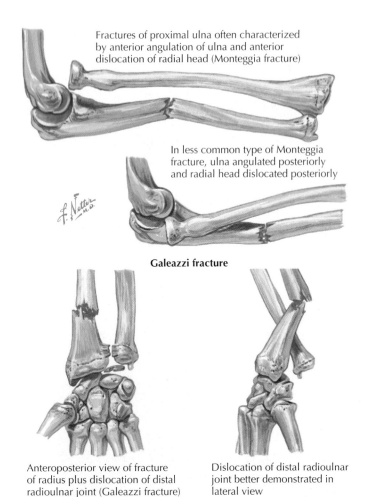

Anteroposterior view of fracture of radius plus dislocation of distal radioulnar joint (Galeazzi fracture)

Dislocation of distal radioulnar joint better demonstrated in lateral view

Figure 22-7 *Monteggia fracture.*

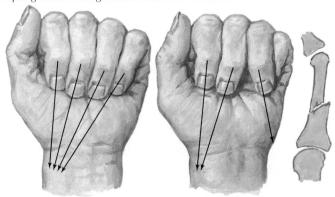

Transverse fractures of proximal phalanx tend to angulate volarly because of pull of interosseous muscles on base of proximal phalanx and collapsing action of long extensor and flexor tendons.

Reduction of fractures of phalanges or metacarpals requires correct rotational as well as longitudinal alignment. In normal hand, tips of flexed fingers point toward tuberosity of scaphoid, as in hand at left. Hand at right shows result of healing of ring finger in rotational malalignment. Rotational malalignment, usually discernible clinically, may also be evidenced on radiographs by discrepancy in cross-sectional diameter of fragments, as shown at extreme right. Discrepancy in diameter is most apparent in true lateral radiograph but is visible to some extent in anteroposterior view.

Figure 22-8 *Fracture of the proximal phalanx.*

discussed in more detail in Chapter 8. Acetabular fractures are also rare in children and are often associated with hip dislocation. Avulsion fractures are described earlier in this chapter and in Chapter 25.

Fractures of the Femur

Femur fractures occur commonly in children. The majority of femur fractures result from low-energy events, such as falls from playground equipment or sports-related injuries. These occur primarily in children age 5 to 10 years old. Femur fractures in children younger than 2 years old should raise concern for non-accidental trauma (see Chapter 12). Femur fractures can also result from high-energy events such as motor vehicle collisions.

Because femur fractures can result in significant blood loss, the patient's hemodynamic status must be assessed, and a thorough neurovascular evaluation should also be performed. Immediate management consists of traction and splinting to minimize blood loss. Definitive management of femur fractures most often includes a period of hospitalization for skeletal traction followed by application of a spica body cast.

Stress fractures of the femoral neck are becoming increasingly recognized in young athletes. See Chapter 25 for a discussion of these fractures.

Fractures of the Tibia and Fibula

Tibial and fibular shaft fractures are the most common fractures of the lower extremity in children. These types of fractures result from low-energy injuries such as falls or athletics or from high-energy injuries such as motor vehicle collisions or automobile–pedestrian injuries. Adolescent athletes performing in activities that involve jumping can occasionally present with tibial tuberosity fractures, which are avulsion fractures of the tibial tuberosity apophysis.

Patients with lower leg injuries may present with pain, swelling, deformity, and inability to bear weight on the affected limb. Evaluation of these injuries includes performing a thorough neurovascular examination. Diagnosis is confirmed with radiographs. Most of these injuries can be managed with immobilization and orthopedic referral as long as the neurovascular status is normal, but orthopedic consultation is often indicated to determine whether emergent reduction is necessary. Patients with significant tibial and fibular fractures are also at risk for compartment syndrome, which mandates an emergent orthopedic consultation.

TODDLER'S FRACTURE

Toddler's fractures occur in young ambulatory children, usually from 1 to 4 years of age. These injuries often occur after a seemingly insignificant fall, which is often unwitnessed. Young children often present with limp or refusal to walk. Most patients have no obvious deformity or swelling on examination, although gentle twisting of the lower leg or heel tapping may elicit pain. Radiography may reveal a spiral or oblique fracture through the distal third of the tibia on anteroposterior or lateral views, but oblique views are sometimes required to visualize the fracture if clinical suspicion is strong. Treatment consists of immobilization with a long leg cast for 3 to 4 weeks. With a high clinical suspicion but negative radiographs, a long leg splint or cast may still be considered.

Fractures of the Ankle and Foot

DISTAL TIBIAL AND FIBULAR FRACTURES

Ankle fractures often result from inversion and eversion injuries. Unlike adults, in whom ankle sprains are more common than fractures, in children, the strength of the ankle ligaments makes injury to the distal tibial and fibular epiphyses more likely than a ligamentous disruption. Patients often present with painful, swollen ankles and limited ability to bear weight.

Although any Salter-Harris type injury can be seen in ankle injuries, because the distal tibial epiphysis is the weakest structure in the ankle, Salter-Harris type II fractures of the distal tibia are the most common fractures of the ankle. Of the

fractures of the distal fibula, a Salter-Harris type I injury is the most common. Management of both these types of injuries consists of splinting followed by orthopedic referral and casting.

A Tillaux fracture is a Salter-Harris type III injury of the ankle that occurs as the medial distal tibial physis begins to close in adolescents who are nearing skeletal maturity, usually between the ages of 11 and 15 years. Forced external rotation of the foot leading to external rotation of the distal fibula causes the anterior tibiofibular ligament to avulse a piece of the anterolateral tibial epiphysis (Figure 22-9). This injury usually results from low-energy trauma such as in skateboard and baseball sliding injuries. Diagnostic work-up should begin with radiography, but after diagnosis has been made, a CT or MRI scan should be obtained to determine whether the fracture requires closed or open reduction.

Another fracture of the ankle unique to adolescent patients is the triplane fracture, a multiplanar fracture in which the fracture extends through the growth plate (transversely), epiphysis (sagittally), and distal tibial metaphysis (coronally) resulting in a Salter-Harris type IV fracture with three classically described fragments (see Figure 22-9). These fractures also occur in adolescents between the ages of 11 and 15 years before completion of the distal tibial physis closure. As with Tillaux fractures, the diagnostic workup should begin with radiography followed by CT or MRI to delineate the amount of displacement because many of these fractures require operative management.

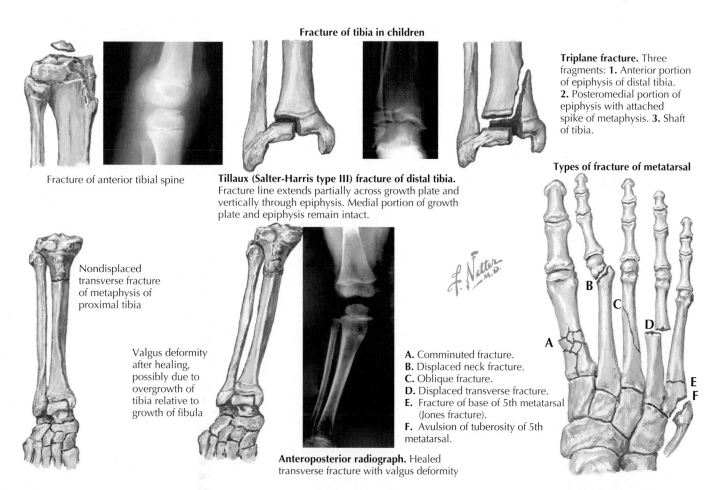

Figure 22-9 *Fractures of the ankle and foot.*

FRACTURES OF THE FOOT

Metatarsal and phalangeal fractures are common in children and account for the majority of fractures in children's feet. Most metatarsal and phalangeal fractures present with pain and swelling, occasionally accompanied by deformity. These injuries should be evaluated radiographically, and most can be treated with bulky splints and crutches. The fifth metatarsal fracture is the most common midfoot fracture. Proximal avulsion fractures of the tuberosity at the base of the fifth metatarsal are very common. They are usually associated with lateral ankle strain and heal well with brief immobilization. It is important to distinguish these fractures from Jones fractures, which can look very similar. Jones fractures are transverse fractures of the fifth metatarsal. Although far less common than avulsion fractures, they are associated with greater morbidity. If unrecognized, they have a high rate of nonunion, which can require bone grafting and internal fixation (see Figure 22-9).

FUTURE DIRECTIONS

Despite prevention efforts, the overall rate of fractures is increasing, largely because of the growth of organized sports. Therefore, pediatricians must maintain a focus on injury prevention.

Moreover, as childhood exposure to radiation continues to face increasing scrutiny, the utility of ultrasonography for the diagnosis of many fractures is currently being explored.

SUGGESTED READINGS

Eiff MP, Hatch RL: Boning up on common pediatric fractures, *Contemp Pediatr* 20:30-42, 2003.

Fleisher GR, Ludwig S, Henretig FM: Orthopedic trauma. In *Textbook of Pediatric Emergency Medicine*, Philadelphia, 2006, Lippincott Williams & Wilkins, pp 1525-1570.

Hart ES, Albright MB, Rebello GN, Grottkau BE: Broken bones: common pediatric fractures—part I, *Ortho Nurs* 25(4):251-256, 2006.

Hart ES, Grottkau BE, Rebello GN, Albright MB: Broken bones: common pediatric upper extremity fractures—part II, *Ortho Nurs* 25(5):311-323, 2006.

Hart ES, Luther B, Grottkau BE: Broken bones: common pediatric lower extremity fractures—part III, *Ortho Nurs* 25(6):390-407, 2006.

Jadhav SP, Swischuk LE: Commonly missed subtle skeletal injuries in children: a pictorial review, *Emerg Radiol* 15(6):391-398, 2008.

Nofsinger CC, Wolfe SW: Common pediatric hand fractures, *Curr Opin Pediatr* 14(1):42-45, 2002.

Shrader MW: Pediatric supracondylar fractures and pediatric physeal elbow fractures, *Orthop Clin North Am* 39(2):163-171, 2008.

Disorders of the Hip and Lower Extremity

23

Jessica Sparks Lilley and Mercedes M. Blackstone

*T*he pediatrician's knowledge of orthopedic disorders must be broad because the clinical presentation and diagnostic approach vary widely with age. Although many of the disorders discussed here are managed in conjunction with orthopedic surgeons, they can often be diagnosed by history and physical examination alone, and some do not require surgical intervention. In addition, delayed diagnosis of relatively common disorders such as developmental hip dysplasia remains one of the largest causes of litigation against primary care pediatricians, and more importantly, results in preventable long-term disability. Furthermore, mismanagement of disorders of rapidly changing bones may lead to chronic morbidity.

We divide several common disorders of the hips and lower extremities into one of three categories: congenital, developmental, or acquired.

CONGENITAL

A vast array of genetic diseases may present with lower limb anomalies at birth. In utero teratogen exposure can also lead to limb deformities. For instance, thalidomide has been off the market in the United States for many years secondary to its association with severe limb deformities. Illicit drugs or alcohol can also cause limb foreshortening. Amniotic bands can also cause structural changes, leading to amputation or dysplasia of limbs.

Clubfoot

Clubfoot, or talipes equinovarus, affects one in 1000 live births and is often diagnosed in utero. The condition is characterized by a smaller foot on the affected side, rigidity to plantar flexion, adductus of the forefoot, and inward angulation of the hindfoot (Figure 23-1). Half of cases are bilateral. Although many cases are idiopathic, maternal smoking, certain ethnic backgrounds, and genes affecting both the musculoskeletal and nervous systems have been identified as risk factors. Some believe that disordered development of the talus in utero causes the disorder.

Management of clubfoot has trended away from immediate surgical reconstruction because of the need for multiple corrective procedures, which can result in muscle weakness or stiffening. Currently, patients with the disorder are treated by progressive treatments that include more specific surgical repair if indicated to prepare for normal ambulation. The Ponseti method is typically used, which begins with tenotomy in most cases and is followed by serial casting and manipulation procedures. The less common French method involves daily physical therapy and binding over the first 2 months of life. Both methods are started early in the neonatal period, so early referral to a pediatric orthopedist is necessary. This visit may be arranged prenatally if the diagnosis is known. Clubfeet that do not respond to these conservative measures necessitate operative management.

DEVELOPMENTAL

In utero packaging causes some expected changes in every infant; some of these variations may take 3 to 4 years to resolve. Some of the more common disorders associated with packaging include rotational problems of the lower extremities such as in-toeing and out-toeing, which are often noted when a child begins to walk.

In-toeing

In-toeing is expected in children until the lower limbs laterally rotate with time; adult walking patterns are not observed until about 7 or 8 years of age. The cause of in-toeing varies by age, often caused by metatarsus adductus in infants, internal tibial torsion in toddlers, and excessive femoral anteversion in preschool-aged children.

METATARSUS ADDUCTUS

Metatarsus adductus is the medial deviation of the tarsometatarsal joints in the transverse plane. This variant is observed in 1% to 2% of infants. Metatarsus adductus is observed in infants who were crowded in utero, such as with oligohydramnios or twin gestation, and soon self-corrects; 85 to 90% resolve by 1 year of age. Indeed, the majority of children with metatarsus adductus have no long-term functional impairment and do not require surgical repair. Severe cases can increase development of bunions and hammertoes, so serial casting or bracing is helpful when the deformity does not resolve on its own.

INTERNAL TIBIAL TORSION

Internal tibial torsion is the most common cause of in-toeing and can be associated with metatarsus adductus. It is usually noted in toddlerhood when children begin to walk. It affects boys and girls equally and is bilateral in about two-thirds of cases. On examination, the knee remains in neutral position while the foot is medially rotated (Figure 23-2). Most cases self-resolve as children begin to walk independently, with normal alignment noted as early as 4 years or as late as 10 years of age.

FEMORAL ANTEVERSION

Excessive femoral anteversion is seen in preschool-aged children and is thought to be either a remnant of in utero positioning or increased ligamentous laxity. It is more common in girls and is almost universally bilateral. On physical examination, the knees are medially rotated, distinguishing this entity from internal tibial torsion. Normal growth usually leads to resolution by 8 to 10 years of age. For all causes of in-toeing, surgery may be

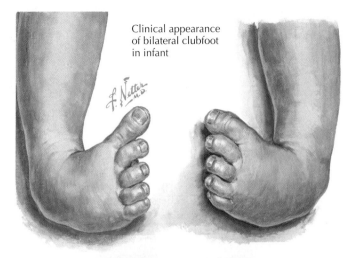

Clinical appearance of bilateral clubfoot in infant

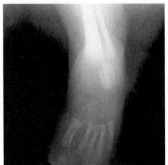

Anteroposterior (above) and lateral (below) radiographs show congenital clubfoot in newborn.

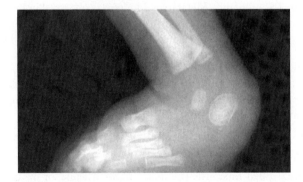

Figure 23-1 *Congenital clubfoot.*

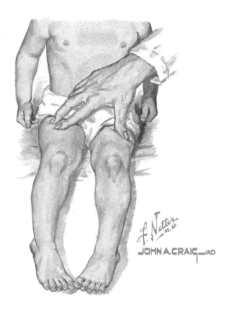

Child seated with knees flexed 90°. Patellae point directly forward, indicating that femurs are in neutral position, but feet point inward, suggesting tibial torsion. Measure tibial torsion by positioning the thigh in neutral rotation, then placing the thumb of one hand over the tibial tuberosity and with the other hand placing the thumb over the prominence of the medial malleolus and the long finger over the prominence of the lateral malleolus. The degree of tibial torsion is the estimate of the angle made by the transmalleolar axis and the axis of the coronal plane of the proximal tibia.

Figure 23-2 *Internal tibial torsion.*

considered for persistent cases or those causing functional impairment.

Bowlegs

Bowlegs, or genu varum, are noted when children begin walking and can be considered normal until about 3 years of age. Past this age group, however, bowing of the legs is pathologic, and other causes must be considered to establish proper treatment plans.

BLOUNT'S DISEASE AND ADOLESCENT TIBIA VARA

Blount's disease, also known as osteochondrosis deformans tibia or tibia vara, is an abnormality seen more frequently in obese

African American girls younger than 3 years of age and can be inherited in an autosomal recessive fashion. A less aggressive cause of progressive bowing is adolescent tibia vara, seen in boys older than 8 years of age. Similar to Blount's disease, adolescent tibia vara is observed more commonly in obese African Americans. Both disorders are associated with early walking. Starting corrective bracing early may prevent progressive deformity, and this additional support is especially crucial while walking. Tibial osteotomy may be considered for correction of bowlegs based on symptoms such as pain or asymmetry despite proper bracing for 1 year.

RICKETS

Rickets is a correctible cause of bowlegs that can be differentiated from tibia vara by family history, radiographic stigmata, and laboratory assessment. Rickets is an anomaly of bone mineralization that develops gradually in growing children because of calcium, phosphate, or vitamin D deficiency or resistance. Bowing of the legs, flaring of metaphyses, and "rachitic rosary" deformity of the ribs may all be seen on physical examination or plain films. The American Academy of Pediatrics (AAP) recommends 400 IU of vitamin D supplementation for all infants receiving less than 1 L of formula daily to prevent rickets. Metabolic bowing usually resolves with metabolic control and rarely requires surgical correction. See Chapter 69 for a more complete discussion of rickets.

Developmental Dysplasia of the Hip

Developmental dysplasia of the hip (DDH) bears special mention because it must be diagnosed promptly and does not resolve without intervention. DDH is a rare disorder with high morbidity when the diagnosis is made after 6 months of age. It is

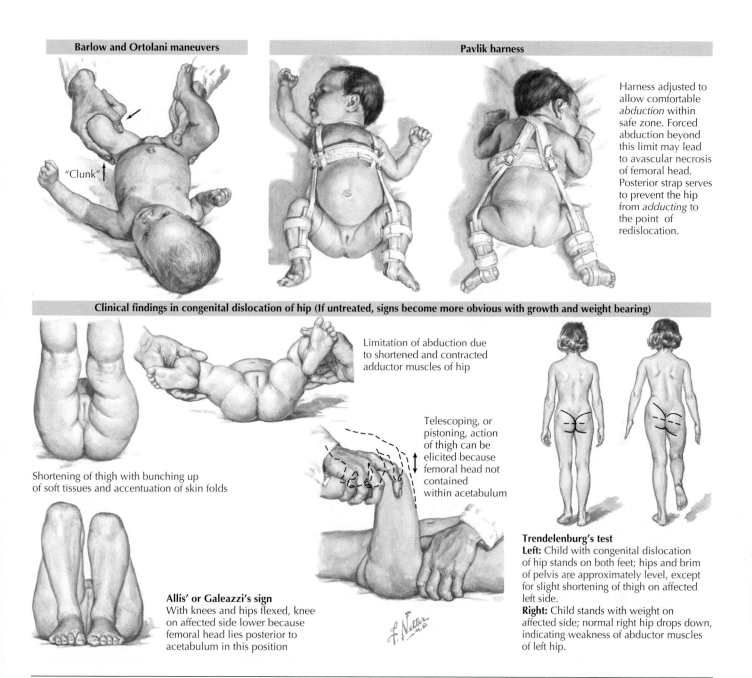

Barlow and Ortolani maneuvers

"Clunk"

Pavlik harness

Harness adjusted to allow comfortable *abduction* within safe zone. Forced abduction beyond this limit may lead to avascular necrosis of femoral head. Posterior strap serves to prevent the hip from *adducting* to the point of redislocation.

Clinical findings in congenital dislocation of hip (If untreated, signs become more obvious with growth and weight bearing)

Limitation of abduction due to shortened and contracted adductor muscles of hip

Telescoping, or pistoning, action of thigh can be elicited because femoral head not contained within acetabulum

Shortening of thigh with bunching up of soft tissues and accentuation of skin folds

Allis' or Galeazzi's sign
With knees and hips flexed, knee on affected side lower because femoral head lies posterior to acetabulum in this position

Trendelenburg's test
Left: Child with congenital dislocation of hip stands on both feet; hips and brim of pelvis are approximately level, except for slight shortening of thigh on affected left side.
Right: Child stands with weight on affected side; normal right hip drops down, indicating weakness of abductor muscles of left hip.

Figure 23-3 *Developmental dysplasia of the hip.*

characterized by an abnormal relationship between the hip socket, or acetabulum, and the femoral head. DDH represents a spectrum of disorders ranging from mild ligamentous laxity of the hip joint to a fully displaced femoral head. Diagnosis is made by physical examination of the neonate; finding a hip clunk on the Barlow or Ortolani maneuvers warrants immediate orthopedics referral. Whereas the Barlow test can identify a dislocatable hip, the Ortolani test attempts to reduce a dislocation (Figure 23-3). After the first few months of life, limitation or asymmetry of hip abduction is a more reliable examination finding.

Babies who are born in the breech presentation have additional stress placed on the developing hip joint and are therefore at higher risk for the disorder. Further risk factors include female gender, positive family history, and high birth weight.

The AAP recommends consideration of this constellation of risk factors for ultrasound screening of infants with no clear dislocation on examination. For instance, breech girls have two risk factors and are at relatively high risk for DDH, so screening is warranted. Plain radiographs are more accurate as ossification centers form and are the imaging modality of choice when the infant is older than 6 months of age.

Very mild abnormalities of the hip joint often resolve spontaneously in the first few months of life. When a true dislocation is diagnosed before 6 months of age, the Pavlik harness is the treatment of choice. It is a splint that prevents hip extension and adduction, which can be adjusted as the child grows (see Figure 23-3). Triple diapering or other measures to force the hip into place are no longer seen as effective treatment measures.

Diagnosis after age 6 months usually requires surgical repair. When not diagnosed in infancy, parents or pediatricians may notice that the affected child has a waddling or Trendelenburg gait when beginning to walk (see Figure 23-3). DDH may be more difficult to detect in older children because they often have bilateral involvement and therefore may not have a markedly asymmetric gait. These children require an urgent orthopedic referral because they are at high risk for long-term morbidity.

ACQUIRED

The majority of acquired disorders of the lower extremity are traumatic in origin. Common fractures of the lower extremity are discussed in Chapter 22, and injuries frequently encountered in young athletes are discussed in Chapter 25. Children who present with lower extremity pain or limp and have no history of trauma can be the cause of much anxiety to pediatric practitioners. The differential diagnosis for acquired limp in the child is vast and includes infectious, oncologic, rheumatologic, metabolic, and inflammatory processes. We focus here on several acquired processes not covered elsewhere in this textbook.

Slipped Capital Femoral Epiphysis

Slipped capital femoral epiphysis (SCFE) refers to an instability of the proximal femoral growth plate in which the femoral head slips posteriorly and inferiorly relative to the femoral neck (Figure 23-4). Although rare, SCFE is an extremely important diagnosis to make because prompt surgical repair is required, and a delay in diagnosis can lead to avascular necrosis. Patients with SCFE are typically obese children in their preadolescent and early adolescent years. A recent study found an incidence of 10.8 SCFE cases per 100,000 children. This incidence is higher in boys than girls and African Americans than whites. Obesity places increased force on the proximal femoral growth plate, putting children at risk for slippage.

Children with SCFE may complain of hip, knee, thigh, or groin pain. Hip pain can refer to the knee via the obturator nerve, so it is imperative to examine the hip in children complaining of isolated knee pain. The most common presentation is that of insidious pain over weeks or months that has gradually worsened and may cause an intermittent limp. SCFE can, however, present acutely as well, often in the setting of minor trauma.

On physical examination, patients with SCFE often hold the affected limb in passive external rotation and have pain with internal rotation. When asked to walk, they may have an antalgic gait. Both hips should be examined to allow for a comparison of range of motion of the two sides. Furthermore, about 20% of SCFEs are bilateral at the time of presentation, and another 20% will progress to bilateral slips if not prevented. Patients diagnosed with SCFE at younger ages are more likely to develop a contralateral slip over time.

Diagnosis is made on anteroposterior (AP) and frog-leg radiographs of the pelvis. The AP view can show widening of the physis and misalignment of the femoral capital epiphysis. On the AP view, the lack of intersection of a line drawn along

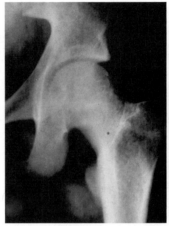
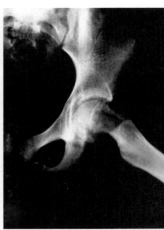

Slipped capital femoral epiphysis not readily apparent on anteroposterior radiograph because slip is usually posterior

Frog-leg radiograph, which demonstrates slipped epiphysis more clearly, always indicated when disorder is suspected

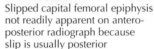

Classification

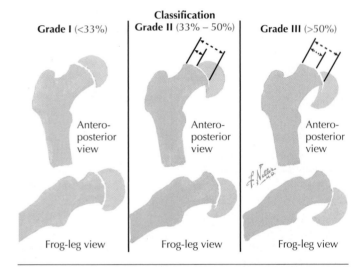

Grade I (<33%)	Grade II (33% – 50%)	Grade III (>50%)
Anteroposterior view	Anteroposterior view	Anteroposterior view
Frog-leg view	Frog-leg view	Frog-leg view

Figure 23-4 *Slipped capital femoral epiphysis.*

the femoral neck (Klein's line) and the femoral epiphysis can confirm the diagnosis. On the frog-leg view, the posterior portion of the femoral head becomes medial, making the slippage more apparent and giving a slipped "ice cream cone" appearance (see Figure 23-4). Patients found to have SCFE should be made non–weight bearing and need to see an orthopedist emergently. Treatment consists of internal fixation using a single cannulated screw, which prevents further slippage and provides symptom relief. There is a great deal of controversy surrounding the role of prophylactic fixation of the unaffected hip in unilateral SCFE.

Legg-Calvé-Perthes Disease

Legg-Calvé-Perthes (LCP) is the eponym given to a disease of idiopathic osteonecrosis of the femoral head. LCP affects children age 3 to 12 years and peaks in the early school years. As with SCFE, there is a male predominance, with males afflicted

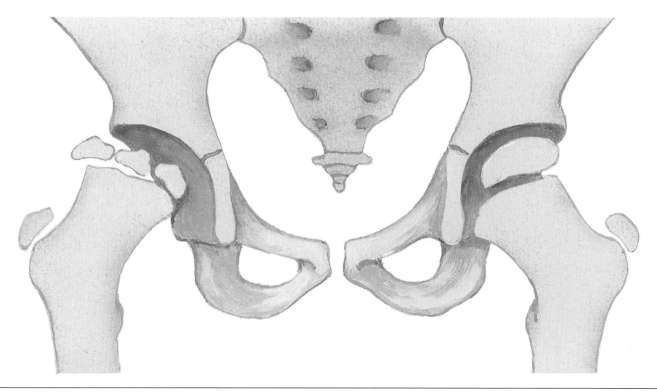

Figure 23-5 *Legg-Calvé-Perthes disease: ancillary prognostic indicators.*

four times as often as females. Unlike SCFE, however, whites are far more likely to have LCP.

These patients usually have an insidious onset of mild pain worsened by activity that may refer to the thigh or knee. On examination, patients may have a Trendelenburg gait, pain, or decreased range of motion with internal rotation and abduction and even atrophy of the muscle groups in the thighs and buttocks. In advanced disease, radiographs can be helpful and may show fragmentation of the femoral head (Figure 23-5). In early cases, however, radiographic changes can be subtle or nonexistent. A significant concern for LCP may mandate further imaging such as a bone scan or MRI.

As in SCFE, patients with LCP should be made non–weight bearing and referred to an orthopedic surgeon. Treatment consists of conservative management, including administration of nonsteroidal antiinflammatory drugs (NSAIDs), crutches, and immobilization with the goal of containing the femoral head within the acetabulum. Older children with LCP have a worse prognosis because of the decreased potential for bone remodeling and may experience disabling osteoarthritis in the adult years.

Transient Synovitis

Transient synovitis (TS) is characterized by inflammation of the hip synovium and is the most common cause of acute hip pain in young children. Children with TS are generally well appearing but have hip pain, a limp, or both. They often have low-grade fevers as well. TS typically presents at 3 to 8 years of age, and boys are affected twice as often as girls. It is often attributed to an infectious cause because many children have a history of a preceding upper respiratory infection. The principal concern with TS is distinguishing it from septic arthritis, which can result in significant morbidity if not promptly diagnosed and treated. To this end, inflammatory markers can be helpful. Children with high fevers or elevated inflammatory markers often require hip ultrasonography and aspiration of hip fluid if effusion is identified. The difference between TS and septic arthritis is discussed in greater detail in Chapter 88. TS is self-limited, but NSAIDs have been shown to shorten the duration of symptoms.

Osteoid Osteoma

Osteoid osteoma is a relatively common benign skeletal neoplasm that typically occurs in the femur, although it can occur anywhere. Most cases of osteoid osteoma occur in children and young adults, and males are affected twice as often as females. They typically present with localized pain at the site of the lesion, which is worse at night and responds well to NSAIDs. A limp may be observed as well. Osteoid osteomas usually appear as a dense central nidus smaller than 2 cm surrounded by a well-circumscribed lucency on plain radiographs or CT. Osteoid osteomas have no malignant potential and usually regress or become dormant spontaneously. If pain persists, the lesion can be surgically excised or ablated.

FUTURE DIRECTIONS

The majority of lower extremity disorders discussed here can be fully treated after they are recognized; prompt diagnosis coupled with appropriate orthopedic referral on the part of primary care physicians is critical. Advanced imaging modalities cannot replace a thorough history and physical examination. Several of the disorders discussed here merit further study of treatment outcomes in a randomized, controlled fashion to determine optimal medical or surgical management.

SUGGESTED READINGS

Clinical practice guideline: early detection of developmental dysplasia of the hip. Committee on Quality Improvement, Subcommittee on Developmental Dysplasia of the Hip. American Academy of Pediatrics, *Pediatrics* 105 (4 Pt 1):896-905, 2000.

Gholve PA, Cameron DB, Millis MB: Slipped capital femoral epiphysis update, *Curr Opin Pediatr* 21(1):39-45, 2009.

Disorders of the Neck and Spine

Mark R. Zonfrillo

24

Pediatric disorders of the neck and spine are generally rare. The majority of these conditions can be treated with rest, antiinflammatory medications, targeted physical therapy, and orthotics. Operative management is typically reserved for severe or refractory pathology and symptoms.

CONGENITAL MUSCULAR TORTICOLLIS

Torticollis, from the Latin words for "twisted neck," is lateral neck flexion with contralateral head rotation (Figure 24-1). Although the majority of torticollis cases result from sternocleidomastoid muscle (SCM) shortening, other causes include neurologic conditions, cervical spine abnormalities, and vision or hearing deficits.

Congenital muscular torticollis (CMT) occurs in 0.3% to 2% of newborns. Although the cause is unknown, intrauterine crowding or birth trauma may cause muscle damage. More than half of infants with CMT are firstborn or had a history of difficult delivery, including use of forceps or breech presentation. Magnetic resonance imaging (MRI) and surgical histopathology have demonstrated muscle atrophy and fibrosis similar to the vascular complications of compartment syndrome. Abnormal head positioning in CMT can cause plagiocephaly and facial asymmetry.

Evaluation of CMT should include a thorough birth history and description of presenting symptoms. The physical examination classically demonstrates an infant with the head tilted towards the side of SCM contraction with the chin pointed in toward the opposite shoulder (see Figure 24-1). A soft, nontender mass may be palpable in the body of the SCM. Visual tracking, hearing, and neurologic function should also be assessed to rule out nonmuscular causes. Patients should be evaluated for other associated conditions such as developmental dysplasia of the hip and referred for diagnostic imaging or surgical consultation as necessary.

Cervical spine radiographs can rule out osseous causes, including congenital spinal fusion (e.g., Klippel-Feil syndrome, unilateral atlantooccipital fusion), hemivertebrae, and rotational cervical instability. Ultrasonography, the diagnostic modality of choice, demonstrates a hyperechogenic muscle mass. Computed tomography (CT) and MRI can help exclude suspected neurologic or osseous etiologies of torticollis. However, these modalities may not be as sensitive as ultrasonography in diagnosing CMT, and exposure to radiation or sedation limits their role in routine evaluation of torticollis.

The majority of CMT resolves spontaneously or with regular physical therapy. If muscle shortening persists beyond 6 months of therapy or 12 months of life, orthopedic referral is necessary for surgical SCM lengthening. Although successful CMT therapy typically resolves the associated plagiocephaly and facial asymmetry, patients with residual symptoms may require referral for further evaluation and treatment.

SCOLIOSIS

Scoliosis is a lateral curvature and rotation of the spine (Figure 24-2). Although most cases of scoliosis are idiopathic, it can also arise from congenital or neuromuscular disorders and is associated with various syndromes.

Idiopathic disease accounts for 80% of all scoliosis cases and is divided by age into infantile (0–3 years), juvenile (3–10 years), and adolescent (>10 years) groups. Infantile idiopathic scoliosis is rare and is unique in that it is more likely to occur in boys, have left-sided curvature, and spontaneously resolve. Juvenile idiopathic scoliosis is similar to the adolescent type; girls are predominantly affected, and the curvature is typically right-sided. Although juvenile idiopathic scoliosis does not occur during a period of rapid spine growth, it is more likely to be progressive than other types. Idiopathic scoliosis most commonly presents in adolescence (70%). Although the cause and pathogenesis of idiopathic scoliosis are largely unknown, there are multiple theories, including genetic factors; lack of melatonin; and abnormalities of platelets, nerves, and muscles.

The evaluation of idiopathic scoliosis should include a careful history and physical examination. Patients are screened for thoracolumbar asymmetry with an Adam's forward bend test and scoliometer (see Figure 24-2). Examination should include comparison of the shoulders, scapulae, trunk, pelvis, and legs. Because idiopathic scoliosis is a diagnosis of exclusion, a careful assessment of neurologic function and signs of associated orthopedic disorders should be assessed. Congenital scoliosis should not be mistaken for infantile idiopathic scoliosis because the former is associated with other osseous and visceral anomalies. Definitive diagnosis and disease severity are determined by measuring the Cobb angle on a posteroanterior spinal radiograph, with any curvature more than 10 degrees being diagnostic. MRI is typically reserved for an atypical presentation or patients with focal neurologic findings.

Treatment of patients with idiopathic scoliosis depends on the age of onset and degree of curvature. Children with mild to moderate curves (<25 degrees), especially in the skeletally mature, can be observed clinically and with serial spinal radiographs. Physical therapy may also be used for minor disease. Patients with more severe curves, particularly younger children, may require bracing to minimize curve progression and prevent potential surgical correction. Unfortunately, the evidence for physical therapy and orthosis is equivocal, and their use is variable. Surgical correction is reserved for patients with severe curvatures (>45 degrees) or progressive disease that could compromise pulmonary or musculoskeletal function. Surgery can improve both the physical and psychological sequelae of idiopathic scoliosis. However, patients and their parents should be cautioned that although operative management can provide permanent structural correction, there are risks of surgical side effects or persistent symptoms.

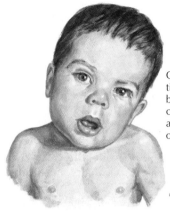

Child with muscular torticollis. Head tilted to left with chin turned to right because of contracture of left sterno-cleidomastoid muscle. Note facial asymmetry (flattening of left side of face)

Figure 24-1 *Torticollis.*

KYPHOSIS

Normal sagittal, thoracic vertebral kyphosis is 20 to 45 degrees by the Cobb angle on a lateral radiograph. Larger angles are pathologic and result in a rounding of the upper back or "hunchback deformity." The most common causes are postural kyphosis and Scheuermann's disease (Figure 24-3). Rare causes include congenital kyphosis, infection, malignancy, and other neuromuscular or osseous disorders. Postural kyphosis is mostly seen in adolescent boys as a result of slouching. There is typically no back pain nor any radiographic abnormality. Scheuermann's disease is an idiopathic osteochondritis that is a common cause of back pain in older children and adolescents. By definition, Scheuermann's disease results in anterior wedging of at least 5 degrees in at least three adjacent vertebral bodies.

Treatment of kyphosis is based on the cause. Because there are no structural irregularities in postural kyphosis, positional exercises are sufficient. The natural history of Scheuermann's disease is not well described, but physical therapy may improve symptoms. Orthotics may be useful for curves between 45 and 60 degrees, partial-angle correction, and pain relief. Operative repair is indicated for severe angles more than 75 degrees or curvature and pain refractory to bracing.

SPONDYLOLYSIS AND SPONDYLOLISTHESIS

Spondylolysis is a fracture or other defect in the pars interarticularis of the vertebra. Spondylolisthesis is anterior vertebral slippage caused by spondylolysis or other vertebral trauma, degeneration, or pathology.

Spondylolysis is a sequela of lumbar hyperextension from sports-related repetitive impacts (e.g., football, gymnastics, wrestling) or congenital vertebral abnormalities (e.g., thoracolumbar kyphosis in Scheuermann's disease). Patients may present with lumbar back pain, radiated buttock pain, or hamstring spasms. Spondylolysis is the most common cause of back pain in children after "idiopathic overuse." Physical examination may be normal or may reveal ipsilateral lateral spine flexion,

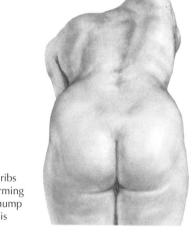

Posterior bulge of ribs on convex side forming characteristic rib hump in thoracic scoliosis

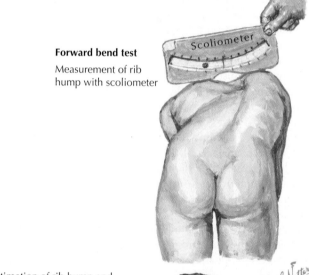

Forward bend test
Measurement of rib hump with scoliometer

Estimation of rib hump and evaluation of curve unwinding as patient turns trunk from side to side

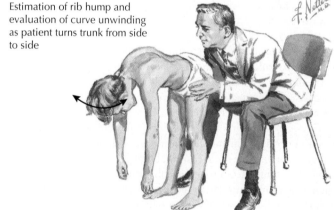

Figure 24-2 *Scoliosis.*

tenderness over the affected vertebra, or limited lumbar flexibility due to pain.

Oblique vertebral radiographs in an unaffected patient demonstrate a "Scottie dog" with the transverse process as the nose, the superior articular process as the ear, the spinous process and lamina as the body, and the inferior articular process as the front

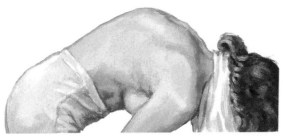

Unlike postural defect, kyphosis of Scheuermann's disease persists when patient is prone and thoracic spine extended or hyperextended and accentuated when patient bends forward (above)

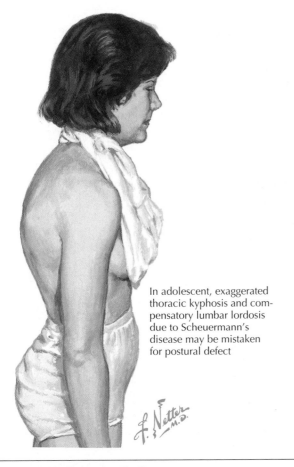

In adolescent, exaggerated thoracic kyphosis and compensatory lumbar lordosis due to Scheuermann's disease may be mistaken for postural defect

Figure 24-3 *Scheuermann's disease.*

leg. In spondylolysis, the dog has a fracture line through the neck (Figure 24-4). In spondylolisthesis, the entire head of the dog is displaced, with or without spondylolysis, on a scale graded from I (<25% slip) to V (complete spondylolisthesis) (see Figure 24-4). Spondylolysis and spondylolisthesis most commonly occur at L5 on S1, which can be seen on anteroposterior and lateral radiographs. Radiographs are also useful in identifying the degree of slip and any associated anomalies. CT and MRI are helpful if there is an atypical presentation, if the degree of slip is severe, or for preoperative planning. A single photon emission CT scan can help distinguish an acute from a chronic pars interarticularis defect, with the latter typically requiring operative repair.

Medical treatment of patients with spondylolysis and spondylolisthesis includes rest, oral nonsteroidal antiinflammatory medications, and physical therapy. Rehabilitation should focus on reduction of the lumbar lordosis and hamstring stretching. Orthotics may be useful for more symptomatic spondylolysis patients to reduce lumbar lordosis. The majority of lesions heal with medical therapy alone. Surgery is usually reserved for chronic spondylolysis or severe (>grade III), symptomatic spondylolisthesis.

VERTEBRAL COMPRESSION FRACTURES

Most compression fractures result from an axial or flexion load on the vertebral body, such as falls from a height, diving, and other sports injuries. Compression fractures represent the most common pediatric thoracic spine injury and are far more common in the thoracolumbar region than the cervical spine. Multiple fractures or an atypical mechanism should alert the provider to alternative diagnoses, including malignancy and nonaccidental trauma. In the absence of neurologic symptoms, treatment is usually conservative with rest, antiinflammatory medications, and use of orthotics. Many cervical injuries may require halo stabilization, and all unstable fractures require vertebral fusion.

INTERVERTEBRAL DISK HERNIATION

Pediatric intervertebral disk herniation is rare but potentially disabling. Most cases are lumbar, typically L4–L5 or L5–S1, with posterolateral herniation. In contrast to adult disease, pediatric disk herniation is more likely to occur in the setting of trauma, with or without prior disk degeneration. Particularly, sports with axial load (e.g., gymnastics, diving) or torsion (e.g., wrestling, football, hockey) confer a higher herniation risk. Patients typically present with acute-onset lower back pain and associated radiculopathy, although the degree of pain varies widely. There are a number of acute and chronic conditions that may present similarly to disk herniation, including muscle strain, vertebral fracture, spondylolysis, spondylolisthesis, ankylosing spondylitis, slipped capital femoral epiphysis, diskitis, and intraspinal tumor. Schmorl's nodes, a variant of disk herniation through the vertebral end plate instead of posterolaterally, should also be considered.

Examination commonly reveals limitation of movement and pain exacerbated by back flexion and straight-leg raises. There may also be a compensatory scoliosis that serves to alleviate nerve root pressure. Although spinal radiographs can show abnormalities consistent with herniation or other conditions, MRI is the study of choice. Nonoperative management is similar to that for other pediatric spine conditions and consists of rest, pain control, and physical therapy. Epidural steroid injections may provide additional pain relief. Unfortunately, pediatric disk histopathology demonstrates higher water content and elasticity compared with the condition in adults, which increases the likelihood of persistent herniation and need for surgical diskectomy in children. Operative repair is also indicated for debilitating neurologic deficits (e.g., severe motor impairment,

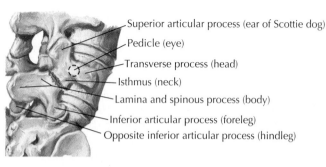
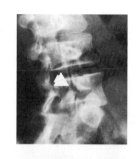

Superior articular process (ear of Scottie dog)
Pedicle (eye)
Transverse process (head)
Isthmus (neck)
Lamina and spinous process (body)
Inferior articular process (foreleg)
Opposite inferior articular process (hindleg)

Spondylolysis without spondylolisthesis. Posterolateral view demonstrates formation of radiographic Scottie dog. On lateral radiograph, dog appears to be wearing a collar

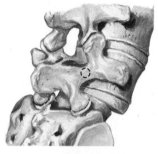
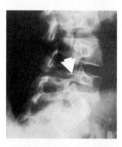

Dysplastic (congenital) spondylolisthesis. Luxation of L5 on sacrum. Dog's neck (isthmus) appears elongated

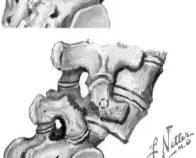
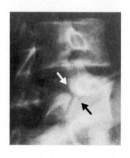

Isthmic type spondylolisthesis. Anterior luxation of L5 on sacrum due to fracture of isthmus. Note that gap is wider and dog appears decapitated

Figure 24-4 *Spondylolysis and spondylolisthesis.*

incontinence), although these are rare. Long-term outcomes of disk herniation are generally favorable.

FUTURE DIRECTIONS

Disorders of the neck and spine are uncommon in children but are potentially debilitating. Although many disorders are benign and self-limiting, patients must be adequately assessed for comorbidities, persistent pathology, or symptoms that affect cosmesis and quality of life. Further study of treatment outcomes in a randomized, controlled fashion is paramount to evaluate the most minimally invasive and maximally effective therapies.

SUGGESTED READINGS

Crawford AH: Orthopedics. In Rudolph CD, Rudolph AM, Hostetter MK, et al editors: *Rudolph's Pediatrics*, New York, 2003, McGraw-Hill.

Do TT: Congenital muscular torticollis: current concepts and review of treatment, *Curr Opin Pediatr* 18(1):26-29, 2006.

Hu SS, Tribus CB, Diab M, Ghanayem AJ: Spondylolisthesis and spondylolysis, *J Bone Joint Surg Am* 90(3):656-671, 2008.

Slotkin JR, Mislow JM, Day AL, Proctor MR: Pediatric disk disease, *Neurosurg Clin North Am* 18(4):659-667, 2007.

Weinstein SL, Dolan LA, Cheng JC, et al: Adolescent idiopathic scoliosis, *Lancet* 371(9623):1527-1537, 2008.

Sports Medicine

Erin Pete Devon and Mercedes M. Blackstone

25

Sports participation among children and adolescents has risen dramatically over the past few decades, with 30 to 45 million preadolescents and adolescents taking part in some form of structured athletic activity. In addition to providing physical exercise, involvement in organized sports can enhance self-confidence, coordination, and team-building skills. Despite these benefits, the relative lack of gross motor skills combined with the unique anatomy of developing children can place skeletally immature athletes at risk of injury. Not only are children at risk for acute injuries, but the increasing trend toward sports specialization at young ages puts them at risk for overuse injuries as well. High school athletes account for an estimated 2 million injuries, 500,000 doctor visits, and 30,000 hospitalizations annually. Primary care physicians must be prepared to treat injuries and to counsel on prevention, rehabilitation, and return to play.

This chapter provides a brief overview of several of the more common sports-related injuries.

ETIOLOGY AND PATHOGENESIS

Pediatric athletes are anatomically and physiologically different from their adult counterparts. Developing bone is structurally weaker than adult bone. The physis, or growth plate, is between the metaphysis and epiphysis in the long bones of children. It is weaker than adjacent ligaments and thus more prone to fracture under high energy transfer. Physeal fractures are unique to children and account for 15% to 20% of all pediatric fractures (see Chapter 22).

Pediatric joints have a higher percentage of cartilage. Growth cartilage is present at the epiphyseal plate, articular surface, and apophysis, which is the insertion site of major tendons. Articular cartilage is susceptible to repetitive microtrauma. Apophyseal injuries, unique to adolescents, occur at tendon insertion sites. Despite these anatomic vulnerabilities, children are also more capable of remodeling and heal better and faster than adults.

INJURIES BY BODY SYSTEM

Shoulder Injuries

The shoulder girdle is composed of three joints: the sternoclavicular joint, acromioclavicular (AC) joint, and glenohumeral joint. The shoulder is the loosest joint in the body, with a shallow glenoid fossa and little bony support (Figure 25-1). Both acute traumatic and chronic overuse injuries are common.

ACROMIOCLAVICULAR SEPARATION

The AC joint is composed of the acromion of the scapula and the distal clavicle. The AC and coracoclavicular ligaments stabilize the joint (see Figure 25-1). AC joint injuries, including sprains, subluxations and dislocations, are referred to as shoulder separations and account for 10% of all shoulder injuries. Injury to the AC joint is usually caused by a fall onto the top of the shoulder, causing the scapula and acromion to be pushed inferiorly, and the clavicle, with its medial end attached to the sternum, to be elevated. AC separations have a 5 : 1 male-to-female ratio and are encountered most frequently in hockey, wrestling, and the martial arts. Examination reveals asymmetric enlargement of the AC joint with localized tenderness to the joint. Forward flexion, extension, and cross-chest adduction results in AC joint pain. Diagnosis is made clinically or by plain radiographs dedicated to the AC joint. Milder separations are typically treated nonoperatively with rehabilitation, and the far less common severe separations may require surgical repair.

ANTERIOR SHOULDER DISLOCATION

Anterior dislocation of the glenohumeral joint accounts for 90% of shoulder dislocations. Common mechanisms are falling onto an outstretched hand with a straight arm or making contact with another player with the shoulder abducted to 90 degrees and forcefully rotated externally. These patients experience the sudden onset of pain, a "pop," and an inability to use the arm. This diagnosis is uncommon in pediatric athletes younger than 10 years of age; a shoulder deformity in younger patients often represents a proximal humeral fracture rather than an acute glenohumeral dislocation.

Examination reveals flattening of the deltoid prominence, prominence of the acromion, fullness of the subcoracoid region, and downward displacement of the axillary fold (Figure 25-2). It is also important to test for axillary and musculocutaneous nerve injury (see Figure 25-2).

Evaluation requires axillary, anteroposterior (AP), and scapular Y radiographs both before and after reduction to rule out associated fracture. An acute glenohumeral joint dislocation is an orthopedic emergency and requires closed reduction. There are many techniques for closed reduction; two of the more common are the traction–countertraction technique and Stimson's maneuver (see Figure 25-2). It is important to reexamine the neurovascular integrity of the arm after reduction. Surgical reduction is rarely indicated. After reduction, the arm is immobilized for 2 to 4 weeks followed by gradual rehabilitation. Up to 90% of patients with shoulder dislocations before age 20 years have a recurrence.

Elbow Injuries

The elbow flexes, extends, pronates, and supinates, serving as the origin and insertion of several muscle groups. The wrist and finger extensors arise from the lateral epicondyle, the forearm flexors-pronators from the medial epicondyle, and the triceps insert into the olecranon process. A thorough understanding of the anatomy and development of the pediatric elbow greatly facilitates the diagnosis of sports-related injuries.

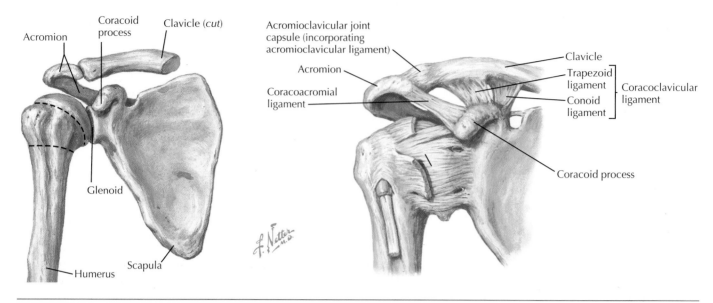

Figure 25-1 *Anterior view scapula and proximal humerus.*

ELBOW DISLOCATION

The elbow is the most commonly dislocated joint in children. Posterior dislocations are more common because of the shape of the olecranon process. They occur in older children, whose physes have closed, after falling backward onto an outstretched hand with the shoulder abducted. Simple dislocations can be seen in conjunction with associated fractures. On examination, an obvious deformity is noted, with the olecranon process displaced prominently behind the distal humerus (Figure 25-3). A careful neurovascular examination must be performed before and after reduction, paying particular attention to the median nerve. AP and lateral radiographs are useful in diagnosis. Isolated dislocation is treated by closed reduction. Unlike a

shoulder dislocation, the greatest risk for an elbow dislocation is stiffness rather than recurrence. For this reason, immobilization is required for a short period of time, and return to full use is closely supervised.

ELBOW OVERUSE INJURIES

"Little League elbow" is a broad term for several different elbow problems. Medial elbow pain is a common complaint of overhand throwers caused by repeated valgus stress on the joint, which can be exacerbated by improper throwing mechanics. In preadolescents, traction apophysitis of the medial epicondyle is most likely. Patients have tenderness along the medial epicondyle that is aggravated by resisted wrist flexion. Treatment

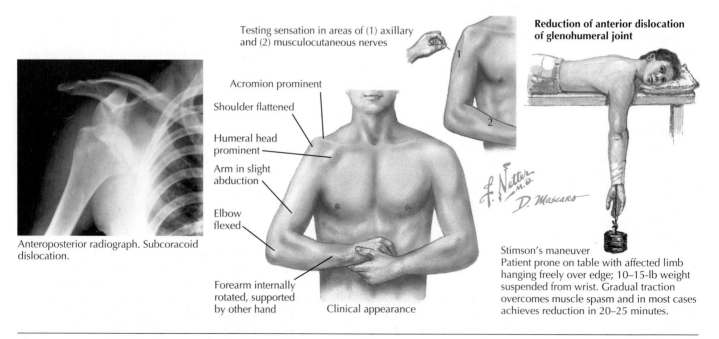

Testing sensation in areas of (1) axillary and (2) musculocutaneous nerves

Acromion prominent

Shoulder flattened

Humeral head prominent

Arm in slight abduction

Elbow flexed

Forearm internally rotated, supported by other hand

Clinical appearance

Anteroposterior radiograph. Subcoracoid dislocation.

Reduction of anterior dislocation of glenohumeral joint

Stimson's maneuver
Patient prone on table with affected limb hanging freely over edge; 10–15-lb weight suspended from wrist. Gradual traction overcomes muscle spasm and in most cases achieves reduction in 20–25 minutes.

Figure 25-2 *Anterior dislocation of glenohumeral joint.*

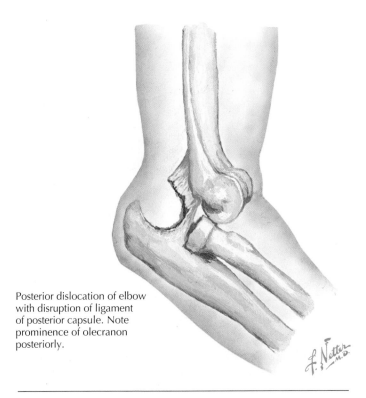

Posterior dislocation of elbow with disruption of ligament of posterior capsule. Note prominence of olecranon posteriorly.

Figure 25-3 *Elbow dislocation.*

includes restricting throwing for 4 to 6 weeks, pain-free strengthening, and gradual reintroduction of throwing with proper instruction.

In an adolescent athlete with medial elbow pain, avulsion fracture of the medial epicondyle must be considered. These can typically be treated with immobilization, but avulsions with significant displacement or neurovascular compromise often require surgical intervention. In young adults with a fused growth plate, ulnar collateral ligament tears are more common.

Lateral epicondylitis, or "tennis elbow," is caused by repetitive contraction of the extensor muscles at their origin on the lateral epicondyle. Tenderness is elicited over the lateral epicondyle, and pain is felt with passive wrist flexion and resisted wrist extension. Initial treatment includes conservative therapy, rehabilitation, and limitation of activity.

Hip Injuries

The hip joint is a "ball and socket" joint in which the femur articulates with the acetabulum. The femur is the longest bone in the body and is subjected to substantial forces transmitted through the hip that can reach three to five times the body's weight during running and jumping. About 10% to 24% of athletic injuries in children are hip related.

AVULSION FRACTURES

Avulsion fractures occur because of a sudden contraction of a muscle pulling on a developing apophysis and are commonly seen in sports such as soccer, ice hockey, gymnastics, and sprinting. The combination of intensive training at an inherently weak

epiphyseal plate predisposes an athlete to an avulsion fracture. Athletes often describe a pop after a forceful kick followed by sudden pain. The most common sites of pelvic avulsion injuries are the anterior inferior iliac spine and the ischial tuberosity caused by the powerful contraction of the sartorius and rectus femoris muscles, respectively. Although commonly seen in the hip, developing athletes can sustain avulsion fractures at other sites as well (see the Elbow Injuries section above). Plain radiographs of the pelvis should be carefully examined when avulsion fractures are suspected, since they can often be quite subtle radiographically.

FEMORAL NECK STRESS FRACTURES

Stress fractures are relatively common among runners and military trainees, and roughly 10% of them occur in the femoral neck. Femoral neck stress fractures are often overlooked or misdiagnosed, with dire consequences. Intensive or improper training regimens and hard running surfaces place patients at risk. Patients with femoral neck stress fractures present with a deep pain in the hip, groin, or thigh that is initially present only with activity and later becomes continuous. They have pain with internal and external rotation, as well as axial loading. Because initial radiographic findings are often negative, this diagnosis requires a high index of suspicion; a bone scan or magnetic resonance imaging scan (MRI) may be necessary. Initial treatment consists of rest, non–weight bearing, and conservative management, but certain types require surgical repair. These fractures can lead to avascular necrosis of the femoral head if not properly treated.

Knee Injuries

The knee is the largest joint in the body. It is a modified hinge joint that primarily permits flexion and extension. The knee is made up of four bones: the femur, patella, tibia, and fibula. Important ligamentous structures include the medial and lateral collateral ligaments and the anterior and posterior cruciate ligaments. The medial and lateral menisci, joint capsule, quadriceps, and hamstrings all act as stabilizing structures. Acute and chronic injuries are very common causes of knee pain, especially in young athletes; however, other causes of knee pain must be included in the differential diagnosis, including malignancy, infection, arthritis, and referred pain from the hip.

PATELLAR DISLOCATION

Patellar dislocations occur when the quadriceps contract to extend the knee but the patella is not in the intercondylar groove and gets displaced laterally. These dislocations typically occur in sports such as dance and gymnastics that involve a lot of jumping, twisting, and pivoting. This dislocation occurs more commonly in girls. Patients present with the knee flexed in intense pain and may describe a popping sensation (Figure 25-4). The examination reveals effusion, limited range of motion, the inability to bear weight, and a laterally displaced patella. Reduction should be performed promptly. With the patient supine with the hips flexed, the knee should be gently extended while medial pressure is applied to the dislocated patella. The practitioner performing the reduction will typically feel the patella

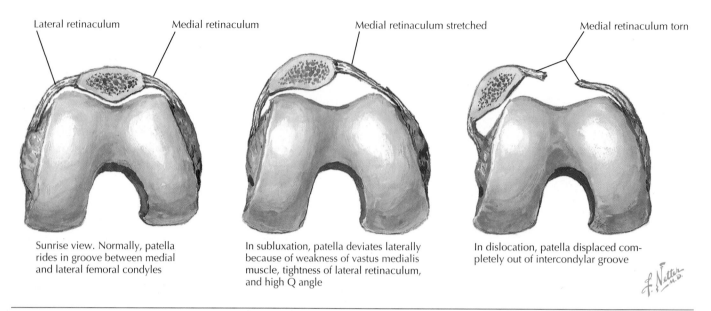

Lateral retinaculum   Medial retinaculum

Medial retinaculum stretched

Medial retinaculum torn

Sunrise view. Normally, patella rides in groove between medial and lateral femoral condyles

In subluxation, patella deviates laterally because of weakness of vastus medialis muscle, tightness of lateral retinaculum, and high Q angle

In dislocation, patella displaced completely out of intercondylar groove

Figure 25-4 *Subluxation and dislocation of patella.*

return to the tibiofemoral tract. After reduction, radiographs should be taken to rule out a concomitant fracture, and the knee should be immobilized. Patellar subluxation may be observed if the history is consistent with dislocation but the pain has improved and the examination results are normal. Patellar dislocations commonly recur, with up to 15% of pediatric patients having a second event.

OSGOOD-SCHLATTER DISEASE

Osgood-Schlatter disease, the most common overuse injury of the adolescent knee, occurs at the anterior tibial tubercle. Athletes involved in sports that involve substantial cutting, running, and jumping are at risk, and they typically present with pain, swelling, and prominence of the tibial tubercle (Figure 25-5). On physical examination, tenderness at the tibial tubercle can

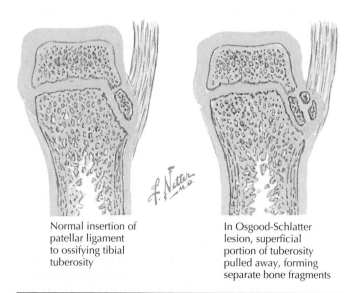

Normal insertion of patellar ligament to ossifying tibial tuberosity

In Osgood-Schlatter lesion, superficial portion of tuberosity pulled away, forming separate bone fragments

Figure 25-5 *Osgood-Schlatter lesion.*

be elicited. Radiographs are not necessary to make this clinical diagnosis, but when obtained, they can demonstrate soft tissue swelling over the tibial tubercle or fragmentation of the tubercle. Osgood-Schlatter disease is typically a self-limited disease and usually resolves with closure of the tibial growth plate. Treatment involves symptomatic control with nonsteroidal anti-inflammatory drugs and may involve limitation of activity until improvement of the pain and limp. Stretching of the quadriceps and hamstrings as well as physical therapy to strengthen the quadriceps can be helpful.

PATELLOFEMORAL PAIN SYNDROME

Patellofemoral pain syndrome (PFPS) is the most common cause of knee pain in the outpatient setting and is the cause of up to 25% of all injuries in runners. Affecting one or both knees, PFPS occurs most commonly in adolescents and young adults, and affects females more often than males. PFPS is multifactorial resulting from overuse or overload of the knee, abnormal tracking of the patella, and muscular causes such as imbalances between the quadriceps. Patients with PFPS often have anterior knee pain or pain behind the patella. They typically complain of pain during running, going down stairs or inclines, or with prolonged sitting, which improves with ambulation. The patient may note a recent change in activity, such as an increase in a training regimen. Physical examination may reveal a medially displaced patella, tenderness of the articular surface of the patella while the knee is extended, crepitus, or a positive patellar stress test result. This test involves the physician fixing the patella against the femur and asking the patient to contract the quadriceps. This maneuver causes pain in patients with PFPS. PFPS is a clinical diagnosis, and radiographs are unnecessary before the initiation of care. Treatment includes avoiding activities that cause pain. Exercises to increase the strength of the quadriceps and flexibility of the hip, hamstring, calf, and iliotibial band are important in the recovery phase. Adjunctive therapies include foot orthosis, bracing, and patellar taping.

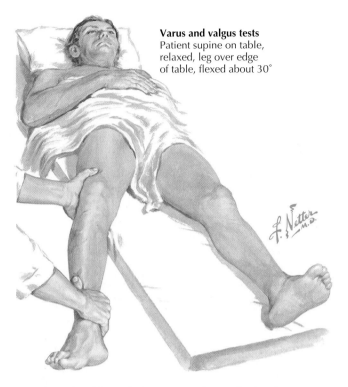

Varus and valgus tests
Patient supine on table, relaxed, leg over edge of table, flexed about 30°

With one hand fixing thigh, examiner places other hand just above ankle and applies valgus stress. Degree of mobility compared with that of uninjured side, which is tested first. For varus stress test, direction of pressure reversed

Figure 25-6 *Abduction stress (forced valgus) test and adduction stress (forced varus) test.*

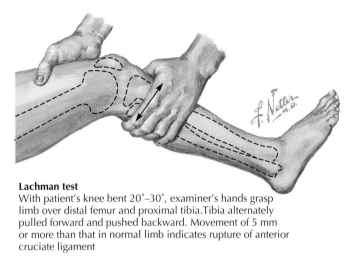

Lachman test
With patient's knee bent 20°–30°, examiner's hands grasp limb over distal femur and proximal tibia. Tibia alternately pulled forward and pushed backward. Movement of 5 mm or more than that in normal limb indicates rupture of anterior cruciate ligament

Figure 25-7 *Lachman test of the knee.*

OSTEOCHONDRITIS DISSECANS

Osteochondritis dissecans is a osteochondral lesion that affects subchondral bone and overlying articular cartilage. A fragment of bone or cartilage partially or completely separates from the joint surface. This disease process occurs most commonly in teenagers and usually affects one joint, most often the knee. The cause is not completely known but is likely a combination of factors, including genetic predisposition, trauma, and interruptions in the blood supply. The usual presentation is generalized pain, which worsens with a twisting motion, and swelling. Patients may complain of stiffness, weakness, or a mechanical sensation such as a popping, locking, or clicking in the knee. Radiographs can be helpful in determining the location of the lesion, but a bone scan or MRI may be necessary. Low-grade lesions heal spontaneously with conservative treatment. If a lesion loosens, internal fixation or debridement may be required.

SOFT TISSUE INJURIES

Medial collateral ligament or lateral collateral ligament injuries are rare when the epiphysis is open because the involved ligaments are stronger than the growth plate. When present, swelling may be minimal, but tenderness will be present over the involved ligament. The knee should be tested for laxity with varus and valgus testing, as shown in Figure 25-6. Anterior cruciate ligament injuries involve rotational forces on a fixed

foot. The patient will report a "pop" and rapid swelling with decreased range of motion. The Lachman test (Figure 25-7) is a method of detecting this injury. Arthroscopy or MRI is often needed for definitive diagnosis.

Leg, Ankle, and Foot Injuries

SHIN SPLINTS

Shin splints are a common overuse injury of the lower leg, presenting with pain along the medial tibia. Pain starts toward the end of exercise and begins earlier and lasts beyond the cessation of exercise if continued exercise occurs. Diagnosis can be made by history and physical examination. Radiographic studies are sometimes necessary to rule out a stress fracture. Treatment involves relative rest and correcting training errors. Fitness can be maintained with alternative exercises such as swimming or cycling.

ANKLE SPRAINS

The ankle is a hinge joint formed by the distal tibia, distal fibula, and talus. Ankle injuries are extremely common in athletes. About 85% are sprains and, of those, 85% percent are inversion injuries. However, in a preadolescent patient, growth plate injuries (Salter-Harris fractures) are more common than sprains. A detailed history about the position of the ankle at the time of injury and the direction of forces are useful in making an assessment. If no deformity is obvious, the clinician should inspect for bruising and swelling and palpate the bony structures of the ankle, including the fibula, distal tibia, and proximal fifth metatarsal. The more common inversion mechanism produces injury to the lateral portion of the foot and ankle, usually the anterior talofibular ligament. The anterior draw test helps to assess the status of the ankle ligaments. A significant difference between the affected and unaffected ankle may suggest a tear of the anterior talofibular ligament. Passive and active range of motion should also be assessed.

Radiographs of the ankle should be obtained when patients are unable to bear weight or have malleolar tenderness. Children with point tenderness who are likely to have open growth plates should have radiographs to rule out Salter-Harris fractures. Early treatmen of ankle sprains includes RICE (rest, ice, compression, elevation) and early mobilization. Functional rehabilitation should begin on the day of injury. It includes range of motion exercise, muscle strengthening, and then activity-specific training.

SEVER DISEASE

Sever disease is an inflammation of the apophysis at the posterior aspect of the calcaneus. It is twice as common in boys and occurs bilaterally 60% of the time. The presentation is between 8 and 13 years of age. Patients complain of heel pain related to activity. Sports involving running and jumping predispose children to Sever disease. There is tenderness to palpation at the insertion of the Achilles tendon into the calcaneus, and the heel cords are tight. Treatment includes relative rest, ice, massage, stretching, and strengthening of the Achilles tendon.

FUTURE DIRECTIONS

Although this chapter focuses on the recognition, evaluation, and management of common sports injuries, efforts should focus on the prevention of sports injuries. Proper education of parents, athletes, coaches, and physicians can prevent overly intensive or improper training and sports specialization at too young an age, all of which can lead to overuse injuries. Physician education in the area of sports medicine should likewise be enhanced to allow for prompt recognition of such injuries.

SUGGESTED READINGS

Brenner JS: Overuse injuries, overtraining, and burnout in child and adolescent athletes, *Pediatrics* 119(6):1242-1245, 2007.

Demorest RA, Bernhardt DT, Best TM, Landry GL: Pediatric residency education: is sports medicine getting its fair share? *Pediatrics* 115(1):28-33, 2005.

Holly BJ, Hang BT: Common acute upper extremity injuries in sports, *Clin Pediatr Emerg Med* 8(1):15-31, 2007.

Intensive training and sports specialization in the young athlete. American Academy of Pediatrics. Committee on Sports Medicine and Fitness, *Pediatrics* 106(1 Pt 1):154-157, 2000.

Sciascia A, Kibler WB: The pediatric overhead athlete: what is the real problem? *Clin J Sports Med* 16(6):471-477, 2006.

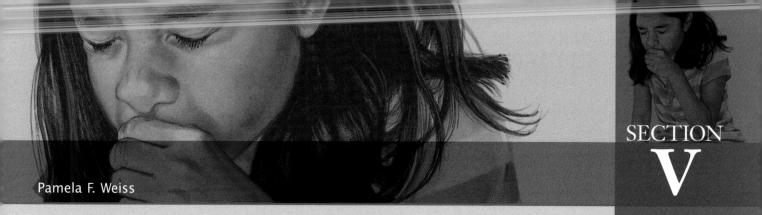

Pamela F. Weiss

SECTION
V

Rheumatologic Disorders

Chronic Arthritis

Julie M. Linton and Pamela F. Weiss

26

Juvenile idiopathic arthritis (JIA) is the most common rheumatologic disease among children. The term JIA describes a clinically heterogeneous group of diseases characterized by arthritis that begins before age 16 years, involves one or more joints, and lasts at least 6 weeks. Prevalence estimates for JIA range from 8 to 150 per 100,000; specific epidemiologic characteristics vary by JIA subtype.

ETIOLOGY AND PATHOGENESIS

Similar to many chronic illnesses, JIA is likely caused by genetic and environmental factors. Although discussion of the full extent of genetic associations identified to date is beyond the scope of this chapter, human leukocyte antigen (HLA) associations exist for each of the JIA subtypes, with the greatest number for oligoarticular disease. Among patients with enthesitis-related JIA, the presence of HLA-B27 may contribute to disease pathogenesis. Non-HLA candidate genes, including *PTPN22*, *MIF*, *SLC11A6*, *WISP3*, and *TNFA*, have been independently confirmed to be associated with various JIA subtypes. Additionally, the presence of autoantibodies such as antinuclear antibody (ANA, found in ≈40% of patients) and rheumatoid factor (RF, present in approximately 5%-10%) gives evidence for immune dysfunction in JIA. The presence of multilineage cells and associated cytokines in the synovium indicate involvement of all levels of the immune system in disease pathogenesis, including innate immunity (via inflammatory cells and cytokines), cell-mediated immunity (via activated T-lymphocytes), and humoral immunity (via autoantibodies).

CLINICAL PRESENTATION

The diagnosis of JIA is made from a detailed history, comprehensive physical examination, directed laboratory tests and imaging, and following the child over time. Distinct clinical features characterize each of the JIA subtypes during the first 6 months of disease.

OLIGOARTICULAR JUVENILE IDIOPATHIC ARTHRITIS

Oligoarticular JIA is defined by arthritis in four or fewer joints during the first 6 months of disease. Oligoarticular JIA is the most common form of JIA, typically occurs before age 4 years, and affects girls more often than boys at a ratio of 4:1. The knee is the most commonly affected joint followed by the ankles and small joints of the hand (Figure 26-1). The temporomandibular joint (TMJ) is also commonly affected. Children often experience morning stiffness, gelling (transient stiffness), and pain, but up to 25% may have painless arthritis. There are two subsets of oligoarthritis; *persistent oligoarthritis* affects a maximum of four joints throughout the disease course, and *extended oligoarthritis* affects more than four joints after the first 6 months of disease. Extended disease is associated with a worse prognosis.

Although children with oligoarticular JIA have the greatest likelihood of remission among the JIA subtypes, complications can cause long-lasting morbidities. Asymmetric joint disease (particularly at the knee) can lead to leg length discrepancy caused by hyperemia of inflammation. Severe disease of the TMJ can lead to difficulty chewing, malocclusion, or micrognathia. Asymptomatic iridocyclitis (anterior uveitis that affects the iris and ciliary body) is common in oligoarthritis, particularly among young girls who are ANA positive, and must be screened for at disease presentation and serially thereafter. Complications of uveitis include visual impairment, posterior synechiae, cataracts, band keratopathy, and glaucoma (Figure 26-2).

POLYARTICULAR JUVENILE IDIOPATHIC ARTHRITIS

Polyarticular JIA, defined by arthritis in five or more joints during the first 6 months of disease, is the second most frequent subtype of JIA. It is divided into two subtypes: RF-negative and RF-positive disease. Seronegative disease affects girls more frequently than boys. Seropositive patients are often adolescent girls who experience an insidious disease onset involving primarily the large and small joints of the hands and feet, the cervical spine, and TMJ. Rheumatoid nodules, boutonniere deformities (proximal interphalangeal joint flexion and distal interphalangeal joint hyperextension), and swan-neck deformities (proximal interphalangeal joint hyperextension and distal interphalangeal joint flexion) are frequently seen in seropositive patients. Mild systemic symptoms, such as low-grade fevers, lymphadenopathy, and hepatosplenomegaly, are common.

SYSTEMIC JUVENILE IDIOPATHIC ARTHRITIS

Systemic JIA is defined by arthritis; fever for at least 2 weeks with high quotidian spikes for at least 3 days; and at least one of the following: evanescent and erythematous rash, lymphadenopathy, hepatosplenomegaly, and serositis (often pericarditis or pleuritis). The disease affects boys and girls equally and can occur at any age but most commonly in early childhood. Children often appear ill during fevers and appear well when afebrile. Arthritis is generally symmetric and polyarticular but may be absent at onset. The rash consists of discrete, salmon-pink macules that are more pronounced during fever and may be associated with the Koebner phenomenon (linear streaks on the skin elicited by scratching) (Figure 26-3).

Complications of systemic JIA include macrophage-activating syndrome (MAS), systemic amyloidosis, infections caused by immunosuppression, and the effects of chronic corticosteroids. Approximately 5% to 8% of children with systemic JIA develop MAS. This life-threatening complication is characterized by acute onset of sustained fever, hepatosplenomegaly, and lymphadenopathy. Associated laboratory abnormalities may include pancytopenia, elevated fibrin split products, transaminitis,

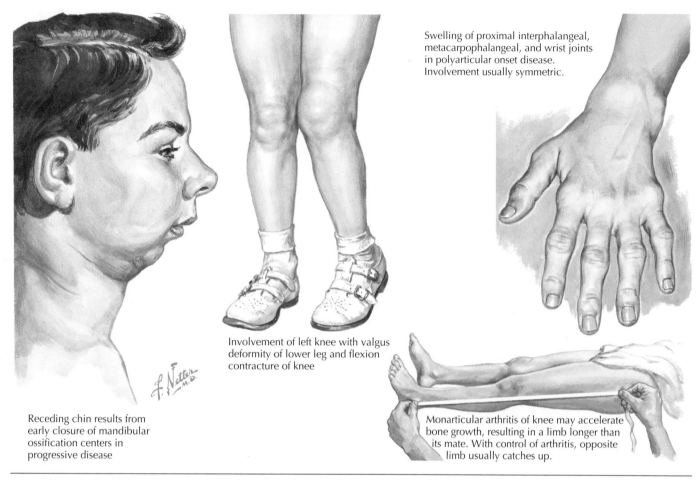

Swelling of proximal interphalangeal, metacarpophalangeal, and wrist joints in polyarticular onset disease. Involvement usually symmetric.

Involvement of left knee with valgus deformity of lower leg and flexion contracture of knee

Receding chin results from early closure of mandibular ossification centers in progressive disease

Monarticular arthritis of knee may accelerate bone growth, resulting in a limb longer than its mate. With control of arthritis, opposite limb usually catches up.

Figure 26-1 *Clinical signs of oligoarticular and polyarticular juvenile idiopathic arthritis.*

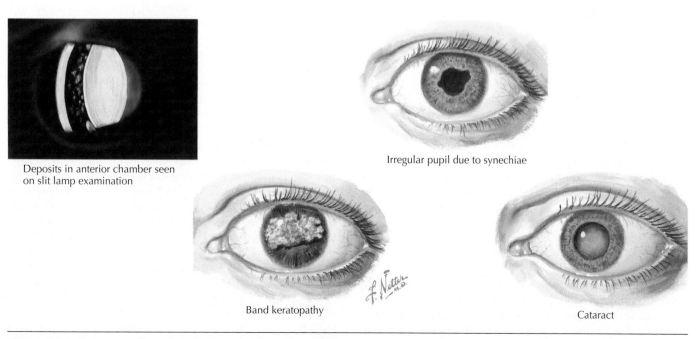

Deposits in anterior chamber seen on slit lamp examination

Irregular pupil due to synechiae

Band keratopathy

Cataract

Figure 26-2 *Ocular manifestations in juvenile idiopathic arthritis.*

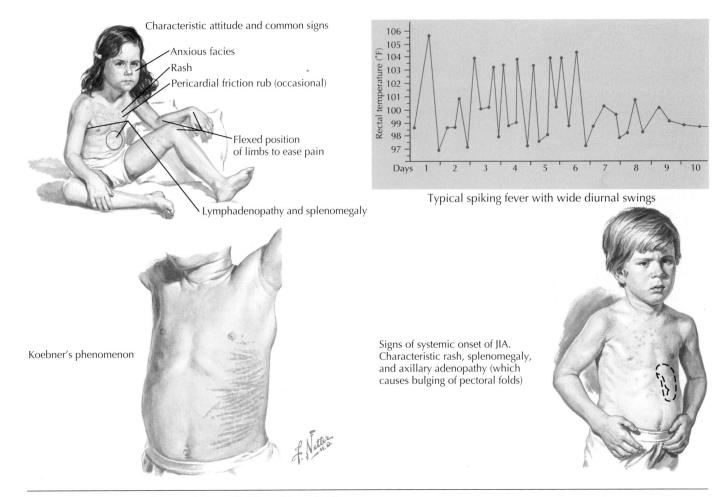

Characteristic attitude and common signs
- Anxious facies
- Rash
- Pericardial friction rub (occasional)
- Flexed position of limbs to ease pain
- Lymphadenopathy and splenomegaly

Typical spiking fever with wide diurnal swings

Koebner's phenomenon

Signs of systemic onset of JIA. Characteristic rash, splenomegaly, and axillary adenopathy (which causes bulging of pectoral folds)

Figure 26-3 *Features of systemic juvenile idiopathic arthritis.*

hypertriglyceridemia, hyperferritinemia, *low* erythrocyte sedimentation rate (ESR) (secondary to hypofibrinogenemia), and elevated coagulation factors. Bone marrow examination reveals active phagocytosis of hematopoietic cells.

PSORIATIC ARTHRITIS

Psoriatic arthritis is defined by presence of arthritis and psoriasis, or if the rash is absent, arthritis and at least two of the following: dactylitis, nail pitting or onycholysis, and psoriasis in a first-degree relative (Figure 26-4). The disease affects girls slightly more often than boys and has a bimodal onset, with peaks in the preschool years and early adolescence. The arthritis is usually an asymmetric monoarthritis or polyarthritis affecting large and small joints and may develop several years before the rash. Patients may be ANA positive and are at risk for developing uveitis.

ENTHESITIS-RELATED ARTHRITIS

Enthesitis-related arthritis (ERA) overlaps with spondyloarthropathies, juvenile ankylosing spondylitis (JAS), and inflammatory bowel disease (IBD)–associated arthritis. Enthesitis is inflammation around the enthesis, the insertion site of ligaments, tendons, joint capsule, or fascia to bones. This disease spectrum is defined

by arthritis and enthesitis *or* either arthritis or enthesitis with at least two of the following: the presence or a history of sacroiliac tenderness or lumbosacral pain; HLA-B27 antigen positivity; onset of arthritis in a male after age 6 years; acute anterior uveitis; and a first-degree relative with ankylosing spondylitis, ERA, sacroiliitis with IBD, reactive arthritis, or acute anterior uveitis.

On physical examination, enthesitis is identified by tenderness where the tendons insert into the bones. Some common enthesitis sites include the inferior pole of the patella, Achilles tendon insertion, plantar fascia insertion, and sacroiliac joints. Progression to JAS is most likely among children with episodic arthritis of the lower extremity large joints, enthesitis, and tarsitis within 1 year of ERA symptom onset. Extraarticular manifestations of ERA include symptomatic anterior uveitis (red, painful, photophobic eye), aortic insufficiency, aortitis, muscle weakness, and low-grade fever. ERA can also be the initial manifestation of IBD (see Chapter 110). Thus, it is important to screen for gastrointestinal symptoms, growth failure, erythema nodosum, and aphthous stomatitis.

UNDIFFERENTIATED ARTHRITIS

Undifferentiated arthritis includes patients who do not meet criteria for any category or who meet criteria for more than one.

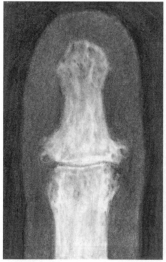
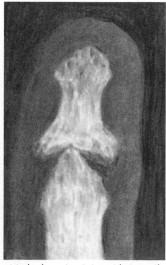

Erosion of cartilage and marginal erosion and osteophytes

Marked erosion joint with "pencil point-in-cup" appearance

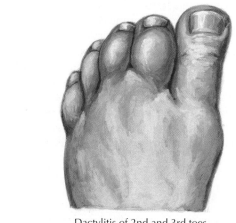

Dactylitis of 2nd and 3rd toes

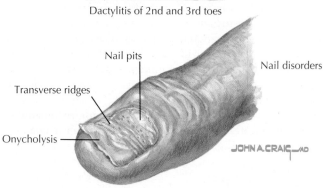

Nail pits

Nail disorders

Transverse ridges

Onycholysis

JOHN A. CRAIG—AD

Figure 26-4 *Psoriatic juvenile idiopathic arthritis.*

Differential Diagnosis

The differential diagnosis of children with suspected JIA is broad given the heterogeneity of disease subsets. The most common classes of disorders that must be considered in the differential diagnosis of JIA include other rheumatologic diseases such as sarcoidosis, infection or postinfectious phenomena, malignancies, orthopedic conditions, and other inflammatory arthropathies (Box 26-1). The differential diagnosis of JIA is

Box 26-1 Differential Diagnosis of Chronic Arthritis

Infectious or Postinfectious
• Viral arthritis (rubella, parvovirus B19, hepatitis B)
• Bacterial infections (Lyme disease, tuberculosis, gonorrhea)
• Toxic synovitis
• Rheumatic fever
• Poststreptococcal arthritis
• Serum sickness
• Osteomyelitis
Oncologic
• Leukemia
• Osteosarcoma
• Ewing's sarcoma
• Metastatic neuroblastoma
Orthopedic
• Legg-Calvé-Perthes disease
• Avascular necrosis from chronic corticosteroids
• Slipped capital femoral epiphysis
Rheumatologic
• Juvenile idiopathic arthritis
• Systemic lupus erythematosus
• Sarcoidosis
• Sjögren's syndrome
• Dermatomyositis
• Vasculitis
Other
• Hemarthrosis
• Avascular necrosis
• Cystic fibrosis-associated arthritis
• Foreign body synovitis
• Pigmented villonodular synovitis

influenced by whether the presentation is acute, subacute, or chronic; whether the child has monoarticular or polyarticular arthritis; and the presence of systemic features.

EVALUATION AND MANAGEMENT

Laboratory Analysis

There are no diagnostic laboratory tests confirmatory for JIA. When evaluating a child with suspected arthritis, a complete blood count with differential, C-reactive protein (CRP), and ESR should be part of the initial evaluation. These tests will document the presence or absence of systemic inflammation and identify hematologic abnormalities that may raise suspicion of malignancy. In the setting of infection, ESR may continue to increase despite antibiotics, but CRP often rapidly declines with appropriate therapy because of its short half-life. In Lyme disease endemic areas, serologic testing for Lyme disease is recommended in children with oligoarthritis.

Among children with confirmed JIA, ANA positivity represents an increased risk for anterior uveitis. ANA can be positive in up to 20% of the normal population; thus, an elevated ANA is *not* diagnostic of JIA. RF is infrequent in JIA; therefore, it is not a good screening test for diagnosis. However, RF positivity is associated with erosive synovitis and poorer prognosis. HLA-B27 is not diagnostic but is strongly associated with reactive arthritis, IBD, and ERA.

Synovial Fluid Analysis

Synovial fluid analysis and culture should be performed in children with acute joint swelling that is accompanied by fever or for whom the diagnosis is uncertain. In JIA, the synovial fluid is usually yellow and cloudy and has decreased viscosity. Synovial fluid leukocyte counts are elevated (typically between 15,000 and 20,000 cells/mm^3 but can be higher) with neutrophil predominance.

Imaging

Plain radiographs are useful as part of the initial evaluation of arthritis to evaluate for periarticular osteopenia, erosions, fractures or other bony abnormalities. Among children with JIA, radiographic features include soft tissue swelling, widening or narrowing of the joint space, osteoporosis, erosions, subluxation, or ankylosis. Erosive changes are uncommon before 2 years of active disease. Children with JIA are at risk for atlantoaxial instability, particularly in the setting of active cervical disease. If instability is suspected, flexion and extension films of the cervical spine should be obtained before anesthesia.

Other imaging modalities that may be useful in the evaluation of JIA include ultrasonography, bone scans, and magnetic resonance imaging (MRI). Ultrasonography is a noninvasive, quick, and inexpensive method to confirm a joint effusion. Bone scans are helpful to detect osteomyelitis, malignancy, and joints with subclinical inflammation. MRI is the most sensitive technique to identify early erosions and TMJ arthritis.

Clinical Management

Treatment of JIA varies based on disease subtype, severity of disease, prior response to therapy, and unique patient circumstances. All patients with JIA should be screened for certain complications, including iridocyclitis, generalized growth impairment, asymmetric growth patterns of the limbs and TMJ, and osteopenia or osteoporosis.

PHARMACOLOGIC INTERVENTIONS

The purpose of pharmacologic therapy is to reduce pain, inflammation, and permanent joint destruction and to maintain remission. Nonsteroidal antiinflammatory drugs (NSAIDs), which have both analgesic and antiinflammatory properties, are often the initial intervention. However, most children with JIA require additional therapy. Intraarticular corticosteroid injections are often used to control disease locally, particularly in the setting of oligoarthritis. In children with polyarticular disease or oligoarticular disease that requires repeated intraarticular injections, disease-modifying antirheumatic agents and biologics are used. The most common of these medications include methotrexate, sulfasalazine, etanercept, infliximab, and adalimumab. Systemic corticosteroids are used for rapid control of severe arthritis and for children who have severe arthritis or systemic features that do not respond to other interventions. In cases of systemic JIA not adequately controlled with corticosteroids, biologic or chemotherapeutic agents may be used.

SURGICAL MANAGEMENT

Orthopaedic surgery has a limited role in the management plan for most children with JIA. However, in cases of refractory disease or persistent leg length discrepancy, an experienced orthopedic surgeon can help to design an individualized surgical intervention. Possible interventions include arthroscopic synovectomy, soft tissue release, epiphysiodesis (growth plate fusion), total arthroplasty (joint replacement), and arthrodesis (joint fusion).

PHYSICAL AND OCCUPATIONAL THERAPY

All children with prolonged arthritis should be evaluated by a physical or occupational therapist to maximize musculoskeletal health and function and to prevent flexion contractures. Among children with JIA, decreased physical activity, fitness, and function not only increase the risk of disability but also place these children at risk for long-term cardiovascular and obesity-related morbidity. Regular exercise programs will not exacerbate the disease and may even reduce disease symptoms. In cases of active joint disease in the upper extremities, occupational therapy can improve the capacity to perform activities of daily living and academic responsibilities.

FUTURE DIRECTIONS

Further research is necessary regarding the correlation between genetic variants associated with JIA, presumed genetic susceptibility, and translation of these findings to disease incidence and clinical care of patients with JIA. As scientists work to better understand the genetics and immunopathogenesis of JIA, there is potential for more directed biologic therapies. In addition, more randomized clinical trials are needed to better understand how advanced therapies used in adults with rheumatologic disease can be safely and effectively used to maximize quality of life and minimize disability among children with JIA.

SUGGESTED READINGS

Ravelli A, Martini A: Juvenile idiopathic arthritis, *Lancet* 369:767-778, 2007.

Wallace CA: Current management of juvenile idiopathic arthritis, *Best Pract Res Clin Rheumatol* 20(2):279-300, 2005.

Weiss JE, Ilowite NT: Juvenile idiopathic arthritis, *Pediatr Clin North Am* 52:413-442, 2005.

Juvenile Dermatomyositis

27

Naomi Brown and Pamela F. Weiss

Juvenile dermatomyositis (JDMS) is the most common inflammatory myositis during childhood, accounting for more than 80% of cases. Endothelial injury of the capillaries, venules, and small arteries of the muscle, skin, and gastrointestinal tract characterize JDMS. It is a distinct disease from adult-onset dermatomyositis because it is not associated with malignancy and tends to remit after several years.

ETIOLOGY AND PATHOGENESIS

The cause of JDMS is unclear; however, roles for genetics, environmental exposures, and infections have been postulated. Certain human leukocyte antigen (HLA) alleles are more common in patients with JDMS, including HLA-DQA1*0501 and HLA-DQA1*0301. Genetic polymorphisms in non–HLA-associated genes, such as tumor necrosis factor-α (TNF-α) and interleukin-1 receptor antagonist, have also been associated with JDMS. The presence of antinuclear antibodies (ANA) in 50% to 70% of patients provides some evidence for immune dysregulation. It has been suggested that viral infections, such as Coxsackie B or echovirus, may trigger an unusual immune response in a genetically susceptible host. However, this theory has yet to be substantiated.

CLINICAL PRESENTATION

JDMS is a rare inflammatory myopathy with an incidence of two to four cases per million per year in children ages 16 years and younger. The mean age of onset is 7 years. However, there is a bimodal distribution with peaks at 2 to 5 years and 12 to 13 years. It is more common in girls than boys by a ratio of 2 : 1. There is no racial predominance.

Cutaneous Features

Dermatomyositis has several classic cutaneous findings (Figure 27-1). Gottron's papules are erythematous, raised, scaling plaques on the dorsal surface of the knuckles, elbows, and knees that are present in more than 90% of children at the time of diagnosis. Gottron's papules are frequently confused with severe eczema if JDMS is not suspected. The classic heliotrope rash is a violaceous discoloration of the eyelids with associated eyelid edema; this is present in approximately 80% of children at diagnosis. About 40% of children also have a prominent erythematous malar rash. This rash can be ulcerative, cross the nasolabial folds, and extend onto the forehead. Raynaud's phenomenon (Figure 27-2) and associated nailfold capillary changes are seen in up to 80% of patients. Nailfold changes are characterized by proximal nailfold erythema, capillary dilatation, tortuosity, or dropout. The measured density of capillaries per millimeter may be a useful tool for monitoring clinical activity. Skin ulcerations reflect significant vasculopathy of the skin and may be a sign of internal organ vasculopathy. Ulcerative

skin lesions are associated with more severe disease and worse prognosis.

Calcinosis, or calcium deposition in the skin and subcutaneous tissues, occurs in up to 40% of patients within a few years of diagnosis. Risk factors for the development of calcinosis include delayed diagnosis or treatment, TNF-α-308a genotype, and an age younger than 5 years at the time of diagnosis. Calcinosis may regress after disease remission, but complete resolution may take years. The calcinosis associated with JDMS occurs in five distinct patterns: (1) superficial calcinosis on the extremities that does not interfere with function and often regresses spontaneously; (2) deep tumoral muscle calcification in the proximal muscle groups that may interfere with joint motion, may ulcerate, and may require surgical debridement; (3) diffuse and painful calcinosis along myofascial planes that limits joint motion; (4) mixed forms of the former three types; and (5) extensive exoskeleton-like calcium deposits that result in severe functional limitations.

Other less common skin manifestations associated with JDMS are "mechanics' hands" (thickening of the margins of the palms and radial surfaces of the hands), the shawl sign (macular erythema on the posterior neck and shoulders), the V sign (macular erythema on the anterior neck and chest), and poikiloderma vasculare atrophicans (circumscribed violaceous erythema with associated telangiectasia, hypopigmentation or hyperpigmentation, and superficial atrophy). The scalp may also be involved with seborrhea-like scaling, atrophy, and alopecia. Lipodystrophy is often underappreciated and may be present in 20% to 50% of children; it may be associated with insulin resistance, decreased glucose tolerance, acanthosis nigricans, and elevated triglycerides.

Musculoskeletal Features

Classic JDMS is manifested by symmetric, proximal muscle weakness especially in the neck, hip flexors, and abdominal wall (Figure 27-3). Targeted muscle testing is necessary because children are often able to compensate well for their weaknesses. Children may have functional limitations at the time of presentation secondary to muscle involvement. For example, affected children may report problems with brushing or washing their hair, climbing stairs, and standing from a seated position (Gower's sign). Dysphonia, difficulty swallowing, dysphagia, and reflux of food into the nasopharynx may be present due to weakness of the palate, cricopharyngeal muscles, and upper esophagus. Rarely, the myocardium can be involved. Joint contractures may be present as a result of muscle shortening. Muscle tenderness may also be a prominent feature.

Amyopathic JDMS has the cutaneous manifestations of JDMS in the absence of clinically apparent muscle disease. Often, imaging by magnetic resonance imaging (MRI) and detailed muscle testing reveals subtle subclinical disease in these cases.

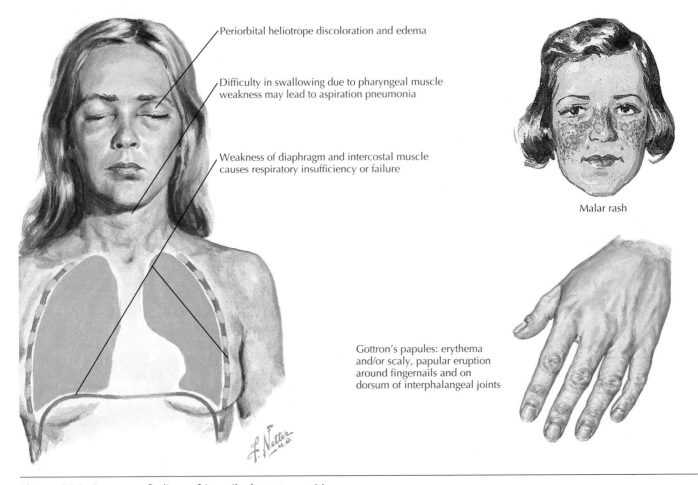

Periorbital heliotrope discoloration and edema

Difficulty in swallowing due to pharyngeal muscle weakness may lead to aspiration pneumonia

Weakness of diaphragm and intercostal muscle causes respiratory insufficiency or failure

Malar rash

Gottron's papules: erythema and/or scaly, papular eruption around fingernails and on dorsum of interphalangeal joints

Figure 27-1 *Cutaneous findings of juvenile dermatomyositis.*

Other Disease Manifestations

Pulmonary involvement is less common in children than adults and is associated with the presence of anti-Jo-1 antibody. Interstitial lung disease and spontaneous pneumothorax may rarely occur. Gastrointestinal vasculopathy is also a rare, but life-threatening, complication that can cause multiple perforations of the gastrointestinal tract. Involvement of the central nervous system may be manifested by edema, seizures, and hallucinations. Anasarca is a poor prognostic sign indicating severe disease that may respond very slowly to treatment and may not respond to corticosteroids alone.

DIFFERENTIAL DIAGNOSIS

The diagnosis of JDMS is relatively straightforward in the presence of the characteristic rash and symmetric proximal weakness. However, the common rashes of JDMS can mimic other diseases. Gottron's papules can be mistaken for psoriasis or seborrheic dermatitis. Malar rash is one of the diagnostic criteria for systemic lupus erythematosus (SLE); however, in contrast to JDMS, the malar rash associated with SLE does not cross the nasolabial folds. Dermatitis, pityriasis rubra pilaris, sunburn, and other sun-induced eruptions may also mimic the rashes of JDMS. Nailfold capillary changes and Raynaud's phenomenon

can be seen with systemic scleroderma, mixed connective tissue disease, CREST syndrome (**c**alcinosis, **R**aynaud's phenomenon, **e**sophageal dysmotility, **s**clerodactyly, **t**elangiectasias), and SLE. Juvenile polymyositis presents with similar proximal muscle weakness but lacks cutaneous manifestations.

In the absence of cutaneous manifestations, JDMS can be difficult to distinguish from other causes of muscle weakness, such as muscular dystrophy, metabolic myopathies, and infectious myositis. Muscle tenderness helps to distinguish myositis from myopathy secondary to metabolic and genetic conditions. Myositis can also be a manifestation of other connective tissue diseases such as SLE, systemic scleroderma, and mixed connective tissue disease. Lesions of the brain, spinal cord, anterior horn cell, lower motor neuron, and neuromuscular junction may also present with muscle weakness.

EVALUATION AND MANAGEMENT

JDMS is defined by the presence of characteristic skin findings plus three of the following: symmetric proximal muscle weakness, elevation of muscle enzymes, typical electromyogram (EMG) changes, and perifascicular atrophy and necrosis on muscle biopsy. To evaluate weakness, the following muscle enzymes should be measured: alanine aminotransferase (ALT), aspartate aminotransferase (AST), lactate dehydrogenase (LDH),

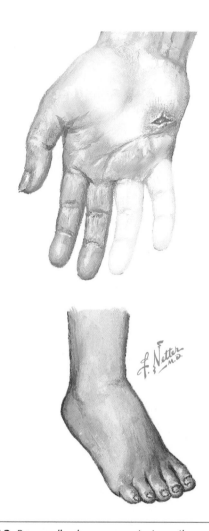

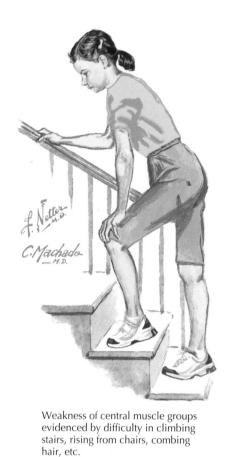

Weakness of central muscle groups evidenced by difficulty in climbing stairs, rising from chairs, combing hair, etc.

Figure 27-3 *Proximal muscle weakness in juvenile dermatomyositis.*

Figure 27-2 *Raynaud's phenomenon in juvenile dermatomyositis.*

aldolase, and creatine kinase (CK). All five enzymes should be checked because it is common for only a few to be elevated. CK levels are typically the first to increase and are usually five to 20 times the normal value; if CK levels are very high, then alternate diagnoses, such as rhabdomyolysis and muscular dystrophy, should be considered. EMG and muscle biopsy are invasive and painful diagnostic procedures reserved for the cases that are more difficult to diagnose. If subclinical myositis is suspected, MRI and ultrasonography are alternate sensitive methods to detect myositis. ANA is often elevated in patients with JDMS, but its significance is uncertain. All patients should have myositis-specific antibodies sent at the time of diagnosis because they may help predict the clinical course and direct therapy: anti-Jo-1 is associated with lung disease, anti-Mi-2 is associated with a good prognosis and response to therapy, and anti-SRP is associated with a poor prognosis and response to therapy. A swallowing study should be performed if neck flexor weakness is present.

Treatment with high-dose systemic corticosteroids is the mainstay of therapy. Typically, corticosteroids are started at high doses (2 mg/kg/d) and weaned slowly over several months.

Steroid-sparing agents, such as methotrexate and cyclosporin A, are frequently initiated at the time of diagnosis. Intravenous immunoglobulin is particularly helpful for myositis and skin lesions that are not responsive to initial treatment with corticosteroids. Hydroxychloroquine is a mainstay of therapy in most patients and can help with skin manifestations; however, it takes about 3 months to reach steady state in the blood and for its effects to be seen. Cyclophosphamide is reserved for patients with severe, life-threatening disease. Quinacrine and topical tacrolimus are secondary options for skin manifestations. It is critical to avoid sun exposure because ultraviolet light exacerbates skin and muscle disease. If the esophagus is involved, patients may need nasogastric tube feeding temporarily.

FUTURE DIRECTIONS

Our improved understanding of the pathogenesis of JDMS will lead to more targeted therapies in the near future. Currently, studies are underway to investigate rituximab, a drug that targets CD-20+ B cells. Preliminary results in adults are encouraging. Additionally, standard criteria to assess JDMS disease activity and damage and response to therapy are being validated prospectively by the Pediatric Rheumatology International Trials Organization; these criteria will allow for comparison of different studies and greater generalizability of results.

SUGGESTED READINGS

Brown VE, Pilkington CA, Feldman BM, Davidson JE: An international consensus survey of the diagnostic criteria for juvenile dermatomyositis, *Rheumatology (Oxford)* 45(8):990-993, 2006.

Feldman BM, Rider LG, Reed AM, Pachman LM: Juvenile dermatomyositis and other idiopathic inflammatory myopathies of childhood, *Lancet* 371(9631):2201-2212, 2008.

Ramanan AV, Feldman BM: Clinical features and outcomes of juvenile dermatomyositis and other childhood onset myositis syndromes, *Rheum Dis Clin North Am* 28(4):833-857, 2002.

Vasculitis

Homaira Rahimi and Pamela F. Weiss

28

Vasculitis is inflammation of a blood vessel, which can occur as a primary process or may be secondary to another disease. For example, rheumatic illnesses, such as systemic lupus erythematosus (SLE) or juvenile dermatomyositis, may have vasculitis as a secondary process. Overall, the childhood vasculitides are a rare group of disorders. The occurrence of vasculitis in patients younger than 17 years old is approximately 20 per 100,000 children. However, specific diseases, such as Churg-Strauss syndrome, can be even rarer. In addition, the prevalence of diseases may be different based on the population studied. For example, Behçet's disease occurs more frequently in the Turkish or Japanese populations (i.e., origins along the "Silk Road").

This chapter focuses on the primary vasculitides. A general overview is presented followed by a more detailed discussion of Henoch-Schönlein purpura (HSP) and Kawasaki disease (KD), the two most common childhood vasculitides.

ETIOLOGY AND PATHOGENESIS

The underlying cause of vasculitis has yet to be elucidated; however, similar to many chronic diseases, there is likely a complex interplay of genetic and environmental factors. Some theories suggest that the inflammation is attributable to the involvement of humoral factors, as seen in the antineutrophil cytoplasmic antibodies (ANCA)–associated vasculitides. Others suggest abnormal regulation of immune complex formation is contributory, as in HSP. Lymphocyte involvement has also been implicated, specifically T-regulatory cell dysfunction. Additionally, antecedent infections, particularly streptococcal infections, have been suggested as a cause in many of the vasculitides such as HSP, Wegener's granulomatosis, and polyarteritis nodosa (PAN).

Classification

Vasculitis can be classified based on the involvement of primarily large, medium, or small vessels (Figure 28-1). In addition, certain vasculitides have a predilection for arteries, veins, or both. The vasculitides can be further classified as granulomatous or nongranulomatous. The granulomatous diseases include Takayasu arteritis, Wegener's granulomatosis, and Churg-Strauss syndrome (see Chapter 30). The nongranulomatous vasculitides include PAN, KD, microscopic polyangiitis, HSP, cutaneous leukocytoclastic vasculitis, and essential cryoglobulinemic vasculitis.

CLINICAL PRESENTATION

Vasculitis often presents with vague symptoms and multiorgan involvement. Nonspecific systemic features may include prolonged fever without any clear source, hypertension, fatigue, malaise, weight loss, and rash. As a consequence, the diagnosis is often delayed and requires a high index of suspicion.

Definitive diagnosis often relies on imaging (angiography) and tissue biopsy. The history should include questions about recent infections, medication exposures, and a detailed family history.

Certain patterns of clinical symptoms and organ involvement may be suggestive of a specific vasculitis (Box 28-1). For example, whereas palpable purpura, arthralgias, abdominal pain, and renal disease suggest HSP, persistent fever, conjunctivitis, cervical lymphadenopathy, extremity swelling, mucocutaneous changes, and rash suggest KD (see below). Microscopic polyangiitis is associated with high titers of pANCA (protoplasmic-staining antineutrophil cytoplasmic antibodies) and affects mainly the pulmonary and renal systems. Hypersensitivity vasculitis is a necrotizing vasculitis that presents with a papular rash that may be red or blistering and is often associated with infection or medication exposure. Hypocomplementemic urticarial vasculitis presents with urticarial skin lesions and low serum complement levels of C4 and C3. Behçet's disease is a unique systemic vasculitis that affects both arteries and veins. The classic triad of Behçet's disease includes oral ulcers, uveitis, and genital ulcers; however, any organ system can be affected.

PAN is a necrotizing vasculitis affecting the medium-sized arteries and can present with systemic disease or in a limited form that only involves the skin and joints. It occurs in school-aged children, and there is typically a history of a preceding upper respiratory infection or streptococcal pharyngitis. In unvaccinated children, hepatitis B can be causative. Symptoms include prolonged fevers, malaise, calf pain, testicular pain, and weight loss. Physical examination findings include painful nodules (particularly on the feet), livedo reticularis (see Figure 29-2), myalgias, and arthritis of large joints. In the systemic form, any organ system can be affected; thus, hypertension, renal abnormalities, gastrointestinal involvement, and coronary disease can be seen. Of the large vessel diseases, temporal arteritis is not seen in childhood. Takayasu arteritis, the third most common childhood vasculitis, preferentially affects the large branches of the aorta. Examination may reveal bruits, hypertension, and absent pulses.

Physical Examination

Hypertension is common with many of the vasculitides. Furthermore, Takayasu arteritis classically presents with a blood pressure difference of greater than 10 mm Hg between arms. Thus, the physical examination should include evaluation of blood pressure in all four extremities. Careful auscultation for bruits (carotid, aortic, and abdominal vessels) and palpation of all peripheral pulses is vital; absent peripheral pulses (claudication) may help narrow the differential diagnosis and areas of vessel involvement. A thorough skin examination is warranted, since the presence of nodules, vasculitis lesions, ulcerations, microinfarctions, or livedo reticularis may help aid in diagnosis. A neurological examination should focus on evidence of neuropathy; some of the vasculitides, such as PAN, are associated

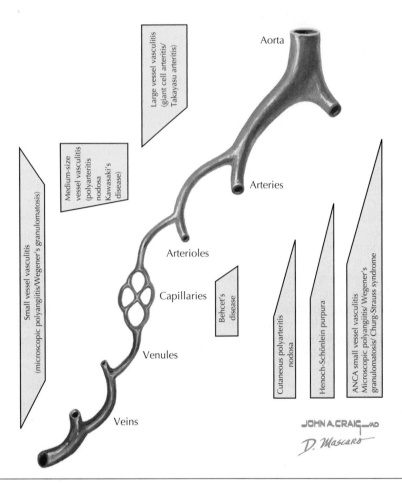

Aorta

Arteries

Arterioles

Capillaries

Venules

Veins

Large vessel vasculitis (giant cell arteritis/ Takayasu arteritis)

Medium-size vessel vasculitis (polyarteritis nodosa Kawasaki's disease)

Small vessel vasculitis (microscopic polyangiitis/Wegener's granulomatosis)

Behcet's disease

Cutaneous polyarteritis nodosa

Henoch-Schönlein purpura

ANCA small vessel vasculitis Microscopic polyangiitis/ Wegener's granulomatosis/ Churg-Strauss syndrome

JOHN A. CRAIG—MD
D. Mascaro

Figure 28-1 *Distribution of specific vasculitis syndromes.*

with mononeuritis multiplex. Two specific areas where blood vessels can be directly visualized are the ocular examination and the nailfold capillaries. As disease progresses, more specific signs may develop, but morbidity also increases. Therefore, a high clinical suspicion for vasculitis is important.

EVALUATION AND MANAGEMENT

Laboratory Evaluation

The laboratory evaluation for vasculitis should include inflammatory markers, such as the erythrocyte sedimentation rate (ESR) and C-reactive protein (CRP), which can be markedly elevated, and a complete blood count (CBC). Liver enzymes, blood urea nitrogen, creatinine, and urinalysis help to evaluate liver and renal involvement. Antibody tests, such as ANA and ANCA, and complement levels should be sent depending on the type of vasculitis being considered. When clinical suspicion is high, imaging examinations, such as computed tomography angiography, magnetic resonance angiography, or conventional angiography, may help identify blood vessel abnormalities. Imaging may also reveal certain patterns of vessel involvement, such as "beading" seen in PAN and aneurysms found in Takayasu arteritis. Typically, these examinations are especially useful when there is concern for large vessel disease. The diagnostic gold standard is tissue biopsy.

Management

Management depends on the specific type of vasculitis and should be done in consultation with a rheumatologist (Table 28-1). Corticosteroids are the cornerstone of treatment for almost all of the vasculitides. In addition, depending on severity of disease, use of immunosuppressive agents such as methotrexate, azathioprine, cyclosporine, and cyclophosphamide may be warranted. In immune complex–mediated disease, plasmapheresis may have a role.

HENOCH SCHÖNLEIN PURPURA

HSP is the most common vasculitis in childhood (Figure 28-2). It is a leukocytoclastic vasculitis (leukocytes infiltrate the vessel walls and cause necrosis) predominantly affecting the small blood vessels. The classic triad is described as nonthrombocytopenic palpable purpura, arthritis, and abdominal pain. The most feared long-term morbidity of HSP is chronic renal disease. It affects boys more often than girls and most cases occur in winter and spring. Although HSP can affect adults, the peak age of onset is between 3 and 15 years.

The pathophysiology of HSP is associated with immunoglobulin A (IgA) deposition; circulating IgA forms immune complexes and activates the alternative complement pathway. IgA is then deposited in affected organs and small vessels,

Table 28-1 Vasculitides in Childhood

	Histopathology	Clinical Findings	Associated Laboratory Findings	Treatment
Small Vessel				
Microscopic polyangiitis	Nongranulomatous necrotizing vasculitis; few or no immune deposits	Fever, weight loss, lower respiratory tract symptoms	pANCA, anti-mpo, hematuria, proteinuria, ↑creatinine	Corticosteroids (2 mg/kg/d) Cyclophosphamide
Wegener's granulomatosis	Granulomatous inflammation of the respiratory tract; necrotizing vasculitis of small and medium vessels; renal: extracapillary proliferation and crescent formation (renal granuloma are rare)	Fever, weight loss, upper respiratory tract signs (epistaxis, sinus pain, hoarseness, nasal ulceration), lower respiratory disease; hearing loss, dacryocystitis, purpura	↑↑ESR, ↑CRP, ↑platelets, mild leukocytosis, anemia, cANCA, anti-pr3, hematuria, proteinuria, ↑creatinine	Corticosteroids (30 mg/kg/d initially; then 2 mg/kg/d) Cyclophosphamide Trimethoprim–sulfamethoxazole (daily)
HSP	IgA deposition in vessel walls	Hypertension, palpable purpura, arthritis, abdominal pain, testicular swelling	↑ESR, ↑CRP, mild leukocytosis, hematuria, proteinuria	NSAIDs Corticosteroids (2 mg/kg)
Medium Vessel				
PAN	Necrotizing vasculitis with aneurysm formation	Hypertension, painful skin nodules (especially soles of feet), arthritis, testicular pain, calf pain, livedo reticularis, maculopapular rash	↑↑ESR, ↑platelets, mild leukocytosis, anemia, hematuria, proteinuria, ↑creatinine	Corticosteroids (2 mg/kg/d) Cyclophosphamide Methotrexate
KD	Necrotizing vasculitis with fibrinoid necrosis; coronary artery aneurysms	Fever, nonpurulent conjunctivitis, cervical lymphadenopathy, extremity changes, strawberry tongue, skin exanthem	↑ESR, ↑CRP, ↑platelets, sterile pyuria, transaminitis, aseptic meningitis	Aspirin (80-90 mg/kg/d) until afebrile; then 3-5 mg/kg/d IVIG (2 g/kg)
Large Vessel				
Takayasu arteritis	Spotty granulomatous inflammation of the vessel walls; aneurysms; vessel dissection	Hypertension, blood pressure difference of >10 mm Hg between arms, subclavian bruit, decreased peripheral pulses, claudication	↑↑ESR, anemia, mild leukocytosis, hypergammaglobulinemia	Corticosteroids (2 mg/kg) Cyclophosphamide Infliximab

anti-mpo, anti-myeloperoxidase antibodies; anti-pr3, anti-proteinase 3; cANCA, cytoplasmic antineutrophil cytoplasmic antibodies; CRP, C-reactive protein; ESR, erythrocyte sedimentation rate; HSP, Henoch-Schönlein purpura; Ig, immunoglobulin; IVIG, intravenous immunoglobulin; KD, Kawasaki disease; NSAID, nonsteroidal antiinflammatory drug; PAN, polyarteritis nodosa; pANCA, perinuclear antineutrophil cytoplasmic antibodies; PO, orally.

resulting in inflammation. In more than 75% of cases, there is a history of preceding upper respiratory illness, and many organisms have been implicated, including group A *Streptococcus*. HSP has also been seen after administration of vaccines and medications.

There are proposed classification criteria to guide the diagnosis of pediatric HSP (Box 28-1). The purpuric rash has raised, nontender, nonpruritic, deep red to purple lesions that are most often found in dependent areas such as the buttocks and lower extremities (with most crops at the feet and ankle area). However,

they can also be on the face, trunk, and upper extremities. Abdominal pain occurs in approximately two-thirds of patients. More severe gastrointestinal symptoms include gastrointestinal hemorrhage and intussusception. Rare gastrointestinal complications include pancreatitis and ulcerative colitis. Up to 25% of children may have abdominal symptoms of HSP before the onset of rash, making the diagnosis a challenge. Arthritis affects 50% to 80% of children with HSP. It usually affects large joints, such as the knee or ankle, but small joints can also be involved. It is often painful but not usually erosive. Fortunately, the arthritis

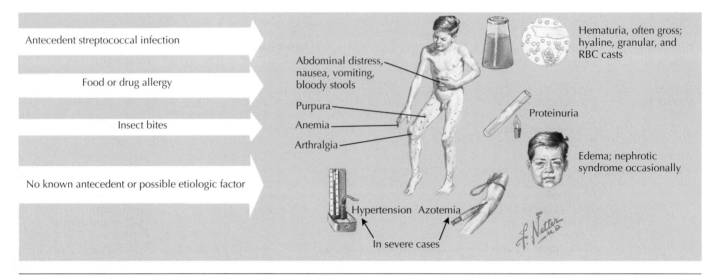

Figure 28-2 *Signs and symptoms of Henoch-Schönlein purpura.*

Box 28-1 Henoch-Schönlein Purpura Classification
Criteria

Must have *palpable purpura* and *at least one* of the
following:
- Abdominal pain (diffuse)
- Arthritis or arthralgia
- Renal involvement (hematuria or proteinuria)
- Predominant IgA deposition seen in any biopsy

---

of HSP is usually transient, lasting a few days to 1 week. Renal manifestations are seen in about one-third of patients with HSP. Symptoms range from microscopic hematuria or proteinuria to acute renal failure. Of the children who develop renal involvement, most do so within the first 3 months of disease.

Laboratory findings in HSP are typically nonspecific. Evaluation should include a CBC (thrombocytopenia indicates an alternative diagnosis), electrolytes (to assess for renal insufficiency), and a urinalysis (to check for blood or protein). Complement levels are normal, and ANA and ANCA are not found. Blood pressure is also important to monitor both at diagnosis and throughout the acute phase of illness. Renal biopsy may be warranted to determine the severity of renal disease.

The prognosis for patients with mild manifestations is very good. In general, nonsteroidal antiinflammatory drugs are used for the arthralgias of HSP. Corticosteroids have been shown to be useful in HSP with regards to abdominal and renal manifestations. Recurrences are seen in up to one-third of children, usually within 4 to 6 months of initial diagnosis, and more often in patients with renal involvement. Long-term morbidity usually depends on the severity of renal disease, with worse disease predicting worse outcome.

KAWASAKI DISEASE

KD is the second most common vasculitis seen in children (Figure 28-3). It is considered an acute vasculitis of medium-sized arteries. The peak age of onset is 2 years old, with 80%

to 90% of cases occurring in children younger than 5 years old. Unlike most vasculitides, it is more common in boys than girls (about 1.5:1), and it has a higher incidence in the Japanese and Korean populations. Although the cause of KD is unknown, studies have suggested a transmissible agent causing a dysfunctional immune response; however, a specific agent has yet to be discovered.

Diagnosis is based on clinical criteria (Table 28-2). The fever, which is usually greater than 38.5°C, must be present for more than 5 days. It is typically minimally responsive to antipyretic medications. The conjunctivitis is nonexudative and limbic sparing. In some cases, patients can develop anterior uveitis, so a slit-lamp examination may be helpful if the diagnosis is unclear. Oral mucous membrane changes occur with continued inflammation and may include dry, red, cracked lips, a "strawberry" tongue; and pharyngitis. Swelling or erythema of the hands and feet usually occurs late in the acute phase. During the convalescent phase, desquamation of the tips of the toes and fingers may be noticeable. A transient arthritis is noted in about one-third of patients and can involve large or small joints. The rash of KD is nonspecific and ranges from erythema at the perineal area or a morbilliform exanthem on the trunk or extremities. Vesicular or pustular lesions are not typical. The final criterion is lymphadenopathy, which is usually the least common finding of KD.

The laboratory evaluation for KD should include a CBC (there is often marked thrombocytosis, sometimes >1 million platelets/microliter), inflammatory markers (ESR and CRP), complete metabolic panel, urinalysis (sterile pyuria can be seen), and tests to exclude infection (adenovirus and Epstein-Barr virus may be present in a similar fashion). Complement and ANA levels are usually normal.

When the diagnosis of KD is suspected based on the clinical examination, electrocardiography and echocardiography must be performed because coronary abnormalities are the major cause of morbidity and mortality in this disease. If an echocardiogram shows evidence of coronary aneurysm, a diagnosis of KD can be made even if the patient has fewer than four criteria. In fact, the population most at risk for coronary abnormalities

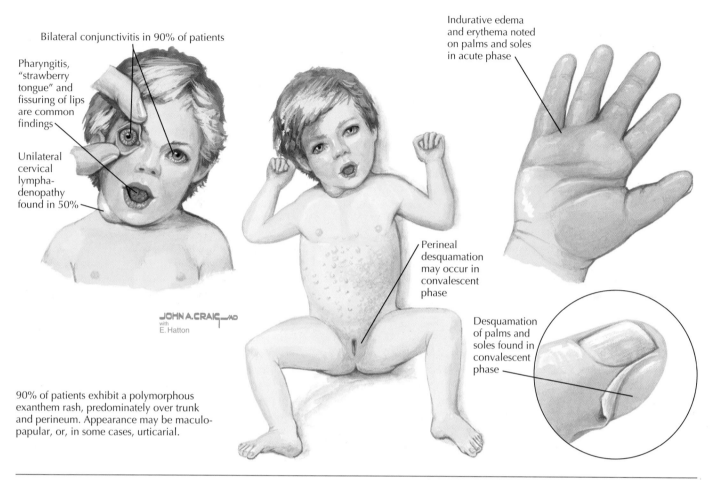

Bilateral conjunctivitis in 90% of patients

Pharyngitis, "strawberry tongue" and fissuring of lips are common findings

Unilateral cervical lympha- denopathy found in 50%

Indurative edema and erythema noted on palms and soles in acute phase

JOHN A.CRAIG—AD
with
E. Hatton

Perineal desquamation may occur in convalescent phase

Desquamation of palms and soles found in convalescent phase

90% of patients exhibit a polymorphous exanthem rash, predominately over trunk and perineum. Appearance may be maculo-papular, or, in some cases, urticarial.

Figure 28-3 *Clinical features of Kawasaki disease.*

is infants, who usually do not meet the criteria for classic KD. The echocardiogram is repeated 6 to 8 weeks after diagnosis to monitor the patient's response to treatment.

After a diagnosis is made, treatment must be initiated because early intervention (within 10 days of onset of fever) has been shown to decrease the occurrence of coronary artery aneurysms by fivefold. Treatment consists of intravenous immunoglobulin (2 g/kg) and high-dose aspirin (80-100 mg/kg/d). Low-dose aspirin is started when the patient has been afebrile for 48 hours. Aspirin therapy is discontinued after inflammatory markers and platelet count have normalized unless there is evidence of coronary artery disease.

The overall outcome for KD is excellent in the majority of patients without cardiac involvement. Because of the monocyclic nature of the disease, most patients have a full recovery. Of patients who develop coronary artery abnormalities, lifelong cardiology monitoring is needed because of the increased risk of heart disease.

FUTURE DIRECTIONS

Vasculitis is a rare childhood condition but should be considered in any child with unexplained constitutional symptoms, significant inflammation, and multiorgan involvement. Newer biologic agents are promising, but large-scale studies of these agents have not been performed in children. Given the rarity of these conditions, large clinical trials are extremely challenging to conduct. Instead, the development of patient registries is likely the key to being able to study these diseases in children in a systemic fashion.

Table 28-2 Kawasaki Disease Diagnostic Criteria

Fever greater than or equal to 5 days duration with *at least four* of the following clinical signs

Sign	Children with Kawasaki Disease (%)
1. Bilateral conjunctival injection with limbic sparing	80-90
2. Oral mucosal membrane changes (e.g., injected or fissured lips, strawberry tongue, injected pharynx)	80-90
3. Peripheral extremity changes (e.g., erythema or edema of hands and feet in the acute phase or desquamation in the convalescent phase)	80
4. Polymorphous, nonvesicular exanthema, usually on the trunk	>90
5. Cervical lymphadenopathy with anterior cervical lymph node ≥1.5 cm in diameter	50

SUGGESTED READINGS

Cabral D, Morishita K: Approach to evaluating childhood vasculitis, *UpToDate* November 12, 2008.

Dedeoglu F, Sundel RP: Vasculitis in children, *Rheum Dis Clin North Am* 33:555-583, 2007.

Ozen S, Ruperto N, Dillon MJ, et al: EULAR/PreS endorsed consensus criteria for the classification of childhood vasculitides, *Ann Rheum Dis* 65:936-941, 2006.

Woo P, Laxer RM, Sherry DD: Vasculitis. In Pediatric Rheumatology in Clinical Practice, ed 1. London, Springer-Verlag, 2007, pp 97-117.

Systemic Lupus Erythematosus

Christopher P. Bonafide and Pamela F. Weiss

29

Systemic lupus erythematosus (SLE) is a chronic autoimmune disease that that can affect numerous organ systems, including the skin, eyes, kidneys, joints, brain, and blood. The overall prevalence of SLE is one in 4000. The prevalence of SLE is higher in females, those who live in urban areas, Asians, African Americans, and Hispanic Americans. Twenty percent of SLE patients are diagnosed before age 16 years. The primary treatment goal in SLE patients is reducing long-term, life-limiting complications.

ETIOLOGY AND PATHOGENESIS

The cause of SLE involves a complex interplay of genetic, environmental, and immunologic factors. Several genes have been identified that confer susceptibility to SLE, including human leukocyte antigen haplotypes, complement component and receptor genes, cytokine polymorphisms, Fc receptors, and T-cell receptor polymorphisms. It is likely that a combination of these genes provides a genetic risk profile that allows the subsequent development of SLE under the appropriate conditions. Familial clustering has been reported, and the concordance rates among monozygotic and dizygotic twins are 25% and 2%, respectively

The immune dysregulation in SLE is multifactorial and includes abnormal clearance of apoptotic debris, B- and T-cell abnormalities, and autoantibody and immune complex formation. In SLE, the system of apoptotic particle removal is dysfunctional, allowing for the presentation of autoantigens to T cells. These T cells stimulate B cells to produce high-affinity autoantibodies that bind directly to cells in end organs, causing injury, or form immune complexes in the circulation that deposit in tissues and cause inflammation. Additionally, early classical complement deficiencies are associated with SLE; this association is probably secondary to delayed clearance of apoptotic debris and immune complexes.

Other factors have been hypothesized to play a role in the cause of SLE, including hormonal influences, Epstein-Barr virus and other infections, exposure to ultraviolet light, L-canavanine (a chemical in alfalfa sprouts), and silica dust inhalation. Although the precise cause of SLE is unknown, it is clear that genetic susceptibility, immunologic dysregulation, and environmental influences all contribute.

CLINICAL PRESENTATION

SLE is rare in children younger than age 5 years and is uncommon before adolescence. In childhood, girls are affected approximately four times more often than boys. The presenting symptoms are widely variable. Constitutional signs and symptoms, including fever, fatigue, lymphadenopathy, hepatosplenomegaly, and weight loss, are commonly seen. The most frequently involved specific sites affected by SLE are the skin, joints, and kidneys. Symptoms often precede the diagnosis by several months and may be insidious or acute in onset. The American College of Rheumatology provides criteria which are used clinically to aid in the diagnosis of SLE (Table 29-1, Figure 29-1). The diagnosis of SLE is made if at least four of the criteria are present or have been present in the past without another diagnosis that explains the findings. The antinuclear antibody (ANA), one of the criteria for diagnosis of SLE, is not a useful general screening test for rheumatologic disease and should not be sent routinely in the absence of other criteria for SLE.

Skin and Mucus Membrane Manifestations

There are four skin and mucocutaneous criteria: malar rash, discoid rash, oral or nasal ulcers, and photosensitivity. The malar rash, or classic "butterfly rash," is typically maculopapular and photosensitive. Additionally, it classically extends across the nasal bridge, spares the nasolabial folds, and is nonscarring (Figure 29-2). Depending on the race of the child, it may be either hyper- or hypopigmented. A discoid rash is less common. These inflammatory lesions are coin shaped, raised, and erythematous. They are most commonly located on the face (especially the ears), scalp, and extremities. These lesions are scarring and lead to permanent alopecia when they occur on the scalp. The oral and nasal ulcers associated with SLE are usually painless; oral ulcers are classically located on the hard palate (see Figure 29-2). Other common skin manifestations include livedo reticularis (see Figure 29-2), alopecia, Raynaud's phenomenon (see Figure 27-2), and digital ulcerations.

Musculoskeletal Manifestations

Nonerosive arthritis affecting both the small and large joints is common in pediatric patients with SLE. It is generally symmetric and involves two or more joints. Frequently affected joints include the knees, wrists, and fingers. Although the joint effusions are often small, the arthritis is painful with substantial joint-line tenderness and impaired range of motion. As in juvenile idiopathic arthritis, morning stiffness is common.

Renal Manifestations

Renal disease is present in a majority of pediatric SLE and is a strong determinant of long-term prognosis. Its severity ranges from microscopic hematuria to chronic renal failure. Lupus nephritis usually develops within 2 years of diagnosis (see Chapter 62). SLE patients with significant proteinuria or abnormal renal function should undergo renal biopsy to classify their degree of renal involvement to aid in treatment decision making. The classification of lupus nephritis includes six classes, ranging from minimal mesangial involvement to diffuse involvement and glomerulosclerosis (Figure 29-3).

Table 29-1 American College of Rheumatology 1997 Revised Classification Criteria for Systemic Lupus Erythematosus

Criterion	Description
Malar rash	"Butterfly" erythematous rash over malar eminences; spares nasolabial folds (see Figure 29-2)
Discoid rash	Raised erythematous patches with scaling and follicular plugging on the face, scalp, and extremities; may lead to scarring
Photosensitivity	Any rash that occurs as an unusual reaction to sunlight
Oral or nasal ulcerations	Painless ulcerations of the oral or nasal mucosa (see Figure 29-2)
Arthritis	Nonerosive arthritis of two or more peripheral joints
Nephritis	Persistent proteinuria >0.5 g/d or cellular casts (red blood cell, hemoglobin, granular, tubular, or mixed)
Serositis	Pleuritis or pericarditis
Neurologic disorder	Seizures or psychosis (in the absence of offending drugs or metabolic disturbances)
Cytopenia	Hemolytic anemia with reticulocytosis or leukopenia (<4000/mm^3) or lymphopenia (<1500/mm^3) or thrombocytopenia (<100,000/mm^3)
Positive immunoserology	Antibodies to dsDNA or antibodies to Sm nuclear antigen or anticardiolipin antibodies or presence of lupus anticoagulant or false-positive serologic test for syphilis (known to be positive for ≥6 months and confirmed by *Treponema pallidum* immobilization or fluorescent treponemal antibody absorption test)
Positive antinuclear antibody	Abnormal titer of antinuclear antibodies at any point in time

Adapted from Hochberg MC: Updating the American College of Rheumatology revised criteria for the classification of systemic lupus erythematosus. Arthritis Rheum 40(9):1725, 1997.

Neuropsychiatric Manifestations

The most common neuropsychiatric manifestations of SLE are headache, cognitive dysfunction, psychosis, and seizures. Headache occurs frequently and may result in presentation to the emergency department because of difficulty managing the pain with over-the-counter analgesics. Cognitive dysfunction in SLE patients may be subtle and should be screened for carefully. Because SLE patients often present during adolescence, deteriorating school performance, concentration difficulties, and changes in mood secondary to SLE may be wrongfully attributed to normal teenage behavior. Children with psychosis may experience hallucinations, confusion, and suicidal ideation. Seizures may also occur as a manifestation of SLE and are usually generalized. Acute causes of severe headache, seizure, psychosis, and behavioral changes in lupus patients should be considered, including central nervous system (CNS) vasculitis, increased intracranial pressure, CNS infection, and cerebral vein thrombosis. Other less common neuropsychiatric manifestations of SLE include movement disorders such as unilateral chorea and parkinsonism, cranial neuropathies, and stroke.

Hematologic Manifestations

Cytopenias seen in patients with SLE include Coombs-positive hemolytic anemia, leukopenia, lymphopenia, and thrombocytopenia. Coagulation abnormalities are also frequently present. The presence of lupus anticoagulant predisposes patients to cerebral vein thrombosis and deep vein thrombosis, which may lead to thromboemboli.

Cardiopulmonary Manifestations

Pleuritis and pericarditis are common manifestations of SLE in children. These patients often complain of chest pain that may worsen on inhalation. Cardiac issues that may arise less commonly are valvular heart disease, Libman-Sachs endocarditis, and myocarditis. Pulmonary involvement may also include pneumonitis, pneumothorax, and pulmonary hemorrhage.

Differential Diagnosis

The differential diagnosis of SLE is broad and includes acute and chronic diseases that affect many organ systems (Box 29-1). Broad categories most important to consider include infectious, oncologic, rheumatic, and drug-induced causes.

At least four should be present for diagnosis

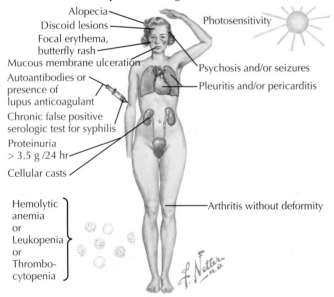

Alopecia
Discoid lesions
Focal erythema, butterfly rash
Mucous membrane ulceration
Autoantibodies or presence of lupus anticoagulant
Chronic false positive serologic test for syphilis
Proteinuria > 3.5 g /24 hr
Cellular casts
Hemolytic anemia or Leukopenia or Thrombocytopenia
Photosensitivity
Psychosis and/or seizures
Pleuritis and/or pericarditis
Arthritis without deformity

Figure 29-1 *Criteria used for the diagnosis of systemic lupus erythematosus.*

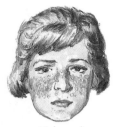

Malar rash

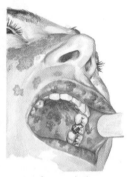

Painless oral ulcers

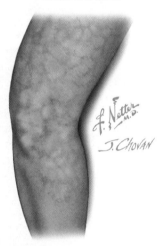

Livedo reticularis

Figure 29-2 *Skin and mucous membrane manifestations of systemic lupus erythematosus.*

Morbidity and Mortality

Renal, neurologic, hematologic, and cardiovascular disease processes are the main sources of morbidity and mortality in patients with SLE. SLE is a lifelong illness that was considered uniformly fatal within 2 years as recently as the 1960s. The long-term survival of children with SLE has improved significantly over the years with earlier diagnosis, the use of immunosuppressant therapies early in the disease course, and better understanding of the appropriate management of end stage renal disease. Five-year survival rates are now near 100%, and 10-year survival rates are greater than 85%.

The morbidity and mortality attributed to renal disease is related to the histology of the lupus nephritis seen on the kidney biopsy (Figure 29-3). End-stage renal disease is most strongly associated with focal lupus nephritis (class III) and diffuse lupus

---

Box 29-1 Differential Diagnosis of Systemic Lupus Erythematosus

Infectious
• HIV
• Epstein-Barr virus
• Parvovirus B19
• Sepsis
• Poststreptococcal glomerulonephritis
• Acute rheumatic fever
Oncologic
• Leukemia
• Lymphoma
• Central nervous system tumor
Rheumatologic
• Systemic-onset juvenile idiopathic arthritis
• Mixed connective tissue disease
• Other systemic vasculitis
Drug Induced
• Hydralazine
• Phenytoin
• Carbamazepine
• Isoniazid
• Penicillin
• Sulfonamides
• Minocycline

---

nephritis (class IV). The most frequent cause of death for children with SLE is infection. Factors including leukopenia, hypocomplementemia, and immunosuppressive therapy contribute to an immunocompromised state that can result in death if a serious infection is not recognized.

Over the long term, the renal disease, vasculitis, hypercoagulable state, lipid abnormalities, and steroid therapy can all contribute to life-limiting accelerated cardiovascular disease, including atherosclerosis, stroke, and myocardial infarction during adolescence and young adulthood.

EVALUATION AND MANAGEMENT

The diagnosis of SLE is established using the classification criteria, with consideration of important possibilities in the differential diagnosis based on the presenting signs and symptoms (see Table 29-1). In addition to the laboratory evaluation necessary to determine the criteria met by the patient, several other laboratory studies should be considered as part of the evaluation of a child with suspected SLE. Inflammatory markers (C-reactive protein [CRP] and erythrocyte sedimentation rate [ESR]) are helpful as a general screen of the degree of inflammation present. Classically, the ESR is markedly elevated, and the CRP is normal or mildly elevated in patients with SLE. Complement levels (C3, C4) are decreased when active nephritis is present. The partial thromboplastin time (PTT) is prolonged when the lupus anticoagulant is present. Despite the prolongation of the PTT in the laboratory, the lupus anticoagulant leads to a hypercoagulable state clinically as described above. A complete urinalysis should be performed in all SLE patients. If proteinuria is present, a first-morning urine protein to creatinine ratio and a 24-hour urine collection should follow. If proteinuria is significant (>1 g/24 h), then a renal biopsy is warranted before therapy

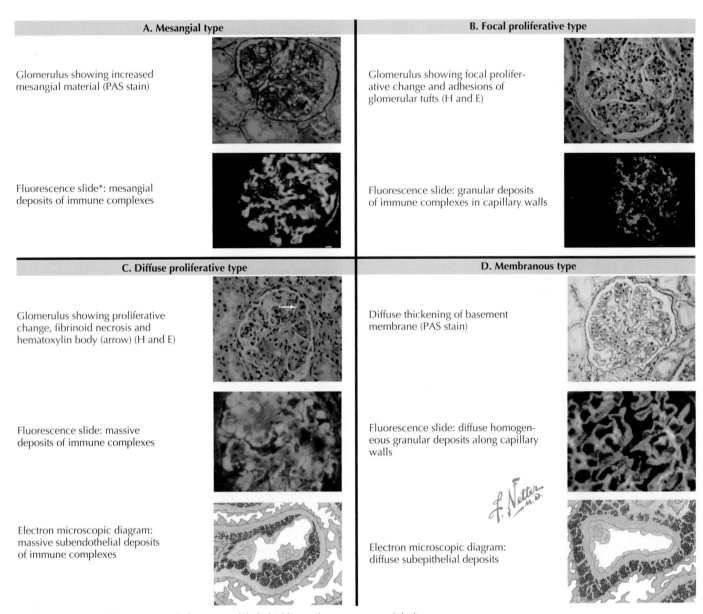

A. Mesangial type

Glomerulus showing increased mesangial material (PAS stain)

Fluorescence slide*: mesangial deposits of immune complexes

B. Focal proliferative type

Glomerulus showing focal prolifer-ative change and adhesions of glomerular tufts (H and E)

Fluorescence slide: granular deposits of immune complexes in capillary walls

C. Diffuse proliferative type

Glomerulus showing proliferative change, fibrinoid necrosis and hematoxylin body (arrow) (H and E)

Fluorescence slide: massive deposits of immune complexes

Electron microscopic diagram: massive subendothelial deposits of immune complexes

D. Membranous type

Diffuse thickening of basement membrane (PAS stain)

Fluorescence slide: diffuse homogen-eous granular deposits along capillary walls

Electron microscopic diagram: diffuse subepithelial deposits

* All fluorescence slides stained with fluorescein-labeled rabbit antihuman gamma globulin

Figure 29-3 *Renal manifestations of systemic lupus erythematosus.*

initiation to stage the lupus nephritis and aid in treatment deci-sion making. It is also recommended that children with a new diagnosis have a baseline electrocardiogram, echocardiogram, and chest radiograph.

Management

The chronicity, waxing and waning course, and multisystem effects of SLE make it challenging to treat. The benefits of therapies must be weighed against the side effects, risks, and impact on quality of life for adolescents who are already expe-riencing a period in their lives that can be socially challenging. Long-term compliance with therapies is key to improving sur-vival. Development of a system of patient and family education about the disease process, putting school support measures in place, and providing robust support systems for families with

low socioeconomic status are critical to the success of each patient's treatment.

General recommendations for all children with SLE regard-less of disease severity include sun protection (use of sunscreen, hats, and light clothing in the summer), a healthy diet and an exercise regimen to decrease cardiovascular risk factors, smoking avoidance, multivitamin therapy (especially vitamin D and calcium to prevent osteoporosis), and vaccination (inactivated vaccines only for patients with active disease or receiving immu-nosuppressive therapy).

The approach to pharmacologic therapy depends on the disease severity and the organ systems affected. The overall model of treatment is similar to the approach used in treating patients with oncologic disease, with induction treatment ini-tially to induce remission followed by maintenance therapy to sustain remission.

MILD DISEASE

For disease that is limited to the skin and musculoskeletal systems, treatment with nonsteroidal antiinflammatory drugs (NSAIDs) and the antimalarial drug hydroxychloroquine (HCQ), a disease-modifying agent, may be sufficient. Many children with arthritis refractory to NSAIDS and HCQ will need low-dose oral corticosteroid therapy to induce remission.

MODERATE TO SEVERE DISEASE

Patients with arthritis or organ involvement, including neuropsychiatric, renal, and hematologic manifestations, are treated with a combination of corticosteroids and disease-modifying antirheumatic agents (DMARDs) that may include methotrexate, azathioprine, cyclosporine, and mycophenolate mofetil. Cyclophosphamide and rituximab are typically reserved for organ-threatening disease. Although the DMARDs and cytotoxic agents reduce inflammation and the need for long-term corticosteroid use, they may also introduce other toxicities, including immunosuppression, infertility, and future malignancy risk.

In addition to medication to modify the course of the disease, symptomatic therapy is also very important in the management of children with SLE. Aggressive treatment of hypertension and early consultation with a pediatric nephrologist are critical in preserving renal function. Consultation with a pediatric neurologist is recommended if neuropsychiatric manifestations are present. Psychiatric evaluation may be necessary to aid in the decision to treat with antidepressant or antipsychotic mediations.

FUTURE DIRECTIONS

Our improved understanding of the pathogenesis of SLE will lead to more precise, targeted therapies with more favorable adverse effect profiles in the coming years. Targets of particular interest for pharmacologic intervention include other B-cell surface markers, the antigen-presenting cell–T-cell interaction, components of the complement cascade, and cytokines known to be elevated in SLE. Continued progress in our understanding of the mechanism of disease and rigorous prospective evaluation of disease-modifying agents may indicate that a cure for SLE will soon be within reach.

SUGGESTED READINGS

Ginzler EM, Dooley MA, Aranow C, et al: Mycophenolate mofetil or intravenous cyclophosphamide for lupus nephritis, *N Engl J Med* 353(21): 2219-2228, 2005.

Macdermott EJ, Adams A, Lehman TJ: Systemic lupus erythematosus in children: current and emerging therapies, *Lupus* 16(8):677-683, 2007.

Rahman A, Isenberg DA: Systemic lupus erythematosus, *N Engl J Med* 358(9):929-939, 2008.

Granulomatous Disease

Scott M. Lieberman and Pamela F. Weiss

30

Noninfectious granulomatous disease is rare in children, with the exception of Crohn disease (see Chapter 110). This group of diseases includes sarcoidosis, granulomatous vasculitides (Wegener granulomatosis [WG] and Churg-Strauss syndrome [CSS]), and familial juvenile systemic granulomatosis (Blau syndrome).

SARCOIDOSIS

Sarcoidosis is an uncommon multisystem disorder of uncertain etiology involving granulomatous infiltrates in affected organs. Sarcoidosis occurs in children worldwide without gender predominance. The incidence ranges from 0.22 to 0.9 per 100,000 children in Denmark and Japan, respectively. Race predilection follows the predominant race of the country (e.g., whites in Scandinavian countries and Asians in Japan); however, there is a higher prevalence in 8- to 15-year-old black children of the southeastern United States. The incidence in children in the United States is unclear owing to lack of systematic evaluation.

Etiology and Pathogenesis

Despite considerable research, the cause of sarcoidosis is unknown. Inheritance is multigenic with relatively weak human leukocyte antigen associations varying with populations studied. An infectious cause has been considered but not confirmed. Interestingly, mycobacterial DNA has been detected by polymerase chain reaction in sarcoidosis lesions. A candidate mycobacterial antigen, *Mycobacterium tuberculosis* catalase-peroxidase protein (mKatG), has been proposed as a trigger for an adaptive immune response that leads to granuloma formation. Other microbes, including *Propionibacterium acnes*, have been implicated, but not confirmed, by independent studies.

Sarcoidosis is characterized by granulomas consisting of tightly packed epithelioid cells and macrophages surrounded by lymphocytes (Figure 30-1). In the lung, CD4+ T cell-mediated alveolitis occurs early followed by granuloma formation. Granulomas may resolve without sequelae or may heal with residual fibrosis.

Clinical Presentation

Sarcoidosis in children occurs in two distinct forms. Older children (age 8-15 years) typically present with symptoms resembling the adult form of disease, including lymphadenopathy, lung involvement (often asymptomatic), systemic signs (fever, weight loss), and hypercalcemia, but rarely with joint involvement. In children younger than 5 years, the onset typically consists of the triad of rash, arthritis, and uveitis. Sarcoidosis commonly presents with lymphadenopathy and may affect a wide range of organs (Figure 30-2).

LYMPHORETICULAR SYSTEM MANIFESTATIONS

Lymphadenopathy is the most common presenting sign in childhood sarcoidosis. Enlarged nodes are generally nontender, firm, and mobile. Hepatosplenomegaly occurs less commonly.

PULMONARY MANIFESTATIONS

Pulmonary involvement is often asymptomatic, consisting of hilar adenopathy and pulmonary infiltrates. Chronic dry cough is the most common pulmonary symptom, but children are often asymptomatic despite having restrictive disease on pulmonary function testing (PFT).

OCULAR MANIFESTATIONS

Uveitis (anterior, posterior, or panuveitis) is the most common ocular manifestation and is typically bilateral and asymptomatic, with occurrence of redness, pain, photophobia, or blurry vision in fewer than 30% of patients with uveitis. Keratic precipitates (tightly packed lymphocytic accumulations) are characteristic and occur at the corneal edge or pupil–iris junction. Synechiae may occur, typically between the lens and iris, resulting in irregular pupils. Conjunctival granulomas (small, pale yellow, translucent nodules), keratitis, glaucoma, or retinitis may also occur.

SKIN MANIFESTATIONS

Typical rashes include yellow-brown erythematous papules on the face or larger violaceous plaques on the trunk, extremities, and buttocks. Other skin involvement includes nodular (e.g., erythema nodosum), papular, macular, or ichthyosiform lesions; hypopigmentation; hyperpigmentation; or ulceration.

MUSCULOSKELETAL MANIFESTATIONS

The arthritis of sarcoidosis is characterized by boggy tenosynovitis with effusion that is minimally painful or painless. Joint involvement may be oligoarticular (i.e., in few joints) initially but frequently progresses to polyarthritis over time. Associated stiffness and limited range of motion, typical in other forms of chronic arthritis, are generally minimal at diagnosis; however, with increased duration of disease, they become more apparent. Bony involvement is rare, but in the right setting, vertebral sarcoidosis should be considered in a child with back pain. Additionally, the small bones of the hands and feet may be involved. Nodular or inflammatory muscle lesions are rare.

CENTRAL NERVOUS SYSTEM MANIFESTATIONS

Central nervous system (CNS) disease includes cranial nerve abnormalities (e.g., optic neuritis or facial nerve palsy), encephalopathy, seizures, and mass lesions.

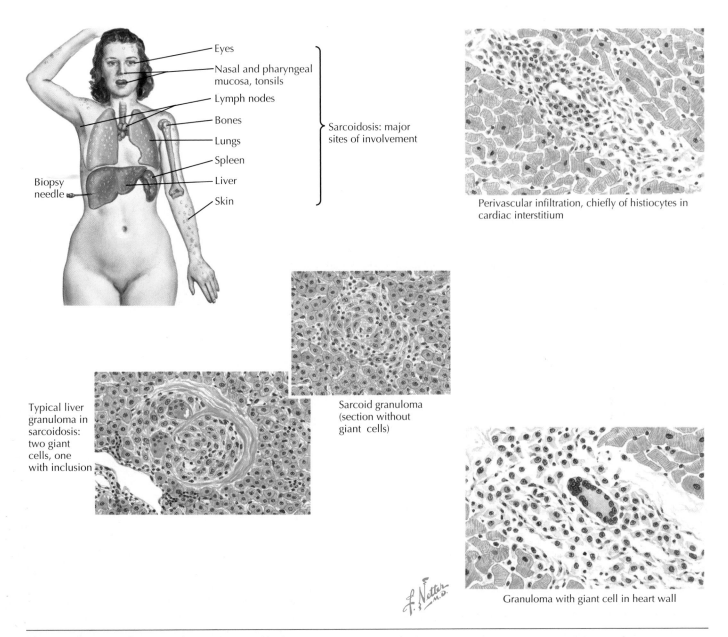

Sarcoidosis: major sites of involvement

- Eyes
- Nasal and pharyngeal mucosa, tonsils
- Lymph nodes
- Bones
- Lungs
- Spleen
- Liver
- Skin

Biopsy needle

Perivascular infiltration, chiefly of histiocytes in cardiac interstitium

Typical liver granuloma in sarcoidosis: two giant cells, one with inclusion

Sarcoid granuloma (section without giant cells)

Granuloma with giant cell in heart wall

Figure 30-1 *Granulomatous disease in sarcoidosis.*

OTHER MANIFESTATIONS

Salivary or lacrimal gland involvement may present similarly to Sjögren syndrome (recurrent parotitis, sicca syndrome, or lacrimal gland enlargement). Pancreatitis is very rare. Renal involvement is usually the result of nephrocalcinosis and nephrolithiasis rather than direct granulomatous inflammation. Heart block, cardiomyopathy, or ventricular arrhythmias may occur but are less common in children. Cytopenias may result from granulomatous infiltrates in bone marrow. Vasculitis affecting any sized vessel has been reported but is rare.

Differential Diagnosis

Sarcoidosis should be considered in any child presenting with nonspecific findings, including fever, weight loss, and lymphadenopathy, especially if accompanied by rash, arthritis, or hilar adenopathy, or in any child with fever of unknown origin (see Chapter 86, Figure 86-1). Other conditions that must be considered in a child suspected of having sarcoidosis include infections, malignancies, and other rheumatic illnesses (vasculitides, systemic lupus erythematosus [SLE], mixed connective tissue disease [MCTD], Sjögren syndrome, juvenile idiopathic arthritis [JIA]). Hilar adenopathy with constitutional symptoms may mimic lymphoma. After granulomatous inflammation has been established, infections must be ruled out before initiation of immunosuppressive medications (Box 30-1).

Evaluation and Management

BLOOD AND URINE STUDIES

No diagnostic tests specific for sarcoidosis exist. Many children have increased nonspecific inflammatory markers (e.g.,

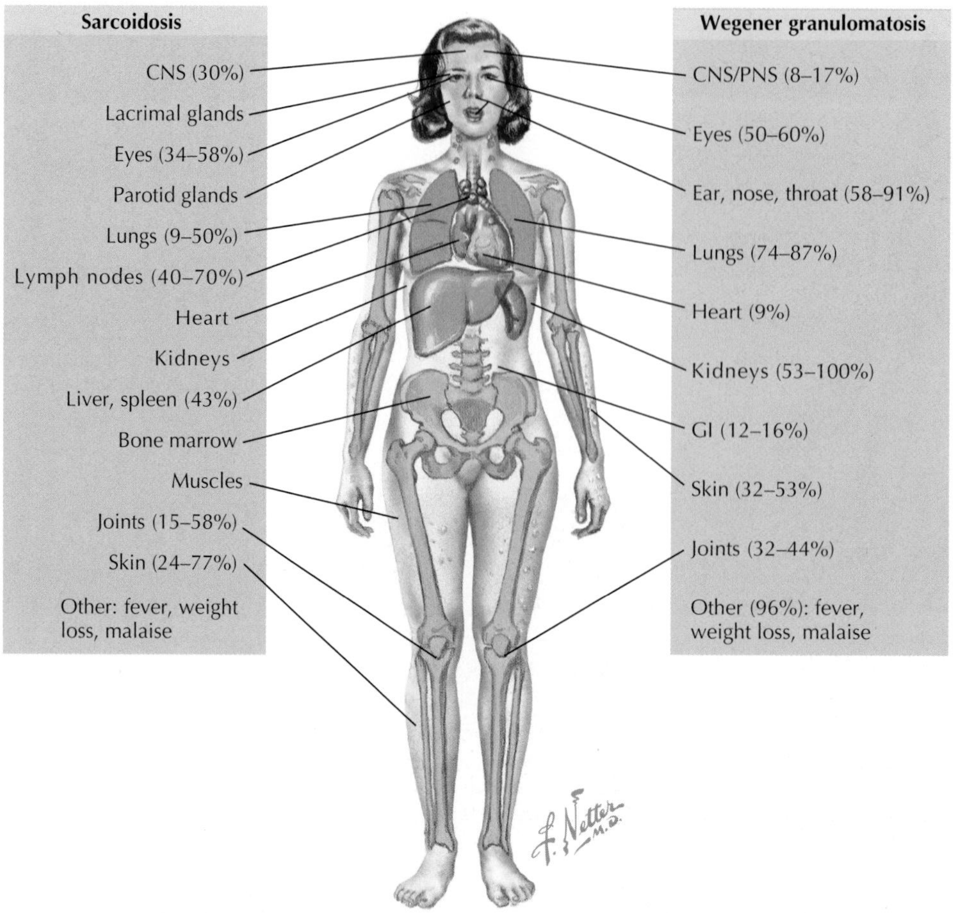

Figure 30-2 *Clinical features in sarcoidosis and Wegener granulomatosis.*

erythrocyte sedimentation rate [ESR], C-reactive protein [CRP], and platelets). Serum angiotensin-converting enzyme (ACE) is elevated in up to 80% of children with sarcoidosis because of production of ACE by granuloma epithelial cells, and levels often correlate with disease activity. Sarcoid granuloma

---

Box 30-1 Differential Diagnosis for Granulomatous Inflammation

Infection
- Mycobacterial (tuberculous or nontuberculous)
- Fungal (histoplasmosis, blastomycosis, coccidioidomycosis, aspergillosis)
- Parasites (schistosomiasis, toxoplasmosis, leishmaniasis, toxocariasis)
- Bacteria (brucellosis, actinomycosis, melioidosis, listeriosis, tularemia, *Bartonella henselae*)
- Viral (Epstein-Barr virus, cytomegalovirus, measles, mumps)
- Other (syphilis, *Coxiella burnetii*, *Chlamydia* spp.)

Noninfectious
- Sarcoidosis
- Wegener granulomatosis
- Churg-Strauss syndrome
- Blau syndrome
- Crohn disease
- Chronic granulomatous disease

---

macrophages express 25-hydroxyvitamin D3-1α and are able to synthesize 1,25-dihydroxyvitamin D, resulting in increased intestinal calcium absorption and bone resorption. Calciuria is present in most children with sarcoidosis and commonly occurs in the absence of hypercalcemia. Thus, the urine calcium/creatinine ratio should be obtained. Other common nonspecific findings include leukopenia, anemia, eosinophilia, hypergammaglobulinemia, and positive rheumatoid factor (RF). In early-onset sarcoidosis, genetic tests for *NOD2/CARD15* mutations should be performed (see Blau Syndrome below).

IMAGING

Chest radiography should be performed to evaluate for hilar adenopathy or other pulmonary involvement suggestive of, but not specific for, sarcoidosis. Chest computed tomography (CT) may be considered to further characterize abnormalities found on chest radiographs. Plain radiographs of the hands and vertebrae may demonstrate characteristic lytic bone lesions in up to 19% of children with sarcoidosis. A gallium scan or ^{18}F-fluorodesoxyglucose-positron emission tomographic (FDG-PET) scan is useful in determining extent of pulmonary and extrapulmonary involvement. Lacrimal and parotid gland involvement results in the so-called "panda" pattern, in which gallium uptake is noted in the nasopharynx and lacrimal and parotid glands, resulting in a PET image that resembles the face of a panda. Magnetic resonance imaging (MRI) is preferred for evaluation of CNS or bone involvement.

HISTOLOGY

Biopsy-proven granulomatous inflammation is vital to the diagnosis of sarcoidosis. Tissue should be sampled from the most accessible site (preferably superficial lymph nodes), which may be determined by imaging (e.g., FDG-PET) if not clinically apparent. Typical histology includes noncaseating epithelioid cell granulomas; however, this is not specific and does not distinguish sarcoidosis from other granulomatous diseases, including infections. Specific stains and cultures for granulomatous infections should be performed (see Box 30-1).

PULMONARY FUNCTION TESTING

PFTs should be performed to evaluate for subclinical pulmonary involvement.

OPHTHALMOLOGIC EVALUATION

Ophthalmologic evaluation, including a slit-lamp examination, should be sought early in the diagnostic workup because ocular lesions typical of sarcoidosis are not common in infections or malignancy.

Management

Sarcoidosis is often quite responsive to corticosteroid therapy and may be controlled on low daily doses. For cases in which low-dose corticosteroids are not adequately effective because of persistent disease or side effects, immunomodulatory therapies, such as methotrexate or anti–TNF-α (tumor necrosis factor-α) monoclonal antibodies (infliximab or adalimumab), may be used. Other immunomodulatory agents that have been used include azathioprine, cyclophosphamide, chlorambucil, and cyclosporine.

WEGENER GRANULOMATOSIS

WG is a systemic disease characterized by granulomatous inflammation and necrotizing vasculitis predominantly involving small vessels. A rare disease, the incidence is approximately 0.1 in 100,000 children, with a female predominance (4:1) and a median age at onset of 14.5 years (range, 9-17 years).

Etiology and Pathogenesis

The cause of WG is unknown, but a pathogenic role for antineutrophil cytoplasmic antibodies (ANCAs), specifically antiproteinase 3 (anti-PR3, the main component of cytoplasmic ANCA or c-ANCA), has been proposed in the mechanism of initial endothelial cell damage. A correlation with *Staphylococcus aureus* infections and WG flares suggests that extrinsic factors play a role.

Clinical Presentation

The triad of pulmonary, renal, and sinus involvement characterizes classic WG; however, the most common presentation is nonspecific constitutional symptoms (fever, weight loss) and arthralgias. Limited WG involves the upper airway and spares the kidneys.

PULMONARY MANIFESTATIONS

Pulmonary involvement ranges from asymptomatic pulmonary nodules to hemorrhage and respiratory failure. Common symptoms include cough, dyspnea, and hemoptysis.

RENAL MANIFESTATIONS

Necrotizing glomerulonephritis is a serious manifestation and may initially be asymptomatic with progression to renal failure necessitating hemodialysis or transplantation.

EAR, NOSE, AND THROAT MANIFESTATIONS

Upper airway manifestations typically involve sinusitis or recurrent epistaxis but may also include oral or nasal ulcers, recurrent otitis media, hearing loss (conductive or sensorineural), subglottic stenosis, or granulomatous inflammation of nasal cartilage resulting in nasal septal perforation or saddle nose deformity.

OCULAR MANIFESTATIONS

Ocular involvement includes scleritis, episcleritis, conjunctivitis, or uveitis and may present as blurry vision, eye pain, or without symptoms. Before establishment of the diagnosis, the eye involvement is frequently misdiagnosed as allergic conjunctivitis.

MUSCULOSKELETAL MANIFESTATIONS

Arthritis may occur with active disease but is usually not chronic. Myalgias and arthralgias are common.

SKIN MANIFESTATIONS

The rash of WG most commonly presents as palpable purpura (often misdiagnosed as Henoch-Schönlein purpura) or erythematous nodules, but necrotizing vasculitic lesions and ulcerations may occur.

CNS MANIFESTATIONS

Cerebral vasculitis, seizures, optic neuritis, and cranial nerve palsies are rare.

OTHER MANIFESTATIONS

Less common manifestations include cardiac involvement (infarction, arrhythmia, or valvulitis), gastrointestinal tract involvement (nausea, vomiting, or pain), and venous thromboembolism.

Differential Diagnosis

The differential diagnosis depends on presentation and often requires evaluating for other causes of nonspecific systemic symptoms, such as fever and malaise or fever of unknown origin (see Chapter 86, Figure 86-1). Infectious causes of granulomatous vasculitis must be considered (see Box 30-1). Other rheumatologic illnesses (sarcoidosis, CSS, microscopic polyangiitis, SLE, MCTD, Sjögren syndrome, and Goodpasture syndrome) and chronic granulomatous disease (especially in young children) should be considered.

Evaluation and Management

BLOOD AND URINE STUDIES

No diagnostic laboratory tests exist for WG, though 90-95% of children are ANCA positive, with cANCA (cytoplasmic antineutrophil cytoplasmic antibodies) occurring more frequently than pANCA (perinuclear antineutrophil cytoplasmic antibodies) (87% vs. 13%, respectively). Anti-PR3 antibodies should also be evaluated. RF is positive in up to 63% of children with WG. Inflammatory markers (ESR and CRP) and other acute-phase reactants (e.g., platelets) are typically elevated, and a mild anemia is often present. Elevated serum creatinine occurs in up to 44% and abnormal urine analysis (proteinuria, microscopic hematuria, and red blood cell casts) in up to 50%.

IMAGING

Chest radiograph abnormalities, typically nodular infiltrates, are present in up to two-thirds of children, half of whom are asymptomatic. Pleural effusions and pneumothoraces may occur. Chest and sinus CTs should be obtained to characterize the extent of pulmonary and sinus involvement. FDG-PET scan may help to characterize the extent of extrapulmonary involvement and to determine the least invasive biopsy site.

PULMONARY FUNCTION TESTS

Decreased diffusion capacity of the lung for carbon monoxide (DLCO) suggests early pulmonary hemorrhage.

OPHTHALMOLOGIC EVALUATION

Because ophthalmologic manifestations are common in WG, ophthalmologic evaluation should be sought early in the diagnostic workup.

HISTOLOGY

Classic granulomas include central necrosis, histiocytes, lymphocytes, and giant cells. The pathology varies by biopsy site. Typical kidney lesions include pauciimmune crescentic necrotizing glomerulonephritis, with granulomas or vasculitis rarely noted. Biopsies from the upper respiratory tract (sinus or nasal septum) may reveal granulomas with giant cells or necrotizing vasculitis. Whereas lung nodules typically show granulomas, other air-space disease may reveal vasculitis or posthemorrhage changes.

Management

Corticosteroids are the mainstay of management of patients with WG. Other immunomodulatory therapy choices depend on the extent of organ involvement. For life-threatening disease, cyclophosphamide is warranted; for more limited disease, azathioprine or mycophenolic acid have been used. Trimethoprim–sulfamethoxazole is often used as adjunct treatment; whether the benefit is attributable to antimicrobial properties (i.e., in limiting S. aureus–associated WG flares) or to other antiinflammatory properties is unclear. Newer biologic agents, such as anti–TNF-α monoclonal antibodies, provide a promising alternative, but large-scale studies of these agents have not been performed in children. Plasmapheresis has been used for severe, life-threatening disease. WG is generally well controlled with therapy; however, relapse is common, especially as medication is weaned or discontinued. Notably, approximately one-third of children with WG develop irreversible renal insufficiency.

CHURG-STRAUSS SYNDROME

CSS, also known as allergic granulomatosis, is a granulomatous small vessel vasculitis associated with asthma, eosinophilia, and allergic rhinitis. Classification criteria include asthma, eosinophilia (>10% of white blood cells), allergy history, peripheral neuropathies (mono-, poly-, or mononeuritis multiplex), transient pulmonary infiltrates, paranasal sinus abnormalities, and extravascular eosinophils. The presence of four of these criteria achieves 85% sensitivity and 99.7% specificity. CSS is extremely rare in children, with 33 cases reported in the literature between 1951 and 2007. The mean age of onset is 12 years, ranging from 2 to 18 years, with a slight female predominance (1.35 : 1). The cause and pathogenesis are currently unknown.

Clinical Presentation

At diagnosis, there is a history of asthma in 91% of children and of sinusitis in 77%. Nonfixed pulmonary infiltrates occur in 85% and pleural effusions in 12%. Skin involvement occurs in 66%, typically with leukocytoclastic vasculitis manifesting as purpura, but other rashes (maculopapular, cutaneous nodules, livedo reticularis, ulcers, and bullae) occur as well. Pericardial effusion occurs in 27% and cardiomyopathy in 42%. Other manifestations include peripheral neuropathy (39%), gastrointestinal (40%) or musculoskeletal (20%) involvement, and mild nonprogressive renal disease (20%). Involvement of the lymph nodes, mammary glands, orbits, salivary glands, testes, and thymus has also been noted.

Evaluation and Management

No tests are diagnostic, but eosinophilia, high immunoglobulin E (IgE), and elevated inflammatory markers are common. ANCAs are detected in 25%, with one-third having cANCA and two-thirds having pANCA. On histology, affected tissues demonstrate vasculitis of small arteries, veins, or both with associated extravascular eosinophilic infiltrates and necrotizing granulomas. High-dose corticosteroids in combination with other immunomodulatory therapies, such as cyclophosphamide or azathioprine, are the mainstays of treatment. Overall prognosis is guarded, with relapse common (≈50%) and mortality from disease manifestations (intestinal perforation, cardiac failure, and respiratory insufficiency) occurring in 18% within 1 to 2 years of diagnosis.

FAMILIAL JUVENILE SYSTEMIC GRANULOMATOSIS (BLAU SYNDROME)

Blau syndrome is an autosomal dominant disease characterized by the triad of arthritis, uveitis, and dermatitis along with evidence of noncaseating granulomas and mutations in *NOD2/CARD15*. This disease is rare, typically occurs in infants and young children (median age, 2 years; range, 2 months–14 years), and is more common among whites. The cause and pathogenesis are unknown. Arthritis is polyarticular in 96% and oligoarticular in 4%. Similar to sarcoidosis, the arthritis is boggy in the majority (74%), but tenosynovitis is less common. Dermatitis consists of nonerythematous, scaly, ichthyosiform rash. Erythema nodosum, liver granulomas, and large vessel vasculitis have also been reported. The lungs are not affected.

Diagnostic and management considerations for Blau syndrome are similar to those for sarcoidosis (with the addition of genetic testing for *NOD2/CARD15* mutations), and some regard Blau syndrome and early onset sarcoidosis as a single entity. Ocular outcomes in children with Blau syndrome are frequently worse than in sarcoidosis.

FUTURE DIRECTIONS

Noninfectious granulomatous diseases are rare in children but should be considered in any child with multisystem manifestations or unexplained constitutional symptoms (e.g., fever of unknown origin). If undiagnosed and untreated, these conditions result in serious disabilities or death. Newer immunomodulatory agents are promising in the treatment of patients with these diseases. The greatest hurdle in determining optimal therapy for noninfectious granulomatous disease in children is the lack of systematic evaluation owing to the low incidence of these diseases. Establishment of registries for these rare conditions will allow for a more systematic and comprehensive evaluation of their characteristics, pathogenesis, genetics, and outcomes, which are prerequisites for improving therapeutic management.

SUGGESTED READINGS

Lindsley CB, Laxer RM: Granulomatous vasculitis, giant cell arteritis, and sarcoidosis. In Cassidy JT, Petty RE, Laxer RM, Lindsley CB, editors: *Textbook of Pediatric Rheumatology*, ed 5, Philadelphia, 2005, Elsevier, pp 539-560.

O'Neil KM: Progress in pediatric vasculitis, *Curr Opin Rheumatol* 21(5):538-546, 2009.

SARCOIDOSIS

Ianuzzi MC, Rybicki BA, Teirstein AS: Sarcoidosis, *N Engl J Med* 357:2153-2165, 2007.

Shetty AK, Gedalia A: Childhood sarcoidosis: a rare but fascinating disorder, *Pediatr Rheumatol Online J* 6:16-25, 2008.

WEGENER GRANULOMATOSIS

Akikusa JD, Schneider R, Harvey EA, et al: Clinical features and outcome of pediatric Wegener's granulomatosis, *Arthritis Rheum* 57:837-844, 2007.

Frosch M, Foell D: Wegener granulomatosis in childhood and adolescence, *Eur J Pediatr* 163:425-434, 2004.

CHURG-STRAUSS SYNDROME

Zwerina J, Eger G, Englbrecht M, et al: Churg-Strauss syndrome in childhood: a systematic literature review and clinical comparison with adult patients, *Semin Arthritis Rheum* 39(2):108-115, 2009.

BLAU SYNDROME

Rose CD, Wouters CH, Meiorin S, et al: Pediatric granulomatous arthritis: an international registry, *Arthritis Rheum* 54:3337-3344, 2006.

Christina L. Master

Disorders of the Head, Neck, and Upper Airway

Otitis

*O*titis is defined as inflammation of the ear. Otitis media is inflammation of the middle ear, and otitis externa is inflammation of the outer ear and canal.

To first review basic anatomy, the ear is divided into three parts: the outer, middle, and inner ear. The outer ear consists of the auricle and ear canal up to the tympanic membrane (TM). The middle ear is bounded by the TM and the round window. The middle ear contains three bones that conduct sound—the malleus, the incus, and the stapes—and the Eustachian (pharyngotympanic) tube that connects the middle ear cavity to the pharynx. The inner ear contains the cochlea and semicircular canals (Figure 31-1).

OTITIS EXTERNA

Acute otitis externa (AOE), more commonly known as "swimmer's ear," is a condition of diffuse inflammation in the external auditory canal. The estimated yearly incidence is 1 in 100 to 250, and although costs have not been reported, they are likely considerable because the condition is so widespread.

ETIOLOGY AND PATHOGENESIS

The lateral two-thirds of the ear canal is composed of epithelium with glands producing cerumen; in the medial third, the epithelium is tightly adherent to the periosteum and there are no glands. Uniquely, the cells and cerumen migrate laterally to self-cleanse. Cerumen has antimicrobial activity with a low pH and lysozymes; therefore, insufficient cerumen may predispose to AOE. With a combination of moist conditions (from swimming, humidity, sweating, and so on) and local trauma to the ear canal, organisms invade the epithelium, causing cellulitis.

In the United States, between 90% and 98% of cases of AOE are bacterial in origin. The most common bacterium by far is *Pseudomonas aeruginosa*. The second most common bacteria are *Staphylococcus* species, including *S. aureus*. Other gram-negative and -positive bacteria are often cultured. Fungi, either *Candida* or *Aspergillus* spp., and some other organisms cause the remaining cases of canal inflammation. It is common to have polymicrobial infections.

CLINICAL PRESENTATION

The patient presents with symptoms that are rapid in onset over days, including ear pain and pruritus, or "fullness" in the ear canal. Some families may also note redness, discharge, or even hearing loss if the condition has progressed sufficiently to block the ear canal.

The peak incidence of AOE occurs in children age 7 to 12 years. There has often been significant water exposure, and even if swimming pool water quality is high, causative organisms are generally still present. Some parents or patients may admit to

canal trauma with cotton swabs or bobby pins when questioned on history.

In AOE, the physical examination is critical in diagnosis. Debris and cerumen must be cleared from the canal to ensure accurate otoscopy of the TM as well as to improve the ability of topical treatment to reach the area of infection. The hallmark sign of AOE is tenderness of the tragus or the pinna when manipulated. The clinician will see diffuse edema and erythema of the canal, possibly with otorrhea or other debris present (Figure 31-2). The TM may be erythematous, but this should not imply a definite diagnosis of otitis media. On pneumatic otoscopy, if there is normal movement of the TM without visible effusion, the erythema may be attributed to the AOE.

On differential diagnosis, other conditions that should be considered include otitis media with perforation, malignant otitis externa (necrotizing osteomyelitis), furunculosis, contact otitis of the ear canal (largely from nickel jewelry, but also topical antimicrobials, chemicals, plastics, and so on), and other generalized dermatologic conditions occurring in or around the ear canal.

EVALUATION AND MANAGEMENT

After the diagnosis of AOE has been made by history and physical examination, it is rare that further evaluation is warranted. Only if an initial presentation has not resolved with prescribed therapy should a culture be taken for bacterial and fungal identification. On suspicion that the patient could have malignant otitis externa, further imaging may be needed to clarify the diagnosis. This serious condition should be suspected if the patient has a high temperature or necrotic tissue, facial paresis, meningeal signs, or mastoid involvement.

Appropriate management of AOE includes treating the causative organism as well as the debilitating pain. Topical therapy should be the initial treatment for uncomplicated AOE, and systemic antibiotics are not warranted. No studies have reliably proven one topical agent to work better than another. Acetic acid (2.0%) and alcohol (90%-95% isopropyl) solutions work as well as antimicrobial drops to clear AOE; however, they may be irritating. Aminoglycosides and fluoroquinolones with and without steroids have been approved for treatment of AOE. Examples include combinations of ciprofloxacin and hydrocortisone or dexamethasone, the combination of neomycin, polymyxin B, and hydrocortisone, and ofloxacin.

Because none of these treatments has proven best, an important consideration is the side effect profile. With a perforated TM or a myringotomy tube present, agents with ototoxicity should be strictly avoided, including the aminoglycosides and alcohol-based products. Contact dermatitis commonly (5%-15% prevalence) occurs with aminoglycoside otic drops. Other factors to consider include cost and compliance. Currently, fluoroquinolone drops are much more costly than other

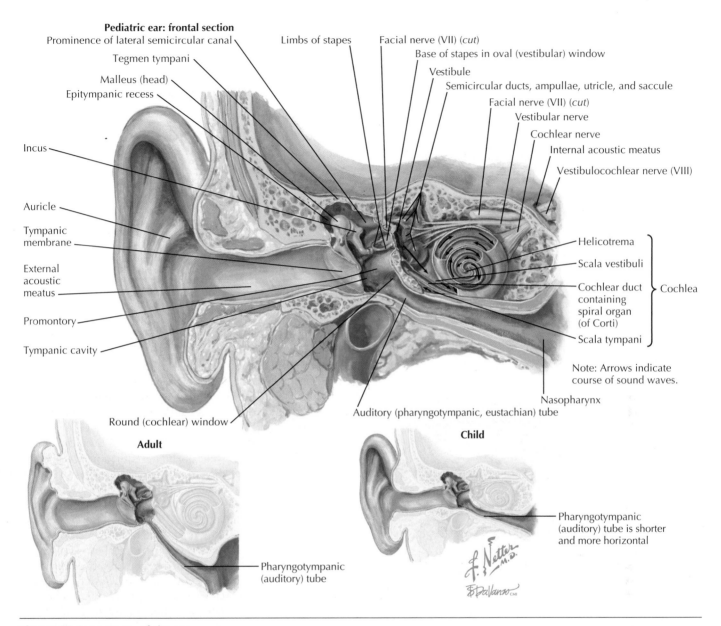

Pediatric ear: frontal section

Prominence of lateral semicircular canal

Tegmen tympani

Malleus (head)

Epitympanic recess

Incus

Auricle

Tympanic membrane

External acoustic meatus

Promontory

Tympanic cavity

Limbs of stapes

Facial nerve (VII) (*cut*)

Base of stapes in oval (vestibular) window

Vestibule

Semicircular ducts, ampullae, utricle, and saccule

Facial nerve (VII) (*cut*)

Vestibular nerve

Cochlear nerve

Internal acoustic meatus

Vestibulocochlear nerve (VIII)

Helicotrema

Scala vestibuli

Cochlear duct containing spiral organ (of Corti)

Scala tympani

Cochlea

Note: Arrows indicate course of sound waves.

Nasopharynx

Auditory (pharyngotympanic, eustachian) tube

Round (cochlear) window

Adult

Child

Pharyngotympanic (auditory) tube is shorter and more horizontal

Pharyngotympanic (auditory) tube

Figure 31-1 *Anatomy of the ear.*

preparations. Conversely, patients may be more compliant with the fluoroquinolone drops because they need only be administered twice daily compared with four times daily for aminoglycosides.

Systemic oral antimicrobials should be reserved for cases in which cellulitis is extending onto the external ear or face, necrotizing disease is discovered, a concomitant middle ear infection exists, or the patient has an underlying immunodeficiency that makes him or her more susceptible to disease progression.

If a fungal cause of AOE is suspected, the clinician will see white strands with or without black or white fungal balls. Mild fungal infections respond to acid or alcohol solutions, but more advanced infections may require a topical antifungal such as clotrimazole.

Appropriate drug delivery is paramount. If the canal debris cannot be cleared by the physician, a wick should be inserted so

that topical treatment can reach the infection. The parents should be instructed on how to correctly administer drops with the patient lying down, drops applied until filling the ear canal, and the patient maintaining this position for 3 to 5 minutes. Children should avoid submerging their heads underwater for 7 to 10 days while being treated, and beneficial effects from treatment should be seen in 48 to 72 hours.

Pain should be evaluated and treated for each patient. Most patients will benefit simply from a nonsteroidal antiinflammatory drug (NSAID). Topical anesthetic agents such as benzocaine may be used, but the relief they provide may mask progression of disease.

FUTURE DIRECTIONS

Topics that greatly need further exploration for AOE include determining which topical agents are superior to others,

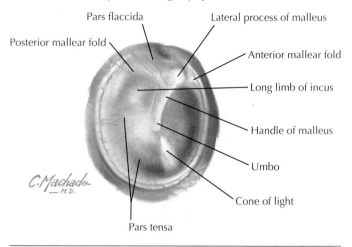

Otoscopic view of right tympanic membrane

In otitis externa, inflammation, edema, and discharge are limited to external auditory canal and its walls

Figure 31-3 *Right tympanic membrane.*

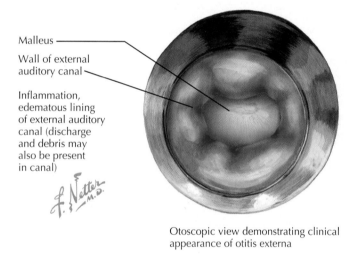

Otoscopic view demonstrating clinical appearance of otitis externa

Figure 31-2 *Acute otitis externa.*

determining outcome differences when topical steroids are added to antimicrobials, and studying the efficacy of home remedy solutions.

OTITIS MEDIA

Otitis media is inflammation in the middle ear. Otitis media should be further delineated into either acute otitis media (AOM) or otitis media with effusion (OME). Both of these conditions are extremely prevalent; AOM is the most common illness pediatricians encounter and the most common reason for antibiotic prescriptions in children. OME is reported to occur in 90% of children before they reach school age.

ETIOLOGY AND PATHOGENESIS

AOM and OME both may occur through similar mechanisms. In young children, the Eustachian tube exists more horizontally than the final oblique direction. This immature orientation predisposes to fluid accumulation in the middle ear. Furthermore, when there is inflammation in the pharynx because of viral or other causes, the edema causes swelling of the Eustachian tube, blocking the physiologic tube opening, ventilation, and pressure equalization of the middle ear that occurs during swallowing. When pressure is not equalized, a negative pressure builds in the cavity that allows aspiration of contents and bacteria from the pharynx into the middle ear. OME may also occur as an inflammatory response after an episode of AOM.

OME does not imply a specific bacterial or viral cause; however, AOM is classically defined by the causative organisms. The most common bacteria implicated are *Streptococcus pneumoniae*, nontypeable *Haemophilus influenzae*, and *Moraxella catarrhalis*. Viral pathogens are often found in combination with bacteria, and viruses are found in 5% to 22% of cases as the sole cause.

CLINICAL PRESENTATION

Acute Otitis Media

AOM is common in children of all ages. Parents will generally bring their child to the office with a complaint of pain, pulling on the ear, fever, and/or ear drainage. Before examining a child for AOM or OME, the physician must be comfortable with otoscopy of the normal ear and TM. The most common TM landmarks visible on a normal examination include the umbo and handle of the malleus, the shadow of the incus, and the cone of light reflex (Figure 31-3). On pneumatic otoscopy, the physician should appreciate the back-and-forth motion of the normal TM with gentle squeezing and releasing of the bulb.

A physical examination is required to determine the presence of a middle ear effusion (MEE). On inspection of the TM, it may be bulging, or an air-fluid level or bubble will be visible. The normal landmarks may be obscured and the light-reflex

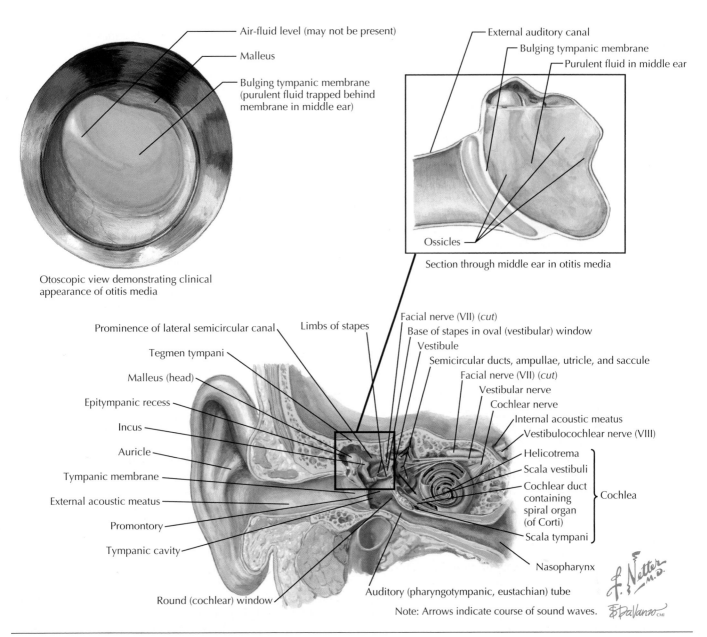

Air-fluid level (may not be present)

Malleus

Bulging tympanic membrane
(purulent fluid trapped behind
membrane in middle ear)

Otoscopic view demonstrating clinical
appearance of otitis media

External auditory canal

Bulging tympanic membrane

Purulent fluid in middle ear

Ossicles

Section through middle ear in otitis media

Prominence of lateral semicircular canal

Tegmen tympani

Malleus (head)

Epitympanic recess

Incus

Auricle

Tympanic membrane

External acoustic meatus

Promontory

Tympanic cavity

Round (cochlear) window

Limbs of stapes

Facial nerve (VII) (*cut*)
Base of stapes in oval (vestibular) window
Vestibule
Semicircular ducts, ampullae, utricle, and saccule
Facial nerve (VII) (*cut*)
Vestibular nerve
Cochlear nerve
Internal acoustic meatus
Vestibulocochlear nerve (VIII)
Helicotrema
Scala vestibuli
Cochlear duct
containing
spiral organ
(of Corti)   } Cochlea
Scala tympani
Nasopharynx

Auditory (pharyngotympanic, eustachian) tube

Note: Arrows indicate course of sound waves.

Figure 31-4 *Acute otitis media.*

absent or distorted. The movement of the TM will be decreased or absent. Sometimes purulent material will be seen behind the TM (Figure 31-4). In the case of a perforated TM, the perforation itself may be visible or the canal may be filled with debris, fluid, or exudate. Erythema of the TM alone is nondiagnostic because the TM may be red in many other conditions, including AOE and OME and during a child's crying. In children, lack of cooperation often impedes a complete examination. Treatment recommendations for a nondiagnostic, uncertain examination are discussed further below.

Otitis Media with Effusion

In some cases of OME, a child may present with mild ear pain, but often, OME is seen on a routine well-child examination or on examination for follow-up of AOM. Generally, this condition is asymptomatic, but effects of persistent effusion such as hearing loss, speech/language delay, behavioral difficulties, or difficulty sleeping may be noticed and reported by parents.

On examination, as in AOM, an air-fluid level or fluid bubble may be seen. Generally, the fluid visualized is clear. There is no distinct erythema to the TM. There will be decreased movement of the TM with pneumatic otoscopy.

The differential diagnosis of ear pain is broad, but when considering otitis media as a diagnosis, some common conditions that should be considered in children include AOE, mastoiditis, sinusitis, pharyngitis, foreign body, and dental caries.

EVALUATION AND MANAGEMENT

The most recent clinical guidelines by the American Academy of Pediatrics (AAP) detail a certain diagnosis of AOM when there is a history of acute onset, signs of MEE, and signs or symptoms of middle ear inflammation such as severe otalgia or severe erythema. A certain diagnosis of OME is made if a MEE is visible but the other conditions are not present. If the TM cannot be visualized for any reason, a physician could consider tympanometry, if available, to determine the presence or absence of an effusion.

In almost all cases of AOM and OME, after a complete history and physical examination, further testing is not necessary. Rarely, a culture may be taken from a chronically draining ear or radiologic studies may be ordered if there is a suspicion of mastoiditis. In children with OME at risk for developmental disabilities, such as those with underlying developmental syndromes, hearing and language testing should be considered early in the course of disease. For otherwise healthy children with OME, any concern for developmental delay or hearing loss or the persistence of effusion for longer than 3 months should prompt testing.

Acute Otitis Media Treatment

The goals of treatment for AOM include relieving pain, eradicating infection, and preventing complications. Pain should be evaluated and treated in all patients either with an NSAID or acetaminophen. Topical anesthetic otic drops such as benzocaine may provide additional, brief pain relief.

In recent years, there has been a shift in the treatment recommendations for AOM from universal antibiotic use to include the option of observation before requiring antibiotics. Clinical research has shown that most children older than 2 years of age have spontaneous resolution of AOM without antibiotic therapy. There also appears to be no increased risk for complications such as mastoiditis with watchful waiting of older children. Importantly, the observation option helps to limit further emergence of resistant bacteria. The decision to observe or treat should be based on the child's age, diagnostic certainty, and disease severity (Table 31-1). The treatment guidelines proposed by the New York Regional Otitis Project, the AAP, and the American Academy of Family Physicians recommend treatment differences based on age because severe complications are most common in infants and the youngest children.

In choosing antimicrobial therapy for AOM, amoxicillin is the antibiotic of choice even though a large percentage of *S. pneumoniae* are resistant. The mechanism of resistance is via a penicillin-binding protein that may be overcome by "high-dose" amoxicillin at 80 to 90 mg/kg/d in two divided doses. Even though half of all *H. influenzae* and all of *M. catarrhalis* are β-lactamase positive, more of these infections clear spontaneously than infections with *S. pneumoniae*. In patients with severe illness or recurrent AOM, a broader antibiotic should be used such as amoxicillin–clavulanate, a third-generation cephalosporin, or azithromycin in a penicillin-allergic patient. The length of treatment has traditionally been 10 days, but newer studies conclude that 5 days of treatment may be sufficient for older children. Intramuscular ceftriaxone may also be used if the patient cannot tolerate oral antibiotics or has failed initial treatment.

If a perforation of the TM exists or a draining tympanostomy tube is present, only a topical antimicrobial agent is necessary.

Table 31-1 Criteria for Initial Antibiotic Treatment versus Observation in Children with Acute Otitis Media

Age	Certain Diagnosis	Uncertain Diagnosis
<6 months	Antibiotic therapy	Antibiotic therapy
6 months–2 years	Antibiotic therapy	Antibiotic if severe; observation option if not*
>2 years	Antibiotic if severe; observation option if not*	Observation option*

*Observation option is appropriate only when follow-up can be ensured within 48 to 72 hours and antibiotics started if symptoms persist or worsen. Nonsevere illness is defined as only mild otalgia and fever below 39°C. A history of acute symptom onset, middle ear effusion, and signs of middle ear inflammation make a certain diagnosis.

Modified Rosenfeld R: Observation option toolkit for acute otitis media. Int J Pediatr Otorhinolaryngol 58(1):1-8, 2001; New York Regional Otitis Project: Observation Option Toolkit for Acute Otitis Media. State of New York, Department of Health, Publication #4894, March 2002; and American Academy of Pediatrics Subcommittee on Management of Acute Otitis Media. Diagnosis and management of acute otitis media. Pediatrics 113(5):1451-1465, 2004.

Possible choices include ofloxacin or ciprofloxacin with dexamethasone. Decongestants, antihistamines, and oral steroids have not shown any clinical benefit and should not be recommended for AOM treatment.

Referral to an otolaryngologist should be considered if the child has had AOM four times in 6 months or six times in 1 year, there is worsening of symptoms despite antibiotic therapy, or there is any complication of AOM. Tympanostomy tubes may be considered for recurrent AOM because they have been shown to decrease the number of episodes of AOM per year.

Otitis Media with Effusion Treatment

The management of children with OME has trended toward "watchful waiting." Antibiotic therapy is not effective for long-term treatment of OME. Furthermore, most cases (75%-90%) of OME resolve spontaneously within 3 months. In a healthy child with persistent OME and normal hearing and language testing results, the period of watchful waiting may continue with primary care visits every 3 months to follow the effusion and assess for developmental difficulties.

Referral to an otolaryngologist should occur when OME is associated with hearing or language delay or there are physical changes to the TM such as retraction pockets. The primary surgery is tympanostomy tube placement, although adenoidectomy with myringotomy may be considered for children older than age 4 years as a second surgery. Data regarding beneficial outcomes for tympanostomy tube placement to treat OME are lacking but have shown that tube presence does decrease effusions and raise hearing levels. It has been clearly shown, though, that using early tympanostomy tubes to treat OME does not improve long-term developmental outcomes at 6 years and 9 to 11 years.

A link between allergic rhinitis and OME makes physiologic sense but has not proven true in research studies. As with

AOM, antihistamines and decongestants have not shown benefit in treating or preventing OME and may cause harm in children; these agents should not be prescribed for children with OME.

FUTURE DIRECTIONS

For AOM, an important research question is whether or not amoxicillin will remain a first-line antibiotic as the *Pneumococcal* vaccine continues to change the prevalence of *S. pneumoniae.* Continual monitoring of outcomes in the United States is a necessity to ensure that serious bacterial infectious complications do not increase as more physicians adopt the observation option before treatment. Because the most recent and conclusive data have shown no developmental advantage to healthy children receiving tympanostomy tube placement for persistent OME, future research should focus on other modifiable risk factors for delayed language development.

SUGGESTED READINGS

OTITIS EXTERNA

Osguthorpe JD, Nielsen DR: Otitis externa: review and clinical update, *Am Fam Phys* 74(9):1510-1516, 2006.

Roland PS, Stroman DW: Microbiology of acute otitis externa, *Laryngoscope* 112(7 Pt 1):1166-1177, 2002.

Rosenfeld RM, Brown L, Cannon CR, et al: Clinical practice guideline: acute otitis externa, *Otolaryngol Head Neck Surg* 134(Suppl 4):S4-S23, 2006.

Rosenfeld RM, Singer M, Wasserman JM, Stinnett SS: Systematic review of topical antimicrobial therapy for acute otitis externa, *Otolaryngol Head Neck Surg* 134(Suppl 4):S24-S48, 2006.

OTITIS MEDIA

American Family Physicians; American Academy of Academy of Otolaryngology-Head and Neck Surgery; American Academy of Pediatrics Subcommittee on Otitis Media With Effusion: Otitis media with effusion, *Pediatrics* 113(5):1412-1429, 2004.

American Academy of Pediatrics Subcommittee on Management of Acute Otitis Media: Diagnosis and management of acute otitis media, *Pediatrics* 113(5):1451-1465, 2004.

Griffin GH, Flynn C, Bailey RE, Schultz JK: Antihistamines and/or decongestants for otitis media with effusion (OME) in children, *Cochrane Database Syst Rev* (4):CD003423, 2006.

Lous J, Burton MJ, Felding JU, et al: Grommets (ventilation tubes) for hearing loss associated with otitis media with effusion in children, *Cochrane Database Syst Rev* (1):CD001801, 2005.

New York Regional Otitis Project: *Observation Option Toolkit for Acute Otitis Media,* State of New York, March 2002, Department of Health, Publication #4894.

Paradise JL, Campbell TF, Dollaghan CA, et al: Developmental outcomes after early or delayed insertion of tympanostomy tubes, *N Engl J Med* 353(6):576-586, 2005.

Paradise JL, Feldman HM, Campbell TF, et al: Tympanostomy tubes and developmental outcomes at 9 to 11 years of age, *N Engl J Med* 356(3):248-261, 2007.

Rosenfeld R: Observation option toolkit for acute otitis media, *Int J Pediatr Otorhinolaryngol* 58(1):1-8, 2001.

Disorders of the Eye

32

Eden Kahle

General pediatricians must be able to identify common ocular problems in infants and children. Many of these conditions can be managed by the pediatrician, but others require referral to an ophthalmologist. Evaluation of the eye and adnexa involves inspection of the eyelids and preauricular lymph nodes; the extraocular movements, confrontational fields, and pupils; red light reflex in young children and fundus examination if indicated; and the globe itself, noting the conjunctiva, cornea, and sclera. Visual acuity can be assessed using several instruments, most commonly the Snellen eye chart. Corneal epithelial defects can be detected by applying fluorescein dye and then illuminating the cornea with a blue-filtered light or Wood's lamp. Further evaluation by slit lamp and tonometry can be performed by an ophthalmologist if required.

ABNORMAL RED LIGHT REFLEX

All children should have an examination of the red reflex within the first 2 months of life. Children with dark spots in the red reflex, a blunted or absent red reflex, or a white reflex (leukocoria) should be referred to an ophthalmologist. An abnormal red reflex can result from corneal opacities, aqueous opacities, vitreous opacities, and retinal lesions. Leukocoria may indicate pathology, including metabolic, inflammatory, infectious, toxic, oncologic, and traumatic causes; the most common are congenital cataracts and retinoblastoma.

Cataracts

Congenital cataracts occur in two in 10,000 births (Figure 32-1). Of these, 20% to 25% of cases occur secondary to a congenital infection (rubella, cytomegalovirus, or toxoplasmosis) or as a component of a genetic or metabolic condition, such as Turner syndrome, Down syndrome, trisomy 13 and 18, galactosemia, and peroxisomal disorders. Children exposed to high-dose long-term corticosteroid therapy are also at risk, as are children with uveitis or who sustain ocular trauma.

Retinoblastoma

Retinoblastoma occurs in one in 15,000 live births, and 250 to 300 new cases are diagnosed annually in the United States. The hereditary form is caused by a mutation in the retinoblastoma gene, a tumor suppressor gene. A second mutation is then necessary for tumor growth. In the hereditary form, approximately 60% of cases are bilateral and are associated with other cancers, notably osteosarcoma. Retinoblastoma can present with leukocoria and strabismus, and in more advanced cases, proptosis, eye pain, or hyphema. The extent of the disease should be evaluated by computed tomography (CT) or magnetic resonance imaging and orbital ultrasonography. The average age at diagnosis is 1 year for bilateral cases and 2 years for unilateral cases. Urgent referral to an ophthalmologist for potentially vision-sparing and lifesaving treatment is imperative.

DISORDERS OF EYE MOVEMENT

Strabismus

Misalignment of the eyes affects approximately 4% of children younger than 6 years of age (Figure 32-2). Heterophoria is the intermittent tendency for eyes to deviate, and heterotropia is a constant misalignment. The prefixes eso- (inward), exo- (outward), hyper- (upward), and hypo- (downward) indicate the direction of the misaligned eye. Other causes of eye deviations are cranial nerve palsies, intracranial or intraorbital mass, increased intracranial pressure (ICP), and myasthenia gravis.

Heterophorias are usually not apparent; however, under certain conditions such as stress, fatigue, or illness, this latent deviation can be detected. If the deviation is large, patients may experience double vision (diplopia), headache, or eye strain. Heterotropias are present at all times.

Tropias can be tested using the corneal light reflex. The examiner shines a light onto both cornea and notes the placement of the light reflex. If strabismus is present, the reflected light is asymmetric on the cornea. To further test for strabismus, the examiner can perform a cover test. The child should look at an object in the distance. The examiner covers one eye and watches for movement in the uncovered eye. If movement occurs in the uncovered eye, then a misalignment exists in that eye. Phorias can be detected by covering the affected eye; when the eye is uncovered, the practitioner will note the eye moving back into alignment.

Early detection of strabismus is essential because amblyopia can develop if misalignment persists, resulting in permanent visual impairment. Strabismus that is constant or intermittent strabismus that does not correct by age 3 months should prompt ophthalmology referral to begin treatment. The unaffected eye is patched or blurred (with glasses or drops), thereby forcing the strabismic eye to provide a retinal image to the brain and stimulate the proper visual development. In some cases, surgery on the extraocular muscles is necessary to achieve proper alignment.

Amblyopia

Amblyopia is vision impairment caused by an interference with a clear retinal image in one or both eyes during the development of visual acuity in infancy and early childhood. Amblyopia occurs during the critical period of development before the cortex has become visually mature, mainly within the first decade of life. It can be caused by a deviated eye (strabismus), refractive error, or opacity within the visual axis. Treatment is specific to the cause such as strabismus correction, corrective glasses, or removal of the opacity.

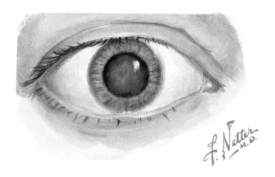

Figure 32-1 *Cataract.*

RED EYE

Red eye is a common pediatric complaint. The differential diagnosis is broad, including infectious, allergic, and inflammatory causes, as well as trauma, glaucoma, and Kawasaki disease. The most common cause is conjunctivitis, inflammation of the conjunctivae, the mucous membrane that covers the surface of the eye up to the limbus (the junction of the sclera and the cornea) and continues onto the inside surface of the eyelids.

Viral Conjunctivitis

Viral conjunctivitis presents with watery or mucopurulent discharge, eye irritation, and scleral injection (Figure 32-3). Both eyes are usually affected simultaneously or in sequence. More serious infection causes pseudomembranes (inflammatory debris and fibrin) or true conjunctival membranes. Punctate keratitis

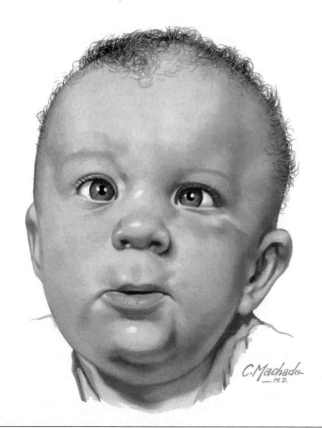

Figure 32-2 *Strabismus.*

Conjunctivitis

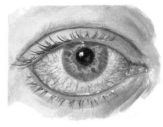

Cobblestoning of tarsal conjunctiva

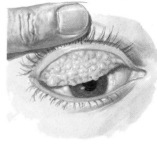

Fluorescein staining and HSV keratitis

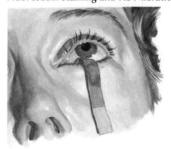

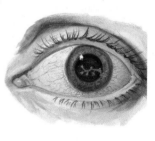

Technique of applying fluorescein strip in previously anesthetized eye

Dendritic keratitis (herpes simplex) demonstrated by fluorescein

Figure 32-3 *Red eye.*

and subepithelial opacities may also occur, causing decreased vision, photosensitivity, or glare and haloes around bright lights.

Adenovirus is the most common pathogen causing viral conjunctivitis. Other symptoms include fever, pharyngitis, rhinitis, cough, and preauricular lymphadenopathy. This infection is highly contagious, and those who are infected should avoid sharing towels and touching their eyes and should wash their hands frequently. Treatment is symptomatic, including cool compresses or antiallergy drops for itchiness. Topical antibiotics should be used if large epithelial defects are present.

Other agents such as measles (rare because of widespread immunization), influenza, enterovirus, and herpes simplex virus (HSV) can cause conjunctivitis. Primary or recurrent HSV can also cause keratitis (corneal inflammation) with a dendrite pattern seen on fluorescein staining (see Figure 32-3). Treatment of ocular HSV includes topical antivirals (trifluridine, vidarabine, or iododeoxyuridine) and, depending on the extent of infection, oral or intravenous acyclovir. Consultation with an ophthalmologist is recommended.

Bacterial Conjunctivitis

Bacterial conjunctivitis presents with hyperemia, edema, mucopurulent discharge, and ocular pain. Common organisms involved are nontypeable *Haemophilus influenzae* (often associated with ipsilateral otitis media), staphylococcus and streptococci species, and *Moraxella catarrhalis*. Gram stain and culture can be performed to identify the organism. Treatment involves topical antibiotic drops or ointment such as polymyxin–trimethoprim, erythromycin, or bacitracin, and patients who wear contact lens should be treated for *Pseudomonas aeruginosa* with fluoroquinolone drops.

Practitioners should suspect *Neisseria gonorrhoeae* or *Chlamydia trachomatis* infection when symptoms of conjunctivitis are present in an infant in the first 2 weeks of life, termed *ophthalmia neonatorum* (see Chapter 105 for a detailed discussion).

Allergic Conjunctivitis

The hallmark of allergic conjunctivitis is itching along with clear tearing, injected conjunctivae, and conjunctival edema (chemosis) in both eyes. In more severe cases, cobblestoning of the tarsal conjunctivae is present (see Figure 32-3). Allergic conjunctivitis occurs as a seasonal disorder accompanied by allergic rhinitis or can occur perennially if associated with allergens such as cat dander, dust mites, mold spores, and other environmental allergens. Elimination of the offending agent and symptomatic treatment with cold compresses is recommended. Topical therapy with mast cell stabilizers or antihistamines can be used, as can oral antihistamines. More severe cases may require referral to an allergist, who may prescribe topical corticosteroids or immunotherapy.

Chemical Conjunctivitis

Various substances can cause a chemical conjunctivitis. Alkali exposure lingers in the conjunctival tissues and continues to cause damage for hours or days. Acids precipitate proteins and produce their effect immediately. In every patient with a chemical exposure, the eyes should be irrigated thoroughly with normal saline to remove the noxious substance. Irrigation should continue until a neutral pH ($\approx$7.4) of the eye is achieved.

Uveitis

Uveitis is inflammation of the inner vascular coat of the eye (iris, ciliary body, and choroids). Posterior uveitis involves the choroid and presents with visual changes such as floaters and decreased vision. Anterior uveitis is synonymous with iritis and involves inflammation of the iris and ciliary body. Patients may have circumlimbal redness, eye pain, headache, photophobia, decreased vision, miosis, hypopyon (layering of white blood cells in the anterior chamber), and keratic precipitates. Uveitis can be seen in systemic immune-mediated diseases such as juvenile idiopathic arthritis, inflammatory bowel disease, and sarcoid and certain infections such as toxoplasmosis, tuberculosis, cytomegalovirus, and syphilis. Patients should be referred to an ophthalmologist for management.

DISORDERS OF ADNEXAL STRUCTURES

Nasolacrimal Duct Obstruction

Nasolacrimal duct obstruction occurs in 2% to 4% of full-term babies and is even more common in premature babies. Congenital obstruction is usually caused by an imperforate membrane at the distal end of the nasolacrimal duct (Figure 32-4). Patients present with tears overflowing the eyelid (epiphora) and mucoid matter crusting the eyelashes.

If the patient has excessive tearing associated with photophobia, blepharospasm, or corneal and ocular enlargement, the physician should consider glaucoma as a cause of the symptoms and refer the patient to an ophthalmologist immediately. Glaucoma is a rare entity in infancy but can be vision threatening. Other causes of excessive tearing are corneal abrasion, intraocular inflammation, and foreign body.

Treatment of nasolacrimal duct obstruction involves applying digital pressure with downward strokes several times a day. Approximately 90% of cases resolve before 1 year of age. Patients can be referred to an ophthalmologist if symptoms do not resolve, in which case probing of the duct may be necessary. If mucopurulent discharge is expressible with palpation of the lacrimal sac and the sac is swollen, red, and tender, the patient may have an associated dacryocystitis, or inflammation of the lacrimal sac, which would require treatment with topical and often oral or intravenous antibiotics.

Hordeolum and Chalazion

A hordeolum is inflammation or impaction of a sebaceous gland of the eyelid. Whereas an internal hordeolum involves the meibomian glands and occurs on the conjunctival surface, infection of the glands of Zeiss or Moll causes an abscess on the eyelid margin known as an external hordeolum (stye). A chalazion is a chronic granulomatous inflammation of a meibomian gland, which is noted as a small, rubbery nodule located more centrally on the eyelid (see Figure 32-4).

Treatment of an external hordeolum involves warm compresses to encourage drainage and rarely incision and drainage. Topical antibiotics can be used for lesions that appear infected or are accompanied by discharge. Resolution may take several weeks. If infection spreads further, causing preseptal cellulitis, oral or intravenous antibiotics are required. A chalazion, if persistent, can be removed by an ophthalmologist by incision and curettage or steroid injection.

Preseptal (Periorbital) Cellulitis

Preseptal cellulitis is inflammation of the eyelids and periorbital tissues anterior to the orbital septum (see Figure 32-4), usually caused by contiguous infection of the periorbital soft tissues of the face. The most common pathogens are *Staphylococcus aureus*, group A β-hemolytic streptococcus, and *Streptococcus pneumoniae*. Patients present with erythema and swelling of the eyelids and conjunctival injection but will not have proptosis or limited ocular movements as in orbital cellulitis (see below).

Mild cases can be managed on an outpatient basis with broad spectrum antibiotics such as amoxicillin-clavulanate or clindamycin while more severe cases require intravenous antibiotics. If there is no clinical response within 24 hours or any suspicion for orbital cellulitis, the patient should have a CT scan of the sinuses and orbits and receive parenteral antibiotics.

Orbital Cellulitis

Orbital cellulitis presents with the previously described symptoms of periorbital cellulitis, but also with proptosis, limitation of eye movement, and sometimes decreased visual acuity, which distinguish it from a preseptal infection. Paranasal (ethmoid) sinusitis is the most common cause, but may also result from

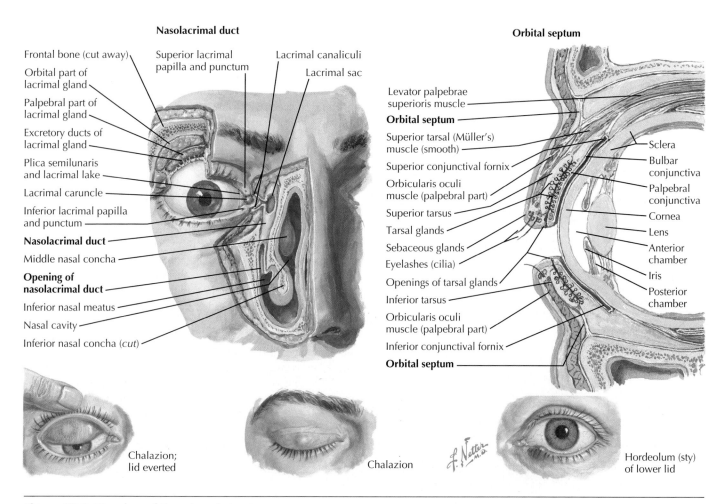

Figure 32-4 *Disorders of the adnexal structures.*

seeding from bacteremia as well as direct extension or venous spread of infection from contiguous sites such as the eyelids, conjunctiva, globe, lacrimal gland, and nasolacrimal sac. *S. aureus*, group A streptococcus, *S. pneumoniae*, *Haemophilus influenzae*, and anaerobes are commonly implicated as pathogens. Fungal infection should be considered in immunocompromised hosts. More serious cases may involve the optic nerve and cause loss of vision or extend intracranially and result in complications such as cavernous sinus thrombosis, meningitis, epidural and subdural empyema, or brain abscesses.

Treatment with broad-spectrum parenteral antibiotics such as high-dose ampicillin–sulbactam is indicated. Clindamycin or vancomycin may be used as well to ensure coverage of methicillin-resistant *S. aureus* (MRSA), and metronidazole can be added for additional anaerobe coverage. A CT of the sinuses and orbits with contrast should be performed to confirm infection within the orbit and to detect subperiosteal abscess or intracranial extension. Neurosurgical intervention may be necessary in cases with abscess or empyema formation.

OCULAR TRAUMA

Pediatricians can treat some minor ocular injuries. Injuries that require immediate referral to an ophthalmologist are penetrated or ruptured globe, laceration of the eyelid margin, or entrapment of the extraocular muscles after orbital fracture.

Corneal Abrasion

Corneal abrasion presents with the sensation of a foreign body in the eye, pain, scleral injection, tearing, and photophobia. Pediatricians can detect corneal epithelial defects with fluorescein dye (see Figure 32-3). The eyelid should be everted to check for retained foreign body. Vision testing should also be performed, and if vision changes are present, the patient should be referred to an ophthalmologist. Topical antibiotic ointment is prescribed for infection prophylaxis and lubrication of the eye. Patients who wear contact lenses should be treated with topical fluoroquinolones for *Pseudomonas* spp. Without treatment, an infection could progress to a corneal ulcer. Oral analgesics can be used for pain. Topical anesthetics are no longer recommended because they slow epithelial healing and decrease the protective blinking reflex.

Hyphema

Hyphema is blood in the anterior chamber that is usually caused by blunt injury. Layering of blood cells can be seen by penlight

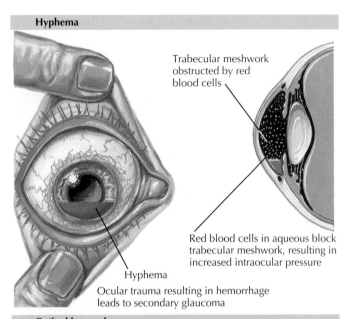

Hyphema

Trabecular meshwork obstructed by red blood cells

Red blood cells in aqueous block trabecular meshwork, resulting in increased intraocular pressure

Hyphema

Ocular trauma resulting in hemorrhage leads to secondary glaucoma

Retinal hemorrhage

Retinal hemorrhage

Papilledema

In older children, frank papilledema may accompany increased intracranial pressure caused by subdural bleeding

Subconjunctival hemorrhage

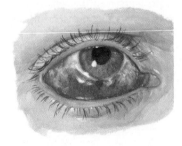

Figure 32-5 *Ocular trauma.*

or slit lamp (Figure 32-5). Increased ocular pressure may develop if the trabecular meshwork is affected either by the original injury or by red blood cells causing a blockage. Patients are at risk for rebleeding 3 to 5 days later. Patients with sickle cell disease or trait are at higher risk for complications and require more aggressive intervention.

An ophthalmology evaluation is required urgently. Treatment involves wearing an eye shield and maintaining a 30-degree angle of the head to promote drainage and prevent secondary bleeding. The ophthalmologist may prescribe topical mydriatics, topical or oral corticosteroids, or aminocaproic acid to prevent rebleeding. Nonsteroidal antiinflammatory drugs and aspirin should be avoided.

Retinal Hemorrhage

Retinal hemorrhages can be caused by increased intrathoracic pressure or by acceleration–deceleration injuries. They are common in newborns delivered vaginally and resolve within 2 to 6 weeks without sequelae. They can also occur during trauma and are present in 85% of cases of shaken babies. The hemorrhages seen in non-accidental trauma have a distinctive pattern and are often bilateral, flame-shaped, and include preretinal structures and the macula (see Figure 32-5).

Subconjunctival Hemorrhage

Subconjunctival hemorrhage is the presence of blood between the conjunctiva and sclera (see Figure 32-5), is extremely common in newborns after vaginal birth, and resolves spontaneously within 2 weeks. In older children and adults, these hemorrhages are usually caused by increased intraocular pressure from coughing or sneezing or result from infection such as adenoviral conjunctivitis. Patients should be carefully examined to rule out a perforating injury.

FUTURE DIRECTIONS

Advances continue to be made in diagnostic techniques and treatments of pediatric ophthalmologic conditions. Ocular ultrasonography is an emerging technique for evaluating patients in the emergency department. For traumatic eye injuries, ultrasound can identify penetrating globe injury and intraocular foreign body. Ultrasound can also be used to measure the optic nerve sheath diameter, which correlates with ICP.

For children with a refractive error that is resistant to conventional therapy, refractive surgery such as laser in situ keratomileusis (LASIK) is now becoming an accepted treatment option. It can be particularly beneficial in children with amblyopiogenic refractive errors who have poor compliance wearing glasses or contact lenses and in children with neurobehavioral impairment who cannot tolerate wearing corrective lenses.

SUGGESTED READINGS

American Academy of Pediatrics; Section on Ophthalmology; American Association for Pediatric Ophthalmology And Strabismus; American Academy of Ophthalmology; American Association of Certified Orthoptists: Red reflex examination in neonates, infants, and children, *Pediatrics* 122(6):1401-1404, 2008.

Binenbaum G, Mirz-George N, Christian CW, Forbes BJ: Odds of abuse associated with retinal hemorrhages in children suspected of child abuse, *J AAPOS* 13(3):268-272, 2009.

Blaivas M, Theodoro D, Sierzenski PR: A study of bedside ocular ultrasonography in the emergency department, *Acad Emerg Med* 9(8):791-799, 2002.

Daoud YJ, Hutchinson A, Wallace DK, Song J, Kim T: Refractive surgery in children: treatment options, outcomes, and controversies, *Am J Ophthalmol* 147(4):573-582, 2009.

Pieramici DJ, Goldberg MF, Melia M, et al: A phase III, mulitcenter, randomized, placebo-controlled clinical trial of topical aminocaproic acid (Caprogel) in the management of traumatic hyphema, *Ophthalmology* 110(11):2106-2112, 2003.

Togioka BM, Arnold MA, Bathurst MA, et al: Retinal hemorrhages and shaken baby syndrome: an evidence-based review, *J Emerg Med* 37(1):98-106, 2009.

Sinusitis

33

Pamela A. Mazzeo

*S*inusitis is a frequently diagnosed but incompletely under- stood condition in pediatrics. Young children are estimated to have at least six to eight colds per year, and an estimated 5% to 13% of those infections are thought to be complicated by acute bacterial sinusitis (ABS). Other conditions that predispose to sinusitis include allergic rhinitis, adenoiditis, cystic fibrosis, immunodeficiency, ciliary dyskinesia, and anatomic or mechani- cal obstructions of normal sinus clearance. Diagnosis can be difficult because the symptoms of sinusitis overlap with those of some of its predisposing conditions; however, it is a clinically important diagnosis because of significant associated morbidity and potentially life-threatening complications.

ETIOLOGY AND PATHOGENESIS

Paranasal sinus development begins in utero and continues until adolescence. The ethmoid and maxillary sinuses are present at birth, although the maxillary sinuses are not pneumatized until approximately 4 years of age. The sphenoid sinus is pneuma- tized by about 5 years of age. The frontal sinuses are present at 7 to 8 years of age, but they do not fully develop until adoles- cence (Figure 33-1).

The frontal, anterior ethmoid, and maxillary sinuses drain into the middle meatus of the nasal cavity through the osteo- meatal complex. This structure forms a direct communication between the sinuses, which are normally sterile, and the naso- pharynx, which is heavily colonized with bacteria. Under normal circumstances, sinus sterility is maintained by the mucociliary apparatus of the sinuses, which mobilizes secretions (and any bacteria that may have entered the sinus cavity) in the direction of the sinus ostia (Figure 33-2). This clearance mechanism may be compromised when the ostia are obstructed (because of mucosal inflammation and swelling, as in viral or allergic rhinitis or mechanical obstruction). The cilia do not function properly, resulting in stasis of secretions and hypoxia, which worsens edema and inflammation and creates an ideal environment for the overgrowth of bacteria (Figure 33-3).

The pathogens most commonly responsible for ABS are similar to those for acute otitis media (AOM): *Streptococcus pneu- moniae*, *Haemophilus influenzae*, and *Moraxella catarrhalis*. The microbiology of ABS, as of AOM, is thought to be changing in the era of the pneumococcal conjugate vaccine and an increasing prevalence of penicillin-resistant *S. pneumoniae*.

Chronic sinusitis is a poorly understood phenomenon, defined by symptoms lasting for longer than 90 days without interval improvement. It is unclear how significant a role is played by bacterial infection in chronic sinusitis, with some theorizing that an inciting infection causes a prolonged inflammatory response. No clear data exist as to the most common causative agents; these infections are generally considered polymicrobial.

Rhinitis without sinus involvement is also an extremely common pediatric complaint and may be confused with sinus- itis. The majority of these cases result from infection or allergy.

Infectious rhinitis is caused by a number of common viruses, including rhinovirus, respiratory syncytial virus, and adenovirus, among others. Allergic rhinitis results from an immunoglobulin E–mediated response to allergens in the nasal airway, in which mast cell degranulation effects an inflammatory response result- ing in edema of the nasal mucosa and the characteristic symp- toms of rhinorrhea, congestion, and pruritus.

CLINICAL PRESENTATION

ABS most commonly presents in a patient with a preceding upper respiratory infection (URI), and the signs and symptoms of the two conditions are similar. Although most uncomplicated URIs will at least have begun to resolve by the tenth day of illness, however, a URI complicated by an evolving bacterial sinusitis will not have lessened in severity by day 10.

Nasal discharge in ABS is typically consistently purulent and without improvement, in contrast with the nasal discharge in a typical URI, which may become purulent but usually turns clear again before resolving. Nasal congestion or obstruction, fever, and cough (which may be worse at night) are also generally present in URIs but are more persistent in ABS. Halitosis, headache, ill appearance, reproducible facial pain or tenderness, and eye swelling are commonly seen in ABS (Figure 33-4). A thorough physical examination of the nasopharynx may reveal a foreign body, nasal polyps, a deviated septum, or other struc- tures causing mechanical obstruction; more commonly in ABS, mucosal erythema and edema and purulent nasal discharge are seen. Periorbital swelling may be noted. Sinus tenderness may be reproduced over the frontal and maxillary bones, although this sign is difficult to elicit in small children. Transil- lumination, classically taught to demonstrate the presence of fluid in the sinuses, is also difficult to perform and interpret in children.

EVALUATION AND MANAGEMENT

Evaluation

The clinical diagnosis of ABS is based on history and physical examination, and it is distinguished from URI on the basis of either persistence or severity of symptoms. Persistent symptoms are defined as respiratory symptoms (nasal discharge, conges- tion, obstruction, or cough) lasting for more than 10 but fewer than 30 days without improvement. Severe symptoms are defined as a temperature greater than 39°C and purulent nasal discharge for 3 or 4 days in an ill-appearing child.

Radiographic imaging has a limited role in the diagnosis of ABS. Plain radiographs of the paranasal sinuses are difficult to perform and interpret in young children, and clinical history has been shown to be highly predictive of abnormal radiographs. Therefore, their routine use is not recommended in children younger than 6 years of age. Computed tomography (CT) of

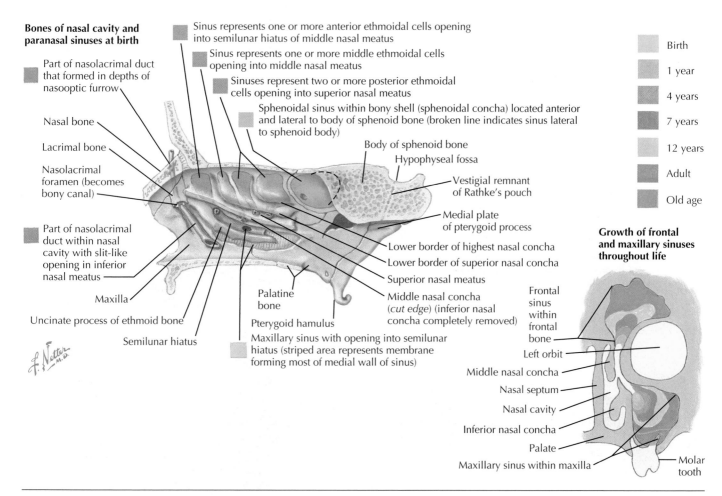

Bones of nasal cavity and paranasal sinuses at birth

Part of nasolacrimal duct that formed in depths of nasooptic furrow

Nasal bone

Lacrimal bone

Nasolacrimal foramen (becomes bony canal)

Part of nasolacrimal duct within nasal cavity with slit-like opening in inferior nasal meatus

Maxilla

Uncinate process of ethmoid bone

Semilunar hiatus

Sinus represents one or more anterior ethmoidal cells opening into semilunar hiatus of middle nasal meatus

Sinus represents one or more middle ethmoidal cells opening into middle nasal meatus

Sinuses represent two or more posterior ethmoidal cells opening into superior nasal meatus

Sphenoidal sinus within bony shell (sphenoidal concha) located anterior and lateral to body of sphenoid bone (broken line indicates sinus lateral to sphenoid body)

Body of sphenoid bone

Hypophyseal fossa

Vestigial remnant of Rathke's pouch

Medial plate of pterygoid process

Lower border of highest nasal concha

Lower border of superior nasal concha

Superior nasal meatus

Middle nasal concha (cut edge) (inferior nasal concha completely removed)

Palatine bone

Pterygoid hamulus

Maxillary sinus with opening into semilunar hiatus (striped area represents membrane forming most of medial wall of sinus)

Birth
1 year
4 years
7 years
12 years
Adult
Old age

Growth of frontal and maxillary sinuses throughout life

Frontal sinus within frontal bone

Left orbit

Middle nasal concha

Nasal septum

Nasal cavity

Inferior nasal concha

Palate

Maxillary sinus within maxilla

Molar tooth

Figure 33-1 *Paranasal sinuses: changes with age.*

inflamed sinuses may demonstrate air-fluid levels, mucosal thickening, and sinus opacification; however, this modality cannot distinguish between inflammation caused by ABS and that caused by viral rhinosinusitis. The use of CT scanning in clinically diagnosed sinusitis should be reserved for patients in whom surgery is being considered, complications are suspected, or medical treatment has failed.

The gold standard for diagnosis of ABS is culture of sinus secretions obtained by maxillary sinus aspiration. This invasive procedure, which is accomplished via a transnasal approach by an otolaryngologist, is indicated only in patients with severe symptoms, failure to respond to antibiotic therapy, immunosuppression, or life-threatening complications.

Although most of this discussion has centered around acute sinusitis, other categories of diagnosis are worth mentioning. Unlike ABS, which resolves completely within 30 days, subacute sinusitis is characterized by mild to moderate symptoms, often intermittent, lasting for between 30 and 90 days, and it is caused by the same organisms as ABS. Recurrent sinusitis is characterized by three episodes of ABS within 6 months or four episodes within 12 months. Episodes of recurrent sinusitis are antibiotic responsive, and resolution of symptoms is complete between episodes. Chronic sinusitis is that lasting for more than 90 days without resolution of symptoms.

Management

ANTIMICROBIAL THERAPY

Although their use is a matter of controversy, antibiotics remain the mainstay of treatment for ABS, with the goal of speeding recovery and preventing suppurative complications. When treated with an appropriate antibiotic, most patients experience improvement in respiratory symptoms within 2 to 3 days.

The first line of therapy, based on the American Academy of Pediatrics current clinical practice guidelines for sinusitis, is typically amoxicillin, at high (90 mg/kg/d divided twice daily) dosing. For patients with penicillin allergy but not a type 1 hypersensitivity reaction, cefdinir, cefuroxime, or cefpodoxime is recommended. In patients with history of type 1 hypersensitivity reaction to penicillin, clarithromycin or azithromycin is recommended.

Patients in certain populations should receive an alternative regimen. These patients include those with illness refractory to first-line therapy, moderate or more severe illness, history of recent antimicrobial therapy, or attendance at day care. For this group, amoxicillin–clavulanate is recommended (80-90 mg/kg/d of amoxicillin component divided twice daily). Cefdinir, cefuroxime, and cefpodoxime may be used as alternatives in these patients.

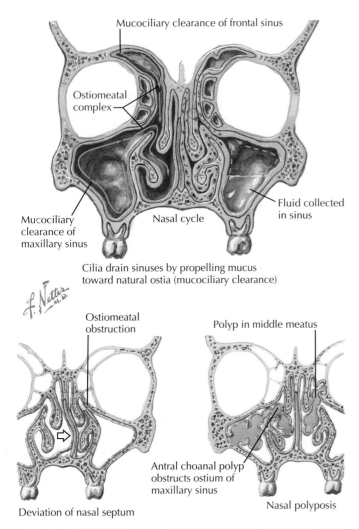

Figure 33-2 *Histology and physiology of nasal cavity and sinuses.*

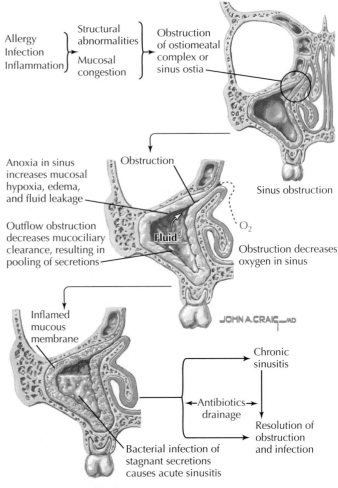

Figure 33-3 *Pathogenesis of sinusitis.*

Patients who fail to improve with a second course of antibiotics and those who are acutely ill may be treated with intravenous cefotaxime or ceftriaxone. They may also be referred to an otolaryngologist at this point for evaluation for sinus aspiration.

At this time, there are no definitive recommendations about the length of antibiotic treatment for patients with ABS. Some clinicians empirically treat for 10, 14, 21, or 28 days; others prescribe therapy until the patient is symptom free and then for an additional 7 days. Similarly, there is little consensus about the appropriate length of treatment for patients with chronic sinusitis, with most practitioners opting for long courses of antibiotics, generally at least 4 to 6 weeks.

ADJUVANT AND SURGICAL THERAPY

The use of adjunctive medical therapies for ABS is also an incompletely studied area. Although nasal saline washes appear to be potentially helpful, no substantial data support the use of decongestants, antihistamines, mucolytic agents, or topical intranasal steroids.

As already described, an otolaryngologist can perform sinus aspiration to help direct antimicrobial therapy. Another important consideration for referral to an otolaryngologist is the possibility of surgical correction of underlying abnormalities, such as nasal polyps or a deviated septum, which may contribute to morbidity.

Patients who have failed medical therapy and have CT evidence of sinusitis may also be candidates for surgical intervention. Adenoidectomy is thought to be helpful because it alleviates a likely bacterial reservoir. Endoscopic sinus surgery, performed at least 3 months after adenoidectomy, usually involves maxillary antrostomy with anterior ethmoidectomy as a means of relieving osteomeatal obstruction.

RHINITIS WITHOUT SINUSITIS

When a patient's symptoms are clearly more consistent with a viral infectious rhinitis, antibiotics are not indicated, and treatment is supportive. In the case of allergic rhinitis, therapy depends on the use of antihistamines, decongestants, and mast-cell mediators; referral to an allergist for desensitization therapy may also be indicated.

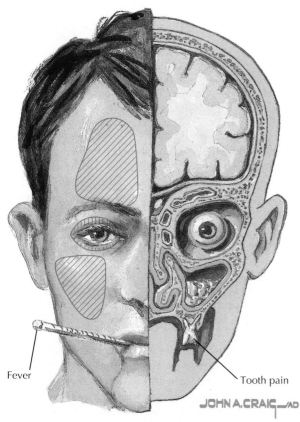

Fever

Tooth pain

JOHN A.CRAIG—AD

Areas of pain and tenderness (*green*). Pain
caused by pressure in obstructed sinus

Figure 33-4 *Sinusitis.*

COMPLICATIONS

The common orbital and central nervous system (CNS) complications of ABS include periorbital or orbital cellulitis, orbital abscess, subperiosteal abscess, Pott's puffy tumor (osteomyelitis of the frontal bone), epidural or brain abscess, subdural empyema, meningitis, and cavernous sinus thrombosis. Patients with suspected orbital or CNS complications should receive appropriate and timely imaging and should be treated aggressively. Appropriate referrals should be made to otolaryngology, ophthalmology, neurosurgery, and infectious disease specialists.

FUTURE DIRECTIONS

More randomized, placebo-controlled studies are needed to direct the clinical approach to acute and chronic sinusitis. Antimicrobial treatment for ABS is an area of active research, with conflicting results among the few studies available. Studies are also needed to determine the benefit, if any, of adjuvant therapies and prophylactic antibiotics in patients with recurrent sinusitis. Chronic sinusitis is a particularly poorly understood condition, and more data are needed to elucidate its pathophysiology and help guide therapy.

SUGGESTED READINGS

Ahovuo-Saloranta A, Borisenko OV, Kovanen N, et al: Antibiotics for acute maxillary sinusitis, *Cochrane Database Syst Rev* (2):CD000243, 2008.

American Academy of Pediatrics: Subcommittee on Management of Sinusitis and Committee on Quality Improvement. Clinical practice guideline: management of sinusitis, *Pediatrics* 108(3):798-808, 2001.

Bluestone CD, Stool SE, Alper CM, et al: *Pediatric Otolaryngology*, ed 4, Philadelphia, 2003, Saunders.

Garbutt JM, Goldstein M, Gellman E, Whannon W, Littenberg B: A randomized, placebo-controlled trial of antimicrobial treatment for children with clinically diagnosed acute sinusitis, *Pediatrics* 107(4):619-625, 2001.

Wald ER, Chiponis D, Ledesma-Medina J: Comparative effectiveness of amoxicillin and amoxicillin-clavulanate potassium in acute paranasal sinus infections in children: a double-blind placebo-controlled trial, *Pediatrics* 77(6):795-800, 1986.

Wald ER, Nash D, Eickhoff J: Effectiveness of amoxicillin/clavulanate potassium in the treatment of acute bacterial sinusitis in children, *Pediatrics* 124(1):9-15, 2009.

34

Dentition and Common Oral Lesions

Pamela A. Mazzeo

DENTITION

The development of the teeth begins in utero and continues well into adolescence. The 20 primary teeth (also known as deciduous or milk teeth) typically erupt between the ages of 6 months and 2 years. The exfoliation of the primary dentition and the eruption of the 32 permanent teeth usually begin at around age 6 years. On each side of the mouth, the mature permanent dentition consists of maxillary and mandibular central incisors, lateral incisors, canines, two premolars, and three molars (Figure 34-1).

Normal Tooth Anatomy

The visible portion of the tooth, which protrudes from the gingiva, is the crown, and its hard surface is an enamel made of hydroxyapatite crystals. The portion of the tooth that connects to the maxillary and mandibular alveolar bones is the root, and its hard covering is called cement. The neck of the tooth is the portion that connects the crown and the root. The periodontal ligament, or periodontal membrane, holds the root in place by attaching the cement to the periosteum of the alveolar bone. Beneath the protective overlying enamel and cement, a layer known as dentin provides the bulk of the body of the tooth. The innermost portion of the tooth, surrounded and protected by dentin, is the pulp chamber, which contains nerves, blood vessels, and connective tissue (Figure 34-2).

Dental Trauma

The most common traumatic injuries in pediatric dentistry are luxation injuries to the maxillary central incisors followed by the maxillary lateral incisors and mandibular incisors. Luxation injuries range from simple concussion, in which the tooth and ligament may be injured without being displaced or knocked loose, to avulsion, in which the tooth in its entirety is displaced from the socket. They also include intrusion, extrusion, subluxation, and lateral luxation injuries in which the tooth may be displaced in any direction with varying degrees of injury to the periodontal ligament.

The most common mechanism of injury for dental trauma is falls, especially in toddlers who are learning to walk. Fractures are also common sequelae of dental trauma, and they may be uncomplicated (involving only enamel or enamel and dentin) or complicated (involving pulp) and involve the crown or the root. Dental fractures are more common in boys and in children whose maxillary teeth more substantially override the mandibular teeth.

A thorough physical examination of the mouth in dental trauma should reveal evidence of soft tissue injury (to the lips, frenula, tongue, buccal and lingual mucosa, hard and soft palate); fracture of the teeth (with attention to whether enamel, dentin, or pulp is exposed); loose, displaced, or missing teeth; pain, tenderness, or sensitivity; or malocclusion. The clinician must always consider the possibility of child abuse and be alert for suspicious signs such as bruising or a torn upper labial frenulum. Radiographic imaging may be appropriate to reveal fractures to the teeth and supporting bone or to locate missing tooth fragments (which may have been swallowed, aspirated, or completely intruded into the alveolar socket).

The focus of management in dental trauma is to prevent aspiration, infection, and injury to the permanent dentition. In injuries of the primary teeth, children with fractured, loose, or severely displaced teeth should be referred for immediate dental management; for most, however, routine follow-up is appropriate. For children with injuries to permanent teeth, maintaining the viability of the periodontal ligament is of paramount importance; thus, most children with luxation injuries of the permanent teeth require immediate referral to a pediatric dentist. In the case of an avulsed permanent tooth, the viability of the tooth is inversely proportional to the time to reimplantation. Parents should be advised to handle the tooth by the crown, gently rinse it with tap water or saline, place it back into the socket, and ask the child to maintain pressure with a finger or by biting on gauze or a clean cloth to keep the tooth in place. Transporting the tooth in milk or Hank's balanced salt solution will also keep the tooth viable.

Dental Infections

CARIES

Dental caries remains a highly prevalent disease among children, both in the primary and permanent dentition. The risk of early childhood caries is increased in babies who sleep with bottles, who graze (rather than eating at discrete mealtimes), and whose parents have untreated caries.

Bacteria, especially the *Streptococcus mutans* group, are typically transmitted from mother to infant soon after the eruption of the primary teeth. These bacteria colonize tooth surfaces and form plaques above and below the gingival margin. Caries result when these bacteria ferment sucrose from ingested dietary carbohydrate, producing organic acids on the tooth surface. These acids lead to the destruction of the hydroxyapatite crystals that give the enamel its structure, making the enamel more and more porous and eventually causing breakdown of the tooth surface (Figure 34-3). These areas of breakdown can erode through the enamel and dentin into the pulp, where an inflammatory response raises the pressure in the pulp chamber and can cause compression, and thus ischemia, of the pulp vessels. This is known as pulp necrosis.

When pulp necrosis extends into the periapical region, a periapical abscess can form and can erode the alveolar bone

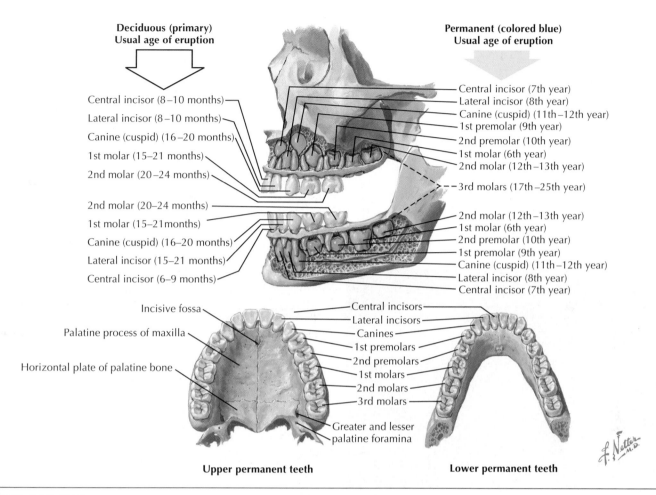

Deciduous (primary)
Usual age of eruption

Central incisor (8–10 months)
Lateral incisor (8–10 months)
Canine (cuspid) (16–20 months)
1st molar (15–21 months)
2nd molar (20–24 months)

2nd molar (20–24 months)
1st molar (15–21months)
Canine (cuspid) (16–20 months)
Lateral incisor (15–21 months)
Central incisor (6–9 months)

Permanent (colored blue)
Usual age of eruption

Central incisor (7th year)
Lateral incisor (8th year)
Canine (cuspid) (11th–12th year)
1st premolar (9th year)
2nd premolar (10th year)
1st molar (6th year)
2nd molar (12th–13th year)

3rd molars (17th–25th year)

2nd molar (12th–13th year)
1st molar (6th year)
2nd premolar (10th year)
1st premolar (9th year)
Canine (cuspid) (11th–12th year)
Lateral incisor (8th year)
Central incisor (7th year)

Incisive fossa
Palatine process of maxilla
Horizontal plate of palatine bone

Central incisors
Lateral incisors
Canines
1st premolars
2nd premolars
1st molars
2nd molars
3rd molars
Greater and lesser palatine foramina

Upper permanent teeth

Lower permanent teeth

Figure 34-1 *Teeth.*

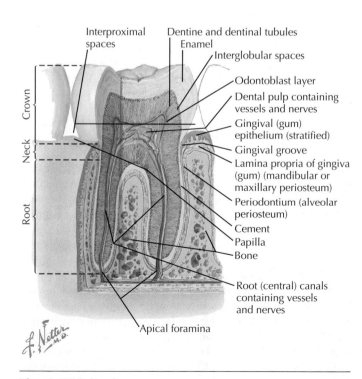

Interproximal spaces
Dentine and dentinal tubules
Enamel
Interglobular spaces
Odontoblast layer
Dental pulp containing vessels and nerves
Gingival (gum) epithelium (stratified)
Gingival groove
Lamina propria of gingiva (gum) (mandibular or maxillary periosteum)
Periodontium (alveolar periosteum)
Cement
Papilla
Bone
Root (central) canals containing vessels and nerves
Apical foramina

Crown
Neck
Root

Figure 34-2 *Tooth anatomy.*

or involve other teeth. An abscessed tooth may be tender and mobile, with soft tissue swelling or purulence. It can result in cellulitis and impair development of an underlying permanent tooth.

Caries prevention can be accomplished through appropriate anticipatory guidance. In addition to promoting healthy dietary habits (minimal juice at meals only, no carbonated beverages, discontinuing bottle use at 1 year of age, and never putting baby to bed with a bottle), providers can educate parents on proper dental hygiene and fluoride supplementation. From the first tooth eruption to age 24 months, parents should clean the child's teeth twice a day without toothpaste. Starting at age 2 years, the teeth may be brushed using standard fluoride-containing toothpaste. Children younger than 6 years of age may swallow too much toothpaste and should be supervised while brushing.

In low concentrations, fluoride protects against caries by promoting enamel mineralization; in addition to fluoridated toothpaste, many children are exposed to fluoride supplementation in community water supplies. This supplementation is thought to have dramatically reduced the prevalence of caries among children. However, in higher concentrations in children, fluoride can cause fluorosis, a condition in which the enamel is hypomineralized, increasing its porosity. The clinical

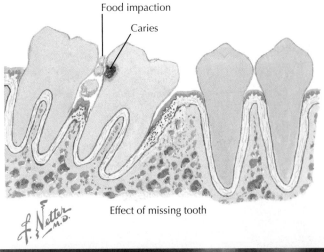

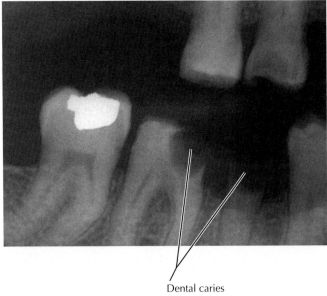

Figure 34-3 *Dental caries.*

manifestations range in severity from white flecks to severe pitting and mottling.

PERIODONTAL INFECTIONS

Gingivitis is an inflammatory response to bacteria that live in the sulcus between the enamel and the gingiva. The gingiva may be edematous and erythematous and may also bleed and ulcerate. Long-term gingivitis may result in tissue hypertrophy. It is highly prevalent in children and adolescents, and poor dental hygiene is usually causative.

Periodontitis evolves from gingivitis with bacterially induced destruction of the tooth's surrounding and supportive structures. There are several forms of periodontitis. Chronic periodontitis is the most common, but it is not usually diagnosed until adulthood. Several rare but aggressive forms exist in children. Clinical manifestations include tooth mobility and loss of attachment, gingival recession, periodontal bone loss, and tooth loss.

LESIONS OF THE ORAL SOFT TISSUES

Anatomic Lesions of the Oral Cavity

ANKYLOGLOSSIA

Uncommonly, children may be born with a short lingual frenulum, known as ankyloglossia or "tongue-tie" (Figure 34-4). Tongue movement may be restricted, and the close attachment of the frenulum to the tongue may cause the tip of the tongue to appear to have a mild cleft ("heart-shaped tongue"). The condition is more prevalent in boys than in girls. It does not usually affect speech or feeding, and the frenulum often lengthens as the child grows. In some cases, the short lingual attachment may impair a child's ability to clear food from the buccal side of the teeth, which may promote bacterial growth and tooth decay. A frenulectomy may be required in the case of true disability.

GEOGRAPHIC TONGUE

This benign condition is characterized by irregular red patches on the tongue, with yellow, gray, or white margins (see Figure 34-4). The filiform papillae are absent in these areas. The lesions typically spontaneously resolve and then subsequently appear elsewhere on the tongue, giving the condition its other name of "migratory glossitis."

Common Soft Tissue Lesions of the Oral Cavity

MUCOCELE

This painless pseudocyst results from trauma to the duct of a minor salivary gland, usually in the lower lip or cheek (e.g., from lip biting). Ranging in size from 1 mm to several centimeters, it is usually smooth, soft, and bluish to translucent, filled with mucin from the damaged duct (see Figure 34-4). It may spontaneously drain as a result of the patient's unroofing the lesion with his or her teeth; however, surgical excision may be required, in which case the entire underlying gland must be removed to prevent recurrence.

RANULA

Similar in appearance and pathophysiology to a mucocele, a ranula is a mucous cyst on the floor of the mouth. Rarely, it may herniate through the mylohyoid muscle to involve the submandibular region and neck. It must be removed by surgical excision.

TRAUMATIC ULCERS

These lesions are usually single, painful, and located on the lateral tongue, buccal mucosa, lips, or gingiva. Treatment is symptomatic relief, and healing is usually complete within 1 to 3 weeks. A special case is Riga-Fede disease in infants, who sustain traumatic ulceration on the ventral surface of the tongue as a result of rubbing the tongue against the mandibular incisors.

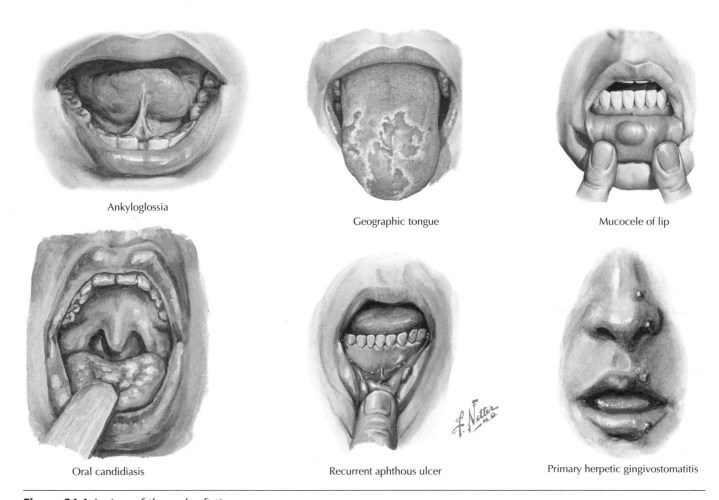

Ankyloglossia

Geographic tongue

Mucocele of lip

Oral candidiasis

Recurrent aphthous ulcer

Primary herpetic gingivostomatitis

Figure 34-4 *Lesions of the oral soft tissues.*

APHTHOUS ULCERS

These recurrent and painful ulcers, also known as canker sores, occur in up to one-third of children. Their cause is unclear, but viruses, T-cell dysfunction, trauma, and genetic predisposition have been implicated. They appear as white necrotic areas surrounded by a red margin, usually on the buccal and labial mucosa (see Figure 34-4). They usually resolve completely within 10 to 14 days. Differential diagnosis consideration should include recurrent traumatic ulcers from child abuse, oral manifestations of inflammatory bowel disease, secondary herpetic ulcers, neutropenic ulcers, and PFAPA (periodic fever, aphthous stomatitis, pharyngitis, cervical adenitis) syndrome.

Soft Tissue Infections of the Oral Cavity

CANDIDIASIS

Thrush caused by the overgrowth of *Candida* spp. (mostly *Candida albicans*) occurs in 2% to 5% of normal newborns; it is also common in immunocompromised children and those who have used antibiotics or steroids. It presents as pseudomembranous white plaques on the buccal mucosa, palate, and tongue (see Figure 34-4). These plaques may be wiped away to reveal underlying raw, painful, erythematous mucosa. Treatment with an oral suspension of nystatin is usually effective; most clinicians

recommend a course of 2 weeks or until 2 to 3 days after symptoms have resolved. For immunocompromised children or those who do not respond to nystatin, systemic fluconazole should be considered. Any objects that the infected child has regularly put in his or her mouth, such as pacifiers and toothbrushes, should be discarded.

PRIMARY HERPETIC GINGIVOSTOMATITIS

Primary herpes simplex virus (HSV) infection presents with clusters of painful vesicles surrounded by erythema, which are primarily located on the gingiva, hard palate, and anterior tongue and extend to the vermilion border of the lips (see Figure 34-4). These vesicles may have a red halo, may ulcerate, and may become secondarily infected with bacteria. Other symptoms may include fever, lymphadenopathy, arthralgia, headache, and drooling or dehydration resulting from the pain associated with swallowing. Diagnosis is made by unroofing a vesicle with a sterile needle and sending vesicular fluid for viral culture, polymerase chain reaction, direct immunofluorescence, or Tzanck smear. Treatment with acyclovir within 3 days of symptom onset shortens the length of symptoms and the period of viral shedding. After primary HSV infection, recurrence may occur because the virus remains latent within the trigeminal ganglion until a flare is triggered by stress, sunlight, cold, trauma, or immunosuppression.

ENTEROVIRUS INFECTIONS

Herpangina, usually caused by the Coxsackie A virus in summer and early fall, manifests as painful vesicles on the tonsils and soft palate. It is distinguished from HSV stomatitis by its predilection for the posterior oropharynx. It can be associated with headache, vomiting, abdominal pain, and fever. Treatment is supportive, and resolution is usually spontaneous after 3 to 5 days.

Hand, foot, and mouth disease, often caused by the Coxsackie A and B viruses in the spring and early summer, manifests with vesicles similar in appearance to herpangina; however, children may also have vesicles on the palate, tongue, buccal mucosa, hands, feet, buttocks, and sometimes genitalia. It may also be associated with fever and resolves spontaneously in several days.

FUTURE DIRECTIONS

Access to dental care for underserved populations continues to be a challenge for dentists and primary care physicians. Medically complex children are at particularly high risk of dental caries and associated complications, and both preventive and regular dental care are paramount for this population. A public health focus on injury prevention is also important in preventing damage to the teeth.

SUGGESTED READINGS

Cameron AC, Widmer RP: *Handbook of Pediatric Dentistry*, ed 3, Edinburgh, 2008, Mosby Elsevier.

Feigin RD, Cherry JD: *Textbook of Pediatric Infectious Diseases*, ed 5, Philadelphia, 2004, Saunders.

McTigue DJ: Diagnosis and management of dental injuries in children, *Pediatr Clin North Am* 47(5):1067-1084, 2000.

Norton NS: *Netter's Head and Neck Anatomy for Dentistry*, Philadelphia, 2007, Saunders Elsevier.

Pinkham J, Casamassimo P, Fields HW, et al: *Pediatric Dentistry: Infancy through Adolescence*, ed 4, St. Louis, 2005, Elsevier Saunders.

Zitelli BJ, Davis HW: *Atlas of Pediatric Physical Diagnosis*, ed 5, Philadelphia, 2007, Mosby Elsevier.

Melissa Desai

Pharyngitis is an inflammation of the mucous membranes and submucosal structures of the pharynx, including the nasopharynx, oropharynx, and laryngopharynx (Figure 35-1). It accounts for approximately 7.3 million outpatient childhood doctor's visits each year, and it remains one of the most common reasons for which children and adolescents seek medical attention. The cause of pharyngitis can vary widely depending on a person's comorbidities, season of year, and exposure history, and the goals of diagnosis and management are to correctly treat the cases that require medical intervention and minimize the risk of long-term complications that may result from a primary pharyngitis. Yet despite the fever, sore throat, malaise, and associated symptoms that are often distressing to patients and their families, most cases of pharyngitis are benign and self-limited.

ETIOLOGY AND PATHOGENESIS

There are numerous causes of pharyngitis, including infection, allergic rhinitis, environmental exposures, gastroesophageal reflux, and malignancy. The most common type of pharyngitis, however, is acute infectious pharyngitis, which is the focus of this chapter (Table 35-1). Viral infectious account for 40% to 60% of pediatric pharyngitis and usually present as part of a larger viral syndrome. Rhinovirus, adenovirus, and coronavirus, for example, present with sore throat along with fever, rhinorrhea, and other cold symptoms. Pharyngitis secondary to Epstein-Barr virus (EBV), on the other hand, commonly presents in adolescents and young adults as a symptom of mononucleosis syndrome.

Alternatively, various bacteria may cause acute infectious pharyngitis. *Streptococcus pyogenes*, also known as group A β-hemolytic streptococci (GABHS), is the most common bacterial cause of pharyngitis. It accounts for 15% to 30% of pediatric pharyngitis and is an important pathogen to identify because treatment is essential in reducing the risk of postinfectious complications. Other common bacterial pathogens as well as a few fungal pathogens that can cause pharyngitis are listed in Table 35-1.

Most infectious pathogens, including GABHS, cause pharyngitis by directly invading the pharyngeal mucosa and causing a local inflammatory response. A few pathogens, however, such as rhinovirus, respiratory syncytial virus (RSV), and coronavirus, primarily affect the nose by increasing secretions and mucus production, which then causes a secondary irritation of the pharyngeal mucosa and resulting pharyngitis symptoms.

CLINICAL PRESENTATION

The presenting signs and symptoms surrounding pharyngitis can vary from one patient to another, yet some clinical findings are fairly typical of acute infectious pharyngitis. The most common findings in those with infectious pharyngitis include a history of fever; cervical lymphadenopathy; and oropharyngeal or tonsillar erythema, enlargement, or exudates (Figure 35-2). Although no definitive clinical presentations can correctly identify the cause of an individual's pharyngitis, various signs and symptoms are more characteristic of one pathogen than another. These common presentations include:

- Rhinovirus, coronavirus: rhinorrhea, congestion, sore throat as secondary symptom
- Adenovirus: conjunctivitis, rhinorrhea, exudative pharyngitis
- Influenza: fever, myalgia, nonexudative pharyngitis
- EBV and cytomegalovirus (CMV): prodrome of fever, chills, and malaise; posterior cervical lymphadenopathy; splenomegaly or hepatomegaly; palatal petechiae
- Herpes simplex virus (HSV) and Coxsackievirus: oral ulcers or vesicles, gingivitis, stomatitis
- HIV-1: aphthous ulcers, fatigue, fever, lymphadenopathy
- GABHS: sudden onset, lack of cough, anterior cervical lymphadenopathy, headache, fever, palatal petechiae, scarlatiniform rash, nausea and vomiting
- *Neisseria gonorrhoeae*: history of recent orogenital sexual contact
- *Mycoplasma* and *Chlamydia*: nonproductive cough, lower respiratory infection
- Diphtheria: gray pseudomembranes in the oropharynx and nares, bull-shaped neck secondary to diffuse lymphadenopathy
- *Candida albicans*: whitish plaques on the tongue and oropharynx

Finally, epiglottitis, croup, retropharyngeal abscesses, and peritonsillar abscesses can present similarly to pharyngitis but usually have other differentiating signs such as asymmetric tonsils (peritonsillar abscess), limited extension of the neck (retropharyngeal abscess), stridor and barky cough (croup), and toxic appearance with tripod positioning (epiglottitis). These diseases often require more acute intervention at the time of presentation and are discussed in more detail in other chapters of this textbook.

EVALUATION AND MANAGEMENT

As with any patient, airway management is paramount and airway patency should be the first step in assessing a patient with pharyngitis. Additionally, hydration status should be evaluated because patients with severe odynophagia may have minimal oral intake and become severely hydrated. After management of these potentially life-threatening complications, attention can be turned to management of the pharyngitis itself.

Most cases of infectious pharyngitis are self-limited, and supportive measures provide adequate treatment. Management often includes pain and fever control with acetaminophen, ibuprofen, or both; maintaining adequate hydration status; and clearing secretions through nasal suctioning and chest

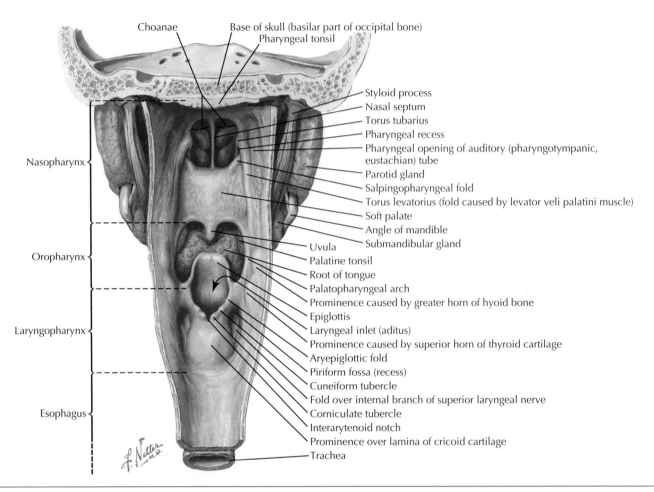

Choanae
Base of skull (basilar part of occipital bone)
Pharyngeal tonsil

Styloid process
Nasal septum
Torus tubarius
Pharyngeal recess
Pharyngeal opening of auditory (pharyngotympanic, eustachian) tube
Parotid gland
Salpingopharyngeal fold
Torus levatorius (fold caused by levator veli palatini muscle)
Soft palate
Angle of mandible
Submandibular gland
Uvula
Palatine tonsil
Root of tongue
Palatopharyngeal arch
Prominence caused by greater horn of hyoid bone
Epiglottis
Laryngeal inlet (aditus)
Prominence caused by superior horn of thyroid cartilage
Aryepiglottic fold
Piriform fossa (recess)
Cuneiform tubercle
Fold over internal branch of superior laryngeal nerve
Corniculate tubercle
Interarytenoid notch
Prominence over lamina of cricoid cartilage
Trachea

Nasopharynx

Oropharynx

Laryngopharynx

Esophagus

Figure 35-1 *Pharynx: opened posterior view.*

Table 35-1 Common Causes of Acute Infectious Pharyngitis

Viral	Bacterial	Other Pathogens
Rhinovirus	GABHS	Mycobacterium tuberculosis
Adenovirus	Non-GABHS (group C and G)	*Candida albicans*
Coronavirus	*Neisseria gonorrhoeae*	*Mycoplasma pneumoniae*
RSV	*Corynebacterium diphtheriae*	
HSV	*Arcanobacterium haemolyticum*	
Parainfluenza	*Francisella tularensis*	
Influenza	*Chlamydia pneumoniae*	
Enterovirus		
EBV		
CMV		
HIV		

CMV, cytomegalovirus; EBV, Epstein-Barr virus; GABHS, group A β-hemolytic streptococci; HSV, herpes simplex virus; RSV, respiratory syncytial virus.

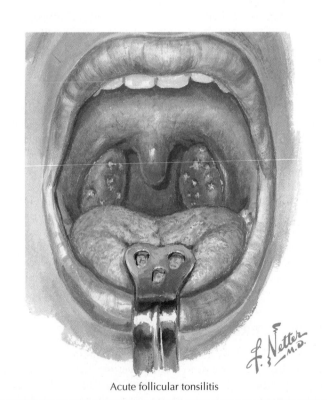

Acute follicular tonsilitis

Figure 35-2 *Tonsillitis.*

Table 35-2 Diagnostic Testing for Infectious Pharyngitis

Pathogen	Diagnostic Test
GABHS	RADT, throat culture
Neisseria gonorrhoeae	Thayer-Martin culture medium
Chlamydia pneumoniae	Fluorescent monoclonal antibody
Corynebacterium diphtheriae	Loeffler agar, tellurite agar
Influenza	Rapid diagnostic testing, PCR, culture
EBV	Heterophile antibody, EBV serology, peripheral smear (atypical lymphocytosis)
CMV	CMV antibody titers
Herpes virus	HSV PCR
HIV	HIV RNA or HIV antibody

CMV, cytomegalovirus; EBV, Epstein-Barr virus; GABHS, group A β-hemolytic streptococci; HSV, herpes simplex virus; PCR, polymerase chain reaction; RADT, rapid antigen detection test.

physiotherapy. Some physicians may use a short course of steroids for patients with potential airway compromise or to provide symptomatic relief in those with extreme pain, but there is little evidence supporting the effectiveness of steroids in the management of acute pharyngitis.

Although most cases of acute infectious pharyngitis resolve spontaneously within 3 to 7 days, the purpose of a diagnostic workup is to identify and treat pathogens that have potentially harmful sequelae (see Table 35-2 for common diagnostic testing). In particular, GABHS is the only common form of pharyngitis for which antimicrobial therapy is definitively indicated because it can prevent complications of the illness, most importantly, acute rheumatic fever (Figure 35-3). The additional benefits that come from antimicrobial treatment of GABHS are a reduction in the incidence of toxic shock syndrome, peritonsillar or retropharyngeal abscesses, cervical lymphadenitis, and mastoiditis. The one sequela of GABHS that is not prevented by adequate treatment of strep pharyngitis is poststreptococcal glomerulonephritis.

The two tests most commonly used to diagnose GABHS are rapid antigen detection testing (RADT) and throat culture. When the swab is performed correctly, throat culture is the gold standard for diagnosis and has a sensitivity of greater than 90% and specificity close to 99%. RADT, however, has a high specificity of approximately 95% but a relatively low sensitivity of 80% to 90%. Because of the high rate of false-negative results with RADT compared with throat culture, the American Academy of Pediatrics, the Infectious Disease Society of America, and the American Heart Association recommend that all negative RADT results be confirmed by throat culture.

If RADT or throat culture results are positive, the first line treatment for GABHS is penicillin V taken orally two or three times per day for 10 days, a single intramuscular dose of penicillin G, or a single 50-mg/kg daily dose of amoxicillin for 10 days. Alternative therapies in penicillin-allergic patients include cephalosporins, erythromycin, azithromycin, and clindamycin. Because there has not yet been a documented case of penicillin-resistant GABHS around the world, penicillin remains the treatment of choice in those who are not allergic to the medication.

Throat cultures can also be used to identify other bacterial causes of pharyngitis, but many laboratories will not look for additional organisms unless specifically asked to do so. If a child's history and clinical presentation raise suspicion for an alternative source of infection, clinicians must remember that culture requirements may be different for the various pathogens (see Table 35-2). *N. gonorrhoeae*, for instance, requires Thayer-Martin culture medium for growth and *Corynebacterium diphtheria* grows on Loeffler agar or tellurite agar. *Chlamydia pneumoniae*, on the other hand, is most commonly detected by fluorescent monoclonal antibody testing.

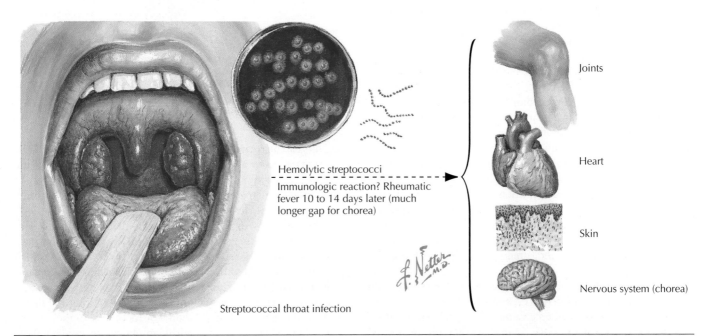

Joints

Heart

Skin

Nervous system (chorea)

Hemolytic streptococci

Immunologic reaction? Rheumatic fever 10 to 14 days later (much longer gap for chorea)

Streptococcal throat infection

Figure 35-3 *Rheumatic fever.*

Table 35-3 Pharmacologic Management of Acute Infectious Pharyngitis

Bacterial Pathogens	Treatment
GABHS	Penicillin–amoxicillin (second line: azithromycin, erythromycin, or clindamycin)
Neisseria gonorrhoeae	Ceftriaxone (with azithromycin or doxycycline for Chlamydia co-infection)
Chlamydia pneumoniae	Azithromycin (1 g single dose) or doxycycline (for 7 days)
Corynebacterium diphtheriae	Penicillin or erythromycin and equine hyperimmune diphtheria antitoxin
Arcanobacterium haemolyticum*	Azithromycin–erythromycin or cephalosporins
Non-GABHS (group C and G)*	Penicillin (typically shorter duration than with GABHS treatment)

Viral Pathogens	Treatment
HSV	Acyclovir or valacyclovir
Influenza*	Oseltamivir–zanamivir or amantadine–rimantadine
HIV	Antiretrovirals

Other Infectious Pathogens	Treatment
Mycoplasma pneumoniae	Azithromycin or doxycycline

GABHS, group A β-hemolytic streptococci; HSV, herpes simplex virus.
*Treatment is not routinely indicated but may be used in children with specific comorbidities or clinical presentations.

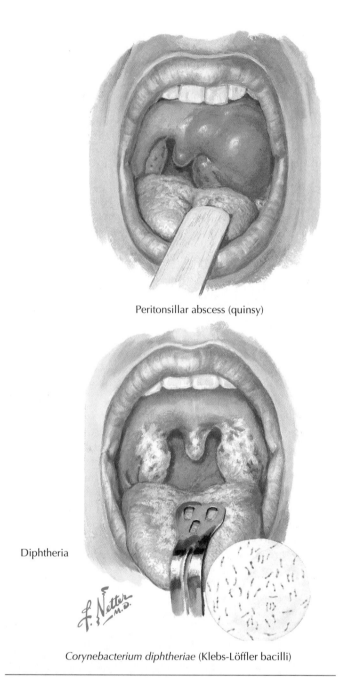

Peritonsillar abscess (quinsy)

Diphtheria

Corynebacterium diphtheriae (Klebs-Löffler bacilli)

Figure 35-4 Infections of pharynx.

The treatment of patients with bacterial pharyngitis differs based on the causative pathogen (Table 35-3). *Neisseria* spp. are most commonly treated with a single dose of intramuscular ceftriaxone along with azithromycin or doxycycline for empiric treatment of possible *Chlamydia* co-infection. Diphtheria, a disease more commonly found in unimmunized children, can lead to severe respiratory obstruction depending on the location of the pseudomembranes (Figure 35-4). Additionally, the toxin released by the bacteria can cause life-threatening neurotoxicity and cardiac toxicity. Therefore, the treatment for diphtheria includes both an antitoxin to counter the toxin in conjunction with penicillin or erythromycin to reduce the bacterial load. Other bacteria such as non-GABHS and *Arcanobacterium haemolyticum* rarely require antimicrobial treatment.

With respect to viral pathogen identification, testing for the common viruses such as rhinovirus or coronavirus is not routinely indicated because identification of the pathogen will not change management of the patient. In immunocompromised patients or those with certain comorbid conditions, however, identification of adenovirus, influenza, or RSV can be useful because treatment may be indicated in these high-risk populations (see Table 35-3).

Unlike identification of the viruses that cause common cold symptoms, diagnosis of HSV, HIV, and EBV is important in all populations so patients can receive the appropriate anticipatory guidance and treatment. HSV is most commonly diagnosed with polymerase chain reaction or viral culture, and infected patients can be treated with either acyclovir or valacyclovir. HIV testing is done by antibody testing or RNA analysis, and if the results are positive, treatment with antiretrovirals as well as appropriate anticipatory guidance for reducing the risk of transmission are imperative.

The diagnosis of EBV is unique in that workup can vary based on stage of illness. Heterophile antibody testing (monospot test) is up to 95% sensitive and should be considered for all patients presenting with a high clinical suspicion of infectious mononucleosis. Unfortunately, monospot may be falsely negative in those presenting early in their illness (during the first 2 weeks) and in those younger than 4 years of age. In these cases, a peripheral smear with an atypical lymphocytosis can be indicative of mononucleosis, and EBV serology may be diagnostic.

For children and adolescents diagnosed with EBV, it is imperative to give patients appropriate anticipatory guidance to reduce the risk of splenic injury. But as with most cases of pharyngitis, the mainstay of treatment is supportive care.

FUTURE DIRECTIONS

Although pharyngitis tends to be a fairly benign process, the morbidity and cost to society resulting from pain, clinical visits, missed school days, and missed work is significant. Therefore, finding a way to decrease the pathologic burden of disease could be beneficial in reducing the cost to society. One potential method, the development of a vaccine against GABHS, would minimize not only the incidence of disease but also the suppurative and nonsuppurative complications that can follow GABHS pharyngitis. Another potential area for improvement arises in the context of antibiotic use. Because 10% to 15% of children are asymptomatic carriers of GABHS, clinicians need a better algorithm to discern which patients have a high pretest probability of GABHS pharyngitis so that GABHS carriers with viral pharyngitis are not receiving unnecessary antibiotics. Such a decision rule would reduce overtreatment and in turn minimize antibiotic exposure and the potential for antibiotic resistance.

SUGGESTED READINGS

Altamimi S, Khalil A, Khalaiwi KA, et al: Short versus standard duration antibiotic therapy for acute streptococcal pharyngitis in children, *Cochrane Database Syst Rev* (1):CD004872, 2009.

Bisno AL: Acute pharyngitis, *N Engl J Med* 44(3):205-211, 2001.

Jaggi P, Shulman ST: Group A streptococcal infections, *Pediatr Rev* 27(3):99-105, 2006.

Merrill B, Kelsberg G, Jankowski A: What is the most effective diagnostic evaluation of streptococcal pharyngitis, *J Fam Pract* 53(9)734-739, 2004.

Pfoh E, Wessels MR, Goldman D, Lee GM: Burden and economic cost of group A Streptococcal pharyngitis, *Pediatrics* 121(2):229-234, 2008.

Tanz RR, Gerber MA, Kabat W, et al: Performance of a rapid antigen-detection test and throat culture in community pediatric offices: implications for management of pharyngitis, *Pediatrics* 123(2):437-444, 2009.

Stridor

Soorena Khojasteh and Paul L. Aronson

36

Stridor is a clinical finding reflecting partial extrathoracic airway obstruction. Although it is not pathognomonic for any single disease process, its presence can indicate a life-threatening upper airway obstruction. In addition, although stridor is traditionally thought to be inspiratory in nature, it can also be expiratory or biphasic, presenting in both phases of the respiratory cycle.

ETIOLOGY AND PATHOGENESIS

Stridor can be caused by any upper airway obstruction. When thinking about the causes of stridor, it is helpful to first understand the anatomy of the larynx (Figure 36-1) and then to separate the causes of stridor into chronic and acute processes.

Chronic Stridor

The most common cause for inspiratory stridor is laryngomalacia, which accounts for approximately 75% of all cases of neonatal stridor. Laryngomalacia results from the immature cartilage of the upper larynx collapsing inward during inhalation, causing airway obstruction. Vocal cord dysfunction, the second leading cause of stridor in the neonatal period, can be congenital or iatrogenic, such as from damage to the left recurrent laryngeal nerve during ligation of a patent ductus arteriosus or from direct injury to the vocal cord during endotracheal intubation. Congenital subglottic stenosis occurs when there is incomplete canalization of the subglottic airway and cricoid rings. Subglottic stenosis is most often acquired after prolonged intubation in the neonatal period, usually in the setting of extreme prematurity. Tracheomalacia results from a defect in the tracheal cartilage that causes a "floppy" airway lacking the rigidity necessary to maintain patency. Tracheomalacia is the leading cause of expiratory stridor. Tracheal stenosis can be caused by the presence of complete tracheal rings instead of the normally C-shaped rings. Stridor can also result from tracheal compression caused by vascular rings such as a double aortic arch. Other less common causes of chronic stridor include laryngeal papillomas caused by maternal human papillomavirus infection, webs, cysts, hemangiomas, and laryngeal dyskinesia.

Acute Stridor

The causes of acute stridor are primarily infectious in cause with two notable exceptions, foreign body aspiration and allergic reaction. The most common cause of acute stridor is laryngotracheobronchitis, or croup (Figure 36-2). Croup is classically caused by parainfluenza virus but can also be caused by respiratory syncytial virus, influenza, adenovirus, and *Mycoplasma pneumoniae*. Bacterial tracheitis, usually caused by *Staphylococcus aureus*, is an uncommon but life-threatening condition that occurs most frequently as a bacterial superinfection in patients who have viral croup.

Retropharyngeal and peritonsillar abscesses are common infections that can present with acute stridor. Both infections are usually polymicrobial, including β-hemolytic streptococci; oral anaerobic bacteria; and in retropharyngeal abscess, *S. aureus*. Finally, epiglottitis, traditionally caused by *Haemophilus influenzae* type B (Hib), is now a rare cause of stridor as a result of the widespread use of the conjugated Hib vaccine.

CLINICAL PRESENTATION

Chronic Stridor

Laryngomalacia can present at birth but usually presents at 2 to 4 weeks of age. The inspiratory stridor of laryngomalacia is exacerbated when the infant lies supine, cries, or when feeding and is alleviated when the infant is prone.

Vocal cord paralysis can be unilateral or bilateral. Bilateral vocal cord paralysis results in aphonia and high-pitched biphasic stridor, with significant respiratory distress. Unilateral paralysis can cause inspiratory or biphasic stridor, as well as a weak or hoarse cry.

Whereas subglottic stenosis and vascular rings may likewise present with inspiratory or biphasic stridor, tracheomalacia usually presents with expiratory stridor. Tracheomalacia may present with a monophonic wheeze if the obstruction is intrathoracic.

Acute Stridor

Croup occurs most commonly in children age 6 months to 2 years and is characterized by a harsh cough described as "barky" or "seal-like." Associated upper respiratory symptoms are common, and stridor can be mild, occurring only with crying, or in severe cases, can occur at rest with severe respiratory distress. Bacterial tracheitis is a rare complication of croup, and in addition to stridor. the child also will have high fever and a toxic appearance.

Retropharyngeal abscess usually occurs in children younger than 6 years old before the retropharyngeal lymph nodes atrophy. Patients often have a viral prodome followed by the abrupt onset of high fever, limited neck movement (especially resistance to extension), and occasionally stridor. Unilateral neck swelling may occur as the infection tracks from the retropharyngeal space, and a bulge of the posterior oropharynx may sometimes be present on physical examination. Peritonsillar abscess occurs in preadolescents and adolescents and can present with sore throat, trismus, dysphagia, a "hot potato" or muffled voice, and tender unilateral neck swelling. Asymmetric tonsils, deviation of the uvula, and a fluctuant area are present on physical examination (Figure 36-3). Stridor may be heard if tracheal compression is present. Epiglottitis classically presents with the

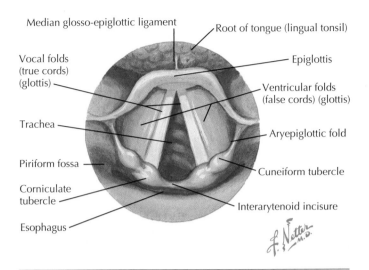

Figure 36-1 *Normal larynx: inspiration.*

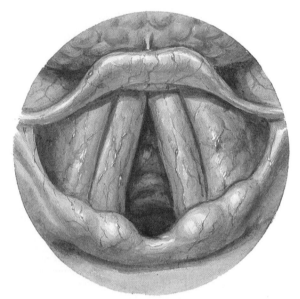

Acute laryngitis

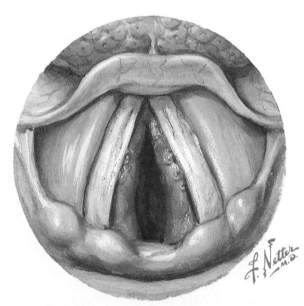

Subglottic inflammation and swelling in inflammatory croup

Figure 36-2 *Croup.*

abrupt onset of high fever, stridor, drooling, "tripod" positioning, and toxicity.

Foreign body aspiration should be suspected when stridor occurs acutely in an unobserved toddler. A history of choking or coughing preceded by eating or playing with small objects may be present. Focal wheezing or reduced breath sounds can be heard if the object is lodged in the smaller airways.

Allergic reactions, or anaphylaxis, may present with stridor or wheeze after exposure to a known food or drug allergen but should be suspected in any patient who presents with the acute onset of respiratory distress occurring within 30 minutes of food ingestion. Other signs of anaphylaxis include urticaria, gastrointestinal distress, and hypotension.

EVALUATION AND MANAGEMENT

Evaluation

Although taking a thorough history is an essential part of elucidating the cause of stridor, initial rapid assessment of airway, breathing, and circulation (the ABCs) can be lifesaving. The practitioner must assess first for impending complete airway obstruction or respiratory failure; observing the patient for severity of work of breathing, intercostal and suprasternal retractions, cyanosis, perfusion, and responsiveness will guide initial management. Although a complete blood count, inflammatory markers (C-reactive protein, erythrocyte sedimentation rate), and blood culture may help guide treatment, none are essential to the initial care of patients with stridor. Arterial blood gas analysis may be helpful in assessing the degree of respiratory compromise, but the physical examination and pulse oximetry are the best tools for developing an immediate treatment plan.

Anteroposterior and lateral radiographs of the neck and chest will allow evaluation of both the upper and lower airways and may be indicated for specific diagnoses. Other imaging modalities such as contrast-enhanced computed tomography and fluoroscopy may also be used. Further imaging may be indicated for specific cases (Table 36-1).

Management

Congenital causes of stridor often self-resolve but may necessitate surgical intervention. Laryngomalacia usually resolves spontaneously by 2 years of age. Surgical intervention such as supraglottoplasty or laryngeal reconstruction is indicated if obstruction is significant or if the patient exhibits severe failure to thrive. Similarly, unilateral vocal cord paralysis in infancy usually resolves by age 2 years with no intervention. However, in the setting of bilateral vocal cord paralysis or persistent aspiration, tracheostomy is often indicated. The presence of subglottic stenosis may necessitate tracheostomy, particularly if the patient has persistent respiratory compromise. Definitive

Table 36-1 Diagnostic Approach to Stridor

Cause of Stridor	Diagnostic Imaging
Laryngomalacia	DL will show inspiratory collapse of the epiglottis. Redundant arytenoids may be present. DL is also the test of choice for diagnosing laryngeal webs, cysts, and subglottic hemangiomas.
Subglottic stenosis	DL or bronchoscopy
Tracheomalacia	Airway fluoroscopy or bronchoscopy. Barium swallow to determine the presence of coexisting conditions.
Vascular ring	Barium swallow may show an indentation on the esophagus. Echocardiography is often diagnostic.
Croup	Usually a clinical diagnosis. Lateral neck radiograph, if obtained, demonstrates normal epiglottis but with subglottic narrowing (steeple sign).
Epiglottitis	Lateral neck radiograph demonstrates edematous epiglottis (thumb sign)
Retropharyngeal abscess	Lateral neck radiograph shows widening of the prevertebral soft tissues to greater than half the width of the adjacent vertebral body.
Peritonsillar abscess	Usually a clinical diagnosis. Contrast-enhanced CT scan of the neck may delineate abscess versus phlegmon and degree of airway impingement.
Foreign body aspiration	Lateral neck or chest radiograph may show the foreign body if radiopaque. Inspiratory and forced expiratory or lateral decubitus chest radiographs may demonstrate hyperinflation and air trapping on the affected side. Bronchoscopy is often required for definitive diagnosis.

CT, computed tomography; DL, direct laryngoscopy.

surgical correction with laryngeal reconstruction is often needed in severe cases.

Similar to other viral processes, croup self-resolves in approximately 7 days with maximal severity of symptoms usually occurring on the third or fourth day of illness. A single dose of oral or intramuscular dexamethasone has been shown to improve symptoms and prevent return to medical care. If the stridor occurs at rest or the patient is in moderate to severe distress, racemic epinephrine can be given via nebulizer for temporary relief.

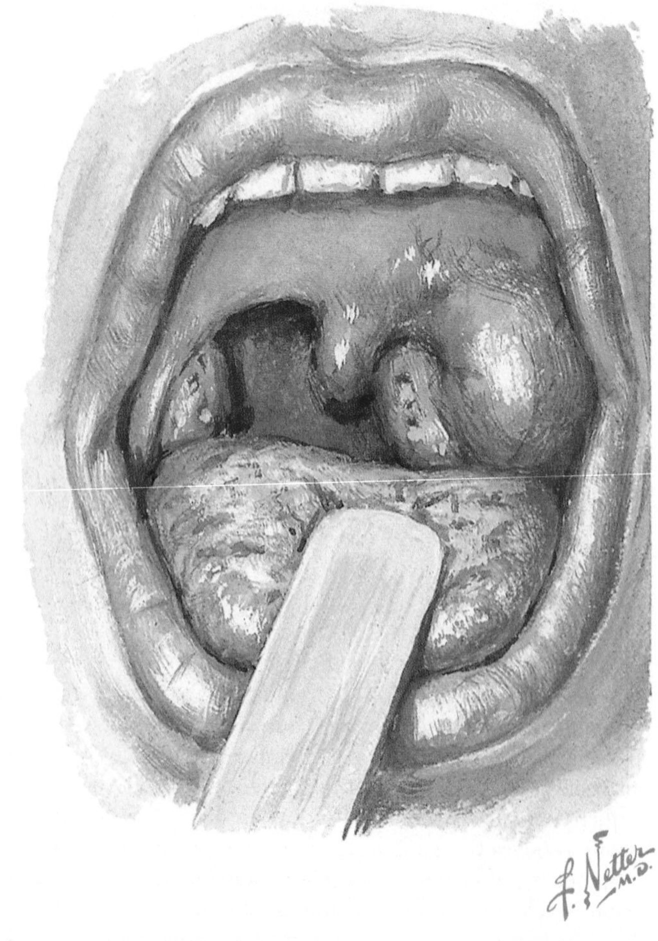

The bacterial infectious causes of stridor all require antibiotics (Table 36-2). Peritonsillar and retropharyngeal abscesses often require drainage as well because antibiotic penetration of the abscess may not be optimal. Epiglottitis is an entity that should be considered a medical emergency necessitating immediate intubation for airway protection.

Stridor caused by anaphylaxis requires the immediate intramuscular injection of epinephrine, which the patient can self-administer at home via EpiPen. Adjunctive treatments include antihistamines and systemic corticosteroids. If foreign body aspiration is strongly suspected or diagnosed on radiography, rigid bronchoscopy is necessary to remove the object, often from the right main stem bronchus.

FUTURE DIRECTIONS

Surfactant therapy and increasing use of noninvasive ventilation in premature neonates should reduce the incidence of prolonged intubation and resultant subglottic stenosis. Societal concerns regarding vaccination have led to reemergence of Hib as a pathogen in certain areas of the country. Educational efforts aimed at the general public on the importance of childhood vaccination are paramount in prevention.

Figure 36-3 *Peritonsillar abscess.*

Table 36-2 Treatment for Bacterial Causes of Stridor

Infectious Causes of Stridor	Empiric Antibiotic Therapy
Epiglottitis	Ceftriaxone
Retropharyngeal abscess	Clindamycin or ampicillin–sulbactam
Peritonsillar abscess	Clindamycin or ampicillin–sulbactam
Bacterial tracheitis	Vancomycin or clindamycin

SUGGESTED READINGS

Bjornson CL, Klassen TP, Williamson J, et al: A randomized trial of a single dose of oral dexamethasone for mild croup, *N Engl J Med* 351(13):1306-1313, 2004.

Craig FW, Schunk JE: Retropharyngeal abscess in children: clinical presentation, utility of imaging, and current management, *Pediatrics* 111(6 Pt 1):1394-1398, 2003.

Masters IB: Congenital airway lesions and lung disease, *Pediatr Clin North Am* 56(1):227-242, xii, 2009.

Sampson HA, Muñoz-Furlong A, Campbell RL, et al: Second symposium on the definition and management of anaphylaxis: summary report—Second National Institute of Allergy and Infectious Disease/Food Allergy and Anaphylaxis Network symposium, *J Allergy Clin Immunol* 117(2):391-397, 2006.

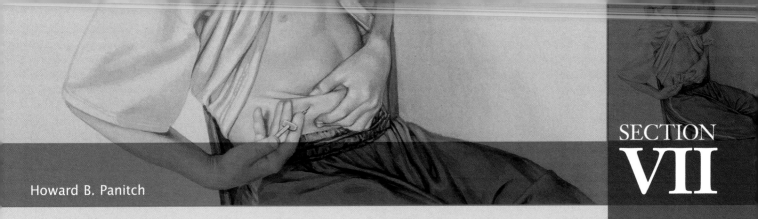

Howard B. Panitch

SECTION
VII

Disorders of the Respiratory System and Lower Airway

Bronchiolitis and Wheezing

37

Gustavo Nino

Wheezing is a high-pitched musical sound produced by air flowing through narrowed airways. Wheezes are heard mostly during the expiratory phase. They are usually a sign of increased airway resistance resulting from obstruction in the intrathoracic airways. The predominance of wheezing during expiration is explained by the normal tendency of the intrathoracic airways to narrow when the intrapleural pressure exceeds intraluminal pressure during this phase of respiration. Narrowing of the intrathoracic airways is accentuated when the expiratory intrapleural pressure becomes positive during forced exhalation or in the setting of small airways obstruction. When obstruction occurs in the extrathoracic airways, it manifests with a distinct harsh inspiratory noise that is referred to as *stridor*.

Wheezing is *heterophonous* or *polyphonic* in nature when there is diffuse narrowing of the airways. This widespread involvement of the airways produces a mixture of sounds associated with various degrees of obstruction to airflow. Multiple varied degrees of obstruction typically occur in the presence of bronchospasm, edema, or intraluminal secretions. The most common causes of heterophonous wheezing in the pediatric population are viral bronchiolitis and asthma (see Chapter 38). Conversely, *homophonous* wheezing refers to a single set of pitches that originates in the larger airways but that can be transmitted widely. Common causes of homophonous wheezing include tracheomalacia, bronchomalacia, foreign body aspiration, and anatomic compression of the airways (Figure 37-1).

ETIOLOGY AND PATHOGENESIS

The majority of wheezing in infants is caused by viral bronchiolitis or asthma, but many other entities can also cause wheezing at this age (Box 37-1).

Bronchiolitis

Bronchiolitis commonly refers to an acute episode of obstructive lower airway disease caused by a viral infection in infants younger than 24 months of age. The peak incidence of severe disease occurs between 2 and 6 months of age. Approximately 1% of infants in the first 12 months of life are hospitalized with bronchiolitis, accounting for more than 125,000 annual hospitalizations in the United States. Hospitalization rates are five times higher in high-risk groups, including premature infants with bronchopulmonary dysplasia and patients with congenital heart disease.

The infectious cause of acute bronchiolitis typically includes viruses with specific tropism for bronchiolar epithelium. Respiratory syncytial virus (RSV) is responsible for more than 50% of cases, but other viruses are increasingly recognized as causes of this clinical entity. Viral infection of the lower airways can induce severe changes in the epithelial cell and mucosal surfaces of the human respiratory tract. Bronchiolar epithelial cell

necrosis, ciliary disruption, and peribronchiolar lymphocytic infiltration are the earliest lesions. Edema of the small airways and mucus secretion, mixed with denuded epithelial cells, elicits obstruction and narrowing of the airways (see Figure 37-2). The generation of atelectasis is often associated with ventilation/perfusion mismatch and consequent hypoxemia. Heterogeneous ventilation and dynamic collapse of the airways during exhalation can lead to air trapping and pulmonary hyperinflation (see Figure 37-2). With severe obstructive lung disease and respiratory muscle fatigue, hypercapnia can also arise.

Many infants with RSV infection do not develop bronchiolitis. Approximately 60% to 70% of RSV-infected infants will have disease confined to the upper respiratory tract. The severity of the clinical syndrome is largely determined by host immunologic and anatomic factors. The presence of immunoglobulin G antibodies to the F (fusion) protein of RSV (whether transplacentally acquired or administered postnatally) attenuates the severity of the RSV infection. Conversely, premature infants are particularly prone to developing significant lower respiratory symptoms. The lungs of newborns with bronchopulmonary dysplasia have alveolar simplification and thus decreased small airways diameter because of lower elastic recoil. Because airflow resistance is inversely related to the radius of the airway to the fourth power, airflow in infants with bronchopulmonary dysplasia can be compromised with minimal changes in the bronchiolar lumen. Bronchiolitis is also more common in boys, in those who have not been breastfed, and in those who live in crowded conditions.

Asthma

Asthma is another important cause of wheezing in infants and children (see Chapter 38). This clinical entity is characterized by recurrent episodes of airway obstruction that are at least partially reversible with bronchodilators. Another pathogenic feature of the disease is chronic inflammation of the airways. Whereas extensive bronchiolar epithelial cell necrosis and T-helper cell type 1 (Th1) cytokines like interferon-γ are present in viral bronchiolitis, inflammation in asthma is often driven by allergic (Th2) cytokines such as interleukin-13 (IL-13), IL-4, and IL-5. Other abnormalities of the asthmatic airway include constriction and hypertrophy of the airway smooth muscle, mucosal edema, hypertrophic mucous glands, and sometimes eosinophilic infiltration.

Viral infections are the most common causes of exacerbations in infantile asthma. As opposed to bronchiolitis, lower respiratory symptoms in asthma tend to recur during exposure to other triggers, such as exercise, allergens, or cold air. Depending on the clinical course of their wheezing, infants may be *early transient wheezers* with at least one episode before the age of 3 years but complete resolution by school age; *persistent wheezers* with episodes before 3 years that are still present at 6 years of age; or *late-onset wheezers* with no history of wheezing by 3 years but

Homophonous "central" wheezing

Uniform sine waves represent a single set of pitches originating in the larger airways.

Extrinsic compression

Foreign body

Intrinsic obstruction

Adenopathy or tumor

Vascular ring

Heterophonous "central" wheezing

Multiple sine waves represent a mixture of sounds produced by several sites and degrees of obstruction to airflow

Bronchoconstriction; airway secretions

Asthma

Cystic fibrosis

Aspiration syndromes (mucosal edema)

Gastro-esophageal reflux

Tracheo-esophageal fistula

Figure 37-1 *Homophonous and heterophonous wheezing.*

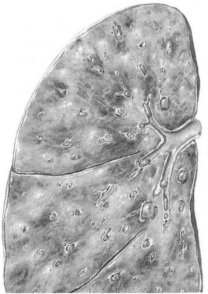
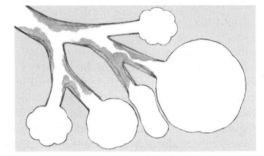
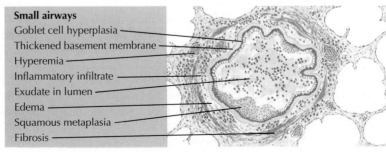

Small airways are partially or completely obstructed by edema, mucous secretions, denuded epithelial cells, and inflammatory infiltrates. These pathologic changes can lead to regional or diffuse air trapping, and nonuniform alveolar ventilation

Small airways

Goblet cell hyperplasia

Thickened basement membrane

Hyperemia

Inflammatory infiltrate

Exudate in lumen

Edema

Squamous metaplasia

Fibrosis

Figure 37-2 *Pathogenesis of bronchiolitis.*

Box 37-1 Differential Diagnosis of Wheezing in Infants and Young Children

I. Infection
  • Respiratory syncytial virus
  • Human metapneumovirus
  • Parainfluenza virus 3
  • Parainfluenza virus 1
  • Parainfluenza virus 2
  • Adenovirus
  • Influenza virus (A or B)
  • Rhinovirus
  • *Mycoplasma pneumoniae*
  • Bacterial bronchitis (e.g., *Haemophilus influenzae*, *Moraxella catarrhalis*)
II. Asthma
III. Aspiration Syndromes
  • Gastroesophageal reflux
  • Swallowing dysfunction
  • Tracheoesophageal fistula or laryngeal cleft
IV. Mucociliary Clearance Disorders
  • Cystic fibrosis
  • Primary ciliary dyskinesia
V. Anatomic Abnormalities
  • Tracheomalacia or bronchomalacia
  • Vascular ring or sling
  • Compressing lymphadenopathy or tumor
  • Airway hemangioma
  • Cystic adenomatoid malformation
  • Bronchial or lung cyst
  • Congenital lobar emphysema
  • Pulmonary sequestration
  • Foreign body aspiration
VI. Immunodeficiency
  • HIV infection
  • Congenital cellular or humoral immunodeficiency
VII. Other Causes
  • Interstitial lung disease (e.g., surfactant protein C deficiency)
  • Bronchiolitis obliterans
  • Pulmonary edema
  • Toxic inhalation

with wheezing by 6 years. Approximately 60% of infants who wheeze will outgrow wheezing by 6 years of age. Risk factors for persistent wheezing include a maternal history of asthma, maternal smoking, elevated immunoglobulin E (IgE) level, and eczema at younger than 1 year of age. In addition, early respiratory viral infections, particularly RSV and rhinovirus, are associated with the presence of subsequent recurrent wheezing and asthma.

Whether bronchiolitis modifies the immune response or airway biology to evoke asthma later in life is still unclear. Experimental studies primarily based on animal models have reported that early RSV infection can upregulate neurokinin-mediated neurogenic inflammation, potentially leading to airway hyperreactivity. Other proasthmatic mechanisms postulated include a viral-induced bias of the host toward allergic Th2 immune responses during early infancy and the production of virus-specific IgE antibodies. Notwithstanding these hypotheses, infants with bronchiolitis may be a select group of patients with an inherent predisposition to asthma that is simply unmasked by an episode of viral respiratory infection. The relationship between early respiratory viral infections and subsequent wheezing and asthma remains a topic of intense investigation and controversy.

Other Causes of Wheezing

Gastroesophageal reflux (GER) is another important cause of acute or chronic wheezing in infants and children. Wheezing in GER is caused by pulmonary aspiration of gastric contents or by a vagal reflex that induces bronchospasm without aspiration. Other conditions associated with widespread involvement of the intrathoracic small airways such as cystic fibrosis (CF), primary ciliary dyskinesia (PCD), or immunodeficiency can present with heterophonous wheezing as well (see Figure 37-1).

The presence of homophonous wheezing is suggestive of narrowing or obstruction in the large central airways. Homophonous wheezing is commonly heard in children with tracheomalacia, bronchomalacia or anatomic abnormalities (i.e., vascular ring). In addition, an isolated homophonous wheeze localized in just one area may signal bronchial obstruction by an extrinsic compression or intraluminal foreign body (see Figure 37-1).

CLINICAL PRESENTATION

When evaluating an infant with an acute respiratory illness a critical question to answer is whether or not there is involvement of the lower airways. In RSV infection, non-specific upper respiratory tract symptoms consisting of nasal discharge and mild cough begin about 3 to 5 days after exposure. The progression of the disease to the lower respiratory tract is characterized by the presence of tachypnea, hypoxemia, nasal flaring and intercostal or subcostal retractions. The typical course for a previously healthy infant older than 6 months is one of improvement over the subsequent 2 to 5 days. Significant hypoxemia, grunting and marked use of accessory muscles are signs of severe disease and impending respiratory failure (Figure 37-3). Central apnea can also be an early manifestation of RSV infection, at times also resulting in respiratory failure.

Viral bronchiolitis is one of several syndromes associated with obstruction of the intrathoracic small airways; thus, the presence of expiratory heterophonous wheezing is a common but non-specific sign of the disease. Wheezing in infants can be better appreciated on pulmonary auscultation when elicited by gentle chest compression (so-called "squeeze the wheeze") to induce forced expiratory flow. A marked reduction in amplitude of breathing sounds suggests very severe disease with nearly complete bronchiolar obstruction. Auscultation in bronchiolitis may also reveal inspiratory crackles as small airways re-open, and prolongation of the expiratory phase. The other cardinal feature of small airways obstruction is pulmonary hyperinflation. This clinical feature helps to localize the disease in the small airways as it is a manifestation of alveolar air trapping. The key signs of hyperinflation are an increase in anteroposterior diameter of the chest wall, the presence of subcostal retractions and the palpation of a normal sized liver below the costal margin (see Figure 37-3).

Given that early respiratory viral infections are associated with the presence of recurrent wheezing and asthma, the initial

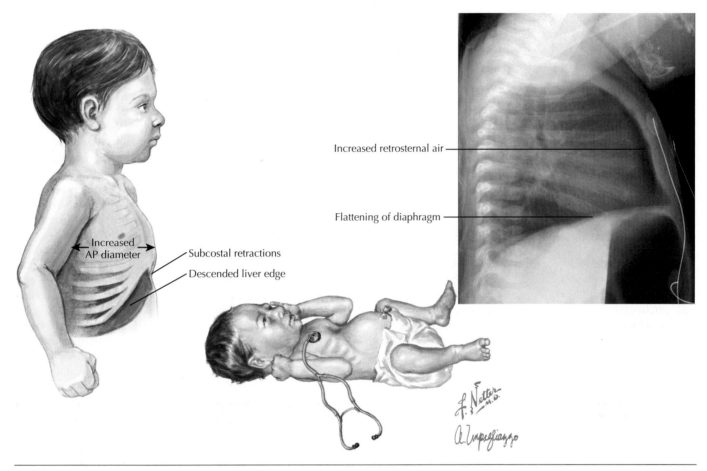

Figure 37-3 *Clinical evaluation of wheezing and bronchiolitis.*

differentiation between these entities is often difficult. Many infants originally diagnosed with viral bronchiolitis are later categorized as asthmatics. In the asthmatic child, the presence of intermittent symptoms such as coughing or wheezing at night or in response to exercise, crying, laughing, mist, or cold air can facilitate the diagnosis. Adequate responses to bronchodilator therapy and typically also to corticosteroids are characteristic features of asthma as well. An atopic phenotype (i.e., eczema or elevated IgE levels) and a positive family history of asthma also point toward the diagnosis of this disease.

The clinical evaluation of wheezing should also include a detailed feeding history. Respiratory symptoms such as cough, cyanosis, or respiratory distress during feeds suggest laryngeal penetration or pulmonary aspiration. Given that aspiration can also be "silent," especially at night, early morning symptoms may be the only clue for the diagnosis. Aspiration of gastric contents or direct penetration of oral liquids during feeding is particularly common in children with neurodevelopmental abnormalities or anatomic defects of the respiratory system such as tracheoesophageal fistula (TEF) or laryngeal cleft.

When wheezing is persistent and nonresponsive to therapy, the consideration of uncommon but serious medical conditions such as CF, PCD, and immunodeficiency is in order. As opposed to asthma, these diseases are often associated with failure to thrive. This is particularly true in patients with CF because of the presence of malabsorption caused by pancreatic insufficiency.

Digital clubbing may be present in patients with CF, PCD, and other causes of bronchiectasis but should never be present in uncomplicated asthma. Recurrent sinusitis and bacterial bronchitis are common features of CF, PCD, and some immunodeficiencies. PCD invariably causes significant abnormalities of the middle ear and is often associated with situs inversus or abdominal heterotaxy. Tachypnea during the neonatal period and persistent purulent rhinorrhea during infancy are also typical features of this disease.

The presence of homophonous wheezing is suggestive of abnormalities in the large rather than the small intrathoracic airways. Tracheal collapse secondary to highly compliant airways can produce homophonous wheezing in infants. This condition, termed *tracheomalacia*, seldom affects respiratory function at rest (infants are often referred to as "happy wheezers"), and isolated congenital tracheomalacia usually resolves after 1 year of age. Nevertheless, infants with significant collapse of the central airways during the expulsive phase of cough, particularly those with congenital or acquired tracheal abnormalities (e.g., TEF), can have inadequate clearance of airway secretions. A harsh "barking" cough is a key clinical sign present in this situation. These patients often have a protracted clinical course accompanied by recurrent lower tract infections and frequent hospital visits.

Congenital malformations cause homophonous wheezing in early infancy when they externally compress the airway or cause intrinsic obstruction of the airway lumen. Vascular rings secondary to abnormal development of the aortic arch can produce considerable constriction of the subjacent trachea (see Figure 37-1). Virtually any type of congenital intrathoracic lesion, depending on its size and location, can potentially cause external compression of the airways. Other causes of external compression include mediastinal lymphadenopathy secondary to infections (e.g., tuberculosis) or malignancies (e.g., lymphoma) (see Figure 37-1). Intrinsic obstruction of the airway lumen may be caused by foreign body aspiration, hemangiomas, and rarely carcinoid tumors (see Figure 37-1). Airway hemangiomas should be suspected particularly when they are present in other areas of the body (e.g., skin).

EVALUATION AND MANAGEMENT

The diagnosis of bronchiolitis is essentially clinical but can be supported by radiographic findings. Typical chest radiographic findings are hyperinflation, increased peribronchial markings, and patchy subsegmental atelectasis. The absence of cystic lesions, pleural effusions, and focal densities suggestive of bacterial infection are other valuable pieces of information obtained from the chest radiograph. Rapid viral detection tests (i.e., immunofluorescence or polymerase chain reaction) are helpful if the diagnosis is uncertain or for epidemiologic purposes.

The management of patients with bronchiolitis largely depends on the severity of the disease. Most infants can be managed at home with supportive care, but hypoxemia or inability to feed adequately requires hospitalization. After an infant is hospitalized, supportive care is the mainstay of therapy and involves appropriate fluid replacement and the use of supplemental oxygen when necessary. Routine use of bronchodilators and corticosteroids is not indicated unless there is a component of airway hyperreactivity or a formal diagnosis of asthma. Severe cases of bronchiolitis may need the initiation of noninvasive ventilation techniques to deliver continuous positive airway pressure (CPAP) or bilevel positive airway pressure (BLPAP) and sometimes endotracheal intubation to provide invasive mechanical ventilatory support.

Several other interventions may be helpful in refractory cases. Pulmonary aspiration is a common complication in infants with bronchiolitis caused by tachypnea and respiratory distress. Enteral feeds via nasogastric tube may be indicated to prevent ongoing lung damage and allow recovery from the acute illness. Nebulized hypertonic saline to facilitate the mobilization of tenacious airway secretions and racemic epinephrine to decrease airway mucosal edema have shown positive results in some clinical trials, but their routine use is not currently recommended. Other small studies have also suggested that exogenous surfactant, helium and oxygen mixtures (heliox), and combination therapies (i.e., corticosteroids and epinephrine and bronchodilators) can offer clinical benefit in some cases. Ribavirin is a nucleoside analogue with in vitro activity against RSV and other viruses, but its usefulness is controversial, and it is rarely used in clinical practice.

In addition to the care of the acute episode, prevention is another important consideration in the management of viral bronchiolitis. Meticulous hand washing is the best measure to prevent the transmission of RSV and most other respiratory viruses. Monthly administration of monoclonal anti-F antibody (palivizumab) throughout the RSV season has become standard of care for infants at high risk for developing severe respiratory illnesses secondary to RSV infection. In general, palivizumab is recommended for infants younger than 6 to 12 months of age born prematurely or those younger than 2 years of age with bronchopulmonary dysplasia or other significant comorbidities, including immunodeficiency, chronic lung disease, and cyanotic congenital heart conditions. Secondhand tobacco smoke is associated with an increased incidence of respiratory infections in infants and young children, so parents should be counseled to avoid exposing their children to this irritant.

Many children develop multiple wheezing illnesses during infancy secondary to viral bronchiolitis or asthma; however, a poor response to therapy, complicated courses, and a nonreassuring clinical evaluation (e.g., failure to thrive) are indications for further evaluation. A sweat test to evaluate for CF and assessment of baseline immune status are simple tests that can rule out serious underlying conditions. Careful clinical observation after administration of a bronchodilator aerosol is often all that is required to demonstrate the presence of bronchospasm and bronchodilator responsiveness. Pulmonary function testing, available for infants at some specialized centers, can also evaluate bronchodilator responsiveness and inform about the degree and location of the obstruction. If there is concern about aspiration, a swallowing study and evaluation for GER should be considered. In addition, visualization of the gastrointestinal (GI) and respiratory tract may be necessary to exclude congenital abnormalities such as laryngeal cleft or TEF. Depending on the clinical suspicion, contrast upper GI studies, laryngoscopy, bronchoscopy, or GI endoscopy may be indicated.

If there is no clear clinical evidence of tracheomalacia, the existence of homophonous wheezing often requires direct visualization of the respiratory system by bronchoscopy to exclude fixed obstruction or foreign body aspiration. This is particularly true when the sound is located in just one area of the chest or when it is present during inspiration and expiration (biphasic wheezing). A chest radiograph provides valuable information about the presence of mediastinal adenopathy, masses, and other space-occupying lesions. Because vascular rings are often associated with a right aortic arch, the chest radiograph can also be used to confirm the normal location of the aortic arch on the left side. Upper GI series can also inform about potential extrinsic vascular compressions of the trachea. If indicated, magnetic resonance imaging or computed tomography (CT) angiography are best to delineate vascular lesions of the chest. Chest CT scan is sometimes necessary to further evaluate the anatomy or to rule out extrinsic obstruction of the airways. The diagnosis of other less common causes of wheezing such as PCD often requires more sophisticated testing. These evaluations may include biopsies of the respiratory tract or genetic-molecular analysis and are indicated only in select cases with high index of clinical suspicion.

FUTURE DIRECTIONS

Significant progress continues in the development of active vaccines and monoclonal antibodies with enhanced neutralizing activity against RSV. Larger clinical trials are being conducted to confirm the utility of new treatments for bronchiolitis, including hypertonic saline and combination therapies. A better understanding of the pathogenesis of asthma is expected to provide new insights about the management and prognosis of wheezing illnesses in infancy as well.

SUGGESTED READINGS

Castro-Rodriguez JA, Rodrigo GJ: Efficacy of inhaled corticosteroids in infants and preschoolers with recurrent wheezing and asthma: a systematic review with meta-analysis, *Pediatrics* 123(3):e519-e525, 2009.

Meissner HC: Bronchiolitis. In Long SS, Pickering LK, Prober CG, editors: *Principles and Practice of Pediatric Infectious Diseases*, ed 3, Philadelphia, 2009, Saunders, pp 241-245.

Panickar J, Lakhanpaul M, Lambert PC, et al: Oral prednisolone for preschool children with acute virus-induced wheezing, *N Engl J Med* 360(4):329-338, 2009.

Panitch HB: The relationship between early respiratory viral infections and subsequent wheezing and asthma, *Clin Pediatr (Phila)* 46(5):392-400, 2007.

Panitch HB: Treatment of bronchiolitis in infants, *Pediatr Case Rev* 3(1):3-19, 2003.

Plint AC, Johnson DW, Patel H, et al: Pediatric Emergency Research Canada (PERC): Epinephrine and dexamethasone in children with bronchiolitis, *N Engl J Med* 360(20):2079-2089, 2009.

Weinberger M, Abu-Hasan M: Pseudo-asthma: when cough, wheezing, and dyspnea are not asthma, *Pediatrics* 120(4):855-864, 2007.

Zhang L, Mendoza-Sassi RA, Wainwright C, et al: Nebulized hypertonic saline solution for acute bronchiolitis in infants, *Cochrane Database Syst Rev* 8(4):CD006458, 2008.

Asthma

James Aaron Feinstein

38

Asthma, a chronic inflammatory disorder of the airways, is one of the most prevalent pediatric pulmonary disorders, affecting an estimated 6.8 million American children younger than 18 years of age. Acute asthma exacerbations are responsible for 700,000 emergency department (ED) visits per year and are the third leading cause of hospitalization in the United States for children younger than 15 years of age. Treatment is expensive—direct health care costs total $14.7 billion per year, of which $6.2 billion is spent on asthma prescriptions. Approximately 12.8 million school days are lost each year secondary to absenteeism from asthma exacerbations.

Instituting proper asthma management—by initiating appropriate therapy, providing patient and parent education, and monitoring patient symptoms and response to therapy—will reduce symptom frequency and severity, improve quality of life, and cut excess healthcare expenditures. This chapter discusses classical atopic asthma as it pertains to children and adolescents.

ETIOLOGY AND PATHOGENESIS

Asthma is characterized by the presence of three airway components: inflammation, obstruction, and hyperresponsiveness. Chronic airway inflammation establishes baseline airway edema and obstruction, which sets the stage for acute exacerbations. During acute exacerbations, inciting triggers (Box 38-1) cause inflammation and bronchoconstriction of already hyperresponsive airways. Key cellular components involved in the pathogenesis of asthma include mast cells; eosinophils; and, to some degree, neutrophils, T cells, macrophages, and epithelial cells (Figures 38-1 and 38-2).

Although downstream symptoms are relatively uniform (e.g., respiratory distress, wheezing), upstream predisposing factors are broader in their scope. Asthma is likely the result of interplay among environmental *and* genetic causes. Environmental factors, such as respiratory pathogens, allergens, and pollutants, can cause airway inflammation and irritation, immune system dysregulation, or both, leading to the development of asthma. Environmental factors can also worsen existing disease. Genetic factors, such as a family history of atopic disease or an altered cytokine profile, can also result in abnormal modulation of the immune system and predispose a patient to developing asthma. For example, a T-helper cell type 2 (Th2)–cytokine profile likely correlates with the development of asthma and allergy. Currently, the genetics of asthma remain complex and multifactorial in nature; in the future, the genetic identification of particular genotypes and phenotypes may allow for the categorization of asthma into distinct subtypes that will aid in tailoring treatment plans.

CLINICAL PRESENTATION

When providing a patient history, parents of a child with asthma often recall symptoms secondary to episodic airway obstruction. The most common reported symptom is persistent cough, which frequently is the *only* symptom, and may occur more often while the child is asleep. Nighttime cough caused by asthma, which occurs several hours into sleep, must be differentiated from cough caused by gastroesophageal reflux (GER) or postnasal drip, which occurs soon after a child is recumbent.

Although wheezing is a hallmark symptom of asthma, parents rarely report hearing an audible wheeze. Other symptoms a parent may recall include shortness of breath, chest pain, exercise intolerance, and variable degrees of respiratory distress. Subacute presentations of any of these symptoms, including the presence of chronic cough, are much more commonly encountered than life-threatening episodes of airway obstruction.

A patient or family history of allergy and atopic skin disease may be present. It is important to inquire about the setting(s) in which symptoms occur because a variety of inciting triggers exist (Box 38-1 and Figure 38-3). A patient should also be assessed for comorbid medical conditions, including GER, allergic rhinitis, sinusitis, and obesity, all of which can exacerbate asthma symptoms. For a patient with a previous asthma diagnosis, it is useful to inquire about the frequency of ED visits and hospital admissions, oral steroid use, and any history of severe complications (e.g., endotracheal intubation or admission to the intensive care unit [ICU]).

The physical examination of a patient with well-controlled asthma is generally unrevealing. The physical examination of a patient with asthma during an acute exacerbation will most frequently demonstrate heterophonous wheezing (inspiratory, or expiratory, or both). To properly assess for the presence of wheezing, adequate airflow is required; it may be necessary to "squeeze the wheeze" and compress the chest wall to ensure forced exhalation or to ask an older child to exhale forcefully with the mouth wide open. Heterophonous or polyphonic wheezing results from turbulent air flow through multiple obstructed small airways; the different "musical" pitches are a consequence of varying degrees of obstruction. Heterophonous wheezing should be differentiated from homophonous or monophonic wheezing, which typically occurs with obstruction of larger airways.

Additionally, a symptomatic patient with asthma is frequently short of breath and tachypneic. The patient may also have other signs of airway obstruction, including decreased air entry, prolongation of the expiratory: inspiratory ratio, and hyperexpansion of the chest (a widened anteroposterior diameter). Nasal flaring and the use of accessory muscles (e.g., the sternocleidomastoid, intercostal, pectoralis major, and abdominal muscles) are also commonly observed.

Careful attention should be paid to the skin examination for signs of atopic disease, such as eczema or atopic dermatitis, and to the upper respiratory exam for signs of allergic rhinitis, including mucosal swelling, nasal polyps, and rhinorrhea. The presence of nasal polyps should trigger evaluation for cystic fibrosis. Digital clubbing is *never* a component of uncomplicated asthma and should prompt further evaluation.

DIFFERENTIAL DIAGNOSIS

If considering a diagnosis of asthma, the time-worn axiom must be remembered that "all that wheezes is not asthma." Before a diagnosis of asthma can be confirmed, alternative diagnoses must be considered (Table 38-1). Furthermore, not all wheezes are equal. For example, monophonic wheezing associated with foreign body aspiration is distinct from polyphonic wheezing associated with asthma.

Within the respiratory system, upper respiratory infections and allergic rhinitis are the most common causes of recurrent cough and wheezing. Other potential causes include foreign

---

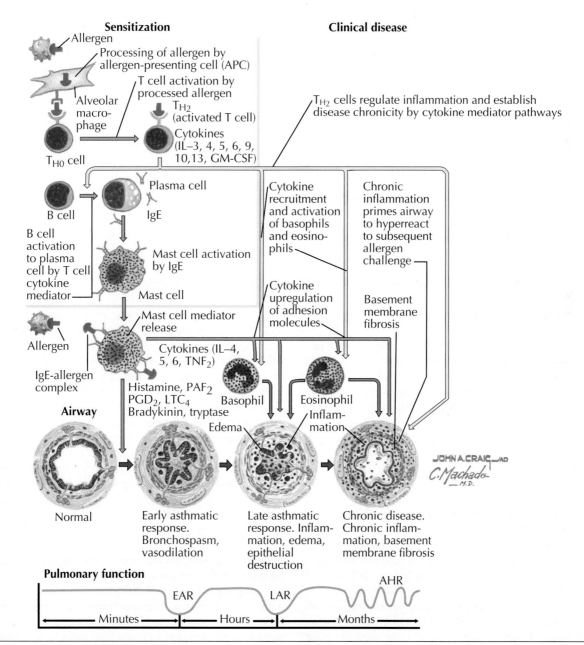

Figure 38-1 *Steps in the pathogenesis of asthma.*

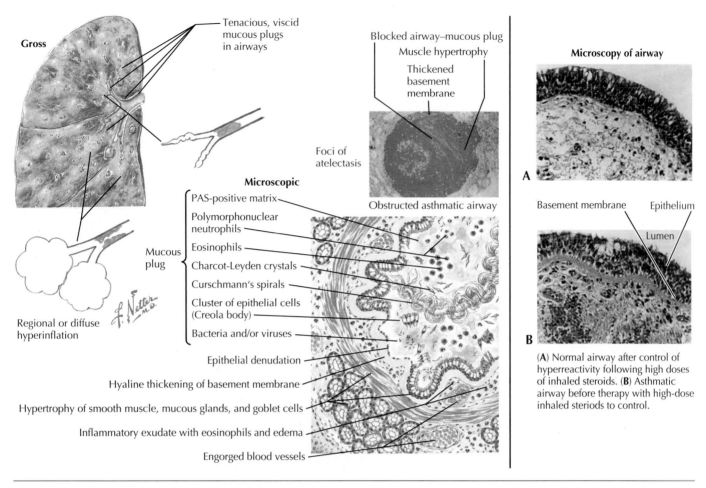

Gross

Tenacious, viscid mucous plugs in airways

Blocked airway–mucous plug
Muscle hypertrophy
Thickened basement membrane

Microscopy of airway

Foci of atelectasis

Microscopic

PAS-positive matrix
Polymorphonuclear neutrophils
Eosinophils
Mucous plug
Charcot-Leyden crystals
Curschmann's spirals
Cluster of epithelial cells (Creola body)
Bacteria and/or viruses

Obstructed asthmatic airway

Basement membrane   Epithelium
Lumen

A

B

Regional or diffuse hyperinflation

Epithelial denudation

Hyaline thickening of basement membrane

Hypertrophy of smooth muscle, mucous glands, and goblet cells

Inflammatory exudate with eosinophils and edema

Engorged blood vessels

(**A**) Normal airway after control of hyperreactivity following high doses of inhaled steroids. (**B**) Asthmatic airway before therapy with high-dose inhaled steriods to control.

Figure 38-2 *Pathology of an acute asthma attack.*

body aspiration, vocal cord dysfunction, tracheal or bronchial compression (by vessels, strictures, or masses), cystic fibrosis, and bronchopulmonary dysplasia (chronic lung disease of prematurity).

Nonrespiratory system causes should be excluded. Cardiac pathology—such as congenital heart disease, pulmonary edema, or vascular abnormalities compressing the respiratory tree—must be considered. GER; aspiration pneumonitis; and less frequently, tracheoesophageal fistula can all cause recurrent wheezing and so mimic asthma.

EVALUATION

Chronic Disease

It is useful to classify a patient's different symptoms into categories of severity (Table 38-2), which can guide stepwise treatment. Historical data provide the most useful information in establishing a diagnosis of asthma. When a tentative diagnosis of asthma is suspected based on a patient's history and physical findings, further evaluation with spirometry is warranted.

Spirometry is useful in quantifying pulmonary function, as well as for demonstrating a response to a trial of bronchodilators in patients who are old enough to cooperate with the test (usually older than 5 years of age, although the reliability of

spirometry is being investigated in younger populations). After a challenge with a bronchodilator, an improvement in a patient's FEV_1 (forced expiratory volume in 1 second) of at least 12% demonstrates significant bronchodilator responsiveness and so is strongly suggestive of asthma in the proper historical context. Additionally, the flow-volume curve will reveal a typical concave obstructive pattern. For a patient with an existing asthma diagnosis, trends in spirometry data can reflect the severity and relative control of a patient's disease.

Depending on the presence of atypical or comorbid symptoms, other studies may be indicated, including a chest radiograph. Although more useful in the acute setting, a chest radiograph can demonstrate hyperinflation and retrosternal air trapping and can aid in ruling out pulmonary infection, heart disease, tumor, and foreign body aspiration.

Acute Exacerbation

A patient experiencing an acute asthma exacerbation should be promptly evaluated and triaged based on the severity of his or her symptoms (Table 38-3). Standardized criteria should be used within an institution, although many different schemes exist. Criteria are primarily based on symptom assessment, and concerning symptoms and signs include tachypnea, breathlessness, increased work of breathing, accessory muscle use, and decreased

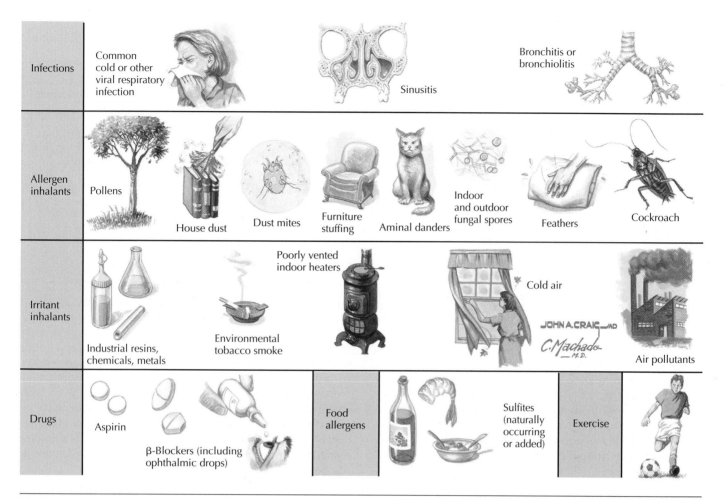

Infections	Common cold or other viral respiratory infection	Sinusitis	Bronchitis or bronchiolitis
Allergen inhalants	Pollens — House dust — Dust mites — Furniture stuffing — Aminal danders — Indoor and outdoor fungal spores — Feathers — Cockroach		
Irritant inhalants	Industrial resins, chemicals, metals — Environmental tobacco smoke — Poorly vented indoor heaters — Cold air — Air pollutants		
Drugs	Aspirin — β-Blockers (including ophthalmic drops)	Food allergens	Sulfites (naturally occurring or added) — Exercise

JOHN A. CRAIC C. Machado M.D.

Figure 38-3 *Asthma triggers.*

Table 38-1 Differential Diagnosis of Asthma in Children

Differential Diagnosis		Suggested Confirmatory Tests
Upper airway diseases	Allergic rhinitis or sinusitis	Physical examination, sinus CT scan
Obstruction of large airways	Foreign body in trachea or bronchus	Chest radiography
	Vocal cord dysfunction	Laryngoscopy
	Vascular rings or laryngeal webs	Barium swallow, chest MRI
	Tracheomalacia	Laryngoscopy, flexible bronchoscopy
	Tracheal- or bronchostenosis	Chest radiography, chest CT scan, bronchoscopy
	Enlarged lymph nodes or tumor	Chest radiography, chest CT scan
Obstruction of small airways	Viral bronchiolitis	History, chest radiography, viral antigen or PCR testing
	Bronchiolitis obliterans	Chest CT scan, lung biopsy
	Cystic fibrosis	Chest radiograph, sweat chloride test, genetic test
	Bronchopulmonary dysplasia	Prenatal history, chest radiography, chest CT scan
	Heart disease	Chest radiograph, ECG, echocardiography
Other causes	Gastroesophageal reflux	pH probe, barium swallow, nuclear milk scan
	Oromotor dysfunction leading to chronic aspiration	Modified barium swallow, speech pathology evaluation
		Chest radiography
	Pulmonary edema	Chest radiography, fluoroscopy, chest CT
	Tracheoesophageal fistula	

CT, computed tomography; ECG, electrocardiography; MRI, magnetic resonance imaging; PCR, polymerase chain reaction.

Adapted from the Expert Panel Report 3 (EPR3): *Guidelines for the Diagnosis and Management of Asthma*. Washington, DC, U.S. Department of Health and Human Resources, 2007, p 12. Available at http://www.nhlbi.nih.gov/guidelines/asthma/asthgdln.htm.

Table 38-2 Classifying Asthma Severity in Children 5 to 12 Years Old

Components of Severity	Intermittent	Persistent		
		Mild	*Moderate*	*Severe*
Symptoms	≤2 days/wk	>2 days/wk but not daily	Daily	Consistently throughout each day
Nighttime awakenings	≤2 times/mo	3-4 times/mo	>1x/wk but not nightly	Often 7x/wk
SABA use	≤2 days/wk	>2 days/wk but not daily	Daily	Several times per day
Interference with daily activity	None	Minor limitations	Some limitations	Severe limitations
Lung function	Normal FEV_1 between exacerbations FEV_1 >80% predicted FEV_1/FVC >85%	FEV_1 >80% predicted FEV_1/FVC >80%	FEV_1 = 60%-80% predicted FEV_1/FVC = 75%-80%	FEV_1 <60% predicted FEV_1/FVC <75%
Risk	0-1 exacerbations/y	>2 exacerbations/y		
Recommended step for initiating therapy	Step 1	Step 2	Step 3	Step 3

FEV_1, forced expiratory volume in 1 second; FVC, forced vital capacity; SABA, short-acting bronchodilator agent.
Adapted from the Expert Panel Report 3 (EPR3): *Guidelines for the Diagnosis and Management of Asthma.* Washington, DC, U.S. Department of Health and Human Resources, 2007, p 45. Available at http://www.nhlbi.nih.gov/guidelines/asthma/asthgdln.htm.

pulse oximetry values. For a child old enough to perform the maneuver, obtaining peak flow measurements can aid in determining the severity of an exacerbation, with peak expiratory flows of less than 40% predicted signaling a severe exacerbation requiring further assessment in an ED. However, peak flows are not a reliable measure because they measure large airway obstruction, and one can experience a 25% decrease in small

airway flow before there is any decrease in peak flow. Spirometry is a much more sensitive measure of both small and large airway function and can also be used in the acute setting to assess both severity of the exacerbation and acute response to therapy.

A child who scores in the severe classification should immediately be placed on cardiorespiratory and pulse oximetry monitors and further acute testing may be indicated, such as

Table 38-3 Classifying Asthma Exacerbation Severity in Children Younger Than 12 Years Old

	Symptoms and Signs	Clinical Course
Mild	• Dyspnea with activity • Tachypnea with activity • Expiratory wheezing • Normal oxygen saturations	• Usually cared for at home • Prompt relief with inhaled SABA • Possible benefit from course of oral corticosteroids
Moderate	• Dyspnea interferes with activity • Tachypnea interferes with activity • Expiratory wheezing • Mild increased work of breathing • Some accessory muscle use • Normal oxygen saturations	• Usually requires office or ED visit • Relief from frequent inhaled SABA • Oral systemic corticosteroids
Severe	• Dyspnea at rest • Tachypnea at rest • Breathlessness or inability to talk • Expiratory and inspiratory wheezing • Significantly increased work of breathing • Decreased air entry • Accessory muscle use • Oxygen saturations <92%	• Usually requires ED visit and hospitalization • Partial relief from frequent inhaled SABA • Oral systemic corticosteroids • Additional therapies often indicated
Life threatening	• As above in severe category • Altered mental status • Sleepiness	• Requires ED visit and hospitalization • Possible ICU admission • Minimal or no relief from frequent inhaled SABA • IV corticosteroids • Additional therapies indicated • Monitor blood gases, electrolyte • Prepare for intubation

ED, emergency department; ICU, intensive care unit; IV, intravenous; SABA, short-acting bronchodilator agent.
Adapted from the Expert Panel Report 3 (EPR3): *Guidelines for the Diagnosis and Management of Asthma.* Washington, DC, U.S. Department of Health and Human Resources, 2007, p 54. Available at http://www.nhlbi.nih.gov/guidelines/asthma/asthgdln.htm.

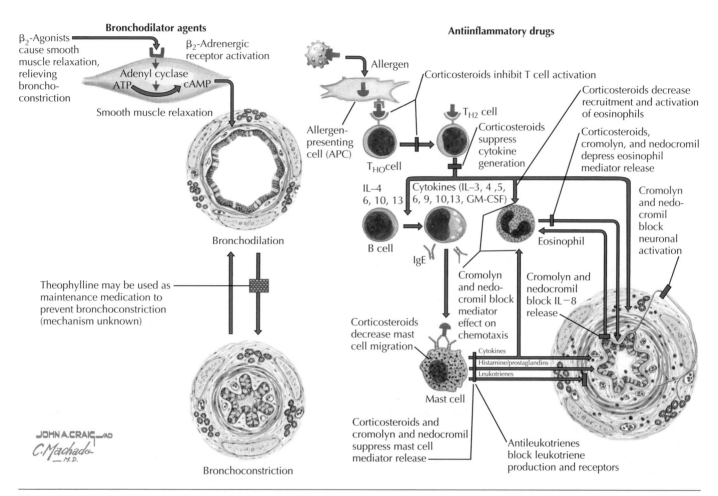

Figure 38-4 *Mechanisms of asthma medications.*

checking serum electrolytes and arterial blood gas values. The medical team must make frequent reassessments of such a patient. The majority of patients who have repeated pulse oximetry values less than 92% or continued symptoms 1 to 2 hours after initiation of acute therapy generally require inpatient hospital admission.

MANAGEMENT

For patients requiring therapy, the mainstays of treatment include administration of bronchodilators and inhaled or systemic corticosteroids (Figures 38-4 and 38-5).

Chronic Disease

For long-term control, an inhaled corticosteroid is the preferred treatment. In general, patients with asthma should receive the minimal therapy indicated to control their symptoms (Table 38-4). If comorbid medical conditions are present, they should also be treated (i.e., a patient with allergic rhinitis should receive intranasal corticosteroids or oral antihistamine therapy). Depending on the severity of a patient's asthma symptoms, he or she should be reassessed at regular intervals after initiation of treatment to evaluate response to therapy and the need for adjustment of therapy.

After being stabilized on a proper regimen, patients should be reevaluated periodically. The most important mitigating factor for future asthma exacerbations is patient adherence to the asthma action plan. The asthma action plan, which outlines both baseline management and the simple steps a patient should follow to escalate treatment during an exacerbation, should be updated at least annually. Patients, parents, and clinicians should review the asthma action plan together, and a written copy should be given to the family to ensure understanding and adherence. When used correctly, asthma action plans have a significant impact on reducing urgent care and ED visits. Additionally, steps should be taken to remove any offending environmental triggers from a patient's daily life, such as exposure to cigarette smoke or other pollutants and allergens. A patient with asthma should receive a yearly influenza vaccination.

Acute Exacerbation

For mild to moderate exacerbations, a patient should increase the frequency of bronchodilator treatments until the patient's symptoms have resolved. A patient who has more severe baseline disease may need to begin a short course of oral steroid therapy (prednisolone or prednisone 1-2 mg/kg/d; maximum, 60 mg/d for 3-10 days). Generally, if symptoms persist for more

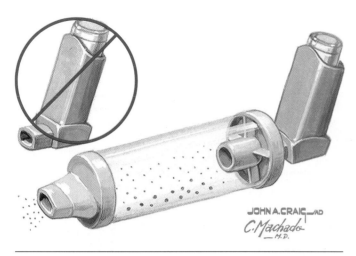

Figure 38-5 *Proper administration of inhaled bronchodilators and corticosteroids.*

than 24 hours or worsen, the patient must be evaluated by a medical caregiver.

In pediatric EDs, immediate therapy usually consists of a nebulized bronchodilator (albuterol 0.15 mg/kg every 20 min for three doses or albuterol 0.5 mg/kg/h by continuous nebulization), nebulized ipratropium (an anticholinergic bronchodilator; 0.25-0.5 mg every 20 minutes for three doses), and oxygen (to keep oxygen saturations above 90%). Oral steroids such as prednisone (loading dose, 2 mg/kg/dose; maximum, 60m g followed by 1 mg/kg/dose twice daily; maximum, 60 mg/d for 3-10 days) should be used to reduce airway inflammation and improve symptoms. If a patient cannot tolerate oral medications because of a worsening respiratory status, intravenous (IV) steroids may be used (loading dose, 2 mg/kg/dose; (maximum, 60 mg followed by 1 mg/kg/dose every 6-12 h; maximum, 60 mg/d for 3-10 days). A steroid taper is indicated in patients requiring a

course lasting more than 10 to 14 days. A patient who fails to respond to treatment within the first 2 hours generally requires inpatient admission and observation.

In severe cases, when a patient is unresponsive to continuous albuterol therapy, additional therapies are used, including subcutaneous epinephrine (0.01 mg/kg every 20 minutes for 3 doses; maximum, 0.5 mg/dose), subcutaneous terbutaline (0.01 mg/kg/dose every 20 minutes for three doses; maximum, 0.4 mg/dose), and IV magnesium (50 mg/kg/dose of magnesium sulfate; maximum, 2000 mg/dose). A patient requiring additional therapy should be treated in an ICU setting and undergo frequent reassessment. Although no additional efficacy over continuous inhaled bronchodilators has been demonstrated, in some cases, IV β-agonists are initiated in the ICU, such as a continuous terbutaline infusion (loading dose, 2-10 μg/kg [0.002-0.01 mg/kg] followed by continuous infusion of 0.1-0.4 μg/kg/min; the dose is titrated by clinical response). A patient receiving IV β-agonist therapy should have continuous electrocardiographic monitoring because of increased myocardial stimulation and should undergo frequent fluid and electrolyte assessments.

For a patient who progresses toward respiratory failure, early controlled endotracheal intubation should occur before complete respiratory failure ensues. Indications for intubation include persistent hypoxemia with maximal noninvasive ventilation, fatigue of the respiratory muscles, altered mental status, or actual respiratory failure.

FUTURE DIRECTIONS

As mentioned in this chapter, recent basic science research at the molecular level has demonstrated that some patients may have different genetic risk factors for the development of asthma. Investigators have used single nucleotide polymorphisms to detect variation in β-adrenergic receptors, cytokine profiles, and

Table 38-4 Stepwise Approach for Managing Asthma Long Term in Children 5 to 12 Years Old						
	Step 1	**Step 2**	**Step 3**	**Step 4**	**Step 5**	**Step 6**
	Intermittent Asthma	**Persistent Asthma: Daily Medications**				
Preferred	SABA PRN	Low-dose ICS	Medium-dose ICS	Medium-dose ICS *and* LABA	High-dose ICS *and* LABA	High-dose ICS *and* Oral corticosteroids *and* LABA
Alternative	None	Cromolyn *or* LTRA *or* Nedocromil *or* Theophylline	Low-dose ICS *and* LABA *or* LTRA *Or* Theophylline	Medium-dose ICS *and* LRTA *or* Theophylline	High-dose ICS *and* LTRA *or* Theophylline	High-dose ICS *and* Oral corticosteroids *and* LTRA *or* Theophylline
	Each step: Patient education, environmental control, and management of comorbidities					
Quick relief medication	Each step: SABA as needed for symptoms with intensity of treatment depending on severity of symptoms					

ICS, inhaled corticosteroid; LABA, long-acting bronchodilator agent; LTRA, leukotriene receptor antagonist; SABA: Short-acting bronchodilator agent.

Adapted from the Expert Panel Report 3 (EPR3): *Guidelines for the Diagnosis and Management of Asthma.* Washington, DC, U.S. Department of Health and Human Resources, 2007, p 43. Available at http://www.nhlbi.nih.gov/guidelines/asthma/asthgdln.htm

antigen responses. The ability to define particular asthma genotypes and phenotypes is especially important given that a growing body of pharmacologic evidence supports the directed use of certain therapies in certain subgroups. For example, several pilot studies have demonstrated that patients homozygous for β-adrenergic receptor gene alleles have altered responses to inhaled long-acting bronchodilators. Although genetic testing is of little use in the acute setting of an initial presentation, as testing becomes more available, it may aid in the management of patients' chronic asthma and long-term control.

CONCLUSION

The overall goal of asthma management is to reduce the morbidity associated with the disease and to decrease the frequency of acute exacerbations. This requires a careful assessment of the patient's symptoms, the institution of an appropriate asthma control regimen, the ongoing education of a patient and his or her family, and interval monitoring to reassess the patient's control of symptoms.

SUGGESTED READINGS

Bhogal S, Zemek R, Ducharme FM: Written action plans for asthma in children, *Cochrane Database Syst Rev* 3:CD005306, 2006.

Bleecker ER, Postma DS, Lawrance RM, et al: Effect of ADRB2 polymorphisms on response to longacting beta2-agonist therapy: a pharmacogenetic analysis of two randomised studies, *Lancet* 370(9605):2118-2125, 2007.

National Heart, Lung, and Blood Institute: Guidelines for the Diagnosis and Management of Asthma, 2007. Available at http://www.nhlbi.nih.gov/guidelines/asthma/index.htm.

Robinson PD, Van Asperen P: Asthma in childhood, *Pediatr Clin North Am* 56(1):191-226, 2009.

Congenital anomalies of the lung are a heterogeneous group of disorders that represent 5% to 18% of all congenital anomalies. All conducting airways are formed by the first 16 weeks of gestation. The gas exchange region of the lung develops after 16 weeks and extends into the first 2 to 4 years of postnatal life. Thus, lesions that cause airway anomalies occur early in lung development. Those that affect the parenchyma usually begin in early gestation during organogenesis, but their impact on lung function can be exacerbated by later gestational events. Many lesions resolve spontaneously antenatally; others are detected only in later life.

This chapter addresses congenital abnormalities in three main components of the respiratory system: airway, parenchyma, and vasculature.

CONGENITAL ANOMALIES OF THE AIRWAY

ETIOLOGY AND PATHOGENESIS

Laryngomalacia is the most common congenital abnormality of the extrathoracic airway. Structural abnormalities that occur in some cases include shortened aryepiglottic folds; a flaccid, omega-shaped epiglottis; and prolapsing arytenoid cartilages. Poor tone and coordination of the laryngeal muscles caused by neuromuscular immaturity contributes to inspiratory collapse of laryngeal structures.

Laryngeal atresia is a life-threatening condition that occurs when the occluded laryngeal lumen fails to recanalize at 10 weeks of gestation. Incomplete recanalization can result in laryngeal webs, which are often associated with DiGeorge or velocardiofacial syndromes. *Congenital subglottic stenosis* is similar in pathogenesis; however, the defect occurs below the glottis at the level of the cricoid cartilage. *Laryngeal clefts* develop between 25 and 35 days in utero because of abnormal separation of the trachea from the foregut.

Tracheomalacia may be either primary or secondary, the latter being more common. In primary tracheomalacia, there is an intrinsic weakness of the tracheal cartilage and sometimes shortening of the cartilage rings so that the posterior membrane comprises a greater proportion of the tracheal circumference. Secondary tracheomalacia results from extrinsic compression of the airway in association with cardiovascular abnormalities such as double aortic arch, or it may be a complication of prolonged intubation, tracheostomy placement, or severe tracheobronchitis.

Tracheoesophageal fistula (TEF) occurs when there is incomplete mesodermal septation of the primitive foregut. The trachea is anatomically abnormal, causing primary malacia. In 85% of cases, there is a proximal blind-ending pouch with a distal fistula (Figure 39-1). The pouch expands and compresses the trachea, thus also causing secondary malacia. Less common types include the H-type fistula and upper esophageal fistula with distal atresia. The fistulae are often small and found between the larynx and the thoracic inlet.

Tracheal stenosis refers to a fixed narrowing of the trachea either from extrinsic compression or from an intrinsic abnormality. Intrinsic tracheal stenosis is usually associated with complete cartilaginous tracheal rings. The rings completely encircle the trachea, and there is absence of the posterior membranous portion. Complete rings are commonly seen in association with a left pulmonary artery sling. The left pulmonary artery arises from the right pulmonary artery and then passes around the right side and behind the carina and then between the trachea and esophagus. *Tracheal atresia* is rare and usually caused by a malformation of the laryngotracheal groove.

Bronchial abnormalities include bronchomalacia, which may be diffuse from intrinsic airway properties, or isolated because of local compression or damage (e.g., after prolonged mechanical ventilation). Williams-Campbell syndrome is a severe form with marked deficiency of airway cartilage. Mounier-Kuhn syndrome is congenital tracheobronchomegaly associated with tracheomalacia and bronchiectasis. Anatomic abnormalities of the bronchi include a tracheal bronchus or "pig bronchus" in which an abnormal bronchus arises from the trachea proximal to the carina rather than from the right main bronchus; it usually supplies a segment of the right upper lobe. An aberrant "bridging bronchus" occurs when the right lower lobe bronchus arises from the left bronchial tree.

CLINICAL PRESENTATION

Airway abnormalities can present with immediate respiratory distress after birth or their presentation may be subtle (e.g., an abnormal cry or difficulty feeding). Inspiratory stridor is often a key feature in laryngeal abnormalities. Increased inspiratory airflow or effort accentuates the stridor (e.g., during crying, feeding or upper respiratory tract infections). Laryngomalacia is associated with other congenital anomalies in 20% of cases. Episodes of recurrent croup in the first 18 months of life or episodes of croup that continue past 5 or 6 years of age should always raise the possibility of a fixed upper airway narrowing such as laryngeal web or subglottic stenosis. Laryngeal clefts can present with the triad of stridor, excessive salivation, and a muted cry. They, similar to the H-type TEF, are also associated with coughing during feedings. Other diagnostic considerations for stridor to consider include congenital hemangiomas and laryngeal cysts.

Patients with tracheomalacia and bronchomalacia may present with a harsh "barking" cough and homophonous wheeze, representing intrathoracic obstruction. Some cases are misdiagnosed as difficult-to-treat asthma. Symptoms of TEF can be varied and include recurrent coughing with feeds, choking or cyanotic spells, and frothing. If symptoms are mild, the diagnosis can be delayed beyond infancy. Recurrent infection in the

A. Tracheoesophageal fistula

Most common form (90% to 95%) of tracheoesophageal fistula. Upper segment of esophagus ending in blind pouch; lower segment originating from trachea just above bifurcation. The two segments may be connected by a solid cord

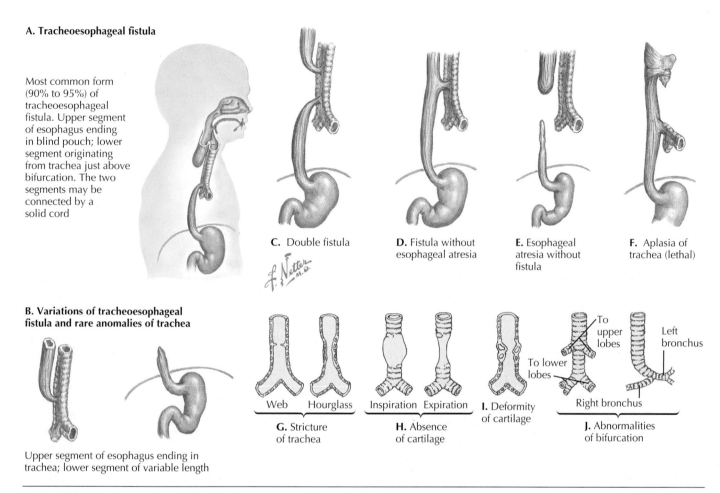

C. Double fistula

D. Fistula without esophageal atresia

E. Esophageal atresia without fistula

F. Aplasia of trachea (lethal)

B. Variations of tracheoesophageal fistula and rare anomalies of trachea

Upper segment of esophagus ending in trachea; lower segment of variable length

Web   Hourglass

G. Stricture of trachea

Inspiration   Expiration

H. Absence of cartilage

I. Deformity of cartilage

To upper lobes

To lower lobes

Left bronchus

Right bronchus

J. Abnormalities of bifurcation

Figure 39-1 *Tracheoesophageal fistula.*

same location of the lung can point to a structural bronchial anomaly, including stenosis or malacia.

EVALUATION AND MANAGEMENT

In most cases of laryngomalacia, a careful history and physical examination are sufficient to make a diagnosis. However, when symptoms are associated with failure to thrive or other laryngeal malformations are being considered, a flexible endoscopy should be performed. Anteroposterior and lateral airway radiographs may also help to localize a fixed anatomic narrowing. If a laryngeal cleft is suspected, a contrast swallow can demonstrate the defect, but a rigid bronchoscopy is also usually necessary. Laryngomalacia is usually a benign entity that resolves without intervention within the first 2 years of life, but aryepiglottoplasty has been used to treat cases associated with severe airway obstruction. Surgical excision or laser ablation is used to treat many laryngeal anomalies, including webs and cysts. Surgery for subglottic stenosis, if warranted, may involve a cricoid split or laryngotracheoplasty. Rarely in these cases or with laryngeal clefts, a tracheostomy is needed to allow for staged repair.

Tracheobronchial abnormalities usually require rigid or flexible bronchoscopy for diagnosis. Areas of extrinsic airway compression should prompt imaging by computed tomography (CT) or magnetic resonance imaging (MRI) to define the offending lesion. Patients with significant obstructive symptoms from tracheomalacia may benefit from an aortopexy, tracheostomy with or without continuous positive airway pressure (CPAP), or use of bronchoconstrictor drugs. Bronchomalacia, if severe, may also require use of CPAP; complications relating to impaired airway clearance often require chest physiotherapy and antibiotic administration.

In suspected cases of TEF, the diagnosis is made by injecting contrast via a nasogastric tube in the prone position and monitoring by fluoroscopy as the tube is withdrawn up from the midesophagus. Surgical repair involves a cervical approach in most cases with ligation of the fistula and either primary or subsequent repair of the atresia. Recurrent laryngeal nerve injury is a risk of the procedure.

CONGENITAL ANOMALIES OF LUNG PARENCHYMA

ETIOLOGY AND PATHOGENESIS

These lesions occur early in lung development, and the degree to which they affect the rest of the lung depends on their size and position. Classification of parenchymal lesions is a controversial topic, but most authors agree that descriptive terms based on

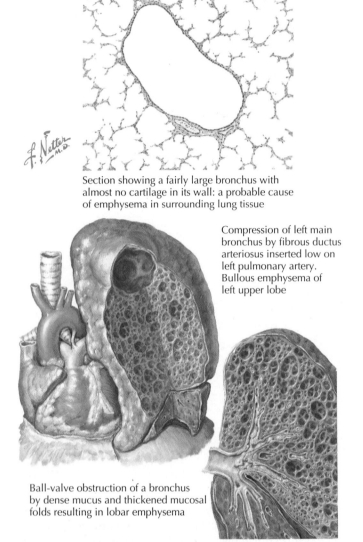

Section showing a fairly large bronchus with almost no cartilage in its wall: a probable cause of emphysema in surrounding lung tissue

Compression of left main bronchus by fibrous ductus arteriosus inserted low on left pulmonary artery. Bullous emphysema of left upper lobe

Ball-valve obstruction of a bronchus by dense mucus and thickened mucosal folds resulting in lobar emphysema

Figure 39-2 *Congenital lobar emphysema.*

imaging (e.g., presence or absence of cysts) are preferable to the assignment of histologic terms until a tissue diagnosis is made.

Congenital lobar emphysema (CLE) describes cases of an overdistended, hyperlucent lobe (Figure 39-2). The most commonly affected region is the left upper lobe (42% of cases). CLE may be caused by partial bronchial obstruction producing a ball-valve effect or a deficiency of bronchial cartilage. Less commonly, alveolar hyperplasia produces a polyalveolar lobe.

Congenital cystic adenomatoid malformation (CCAM) or *congenital pulmonary airway malformation (CPAM)* represents a broad spectrum of hamartomatous defects resulting from developmental arrest during morphogenesis of the bronchial tree. Genetic defects, including mutations in the platelet-derived growth factor B gene, have been proposed to trigger abnormal cell signaling and proliferation resulting in these defects. Histologically, there are five types, although some are not cystic, and only type 3 is adenomatoid. Type 1 is the most common, occurring in 50% of cases. It is usually localized to a single lobe with no

regional predilection (Figure 39-3). The cysts are lined with bronchial cells and hyperplastic mucous cysts. In rare situations, this hyperplasia extends into surrounding parenchyma and is reclassified as bronchoalveolar carcinoma. Type 2 is the next most common histologic pattern consisting of bronchiolar cell hyperplasia within the cysts.

Bronchogenic cysts are a type of foregut duplication cyst produced when a segment of bronchial-type tissue separates from the developing bronchial tree. The cysts are lined with ciliated bronchial epithelium and contain cartilage in their walls, which differentiates them from simple foregut cysts. The majority of these cysts are located in the mediastinum close to the main carina and usually do not communicate with the tracheobronchial tree (see Figure 39-3).

Pulmonary sequestrations are generally thought to be masses of nonfunctioning pulmonary tissue derived from accessory foregut budding. They have no connection with the tracheobronchial tree and receive their arterial supply from the systemic circulation; in 20% of cases, the systemic artery is subdiaphragmatic in origin. Whereas extralobar sequestrations usually have both arterial and venous systemic blood supply, the venous drainage of intralobar sequestrations is by pulmonary veins (Figure 39-4). Extralobar sequestrations are covered by their own pleura; in contrast, intralobar sequestrations are surrounded by the same visceral pleura as the rest of the lung. In 40% of cases of extralobar sequestration, there are associated anomalies, including hindgut duplications or congenital heart defects. Histologically, in both types, there are cystic, nonaerated bronchial and alveolar tissue.

Pulmonary hypoplasia is defined as lung weight more than 2 standard deviations below the normal range for age. Causes include congenital diaphragmatic hernia (CDH), oligohydramnios, thoracic cage anomalies, and giant omphalocele. In cases of CDH, pulmonary hypoplasia most likely occurs before abdominal contents migrate into the thorax, but the additional insult of a space-occupying lesion further contributes to hypoplasia (Figure 39-5).

CLINICAL PRESENTATION

Because of improvements in ultrasound imaging techniques, many parenchymal lung lesions are now detected antenatally at the time of prenatal screening. Postnatally, infants may present early with progressive tachypnea and respiratory distress without signs of upper airway obstruction (no stridor). With large thoracic lesions that interfere with fetal swallowing, there may be a history of polyhydramnios and possible premature labor. In cases of CLE and CCAM, mediastinal shift or pneumothorax may be appreciated on examination. High-output cardiac failure can be present in cases of pulmonary sequestration with significant arteriovenous shunting, but most cases of sequestration are asymptomatic, at least initially. In cases of pulmonary hypoplasia, the precipitating factor may be evident on examination (e.g., a "bell-shaped" chest wall deformity of thoracic dystrophy or scaphoid abdomen of CDH). Other features concerning for possible CDH include mediastinal shift with apparent dextrocardia (90% of cases are left sided), decreased breath sounds over the affected side, and audible bowel sounds in the chest resulting from visceral herniation.

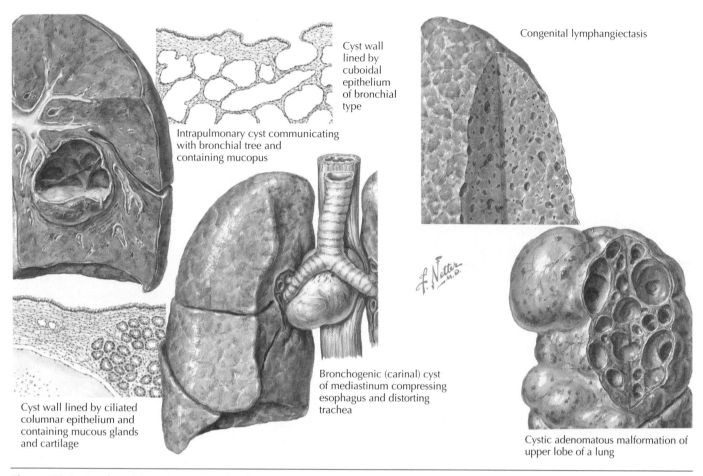

Cyst wall lined by cuboidal epithelium of bronchial type

Intrapulmonary cyst communicating with bronchial tree and containing mucopus

Congenital lymphangiectasis

Cyst wall lined by ciliated columnar epithelium and containing mucous glands and cartilage

Bronchogenic (carinal) cyst of mediastinum compressing esophagus and distorting trachea

Cystic adenomatous malformation of upper lobe of a lung

Figure 39-3 *Congenital bronchogenic and pulmonary cysts.*

Many parenchymal lesions may remain asymptomatic initially but present in later life as recurrent pneumonia in the same location if they become infected; less commonly, an abscess will develop within the lesion. Some lesions will be identified coincidentally on a chest radiograph as a focal solid or cystic mass or area of hyperlucency. Rarely, cystic lesions can present in later life with a pneumothorax or hemothorax or even undergo malignant transformation.

EVALUATION AND MANAGEMENT

Antenatal

Many parenchymal lung lesions can now be diagnosed at least macroscopically on antenatal ultrasonography at the time of screening studies in the second trimester. Lesions are usually identified either by mediastinal shift or the presence of a mass, which may be either cystic or solid. Whereas cysts that are visible on ultrasonography are more suggestive of a CCAM, solid lesions are more consistent with sequestration, especially if they are located in the lower chest. Definitive diagnosis is often not possible until further radiologic imaging such as prenatal ultrafast MRI is performed or histologic testing is done after birth. In addition, many of these lesions can spontaneously involute or remain asymptomatic postnatally; this poses a challenge for management strategies. Intrauterine surgery is

performed in select cases in specialized centers. Fetal tracheal occlusion is an experimental procedure performed in some cases of congenital diaphragmatic hernia in which the airway is occluded in utero in hope that secreted lung fluid will promote further lung growth. In certain cases of CCAM or sequestration, large lesions can be associated with polyhydramnios or hydrops. In these cases, in utero surgical decompression may be considered. Extrauterine intrapartum treatment (EXIT) procedures, in which a surgery is performed with the umbilical circulation left intact to provide gas exchange to a partially delivered fetus, have been performed in circumstances when the lesion or the procedure would render pulmonary gas exchange untenable. In select cases of CCAM, antenatal steroids have been used with moderate success to reduce the size of the lesion and resolve hydrops. In all cases when suspicion for a parenchymal lung lesion persists antenatally, delivery of these infants should be at a center with the necessary neonatal and surgical expertise.

Postnatal

A chest radiograph is the first mode of evaluation whether there was antenatal concern for a lesion or the initial presentation is postnatal respiratory distress. Typical findings in CCAM include the presence of air-filled cystic regions, and in patients with CLE, there may be areas of lobar hyperinflation with mediastinal

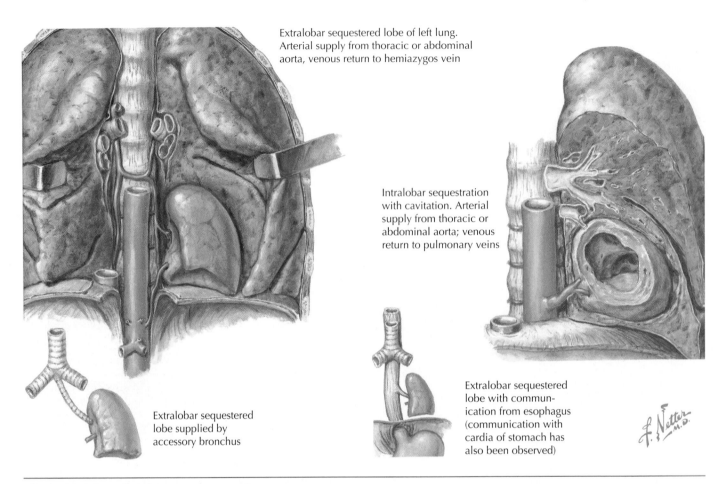

Extralobar sequestered lobe of left lung. Arterial supply from thoracic or abdominal aorta, venous return to hemiazygos vein

Intralobar sequestration with cavitation. Arterial supply from thoracic or abdominal aorta; venous return to pulmonary veins

Extralobar sequestered lobe supplied by accessory bronchus

Extralobar sequestered lobe with communication from esophagus (communication with cardia of stomach has also been observed)

Figure 39-4 *Bronchopulmonary sequestration.*

shift and contralateral atelectasis. A normal chest radiograph does not, however, exclude a significant malformation.

CT scanning can be helpful if radiograph results are normal despite antenatal diagnosis and in cases of older patients with suspected anomalies. CT with contrast is helpful in delineating vascular supply in suspected cases of sequestration. MRI of the chest is becoming more popular because of the lack of radiation exposure to the patient, and it is considered more specific at diagnosing neuroenteric cysts and mucus-containing cysts. Echocardiography can be used to rule out any associated cardiac anomalies. Ultrasonography of the abdomen and chest can be used in suspected cases of diaphragmatic hernia to assess the location, size, and contents of the defect.

Management of a cystic lung lesion, if symptomatic, is usually by surgical resection. This relieves compression of surrounding normal lung and potentially allows for compensatory lung growth in the remaining lung tissue. In cases of CCAM, this can be done either by segmental resection, which is considered for bilateral disease, or by lobectomy if there is localized disease. In CLE, a lobectomy is required unless the lesion is small and asymptomatic; in such cases, it can be monitored for regression. Bronchogenic cysts are typically resected whether symptomatic or not because of the high risk of complications. Sequestrations are also usually resected after the vascular supply has been carefully determined. Embolization of collateral vessels is also sometimes performed.

In cases of asymptomatic CCAM, most institutions propose surgical resection to prevent potential complications of infection and malignancy. However, some authors still support initial observation alone. In infants with CDH, prompt endotracheal intubation with minimal bag-mask ventilation is essential to avoid gaseous distension of the organs in the chest cavity. Many infants will have significant pulmonary hypertension and may require stabilization on extracorporeal membrane oxygenation (ECMO) before surgical repair. Surgical options include primary repair of the diaphragmatic defect and a patch insertion for larger defects.

PULMONARY VASCULAR MALFORMATIONS

ETIOLOGY AND PATHOGENESIS

Pulmonary vascular malformations are rare congenital anomalies, but when present, they can cause significant morbidity. *Pulmonary arteriovenous malformations* (AVMs) can be found as isolated lesions or in association with another parenchymal anomaly (e.g., sequestration). Most commonly, they occur in association with hereditary hemorrhagic telangiectasia. *Alveolar capillary dysplasia* (ACD) is a life-threatening malformation of poorly developed alveolar capillaries often associated with misalignment of the pulmonary veins, which travel in the

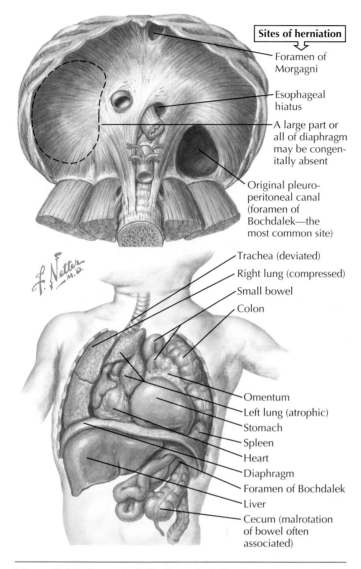

Sites of herniation

Foramen of Morgagni

Esophageal hiatus

A large part or all of diaphragm may be congenitally absent

Original pleuro-peritoneal canal (foramen of Bochdalek—the most common site)

Trachea (deviated)

Right lung (compressed)

Small bowel

Colon

Omentum

Left lung (atrophic)

Stomach

Spleen

Heart

Diaphragm

Foramen of Bochdalek

Liver

Cecum (malrotation of bowel often associated)

Figure 39-5 *Congenital diaphragmatic hernia.*

bronchoarterial bundle rather than in the septae. *Scimitar syndrome* is another rare vascular anomaly involving aberrant pulmonary venous drainage, usually of the right lung to the inferior vena cava below the diaphragm.

CLINICAL PRESENTATION

Large PAVMs present with evidence of right-to-left shunting with cyanosis, exercise limitation, and occasionally cardiac failure. Patients often have evidence of digital clubbing and a systolic murmur. Occasionally, a bruit can be heard over the AVM; this can be accentuated by having the patient inspire against a closed glottis (Mueller maneuver). Hemoptysis is also a concerning feature. There may be evidence of telangiectasias on the lips, under the tongue, between the fingers, or elsewhere. Scimitar syndrome can also present in infancy with cardiac failure and respiratory distress. Here, however, the shunt is left to right, cyanosis is absent, and the respiratory distress is likely the result of associated pulmonary hypoplasia or congenital

heart disease. ACD presents with progressive respiratory failure and pulmonary hypertension in early life that is typically refractory to all forms of treatment. These infants will improve with ECMO but will not tolerate its withdrawal.

EVALUATION AND MANAGEMENT

The chest radiograph can be normal or it may reveal only poorly defined opacities or a "vascular blush." In cases of scimitar syndrome, the typical scimitar sign representing the anomalous vein can be seen. A contrast echocardiogram ("bubble study") in which agitated saline is injected can disclose the late phase shunt typical of PAVMs. High-resolution contrast CT scanning, pulmonary angiography, or cardiac catheterization, however, is usually necessary for definitive diagnosis. PAVMs can often be managed by embolization using coils or sclerosing agents, but surgical resection is occasionally required. The prognosis in cases of multiple AVMs is poor, and lung transplantation may be the only recourse in some instances. Scimitar syndrome can be managed expectantly or initially by coil embolization of the anomalous vessel. If correction is required, however, definitive surgery with redirection of the anomalous vein to the left atrium is eventually required. Diagnosis of ACD can only be made by lung biopsy. If not managed with lung transplantation as soon as possible, the condition is fatal.

FUTURE DIRECTIONS

As antenatal screening has become more routine and imaging techniques have improved, we now know that many of these lesions regress spontaneously. Physicians thus are being faced with the dilemma of when to intervene and how best to follow those lesions treated expectantly. Additionally, some malformations are only diagnosed incidentally. Therefore, there is a need for documentation of long-term outcomes of all cases of congenital lung lesions, including those treated antenatally.

Nomenclature of congenital lung parenchymal lesions remains confusing, with various terms used by different authors; for example, CCAM, CPAM, and cystic congenital thoracic malformation all refer to a similar but unclear diagnosis. A universal classification system needs to be developed to avoid confusion over diagnosis.

Strategies for postnatal diagnosis also continue to be refined with MRI in particular offering an imaging modality free of radiation. Controversy remains also as to whether "compensatory" lung growth occurs in infants with pulmonary hypoplasia. Many infants who are temporized in infancy and early childhood may well outgrow their pulmonary vascular supply as teenagers or young adults, thus rendering them the sickest in this complex group. Ongoing research is addressing methods of stimulating lung growth both in and ex utero for infants with pulmonary hypoplasia.

SUGGESTED READINGS

Abdalla SA, Geisthoff UW, Bonneau D, et al: Visceral manifestations in hereditary haemorrhagic telangiectasia type 2, *J Med Genet* 40:494-502, 2003.

Adzick NS: Management of fetal lung lesions, *Clin Perinatol* 30(3):481-492, 2003.

Azizkhan RG, Crombleholme TM: Congenital cystic lung disease: contemporary antenatal and postnatal management, *Pediatr Surg Int* 24(6):643-657, 2008.

Boogaard R, Huijsmans SH, Pijnenburg MW, et al: Tracheomalacia and bronchomalacia in children: incidence and patient characteristics, *Chest* 128(5):3391-3397, 2005.

Daniel SJ: The upper airway: congenital malformations, *Paeditar Respir Rev* 7(suppl 1):S260-S263, 2006.

Doyle NM, Lally KP: The CDH Study Group and advances in the clinical care of the patient with congenital diaphragmatic hernia, *Semin Perinatol* 28(3):174-184, 2004.

Houben CH, Curry JI: Current status of prenatal diagnosis, operative management and outcome of esophageal atresia/tracheo-esophageal fistula, *Prenat Diagn* 28(7):667-675, 2008.

Kussman BD, Geva T, McGowan FX: Cardiovascular causes of airway compression, *Paediatr Anaesth* 14(1):60-74, 2004.

Langston C: New concepts in the pathology of congenital lung malformations, *Semin Pediatr Surg* 12(1):17-37, 2003.

Masters IB: Congenital airway lesions and lung disease, *Pediatr Clin North Am* 56(1):227-242, 2009.

Wilson RD, Hedrick HL, Liechty KW, et al: Cystic adenomatoid malformation of the lung: review of genetics, prenatal diagnosis and in utero treatment, *Am J Med Genet* 140A:151-155, 2006.

40

Pleural Effusions and Pneumothorax

Jason B. Caboot

Pleural effusions and pneumothoraces occur as a result of structural and mechanical abnormalities of the pleural space. Abnormalities of the pleural space are an important cause of morbidity and mortality in infants and children worldwide, and the number of children who develop clinically significant pleural effusions is increasing. Pleural effusions are the result of excessive fluid accumulation in the pleural space, and pneumothoraces occur as a result of the accumulation of air within the pleural space. To better understand the pathophysiology of pleural effusions and pneumothoraces, it is essential to understand the anatomy of the pleural space. The pleural space is a potential anatomic space, approximately 10 to 20 μm wide, located between the visceral and parietal pleurae. The visceral pleura lines the surface of the lung parenchyma, including the interlobar fissures, and the parietal pleura lines the inner surface of the chest wall, mediastinum, and diaphragm (Figure 40-1). The pleural space contains a small amount of fluid (0.3 mL/kg body weight) that is in equilibrium between the amount of fluid formed (filtered) and the amount removed (absorbed).

PLEURAL EFFUSIONS

Starling forces normally govern the amount of pleural fluid that is formed by the subpleural capillaries of the visceral pleura and the amount that is removed by stomata in the parietal pleura and lymphatic system. If the flow of fluid into the pleural space exceeds the amount absorbed, excess fluid accumulates in the pleural space.

ETIOLOGY AND PATHOGENESIS

Pleural effusions are the result of an imbalance of hydrostatic and oncotic pressures between the blood in the pulmonary capillary bed and fluid in the pleural space, an alteration in permeability of the pleural membranes, or inadequate uptake by the lymphatic system. Pleural effusions can be divided into transudates and exudates. *Exudative* effusions occur from pleural inflammation or lymphatic flow obstruction. *Transudative* effusions occur when there is an imbalance between the formation and reabsorption of pleural fluid. Pleural fluid analysis determines whether the effusion is transudative or exudative. Because exudative effusions result from inflammation of the pleural membranes and leaky capillaries, large molecules such as cholesterol, lactate dehydrogenase (LDH), and proteins enter the pleural space. Conversely, the protein, LDH, and cholesterol levels in transudates are low because the filtration properties of the pleural membranes are not altered.

Typically, small amounts of protein are filtered into the pleural space and are readily absorbed by the parietal pleura via the lymphatic system. If increased amounts of protein enter the pleural space, especially when accompanied by increased capillary permeability (e.g., in pneumonia), the lymphatic system cannot absorb the excessive protein, and an exudative pleural effusion forms. The most common cause of exudative pleural effusions in children is bacterial pneumonia. Additional causes include connective tissue diseases, metastatic intrathoracic malignancy, subdiaphragmatic abscess, and aspiration pneumonitis. Transudative effusions in children are typically associated with overhydration, atelectasis, nephrotic syndrome, and congestive left heart failure. Correcting the oncotic and hydrostatic pressures usually results in resolution of a transudate; drainage of the fluid is only needed for immediate symptomatic relief.

An exudative pleural effusion that is associated with pneumonia is referred to as a *parapneumonic effusion*. Parapneumonic effusions result from the spread of inflammatory cells and infecting organisms into the pleural space. Initially, the pleurae become inflamed, and the leakage of proteins and leukocytes into the pleural space forms the effusion. Initially, the fluid is sterile with a low leukocyte count. As a parapneumonic effusion progresses and bacteria leak into the pleural space, the pleural fluid becomes purulent, and the effusion is referred to as an *empyema*, occurring in approximately 0.6% of childhood pneumonia. Loculations (parietal–visceral pleural adhesions) and septations (fibrous strands) form within parapneumonic effusions as the pleural fluid exudate thickens and deposition of fibrin occurs within the pleural space.

The risk of a child developing an empyema increases in certain underlying diseases, such as immunodeficiencies, malignancy, Down syndrome, congenital heart disease, tuberculosis, and cystic fibrosis (CF). *Streptococcus pneumoniae* remains the most common pathogen causing parapneumonic effusions. Community-acquired methicillin-resistant *Staphylococcus aureus* is an increasingly common cause of both parapneumonic effusions and empyemas. Empyemas can also be caused by the rupture of lung abscesses into the pleural space; by bacteria entering the pleural space from trauma, thoracic surgery, mediastinitis; or through the spread of intraabdominal abscesses. Complications associated with parapneumonic effusions and empyemas are infrequent in children but include bronchopleural fistula, lung abscess, and empyema necessitatis (perforation through the chest wall). Boys and girls are affected equally by empyemas, and the morbidity and mortality are highest in children younger than 2 years of age.

CLINICAL PRESENTATION

The size of the effusion, the underlying cause, and when in the course a child presents all determine the clinical presentation. Children with small pleural effusions may be asymptomatic. As the effusion enlarges, it limits lung inflation, causing a decrease in vital capacity. Furthermore, if present, pleural inflammation is associated with dyspnea, chest tightness, and chest pain that is exaggerated by deep breathing, coughing, and straining; all of these further limit full lung expansion. The pain, resulting from stretching of parietal pleura nerve fibers, is often described as a

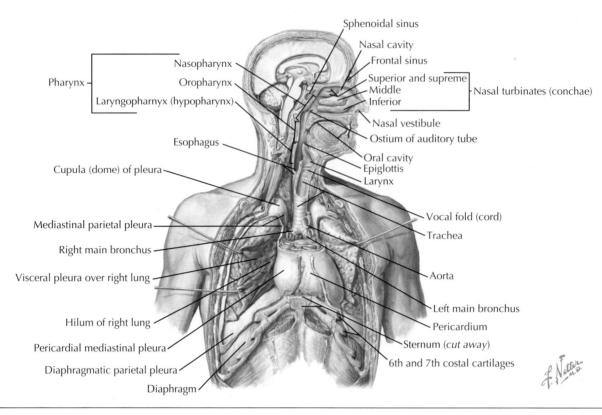

Figure 40-1 *Pleural space.*

dull ache that worsens with inspiration. The pain is often localized over the chest wall and is referred to the shoulder or the back. Often the child will attempt to decrease the pain by lying on the affected side in an attempt to splint it during breathing.

On physical examination, a child with a significant pleural effusion can appear ill but is rarely toxic appearing. Most children are tachypneic with shallow breathing to minimize the pain. It is important to look for signs and symptoms of underlying conditions that predispose to the development of pleural effusions. If the child has an empyema, he or she is usually febrile with a cough and malaise. If a child is being appropriately treated for pneumonia and is not improving within 48 hours, a parapneumonic effusion must be suspected. A malignant effusion must be suspected in a child with an effusion accompanied by a mediastinal mass or lymphadenopathy. A history of recurrent serious bacterial infections, failure to thrive, or chronic diarrhea is suggestive of a primary immunodeficiency.

Because of splinting toward the affected side, the child may appear to have mild scoliosis. There can be ipsilateral bulging of the intercostal spaces and contralateral displacement of the heart and trachea. A pleural friction rub caused by roughened pleural surfaces may be the only physical examination finding early in the course of disease, heard during inspiration and exhalation. As the pleural effusion increases and separates the pleural membranes, the plural rub disappears. Diminished thoracic wall excursion, decreased breath sounds, dullness to percussion, and decreased tactile and vocal fremitus can be observed over the affected area in an older child with a moderate effusion. If pneumonia is present, crackles and rhonchi can also be audible. In infants, the physical signs of an effusion are less noticeable. Breath sounds can be deceptively loud and clear throughout both lungs because of the small lung volume in an infant.

EVALUATION AND MANAGEMENT

Children with the clinical history and findings suggestive of a pleural effusion should be evaluated with an upright chest radiograph and a lateral decubitus view (Figure 40-2). Performing radiographic examinations with the child in multiple positions helps to demonstrate a shift in the effusion with position changes. These radiographic images can help in making the diagnosis of pleural effusion and in determining the need for thoracocentesis or chest tube placement.

Radiographic signs of pleural effusion include a homogenous density overlying the normal markings of the underlying lung, obliteration of the costophrenic angle, the "meniscus sign" or "pleural stripe" (a rim of fluid ascending the lateral chest wall), and possible scoliosis. Infants or children whose radiograph is taken in a recumbent position will not have a meniscus, but instead demonstrate only a denser hemithorax on the affected side. Air-fluid levels within the pleural space suggest the presence of gas-forming organisms, pneumothorax, perforated viscus, or bronchopleural fistula. If there is no shift in the fluid on chest radiograph with a change in position, the effusion is most likely a loculated empyema.

Ultrasonography is useful in confirming the presence of fluid in the pleural space. Additionally, if a child has findings consistent with a parapneumonic effusion, ultrasonography should be undertaken to determine whether loculations are present.

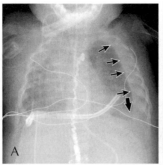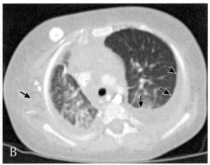

Anteroposterior chest radiograph of a child with congenital lymphangiectasis, demonstrating a prominent left-sided pleural effusion. Note the "pleural stripe" (thin arrows) and blunted costophrenic angle (thick arrow) in the left hemithorax. This child had previously undergone pleurodesis of the right lung, a procedure where the parietal and visceral plurae are mechanically abraded so that they stick together and prevent accumulation of fluid in the pleural space.

Axial computed tomogram of the same patient, demonstrating a prominent rim of fluid in the pleural space in the left hemithrorax (arrows). A smaller effusion is also present in the right hemithorax, where pleurodesis had been performed.

Figure 40-2 *Pleural effusion.*

Chest computed tomography (CT) can also be helpful in determining the presence of pleural fluid; however, CT findings do not typically affect management decisions, and they should not be performed routinely in the evaluation of children with pleural effusions. Chest CT can be useful in the evaluation of complicated cases when more detail about the effusion or the underlying lung parenchyma is desired.

When infection is in the differential diagnosis, pleural fluid aspiration via thoracocentesis should be performed if at least 1 cm of fluid is seen on decubitus radiographs to determine the type of effusion (i.e., infectious exudate, empyema, hydrothorax, hemothorax, or chylothorax) before starting therapy (Figure 40-3). Certain laboratory studies should always be performed on the pleural fluid aspirate. Additional laboratory studies should also be obtained during the evaluation of a child with a parapneumonic effusion or empyema (Table 40-1). Microbiologic studies of the pleural fluid can identify a causative organism, and the analysis of pleural fluid is helpful in guiding

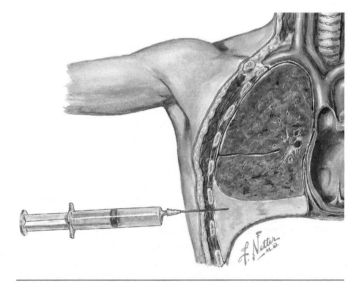

Figure 40-3 *Pleural fluid aspiration.*

Table 40-1 Laboratory Studies Obtained at Time of Pleural Fluid Aspiration	
Pleural fluid	Protein, pH, glucose, LDH, cholesterol Differential cell count Gram stain and cultures (bacterial, fungal, and mycobacterial) Latex agglutination studies (especially if antibiotics have been administered before pleural fluid aspiration) Specific or broad-range PCR studies Cytology (if malignancy is suspected)
Serum	Complete blood cell count with differential Serum LDH (pleural fluid:serum LDH ratio >0.6 is indicative of an exudate) Serum protein (pleural fluid:serum protein >0.5 is indicative of an exudate) Glucose Blood culture (in children with a parapneumonic effusion) CRP (useful in monitoring therapeutic progress)
Miscellaneous	Sputum culture Mantoux testing and sputum (or gastric aspirates) for AFB in patients with risk factors for tuberculosis

AFB, acid-fast bacilli; CRP, C-reactive protein; LDH, lactic dehydrogenase; PCR, polymerase chain reaction.

therapeutic options. Pleural fluid can be obtained through thoracocentesis, aspiration under ultrasonographic guidance, or through video-assisted thoracoscopic surgery (VATS), depending on the presence of loculations or the availability of pediatric surgeons trained in VATS.

There are no definitive management approaches for children with exudative pleural effusions. The aim of treatment is to aspirate the pleural fluid, sterilize the pleural cavity, decrease the duration of symptoms, and ensure full expansion of the lung with return to normal function. Therapeutic options include administration of systemic antibiotics; thoracocentesis; chest tube thoracostomy with or without instillation of fibrinolytic agents; and more invasive techniques, including thoracoscopic surgery (i.e., VATS), mini-thoracotomy, or standard thoracotomy with decortication (removal of fibrinous "peel" from the lungs). Some clinicians have suggested that children with loculated effusions documented on ultrasonography proceed directly to VATS but those with free fluid undergo initial thoracocentesis with administration of systemic antibiotics. Most children improve with antibiotic therapy and simple drainage. However, early, more invasive therapies (i.e., chest tube placement with or without fibrinolytic therapy or VATS) may result in a shorter duration of illness and length of hospital stay.

A chest tube drain should be considered for any of the following pleural fluid findings suggestive of a complicated empyema: frank pus or positive gram stain, pH below 7.0, LDH level above 1000 IU/dL, or glucose level below 40 mg/dL. Additionally, children who have effusions that are enlarging or compromising respiratory function require chest tube insertion and drainage of the pleural effusion.

Supportive care for children with parapneumonic effusions and empyema includes antipyretics, adequate analgesia with nonsteroidal antiinflammatory agents, and early mobilization. Sedatives and analgesics that can cause central respiratory depression should be used cautiously with close monitoring of respiratory status. Intravenous (IV) fluids should be administered if the child refuses oral intake or is unable to drink.

All children with a parapneumonic effusion or empyema should be treated with antibiotics. In mild cases, this can include broad-spectrum oral antibiotics and close observation with chest radiographs on an outpatient basis. Children with empyema should be hospitalized and treated with IV antibiotics in doses adequate to ensure pleural penetration. The choice of antibiotic coverage should be based on the suspected causative organism. Most clinicians agree on continuing IV antibiotic therapy as long as the child is febrile; however, the duration of IV antibiotic therapy after resolution of fever is controversial. Some clinicians continue IV antibiotics for 48 hours after the patient becomes afebrile or after the chest drain is removed; others continue IV therapy for up to 2 weeks.

For both medical and surgical options, the chest tube can be removed when the patient is clinically improved and the chest tube drainage has slowed. Evidence of clinical resolution includes the following: absence of fever, overall sense of well-being, improved chest radiograph and ultrasound appearance, and decrease in white blood cell count and acute-phase reactants.

With appropriate therapy, children with parapneumonic effusions should clinically improve within the first few days of treatment. Those with empyema typically have more protracted courses. If a child with chest tube drain remains febrile or tachypneic and aeration does not improve, the chest tube may be obstructed or fail to drain because of the development of loculations.

Children with a pleural effusion should have a follow-up chest radiograph 1 to 2 months after discharge from the hospital. These children should continue to be followed until they have recovered completely and their chest radiographs have returned to near normal. This usually occurs by 3 to 6 months but may take as long as 16 months. Patients can have residual dullness to percussion and decreased breath sounds over the affected areas related to pleural thickening.

Despite the marked abnormalities at the time of presentation, the majority of children make a complete recovery. Long-term follow-up studies suggest that fewer than 10% of children have residual symptoms. Patients with residual restrictive abnormalities in lung function are usually asymptomatic and have normal exercise tolerance.

PNEUMOTHORAX

Pneumothorax is the accumulation of extrapulmonary air in the pleural space. A pneumothorax typically results from leakage of air from within the lung through the visceral pleura, but air can also enter the pleural space from a defect in the parietal pleura (Figure 40-4). Pneumothoraces are uncommon in children but can be life threatening.

ETIOLOGY AND PATHOGENESIS

A pneumothorax can be classified as spontaneous, traumatic, or catamenial. Spontaneous pneumothorax is the most common type that occurs in children. Traumatic pneumothorax is caused by blunt or penetrating trauma to the chest, by injury from a diagnostic or therapeutic procedure (i.e., subclavian line placement, thoracocentesis, or transbronchial biopsy), or as a consequence of mechanical ventilation. Catamenial pneumothorax (thoracic endometriosis) is a rare disorder that occurs exclusively in women of reproductive age who present with a spontaneous pneumothorax within 24 to 48 hours of the onset of menstruation. The mechanism is uncertain, but this type of pneumothorax is thought to result from the passage of intraabdominal air through diaphragmatic defects. Spontaneous pneumothorax, which occurs in the absence of identified trauma, is subdivided into primary and secondary types.

Primary Spontaneous Pneumothorax

Primary spontaneous pneumothorax occurs in children without trauma or an underlying lung disease that predisposes to air leaking into the pleural space. Primary pneumothorax is more likely to occur in teenagers and young adults who are usually tall and thin and more often in men than women. In particular, children with collagen synthesis defects such as Ehlers-Danlos and Marfan syndromes are prone to pneumothorax. Often, apical blebs can be detected in patients with primary spontaneous pneumothorax by chest CT imaging or during surgical

Pathophysiology

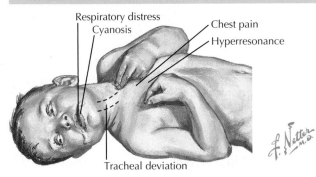

Inspiration

Expiration

Air enters pleural cavity through lung wound or ruptured bleb (or occasionally via penetrating chest wound) with valve-like opening. Ipsilateral lung collapses, and mediastinum shifts to opposite side, compressing contralateral lung and impairing its ventilating capacity

Intrapleural pressure rises, closing valve-like opening, preventing escape of pleural air. Pressure is thus progressively increased with each breath. Mediastinal and tracheal shifts are augmented, diaphragm is depressed, and venous return is impaired by increased pressure and vena caval distortion

Clinical manifestations

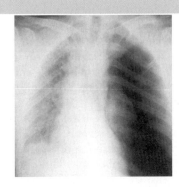

Left-sided tension pneumothorax. Lung collapsed, mediastinum and trachea deviated to opposite side, diaphragm depressed, intercostal spaces widened

Figure 40-4 *Tension pneumothorax.*

procedures. The cause of the blebs is uncertain. Snorting cocaine and smoking marijuana also predispose children to spontaneous pneumothorax.

Secondary Spontaneous Pneumothorax

Secondary spontaneous pneumothorax occurs as a complication of an underlying lung disease, such as chronic obstructive pulmonary disease, in older individuals. Pneumothorax can occur in children with pneumonia complicated by empyema (pyopneumothorax), rupture of an emphysematous bleb during an asthma exacerbation, or with CF. A pneumothorax can also occur in children with underlying malignancies or lymphoma and in children with graft-versus-host disease who develop bronchiolitis obliterans and the subsequent formation of multiple bullae. The incidence is also relatively high in infants with staphylococcal pneumonia.

A small pneumothorax can be well tolerated, and the child will frequently be asymptomatic; in contrast, a large pneumothorax usually causes physiologic abnormalities. When air enters the pleural space as the result of a pneumothorax, the lung collapses because the outward pull of the chest wall is uncoupled from the inward recoil of the lung. The intrapleural pressure may remain atmospheric with a small pneumothorax. However,

when air enters the pleural space during inspiration but cannot exit during exhalation (tension pneumothorax), the continuing air leak causes increased positive pressure in the pleural space that is higher than atmospheric pressure. This results in further compression of the lung, a shift of the mediastinal structures toward the contralateral side, decreased venous return, and decreased cardiac output (see Figure 40-4).

CLINICAL PRESENTATION

The clinical presentation of a pneumothorax depends on the extent of lung collapse and the amount of underlying lung disease. The most common presenting symptom is acute chest pain, which is typically sharp or stabbing and may be preceded by a popping sensation. The pain is diffuse on the affected side with radiation to the ipsilateral shoulder. Dyspnea, cyanosis, tachypnea, and tachycardia are often seen.

Physical examination findings include decreased chest excursion, diminished breath sounds, and hyperresonant percussion on the affected side. The larynx, trachea, and heart can be shifted toward the contralateral side, especially in tension pneumothorax. It may be difficult to diagnose a pneumothorax in infancy because the symptoms and physical signs can be difficult to recognize.

EVALUATION AND MANAGEMENT

The diagnosis of a pneumothorax is verified radiographically (see Figure 40-4). Lateral and anteroposterior views of the chest can confirm the presence of intrapleural air that appears to outline the visceral pleura. Expiratory views accentuate the contrast between lung markings and the hyperlucency of the air in the pleural space. The trachea and mediastinum shift away from the pneumothorax, especially in the case of a tension pneumothorax. However, if both lungs are poorly compliant, as in patients with CF or respiratory distress syndrome, the unaffected lung may not collapse easily, and the shift may not occur.

Often, it is necessary to differentiate a pneumothorax from localized or generalized emphysema, emphysematous blebs, cystic formations (e.g., congenital lobar emphysema), diaphragmatic hernia, compensatory overexpansion with contralateral atelectasis, and gaseous distension of the stomach, which radiographically can mimic air in the pleural space. In most cases, a chest CT or contrast studies differentiate these conditions.

If a patient has significant respiratory distress, an arterial blood gas analysis should be done. Hypoxemia can occur because of alveolar hypoventilation, ventilation/perfusion mismatch, and intrapulmonary shunt. Hypercapnia is usually not present unless the child has underlying lung disease.

Treatment varies with the extent of lung collapse, cause of the collapse, extent of respiratory distress, and severity of underlying lung disease. Therapies are aimed at removal of air from the pleural space and prevention of recurrence. In addition to treating the air leak, the aggressive treatment of underlying pulmonary disease, when present, is essential. A small (<5% of the involved hemithorax) or moderate-sized pneumothorax in an otherwise healthy child can resolve spontaneously, usually within 1 week. These children can be observed in an outpatient setting if serial chest radiographs are obtained and emergency care is available if needed. However, if there is more than a 5% collapse or if the pneumothorax is recurrent or under tension, hospitalization is usually warranted. Analgesia should be used to decrease the pleural pain.

If the communication between the alveoli and pleural space is eliminated, the air in the pleural space is gradually reabsorbed. Administration of 100% supplemental oxygen can hasten the rate of pleural air absorption. Oxygen replaces nitrogen in the extrapulmonary air, allowing for enhanced gas absorption and resolution of the pneumothorax.

The aspiration of pleural air via a needle thoracostomy is necessary for pneumothoraces that occupy more than 15% of the involved hemithorax; if a tension pneumothorax is suspected; or if the child has severe dyspnea, hypoxemia, or significant pain (see Figure 40-4). Needle aspiration is associated with a recurrence risk of 20% to 50%; therefore, close follow-up is required. If a child has failed a needle aspiration, has a large pneumothorax, or is having recurrent spontaneous pneumothoraces, a thoracostomy tube should be placed; pigtail catheters are frequently used. A water seal device or one-way Heimlich valve should be used to prevent reaccumulation of the air.

Surgical intervention in the treatment of spontaneous pneumothorax is controversial. However, good evidence suggests that surgery is warranted to treat persistent air leaks and to prevent recurrence. Surgery for a pneumothorax involves stapling or oversewing ruptured blebs or tears in the visceral pleura and resection of abnormal lung tissue. This procedure is done via VATS, mini-thoracotomy, or open thoracotomy. Repair by VATS is associated with less morbidity than that related to traditional open thoracotomy.

Chemical pleurodesis (intrapleural instillation of a sclerosing agent) can be performed during chest tube placement or at the time of surgery to induce the formation of strong adhesions between the lung and chest wall and decrease the risk of recurrence. Sclerosing agents include talc, tetracycline, doxycycline, fibrin glue, or autologous blood patches. Most studies in adults do not support the use of chemical pleurodesis through a chest tube unless there is a persistent air leak and a patient refuses surgery or a contraindication to surgery exists. Mechanical pleurodesis, accomplished by directly stripping and abrading the pleura with gauze during surgery, leaves inflamed intrapleural surfaces that heal with sealing adhesions.

Information about the prognosis after a spontaneous pneumothorax in children is based on adult patients, in whom there is a substantial recurrence risk. The majority of recurrences develop within 1 year of the initial event, after which the risk decreases. Activities such as deep sea diving and flying in small, unpressurized aircraft are associated with increased risk of pneumothorax and should be avoided in individuals who did not undergo pleurodesis.

FUTURE DIRECTIONS

Despite the improvement in the technology available for diagnosing and treating pleural effusions in children, management remains controversial. This is particularly true in children with parapneumonic effusions or empyema because there is no consensus on the role of medical versus surgical management, and there is no consensus on whether surgery should be the initial treatment of choice or reserved for failed medical management. Although there have been a few prospective, randomized controlled trials comparing the various treatment options, additional trials are necessary before standards based on high-quality evidence for the treatment of pleural effusions in children can be developed.

As with pleural effusions, much of the information about pediatric spontaneous pneumothoraces is limited, and most of the published therapeutic guidelines are based on adult data. Thus, although indications for conservative therapy in children with pneumothoraces are fairly well accepted, the criteria for specific drainage procedures remain controversial. Further studies evaluating the role of surgical management options and outcomes are needed for children with pneumothoraces.

SUGGESTED READINGS

Avansino JR, Goldman B, Sawin RS, et al: Primary operative versus nonoperative therapy for pediatric empyema: a meta-analysis, *Pediatrics* 115:1652-1659, 2005.

Balfour-Lynn IM, Abrahamson E, Cohen G, et al: BTS guidelines for the management of pleural infection in children, *Thorax* 60(Suppl 1):i1-i21, 2005.

Baumann MH: Management of spontaneous pneumothorax, *Clin Chest Med* 27:369-381, 2006.

Baumann MH, Strange C, Heffner JE, et al: Management of spontaneous pneumothorax: an American College of Chest Physicians Delphi consensus statement, *Chest* 119:590-602, 2001.

Jaffé A, Balfour-Lynn IM: Management of empyema in children, *Pediatr Pulmonol* 40:148-156, 2005.

Sahn SA, Heffner JE: Spontaneous pneumothorax, *N Engl J Med* 342:868-874, 2000.

Schultz KD, Fan LL, Pinsky J, et al: The changing face of pleural empyemas in children: epidemiology and management, *Pediatrics* 113:1735-1740, 2004.

Shaw KS, Prasil P, Nguyen LT, et al: Pediatric spontaneous pneumothorax, *Semin Pediatr Surg* 12:55-61, 2003.

Cystic Fibrosis

41

Paul McNally

*C*ystic fibrosis (CF) is the most common fatal hereditary disease of Caucasians. The disease is caused by a defect in the CF transmembrane conductance regulator (CFTR), an epithelial chloride channel. Defective electrolyte transport in epithelial cells of several exocrine organs, including the lungs, pancreas, liver, and gastrointestinal (GI) tract, leads to accumulation of viscid secretions in these organs. The most common clinical manifestations are recurrent respiratory infections and failure to thrive from GI malabsorption. Chronic pulmonary infection and inflammation ultimately result in parenchymal lung damage and respiratory failure, the most common cause of death in patients with CF. The mean survival of patients with CF has markedly improved over the past few decades, and many new therapies are currently in development with the hope of continuing this trend.

ETIOLOGY AND PATHOGENESIS

CF is caused by defects in a single gene on the long arm of chromosome 7, which codes for the CFTR. The protein is a cyclic adenosine monophosphate regulated chloride channel. More than 1400 mutations in the *CFTR* gene have been described to date. Defective *CFTR* function leads to abnormal electrolyte transport at epithelial surfaces, resulting in the net reabsorption of water and dehydration of luminal secretions (Figure 41-1). Accumulation of these viscid secretions results in obstruction, inflammation, tissue damage, and progressive scarring in a number of organs. Despite the discovery of the gene for CF in 1989, much of the pathogenesis of this complicated condition remains to be understood. The disease is inherited in an autosomal recessive manner, with an annual incidence in the United States of approximately one in 3,500 live births. There is a significantly higher carrier frequency in whites compared with other groups.

The bulk of morbidity and mortality associated with CF is related to lung disease. Here, excessive sodium and water resorption from the airway surface leads to dehydrated mucus that is hard to clear effectively. Impaired airway clearance and defects in airway innate defense facilitate chronic bacterial colonization and intermittent acute infection. CF lung disease is thus characterized by a self-perpetuating cycle of airway obstruction, chronic bacterial infection, and airway inflammation. Ultimately, inflammatory destruction of lung tissue results in progressive bronchiectasis, further impairing airway clearance and facilitating this chronic cycle of infection and inflammation (Figure 41-2). A similar cycle of chronic inflammation and infection occurs in the paranasal sinuses of patients with CF causing chronic pansinusitis. Nasal polyps are found commonly in patients with CF and can compound chronic sinusitis.

In the GI system, obstruction of pancreatic ducts with viscid secretions results in exocrine pancreatic insufficiency and intestinal malabsorption in 90% of patients. Pancreatic endocrine function can also be impaired resulting in diabetes. CF-related diabetes (CFRD), which is distinct from both type 1 and type 2 diabetes, rarely occurs in the first decade, but its incidence increases after that with age. Accumulation of viscid secretions can also cause small bowel obstruction, particularly in newborns, a condition known as meconium ileus (Figure 41-3). Bowel obstruction can also occur in older children and adults as a result of mucus impaction in the distal small bowel, a condition known as distal intestinal obstruction syndrome (DIOS) . The liver is also commonly affected in patients with CF. A number of different types of liver disease can be seen, including asymptomatic elevation of liver enzymes, hepatic steatosis, and microgallbladder; however, the most prominent finding is focal biliary cirrhosis. This is likely caused by bile duct obstruction, and disease can progress to widespread cirrhosis with portal hypertension and liver failure in some patients. Other GI problems can occur in CF, including gastroesophageal reflux (GER), which is common in both children and adults, chronic pancreatitis, and rectal prolapse.

The reproductive system is also affected in patients with CF. Men are almost universally infertile because of congenital bilateral absence of the vas deferens, although sperm is normal and can be harvested for in vitro fertilization. Women with CF also have reduced fertility owing to thick cervical mucus, although pregnancy can occur.

Because CF is a lifelong multisystem disease, many complications may occur. In general, these are more common as the disease progresses and include decreased bone mineral density with fractures and osteoporosis, pneumothoraces, hemoptysis, recurrent acute pancreatitis, gallstones, and side effects of medications such as steroids and aminoglycosides.

CLINICAL PRESENTATION

With the increasing number of newborn screening programs for CF, many patients are now diagnosed before the development of symptoms. In the absence of screening, clinical presentation can be quite varied. A total of 10% to 15% of infants will present initially with meconium ileus in the first 48 hours of life and develop small bowel obstruction. The most common early manifestation of CF, however, is failure to thrive caused by intestinal malabsorption. This is often accompanied by a history of greasy or malodorous stools caused by a high content of malabsorbed fat.

Pulmonary involvement in CF most often presents with recurrent respiratory infections, which, in infants and small children, may be accompanied by wheeze. Respiratory symptoms in younger children can be hard to differentiate from those of recurrent viral illnesses or asthma. Patients can have a chronic cough, which is usually productive. Sputum, if it is expectorated, can be yellow or green. Chest examination can reveal hyperinflation, wheezing from lower airway obstruction, or crackles caused by peripheral airspace disease. Children with CF often have digital clubbing, although this can be hard to appreciate in

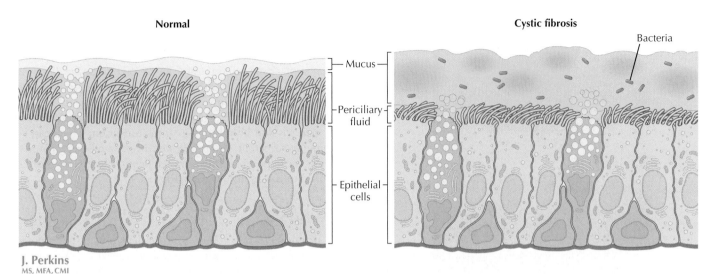

Normal   **Cystic fibrosis**

Bacteria

Mucus

Periciliary fluid

Epithelial cells

J. Perkins
MS, MFA, CMI

Abnormal electrolyte transport at the airway epithelium leads to a net absorption of sodium and water from the periciliary liquid (PCL) layer and airway mucus. The smaller PCL volume leads to trapping of cilia in tenacious mucus, impairing effective mucus clearance.

Figure 41-1 *Abnormal electrolyte transport.*

infants (Figure 41-4). Sinus disease can present as chronic nasal congestion or facial pain, and examination may reveal nasal polyps and sinus tenderness.

Patients with CF characteristically develop chronic lung infections with a limited spectrum of pathogenic bacteria. The predominant organisms include *Staphylococcus aureus, Haemophilus influenzae,* and *Pseudomonas aeruginosa* and to a lesser extent *Burkholderia cepacia, Stenotrophomonas maltophilia,* and *Alcaligenes*

xylosoxidans. Viruses, *S. aureus,* and *H. influenzae* are more commonly seen in younger children with CF but decrease in frequency with age as the incidence of *P. aeruginosa* increases. *P. aeruginosa* organisms in CF lungs often develop a mucoid phenotype and secrete biofilms that help them to avoid host defense

Bilateral extensive bronchiectasis

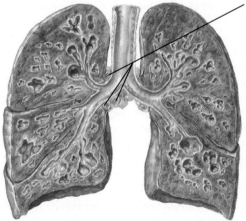

Enlarged hilar lymph nodes

Profuse muco-purulent sputum, foul-smelling, settling into layers characteristic of severe bronchi-ectasis

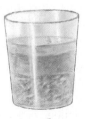

Ongoing infection and inflammation in CF lungs leads to parenchymal lung destruction and ultimately bronchiectasis (shown in figure), where the bronchi lose much of their elasticity. Airway clearance is significantly impaired in the face of bronchiectasis, leading to accumulation of mucus and facilitating the vicious cycle of infection and inflammation.

Figure 41-2 *Ongoing infection and inflammation in cystic fibrosis lungs.*

Cystic fibrosis of the pancreas (hence the name of the disease) and meconium ileus showing distal ileal obstruction and small bowel dilatation

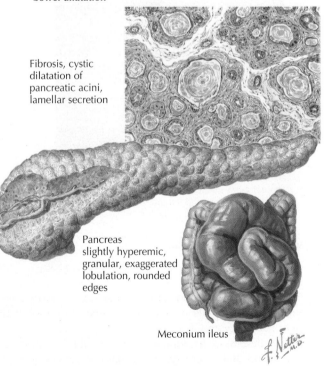

Fibrosis, cystic dilatation of pancreatic acini, lamellar secretion

Pancreas slightly hyperemic, granular, exaggerated lobulation, rounded edges

Meconium ileus

Figure 41-3 *Common gastrointestinal pathology in cystic fibrosis.*

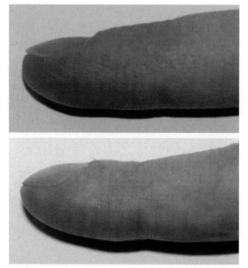

A. The angle between the nailbed and the nailfold (lovibond angle) should normally be <165° as in the upper figure in A. Note the loss of this normal angle in the individual with clubbing (lower image).

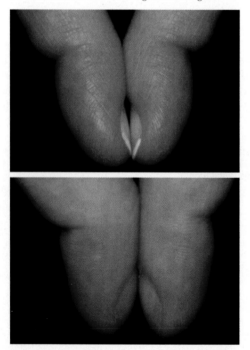

B. Schramroth's sign demonstrated. The diamond shaped space created by both lovibond angles during apposition of right and left index fingers (as seen in the upper figure) is lost in the individual with clubbing.

Figure 41-4 *Digital clubbing.*

and make them almost impossible to eradicate. *P. aeruginosa* is responsible for the bulk of infection-related morbidity in the lungs of patients with CF.

GI manifestations are common in CF. Children can present with frequent bulky, greasy, or malodorous stools from fat malabsorption. This is often accompanied by abdominal pain, bloating, and flatulence. Symptoms of GER are common in patients of all ages with CF and usually respond well to medical

management. Clinical examination commonly reveals fecal masses in the colon, and there can also be epigastric tenderness. Those with CF liver disease may have hepatosplenomegaly or evidence of portal hypertension on examination. Small bowel obstruction is fairly common in CF and can present with abdominal pain, absolute constipation, bilious vomiting, and abdominal distension. Examination can show a distended tender abdomen without bowel sounds. Intussusception, which can be chronic or recurrent, occurs because inspissated fecal material acts as a "lead point" in the terminal ileum. Here, pain is often localized to the right lower quadrant.

DIAGNOSIS

The diagnosis of CF is based on the detection of physiologic evidence of altered epithelial electrolyte transport (e.g., a positive sweat test result), mutations in the *CFTR* gene, and the presence of typical clinical symptoms. In the case of newborn screening, a sample of heel blood is assayed for immunoreactive trypsin (IRT), a pancreatic proenzyme whose serum concentration is elevated because of obstruction of pancreatic ducts. Samples that show high levels of IRT are further analyzed for common CF mutations. Most combined IRT and DNA screening algorithms have high sensitivity and specificity with low rates of false-positive test results. Children identified by newborn screening undergo further confirmatory testing, including a sweat test.

MANAGEMENT

The management of patients with CF is based on actively maintaining health, preventing decline in nutritional status and lung function, and aggressively treating CF-related disease exacerbations. This is best achieved by frequent contact with a skilled multidisciplinary team in an accredited CF center. CF is a progressive lifelong condition with multisystem involvement and onerous treatment schedules. The psychological impact of this on patients cannot be overestimated, and attention must be paid to this aspect of the disease as well if outcomes are to be optimized. Historically, the major advances in treatment of CF have stemmed from provision of adequate nutrition, aggressive antibiotic treatment of pulmonary disease, and use of regular prophylactic airway clearance. These continue to be the mainstays of treatment today. Clinic visits involve the monitoring of nutritional status; lung function; airway colonization; clinical signs of disease complications; and periodic comprehensive assessment including radiographic studies, serum chemistries and blood count, vitamin levels, and other laboratory tests of renal and hepatic function.

As a result of dehydrated airway secretions and airway inflammation, patients with CF have great difficulty in effectively clearing their airways. As infection, inflammation, and lung tissue damage progress, this becomes more and more challenging. Adequate airway clearance cannot be achieved without the use of chest physical therapy (CPT), which should be performed at least on a daily basis when well and more frequently during acute illnesses. Airway clearance treatments can be aimed at decreasing the viscosity and volume of secretions, facilitating their mobilization and helping to expectorate them. DNA derived from the nuclei of dead neutrophils significantly increases the viscosity of sputum in CF. Recombinant human DNAse is an enzyme that breaks down DNA and can significantly improve the vesicoelastic properties of CF sputum when administered by nebulization. It has been shown to improve sputum clearance and lung function in children older than 6 years. Hypertonic saline (7%) can be used to replete airway salt and water in an attempt to reduce mucus viscosity and facilitate airway clearance. It can also stimulate coughing, which may be very helpful in some patients. It has been shown to improve mucociliary clearance and lung function when used regularly in children older than 6 years.

Mobilization of secretions can be facilitated by techniques such as manual percussion with postural drainage, high-frequency chest wall oscillation, and flutter devices. Expectoration of secretions can be enhanced by various physiotherapy techniques such as active cycle of breathing and with exhalation against positive expiratory pressure. In addition to the regular use of physiotherapy, children are encouraged to exercise as much as possible, which is a very effective adjunct to airway clearance.

In patients with chronic airway colonization and impaired airway clearance, the intermittent use of inhaled antibiotics can help to reduce excessive sputum bacterial density and volume of secretions and improve lung function. Agents that are currently available include tobramycin, aztreonam, and colistin. Chronic infection-driven pulmonary inflammation in CF may also respond to regular oral azithromycin and ibuprofen. In the setting of acute exacerbations of CF lung disease, the use of intensive CPT and oral or intravenous antibiotics are the cornerstones of care. The frequency of acute exacerbations tends to increase as lung function declines. In patients who have severe impairment of lung function, frequent pulmonary exacerbations, and impairment in activities of daily living, evaluation for lung transplantation is often considered.

Maintaining adequate nutritional status in patients with CF is vital for overall care. In those with exocrine pancreatic insufficiency, the use of orally administered supplemental pancreatic enzymes has revolutionized CF nutritional management. Adequate intake of enzymes should result in improvement in nutrition; GI symptoms; and the serum levels of the fat-soluble vitamins A, D, E, and K. The use of supplemental vitamins and minerals is often necessary, particularly the fat-soluble vitamins. In those with signs of cholestatic liver disease, the secondary bile acid ursodeoxycholic acid is often used in an effort to slow disease progression.

The development of glucose intolerance and CFRD occurs with increasing frequency in adolescents and young adults and is associated with poorer lung function and worse nutritional status. Close monitoring of glucose levels is necessary, and most patients with CFRD will ultimately need insulin replacement as caloric restriction is not recommended in patients with CF.

FUTURE DIRECTIONS

Advances continue to be made in the symptomatic treatment of disease manifestations, and trials are increasingly being conducted in younger children and infants with a view to intervening as early as possible to prevent clinical decline. More recently, attention has focused on novel small molecules that seek to ameliorate the cellular defects in CFTR processing and function. Several of these agents are in advanced clinical trials. Gene therapy has long been touted as the ultimate corrective solution in CF. Despite many problems with this approach initially, momentum is now gathering again, and extensive preparatory work should result in clinical trials in patients in the next few years.

SUGGESTED READINGS

Amin R, Ratjen F: Cystic fibrosis: a review of pulmonary and nutritional therapies, *Adv Pediatr* 55:99-121, 2008.

Cystic Fibrosis Foundation Patient Registry: *2007 Annual Data Report.* Bethesda, MD.

Cystic Fibrosis Mutation Database at the Hospital for Sick Children, Toronto. www.genet.sickkids.on.ca/home.html.

Flume PA, O'Sullivan BP, Robinson KA, et al: The Cystic Fibrosis Foundation, Pulmonary Therapies Committee: Cystic fibrosis pulmonary guidelines: chronic medications for maintenance of lung health, *Am J Respir Crit Care Med* 176(10):957-969, 2007.

Flume PA, Robinson KA, O'Sullivan BP: The Clinical Practice Guidelines for Pulmonary Therapies Committee: Cystic fibrosis pulmonary guidelines: airway clearance therapies, *Respir Care* 54(4):522-537, 2009.

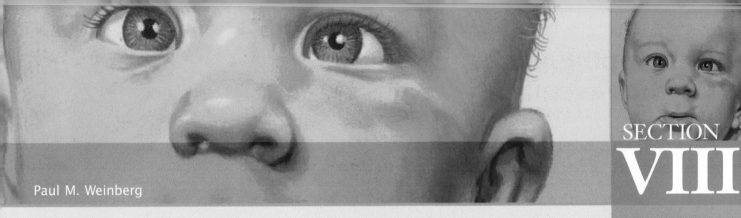

Paul M. Weinberg

Paul M. Weinberg

SECTION
VIII

Disorders of the Cardiovascular System

Development of the Cardiovascular System

42

Kristin N. Ray and Anitha S. John

Embryologic development of the heart requires the coordination of multiple steps, including heart tube formation, cardiac looping, chamber septation, and development of appropriate inflow and outflow tracts. Additionally, the cardiac conduction system and coronary artery system must develop during this time period. After organogenesis is complete, normal fetal circulation is notable for the presence of three levels of communication that normally close after birth, namely the ductus venosus, the foramen ovale, and the ductus arteriosus. Although these communications are vital for fetal circulation, they can be maladaptive in the postnatal period. Functional closure of all three communications generally occurs during the transition to postnatal life. Understanding the complexity of the normal development of the cardiovascular system allows for greater understanding of the development of congenital cardiovascular disease (see Chapters 43 and 44).

EMBRYOLOGIC DEVELOPMENT

Heart Tube Formation

The cardiovascular system is derived primarily from the splanchnic mesoderm, which develops on the 15th day after ovulation. Migrating cells form the cardiogenic crescent, which fuses in the midline as embryonic folding occurs, creating the *heart tube* by day 20 to 21 of development. The heart begins to beat on day 22 of development. At this time, the heart tube segments begin to differentiate, with constrictions demarcating specific segments of the tube (Figure 42-1). Most cranially, the bulbus cordis leads into the truncus arteriosus, which connects to the aortic sac, the aortic arches, and the dorsal aorta. Caudal to the bulbus cordis is the primitive ventricle followed by the primitive atrium, which is connected in turn to the sinus venosus. Between these segments, transitional zones exist that will become septa, valves, conduction tissue, and fibrous skeleton structures.

Cardiac Looping

The crucial process of *cardiac looping* evolves over day 23 to 28 of gestation, with the bulbus cordis of the heart tube bending ventrally, caudally, and toward the right of the embryo, forming a D-looped heart (see Figure 42-1). This positions the proximal bulbus cordis to become the future right-sided right ventricle and the primitive ventricle to become the future left-sided left ventricle while also positioning the atria dorsal to the future ventricles (Figure 42-2). The process and direction of looping appear to be under genetic control within the myocardium, with dysregulation of this process potentially resulting in abnormal positioning of the four chambers of the heart, such as occurs in an L-looped heart (i.e., ventricular inversion). Through looping, the transitional zones are brought together along the inner

curvature, and the primitive chambers are more predominantly located along the outer curvatures. Shortly after the completion of looping, blood begins circulating within the embryo and cardiac septation begins, as does the formation of the aortic arches.

Endocardial Cushion Development and Atrial Septation

After looping has completed, the division of the four chambers and ventricular outflow tract must begin through division of the atrial and ventricular structures via the endocardial cushions, and division of the right and left sided structures through a complex process of septation (Figure 42-3). The endocardial cushions develop early in this process, appearing at the level of the future atrioventricular (AV) valves. Inferior and superior endocardial cushions grow toward each other, dividing the common AV canal into left and right AV openings. In so doing, they establish the site of the future AV valves, which will develop between the fifth and eighth weeks of development through a process of invagination of the cardiac wall.

Around day 26 to 28, atrial septation begins with formation of a crescent-shaped membrane from the posterior-superior wall of the atria, called the septum primum. On day 35, septum primum begins to extend toward the fusing endocardial cushions, gradually separating the left atrium from the right atrium. The endocardial cushions of the AV canal continue to develop and separate the atria, closing the ostium primum (see Figure 42-3). Failure of the aforementioned processes results in AV canal defects, frequently associated with trisomy 21. Classical embryologic teaching has been that before completing the division between the two atria, perforations develop in the septum primum, creating the foramen secundum, allowing continued flow between the two atria. However, virtually all hearts that have a septum primum display a crescentic superior edge with attachments on both ends of the crescent and no remnant of septum primum above the crescent indicating that there is no hole within septum primum but rather that the crescent shape was there originally.

Septum secundum is an infolding of the atrial wall, typically where the truncus arteriosus indents the roof of the embryonic atrium. This structure is thick and muscular unlike the septum primum, which is thin and membrane-like. The septum secundum grows posteriorly and inferiorly and forms the limbus of the fossa ovalis by day 42. The space between these two structures is the foramen ovale, which allows continued right-to-left blood flow between the atria during the fetal period.

During this time, the systemic (superior and inferior venae cavae) and the pulmonary venous connections are also incorporated into the right and left atria, respectively. Abnormal progression of atrial septation can result in ostium secundum atrial

Formation of the heart tube

Seven-somite stage (2.2 mm) at approximately 23 days

Ventral dissection

Oropharyngeal membrane
Left aortic arch I
Aortic sac
Bulbus cordis
Myocardium
Cardiac jelly
Pericardial cavity
Ventricle
Right sinus venosus
Left sinus venosus
Atrium
Foregut

Forebrain
Right aortic arch I
Amnion

Sagittal dissection

Dorsal myocardium
Dorsal mesocardium

Left dorsal aorta
Vitelline veins
Right umbilical vein

Formation of the heart loop

Ten-somite stage (2.5 mm) at approximately 23 days

Buccopharyngeal membrane
Left aortic arch I
Left aortic arch II
Aortic sac
Bulbus cordis
Myocardium
Cardiac jelly
Amnion
Ventricle
Pericardial cavity
AV canal
Left sinus venosus
Septum transversum
Left sinus venosus
Yolk sac
Vitelline veins
Left umbilical vein

Ventral dissection

Forebrain
Right aortic arch I
Right sinus venosus
Atrium

Sagittal dissection

Left carotid artery
Left pharyngeal pouch I
Left anterior cardinal vein
Dorsal mesocardium breaking down to form the transverse sinus
Left dorsal aorta

Fourteen-somite stage (3.0 mm) at approximately 24 days

Oropharyngeal membrane
Left aortic arch I
Left aortic arch II
Aortic sac
Bulbus cordis
Bulboventricular sulcus
Pericardial cavity
Myocardium
Cardiac jelly
Ventricle
AV canal
Atrium
Septum transversum
Hepatic diverticulum
Sinus venosus
Yolk sac
Vitelline veins
Left umbilical vein

Ventral dissection

Right aortic arch I
Truncus arteriosus

Sagittal dissection

Left anterior ⎫
Left common ⎬ Cardinal veins
Left posterior ⎭
Dorsal mesocardium

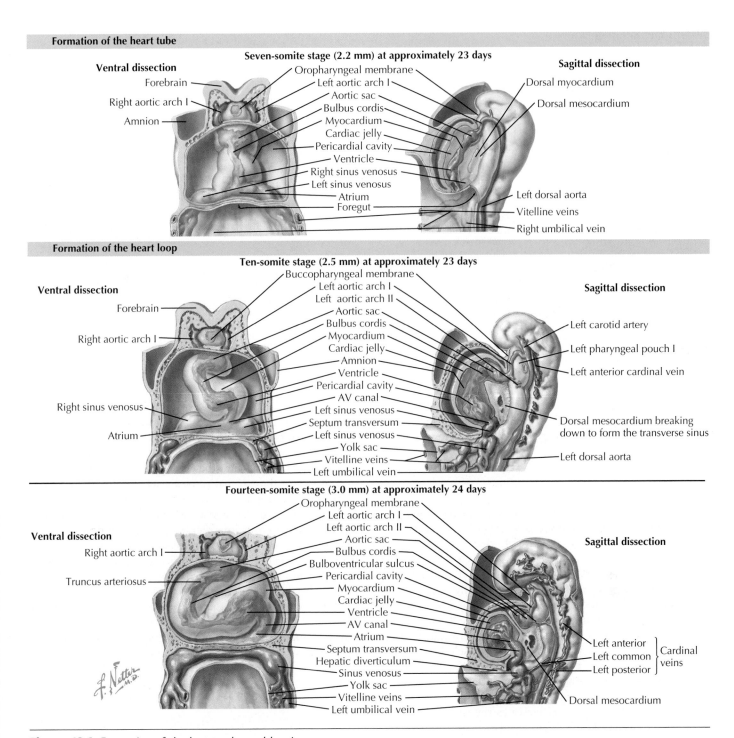

Figure 42-1 *Formation of the heart tube and looping.*

septal defects (defects in the septum primum) and ostium primum atrial septal defects (defects in formation or fusion of the endocardial cushions)

Ventricular Septation

Ventricular septation also involves coordination of multiple converging septal structures (see Figure 42-3). The muscular interventricular septum begins development by day 30 and continues into the seventh week of life. While the muscular ventricular septum is forming, myocardial trabecula develop in both ventricles. The posterior portion of the muscular septum is the inlet ventricular septum, smooth walled and close to the AV canal, and the anterior portion, called the *primary ventricular fold* or *septum*, is trabeculated. The muscular septum growth slows in the seventh week of life, but ventricular septation continues between 36 and 49 days of life with the closure of the infundibular septum (separating pulmonary outflow area from aortic) and closure of the membranous ventricular septum (closed by fusion of the left and right bulbar ridges along with the posterior

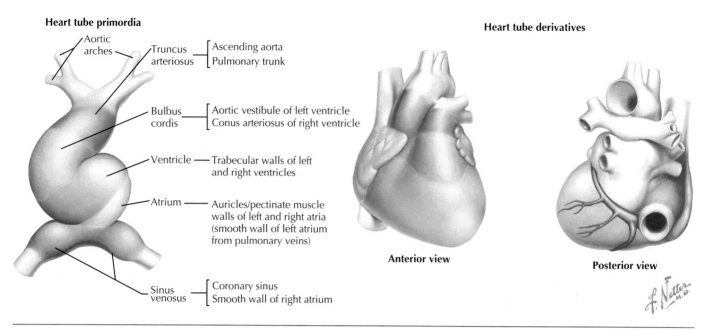

Figure 42-2 *Fate map of looped heart tube.*

endocardial cushion). Depending on the location, defects in ventricular septation can result in five major types of ventricular septal defects, which are further discussed in Chapter 43.

Development of Major Aortic and Pulmonary Outflow Tracts

Development of the ventricular outflow tract and aorticopulmonary septa require division of the associated left and right-sided structures such that the right ventricle flows into the newly developed pulmonary artery and the left ventricle flows into the aorta. The specifics of this process are controversial, with multiple theories currently being explored, generally involving the formation of bulbar and truncal ridges through a process that appears dependent on neural crest cells (Figure 42-4). During this process, expansion of the bulbus cordis beneath the left-sided pulmonary artery with regression of muscle beneath the right-sided aorta while maintaining the fixed position of the superior aorta relative to the pulmonary artery at the level of the bronchus causes the outflow tract to twist around itself, bringing the pulmonary artery closer to the right-sided morphologic right ventricle and the aorta closer to the morphologic left ventricle. Abnormal migration of neural crest cells in certain conditions, such as DiGeorge syndrome, may account for their associated conotruncal anomalies, such as tetralogy of Fallot, truncus arteriosus communis, and interrupted aortic arch with ventricular septal defect.

Development of the Great Arteries

The great arteries are formed through the division of the truncus arteriosus, with more distal portions of the aorta and pulmonary arteries developing from the paired embryonic aortic arches. The aortic arches develop sequentially during early gestation, with the final pair appearing by the sixth week of development

(Figure 42-5). The first aortic arches develop into the maxillary arteries and portions of the external carotid arteries. The second pair of aortic arches provides circulation to the stapes in the inner ear as well as the hyoid artery. The third pair of aortic arch arteries develops into the common carotids and the proximal portion of the internal carotid arteries. The fourth pair of aortic arch arteries has asymmetric development, with the left side developing into the aortic arch and the right side connecting the right seventh intersegmental artery (precursor of the right subclavian artery) to the right carotid to form an innominate artery. The fifth pair regresses without any known remnant structures in normal humans, although a persistent fifth aortic arch has been noted rarely. The sixth pair of aortic arches develops into the ductus arteriosus on the left with involution on the right. Through sequential development and regression, great artery arrangement is evident by the eighth week of development. Abnormal development during this process can result in coarctation of the aorta, double aortic arch, right-sided aortic arch, and anomalous right subclavian artery.

Development of Major Systemic and Pulmonary Veins

The venous inflow tract, the sinus venosus, is originally connected to the common atrium but with asymmetric development such that the right horn is larger. During the fifth week of gestation, the sinus venosus becomes incorporated into the right-sided atrium and develops into recognizable systemic venous structures, including the superior and inferior venae cavae (right horn of sinus venosus) and the coronary sinus (left horn of sinus venosus). The pulmonary veins, in contrast, grow out of the left atrium toward the budding lung, with development beginning as a single vein during week 5 of gestation. Peripheral pulmonary veins develop within the lung and connect to the common pulmonary vein growing out of the heart. The common

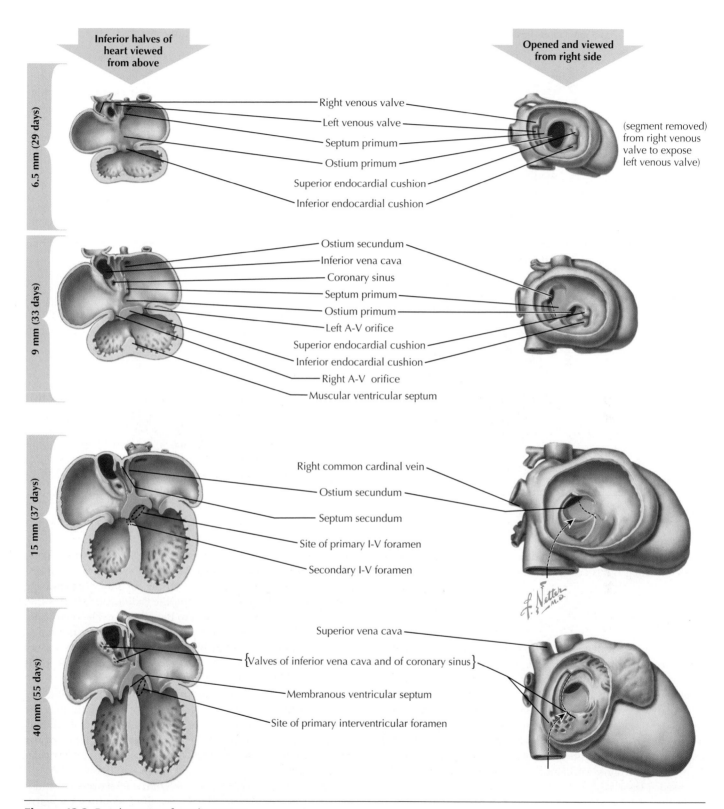

Inferior halves of heart viewed from above

Opened and viewed from right side

6.5 mm (29 days)

Right venous valve
Left venous valve
Septum primum
Ostium primum
Superior endocardial cushion
Inferior endocardial cushion

(segment removed) from right venous valve to expose left venous valve)

9 mm (33 days)

Ostium secundum
Inferior vena cava
Coronary sinus
Septum primum
Ostium primum
Left A-V orifice
Superior endocardial cushion
Inferior endocardial cushion
Right A-V orifice
Muscular ventricular septum

15 mm (37 days)

Right common cardinal vein
Ostium secundum
Septum secundum
Site of primary I-V foramen
Secondary I-V foramen

40 mm (55 days)

Superior vena cava
{Valves of inferior vena cava and of coronary sinus}
Membranous ventricular septum
Site of primary interventricular foramen

Figure 42-3 *Development of cardiac septa.*

pulmonary vein and the proximal individual pulmonary veins are then incorporated into the left atrial wall, accounting for the smooth posterior wall of the left atrium. Failure of some or all of the pulmonary veins to incorporate with the left atrium can result in partial or total anomalous pulmonary

venous connection. Incomplete incorporation of the common pulmonary vein may be the cause of cor triatriatum. Venous structures develop into significant portions of each atrium (including the sinus venosus on the right and the pulmonary veins on the left), resulting in smooth-walled compartments,

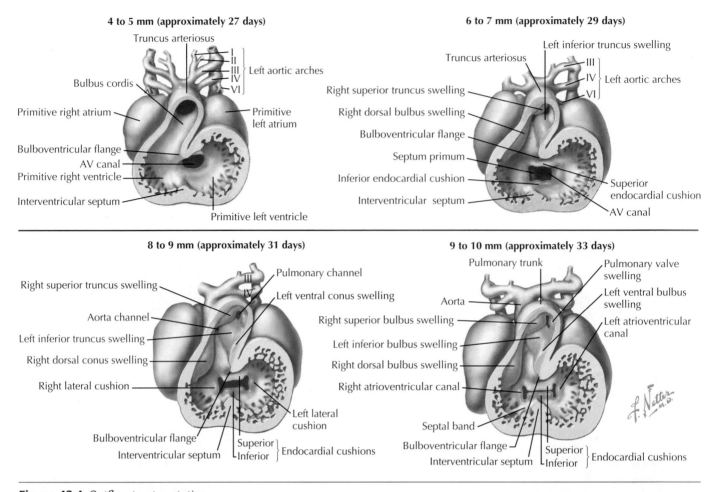

Figure 42-4 *Outflow tract septation.*

with the original embryonic atria becoming the atrial appendages containing the pectinate muscles.

Development of Cardiac Conduction System and Coronary Vessels

The heart tube formed early in gestation has been observed to have peristaltic contraction by the third week of development. As development progresses, however, an organized conduction system must develop as well; this occurs through differentiation of primary myocardial cells into conducting myocardium. Additionally, the developing heart requires more active perfusion as its structure becomes larger and more complex, thus necessitating the development of the coronary vascular system, with cells from the epicardium working into the myocardium to develop the needed vessels.

FETAL CIRCULATION

Because the source of oxygenated blood in fetal life is the placenta, rather than the lung, fetal circulation uses specific mechanisms to preferentially direct more oxygenated blood from the placenta toward specific structures such as the heart and the brain. Specifically, three communications mentioned previously, the ductus venosus, the foramen ovale, and the ductus

arteriosus, are required for normal fetal circulation (Figure 42-6). The right ventricle receives returning deoxygenated systemic blood flow from the brain via the superior vena cava and right atrium. This blood exits via the pulmonary arteries into the ductus arteriosus for return to the placenta. The pulmonary artery also supplies a minimal amount of flow to the lungs. Oxygenated blood from the placenta returns to the right atrium via the ductus venosus and proximal inferior vena cava. This oxygenated blood is directed preferentially to the left atrium through the foramen ovale and is then pumped by the left ventricle into the aorta, where it is delivered primarily into the coronary circulation and upper body, including the developing brain. In fetal circulation, the right ventricular output is slightly larger than that of the left, resulting in relative right ventricular hypertrophy.

Despite completion of formation of the fetal heart structures by 7 weeks of gestation, the myocardium continues to grow by cell division until birth, after which growth is primarily caused by cell enlargement. Genetic and molecular signaling is crucial in this process, but the physical environment, including blood flow, is also vital for ongoing normal development during the fetal period. For example, aortic stenosis may increase left ventricular pressures, resulting in decreased blood flow across the foramen ovale, and subsequent left ventricular hypoplasia.

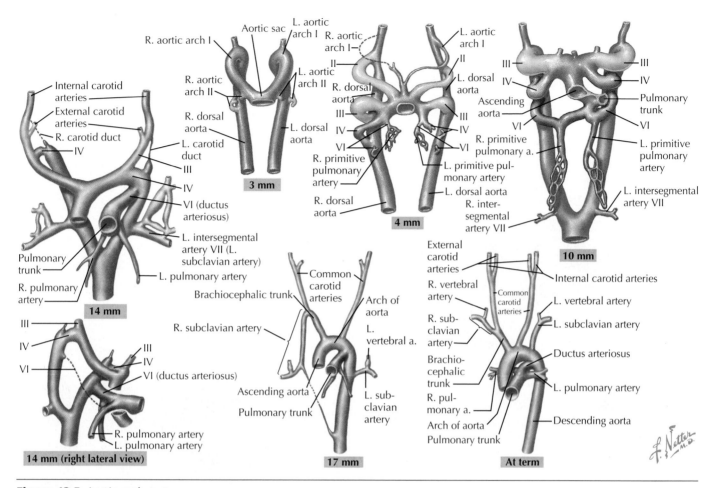

Figure 42-5 *Aortic arch system.*

POSTNATAL TRANSITIONS AND NEONATAL CIRCULATION

After delivery, several transitions must occur because structures required for fetal circulation become maladaptive for extrauterine life. The three previously beneficial communications must close to establish the final configuration of the human cardiovascular system (see Figure 42-6). The foramen ovale, being a flap-valve between the septum primum and septum secundum, functionally closes shortly after delivery when left atrial pressure increases as a result of increased pulmonary venous return after birth. This causes septum primum to become pressed against septum secundum. Anatomic closure of the foramen ovale is a more prolonged process, and it is estimated that 25% to 30% of adults still have a patent foramen ovale. Although this is largely hemodynamically insignificant, it can be a portal for embolic stroke later in life with transient elevation of right atrial pressure.

The ductus arteriosus usually closes in 90% of full-term infants by 48 hours after birth. The ductus arteriosus is maintained in fetal life by endogenous production of prostaglandins in the relatively hypoxic in utero environment. Prematurity is often accompanied by a persistently patent ductus arteriosus, which may require medical or surgical closure because of associated hemodynamic compromise. Some congenital heart defects

with either pulmonary (e.g., pulmonary atresia) or systemic outflow obstruction (e.g., interrupted aortic arch or hypoplastic left heart syndrome) may benefit from a patent ductus. The former may present with severe hypoxemia and the latter with shock at the time of ductus arteriosus closure, and these may temporarily be treated with prostaglandins to maintain ductal patency.

The ductus venosus usually closes 1 to 3 weeks after delivery in term infants (longer in preterm infants and those with persistent pulmonary hypertension or congenital heart disease). Unlike the clear role for oxygen triggering closure of the ductus arteriosus, no specific trigger has been identified for ductus venosus closure. In addition to closure of these three important communications, the umbilical vessels also constrict at birth because they are no longer necessary after the placenta is removed. Finally, although the right ventricle is more hypertrophied at the time of delivery, the left ventricle becomes more hypertrophied by the end of the first month of life because of the differential between pulmonary and systemic pressures after delivery resulting from a decrease in pulmonary vascular resistance with respiration and regression of pulmonary arteriolar smooth muscle. Congenital heart disease, prematurity, and perinatal hypoxemia or stress may disrupt these important physiologic transitions.

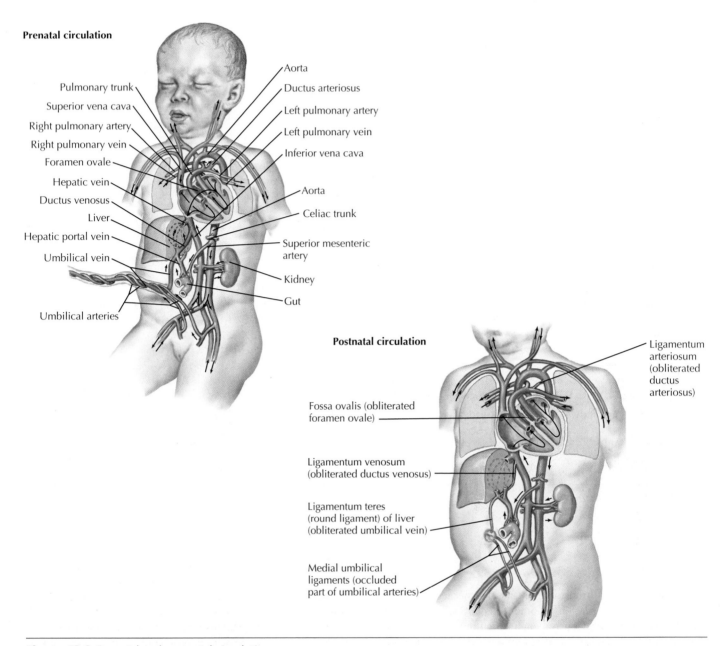

Prenatal circulation

- Pulmonary trunk
- Superior vena cava
- Right pulmonary artery
- Right pulmonary vein
- Foramen ovale
- Hepatic vein
- Ductus venosus
- Liver
- Hepatic portal vein
- Umbilical vein
- Umbilical arteries

- Aorta
- Ductus arteriosus
- Left pulmonary artery
- Left pulmonary vein
- Inferior vena cava
- Aorta
- Celiac trunk
- Superior mesenteric artery
- Kidney
- Gut

Postnatal circulation

- Fossa ovalis (obliterated foramen ovale)
- Ligamentum venosum (obliterated ductus venosus)
- Ligamentum teres (round ligament) of liver (obliterated umbilical vein)
- Medial umbilical ligaments (occluded part of umbilical arteries)
- Ligamentum arteriosum (obliterated ductus arteriosus)

Figure 42-6 *Prenatal and postnatal circulation.*

FUTURE DIRECTIONS

Improving our understanding of normal development allows for further insight into congenital heart disease and its etiology. In strengthening our understanding of normal and abnormal development, we may increase our ability to treat congenital heart disease, such as through gene therapy or fetal interventions. Much work continues into understanding the molecular and genetic components responsible for the development of these diseases.

SUGGESTED READINGS

Abdulla R, Blew GA, Holterman MJ: Cardiovascular embryology, *Pediatr Cardiol* 25:191-200, 2004.

Gittenberger-de Groot AC: Basics of cardiac development for the understanding of congenital heart malformations, *Pediatr Res* 57(2):169-176, 2005.

Kiserud T: Physiology of the fetal circulation, *Semin Fetal Neonat Med* 10:493-503, 2005.

Manner J: The anatomy of cardiac looping: a step towards the understanding of the morphogenesis of several forms of congenital cardiac malformations, *Clin Anat* 22:21-35, 2009.

McFadden DG, Olson EN: Heart development: learning from mistakes, *Curr Opin Genet* 12:328-335, 2002.

Sander TL, Klinkner DB, Tomita-Mitchell A, Mitchell ME: Molecular and cellular basis of congenital heart disease, *Pediatr Clin North Am* 53(5):989-1009, 2006.

Acyanotic Congenital Heart Disease

Marsha Ayzen and Anitha S. John

43

A cyanotic heart lesions can be separated into two categories: shunt lesions and nonshunt lesions. Shunt lesions, such as ventricular septal defects (VSDs), allow oxygenated blood to bypass the systemic circulation and reenter the pulmonary circulation. Nonshunt lesions consist largely of valvular disease and aortic arch anomalies.

SHUNT LESIONS

Atrial Septal Defect

Atrial septal defects (ASDs) constitute 5% to 10% of all congenital heart defects and occur in approximately one in 1500 live births. There are five types of ASDs (Figure 43-1). The most common type is the *ostium secundum ASD*, which results from a deficiency in septum primum, the thin membrane-like septum that normally closes the foramen ovale. The second most common type is the *ostium primum ASD*, which is a defect in the canal septum. This septum normally divides the common atrioventricular (AV) canal and in so doing completes the anterior portion of the atrial septum and the posterior portion of the ventricular septum while dividing the common AV valve into the tricuspid and mitral valve. Defects in this septum result in AV canal defects, which are discussed later in this chapter. The third type is the *sinus venosus defect*, which is not a defect in atrial septum per se but rather a communication between the two atria by way of a "straddling" venous structure, either a pulmonary vein or a vena cava. It is frequently associated with partial anomalous drainage of the right-sided pulmonary veins connected to the superior vena cava (SVC). *Coronary sinus ASDs* are the fourth type and again are not true defects in the atrial septum but rather the physiologic consequence of a partially or completely unroofed coronary sinus with left atrial to right atrial drainage through the coronary sinus ostium. The fifth type of ASD is that seen with *juxtaposition of the atrial appendages*. This is extremely rare and results from an absence or misplacement of septum secundum, which normally closes the foramen ovale.

Children with ASDs are usually asymptomatic unless the defect is very large. Cardiac auscultation reveals a systolic ejection murmur at the left upper sternal border from increased blood flow across the pulmonary valve and a fixed, widely split S2 because of increased venous return to the right heart with both inspiration, when there is normally increased return to the right heart, and expiration when there is increased pulmonary venous return to the left atrium and from there to the right atrium through the ASD. Electrocardiography (ECG) may show right axis deviation and right ventricular hypertrophy because of volume overload (typically an rSR′ pattern, or possibly right bundle branch block. With a significant defect, cardiomegaly may be apparent on chest radiography. Echocardiography is used to confirm the diagnosis.

Ostium secundum defects may spontaneously close within the first 4 years of life, but the other types of ASDs usually do not. Options for repair include surgical closure or transcatheter device closure (Figure 43-2). Secundum defects with well-defined margins are the only type amenable to device closure. If left untreated into adulthood, ASDs can lead to pulmonary hypertension; exercise intolerance; atrial arrhythmias; increased risk of paradoxical embolus or stroke; and, late in life, to heart failure. Even when successfully closed in childhood, atrial arrhythmias may still occur decades later.

Ventricular Septal Defect

Ventricular septal defects (VSDs) account for about 20% of all congenital heart disease and occur in 2-10 of /1000 live births. The ventricular septum consists of the inlet (canal septum) posteriorly and inferiorly, running the full superoinferior length of the septal leaflet of the tricuspid valve; the infundibular, conal, or outlet septum superiorly, the muscular or trabecular septum; and the small, membranous septum at the junction of the other three (Figure 43-3). There are five types of VSDs that result from defects in or between these various components of the ventricular septum.

The most common type of VSDs are the *conoventricular* VSDs, which are defects between the conal or infundibular septum and the rest of the ventricular septum (see Figure 43-3). They may include the membranous septum, in which case they are a type of perimembranous VSD. These VSDs can be partially closed by tissue from the tricuspid valve, and many defects become smaller with time. Rarely, aortic regurgitation may occur because of prolapse of the right or noncoronary cusp into the VSD. *Canal-type* or *inlet defects* are usually seen in common AV canal defects (described more fully below) and occur from absence of the inlet septum; they extend along the full length of the AV valve. They may also be seen in straddling tricuspid valve and in some cases of transposition or double outlet right ventricle without AV valve abnormality. *Malalignment* and *conal septal hypoplasia* defects occur as a result of malalignment or absence of the conal or infundibular septum, respectively. Malalignment defects are seen in patients with tetralogy of Fallot (discussed in Chapter 44) and interrupted aortic arch along with other complex congenital lesions. Conal septal hypoplasia defects (see Figure 43-3) are sometimes referred to as subpulmonary or supracristal VSDs. They occur within the Y-shaped septal band beneath both semilunar valves and may be associated with prolapse of an aortic cusp resulting in aortic regurgitation. The second most common type of VSDs are called *muscular VSDs*, which are defects located anywhere other than those described above. These defects often spontaneously close if they are small to moderate in size (see Figure 43-3).

At 4 to 6 weeks of age, the pulmonary vascular resistance (PVR) decreases, and left-to-right shunting at the ventricular level increases. If the defect is large enough to cause a significant shunt, infants may also show signs of congestive heart failure (CHF) such as sweating with feeds, poor weight gain, tachypnea,

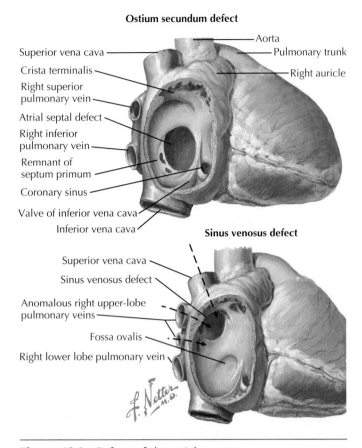

Figure 43-1 *Defects of the atrial septum.*

tachycardia, and hepatomegaly. On cardiac auscultation, moderate to large defects may not produce a murmur early in the newborn period. As the PVR decreases, a harsh, holosystolic murmur can be heard at the left lower sternal border, and large defects can cause a mid-diastolic rumble from an increase in flow across the mitral valve. Children with significant VSDs may also have a hyperactive precordium and a right ventricular heave. If left untreated, larger defects can eventually cause irreversible pulmonary hypertension (Eisenmenger reaction). Eventually, cyanosis results from Eisenmenger's physiology (right-to-left shunting across the defect) when PVR exceeds systemic. At that point, closure of the VSD would not result in a decrease in pulmonary resistance or pressure.

ECG can be normal with small defects or show biventricular hypertrophy in larger defects. Chest radiography can show cardiomegaly and increased pulmonary vascular markings in symptomatic patients. Echocardiography is used to confirm the diagnosis and characterize the type of VSD.

Both small conoventricular and muscular defects often decrease in size and have a high rate of spontaneous closure within the first several years of life. Canal-type, malalignment, and conal septal hypoplasia defects do not spontaneously close and usually require surgical correction. In the absence of symptoms, smaller defects often do not require closure or medical treatment. Treatment is guided by the size of the defect. Large defects (equal to or greater than the size of the aortic valve) require repair, even in the absence of symptoms, to prevent

pulmonary vascular disease. With smaller defects, treatment may depend on the child's symptoms. Medical management includes diuretics, digoxin, higher caloric formula to meet metabolic demands, and iron supplementation if anemia is present. In hemodynamically significant lesions, surgical correction is usually performed before 1 year of age but can be done sooner if the child is symptomatic. Several centers are starting to use a transcatheter approach with an occlusion device for certain muscular VSDs.

Common Atrioventricular Canal

Common AV canal (otherwise known as endocardial cushion defect or AV septal defect) accounts for about 4% to 5% of all congenital heart disease and 40% of heart disease in children with trisomy 21. This results from the failure of the endocardial cushions to fuse (forming the canal septum), preventing separation of the common AV valve into the tricuspid and mitral valves. All cases of common AV canal with two ventricles have deficiency of the anterior portion of the atrial septum and the posterior portion of the ventricular septum. However, there are two frequent combinations of AV valve morphology and attachment to the ventricular septum.

A *complete common AV canal* consists of the above-mentioned septal deficiency, with the common AV valve suspended within the septal defect such that there is space proximal to the valve between the two atria (ostium primum ASD) and space distal to the valve between the two ventricles (canal-type VSD) (see Figure 43-3). An *incomplete (or partial) AV canal* has the same septal deficiency but has leaflet tissue dividing the valve orifice into two orifices and adhering to the crest of the ventricular septum such that there is no direct communication between ventricles. Thus, the entire septal defect, being proximal to the AV valve, is called an ostium primum ASD, and the morphology of the left side of the common AV valve is described as a cleft "mitral" because the two components of what should have formed the anterior leaflet of a mitral valve, remain separate or cleft. A *transitional AV canal*, similar to an *incomplete canal*, occurs when the AV valve attachments to the ventricular septum result in a restrictive VSD. The AV valve in this case also has two orifices. The primary defect in the canal septum remains the same, but the defects vary by degree of VSD closure by valve tissue.

Infants with a complete AV canal have symptoms consistent with large VSDs, as outlined above. Incomplete AV canals develop symptoms more consistent with ASDs but can be compounded by symptomatology from left AV valve regurgitation. Transitional AV canal defects can vary in their presentation and symptoms depending on the size and level of restriction at the VSD and the amount of AV valve regurgitation. The cardiac examination varies with each defect and can reveal a hyperactive precordium, a holosystolic murmur at the lower left sternal border (VSD), a systolic murmur at the apex (left AV valve regurgitation), and a diastolic rumble at the lower left sternal border or the apex (because of increased flow across the AV valves in diastole). An ECG with a "superior QRS axis" (−4- to −150 degrees) is a hallmark of this defect. A chest radiogram can show cardiomegaly with increased pulmonary vascular markings. An echocardiogram will readily identify and characterize the defect.

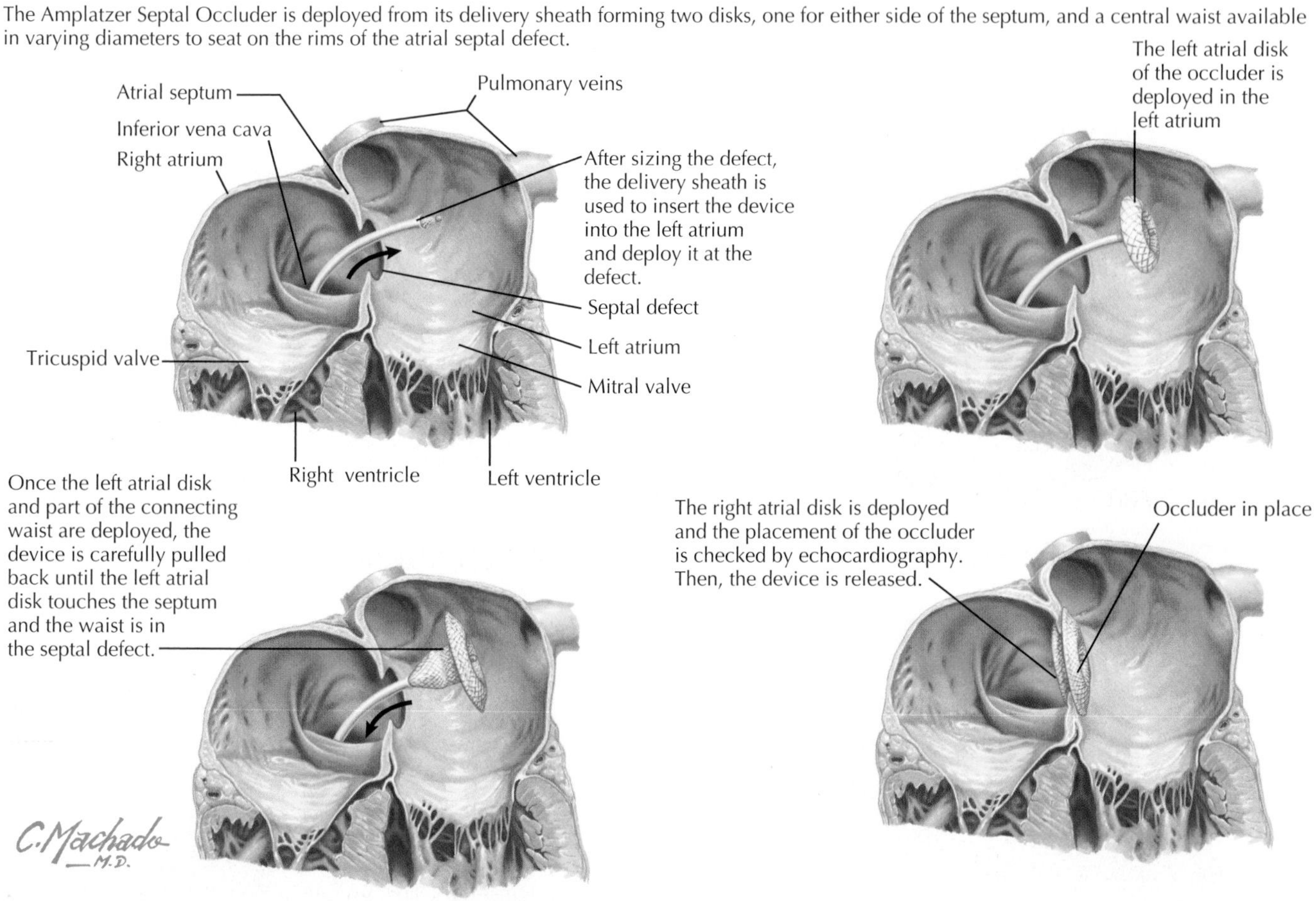

The Amplatzer Septal Occluder is deployed from its delivery sheath forming two disks, one for either side of the septum, and a central waist available in varying diameters to seat on the rims of the atrial septal defect.

Figure 43-2 *Amplatzer septal occluder.*

Medical and surgical management of complete AV canals is similar to that of large VSDs. Surgical repair is usually performed by 4 to 6 months of life with a concern for developing pulmonary vascular disease with delayed closure. Medical management and timing of surgical repair of incomplete AV canals depend largely on the degree of left-sided AV valve regurgitation. Long-term complications of these defects include AV valve regurgitation or stenosis, heart block, and left ventricular outflow tract obstruction. Even with early surgical repair, a subset of patients (especially those with Down syndrome) can still develop pulmonary vascular disease.

Patent Ductus Arteriosus

Patent ductus arteriosus (PDA) accounts for 5% to 10% of all congenital heart disease in term infants. In premature infants weighing less than 1750 g, the incidence is much higher at about 40%.

Failure of the ductus to close after birth results in a left-to-right shunt between the aorta and the pulmonary artery (Figure 43-4). The magnitude and direction of the shunt depend on the size of the open ductus and pulmonary versus systemic vascular resistance. For example, neonates with severe pulmonary hypertension will have a right-to-left shunt (pulmonary artery to aorta).

Infants with small PDAs are asymptomatic; however, those with larger PDAs can present with CHF symptoms. Physical examination reveals bounding pulses, widened pulse pressures, and a continuous murmur on cardiac auscultation. ECG and chest radiography findings are similar to those of a VSD; normal if the ductus is small; and with evidence of cardiomegaly, biventricular hypertrophy, and increased pulmonary markings if the defect is large.

Patients with a suspected PDA should be evaluated with chest radiography and ECG, as well as echocardiography. In premature infants, indomethacin can be used to induce PDA closure. In term infants and children, closure is achieved either through catheter closure with a coil or other ductus occluder or with surgical ligation. If a large ductus is left unrepaired, patients may develop pulmonary vascular disease over time.

NONSHUNT LESIONS

Aortic Valve Disease

Valvar aortic stenosis (AS) comprises about 3% to 8% of congenital heart defects or four in 100,000 live births. There is a strong male predominance (80%). Whereas critical AS (unicuspid aortic valve) presents shortly after birth with symptoms of CHF or shock, noncritical AS (bicuspid aortic valve) is often detected

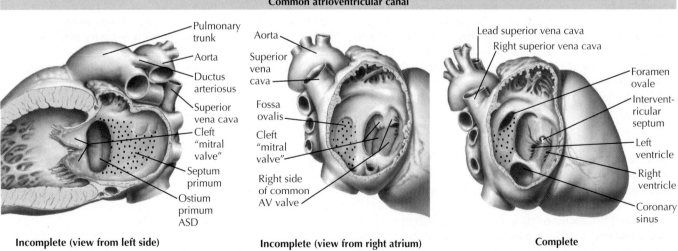

Conoventricular ventricular septal defect

Conal/Infundibular septum

Septal band

Ventricular septal defect

(Left ventricular view)

(Right ventricular view)

Muscular interventricular septal defect

Ventricular septal defect

(Left ventricular view)

Conal septal hypoplasia ventricular septal defect

Ventricular septal defect

Septal band

(Right ventricular view)

Common atrioventricular canal

Pulmonary trunk

Aorta

Ductus arteriosus

Superior vena cava

Cleft "mitral valve"

Septum primum

Ostium primum ASD

Incomplete (view from left side)

Aorta

Superior vena cava

Fossa ovalis

Cleft "mitral valve"

Right side of common AV valve

Incomplete (view from right atrium)

Lead superior vena cava

Right superior vena cava

Foramen ovale

Interventricular septum

Left ventricle

Right ventricle

Coronary sinus

Complete

Figure 43-3 *Ventricular septal defect.*

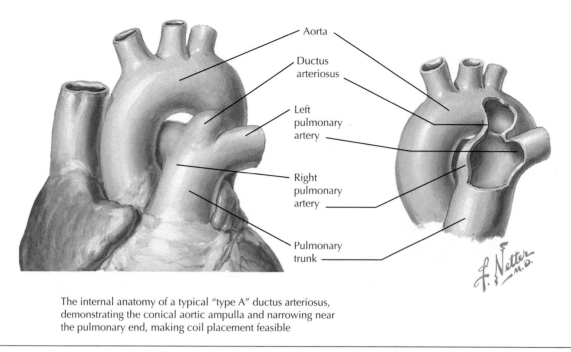

Aorta

Ductus arteriosus

Left pulmonary artery

Right pulmonary artery

Pulmonary trunk

The internal anatomy of a typical "type A" ductus arteriosus, demonstrating the conical aortic ampulla and narrowing near the pulmonary end, making coil placement feasible

Figure 43-4 *Patent ductus arteriosus.*

through physical examination findings of a systolic murmur. *Bicuspid aortic valve* is the most common congenital heart defect and occurs in 1% to 2% of the population. Not all bicuspid aortic valves become stenotic or regurgitant, but patients should continue to be screened periodically throughout life because patients with bicuspid aortic valves can develop aortic regurgitation in later childhood or adulthood and calcific AS or aortic root dilatation and dissection in adulthood.

Supravalvar AS occurs above the level of the aortic valve and is seen in Williams syndrome. It is the least common type of AS and often involves abnormalities in the elastin gene. *Subaortic stenosis* accounts for 10% to 20% of AS in children. It can result from a subaortic membrane (fibrous tissue in the aortic outflow tract), tunnel-like narrowing of the outflow tract or from dynamic obstruction as seen in hypertrophic cardiomyopathy. Subaortic stenosis may be seen with other cardiac defects such as VSDs, common AV canal, and coarctation of the aorta.

AS tends to progress rapidly during the first 2 years of life and during puberty. Most children with AS presenting after infancy are asymptomatic. With severe obstruction, children might present with chest pain on exercise, syncope, heart failure, or sudden death. Exercise restriction to lower intensity sports is extremely important in AS.

Cardiac examination can reveal a thrill at the suprasternal notch and the carotids. In severe cases, the second heart sound can be narrowly or even paradoxically split (rare in children because severe stenosis usually causes an inaudible aortic valve closure). Auscultation reveals a systolic ejection click followed by a crescendo-decrescendo systolic ejection murmur at the right upper sternal border radiating to the carotids. An ECG can show left ventricular hypertrophy (LVH) and, when accompanied by ST changes and T inversion, suggest severe obstruction. ECGs in newborns can be normal. Chest radiography

results are usually normal. Echocardiography is important in the differentiation of valvar, supravalvar, and subvalvar AS and in assessing the gradient across the area of stenosis.

Intervention in the form of surgical valvotomy or balloon valvuloplasty is done for all infants with critical AS regardless of the gradient and in children with noncritical AS with a gradient greater than 50 to 60 mm Hg as measured by cardiac catheterization (Figure 43-5). The gradient upon which intervention is undertaken also depends on the presence of symptoms, changes on rest or exercise ECG, and the desire to play competitive sports. After intervention, the gradient is usually reduced, but resultant aortic regurgitation is not uncommon.

Aortic insufficiency (AI) very infrequently occurs as an isolated lesion. Instead, it can be seen in association with conoventricular VSDs with a prolapsed aortic leaflet, subaortic stenosis, bicuspid aortic valve, connective tissue disorders such as Marfan's disease, or as a result of endocarditis. Rheumatic fever should always be considered in a patient with new-onset AI. The presentation and treatment of AI are discussed in Chapter 49.

Coarctation of the Aorta

Coarctation of the aorta is a discrete narrowing of the distal aortic arch opposite the entrance of the ductus arteriosus or the ligamentum (after ductal closure) (Figure 43-6). In some rare instances, it can be a narrowing of the abdominal aorta. It constitutes about 8% of all congenital heart defects. Boys are affected about four times more frequently than girls. Turner's syndrome should be suspected in any girl with aortic coarctation. Coarctation is also frequently associated with left-sided lesions such as bicuspid aortic valve, AS, mitral valve abnormalities, and VSDs. It can also be associated with noncardiac abnormalities such as intracranial aneurysms.

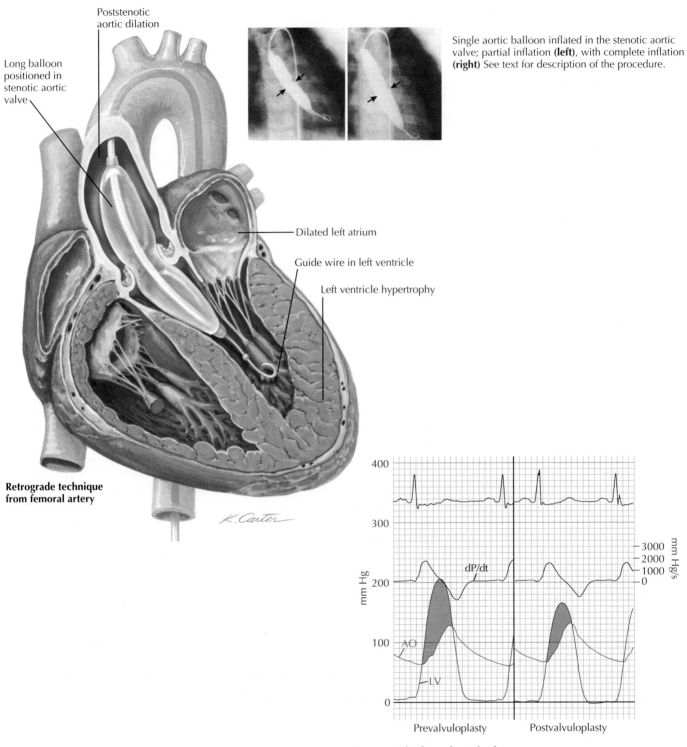

Poststenotic aortic dilation

Long balloon positioned in stenotic aortic valve

Single aortic balloon inflated in the stenotic aortic valve; partial inflation **(left)**, with complete inflation **(right)** See text for description of the procedure.

Dilated left atrium

Guide wire in left ventricle

Left ventricle hypertrophy

Retrograde technique from femoral artery

K. Carter

Representative hemodynamic changes

Representative pressure changes before and after percutaneous balloon aortic valvuloplasty. High-fidelity simultaneous LV and aortic pressures are shown with the accompanying dP/dt before and after the valvuloplasty procedure. The aortic gradient before and after is shaded.

With permission from Bashore TM, Davidson CJ. *Acute Hemodynamics Effects of Percutaneous Balloon Aortic Valvuloplasty and Related Techniques.* Baltimore: Williams and Wilkins; 1991:105.

Figure 43-5 *Balloon aortic valvotomy.*

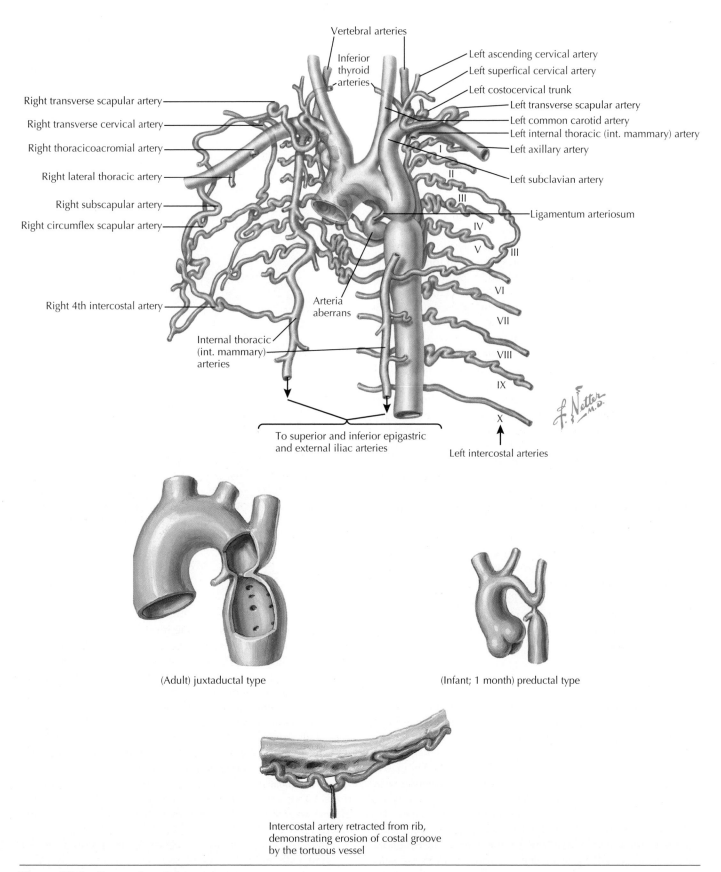

Figure 43-6 *Coarctation of the aorta.*

In neonates with critical or severe coarctation, the presentation is usually shock. Although they too sometimes have discrete juxtaductal coarctation, infants usually have arch hypoplasia proximal to the entrance of the ductus arteriosus (see Figure 43-6) along with intracardiac abnormalities. With slightly less severe coarctation, infants can present with symptoms of CHF, notably feeding intolerance. Children who have adapted to the gradual development of discrete coarctation are often asymptomatic despite upper extremity hypertension but may experience claudication; cold extremities; and rarely, chest pain with exercise.

The typical findings in patients with coarctation are elevated systolic pressures in the upper extremities and lower systolic blood pressures in the lower extremities. However, infants may not have upper extremity hypertension but only a lower extremity hypotension. Therefore, blood pressures in all four extremities should be measured because the blood pressure differential can vary in location based on the area of coarctation and the arch anatomy. Absent or diminished femoral pulses and a delay between the radial pulse and the femoral pulse may be noted. Continuous murmurs from collateral vessels can be auscultated in the back in older children. Children with significant collaterals may not have a significant blood pressure differential. ECG may show right ventricular hypertrophy (RVH) (infants) or LVH (older infants and children) depending on the severity. The chest radiography usually shows increased pulmonary markings and cardiomegaly. In older children, rib notching can be seen in the third through eighth ribs secondary to the erosion by dilated tortuous intercostal arteries connected to collaterals. In younger children, echocardiography may be sufficient for the diagnosis. In older children and adults, further imaging of the distal arch by magnetic resonance imaging (MRI) or computed tomography scan may be required.

Primary surgical repair is recommended in infants and young children because of the high incidence of recoarctation with balloon angioplasty. Older adolescents and adults are candidates for covered stent placement and balloon angioplasty in the cardiac catheterization laboratory. Patients are still at risk for developing hypertension even after repair. The older the patient is at the time of diagnosis, the more likely he or she is to develop chronic hypertension.

Pulmonary Valve Disease

Pulmonary stenosis (PS) occurs in about 8% of children with congenital heart disease or seven in 100,000 live births. PS can be valvular, subvalvular, or supravalvular. Valvular PS is the most common (90%) and is usually seen with varying degrees of leaflet fusion of all three commissures (Figure 43-7). Dysplastic pulmonary valve abnormalities can be seen in association with Noonan's syndrome. Supravalvular stenosis is very rarely an isolated finding and is associated with Williams syndrome, Alagille syndrome, or LEOPARD (lentigines, ECG conduction abnormalities, ocular hypertelorism, pulmonary stenosis, abnormal genitalia, retarded growth, and sensorineural deafness) syndrome. Subvalvar PS is rare in isolation and is typically part of tetralogy of Fallot or is caused by an anomalous muscle bundle of the right ventricle (so-called double-chambered RV) associated with a conoventricular VSD.

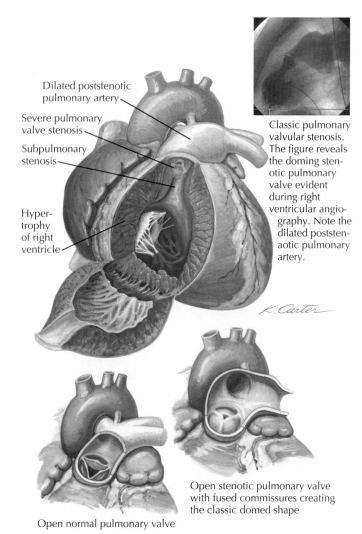

Dilated poststenotic pulmonary artery

Severe pulmonary valve stenosis

Subpulmonary stenosis

Hypertrophy of right ventricle

Classic pulmonary valvular stenosis. The figure reveals the doming stenotic pulmonary valve evident during right ventricular angiography. Note the dilated poststenaotic pulmonary artery.

K. Carter

Open stenotic pulmonary valve with fused commissures creating the classic domed shape

Open normal pulmonary valve

Figure 43-7 *Pulmonary stenosis.*

Infants and children with noncritical PS are rarely symptomatic. In more severe cases, children can have dyspnea with exertion and right-sided heart failure. Newborns with critical or severe PS present with cyanosis from right-to-left shunting through a patent foramen ovale, tachypnea, and poor feeding. On cardiac examination, one should hear a decreased P2 and a harsh systolic ejection murmur radiating to the back. On chest radiography, a dilated pulmonary artery may be evident. RVH is usually present on ECG with moderate to severe cases of PS. Echocardiography will characterize the type of PS and allows for measurement of the gradient across the area of stenosis. Gradients of less than 40 mm Hg are mild, 40 to 70 mm Hg are moderate, and greater than 70 mm Hg is considered severe PS.

No restriction of activity is necessary unless PS is severe. For children with mild degrees of stenosis, periodic echocardiograms are recommended to follow for worsening stenosis. For children with valvar PS with a gradient greater than 50 mm Hg as measured by cardiac catheterization, a balloon valvuloplasty is performed. Newborns with severe or critical PS

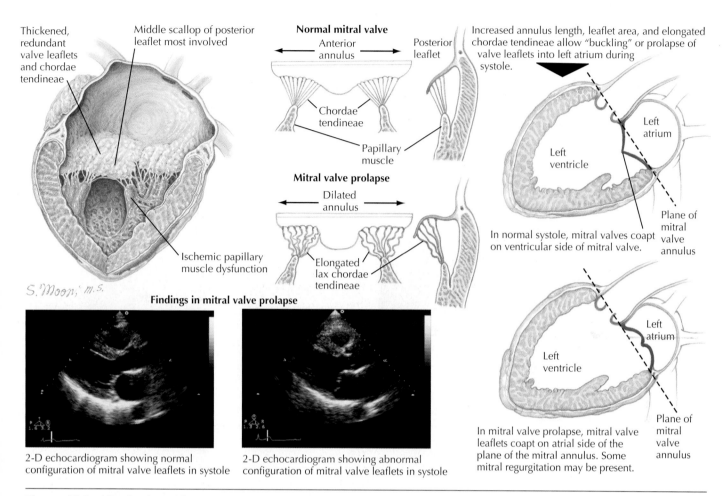

Thickened, redundant valve leaflets and chordae tendineae

Middle scallop of posterior leaflet most involved

Normal mitral valve
Anterior annulus
Posterior leaflet
Chordae tendineae
Papillary muscle

Increased annulus length, leaflet area, and elongated chordae tendineae allow "buckling" or prolapse of valve leaflets into left atrium during systole.

Left atrium
Left ventricle
Plane of mitral valve annulus

In normal systole, mitral valves coapt on ventricular side of mitral valve.

Ischemic papillary muscle dysfunction

Mitral valve prolapse
Dilated annulus
Elongated lax chordae tendineae

S. Moon, M.S.

Findings in mitral valve prolapse

2-D echocardiogram showing normal configuration of mitral valve leaflets in systole

2-D echocardiogram showing abnormal configuration of mitral valve leaflets in systole

Left atrium
Left ventricle
Plane of mitral valve annulus

In mitral valve prolapse, mitral valve leaflets coapt on atrial side of the plane of the mitral annulus. Some mitral regurgitation may be present.

Figure 43-8 *Mitral valve prolapse.*

need balloon valvuloplasty regardless of the gradients because severe PS may result in decrease output across the valve and therefore a lower gradient. (If unsuccessful, a surgical valvotomy can be performed.) Subvalvar PS is corrected by a surgical approach.

Mitral Valve Disease

Mitral stenosis (MS) is an uncommon isolated congenital heart defect but appears more commonly as a complication of rheumatic heart disease. Structural abnormalities that can cause MS include parachute mitral valve (a defect in the mitral valve in which there is only one papillary muscle present), mitral valve arcade (direct attachment of leaflets to the papillary muscles without intervening chordae and therefore absence of interchordal spaces), or a supramitral ring. Any left-sided obstructive lesion warrants evaluation of the mitral valve.

Mitral regurgitation (MR) is also commonly found as a complication of rheumatic heart disease but can occur with structural abnormalities as well. Isolated cleft mitral valve is a rare form of congenital MR. *Mitral valve prolapse* (MVP) may also result in MR caused by posterior movement of one leaflet into the left atrium during systole (Figure 43-8). Although unusual in infants, MVP can be seen in patients with connective tissue

disorders such as Marfan and Ehlers-Danlos syndromes. Bacterial endocarditis of the mitral valve may also result in MR.

Mitral valve disease caused by rheumatic heart disease is discussed in further detail in Chapter 49.

Vascular Ring

Vascular rings are anomalies of the aortic arch that can cause compression of the trachea, esophagus, or both. Infants may present with "noisy breathing" or with stridor. Respiratory distress associated concomitant upper respiratory infections is common. Older children and toddlers might present with swallowing difficulties, although asthma without family history and unresponsive to medical management warrants consideration of a vascular ring. Double aortic arch and right aortic arch with a retroesophageal diverticulum of Kommerell are the two most common types of vascular rings (Figure 43-9). If a vascular ring is suspected, chest radiography can determine arch sidedness and sometimes indentation of the trachea (double aortic arch). In addition, a barium esophagram can reveal a large posterior indentation on the esophagus (virtually all rings). Definitive diagnosis can be made by MRI. Surgical repair is indicated in any symptomatic patient. Symptoms do not always improve immediately and may persist for up to 1 year after repair.

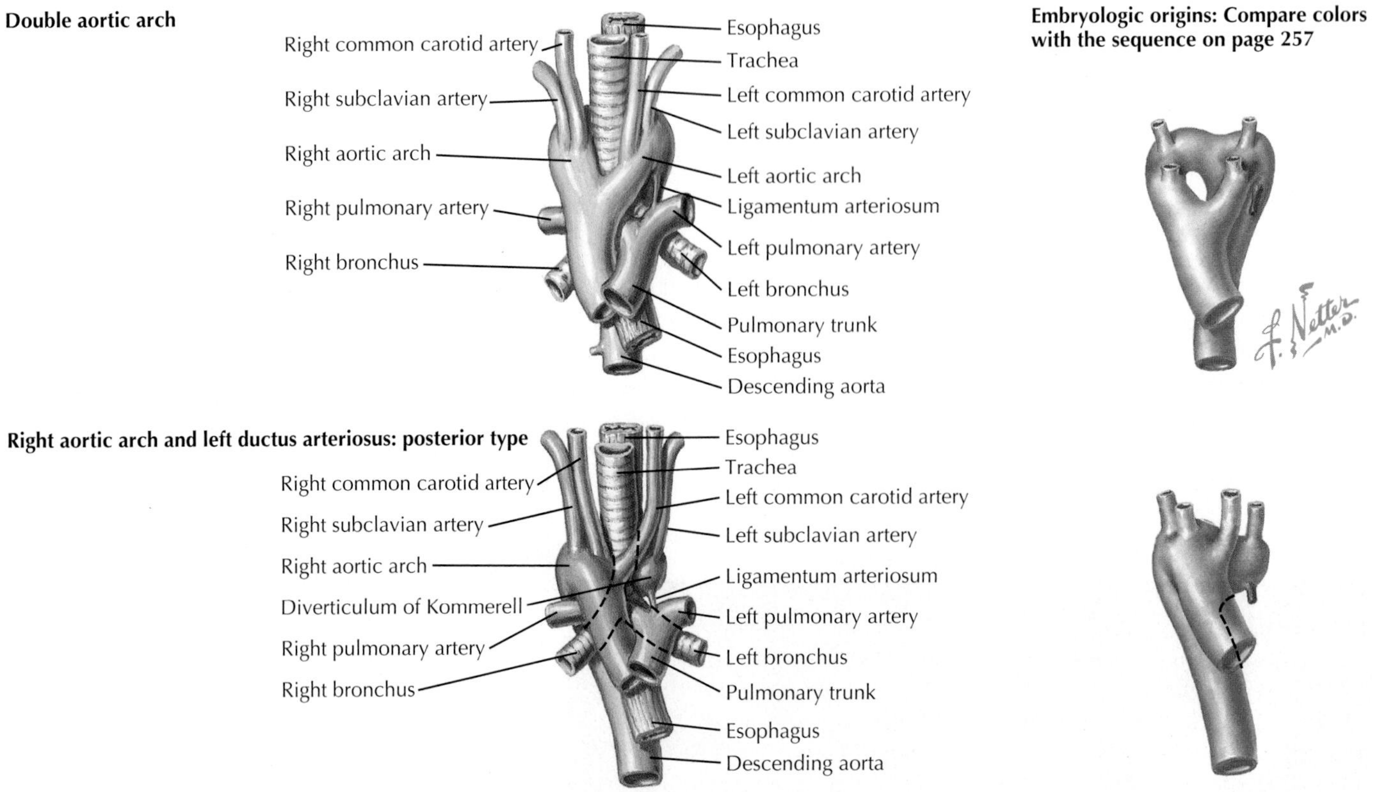

Double aortic arch

Right common carotid artery
Right subclavian artery
Right aortic arch
Right pulmonary artery
Right bronchus

Esophagus
Trachea
Left common carotid artery
Left subclavian artery
Left aortic arch
Ligamentum arteriosum
Left pulmonary artery
Left bronchus
Pulmonary trunk
Esophagus
Descending aorta

Embryologic origins: Compare colors with the sequence on page 257

Right aortic arch and left ductus arteriosus: posterior type

Right common carotid artery
Right subclavian artery
Right aortic arch
Diverticulum of Kommerell
Right pulmonary artery
Right bronchus

Esophagus
Trachea
Left common carotid artery
Left subclavian artery
Ligamentum arteriosum
Left pulmonary artery
Left bronchus
Pulmonary trunk
Esophagus
Descending aorta

Figure 43-9 *Vascular rings.*

FUTURE DIRECTIONS

With the advancements in prenatal diagnosis, imaging technology, cardiac catheterization interventions, and surgical techniques, the diagnosis and management of patients with congenital heart disease continues to be an evolving field. Certainly, the development of cardiac catheterization techniques has allowed for an alternate to surgical treatment for many of these lesions. Fetal intervention is another exciting new area of investigation that may play a role in the future of congenital cardiac treatment. Patients with acyanotic congenital heart lesions have excellent survival rates, but it is important to realize that most patients with these defects require lifelong follow-up by a cardiologist even after surgical palliation.

SUGGESTED READINGS

Allen HD, Driscoll DJ, Shaddy RE, Feltes TF, editors: *Moss and Adams' Heart Disease in Infants, Children, and Adolescents Including the Fetus and Young Adult*, ed 7, Philadelphia, 2008, Lippincott Williams & Wilkins.

Borer JS, Bonow RO: Contemporary approach to aortic and mitral regurgitation, *Circulation* 108(20):2432-2438, 2003.

Campbell M: Natural history of atrial septal defects, *Br Heart J* 32:820-826, 1970.

Chiappa E: The impact of prenatal diagnosis of congenital heart disease on pediatric cardiology and cardiac surgery, *J Cardiovasc Med* 8(1):12-16, 2007.

Graham TP Jr, Bricker JT, James FW, Strong WB: 26th Bethesda conference: recommendations for determining eligibility for competition in athletes with cardiovascular abnormalities. Task Force 1: congenital heart disease, *Med Sci Sports Exerc* 26(10 suppl):S246-S253, 1994.

McMahon CJ, Feltes TF, Fraley JK, et al: Natural history of growth of secundum atrial septal defects and implications for transcatheter closure, *Heart* 87(3):256-259, 2002.

Pinto NM, Marino BS, Wernovsky G, et al: Obesity is a common comorbidity in children with congenital and acquired heart disease, *Pediatrics* 120(5):e1157-e1164, 2007.

Rudolph AM: The effects of postnatal circulatory adjustments in congenital heart disease, *Pediatrics* 36:763-772, 1965.

Cyanotic Congenital Heart Disease

Michael L. O'Byrne and Anitha S. John

44

yanotic heart disease refers to cardiac lesions that result in a characteristic blue discoloration of the skin. Typically, patients with cyanotic heart disease present in infancy. These defects may be detected through prenatal screening echocardiography or by screening pulse oximetry in the newborn period. However, patients with untreated acyanotic lesions can present later in life with cyanosis caused by either progressive subpulmonary stenosis in patients with complex heart disease including a ventricular septal defect (VSD, e.g., tetralogy of Fallot) or development of Eisenmenger physiology.

PATHOPHYSIOLOGY OF CYANOSIS

Cyanosis results from deoxygenated blood entering the arterial circulation. This can result from either abnormal alignment of anatomic segments, resulting in venous drainage being directed to the systemic arterial circulation with limited systemic–pulmonary mixing (e.g., D-transposition) or abundant systemic–pulmonary mixing (e.g., tetralogy of Fallot, single ventricle, total anomalous pulmonary venous connection). The concentration of deoxygenated hemoglobin must exceed 5 g/dL in systemic arterial blood for cyanosis to be manifest, so patients who are anemic may have low oxygen saturations but may not appear cyanotic. Furthermore, clinical cyanosis is often not recognized by parents and even by clinicians, especially in patients who have deeply pigmented skin.

The magnitude of cyanosis depends on which of the two physiologic types mentioned above is present. In the first, the transposition type, cyanosis is independent of the amount of pulmonary blood flow but instead is related to the amount of mixing between the systemic and pulmonary circulations—with more mixing, there is less cyanosis, and with less mixing, there is more cyanosis. In *normal physiology*, the aorta is fully saturated, and the aortic saturation is higher than the pulmonary saturation. The pulmonary and systemic circulations are in series, and oxygenated blood returns from the lungs and exits to the body via the aorta. In *transposition physiology*, the pulmonary artery saturation is higher than the aortic saturation. There are two parallel circulations where the oxygenated blood returns mostly to the lungs and deoxygenated blood mostly to the body. The presence of an atrial septal defect (ASD) (or creating one with a balloon atrial septostomy) allows for some mixing between the two circulations, which results in improved systemic saturation (although still lower than pulmonary saturation). Most of these patients have high pulmonary blood flow.

In the second type of cyanotic heart disease, *tetralogy physiology*, cyanosis depends on the amount of pulmonary blood flow. With much systemic–pulmonary mixing at some level, the greater the amount of pulmonary blood flow, the lesser the degree of cyanosis; the less pulmonary flow, the more cyanosis.

In *differential cyanosis*, the preductal oxygen saturation (right arm) is higher than the postductal (lower extremity). This occurs

when one ventricle delivers the blood to the upper half of the body, and the other ventricle provides some of the blood to the lower half of the body via a patent ductus arteriosus in the absence of complete systemic–pulmonary mixing. This occurs in coarctation of the aorta and interrupted aortic arch and with persistent pulmonary hypertension of the newborn. *Reverse differential cyanosis* (postductal saturation > preductal saturation) occurs with transposition of the great arteries in addition to the above conditions.

Other factors affecting the oxygen content in both the pulmonary venous and systemic venous blood can worsen cyanosis in these lesions. Pulmonary edema, pulmonary parenchymal disease, or increased metabolic demands can result in a greater than expected degree of cyanosis.

CLINICAL PRESENTATION AND EVALUATION

Cyanosis is the most common presenting sign in these newborns when cyanosis is severe. In lesions with abundant mixing and with pulmonary overcirculation, such as truncus arteriosus, total anomalous pulmonary venous connection, and single ventricle without pulmonary stenosis, the cyanosis is less obvious, but tachypnea and respiratory distress may bring the patient to medical attention. Some lesions such as tetralogy of Fallot have a variable presentation depending on the severity of the obstruction to right ventricular outflow. Despite their variability of presentation, these lesions are discussed together because they present at the same age and should all be considered in the differential of a neonate with suspected severe congenital heart disease. It should also be noted that cyanotic congenital heart disease is increasingly diagnosed prenatally via echocardiography, allowing for delivery of infants with the most severe cases in tertiary care hospitals equipped to care for cyanotic heart disease, reducing end-organ damage and complications, and potentially improving overall survival rates.

The differential diagnosis of cyanosis in an infant or young child includes the congenital cardiac lesions described below but also includes acrocyanosis (blue discoloration of extremities caused by peripheral vasoconstriction), pulmonary disease, and methemoglobinemia.

Evaluation of these patients includes a thorough physical examination and pre- and postductal saturations, chest radiography, electrocardiography, and hyperoxia test. Transthoracic echocardiography confirms the anatomy of the lesions and may provide important information regarding cardiac physiology.

The *hyperoxia test* can be a useful tool for differentiating cardiac and noncardiac cyanosis. It relies on the principle that hypoxemia caused by cardiac abnormalities is not corrected by increasing the inspired fraction of inspired oxygen (FiO_2). Therefore, in a child with FiO_2 of 100%, a right radial (i.e.,

External appearance of heart

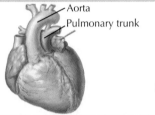

Aorta
Pulmonary trunk

f. Netter m.d.
JOHN A. CRAIG ʌD
C. Machado m.d.

Balloon atrial septostomy (technique)

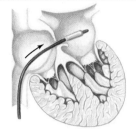 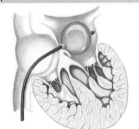 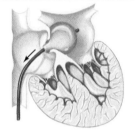 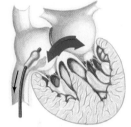

Balloon-tipped catheter introduced into left atrium through
patent foramen ovale

Balloon inflated

Balloon withdrawn
producing large septal defect

Common atrium produced by
septostomy allows mixing of oxygenated and deoxygenated blood

Mustard operation

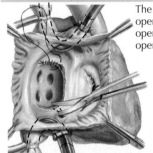

The interatrial septum has been widely excised,
opening into transverse sinus at upper end. This
opening is being sutured and coronary sinus
opened into left atrium.

A patch of pericardium
has been applied to
close incision and
enlarge newly
formed right atrium

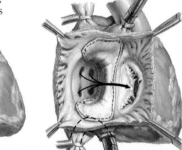

A patch of pericardium has been
applied so as to channel blood
from pulmonary veins through
tricuspid valve to right ventricle,
then out the aorta. Blood from
venae cavae will now pass to
left ventricle and then to
pulmonary artery.

Arterial repair of transposition of the great arteries

First steps

The aorta and the pulmonary artery are
transected. The cut of the aorta is slanted
and above the Valsalva's sinuses. The
pulmonary artery is divided above its
valve at the same level of the transection
of the aorta. Sinuses of the aorta and
pulmonary artery are excised to
translocate the coronary ostia from the
pulmonary artery to the neoaorta.
Pericardium is utilized to reconstruct
the neopulmonary artery sinuses.

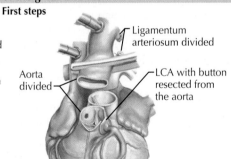

Ligamentum
arteriosum divided

Aorta
divided

LCA with button
resected from
the aorta

Last steps

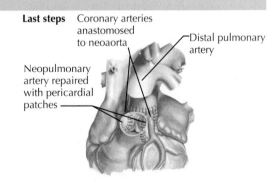

Coronary arteries
anastomosed
to neoaorta

Distal pulmonary
artery

Neopulmonary
artery repaired
with pericardial
patches

Figure 44-1 *Transposition of the great arteries.*

preductal) arterial pAO_2 less than 150 mm Hg suggests cyanotic congenital heart disease. Higher pAO_2s suggest pulmonary disease with rare exceptions. Furthermore, pulmonary disease usually permits a much larger increase in pAO_2 than does structural heart disease.

Transposition of the Great Arteries

Transposition of the great arteries means that the pulmonary artery arises above the left ventricle and the aorta above the right ventricle (Figure 44-1). It is the most common cardiac cause of cyanosis in the neonatal period (0.2-0.4 in 1000 live births), accounting for 7% of congenital heart defects. Its incidence is increased in infants of diabetic mothers. It is not seen in patients with DiGeorge syndrome. Cyanosis results because the pulmonary and systemic circulations flow parallel to one another with minimal mixing: deoxygenated systemic venous blood returns to the right atrium and right ventricle and out the aorta, and oxygenated pulmonary venous blood returns to the left atrium and left ventricle and exits into the pulmonary

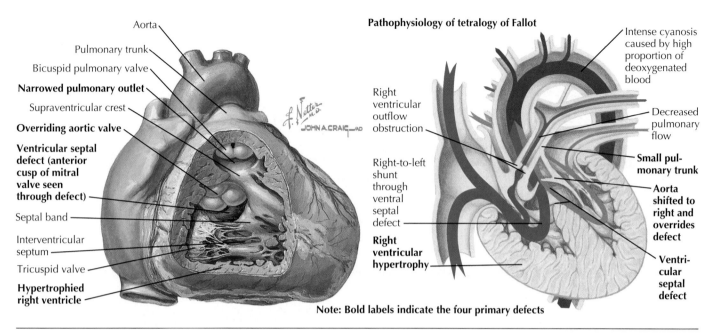

Figure 44-2 *Tetralogy of Fallot.*

arteries. These two parallel circuits are compatible with survival only because there is some point of mixing, usually at the foramen ovale.

Immediate intervention is usually necessary to augment the interatrial shunt. This is accomplished through a Rashkind balloon atrial septostomy (see Figure 44-1). This procedure allows for increased mixing, resulting in tolerable aortic saturations. Surgery remains the definitive therapy. Historically, this was accomplished through an atrial switch operation—Mustard (see Figure 44-1) or Senning procedures—redirecting inflow from the pulmonary veins to the right ventricle and from the venae cavae to the left ventricle. Perioperative mortality was low, but concerns regarding arrhythmia and the durability of the right ventricle (which remains the systemic ventricle) led to a different surgical approach, with a higher degree of technical difficulty but improved physiology. Currently, the preferred method is the arterial switch operation in which (1) the aorta is bisected and the distal aorta is brought beneath the bifurcation of the pulmonary trunk while the pulmonary trunk is displaced anteriorly (the Lecompte maneuver) where the aorta is anastomosed to the former pulmonary trunk and the main pulmonary artery is anastomosed to the former aortic trunk, (2) the coronary arteries are detached from the former aortic trunk and reimplanted on the pulmonary trunk (the new aortic root) with pericardial patches placed on the sites where the coronary arteries were harvested, and (3) the ASD is repaired (see Figure 44-1).

Tetralogy of Fallot

Tetralogy of Fallot is characterized by an abnormally small subpulmonary conus or outflow tract, resulting in anterior and cephalad displacement of the infundibular (outflow tract) septum. This produces the four characteristic findings: (1) subvalvular pulmonic stenosis, (2) VSD caused by malalignment of the infundibular septum relative to the rest of the ventricular septum, (3) "overriding aorta" (i.e., the aortic valve sits above both ventricles), and (4) right ventricular hypertrophy caused by pressure overload from the large VSD (Figure 44-2). It occurs in 0.19 to 0.26 in 1000 live births and represents 8% of congenital cardiac lesions. Tetralogy of Fallot is found in more than 25% of patients with DiGeorge syndrome and chromosome 22q11.2 microdeletion. The incidence of tetralogy of Fallot is higher than the general population in children of mothers with phenylketonuria and occurs more frequently in children with thrombocytopenia absent radii syndrome. Associated cardiac defects include right aortic arch (25% of patients) and ASD (10% of patients).

Cyanosis in tetralogy of Fallot is variable, resulting from extensive systemic–pulmonary mixing and decreased pulmonary blood flow caused by the combination of subpulmonic stenosis and a large VSD.

The earliest surgical treatment was palliative, aimed at increasing pulmonary blood flow without addressing the subpulmonary stenosis or the VSD. The Blalock-Taussig shunt, an end-to-side anastomosis of the subclavian artery to the ipsilateral branch pulmonary artery, was the first operation for cyanotic heart disease. Subsequently, other shunts connecting the aorta to a pulmonary artery branch were devised. Nowadays most shunts for cyanotic heart disease are constructed from polytetrafluoroethylene tube grafts connecting the aorta or an arch vessel to the main pulmonary artery or one of its branches. Currently, surgical therapy is directed at complete repair with (1) effective closure of the VSD by baffling the left ventricle by way of the VSD to the overriding aorta; (2) augmentation of the right ventricular infundibulum; (3) valvotomy of the pulmonary valve, if necessary; and (4) placement of a transannular patch, a continuation of the infundibular incision across the pulmonary valve annulus, if there is significant annular hypoplasia.

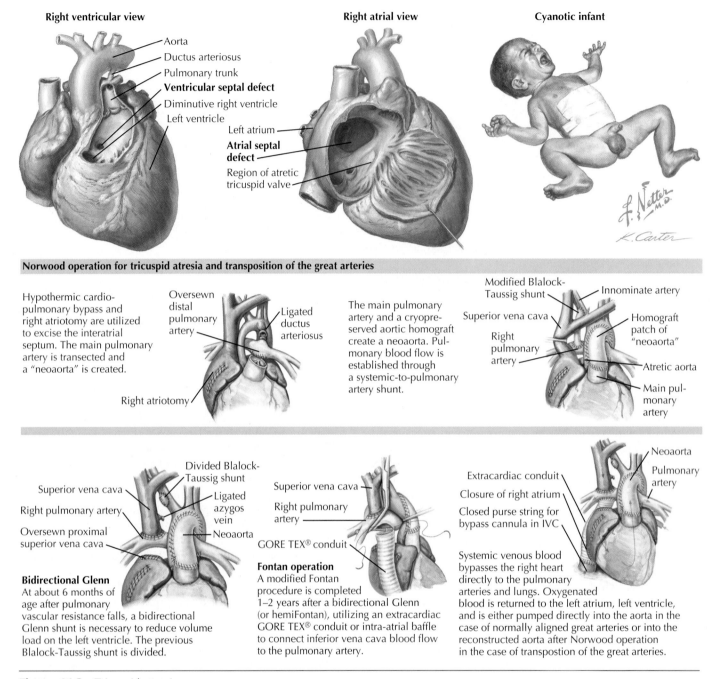

Right ventricular view
- Aorta
- Ductus arteriosus
- Pulmonary trunk
- **Ventricular septal defect**
- Diminutive right ventricle
- Left ventricle

Right atrial view
- Left atrium
- **Atrial septal defect**
- Region of atretic tricuspid valve

Cyanotic infant

Norwood operation for tricuspid atresia and transposition of the great arteries

Hypothermic cardio-pulmonary bypass and right atriotomy are utilized to excise the interatrial septum. The main pulmonary artery is transected and a "neoaorta" is created.

- Oversewn distal pulmonary artery
- Ligated ductus arteriosus
- Right atriotomy

The main pulmonary artery and a cryopre-served aortic homograft create a neoaorta. Pulmonary blood flow is established through a systemic-to-pulmonary artery shunt.

- Modified Blalock-Taussig shunt
- Innominate artery
- Superior vena cava
- Right pulmonary artery
- Homograft patch of "neoaorta"
- Atretic aorta
- Main pulmonary artery

- Superior vena cava
- Right pulmonary artery
- Oversewn proximal superior vena cava
- Divided Blalock-Taussig shunt
- Ligated azygos vein
- Neoaorta

Bidirectional Glenn
At about 6 months of age after pulmonary vascular resistance falls, a bidirectional Glenn shunt is necessary to reduce volume load on the left ventricle. The previous Blalock-Taussig shunt is divided.

- Superior vena cava
- Right pulmonary artery
- GORE TEX® conduit

Fontan operation
A modified Fontan procedure is completed 1–2 years after a bidirectional Glenn (or hemiFontan), utilizing an extracardiac GORE TEX® conduit or intra-atrial baffle to connect inferior vena cava blood flow to the pulmonary artery.

- Neoaorta
- Pulmonary artery
- Extracardiac conduit
- Closure of right atrium
- Closed purse string for bypass cannula in IVC

Systemic venous blood bypasses the right heart directly to the pulmonary arteries and lungs. Oxygenated blood is returned to the left atrium, left ventricle, and is either pumped directly into the aorta in the case of normally aligned great arteries or into the reconstructed aorta after Norwood operation in the case of transpostion of the great arteries.

Figure 44-3 *Tricuspid atresia.*

Double Outlet Right Ventricle with Pulmonic Stenosis

Double outlet right ventricle with pulmonic stenosis has similar physiology to tetralogy of Fallot. The presentation can be similar, with differentiation provided by echocardiography. The surgical approach is similar as well, baffling the left ventricle by way of the VSD to the nearby aorta and either pulmonary outflow augmentation as in tetralogy or placement of an extra-cardiac right ventricle to pulmonary artery conduit. Because the VSD, the effective left ventricular outflow, is surrounded by muscle, it may be necessary to enlarge it before baffling to the aorta to avoid subaortic stenosis.

Tricuspid Atresia

Tricuspid atresia is absence of communication between the right atrium and either ventricle. All blood returning to the right atrium flows across a patent foramen ovale or ASD to the left atrium, left ventricle, and usually through a VSD to the remnant of the right ventricle. In cases with normally aligned great arteries, the size of the VSD affects the amount of pulmonary blood flow and therefore the degree of cyanosis (Figure 44-3). Because many patients have muscular VSDs, it may be large early in life with relatively high pulmonary blood flow and mild cyanosis. Over time, the VSD may become smaller, resulting in decreasing pulmonary blood flow and increasing cyanosis.

Rarely, there is no VSD, and pulmonary blood flow is exclusively from a ductus arteriosus. In cases with transposition of the great arteries, the aorta arises from the small remnant of the right ventricle. These patients usually have high pulmonary blood flow and therefore mild cyanosis. When the VSD is relatively small, there may be additional coarctation of the aorta. These VSDs are rarely muscular and therefore tend to stay about the same relative size over time. High pulmonary blood flow often results in heart failure and, if not surgically addressed, can eventually cause pulmonary vascular disease. In patients with transposition and a restrictive VSD, a Damus-Kaye-Stansel or a Norwood operation is required to effectively bypass the subaortic obstruction by using the pulmonary valve (arising unobstructed from the left ventricle) as an additional (or only) systemic outlet. These operations involve transection of the pulmonary artery above the valve and amalgamation of the pulmonary stump with the ascending aorta and aortic arch, either with (Norwood) (see Figure 44-3) or without (Damus-Kaye-Stansel) supplementary graft material depending on the size difference between the two vessels. The distal pulmonary arteries are then supplied by a systemic-to-pulmonary shunt.

Because all patients with tricuspid atresia, regardless of associated abnormalities, have a functional single ventricle, the ultimate treatment is a Fontan operation, in which all systemic venous return goes directly to the pulmonary arteries (without passing through a ventricle) and pulmonary venous return goes to the left atrium and left ventricle and out the aorta (normally aligned great arteries) or through the VSD to the right ventricular remnant to the aorta (transposition). Because the Fontan operation depends on low pulmonary resistance to allow systemic venous blood to flow without a pump into the pulmonary arteries, it cannot be carried out until the high pulmonary resistance of the normal newborn has resolved. An intermediary operation, superior cavopulmonary anastomosis (bidirectional Glenn [see Figure 44-3] or hemi-Fontan), is typically performed at 4 to 6 months of age. In this operation, the superior vena cava is connected to the right pulmonary artery so that all venous drainage from the upper body goes to the lungs but inferior vena caval blood mixes with pulmonary venous return and goes to the body. One or 2 years later, the inferior vena cava is connected to the pulmonary arteries by way of an intraatrial baffle or extracardiac conduit, completing the Fontan circuit (see Figure 44-3).

Critical Pulmonic Stenosis

Infants with extreme narrowing of the pulmonic valve orifice (critical pulmonic stenosis) (Figure 44-4) can present with hepatomegaly and cyanosis from right-to-left shunting across the foramen ovale because of right ventricular failure or low right ventricular compliance.

Treatment is aimed at relieving obstruction at the pulmonary valve. This is usually accomplished through balloon valvuloplasty in the interventional catheterization laboratory (see Figure 44-4). Before this, patients are often palliated with prostaglandin E$_1$ infusion to maintain ductal patency to increase pulmonary blood flow and reduce cyanosis. If the right ventricular compliance is sufficiently low because of severe hypertrophy or hypoplasia, valvotomy may not be sufficient to provide adequate pulmonary blood flow, and a temporary systemic–pulmonary shunt may be necessary until compliance improves.

Pulmonary Atresia

Pulmonary atresia with intact ventricular septum is a more severe form of critical pulmonary stenosis. This occurs in 0.07 in 1000 live births. Because the severe obstruction occurs during fetal development, the right ventricular hypertrophy causes poor compliance so that the right ventricle stops growing. Thus, patients have a small right ventricle. In many cases, they also have right ventricle-to-coronary artery fistulae. These may lead to perfusion defects of the left ventricle as coronary blood flow is forced retrograde into the aorta from a suprasystemic right ventricle.

The physiology is similar to that of critical pulmonic stenosis, but because the right ventricular size tends to be smaller than that of critical pulmonic stenosis, it is more likely that a systemic-to-pulmonary shunt will be required even when the atretic valve can be perforated and balloon dilated in the catheterization laboratory or when an outflow tract reconstruction can be performed surgically. Many of these patients never achieve significant right ventricular growth and must be treated as functional single ventricles with a Fontan operation (described above with tricuspid atresia).

Ebstein's Anomaly of the Tricuspid Valve

Ebstein's anomaly is a rare anatomic abnormality characterized by displacement of the attachment of the septal and posterior leaflets of the tricuspid valve toward the apex of the right ventricle. The lesion constitutes fewer than 1% of congenital cardiac lesions, representing 0.05 in 10,000 live births. Children of mothers taking lithium have a higher incidence of Ebstein's anomaly. No extracardiac syndromes are associated with it, but it is commonly associated with other cardiac lesions, including interatrial communication (ASD or patent foramen ovale) as well as VSDs, pulmonic stenosis or atresia, and L-transposition of the great arteries.

Downward displacement of the tricuspid valve partitions the right ventricle into an apical right ventricular portion and a proximal atrialized right ventricle (Figure 44-5). The tricuspid valve anterior leaflet becomes large redundant and "sail-like" with variable tricuspid regurgitation. These patients have a high incidence (20%-30%) of preexcitation with accessory pathway.

Hemodynamically, Ebstein's anomaly has a wide range of possible physiologies, depending on the degree of regurgitation or stenosis of the tricuspid valve, the presence of atrial communication, and the degree of right ventricular dysfunction as a result of the dysplastic valve. Thus, patients can present with symptoms of cyanosis, heart failure, or atrial arrhythmias depending on the balance of the aforementioned factors.

Treatment choices depend on the degree of tricuspid regurgitation and presenting symptoms. Patients with mild symptoms do not require intervention and may have a benign natural history. At the other extreme, patients with severe tricuspid regurgitation have high mortality partly related to pulmonary hypoplasia caused by intrauterine cardiomegaly. Survivors past infancy may develop right heart failure in adolescence with

Pulmonary stenosis

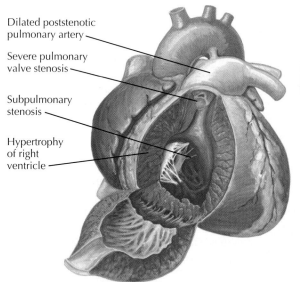

Dilated poststenotic
pulmonary artery

Severe pulmonary
valve stenosis

Subpulmonary
stenosis

Hypertrophy
of right
ventricle

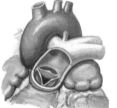

Open normal
pulmonary valve

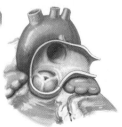

Open stenotic
pulmonary valve
with fused
commissures
creating the
classic domed
shape

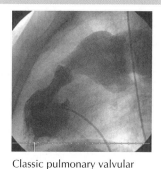

Classic pulmonary valvular
stenosis. The figure reveals the
doming stenotic pulmonary valve
evident during right ventricular
angiography. Note the dilated
poststenotic pulmonary artery.

Pulmonary balloon valvuloplasty

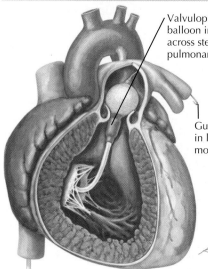

Valvuloplasty
balloon in place
across stenotic
pulmonary valve

Guide wire
in left pul-
monary artery

Percutaneous catheter
from femoral vein

Flouroscopy showing beginning inflation of contrast-
filled balloon (**left**) and full inflation with near dis-
appearance of waist from stenotic valve (**right**).

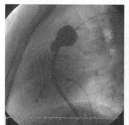

Partially inflated
balloon across
stenotic pulmonary
valve

Fully inflated
balloon across
stenotic pulmonary
valve

Torn valve
cusps after
balloon
inflation

Inoue Balloon Catheter, Toray Industries, Inc., Tokyo, Japan.

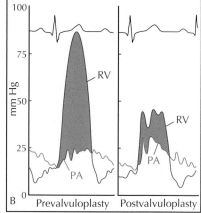

Pressure wave tracings showing difference
between right ventricle and pulmonary artery
before (**left**) and after (**right**) balloon valvotomy

With permission from Bashore TM, Davidson CJ. Acute
hemodynamic effects of percutaneous balloon aortic
valvuloplasty. In: Bashore TM, Davidson CJ, eds.
*Percutaneous Balloon Valvulopasty and Related
echniques.* Baltimore: Williams & Wilkins; 1991:99–111.

Figure 44-4   *Critical pulmonic stenosis.*

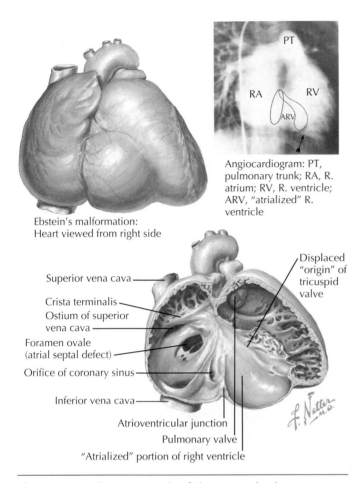

Angiocardiogram: PT, pulmonary trunk; RA, R. atrium; RV, R. ventricle; ARV, "atrialized" R. ventricle

Ebstein's malformation: Heart viewed from right side

Superior vena cava

Crista terminalis

Ostium of superior vena cava

Foramen ovale (atrial septal defect)

Orifice of coronary sinus

Inferior vena cava

Atrioventricular junction

Pulmonary valve

"Atrialized" portion of right ventricle

Displaced "origin" of tricuspid valve

Figure 44-5 *Ebstein anomaly of the tricuspid valve.*

cyanosis if an atrial-level communication exists or may have supraventricular tachycardia.

Early surgical intervention has had poor results, but tricuspid annuloplasty and valvuloplasty have had good results in recent years.

Total Anomalous Pulmonary Venous Connection

Total anomalous pulmonary venous connection means connection of all pulmonary veins to somewhere other than the left atrium. Connections to the innominate vein, the portal system of the liver, and the coronary sinus are representative of the main categories noted below (Figure 44-6). This defect comprises 1% to 3% of congenital cardiac lesions. Anatomically, patients are divided among those whose pulmonary veins connect above the diaphragm (70%), below the diaphragm (25%), or in mixed fashion (i.e., to more than one connection; 5%). Those connecting above the diaphragm are further divided into those connecting to a vein, most often the innominate vein, and those connecting to the heart, either the coronary sinus or the right atrium. The majority of these are unobstructed. Connection below the diaphragm is almost always to the portal vein or one of its branches or to the ductus venosus; hence, they become obstructed when the ductus venosus closes in the first few days of life.

The degree of cyanosis depends on the amount of pulmonary venous obstruction. Patients with significant obstruction present with marked cyanosis from decreased pulmonary blood flow accentuated by pulmonary edema and pulmonary arterial hypertension; they also show tachypnea and respiratory distress. Patients without obstruction have high pulmonary blood flow and initially have minimal cyanosis, but they progress to congestive heart failure because of pulmonary overcirculation.

Therapy is surgical with anastomosis of the pulmonary vein confluence to the left atrium in those with extracardiac anomalous connection, unroofing of the coronary sinus in the coronary sinus type, and repositioning of the atrial septum in the right atrial type. With pulmonary vein obstruction, therapy is urgent. With unobstructed veins, there is no technical surgical advantage in waiting, but increasing evidence suggests that delaying surgery until 1 month of age will improve neurocognitive outcomes. Perioperative mortality remains much higher in patients with pulmonary vein obstruction (20%) versus those without obstruction (<5%).

Truncus Arteriosus Communis

Truncus arteriosus communis denotes a single arterial trunk that serves as the common origin of the aorta, pulmonary artery, and coronary arteries (Figure 44-7). It comprises 2% to 2.8% of congenital cardiac lesions. This condition is almost always associated with a VSD. The truncus is fed by a single truncal valve, most commonly with three cusps, but may have two to five cusps, often myxomatous and asymmetric. This truncal valve typically sits over the VSD but in rare cases arises predominantly above the right ventricle. Associated cardiac defects include right aortic arch (33%) and anomalous coronary artery origins. Extracardiac anomalies associated with truncus include 22q11 microdeletion. The physiology of truncus is usually that of high pulmonary blood flow with minimal cyanosis but commonly tachypnea and respiratory distress. Congestive heart failure is exaggerated by poor coronary perfusion secondary to low diastolic pressures from runoff into the pulmonary arteries.

Treatment is surgical separation of aorta and pulmonary artery, placement of an extracardiac right ventricle to pulmonary artery conduit, and closing the VSD by baffling the left ventricle to the aorta (see Figure 44-7).

FUTURE DIRECTIONS

Progress in the management of patients with cyanotic heart disease is ongoing and reflects the wide range of clinical disciplines involved in the care of these patients. Noninvasive imaging technologies such as magnetic resonance imaging and computed tomography provide increasingly detailed anatomic and physiologic information, directing medical and surgical care without the risk of more invasive modalities. Treatment continues to improve survival after surgical therapy. These include improvements in surgical technique, intensive care unit management, and long-term medical management. Additionally, hybrid procedures combining conventional surgical and percutaneous catheterization techniques (both pre- and postnatally) are being attempted as part of experimental protocols. These

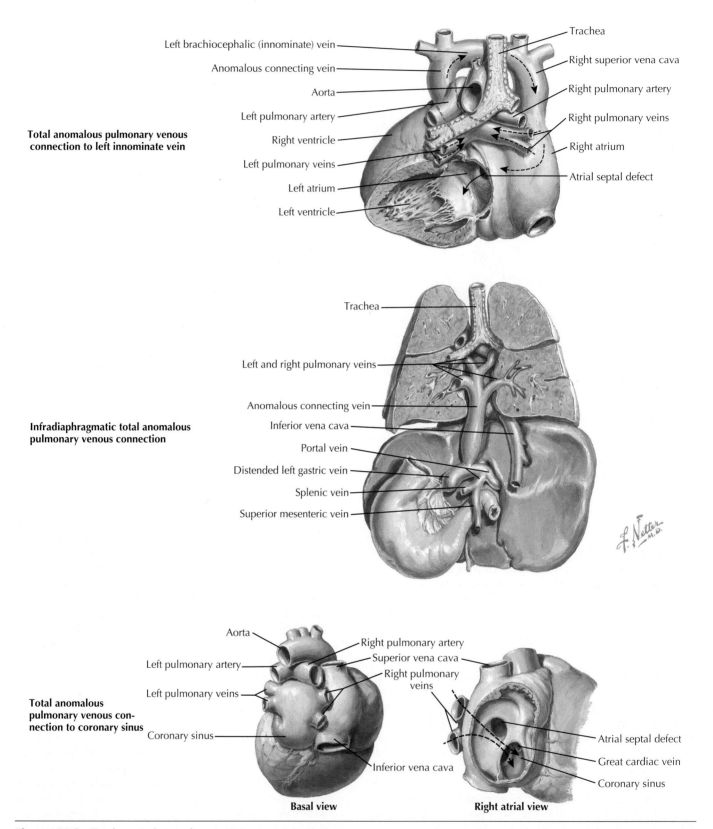

Total anomalous pulmonary venous connection to left innominate vein

Left brachiocephalic (innominate) vein
Anomalous connecting vein
Aorta
Left pulmonary artery
Right ventricle
Left pulmonary veins
Left atrium
Left ventricle

Trachea
Right superior vena cava
Right pulmonary artery
Right pulmonary veins
Right atrium
Atrial septal defect

Infradiaphragmatic total anomalous pulmonary venous connection

Trachea
Left and right pulmonary veins
Anomalous connecting vein
Inferior vena cava
Portal vein
Distended left gastric vein
Splenic vein
Superior mesenteric vein

Total anomalous pulmonary venous connection to coronary sinus

Aorta
Left pulmonary artery
Left pulmonary veins
Coronary sinus

Right pulmonary artery
Superior vena cava
Right pulmonary veins
Inferior vena cava

Atrial septal defect
Great cardiac vein
Coronary sinus

Basal view

Right atrial view

Figure 44-6 *Total anomalous pulmonary venous connection.*

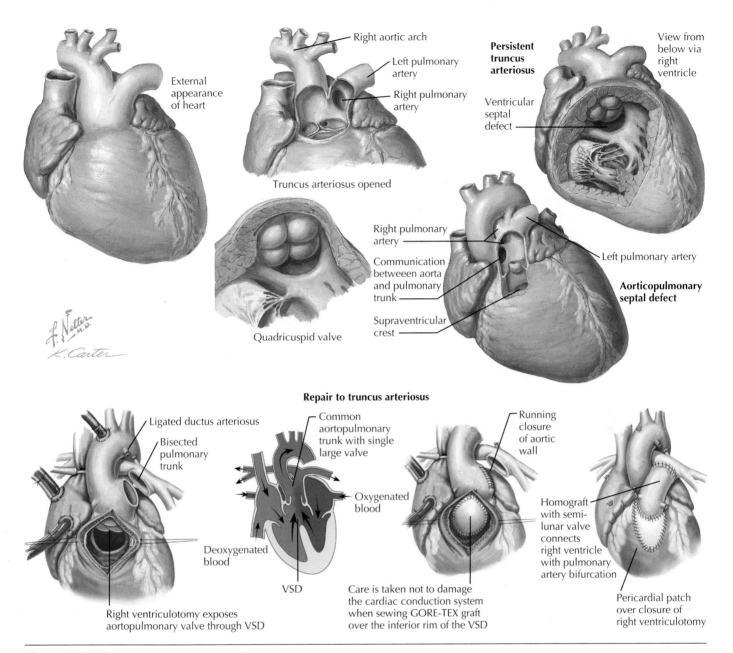

External appearance of heart

Right aortic arch

Left pulmonary artery

Right pulmonary artery

Truncus arteriosus opened

Persistent truncus arteriosus

Ventricular septal defect

View from below via right ventricle

Quadricuspid valve

Right pulmonary artery

Communication betweeen aorta and pulmonary trunk

Supraventricular crest

Left pulmonary artery

Aorticopulmonary septal defect

Repair to truncus arteriosus

Ligated ductus arteriosus

Bisected pulmonary trunk

Common aortopulmonary trunk with single large valve

Oxygenated blood

Deoxygenated blood

VSD

Right ventriculotomy exposes aortopulmonary valve through VSD

Care is taken not to damage the cardiac conduction system when sewing GORE-TEX graft over the inferior rim of the VSD

Running closure of aortic wall

Homograft with semi-lunar valve connects right ventricle with pulmonary artery bifurcation

Pericardial patch over closure of right ventriculotomy

Figure 44-7 *Truncus arteriosus communis.*

interventions appear to hold much promise, but it remains an empiric question whether these procedures will represent an improvement over conventional surgical techniques or have applicability in wider practice. Finally, with dramatically improved postsurgical survival, research has expanded beyond actuarial survival to define characteristics of patients that differentiate the success or failure of therapy far beyond the immediate postsurgical period such as objective measures of quality of life and neurodevelopmental outcomes.

SUGGESTED READINGS

Ballweg JA, Wernovsky G, Gaynor JW: Neurodevelopmental outcomes following congenital heart surgery, *Pediatr Cardiol* 28(2):126-133, 2007.

Beghetti M, Galie N: Eisenmenger syndrome a clinical perspective in a new therapeutic era of pulmonary arterial hypertension, *J Am Coll Cardiol* 53(9):733-740, 2009.

Cohen MS, Frommelt MA: Does fetal diagnosis make a difference? *Clin Perinatol* 32(4):877-890, 2005.

Crean A: Cardiovascular MR and CT in congenital heart disease, *Heart* 93(12):1637-1647, 2007.

Dorfman AT, Marino BS, Wernovsky G, et al: Critical heart disease in the neonate: presentation and outcome at a tertiary care center, *Pediatr Crit Care Med* 9(2):193-202, 2008.

Marino BS, Tomlinson RS, Drotar D, et al: Quality-of-life concerns differ among patients, parents, and medical providers in children and adolescents with congenital and acquired heart disease, *Pediatrics* 123(4):e708-e715, 2009.

Arrhythmias

Javier J. Lasa

45

Although infrequent in the pediatric population, arrhythmias represent potentially significant causes of morbidity and mortality. The diagnosis and management of arrhythmias require an understanding of age-dependent normal variations in heart rate (Table 45-1). This chapter describes the etiology, clinical significance, and treatment options of common arrhythmias found in infants, children, and adolescents, including bradyarrhythmias, tachyarrhythmias, and rhythm disturbances leading to syncope and sudden death.

SINUS ARRHYTHMIAS AND PREMATURE IMPULSES

Sinus Bradycardia

Sinus bradycardia is defined as a heart rate slower than the lower limit of normal for age and originating from the sinus node. Normal individuals and well-trained athletes can have sinus bradycardia without hemodynamic significance. Pathologic conditions in which sinus bradycardia can be present include increased intracranial pressure, increased vagal tone, hypothyroidism, hypothermia, hypoxia, hyperkalemia, and use of drugs or toxins.

Sinus Arrhythmia

Sinus arrhythmia occurs as a normal autonomic response in heart rate to physiologic variations during phases of respiration. During inspiration, heart rate increases secondary to decreased vagal tone. Likewise, heart rate decreases during expiration because of increased vagal tone.

Sinus Pauses

Whereas sinus pauses result from brief inactivity by the sinus node, sinus arrest is of longer duration. Treatment is rarely indicated unless sick sinus syndrome is suspected.

Premature Atrial Contractions

Premature atrial contractions (PACs) are common in the pediatric population and often occur without associated congenital heart disease. PACs result in early QRS complexes that may appear normal in duration and morphology, wide when caused by aberrant conduction, or absent when caused by blocked impulses. Each QRS complex is preceded by a P wave that may have a normal axis or suggest an axis directed from outside the sinus node.

Premature Ventricular Contractions

Premature ventricular contractions (PVCs) result in early and wide QRS complexes without preceding P waves. When multiple PVCs are observed, they should be classified into two categories: unifocal or multifocal. Unifocal or uniform PVCs have the same QRS morphology in a single surface electrocardiographic (ECG) lead and are assumed to arise from a single site in a ventricle. Multifocal PVCs have different morphologies in a single lead and are assumed to arise from multiple ventricular foci. PVCs have been found to occur in up to 50% to 60% of healthy children but can also occur in pathologic conditions such as myocarditis, cardiomyopathy, long QT syndrome, and congenital heart disease. PVCs may have more significance if they are multifocal, occur in pairs (couplets), are incessant, occur with symptoms of syncope, are accompanied by a family history of sudden death, or are associated with underlying heart disease. Benign PVCs generally diminish during exercise, but PVCs associated with cardiac disease persist or become more frequent during exercise.

BRADYARRHYTHMIAS

Primary causes of symptomatic bradyarrhythmias in the pediatric population include sinus node dysfunction and atrioventricular (AV) block. A wide spectrum of clinical presentations can occur. Infants may present with poor feeding, lethargy, or seizures, and older children can have lightheadedness, fatigue, exercise intolerance, or syncope. Severe bradycardia can present with signs of poor perfusion and shock and can lead to death. A complete evaluation of each patient's clinical history is needed to exclude underlying medical conditions that may lead to symptomatic bradyarrhythmias.

Sinus Node Dysfunction

Arrhythmias such as severe sinus pause, sinoatrial exit block, and tachycardia–bradycardia syndrome result from failure of the sinus node to increase the heart rate in response to physiologic stress. Sinus node dysfunction is more commonly caused by secondary causes such as cardiac surgery, infection (myocarditis), trauma, ischemia, or cardioactive drugs rather than a primary arrhythmia. Testing and management strategies are based on clinical symptoms and the presence of coexisting heart disease. In symptomatic cases, permanent pacemaker implantation may be needed for definitive therapy.

Atrioventricular Conduction Abnormalities

Abnormal AV conduction occurs when transmission of the normal sinus node impulses is delayed or blocked because of an abnormality in the conduction system, specifically the AV node or His-Purkinje system (Figure 45-1).

FIRST-DEGREE ATRIOVENTRICULAR BLOCK

Because of an abnormal delay in conduction through the AV node, first-degree AV block results in prolongation of the PR interval above the upper limits of normal for age and heart rate

Table 45-1 Normal Heart Rate for Age

Age	Heart Rate (beats/min)
Newborn	110-160
1-6 months	100-180
6-12 months	95-170
1-3 years	95-150
3-5 years	70-130
5-8 years	65-120
8-12 years	65-120
12-16 years	60-110
>16 years	60-100

(Figure 45-2). It is important to note that bradycardia does not occur because of first-degree AV block alone. This type of block can appear in otherwise healthy children as a benign phenomenon, usually related to increased vagal tone. Other causes may include cardiac surgery, rheumatic fever, Lyme disease, digoxin toxicity, and electrolyte imbalance. Isolated first-degree AV block does not require treatment unless there is progression to more advanced AV block.

SECOND-DEGREE ATRIOVENTRICULAR BLOCK

Intermittent failure of AV conduction results in two forms of second-degree AV block: Mobitz type I and Mobitz type II. Each type of second-degree AV block occurs at a different level within the conduction system, thus yielding different surface ECG morphologies. Pathologic causes include myocarditis, cardiomyopathy, myocardial infarction, digitalis toxicity, congenital heart defects, and cardiac surgery.

Mobitz Type I (Wenckebach phenomenon) occurs at the level of the AV node, yielding progressive lengthening in the PR interval until one QRS complex or ventricular depolarization fails to occur (see Figure 45-2). This may occur in otherwise healthy

children with parasympathetic dominance as well as in trained athletes and is frequently observed during monitoring of heart rates during sleep. After confirmation via surface ECG, management should focus on treating any underlying pathologic causes.

Mobitz type II occurs at the level of the bundle of His and is defined as the intermittent loss of AV conduction without preceding lengthening of the PR interval. This form of second-degree AV block is less common and suggests a more serious form of AV conduction disorder in which progression to complete heart block with hemodynamic compromise is more likely. Although similar causes exist between Mobitz type I and type II, consultation with a pediatric cardiologist is indicated (see Figure 45-2).

THIRD-DEGREE ATRIOVENTRICULAR BLOCK OR COMPLETE ATRIOVENTRICULAR BLOCK

Complete AV block is defined as complete interruption of atrial impulse propagation, resulting in atrial and ventricular activity that is independent of each other (AV dissociation). Surface ECG morphology will show regular P waves at a rate appropriate for age but with QRS complexes occurring at regular and slower rates than the atrial rate with no consistent relationship between P waves and QRS complexes. Both congenital and acquired forms of complete AV block occur and should be suspected in any patient with symptomatic bradycardia (see Figure 45-2).

CONGENITAL COMPLETE HEART BLOCK

Congenital complete heart block has been estimated to occur in about one in 20,000 live births and can occur as an isolated anomaly or with structural heart disease (e.g., L-transposition of the great vessels). However, 90% of all cases occur with associated maternal collagen vascular abnormalities (e.g., systemic lupus erythematosus, Sjögren's syndrome). Patients with fetal

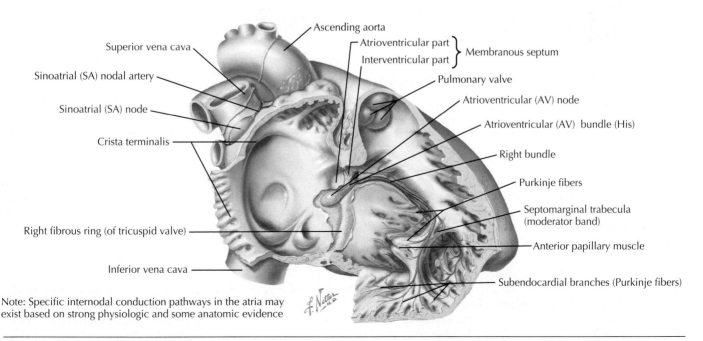

Note: Specific internodal conduction pathways in the atria may exist based on strong physiologic and some anatomic evidence

Figure 45-1 *Cardiac conduction system: right side.*

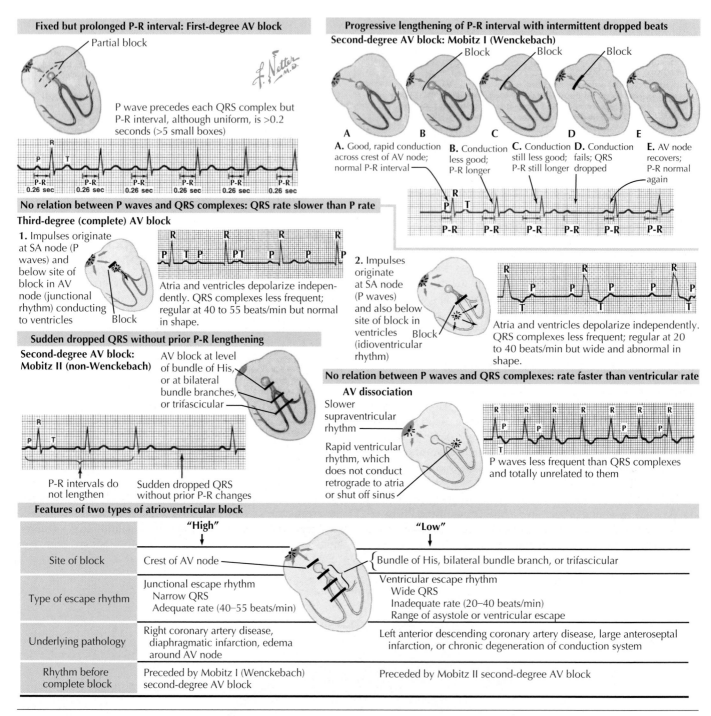

Figure 45-2 *Atrioventricular conduction variations.*

bradycardia may be at risk for hydrops caused by low cardiac output. Likewise, congestive heart failure (CHF) may develop in infancy, although patients with isolated congenital complete heart block can remain asymptomatic through adolescence.

Asymptomatic neonates and infants undergo pacemaker implantation if ventricular rates are less than 70 beats/min with associated congenital heart disease, if ventricular rates are less than 55 beats/min without congenital heart disease, or if ventricular dysfunction or complex ventricular ectopy is present. Infants with in utero hydrops should be delivered as soon as gestational age allows. Some efficacy has been shown by

maternal treatment with steroids and β-agonists during pregnancy. The majority of patients will require pacemaker implantation in the future.

ACQUIRED COMPLETE HEART BLOCK

Acquired complete heart block occurs most commonly in the postoperative patient population. Other causes include severe myocarditis, Lyme disease carditis, acute rheumatic fever, cardiomyopathies, intracardiac tumors, drug overdoses, and myocardial infarction. Symptomatic children and adults should be treated with atropine or isoproterenol until temporary ventricular pacing is available. Permanent pacing is indicated in children and adolescents who have postoperative complete heart block that persists for at least 7 days after cardiac surgery.

TACHYARRHYTHMIAS

Supraventricular Tachycardias

Supraventricular tachycardias (SVT) involve conduction system tissue both above and within the AV node and is the most common tachycardia seen in the pediatric population with published incidence of 1 in 250 to 1000 live births. There are three forms of SVT: reentry tachycardias with an accessory pathway, reentry tachycardias without an accessory pathway (AV nodal and intraatrial), and automatic tachycardias (ectopic).

REENTRY TACHYCARDIA WITH AN ACCESSORY PATHWAY

Wolff-Parkinson-White (WPW) syndrome accounts for 10% to 20% of cases of SVT (Figure 45-3). It is diagnosed by the presence of preexcitation (early depolarization via the accessory pathway) on a surface ECG. This is manifested by a short PR, a widened QRS, and a delta wave. WPW may present at any age and can be associated with Ebstein's anomaly, heterotaxy syndrome, and L-transposition of the great arteries. Sudden death may occur because of rapid ventricular responses with 1:1 conduction in the setting of more rapid atrial tachyarrhythmias such as atrial fibrillation. The risk of sudden death in asymptomatic patients incidentally discovered to have WPW is yet unknown, thus making risk stratification a challenge.

During SVT, impulses may be carried both in an antegrade (orthodromic conduction) or retrograde fashion (antidromic conduction) through the AV node, with an accessory pathway completing the circuit. Orthodromic conduction results in a normal QRS duration with retrograde, inverted P waves after each QRS complex. Antidromic conduction results in a wide QRS duration and is also followed by inverted P waves, although R-P duration is variable.

The SVT associated with WPW occurs with abrupt onset and cessation (paroxysmal) and with a rapid and regular heart rate (usually >200-240 beats/min). Clinical symptoms in young infants and toddlers are often difficult to detect because many children tolerate episodes of SVT very well. If SVT persists or rates are exceptionally elevated, symptoms consistent with CHF may develop (irritability, tachypnea, poor feeding, pallor, fever, and hepatomegaly). Pharmacologic and electrical management strategies are similar to those without an accessory pathway and are discussed below.

REENTRY TACHYCARDIA WITHOUT AN ACCESSORY PATHWAY

AV nodal reentrant tachycardia (AVNRT) occurs when dual conduction pathways exist within the AV node creating substrate for reentry pathophysiology similar to WPW and other accessory pathway SVT (Figure 45-4). Seen more commonly in older children and adolescents, rates can range from 140 to 200 beats/min.

Acute management of hemodynamically unstable patients with reentry tachycardia should seek to restore sinus rhythm

Location of atrioventricular accessory pathways and classification

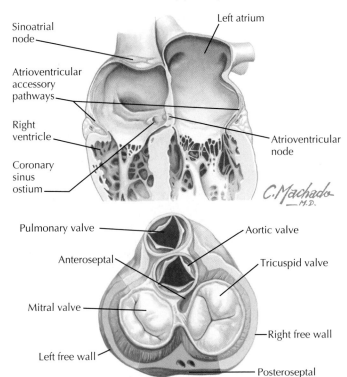

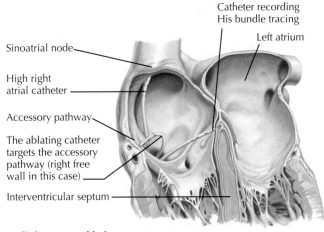

Catheter ablation of accessory pathways

Radiofrequency ablation

Electrocardiogram shows loss of preexcitation after catheter ablation

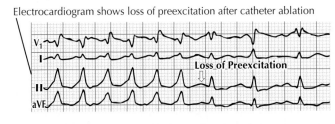

Figure 45-3 *Accessory pathways and the Wolff-Parkinson-White syndrome.*

Location of the atrioventricular node

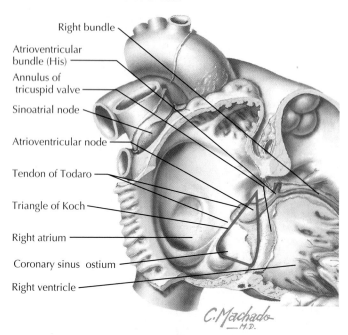

Catheter ablation of atrioventricular nodal reentry tachycardia (AVNRT)

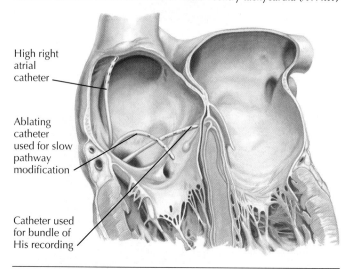

Figure 45-4 *Atrioventricular nodal reentry tachycardia.*

either pharmacologically or electrically with synchronized cardioversion. In non-urgent situations, vagal stimulation by placement of an iced water bag over the face may abort paroxysmal episodes of SVT. Other vagal maneuvers include the Valsalva maneuver, breath-holding, blowing balloons, and even standing upside down. Pharmacologic treatment involves rapid infusion of adenosine, which interrupts reentry circuits by blocking AV conduction. Maintenance medications that can be used include digoxin (contraindicated in patients with WPW), β-blockers, amiodarone, and (less commonly) verapamil. These second-line agents have negative inotropic effects and should be used with caution and only under the supervision of a cardiologist.

Definitive treatment for SVT involves radiofrequency ablation of the accessory pathways, bypass tracts, or ectopic foci in

Atrial flutter

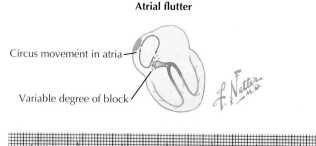

Figure 45-5 *Atrial flutter.*

the heart. Success rates range from 86% to 96% depending on the location of the accessory pathway and type of SVT.

Intraatrial reentrant tachycardia (atrial flutter or fibrillation) is caused by reentrant or "circus" movements within the atria. *Atrial flutter* usually exhibits regular and regularly irregular intervals with atrial rates greater than 250 beats/min. Variable ventricular responses can be observed because of varying degrees of AV block. Risk factors for atrial flutter include structural heart disease with dilated atria, atrial scarring from prior surgery for congenital heart disease (e.g., Fontan, Mustard, or Senning operations), myocarditis, hyperthyroidism, and digitalis toxicity. ECG reveals rapid and regular atrial sawtoothed flutter waves, which are diagnostic for atrial flutter (Figure 45-5).

Evaluation for intraatrial thrombus is required before performing synchronized cardioversion. Radiofrequency ablation in the congenital heart disease population is much more challenging considering multiple reentrant circuits from postoperative scarring, complex atrial anatomy, and thicker atria leading to lower success rates and higher recurrence rates. Long-term anticoagulation with warfarin should be considered in patients with recalcitrant atrial flutter because of the higher incidence of thromboembolic disease.

Atrial fibrillation is much less common in the pediatric population and results from multiple chaotic atrial foci, resulting in an irregularly irregular ventricular response. Risk factors for atrial fibrillation are similar to those for atrial flutter. Acute management of atrial fibrillation in hemodynamically stable patients should focus on ventricular rate control and determination of underlying etiology. Normal sinus rhythm may also be restored with DC synchronized cardioversion after an appropriate evaluation for intracardiac thrombus. As in patients with chronic atrial flutter, long-term anticoagulation with warfarin should be considered for patients with chronic atrial fibrillation.

AUTOMATIC TACHYCARDIAS

Automaticity refers to the ability of conduction tissue to spontaneously depolarize. When present outside of the sinus and AV nodes, automaticity can lead to cells firing repetitively, thus resulting in tachycardia and suppression of dominant pacemaker impulses. Such tachycardias are often susceptible to catecholaminogenic stimulation and have usual "warm-up" and "cool-down" phases compared with paroxysmal forms of reentrant tachycardia. As a group, automatic tachycardias tend to be chronic and incessant with resulting myocardial depression and dysfunction. Therapies target two strategies: slowing the ventricular response rate and decreasing automaticity of the abnormal focus or foci. Three types of automatic tachycardias are observed in the pediatric population:

Ectopic atrial tachycardia accounts for approximately 10% to 20% of all SVT observed in the pediatric population. Heart rates are variable, ranging from 140 to 200 beats/min, with a surface ECG revealing identifiable P waves with an abnormal axis. Vagal maneuvers and adenosine serve as diagnostic tools revealing a gradual slowing in rate with subsequent acceleration after cessation of each maneuver. Spontaneous resolution may occur in some patients, but most patients require chronic therapy with multiple agents.

Multifocal or chaotic atrial tachycardia is a much rarer form of SVT and is characterized by multiple foci of increased automaticity in the atria, resulting in three or more distinct P-wave morphologies on surface ECG. Often confused with atrial fibrillation, this arrhythmia occurs most often in the newborn period without associated cardiac disease. Spontaneous resolution frequently occurs during the first year of life.

Junctional ectopic tachycardia (JET) occurs when a focus of automaticity is present in the region of the AV node. In JET, AV dissociation occurs with a ventricular rate greater than the atrial rate. Congenital, or familial JET often presents in the neonatal period with symptoms of CHF and in association with congenital heart disease. The majority of patients require medical therapy with multiple agents. Radiofrequency ablation has also been used to treat JET but is reserved for more resistant cases because of the high risk of inducing complete heart block from ablation points near the AV node. When occurring in the postoperative period, JET is usually transient and self-limited, lasting from 24 to 72 hours. Although brief in duration, postoperative JET may cause significant hemodynamic compromise and can be fatal if not controlled.

Ventricular Tachycardia

Ventricular tachycardia (VT) is defined as three or more PVCs in series at a heart rate greater than 120 beats/min. These may be self-limited or may present with sudden death (Figure 45-6). Etiologies of VT can be divided into acute and chronic causes. Acute causes include electrolyte imbalance, infections (myocarditis, pericarditis, rheumatic fever), use of toxins or drugs (cocaine, antiarrhythmics, general anesthetics, sympathomimetics, psychotropics), trauma, and myocardial ischemia (infarction, anomalous coronary arteries, Kawasaki disease). Chronic causes of VT include postoperative congenital heart disease (e.g., tetralogy of Fallot), cardiomyopathies (especially hypertrophic cardiomyopathy), tumors or infiltrative processes, primary channelopathies (long QT syndrome, Brugada syndrome), and idiopathic forms. The clinical diagnosis of VT must be distinguished from other arrhythmias that may present with a wide QRS complex tachycardia such as SVT with aberrant conduction. Any wide QRS complex tachycardia, however, should first be considered VT until proven otherwise. Hemodynamically unstable patients with mental status changes or evidence of low cardiac output must be treated promptly with DC synchronized cardioversion. For hemodynamically stable infants and older pediatric patients, intravenous amiodarone and lidocaine are the initial drugs of choice. Ventricular arrhythmias caused by acute etiologies such as electrolyte imbalance, hypoxia, or drug toxicity resolve after the offending abnormality has been corrected. For patients with chronic VT, medical therapies should be aimed at preventing recurrence.

LONG QT SYNDROMES AND SUDDEN DEATH

The long QT syndromes are composed of a group of genetic abnormalities created by ion channel mutations that result in abnormal ventricular repolarization. To date, mutations in 12 genes have been identified involving potassium, sodium, and calcium channels. These alterations in conduction properties are associated with malignant ventricular arrhythmias, exercise- and stress-related syncope, and sudden cardiac death (see Figure 45-6). Approximately half of all cases are familial; the remainder are from sporadic mutations. Initial reports consisted of familial studies by Jervell and Lange-Nielsen, who described QT prolongation with associated deafness (Jervell-Lange-Nielsen syndrome). Romano-Ward also described familial cases of prolonged QT with autosomal dominant transmission and without associated deafness or anomalies (Romano-Ward syndrome).

A wide clinical spectrum can be found in patients with long QT syndromes with presenting features notable for syncope, seizures, sudden death, and associated deafness. Obtaining a family history of unexplained sudden death or long QT is also important in the initial evaluation. However, the diagnosis is based on a combination of ECG findings as well as clinical criteria. Surface ECG will reveal a corrected QT interval greater than 470 msec in the majority of cases, although normal resting QT intervals do not rule out long QT syndrome. Other features include abnormal T-wave morphologies (notched T waves, T-wave alternans), bradycardia for age, and history of torsades de pointes. Holter monitor and outpatient exercise testing are both useful diagnostic tests in evaluating patients with syncope and suspected long QT syndrome. Treatment should aim to eliminate symptoms and reduce the risk of sudden death. Medications such as ß-blockers should be used as first-line therapies. Patients with continued symptoms (syncope) despite medical therapy or those who present with aborted sudden cardiac death should undergo placement of an automatic implantable cardiac defibrillator.

FUTURE DIRECTIONS

The diagnosis and management of arrhythmias in the pediatric population has advanced tremendously in recent years, with progress made in electrophysiologic mapping and pacemaker technologies, as well as ablation strategies. Advances in genetic identification of patients, as well as their relatives, with channelopathies will likely improve morbidity and mortality associated with certain arrhythmias.

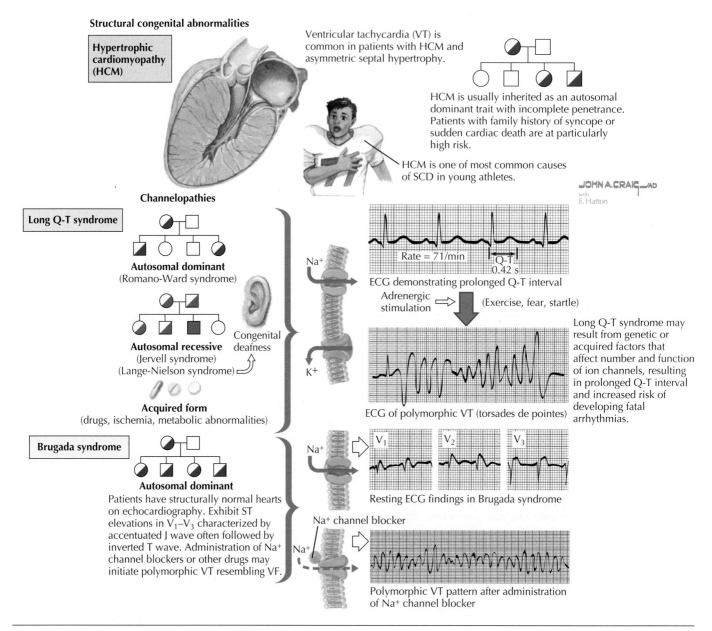

Structural congenital abnormalities

Hypertrophic cardiomyopathy (HCM)

Ventricular tachycardia (VT) is common in patients with HCM and asymmetric septal hypertrophy.

HCM is usually inherited as an autosomal dominant trait with incomplete penetrance. Patients with family history of syncope or sudden cardiac death are at particularly high risk.

HCM is one of most common causes of SCD in young athletes.

JOHN A. CRAIG _AD
with E. Hatton

Channelopathies

Long Q-T syndrome

Autosomal dominant (Romano-Ward syndrome)

Autosomal recessive (Jervell syndrome) (Lange-Nielsen syndrome)

Congenital deafness

Acquired form (drugs, ischemia, metabolic abnormalities)

Na⁺

K⁺

Rate = 71/min   Q-T 0.42 s

ECG demonstrating prolonged Q-T interval

Adrenergic stimulation ⟹ (Exercise, fear, startle)

Long Q-T syndrome may result from genetic or acquired factors that affect number and function of ion channels, resulting in prolonged Q-T interval and increased risk of developing fatal arrhythmias.

ECG of polymorphic VT (torsades de pointes)

Brugada syndrome

Autosomal dominant

Patients have structurally normal hearts on echocardiography. Exhibit ST elevations in V₁–V₃ characterized by accentuated J wave often followed by inverted T wave. Administration of Na⁺ channel blockers or other drugs may initiate polymorphic VT resembling VF.

Na⁺

V₁   V₂   V₃

Resting ECG findings in Brugada syndrome

Na⁺ channel blocker

Na⁺

Polymorphic VT pattern after administration of Na⁺ channel blocker

Figure 45-6 *Sudden cardiac death.*

SUGGESTED READINGS

Ackerman MJ: Molecular basis of congenital and acquired long QT syndromes, *J Electrocardiol* 37(suppl):1-6, 2004.

Delacretaz E: Supraventricular tachycardia, *N Engl J Med* 354:1039-1050, 2006.

Epstein AE, Dimarco JP, Ellenbogen KA, et al: ACC/AHA/HRS 2008 guidelines for device-based therapy of cardiac rhythm abnormalities: a report of the American College of Cardiology/American Heart Association Task Force on Practice Guidelines (Writing Committee to Revise the ACC/AHA/NASPE 2002 guideline update for implantation of cardiac pacemakers and antiarrhythmia devices): developed in collaboration with the American Association for Thoracic Surgery and Society of Thoracic Surgeons, *Circulation* 117(21):e350-e408, 2008.

Kaltman JR, Madan N, Vetter VL, Rhodes LA: Arrhythmias and sudden cardiac death. In Bell LM, Vetter VL, editors: *Pediatric Cardiology: The Requisites in Pediatrics*, Philadelphia, 2006, Elsevier Mosby, pp 171-194.

Kaltman H, Shah M: Evaluation of the child with an arrhythmia, *Pediatr Clin North Am* 51:1537-1551, 2004.

Maron BJ: Sudden death in young athletes, *N Engl J Med* 349:404-410, 2003.

Walsh EP: Clinical Approach to diagnosis and acute management of tachycardias in children. In Walsh EP, Saul JP, Triedman JK, editors: *Cardiac Arrhythmias in Children and Young Adults with Congenital Heart Disease*, Philadelphia, 2001, Lippincott Williams & Wilkins, pp 95-113.

Walsh EP, Cecchin F: Recent advances in pacemaker and implantable defibrillator therapy for young patients, *Curr Opin Cardiol* 19(2):91-96, 2004.

Heart Failure

E. Kevin Hall

A healthy child's heart may beat more than 200,000 times and transport more than 3 tons of blood each day. The heart and vascular systems are primarily responsible for delivering blood to the tissues while providing oxygen and nutrients and withdrawing waste products. Each is involved in the regulation of a perfusing blood pressure, including those homeostatic alterations necessitated with changes in posture. They play a primary role in the circulation of hormones. Heart failure is the inability of the heart to meet the metabolic demands of the body.

The failure of the heart and vascular system to keep up with metabolic requirements may arise from a number of causes, including cellular deficiencies, arrhythmias, metabolic insufficiencies, and congenital defects. Although most frequently a child presents in heart failure because of decompensation from congenital anomalies, the more prevalent of these are discussed elsewhere within this text, and only the principles common to heart failure will be repeated here. It is important to remember "heart failure" as a clinical picture may present in many of these anomalies when the physiology markedly worsens. However, to illustrate the fundamental concepts of pediatric heart failure, the remainder of this chapter focuses on that which may arise in children with normal anatomy. This state of "heart failure" in children may present indolently or very suddenly; in the latter, less-specific symptoms may be present for longer.

Regardless of the source, the goals of treatment are always (1) discovering and addressing the cause of failure along with (2) decreasing myocardial work load and oxygen consumption and (3) augmenting and supporting function and systemic oxygenation. With such interventions, the hope is that the heart will remodel, if not recover. Because of the danger of cardiovascular collapse, which may be very rapid, prompt consultation with pediatric cardiologists and intensivists is important, and early recognition requires diagnostic vigilance. Through a careful history and examination and with tests such as electrocardiography (ECG), echocardiography, and cardiac catheterization, the cause may often be learned and treatment instituted. Invasive arterial or venous monitoring is helpful in some cases if the patient is very ill.

ETIOLOGY AND PRESENTATION

The heart is a pump. It may fail as a pump either from the inability to generate enough contractile force or from structural anomalies that prevent or inappropriately direct blood to the tissues. Examples of the former include myocarditis, an infection of heart muscle cells (myocytes), or a cardiomyopathy, a primary structural or metabolic abnormality of the microscopic elements of a myocyte. Examples of structural anomalies that might lead to heart failure include left-to-right shunt lesions such as ventricular septal defect; patent ductus arteriosus, and, rarely, atrial septal defect, or valvar regurgitation because of the increased volume load on the heart; and severe valvar stenosis

because of the increased pressure load. When the heart is no longer able to compensate, the state of heart failure exists.

When the heart fails to adequately pump blood forward for any reason, venous congestion occurs. On the right side, the liver in particular becomes distended and engorged with blood. This leads to abdominal discomfort or vomiting initially, but in certain prolonged cases, it may lead to liver dysfunction and distension of venous collaterals, some of which may be visible under the skin (Figure 46-1). The signs of peripheral edema and jugular venous distension classically seen in adults are not typically seen in infants or young children. On the left side, pulmonary venous congestion leads to fluid extravasation within the lungs, typically interstitial in infants and intraalveolar in older children and adults (Figure 46-2). This leads to shortness of breath, tachypnea, and dyspnea and can present on chest radiography similar to pneumonia. Indeed, in some cases, a secondary infection may develop superimposed on these wet and stiff lungs.

As the heart begins to fail in the volume of blood it can pump, the sympathetic nervous system seeks to compensate by increasing the heart rate. In these cases, an ECG may be useful in differentiating a sinus tachycardia in response to a failing heart (P-wave axis between 0 and 90 with a one-to-one relationship to the QRS complexes) versus a primary arrhythmia. If prolonged and untreated, some nonsinus heart rhythms can be the cause of heart failure. Finally, upregulation of the sympathetic nervous system may also cause vasoconstriction and diaphoresis, and the child may present as cold, pale, and diaphoretic.

The apex beat may be displaced downward and laterally and may be full and bounding or weak depending on both the cause of the heart failure and how successful the child is compensating. In newborns, anything more than a slight pulsation felt with two fingers placed beneath the xiphisternum is concerning for cardiac involvement. Auscultation may reveal a number of clues as to the cause. Difficult-to-hear heart sounds may signify a pericardial effusion with fluid between the heart and the pericardium that does not permit adequate filling of blood into the heart but more often is caused by poor contraction from a primary cardiomyopathy. A gallop is frequently heard in failing hearts and refers to an extra (third or fourth) heart sound. Third heart sounds may be normal in some children and are thought to be caused by rapid diastolic filling. A fourth heart sound is never normal and is indicative of a poorly compliant ventricle reflecting a high-pressure wave back toward the atrium.

Murmurs may be heard in the setting of heart failure caused by a primary structural abnormality (discussed elsewhere). Some murmurs represent turbulence across an incompetent valve caused by severe left ventricular dilatation seen in some failing hearts.

Evaluation and Management

Because of the high risk of cardiovascular collapse, concerns of heart failure should be managed in close consultation with

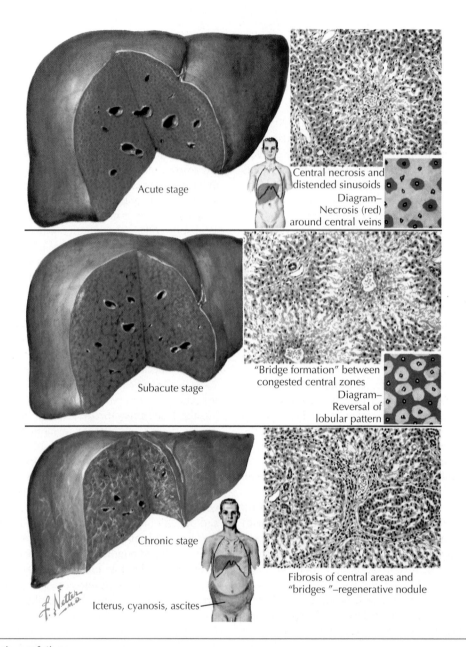

Acute stage

Central necrosis and distended sinusoids
Diagram—
Necrosis (red) around central veins

Subacute stage

"Bridge formation" between congested central zones
Diagram—
Reversal of lobular pattern

Chronic stage

Fibrosis of central areas and "bridges"–regenerative nodule

Icterus, cyanosis, ascites

Figure 46-1 *Liver in heart failure.*

pediatric intensivists and cardiologists. A careful, directed history is important to frame the presentation and learn its time course. Understanding the clinical associations listed above are important in evaluating the vital signs. Resting vital signs, including heart rate, systolic and diastolic blood pressures, and respiratory rate, are of primary importance. High heart rates with borderline or low blood pressures are concerning findings that the cardiovascular system is involved, whether from primary cardiac disease or secondary to another condition such as sepsis. A posteroanterior chest radiograph may be useful in evaluating both the lungs and size of the cardiac silhouette. A child's cardiac shadow should be 50% or less than the diameter of the chest; a larger shadow may indicate a large, overloaded, and potentially failing heart. Evidence of pulmonary infiltration may be of a primary lung cause or secondary to heart failure. An ECG is important to differentiate sinus rhythm from

an arrhythmia. An echocardiogram may be necessary in suspicious cases to evaluate both heart function and structure.

If signs of heart failure are present (tachycardia, borderline or low blood pressure, tachypnea, hepatomegaly), judicious use of fluid replacement along with early support with pressor medications such as milrinone and dopamine and intubation, sedation, and paralysis may be necessary to reduce metabolic demand in the most serious cases. In cases of complete cardiovascular collapse (shock) when the heart function and blood pressure are unable to maintain adequate perfusion despite maximal pharmacotherapeutic support, extracorporeal membrane oxygenation (ECMO) is able to support the child. These large external devices are able to maintain adequate cardiac output to support the patient for a number of weeks. If longer periods are necessary, implantable ventricular assist devices are available and intended to support the child until a heart transplant is available.

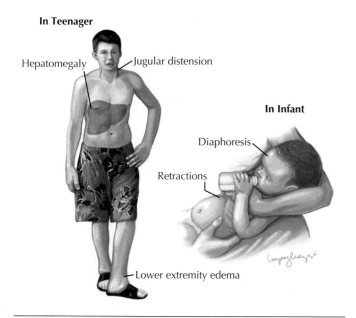

In Teenager

Hepatomegaly

Jugular distension

In Infant

Diaphoresis

Retractions

Lower extremity edema

Figure 46-2 *Clinical presentation of heart failure in a teenager and infant.*

Volume status is critical in the treatment of heart failure because fluid overload and increased myocardial wall stress exert extra strain on a failing heart. A history of recent weight gain, peripheral or (if an infant) periorbital edema, signs of hepatic distension, and electrolyte abnormalities (including hyponatremia) may indicate a picture consistent with heart failure. Increasing central venous pressure along with diminished arterial mean pressure common in this setting will diminish renal perfusion and impair fluid excretion. Inpatient intravenous (IV) diuresis to the patient's estimated dry weight along with the addition of middle-dose milrinone or low-dose dopamine may be necessary. Carefully following orthostatic blood pressures is important and, if possible, measurement of central venous pressure and mixed venous oxygen saturation through a central catheter is often additionally helpful in estimating cardiac output and systemic vascular resistance. Brain-type natriuretic peptide is often used in trending fluid overload and heart failure.

Failing hearts are more prone to arrhythmias, and 24-hour telemetry as an inpatient or 24-hour surveillance Holter monitors should play a routine role in the evaluation of children in heart failure. Finally, hearts that are markedly dilated and hypocontractile are prone to thrombus formation, and such children are at risk for thromboembolism and stroke. Medications to reduce in situ coagulation and platelet function are important in this population.

Because of natural changes in vascular physiology that start at birth, an important clue in the evaluation of a child in heart failure is the patient's age. Infants who present at birth with heart failure most likely have sustained an in utero insult such as asphyxiation, maternal sepsis, intrauterine myocarditis, prolonged fetal arrhythmia, perinatal hemorrhage, or (rarely) primary valvar regurgitation (because shunt lesions are hemodynamically inconsequential before pulmonary resistance falls postnatally). An infant who is presented around 1 week of age typically has structural congenital cardiac anomalies depending on the flow through a patent ductus arteriosus because this

structure typically completes closure between 4 and 10 days of age. Examples of ductal-dependent lesions include hypoplastic left heart syndrome, critical aortic or pulmonary valve stenosis or atresia, severe coarctation of the aorta, and interruption of the aortic arch. Administration of prostaglandin E1 may temporarily reverse the closure of the ductus. Finally, children who present from several weeks to a few months of age in heart failure often have shunt defects because this is the timeframe in which pulmonary vascular resistance decreases, leading to preferential shunting of oxygenated blood back to the lungs. At all of these times or anytime thereafter, genetic, metabolic, or infectious causes of primary myocardial causes of heart failure may present.

CASE EXAMPLE

Myocarditis occurs when there is inflammation of the myocardium with cell damage or death leading to decreased ventricular function and cardiac output. In the United States and Europe, most cases are of viral origin. Although the suspected causative agents have changed over recent decades, today when a successful diagnosis is made, adenovirus and enterovirus are the most frequently isolated viral species. Myocarditis may however arise from a host of other agents, including bacteria, protozoa, pharmaceuticals, and even rheumatologic and autoimmune processes.

There are wildly differing estimations as to the incidence of this disease, but it is likely that many cases remain subclinical and are never discovered. Catheter-based biopsy-proven diagnosis in this disease is often fraught with difficulty. Taking a heart muscle biopsy from an acutely ill child has its dangers, and the result of such a biopsy may not lead to any changes in the acute course of treatment. When biopsy is possible, samples consistent with viral myocarditis will show a lymphocytic infiltrate and cell necrosis. Magnetic resonance imaging may come to play an important role in future diagnoses with tissue characterization suggestive of inflammation, edema, and possibly myocardial scarring.

The decrease in myocardial function caused by myocarditis may present either suddenly or indolently. Paradoxically, patients who present most suddenly (and often in cardiogenic shock, or "fulminant myocarditis") tend to recover most readily if the initial course is supported; more than 90% of these patients survive transplant free 11 years later. But patients in whom function limps along with little recovery rarely regain full function and either develop chronic although stable dilated cardiomyopathy or end-stage heart failure. Of these, fewer than half of patients are alive and transplant free after 11 years. Myocarditis may present at any age.

Infants and children present in varying degrees of heart failure as detailed above, and primary complaints may revolve around chest pain (pericarditis), respiratory distress, or abdominal distress and decreased appetite from increasing venous stasis. There may be a fever or a history thereof from the primary infection; a history of a flulike illness may precede the presentation by 1 to 4 weeks. A resting tachycardia with or without a gallop will be present along with tachypnea or cough. More severe cases may have a signs of cardiogenic shock (hypotension, cool and pale extremities). There may be a systolic murmur of mitral regurgitation, a finding seen when significant left ventricular dilation has occurred. Atrial and ventricular fibrillation along with atrioventricular nodal block are sometimes seen and may lead to sudden death.

The ECG tends to show low-voltage and often markedly widened QRS complexes. There may be inversion of the T waves along with Q waves indicative of myocardial infarction. Cardiomegaly may be present on chest radiography, but its absence does not rule out the disease, particularly in the very beginning of fulminant myocarditis. Echocardiography, the most sensitive of these tests, demonstrates left ventricular dilatation and decreased ventricular function. Global and uniform hypokinesis is the norm, although segmental wall motion abnormality (dyskinesia) may also be present. With increasing left ventricular volume and worsening valve leaflet apposition, color-Doppler ultrasonography will demonstrate mitral regurgitation. Cardiac troponin T will be elevated in patients with myocarditis and is often a useful test in distinguishing myocarditis from cardiomyopathy, in which it is not elevated.

Because of the rapidity with which cardiovascular collapse may ensue, prompt consultation is recommended. Inotropic support with milrinone or dopamine (or both), arterial monitoring, 24-hour telemetry to monitor for ectopy, and ECMO are often needed in the acute fulminant phase of this disease. Lidocaine infusions and magnesium may be necessary if ventricular ectopy develops. Treatment is therefore primarily supportive. Immunosuppressive regimens are controversial, with many studies showing no improvement with combinations of steroids and medications, including cyclosporine and azathioprine. Some evidence has been emerging that IV immune globulin with the possible addition of vitamin C may have a beneficial effect on some forms of myocarditis.

FUTURE DIRECTIONS

One area of rapid improvement in pediatric heart failure is the continuing development of pediatric ventricular assist devices (VADs). Unlike nonpulsatile ECMO, with which a child's heart may be supported for weeks in the hope that it may recover from whatever insult it has sustained, VADs allow much longer support periods and can be used until a child is listed for and receives a heart transplant. Many devices use extrathoracic pneumatic pumps that circulate blood through cannulae introduced through the abdominal wall into the child's circulation. One such device that has found frequent use is the Berlin Heart EXCOR, which just supported its 500th child.

SUGGESTED READINGS

Berlin Heart. *500th Patient Receives Berlin Heart EXCOR Pediatric Ventricular Assist Device*, 2009. Available at http://www.berlinheart.com/500th_EXCOR_Pediatric_Patient_full_story.pdf.

Bowles NE, Ni J, Kearney DL, et al: Detection of viruses in myocardial tissues by polymerase chain reaction. evidence of adenovirus as a common cause of myocarditis in children and adults, *J Am Coll Cardiol* 42:466-472, 2003.

Cooper LT, Baughman KL, Feldman AM, et al: The role of endomyocardial biopsy in the management of cardiovascular disease: a scientific statement from the American Heart Association, the American College of Cardiology, and the European Society of Cardiology Endorsed by the Heart Failure Society of America and the Heart Failure Association of the European Society of Cardiology, *Eur Heart J* 28:3076-3093, 2007.

Gong F, Hu Y, Chen L, Gu W: The therapeutic effect of intravenous immunoglobulins and vitamin C on the progression of experimental autoimmune myocarditis in the mouse, *Med Sci Monit* 13:BR240-246, 2007.

McCarthy RE, Boehmer JP, Hruban RH, et al: Long-term outcome of fulminant myocarditis as compared with acute (nonfulminant) myocarditis, *N Engl J Med* 342:690-695, 2000.

Towbin JA, Bricker JT, Garson A Jr: Electrocardiographic criteria for diagnosis of acute myocardial infarction in childhood, *Am J Cardiol* 69:1545-1548, 1992.

Udi N, Yehuda S: Intravenous immunoglobulin—indications and mechanisms in cardiovascular diseases, *Autoimmun Rev* 7:445-452, 2008.

Hypertension

Michael L. O'Byrne and R. Thomas Collins II

47

*H*ypertension, the abnormal elevation of systolic blood pressure (SBP) or diastolic blood pressures (DBP), is relatively uncommon in children. It is usually divided into primary, or essential, hypertension and secondary hypertension (that which has a clear cause). In either case, elevated BP may result in significant damage to multiple organ systems, proportional to both the magnitude and duration of its elevation.

ETIOLOGY AND PATHOGENESIS

Definitions

Normative BP ranges in adults have been based on long-term, end-organ risk as determined by large-cohort epidemiologic data. In children and adolescents, normal BP ranges have been defined based on data from relatively large cohort studies in presumed-healthy subjects and are stratified by gender, age, and height. The seventh report of the Joint National Committee on Prevention, Detection, Evaluation, and Treatment of High Blood Pressure (JNC7) and the Fourth Report on the Diagnosis, Evaluation, and Treatment of High Blood Pressure in Children and Adolescents (Fourth Report) (NHBPEP) define *hypertension* in children and adolescents as an average SBP or DBP at the 95th percentile or above for gender, age, and height on three or more occasions. BPs (SBP or DBP) between the 90th and 95th percentiles have historically been referred to as "high normal" but in these most recent guidelines have been redefined as *prehypertensive*. This change reflects the addition of prehypertension to the adult diagnostic criteria as defined by JNC7; there is increased risk of developing hypertension in those with prehypertension. *Stage 1 hypertension* is defined as a BP above the 95th and up to 5 mm Hg over the 99th percentile for gender, age, and height. *Stage 2 hypertension* is more than 5 mm Hg higher than the 99th percentile. More timely antihypertensive therapy is recommended for stage 2 hypertension.

White coat hypertension is defined as having a BP consistently above the 95th percentile for age in a physician's office or clinic but being normotensive outside of the clinical setting. This diagnosis usually requires ambulatory BP monitoring for confirmation.

There are many causes of hypertension (Figure 47-1). Whereas BP for which a clear cause can be determined is described as *secondary hypertension*, hypertension without a clear correctable cause is referred to as *primary* or *essential hypertension*. This is necessarily a diagnosis of exclusion.

Physiology

BP is determined by both cardiac output (CO) and systemic vascular resistance (SVR). Factors increasing output or resistance can result in hypertension. The relationship between BP and CO is summarized by the following equations.

$$BP = CO \times SVR$$

$$CO = \text{Heart rate (HR)} \times \text{Stroke volume (SV)}$$

Multiple causes of secondary hypertension are shown in Figure 47-1. Each condition may increase BP via increases in heart rate, SV, or SVR. Considering these three fundamental factors in BP elevation aids in the appropriate therapeutic approach to a given patient.

CLINICAL PRESENTATION

Most children with hypertension have not had years of exposure to elevated BPs. Therefore, unlike their adult counterparts, the clinical signs and symptoms in children and adolescents are generally more indicative of the cause of their disease rather than stigmata of end-organ damage from chronic hypertension. Although hypertensive nephropathy, left ventricular hypertrophy, congestive heart failure, hypertensive retinopathy, and stroke can be seen in children with long-standing, severe hypertension, they are much less common than in adults with chronic hypertension (Figure 47-2).

Still, children with hypertension can present in a number of clinical settings, and the approach to diagnosis and treatment varies accordingly. Presentations may vary from a single asymptomatic BP in an outpatient setting to life-threatening complications in a hypertensive emergency. The differential diagnosis, diagnostic workup, and therapeutic options vary considerably based on the clinical presentation.

EVALUATION

Measurement of Blood Pressure

Accurate and consistent measurement of BP is a precondition to appropriate medical management. BP measurements, even when performed correctly, demonstrate significant variability. As a result, the arithmetic mean of three or more BP measurements on separate occasions is used to diagnose hypertension. The mean BP of multiple measurements most closely approximates those obtained by ambulatory BP monitoring.

Accepted epidemiologic statistics for BP are all based on measurements made by auscultation. Despite this, oscillometric measurements of BP are increasingly used because of their ease of use and the (false) perception that they are more precise. Oscillometric "measurements" of SBP and DBP are based on proprietary algorithms that extrapolate these from measured mean BPs. These estimates have been shown to be consistently at least 5 to 10 mm Hg higher than those measured by auscultation. Because of this, high BPs derived from oscillometric measurements should be repeated by auscultation as a matter of course.

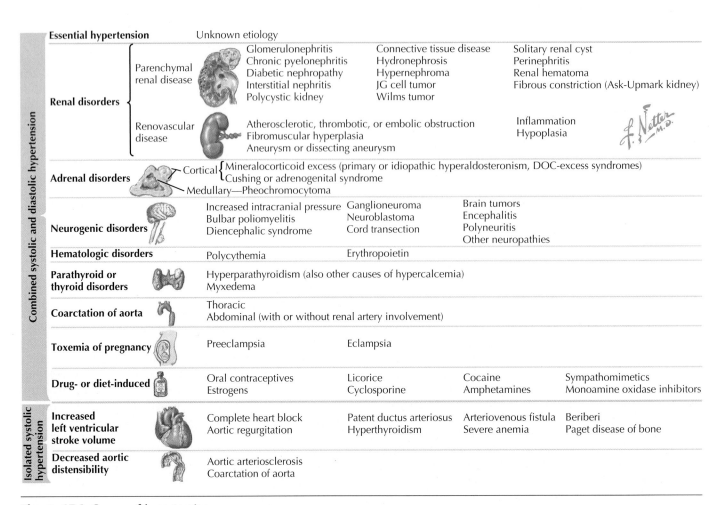

Figure 47-1 *Causes of hypertension.*

Cuff Size and Location

Cuff size also dramatically affects the BP measurement. Cuffs that are too small overestimate BP, and excessively large cuffs may underestimate BP. However, the range of the underestimation with a large cuff is generally smaller in magnitude than errors from very small cuffs. The correct cuff size can be obtained by insuring that the inflatable bladder has (1) a width that is approximately 40% of the arm circumference (or ≈25% greater than the diameter of the arm) at the point midway between the olecranon and acromion and (2) enough length to cover 80% to 100% of the arm circumference. The length-to-width ratio should be approximately 2:1, which is not true of all commercial cuffs.

For appropriate auscultation, the stethoscope should be placed over the site of the brachial pulse proximal and medial to the cubital fossa below the distal border of the cuff. Measurement using the bell (instead of the diaphragm) produces superior discrimination of the Korotkoff sounds. The SBP corresponds to the pressure at which the first Korotkoff sound is audible, and the DBP corresponds to the pressure at which the fifth Korotkoff sound is audible or with obliteration of the last sound. If sounds are still heard at 0 mm Hg, a repeat BP should be attempted with less pressure on the stethoscope head.

The measured BP should be compared against BP tables that have been published by the American Academy of Pediatrics, which are normalized for gender, age, and height percentile.

Diagnostic Approach

Before making a diagnosis of hypertension, it is important to rule out immediate causes of transient BP elevations such as acute pain, anxiety, or medication exposure. After such causes have been ruled out, the diagnostic approach in a patient with hypertension can be organized as follows: (1) define the degree of hypertension, (2) investigate end-organ damage, and (3) evaluate for possible causes of secondary hypertension (see Figure 47-1).

Primary or essential hypertension is generally characterized by stage 1 hypertension, is often associated with family history of hypertension or coronary vascular disease, and frequently coincides with obesity. Because of the well-documented comorbidity of hypertension, obesity, hypercholesterolemia, and insulin insensitivity, screening for these other cardiovascular disease risk factors is sensible. Currently, a fasting lipid profile and fasting glucose are recommended as initial screening tests. There are not sufficient data at present to recommend testing plasma uric acid, homocysteine, or lipoprotein A in children with high BP.

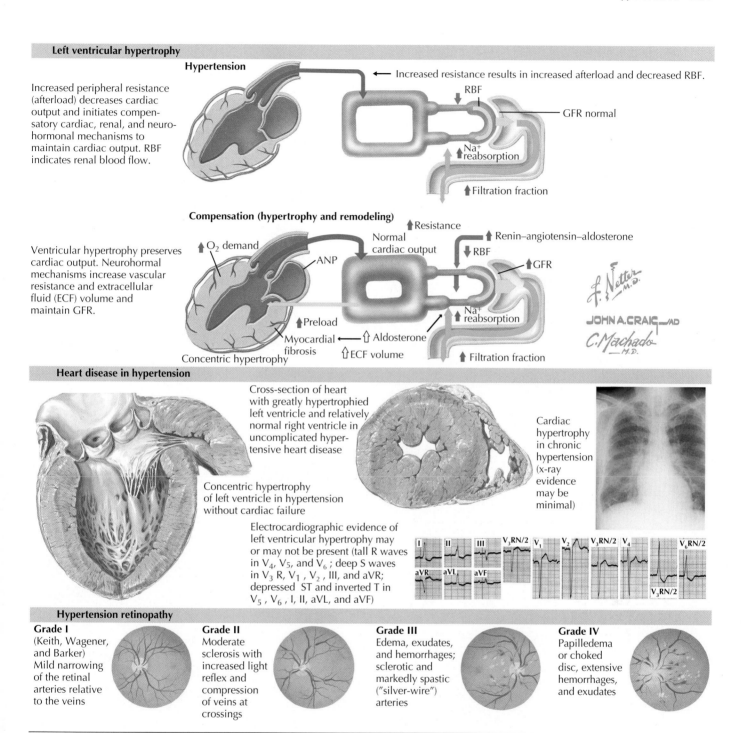

Left ventricular hypertrophy

Hypertension

← Increased resistance results in increased afterload and decreased RBF.

Increased peripheral resistance (afterload) decreases cardiac output and initiates compensatory cardiac, renal, and neurohormonal mechanisms to maintain cardiac output. RBF indicates renal blood flow.

RBF
GFR normal
Na⁺ reabsorption
↑ Filtration fraction

Compensation (hypertrophy and remodeling)

Ventricular hypertrophy preserves cardiac output. Neurohormal mechanisms increase vascular resistance and extracellular fluid (ECF) volume and maintain GFR.

↑ O₂ demand
ANP
↑ Resistance
Normal cardiac output
↑ Renin–angiotensin–aldosterone
↓ RBF
↑ GFR
↑ Preload
Myocardial fibrosis
⇧ Aldosterone
Concentric hypertrophy
⇧ ECF volume
↑ Na⁺ reabsorption
↑ Filtration fraction

Heart disease in hypertension

Cross-section of heart with greatly hypertrophied left ventricle and relatively normal right ventricle in uncomplicated hypertensive heart disease

Cardiac hypertrophy in chronic hypertension (x-ray evidence may be minimal)

Concentric hypertrophy of left ventricle in hypertension without cardiac failure

Electrocardiographic evidence of left ventricular hypertrophy may or may not be present (tall R waves in V₄, V₅, and V₆; deep S waves in V₃R, V₁, V₂, III, and aVR; depressed ST and inverted T in V₅, V₆, I, II, aVL, and aVF)

Hypertension retinopathy

Grade I
(Keith, Wagener, and Barker)
Mild narrowing of the retinal arteries relative to the veins

Grade II
Moderate sclerosis with increased light reflex and compression of veins at crossings

Grade III
Edema, exudates, and hemorrhages; sclerotic and markedly spastic ("silver-wire") arteries

Grade IV
Papilledema or choked disc, extensive hemorrhages, and exudates

Figure 47-2 *Clinical presentation of hypertension.*

Secondary, as opposed to primary, hypertension is more common in children than adults, in whom primary or essential hypertension is overwhelmingly the most common cause. Generally, secondary hypertension is more likely in patients who (1) have stage 2 hypertension, (2) are young (i.e., not adolescents), and (3) have signs or symptoms of systemic disease or have a personal or family medical history of those conditions. As summarized in Figure 47-1, there are numerous causes of secondary hypertension. The history and physical examination should screen for signs and symptoms of causes of secondary hypertension. The physical should include a measurement of height and

weight to calculate body mass index. Upper and lower extremity BPs must always be measured. Additional studies should be tailored to the individual patient based on their presentation. Studies should be divided between those seeking the cause of secondary hypertension and those that identify the stigmata of hypertensive end-organ damage.

In patients with stage 2 hypertension, it is important to immediately screen for signs and symptoms of end-organ damage. *Hypertensive urgency* refers to high BP without evidence of end-organ damage *Hypertensive emergency* is defined as having acute, end-organ dysfunction, such as neurologic symptoms,

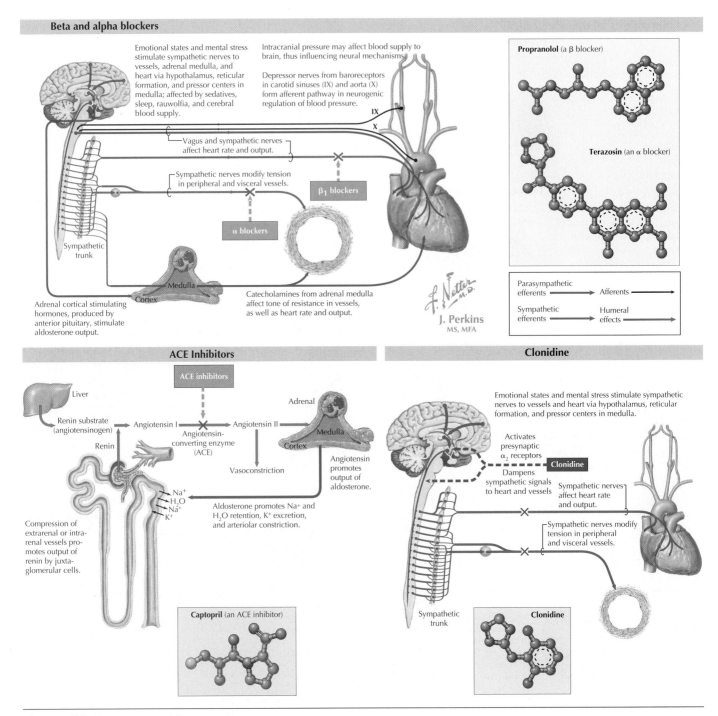

Beta and alpha blockers

Emotional states and mental stress stimulate sympathetic nerves to vessels, adrenal medulla, and heart via hypothalamus, reticular formation, and pressor centers in medulla; affected by sedatives, sleep, rauwolfia, and cerebral blood supply.

Intracranial pressure may affect blood supply to brain, thus influencing neural mechanisms.

Depressor nerves from baroreceptors in carotid sinuses (IX) and aorta (X) form afferent pathway in neurogenic regulation of blood pressure.

Vagus and sympathetic nerves affect heart rate and output.

Sympathetic nerves modify tension in peripheral and visceral vessels.

β₁ blockers

α blockers

Sympathetic trunk

Medulla

Cortex

Adrenal cortical stimulating hormones, produced by anterior pituitary, stimulate aldosterone output.

Catecholamines from adrenal medulla affect tone of resistance in vessels, as well as heart rate and output.

Propranolol (a β blocker)

Terazosin (an α blocker)

J. Perkins
MS, MFA

| Parasympathetic efferents ⟶ | Afferents ⟶ |
| Sympathetic efferents ⟶ | Humeral effects ⟶ |

ACE Inhibitors

Liver

ACE inhibitors

Adrenal

Renin substrate (angiotensinogen) ⟶ Angiotensin I ⟶ Angiotensin-converting enzyme (ACE) ⟶ Angiotensin II ⟶ Medulla / Cortex

Renin

Vasoconstriction

Angiotensin promotes output of aldosterone.

Na⁺ / H₂O / Na⁺ / K⁺

Aldosterone promotes Na⁺ and H₂O retention, K⁺ excretion, and arteriolar constriction.

Compression of extrarenal or intrarenal vessels promotes output of renin by juxtaglomerular cells.

Captopril (an ACE inhibitor)

Clonidine

Emotional states and mental stress stimulate sympathetic nerves to vessels and heart via hypothalamus, reticular formation, and pressor centers in medulla.

Activates presynaptic α₂ receptors

Clonidine

Dampens sympathetic signals to heart and vessels

Sympathetic nerves affect heart rate and output.

Sympathetic nerves modify tension in peripheral and visceral vessels.

Sympathetic trunk

Clonidine

Figure 47-3 *Management of hypertension.*

vision changes, cardiac chest pain, or acute renal failure, in the setting of marked hypertension. Hypertensive urgency and emergency require immediate intervention to control BP.

MANAGEMENT

Long-term outcomes data for hypertension control in children and adolescents are not available, and the degree to which reducing BP will affect morbidity and mortality is unknown. The goal of antihypertensive therapy is to reduce BP to reduce the long-term risk of accumulating end-organ damage without

incurring excessive side effects. Current recommendations are to reduce the BP below the 95th percentile if no other risk factors are present or below the 90th percentile if other risk factors, such as diabetes mellitus, dyslipidemia, or kidney disease, are present.

The first-line therapy for stage 1 hypertension and prehypertension is therapeutic lifestyle change. Data supporting the efficacy of these modifications are limited; however, based on data from studies in adult groups, weight reduction in obese patients, increased intake of vegetables and fruits, increased physical activity, and reduction in dietary sodium intake are all recommended. The recommendations for moderate alcohol consumption are, hopefully, not applicable in children and adolescents. Smoking cessation, if applicable, is also recommended based on the known myriad cardiovascular benefits in adults.

Indications for pharmacologic intervention include insufficient response to therapeutic lifestyle modifications and identification of secondary hypertension, which cannot be corrected otherwise. There is no consensus regarding the choice of antihypertensive medications, although dihydropyridine calcium channel blockers such as amlodipine are frequently first-line medications in many groups. Treatment choice is empiric and generally guided by the cause of the hypertension, especially in secondary hypertension. Medication classes include calcium channel blockers, β-blockers, angiotensin-converting enzyme inhibitors, angiotensin receptor blockers, and diuretics (Figure 47-3). Other agents such as clonidine, prazosin, and minoxidil are primarily used by subspecialists (see Figure 47-3). Data regarding pediatric dosing of most antihypertensive medications are expanding.

The management of hypertensive urgency and emergency must be considered separately. Therapy should be initiated immediately with simultaneous diagnostic workup. The goal of pharmacologic intervention in hypertensive urgency is to reduce the BP to an appropriate level within 24 to 48 hours. In the setting of hypertensive emergency, the goal is to reduce the mean arterial pressure by no more than 25% (within minutes to 2 hours). The BP should then be lowered slowly to a normal level over the next 48 hours. A trial of oral agents (e.g., nifedipine or hydralazine) should be attempted in the setting of hypertensive urgency; however, in hypertensive emergency, intravenous (IV) medications should be used. IV antihypertensive agents, such as nicardipine, esmolol, and nitroprusside, can be given via bolus or continuous infusion, are titratable, and have shorter times to onset. Any patient with a hypertensive emergency or those with hypertensive urgency requiring a continuous infusion should be admitted to a pediatric intensive care unit or other facility with staffing and equipment necessary for BP monitoring. Arterial access for continuous BP monitoring may also be necessary.

In patients with hypertensive nephropathy and severe volume overload, renal replacement therapy with dialysis or ultrafiltration may be an effective intervention. Temporary hemodialysis typically is reserved for patients with hypertensive emergencies that include overt renal failure with resultant volume overload and severe electrolyte imbalances.

FUTURE DIRECTIONS

Pediatric hypertension is an area of active study with a recent focus centered on the increasingly prevalent constellation of obesity and hypertension. The long-term cardiovascular effects of hypertension in children and adolescents are unclear. However, extrapolations from adult data would clearly indicate that prolonged hypertension is a risk factor for increased cardiovascular morbidity and mortality. The risks and benefits of prolonged pharmacotherapy for hypertension in children and adolescents are also unknown. Additionally, the use of population norms to determine goal BPs is not ideal. Prospective studies are necessary to define normative BP ranges based on long-term cardiovascular morbidity and mortality. There is also hope that research into familial and genetic hypertension syndromes will clarify the complex molecular and cellular mechanisms that cause hypertension and will therefore improve therapy.

SUGGESTED READINGS

Chobanian AV, Bakris GL, Black HR, et al: The seventh report of the Joint National Committee on Prevention, Detection, Evaluation, and Treatment of High Blood Pressure: the JNC7 Report, *JAMA* 289:2560-2572, 2003.

National High Blood Pressure Education Program Working Group on High Blood Pressure in Children and Adolescents: The fourth report on the diagnosis, evaluation, and treatment of high blood pressure in children and adolescents, *Pediatrics* 114:555-576, 2004.

Ogden CL, Flegal KM, Carroll MD, Johnson CL: Prevalence and trends in overweight among US children and adolescents, 1999-2000, *JAMA* 288:1728-1732, 2002.

Sorof J, Daniels S: Obesity hypertension in children: a problem of epidemic proportions, *Hypertension* 40:441-447, 2002.

Syncope

Brett R. Anderson and Anitha S. John

48

*S*yncope is defined as a brief, sudden loss of consciousness and *postural tone* as the result of a decrease in cerebral blood flow. Syncope is reported to occur at least once in 15% to 25% of children by age 18 years. The vast majority of cases are benign in etiology. Syncope, however, can be a result of more ominous conditions and should be evaluated critically.

ETIOLOGY AND PATHOGENESIS

Syncope occurs when cerebral blood flow decreases below 30% to 50% of baseline. This decrease may be the result of systemic vasodilation, decreased cardiac output, or both. This results in transient ischemia, causing temporary loss of consciousness and motor tone. Syncope may also be accompanied by brief autonomic movements. Syncope should be distinguished from presyncope (dizziness or lightheadedness without loss of consciousness), vertigo (the sensation of spinning), and syncopal-like events (e.g., seizures, migraines, or conversion disorder). The causes of syncope can be divided into three major categories: neurally mediated, cardiac, and metabolic (Box 48-1). Syncopal-like events are discussed briefly in the following section.

Neurally Mediated Syncope

Neurally mediated syncope (NMS) accounts for more than 80% of cases that present to the emergency department (ED) or primary care physician. Although subtle differences exist among the following subtypes, abnormal regulation of the autonomic nervous system is common to all.

VASOVAGAL SYNCOPE

The most common cause of NMS is vasovagal syncope, otherwise known as the vasodepressor, neurocardiogenic, or reflex syncope. It is believed to be initiated by an exaggerated response to a sudden decrease in ventricular filling pressure. Standing without movement causes a decrease in venous return because of stasis of blood in the lower extremities. In unaffected individuals, the subsequent reduction in left ventricular filling causes a decrease in signaling from ventricular mechanoreceptors to the brainstem, which stimulates sympathetic activity, causing an increase in heart rate and systemic vasoconstriction. In patients with vasovagal syncope, however, stimulation of ventricular mechanoreceptors results in paradoxic central inhibition of peripheral sympathetic tone, and hence, vasodilation and relative bradycardia. The individual experiences a sudden decrease in cardiac output and cerebral blood flow.

Children typically report a prodrome characterized by lightheadedness, dizziness, nausea, pallor, diaphoresis, and visual and auditory changes. Loss of consciousness typically lasts less than 1 minute. The recovery period extends for 5 to 30 minutes, during which time children report fatigue, dizziness, nausea, and

occasionally vomiting. Vasovagal syncope occurs more often in girls. It is most frequently the result of standing for prolonged periods of time, particularly in warm temperatures; rising rapidly from supine or sitting positions; taking hot showers; or emotional stresses such as venipuncture or viewing disturbing images.

SITUATIONAL SYNCOPE

The mechanism of situational syncope is similar to that of vasovagal syncope. Some physicians classify it separately, however, because it occurs only in the setting of a few classic triggers, most of which involve an exaggerated vagal stimulus, including micturition, defecation, coughing, swallowing, hair combing, or pain. In adolescents with new-onset situational syncope, pregnancy and acute or chronic blood loss should be considered in the differential diagnosis.

ORTHOSTATIC SYNCOPE

As already described, the appropriate physiologic response to standing is systemic vasoconstriction. Orthostatic hypotension and syncope occur when there is a disruption in this response immediately upon sitting (from lying down) or standing, resulting in a decrease in systolic blood pressure by greater than 20 or 10 mm Hg within 3 minutes of changing position. This response can be idiopathic or exacerbated by medications, such as diuretics, other antihypertensives, and vasodilators.

POSTURAL ORTHOSTATIC TACHYCARDIA SYNDROME

Postural orthostatic tachycardia syndrome (POTS) is defined as reproducible, exaggerated tachycardia (change >30 beats/min) within 10 minutes of standing associated with modest systemic hypotension. This is likely caused by a collection of disorders, all of which lead to a decrease in cerebral blood flow in the context of lower extremity or splanchnic blood pooling. Although much is still unknown about the cause of this condition, some studies suggest autoimmune or autonomic triggers.

DYSAUTONOMIA

Dysautonomia is a rare cause of syncope in children. When it does occur, it is typically part of a much larger presentation that includes severe orthostatic hypotension, temperature dysregulation, fatigue, bowel and bladder dysfunction, or pain disproportionate to the examination.

BREATH-HOLDING SPELLS

Breath-holding spells typically occur in children age 6 to 24 months. They are classically triggered by emotional insults, such as anger, pain, or fear. Children cry, then forcibly exhale, and

---

Box 48-1 Differential Diagnosis of Presentation for "Syncope"

Neurally Mediated Syncope
Vasovagal syncope
Situational syncope
Orthostatic syncope
Postural orthostatic tachycardia syndrome
Dysautonomia
Breath-holding spells

Cardiac Syncope
Arrhythmias
  Long QT syndrome
  Preexcitation syndromes
  Short QT syndrome
  Brugada syndrome
  Catecholaminergic ventricular tachycardia
  Bradycardias
Structural heart diseases
  Hypertrophic cardiomyopathy
  Arrhythmogenic right ventricular cardiomyopathy
  Dilated cardiomyopathy
  Valvar stenosis
  Aberrant coronary arteries
  Pulmonary hypertension
  Acute myocarditis
  Congestive heart failure

Metabolic
Inborn errors of metabolism
Hypoglycemia
Hypocalcemia
Hyperkalemia
Drug overdose

Syncope-like Events
Seizure
Basilar migraine
Conversion disorder

---

seemingly "forget" to inhale. Cyanosis ensues followed by transient loss of consciousness. Brief posturing or tonic-clonic movements may also occur. Children regain consciousness spontaneously. This condition is typically outgrown by the age of 5 years, and intervention is rarely necessary.

Cardiac Syncope

Although a cardiac cause is found in fewer than 2% of previously healthy children with syncope, it is important to recognize because it can be associated with an increased risk of sudden death. Cardiac syncope results from abrupt decline in cardiac output as the result of obstructive lesions (aortic stenosis, hypertrophic cardiomyopathy [HCM]), myocardial dysfunction (ischemia, cardiomyopathy), or primary arrhythmias (Figure 48-1). Many of these conditions can be asymptomatic until syncope or sudden death occurs. Arrhythmias can also occur secondary to structural heart disease, to myocardial dysfunction, or to postoperative changes in association with congenital heart disease. Any concern for a cardiac syncope warrants a referral to a pediatric cardiologist. Sudden cardiac death (SCD) in the young is estimated to affect between one in 50,000 and one in 200,000 children.

ARRHYTHMIAS

Some of the arrhythmias associated with cardiac syncope are reviewed here. For further discussion of arrhythmias, please refer to Chapter 45.

Long QT Syndrome

Long QT syndrome (LQTs) results from mutations in genes that regulate myocardial repolarization and manifests in prolongation of the corrected QT (QTc) interval on electrocardiography (ECG). It results in a predisposition to life-threatening ventricular arrhythmias, such as torsades de pointes. It is commonly defined as a QTc longer than 460 msec in children younger than 15 years old, longer than 450 msec in men and longer than 470 msec in women, but in some forms, the QTc can be normal on resting ECG.

LQT can be congenital or acquired (as the result of medications or electrolyte disturbances). To date, mutations in 12 genes have been identified, involving potassium, sodium, and calcium channels (LQT1–LQT12). For patients testing positive on genetic studies, LQT1, LQT2, and LQT3 are the most common (45%, 45%, and 7%, respectively). Whereas patients with LQT1 appear to be at a particularly high risk of sudden death with exercise, patients with LQT2 appear to be at most increased risk in the presence of loud noises and emotional stimuli. Treatment with β-blockers has been shown to markedly reduce the incidence of sudden death, especially in patients with LQT1 and to a lesser extent in LQT2. Although there is some benefit of β-blockers in LQT3, these patients may be more likely to require an implantable cardioverter defibrillator.

Preexcitation Syndromes

Preexcitation syndromes are characterized by premature ventricular stimulation. The classic, and most common, preexcitation syndrome is Wolff-Parkinson-White (WPW) syndrome, which is estimated to occur in 0.1% to 0.4% of the population. Preexcitation in WPW syndrome is the result of rapid impulse conduction through an accessory pathway connecting the atria and ventricles and is described in detail in Chapter 45. This predisposes patients to atrioventricular (AV) reentrant tachycardia, atrial flutter, and atrial fibrillation. SCD can occur as a result of 1:1 conduction of an atrial tachycardia (namely atrial flutter or fibrillation) through the accessory pathway, resulting in a rapid ventricular rate.

Short QT Syndrome

Short QT syndrome (QTc <300-340 msec) is a rare condition associated with syncope and sudden death as the result of ventricular fibrillation. This entity is significantly rarer than LQTs. There are increasing numbers of case reports, however, and at least three associated genes have been identified.

Brugada Syndrome

Brugada syndrome is associated with syncope or sudden death at rest or during sleep, often in the setting of elevated body

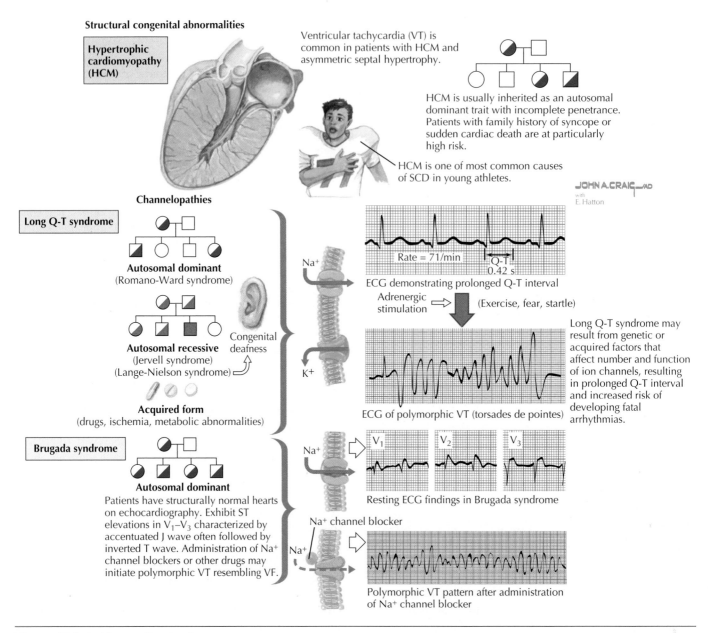

Figure 48-1 *Sudden cardiac death.*

temperature (e.g., with fever or *after* vigorous exercise), or in the early morning. Presentation, therefore, can sometimes be confused with febrile seizures. Patients with this condition have normal QT intervals, ST-segment elevation with a "coved" appearance, and right ventricular conduction delay, although this pattern can be transient or absent (see Figure 48-1). As many as 50% of cases may be sporadic mutations. The other 50%, however, are associated with a positive family history, so special attention should be paid where there is a positive family history of syncope, abnormal ECG, or sudden death.

Catecholaminergic Polymorphic Ventricular Tachycardia

Catecholaminergic polymorphic ventricular tachycardia (CPVT) is caused by abnormalities in calsequestrin and ryanodine receptor (RYR2) genes. It predisposes patients to

exercise-induced polymorphic ventricular tachycardia, syncope, and a high risk of sudden death in the setting of *normal* resting ECGs. CPVT can be diagnosed by stress testing.

Bradycardia

Bradycardia can result from sinus node or AV nodal abnormalities and is reviewed in further detail in Chapter 45. Syncope can sometimes occur from bradycardia because of a decrease in cardiac output and cerebral perfusion pressure.

STRUCTURAL HEART DISEASE

Hypertrophic Cardiomyopathy

HCM is the most common cause of SCD in children and young adults in the United States. Its incidence has been reported to be as high as one in 500 individuals, with an estimated 2% to 8% chance of death per patient per year. In patients with HCM, the left ventricle is hypertrophied but not dilated in the absence of other structural heart disease. It is inherited in an autosomal dominant pattern and results in disordered myocardial architecture with hypertrophied myocytes. Syncope and SCD may result from ventricular tachyarrhythmias because of an abnormal myocardium and increasing left ventricular outflow tract obstruction leading to decreased cardiac output and coronary ischemia. The presence of small vessel disease in intramural coronary arteries may result in ischemia, myocardial death, and intramural scarring, all of which contribute to the electrical instability of the ventricle. Children with a family history of HCM-related deaths, prior cardiac arrest, sustained ventricular tachycardia, syncope, and left ventricular wall thickness 30 mm or larger are at the greatest risk for sudden death. The physical examination in patients with obstruction will reveal a systolic ejection murmur that increases in intensity with Valsalva or moving from sitting to standing. ECGs are abnormal in 90% of patients with HCM.

Arrhythmogenic Right Ventricular Cardiomyopathy/Dysplasia

Arrhythmogenic right ventricular cardiomyopathy (ARVC also known as ARVD) is a primary myocardial disease associated with the replacement of normal myocardium with fibrofatty tissue and is most commonly associated with an autosomal dominant transmission in familial cases. ARVC results in an increased frequency of ventricular arrhythmias, which lead to syncope and sudden death.

Dilated Cardiomyopathy

Dilated cardiomyopathy (DCM) represents another potential cause of syncope and SCD in the young. The disease is characterized by left ventricular dilatation; impaired systolic function; and segmental wall motion abnormalities, which result in cardiac ischemia, leading to myocardial arrhythmias.

Aortic Stenosis

Valvar stenosis, either congenital or acquired, may lead to syncope as the result of insufficient cardiac output to meet demands because of fixed narrowing of the valve orifice or secondary arrhythmias as the result of decreased coronary perfusion in the setting of myocardial thickening or a combination of the two.

Abnormal Origin of the Coronary Arteries

Anomalous origin of the left coronary artery has been associated with syncope and SCD, particularly when the left coronary artery has an intramural course, because this is associated with left coronary ostial stenosis or a "slitlike" orifice of the left coronary. Myocardial ischemia can result predisposing to ventricular arrhythmias. Up to 40% of these patients have symptoms before SCD, and up to 20% to 30% may have ischemic changes on ECG during exercise.

Pulmonary Hypertension

Children with pulmonary hypertension can experience exercise-induced syncope. For these children, however, syncope is a late sign that is associated with decreased cardiac output and hypoxia related to right heart failure.

Acute Myocarditis

Acute myocarditis is the result of inflammation of the myocardium, typically secondary to infection (e.g., enterovirus, adenovirus, or parvovirus) or toxin (e.g., cocaine). As inflammatory cells infiltrate the myocardium, interstitial edema, myocyte death, and fibrotic replacement of myocytes occur. Myocarditis can lead to myocardial electrical instability and left ventricular dysfunction. Children typically present with chest or abdominal pain, exertional dyspnea, palpitations, acute heart failure, or ST changes on ECG. Syncope is associated with the presence of serious ventricular arrhythmias. These children can remain at risk of ventricular arrhythmias, particularly exercise induced, even after resolution of the acute myocarditis.

Congestive Heart Failure

As cardiac output declines, patients with congestive heart failure may experience syncope. This is rarely a presenting sign and is typically accompanied by other signs or symptoms of heart failure, such as exercise intolerance, edema, hepatomegaly, shortness of breath, and respiratory distress.

Metabolic Syncope

Metabolic syncope is rare. More often, disorders of metabolism induce a gradual and prolonged impairment of consciousness. They must also be considered in the evaluation of syncope, however, because they are often easily identified and treated. Metabolic causes of syncope include inborn errors of metabolism, hypoglycemia, and electrolyte abnormalities (e.g., hypocalcemia or hyperkalemia, which can induce arrhythmias). Drug abuse or overdose should also be included in the differential.

Syncope-like Events

Three syncope-like events deserve special mention because they account for an estimated 12% of all presentations for "syncope." These are seizure, basilar migraine, and conversion disorder. These three conditions can often be differentiated from true syncope by history alone. Although myoclonic jerks are common in syncope, they occur after syncope ensues, rarely last more than a few seconds, and are relatively small in amplitude. Tonic-clonic seizures, in contrast, typically are characterized by a longer duration and greater amplitude of movements and a prolonged postictal phase. Basilar migraines may result in syncopal-like episodes, but their prodrome commonly includes vertigo, diplopia, dysarthria, nystagmus, or ataxia. They are typically, but not always, associated with migraine headaches. Conversion disorder can be more difficult to differentiate and is a diagnosis of exclusion. Features that point to this diagnosis include prolonged loss of consciousness (>10 minutes) with a normal metabolic profile, high frequency of episodes, tightly closed or fluttering eyelids,

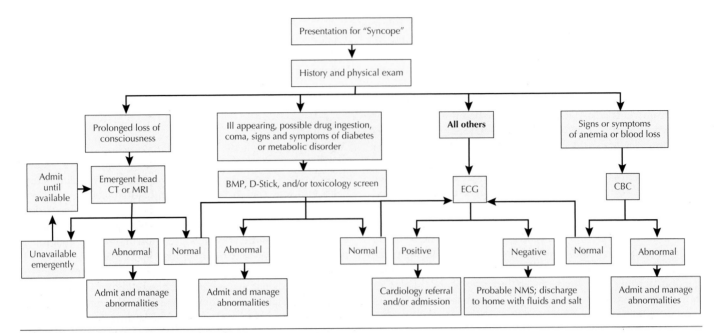

Figure 48-2 *Diagnosis and management of syncope.*

passive lifting and dropping of limbs that demonstrate continued regard for pain, normal or elevated blood pressure, and normal cerebral blood flow. Similar to syncope, conversion disorder occurs more frequently in girls, particularly in high-achieving preteens and teenagers. It is believed to be an unconscious mechanism of sublimating anxiety or depression.

EVALUATION AND DIAGNOSTIC APPROACH

A thorough history and physical examination alone can suggest the diagnosis in the majority of cases of syncope (Figure 48-2). History of the present illness should include a detailed account of the event (including the duration, associated motor activity, and the circumstances surrounding recovery), triggers (including emotional, auditory, and exertional), and prodrome (including palpitations, chest pain, nausea or abdominal pain, diaphoresis, and lightheadedness). Past medical and family histories should focus on previous syncope and cardiac, neurologic, and psychiatric conditions. Family history should also include sudden or unexplained deaths, including sudden infant death syndrome, unexplained motor vehicle accidents, or a history of drowning or near drowning. Physical examination should include orthostatic vital signs and thorough cardiac and neurological examinations. Any patient with suspected cardiac cause should have an ECG as part of the evaluation. Patients with prolonged loss of consciousness, history of seizurelike movements, postepisode lethargy, or neurologic deficit should instead be evaluated with electroencephalography, head computed tomography, or magnetic resonance imaging; patients with suspected metabolic causes should be evaluated with a D-stick, basic metabolic panel, and toxicology screen; and patients with concerns for blood loss or signs of anemia should be evaluated with a complete blood cell count. Any female patient of childbearing age should also undergo a urine pregnancy test because the hemodynamic shifts associated with pregnancy predispose

patients to syncope. If these tests do not reveal a diagnosis, most argue for ECG screening.

MANAGEMENT: INDICATIONS FOR REFERRAL AND ADMISSION

Most patients who present with syncope can be discharged to home from the primary care clinic or ED after evaluation. It is generally recommended that those with focal neurologic signs be admitted to the hospital for further workup and neurologic consult. Similarly, patients with an abnormal ECG; chest pain with exercise; cyanosis; congenital heart disease; syncope triggered by exertion, fright, or noise; or abnormal cardiac examination results should undergo cardiology consult or hospital admission as deemed necessary. Admission should also be considered for children who are ill appearing or have positive toxicology screens, significant electrolyte abnormalities, hypoglycemia not responsive to glucose administration, apnea or bradycardia that resolves only with vigorous stimulation, severe anemia, or orthostatic hypotension that does not resolve with fluid administration.

Children with presumed NMS should be instructed to increase their water (0.25-0.5 oz/kg/d) and salt intake to offset the decreases in blood pressure that occur with stimulation of the autonomic nervous system. Electrolyte-containing fluids can often be helpful. Patients should also avoid caffeine, alcohol, and other diuretics. If presyncopal symptoms (e.g., dizziness, lightheadedness, flushing, or tunnel vision) recur, patients should lie supine with their legs elevated because this will often abort syncope. If syncope is refractory to these interventions, alternate diagnoses should be reconsidered.

FUTURE DIRECTIONS

Continued work is underway to streamline the diagnostic approach and to perfect an evidence-based algorithm. With rising health care costs, much attention has been paid to the large number and low yield of the ancillary studies historically ordered in the evaluation of syncope. Current recommendations remain controversial. It has been found that adding an ECG to a targeted history and physical examination is 96% sensitive for the detection of cardiac abnormalities. Some argue against this because of the low incidence of cardiac abnormalities as the primary cause of syncope in previously healthy children, which leads to a low diagnostic yield and high cost of ECGs per positive result (<0.4% and $28,665/positive result). Prospective cost-effectiveness analyses are necessary to better determine effective patient screening for cardiac causes of syncope.

SUGGESTED READINGS

Corrado D, Basso C, Pavei A, et al: Trends in sudden cardiovascular death in young competitive athletes after implementation of a preparticipation screening program, *JAMA* 296:1593-1601, 2006.

Goldenberg I, Zareba W, Moss AJ: Long QT syndrome, *Curr Probl Cardiol* 33:629-694, 2008.

Johnsrude CL: Current approach to pediatric syncope, *Pediatr Cardiol* 21(6):522-531, 2000.

Lewis DA, Dhala A: Syncope in the pediatric patient. The cardiologist's perspective, *Pediatr Clin North Am* 46(2):205-219, 1999.

Maron BJ, Zipes DP: 36th Bethesda Conference: eligibility recommendations for competitive athletes with cardiovascular abnormalities, *J Am Coll Cardiol* 45(8):1312-1375, 2005.

Maron BJ: Hypertrophic cardiomyopathy: a systematic review, *JAMA* 287:1308-1320, 2002.

Massin MM, Bourguignont A, Coremans C, et al: Syncope in pediatric patients presenting to an emergency department, *J Pediatr* 145(2):223-228, 2004.

Steinberg LA, Knilans TK: Syncope in children: diagnostic tests have a high cost and low yield, *J Pediatr* 146(3):355-358, 2005.

Wieling W, Ganzeboom KS, Saul JP: Reflex syncope in children and adolescents, *Heart* 90(9):1094-1100, 2004.

Acute Rheumatic Fever and Rheumatic Heart Disease

49

Deepika Thacker and Amy L. Peterson

Acute rheumatic fever (ARF) is postulated to be caused by a delayed systemic autoimmune reaction to group A β-hemolytic streptococcal (GAS) pharyngitis. It is a self-limited disease that may involve the heart, skin, brain, joints, and serosal surfaces (Figure 49-1). It is a disease of clinical interest primarily because of its propensity to create heart disease. Rheumatic carditis and valvulitis may be self-limited or may lead to progressive valve deformity.

Since the 1980s, the incidence of ARF has declined in most developed countries to the point where many physicians have little or no practical experience with diagnosis and management of the disease. Credit has been given to improved sanitation and widespread use of antibiotic therapy for GAS pharyngitis. Recently, however, several sporadic outbreaks have been reported in several regions of the United States, which have generally been attributed to new virulent strains of GAS.

In the United States, the incidence of ARF after untreated streptococcal pharyngitis is 0.5% to 3% with a peak frequency in children age 6 to 20 years. The disease is virtually unheard of in children younger than 2 years old and in adults older than 30 years old. The mean age of the first attack of ARF is 8 years. Internationally, however, rheumatic heart disease accounts for 25% to 50% of all cardiac admissions with most major outbreaks occurring in poverty-stricken, overcrowded areas with limited access to antibiotics.

ETIOLOGY AND PATHOGENESIS

The exact cause of ARF and rheumatic heart disease (RHD) is unknown. ARF tends to occur after streptococcal pharyngitis rather than cellulitis. The familial tendency toward ARF is well documented. The HLA-DR2 and DR4 antigens have been linked to an increased incidence of ARF.

The virulence of GAS is related to the bacterial M protein, which structurally resembles human myosin. It is presumed that GAS adheres to the pharyngeal mucosa of the patient and activates antigens and superantigens, which triggers an immune response. In genetically susceptible individuals, antibodies against myosin are produced, which can lead to carditis. Repeated untreated infections with GAS may reactivate antibody production and lead to an autoimmune response that lasts several weeks and eventually damages heart valves (Figure 49-2).

CLINICAL PRESENTATION

The diagnosis of ARF is challenging for several reasons. Pharyngitis is a common complaint in the pediatric population. About 70% of older children and young adults with ARF will recollect an antecedent pharyngitis, but only 20% of young children will. There is an average latent period from the onset of streptococcal pharyngitis to ARF of 18 days (range, 1-5 weeks), which can make recollection during the history challenging. Thus, GAS is rarely isolated from the oropharynx in patients with ARF. Typically, the first manifestation is a painful migratory polyarthritis, but 10% of rheumatic patients will present with pure chorea and no other manifestations of rheumatic fever.

More than 60 years ago, T. Duckett Jones published guidelines for diagnosis of ARF that have been slightly revised by the World Health Organization (Box 49-1 and Figure 49-3). To make a primary diagnosis of ARF, two major or one major and two minor criteria plus evidence of a preceding GAS infection are needed. The exception is rheumatic chorea. Sydenham's chorea (St. Vitus dance) in isolation is considered diagnostic, and no other criteria or evidence of GAS infection are required to make the diagnosis.

Acute carditis is usually clinically manifest by sinus tachycardia without diurnal variation and new onset of a heart murmur of mitral regurgitation with or without aortic regurgitation. With a single attack of ARF, the mitral regurgitation often resolves over months to years, but aortic regurgitation is more likely to persist. In severe cases, signs of heart failure or a friction rub from pericarditis may also be present.

Chronic RHD results when a single or multiple attacks of ARF deform and fuse valve cusps, commissures, or chordae. Stenosis or insufficiency of the valve, and often both, occur. Isolated mitral valve involvement occurs in 60% to 70%, mitral and aortic involvement in 20%, and isolated aortic involvement is rare. The tricuspid valve is involved in 5% to 10% but occurs with mitral or aortic disease. Pulmonary valve involvement is rare.

A history of ARF is obtained in only 60% of patients with RHD. Whereas chronic mitral regurgitation is the most common form of RHD in children and young adults (Figure 49-4), mitral stenosis is more common in older adults. Aortic regurgitation, although less common than mitral regurgitation with ARF, is more likely to persist (see Figure 49-4). Patients with mitral or aortic valve disease may present with an isolated heart murmur or palpitations caused by atrial arrhythmias. They can present with fatigue, decreased exercise tolerance, dyspnea on exertion, orthopnea, and paroxysmal nocturnal dyspnea, which can represent low cardiac output or pulmonary hypertension. However, the onset of symptoms can often be so insidious that patients adapt and are unaware of their significant functional limitations.

The differential diagnosis of ARF is depicted in Box 49-2.

DIAGNOSTIC EVALUATION
Laboratory Studies

With a few exceptions, diagnosis of ARF requires evidence of preceding GAS infection. Throat culture or rapid antigen tests

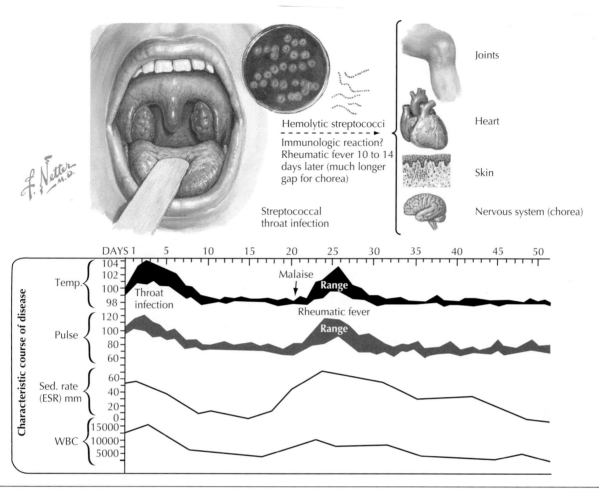

Figure 49-1 *Cardiac manifestations of acute rheumatic fever.*

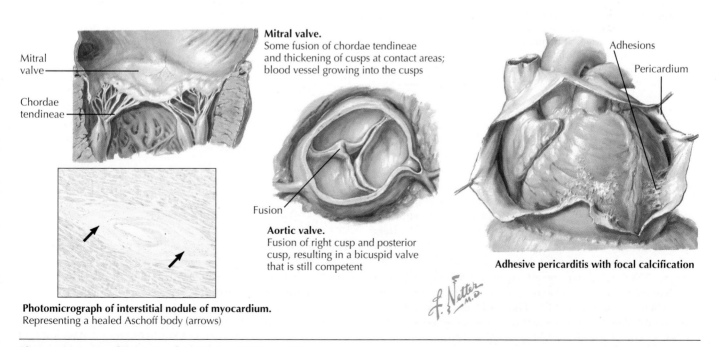

Figure 49-2 *Manifestations of acute rheumatic carditis.*

should be performed, although they have a low yield and do not differentiate between acute infection and a chronic carrier state. Rising titers of antistreptococcal antibodies are more useful in confirming recent GAS infection. The most commonly used antibody test is the antistreptolysin (ASO) titer, which begins to increase approximately 1 week and peaks 3 to 6 weeks after the infection. Anti-DNAse B (anti-deoxyribonuclease B) titers begin to increase after 1 to 2 weeks with a peak after 6 to 8 weeks and may be used if ASO titers are inconclusive.

Other baseline laboratory investigations should include a complete blood count, C-reactive protein (CRP), and erythrocyte sedimentation rate (ESR). The CRP and ESR are both markers of inflammation with high sensitivity but low specificity. They are useful to assess response to antiinflammatory therapy, resolution, and recurrence of the disease process.

Cardiac Evaluation

CHEST RADIOGRAPHY

The chest radiograph may be useful in identifying cardiomegaly and pulmonary congestion in patients with heart failure or valvar heart disease.

ELECTROCARDIOGRAPHY

The most common finding in patients with ARF is sinus tachycardia, although children may have sinus bradycardia because of high vagal tone. First-degree atrioventricular block is also a common finding. Higher degrees of heart block may occasionally be seen, but they resolve with the resolution of the acute process. In patients with chronic RHD, the electrocardiogram (ECG) may suggest chamber enlargement or hypertrophy. It is also invaluable in the diagnosis of complicating arrhythmias such as atrial flutter or fibrillation.

TWO-DIMENSIONAL ECHOCARDIOGRAPHY AND COLOR DOPPLER

All patients with either ARF or chronic RHD must have an echocardiogram. In patients with ARF, echocardiography is necessary to evaluate for signs of acute carditis in the form of pericardial effusion, decreased ventricular function, and mitral regurgitation. In patients with chronic RHD, echocardiography along with color Doppler evaluation is invaluable in identifying the nature and extent of valvar involvement.

CARDIAC MAGNETIC RESONANCE IMAGING

Cardiac magnetic resonance imaging is useful in defining the mechanism and severity of valvar disease in greater anatomic and functional detail. It can be especially useful in planning management strategies and surgical intervention.

Cardiac Catheterization

Cardiac catheterization is not performed in the setting of ARF. In patients with chronic RHD, diagnostic catheterization is now reserved for the few patients in whom the symptoms, clinical findings, and noninvasive imaging are discrepant. However, therapeutic cardiac catheterization and balloon valvuloplasty continue to remain central in management of valvar RHD.

MANAGEMENT AND THERAPY

Acute Rheumatic Fever and Rheumatic Carditis

The age-old adage "rheumatic fever licks the joint but bites the heart" still holds true. The joint disease in rheumatic fever is usually self-limiting. Management is thus focused on treating and preventing the long-term cardiac complications.

Antiinflammatory therapy with either salicylates or steroids is usually started at the time of diagnosis for patients with ARF. They provide prompt symptomatic relief, although their efficacy in altering the natural history of the disease is debatable. Most

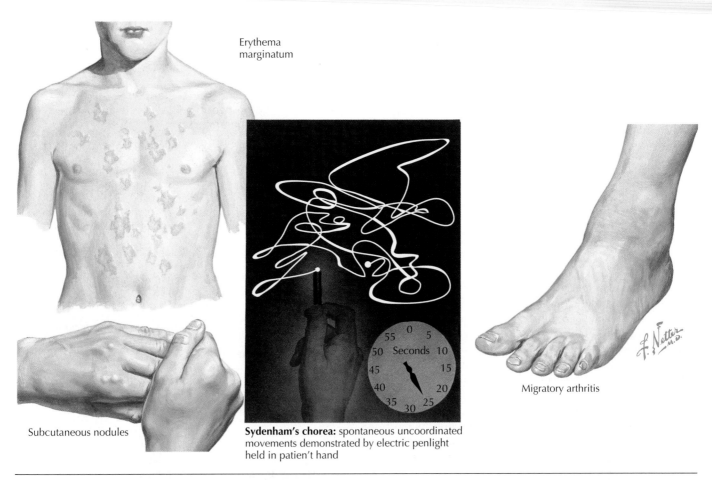

Erythema
marginatum

Subcutaneous nodules

Sydenham's chorea: spontaneous uncoordinated
movements demonstrated by electric penlight
held in patien't hand

55 0 5
50 Seconds 10
45 15
40 20
35 30 25

Migratory arthritis

Figure 49-3 *Noncardiac manifestations of acute rheumatic fever.*

Mitral insufficiency

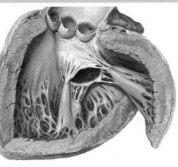

Mitral insufficiency:
mitral valve viewed
from below; marked
shortening of posterior
cusp, with only slight
commissural fusion
and little fusion and
shortening of chordae
tendineae

Calcific plate at anterolateral
commissure of mitral valve,
contributing to insufficiency

Marked enlarge-
ment of left atrium
resulting from mitral
insufficiency

Thickening and shortening
of mitral cusps with
"hamstringing" of posterior
cusp over the musculature
of left ventricle by traction
of enlarged left atrium

Aortic insufficiency

Aortic insufficiency:
Valve viewed from
above; thickened,
short cusps with
triangular deficiency

Concentric hypertrophy with some
dilatation of left ventricle resulting
from aortic insufficiency, causing
chordae tendineae to elongate
and run in a relatively horizontal
direction, thus impeding closure
of mitral valve and leading to
secondary mitral insufficiency

Shortened cusps of
aortic valve with
exposure of sinuses
and dilatation of
aorta: "Jet lesion"
on septal wall of
left ventricle

Figure 49-4 *Rheumatic heart disease: clinical presentation.*

Box 49-2 Differential Diagnosis of Acute Rheumatic Fever

- Myocarditis
- Pericarditis
- Kawasaki disease
- Rheumatoid arthritis
- Other arthritis: traumatic, septic
- Sickle cell disease
- Infective endocarditis
- Systemic lupus erythematosus
- Lyme disease

Table 49-1 Antibacterial Therapy for Group A Streptococcus Pharyngitis and Acute Rheumatic Fever

Penicillin V	Weight ≤27 kg: 250 mg PO BID or TID for 10 days
	Weight >27 kg: 500 mg PO BID or TID daily for 10 days
	or
Amoxicillin	50 mg/kg PO SID (maximum, 1 g) for 10 days
	or
Benzathine penicillin G	Weight ≤27 kg: 0.6 million U IM once
	Weight >27 kg:1.2 million U IM once
Patients Allergic to Penicillin	
Narrow-spectrum cephalosporins: cephalexin, cephadroxil	Dose varies with selection for 10 days
	or
Clindamycin	20 mg/kg/d PO in three doses (maximum, 1.8 g/d) for 10 days
	or
Azithromycin	12 mg/kg PO SID (maximum, 500 mg) for 5 days
	or
Clarithromycin	15 mg/kg/day in two doses (maximum, 250 mg BID) for 10 days
Secondary Prophylaxis After ARF or in Patients with Chronic RHD	
Benzathine penicillin G	Weight ≤27 kg: 0.6 million U IM every 3 to 4 weeks
	Weight >27 kg: 1.2 million U IM every 3 to 4 weeks
	or
Penicillin V	250 mg PO BID
Patients Allergic to Penicillin	
Sulfadiazine or sulfisoxazole	Weight ≤27 kg: 0.5 g PO SID
	Weight >27 kg: 1 g PO SID
	or
Macrolide or azalide	Variable
Duration of Secondary Prophylaxis	
Rheumatic fever with carditis and residual heart disease	10 years or until 40 years of age (whichever is longer), sometimes lifelong
Rheumatic fever with carditis but no residual heart disease	10 years or until 21 years of age (whichever is longer)
Rheumatic fever without carditis	5 years or until 21 years of age (whichever is longer)

ARF, acute rheumatic fever; BID, twice a day; IM, intramuscular; PO, orally; RHD, rheumatic heart disease; SID, once a day; TID, three times a day.

experts recommend that patients with mild degrees of carditis be started on high-dose aspirin, but patients with more severe forms of carditis and heart failure should be initially started on steroids for 2 weeks and later switched to aspirin. The duration of antiinflammatory therapy should be 4 to 6 weeks or until there is laboratory evidence of resolution of inflammatory markers. Other antiinflammatory agents such as immunoglobulins and pentoxifylline may be tried in resistant patients, although neither has been found to be consistently beneficial. Patients with active carditis should have some level of activity restriction. Supportive therapy for heart failure includes the use of diuretics, digoxin, and afterload reduction. In rare cases, mitral valve surgery may be required in the setting of intractable heart failure.

Sydenham's chorea is usually self-limited. Traditionally, it has been treated with sedation and antiseizure and antipsychotic medications. Steroids, immunoglobulins, and plasmapheresis have been tried without conclusive evidence demonstrating a significant benefit.

All patients with ARF should be treated with antibiotics to eliminate GAS from the throat even with negative culture results. Oral penicillin V is the drug of choice. Alternatives include single-dose benzathine penicillin injection or a course of oral ampicillin or amoxicillin. Macrolides or first-generation cephalosporins can be used in patients who are allergic to penicillin. It should be noted that some patients who are allergic to penicillin may also be allergic to cephalosporins. Because the risk of valvar heart disease is greatly increased with each subsequent attack of ARF, all patients should be placed on an antibiotic regimen for secondary prophylaxis to prevent future recurrences (Table 49-1).

Chronic Rheumatic Heart Disease

All patients with established chronic RHD should be placed on secondary prophylaxis to prevent recurrences of ARF. Asymptomatic patients should be followed clinically with periodic echocardiographic evaluation. In symptomatic patients, diuretics may be used for relief of edema or symptoms of heart failure. Anticoagulation with warfarin is recommended for those with chronic atrial fibrillation or a history of previous thromboembolic events. Antiarrhythmic drugs, afterload-reducing agents, and digoxin may be used when indicated.

The American Heart Association (AHA) no longer recommends antibiotic prophylaxis for prevention of infective endocarditis in patients with RHD. However, the AHA and others recognize the increased risk of endocarditis in some groups of patients, including those with prosthetic valves and those with a history of endocarditis, and continue to recommend that these patients receive infective endocarditis prophylaxis.

The AHA also has recommendations regarding the timing of surgical intervention for valvar heart disease based on symptoms and diagnostic testing. Percutaneous balloon valvuloplasty is the

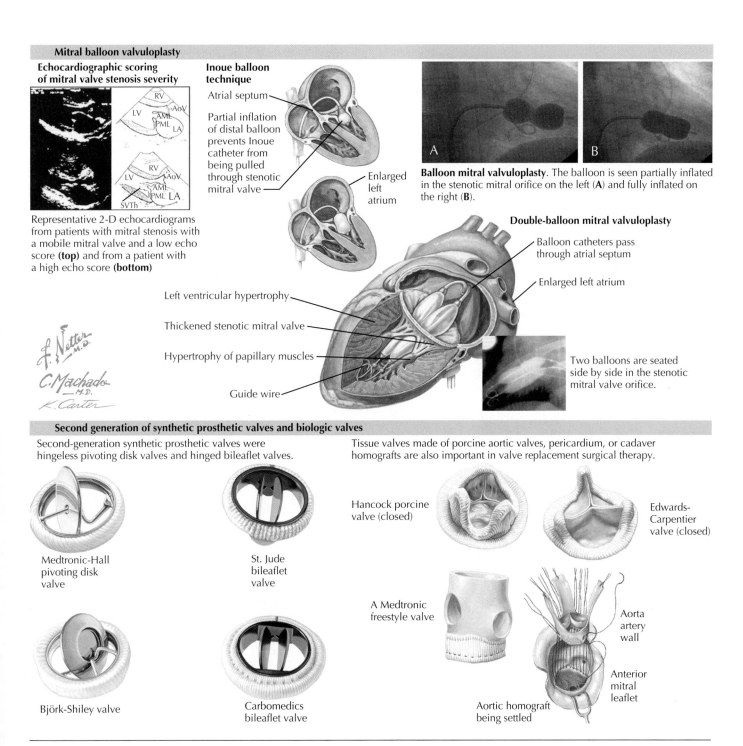

Figure 49-5 *Management and treatment of chronic rheumatic heart disease.*

procedure of choice for patients with mitral stenosis when possible (Figure 49-5). For patients requiring surgical correction, every effort should be made to repair the native valve when feasible. However, a large number of patients go on to require surgical replacement of the valve with a pericardial, bioprosthetic, or a mechanical valve (see Figure 49-5).

FUTURE DIRECTIONS

Vaccine research against GAS, specifically the M protein, has been limited because of the variability of the M protein and the

increased risk of autoimmune complications. However, now that the M protein has been sequenced and different cross-reactive epitopes have been characterized, researchers are closer to creating a vaccine for certain GAS strains. However, much more work must be done before a vaccine is clinically available.

Newer techniques for percutaneous replacement of cardiac valves are being developed. On the surgical front, prosthetic valves with better lifespans and fewer complications are being designed. To reduce the risk of hemorrhage, research involving the use of antiplatelet agents and thrombin inhibitors is underway and shows encouraging results.

SUGGESTED READINGS

Chin TK, Li D: Rheumatic fever, *Emedicine* 2008.

Fyler DC: Rheumatic fever. In Keane JF, Lock JE, Fyler DC, editors: *Nadas' Pediatric Cardiology*, Philadelphia, 2006, Saunders, pp 387-400.

Gerber MA, Baltimore RS, Eaton CB, et al: Prevention of rheumatic fever and diagnosis and treatment of acute Streptococcal pharyngitis: a scientific statement from the American Heart Association Rheumatic Fever, Endocarditis, and Kawasaki Disease Committee of the Council on Cardiovascular Disease in the Young, the Interdisciplinary Council on Functional Genomics and Translational Biology, and the Interdisciplinary Council on Quality of Care and Outcomes Research: endorsed by the American Academy of Pediatrics, *Circulation* 119(11):1541-1551, 2009.

Jones TD: The diagnosis of rheumatic fever, *JAMA* 126:481, 1944.

Tani LY: Rheumatic fever and rheumatic heart disease. In Allen HD, Driscoll DJ, Shaddy RE, Feltes TF, editors: *Moss and Adams' Heart Disease in Infants, Children, and Adolescents Including the Fetus and Young Adult*, Philadelphia, 2008, Lippincott Williams & Wilkins, pp 1256-1280.

World Health Organization: *Rheumatic Fever and Rheumatic Heart Disease*: Report of WHO Expert consultation, Geneva, 2004, World Health Organization, p 923.

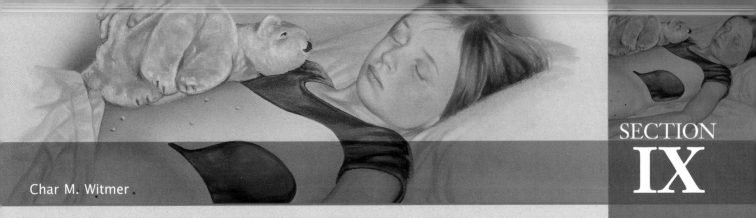

Char M. Witmer

Hematologic Disorders

Howard Topol

R̲ed blood cells (RBC) are non-nucleated cells composed of a cell membrane, complex surface glycoproteins, and hemoglobin (Hb). Hb, the major component of RBCs, facilitates oxygen transport from the lungs to tissue capillaries by reversible binding and releasing oxygen, according to the characteristics of the oxyhemoglobin dissociation curve. As a result, RBC homeostasis is essential to prevent tissue hypoxia and maintain critical organ function.

RBC disorders can be divided into two categories, congenital and acquired disorders. Congenital disorders include membrane defects, thalassemia, hemoglobinopathies, and enzyme defects and aplasia. Acquired disorders include immune destruction, mechanical destruction, anemia of chronic disease, nutritional deficiencies (i.e., deficiency of B12, folate, iron), and aplasia. These disorders have different clinical features and mechanisms of disease, but all result in anemia.

ETIOLOGY AND PATHOGENESIS

Congenital Red Blood Cell Disorders

MEMBRANE DEFECTS

Hereditary spherocytosis (HS) is the most common RBC membrane defect, affecting one in 5000 people of Northern European descent. Two-thirds of cases are inherited by autosomal dominant transmission, but de novo mutations can occur. The disorder arises from abnormalities of RBC membrane proteins. Commonly affected membrane proteins include ankyrin, band 3, and spectrin. These abnormalities lead to an unstable RBC membrane that assumes a spherical shape rather than the biconcave disc shape found in normal RBCs. The spherical RBCs have less deformability and cannot circulate freely through narrow capillaries. As a result, they become trapped in the spleen and are engulfed by macrophages, leading to a shortened RBC lifespan.

Hereditary elliptocytosis (HE) is another RBC membrane defect characterized by elliptical or oval-shaped RBCs on the peripheral blood smear. Unlike HS, HE is more common in people of African and Mediterranean ancestry. It is inherited mostly in an autosomal dominant fashion, although there can be spontaneous mutations. Clinical manifestations are usually similar to HS, but different phenotypic variations exist.

THALASSEMIAS

The predominant adult hemoglobin A molecule is a tetramer formed by two α-globin and two β-globin chains. The thalassemias are a heterogeneous group of inherited disorders in which the production of normal Hb is partly or completely suppressed from the defective synthesis of one of the two globin chains (α or β). The type of thalassemia refers to the specific globin chain that is underproduced and is identified as either α- or β-thalassemia. A decrease in the production of either an α- or β-globin chain results in an excess of free globin chains that precipitate in the RBC and cause RBC membrane damage. The end result is anemia from RBC hemolysis and ineffective erythropoiesis in the bone marrow.

Whereas α-thalassemia is more commonly found in Southeast Asia, β-thalassemia is more common in Mediterranean countries. There are two α-globin genes located on chromosome 16. α-Thalassemias are usually the result of large gene deletions, causing a reduction in α-globin production. The severity of disease is directly related to the number of genes involved (Table 50-1).

There is one β-globin gene located on chromosome 11. Point mutations are the most common type of genetic mutation in β-thalassemia. The β–thalassemia trait occurs when only one gene is affected, resulting in a mild microcytic anemia. The Hb electrophoresis reveals an increased Hb A2 or Hb F level. In contrast the inheritance of two affected β-globin genes results in a broad spectrum of clinical disease. The severity is determined by the residual amount of β-globin synthesis. The clinical phenotype ranges from transfusion dependence (thalassemia major) to a moderate anemia that does not necessitate chronic transfusions (thalassemia intermedia). Severe β-thalassemia is diagnosed between 6 months and 2 years of age. Laboratory analysis reveals a moderate to severe microcytic anemia and 20% to 100% HbF, 2% to 7% HbA2, and 0% to 80% HbA. Clinically, patients present with pallor, failure to thrive, hepatosplenomegaly, and bone deformities from marrow expansion.

HEMOGLOBINOPATHIES

The hemoglobinopathies are a group of autosomal recessive inherited disorders characterized by synthesis of abnormal Hb molecules (i.e., S, and C). The most common and severe hemoglobinopathy is sickle cell disease, in which only HbS is produced. Chapter 53 of this book is dedicated to the in-depth discussion of sickle cell disease.

ENZYME DEFICIENCIES

Glucose-6-phosphate dehydrogenase (G6PD) deficiency is an x-linked recessive disorder characterized by abnormally low levels of the enzyme G6PD. Worldwide it is the most common enzyme deficiency. G6PD is the rate-limiting enzyme of the pentose phosphate pathway, which is crucial for protecting RBCs from oxidative stress. In G6PD deficiency, damage by oxidant free radicals causes RBCs to hemolyze.

The severity of disease is based on the baseline G6PD level. The majority of individuals with G6PD have a moderate deficiency (10% normal activity), and at a steady state, they are hematologically normal. But with exposure to an oxidative stressor, they can develop acute hemolysis with resultant anemia, reticulocytosis, and hyperbilirubinemia or jaundice. Patients with a severe G6PD deficiency (i.e., Mediterranean variant) can

Table 50-1 α-Thalassemia Gene Deletions

Number of α-Globin Genes Mutated	Syndrome	Clinical Features	Hemoglobin Electrophoresis
1 (-α/αα)	Silent carrier	Not anemic, normocytic	Normal levels of HbA2 and HbF. May have low amounts of Hb Barts (γ4) on newborn screen.
2 (–/αα) or (-α/-α)	Thalassemia trait	Mild anemia, microcytosis, and hypochromia	Normal levels of HbA2 and HbF. Hb Barts (γ4) on newborn screen (4%-6%).
3 (-α/–)	HbH disease	Moderate hemolytic anemia (Hb, 7-10 g/dL), splenomegaly, and hemolytic crisis with exposure to oxidant drugs and infections	Hb H (β4) (5%-30%)
4 (–/–)	Hydrops fetalis	Death in utero induced by severe anemia	Hb H (β4)

Hb, hemoglobin.

have baseline mild anemia and reticulocytosis. Drugs that are oxidative stressors and should be avoided in patients with G6PD include antimalarials, sulfonamides and sulfones, quinolones, aspirin, methylene blue, and rasburicase. Other categories of oxidative stressors to avoid include fava beans and naphthalene mothballs. The degree of hemolysis varies with the drug's antioxidant effect, the amount ingested, and the severity of the enzyme deficiency in the patient. The highest prevalence of disease is among persons of African, Asian, and Mediterranean descent.

Pyruvate kinase (PK) deficiency is an inherited metabolic disorder of the enzyme PK, which catalyzes the rate-limiting step in the glycolysis pathway. A deficiency of the enzyme PK compromises RBC adenosine triphosphate production and metabolic energy demand, leading to hemolysis. The inheritance pattern is usually autosomal recessive. Clinically, patients have a moderate to severe hemolytic anemia, reticulocytosis (may be 40%-70%), jaundice, and splenomegaly. Symptoms caused by hemolysis range from mild to severe.

DIAMOND-BLACKFAN ANEMIA

Diamond Blackfan anemia (DBA) is a congenital, lifelong pure RBC aplasia characterized by anemia, reticulocytopenia, and normocellular bone marrow with a paucity of erythroid precursors. The white blood cell count and platelets are usually normal. The anemia can be mildly macrocytic or normocytic and usually manifests after birth or in the first few months of life. DBA is associated with various congenital abnormalities, most commonly short stature, craniofacial abnormalities, and thumb abnormalities (classically triphalangeal thumbs). It is also associated with an increased predisposition to cancer. Inheritance patterns vary, since dominant, recessive, and sporadic mutations can all cause DBA. Approximately 50% of patients with DBA have a single mutation in a gene encoding for a ribosomal protein.

CONGENITAL BONE MARROW FAILURE SYNDROMES

Inherited bone marrow failure syndromes include Fanconi anemia, dyskeratosis congenita, Schwachman-Diamond syndrome, Pearson syndrome, and amegakaryocytic thrombocytopenia. In contrast to DBA, these disorders affect multiple cell lines. These disorders are rare. Presentation can occur at a young age with symptoms of pancytopenia and congenital malformations, which differ by syndrome.

Acquired Red Blood Cell Disorders

MECHANICAL RED BLOOD CELL DESTRUCTION

The previous congenital RBC disorders are caused by abnormalities inherent to RBCs. In contrast, mechanical destruction involves hemolysis caused by extrinsic factors unrelated to the RBCs. Examples of mechanical RBC destruction include vascular lesions (i.e., AVMs), cardiac valvular defects, and microangiopathic damage (i.e., hemolytic uremic syndrome or thrombotic thrombocytopenic purpura). RBCs can also be destroyed by infections, drugs, toxins, and heat (with severe burns).

AUTOIMMUNE HEMOLYTIC ANEMIA

The most common immune-mediated extrinsic anemia is autoimmune hemolytic anemia (AIHA), in which circulating antibodies are directed against the patient's RBCs. AIHA can be primary or secondary to infection, drugs, or an underlying disease process such as lymphoma, systemic lupus erythematosus, or immunodeficiency. Primary AIHA occurs in the majority of children and often occurs after a viral illness. The specific autoantibodies can be either IgG in warm-reactive antibodies or IgM in cold-agglutinin disease. Patients with AIHA require close monitoring because brisk hemolysis can result in a sudden decrease in Hb that can be life threatening.

ANEMIA OF CHRONIC DISEASE

Anemia of chronic disease occurs with a wide range of chronic inflammatory, malignant, autoimmune, and infectious conditions. The theorized primary mechanism involves proinflammatory cytokines disrupting iron homeostasis. An influx of cytokines causes iron sequestration within reticuloendothelial cells, making less iron available in the circulation for erythroid progenitor cells. Anemia of chronic disease is characterized by inadequate RBC production in the setting of low serum iron and low iron-binding capacity. The RBCs are usually normocytic and normochromic, but they also can be mildly hypochromic and microcytic.

NUTRITIONAL DEFICIENCIES

Deficiencies of vitamin B12 (cobalamin) and folate can cause a megaloblastic anemia resulting from inhibition of DNA synthesis during RBC production. The anemia is macrocytic and can be accompanied by leukopenia and thrombocytopenia. Dietary deficiencies of these vitamins are somewhat rare in the pediatric population. Animal products, such as meat and dairy, are the only dietary sources of cobalamin. Even in severely limited diets, vitamin B12 deficiency takes many years to develop because of its long half-life. Folate is more widespread in the human diet and is found in cereal, fruits, vegetables, and meat. Other causes of vitamin B12 deficiency include defective B12 absorption from a failure to secrete intrinsic factor, a failure to absorb B12 in the small intestine, and congenital deficiencies in vitamin B12 transport or metabolism. Other causes of folate deficiency include malabsorption, increased folate requirements in chronic hemolytic anemias, or congenital disorders of folic acid metabolism. Of note, certain drugs (i.e., methotrexate) interfere with folic acid metabolism and can cause folate deficiency.

Iron deficiency is the most common cause of anemia in the pediatric population, affecting approximately 5% to 10% of toddlers and adolescent girls. The prompt diagnosis and treatment of this condition is important because clinical manifestations include poor academic achievement, reduced attention span, and growth retardation. Iron deficiency occurs when an insufficient amount of iron is available to meet the body's requirements. In pediatric patients, it is usually caused by inadequate dietary intake, chronic blood loss (gastrointestinal or menstrual bleeding) or malabsorption (celiac disease or inflammatory bowel disease). High-risk groups include premature infants (who receive less iron from the mother in the third trimester) and infants consuming large amounts of cow's milk (specifically, >24 oz/d) and menstruating women. In children older than 2 years of age, dietary causes of iron deficiency is less likely, and chronic blood loss (heavy menses) or malabsorption (celiac disease or inflammatory bowel disease) need to be considered. Iron-deficiency anemia is microcytic and hypochromic, with a low serum iron and ferritin and an elevated total iron-binding capacity.

TRANSIENT ERYTHROBLASTOPENIA OF CHILDHOOD

Transient erythroblastopenia of childhood (TEC) is a disorder characterized by the temporary cessation of RBC production in previously healthy children. Despite the severity of anemia, patients usually present with slowly developing pallor without other symptoms. Laboratory workup reveals anemia and reticulocytopenia; typically, no other cell lines are affected, but the neutrophil count may be decreased. In TEC, the anemia is transient (unlike DBA). The mean age at diagnosis is 26 months; fewer than 10% are older than 3 years at diagnosis. The cause remains unknown, but a viral cause has been proposed.

TRANSIENT RED BLOOD CELL APLASIA FROM PARVOVIRUS B19

Infection with parvovirus causes a reticulocytopenia for approximately 7 to 10 days. Patients with congenital RBC disorders with increased RBC turnover and decreased RBC life span are at risk for developing a significant anemia during the period of acquired reticulocytopenia (see Chapter 53). Clinically, patients can present with pallor, headache, and a marked decrease in Hb level. The hallmark is a low reticulocyte count, indicating suppression of bone marrow activity. Blood transfusion is indicated in patients with significant anemia who are symptomatic.

CLINICAL PRESENTATION AND DIFFERENTIAL DIAGNOSIS

The clinical presentation of anemia varies greatly depending on the severity of anemia and the time span in which it develops. Frequently, in a process that develops chronically over weeks to months, children will be asymptomatic and may come to medical attention because of an abnormal screening complete blood count (CBC). On the other end of the spectrum, patients with an acute onset of anemia can present with cardiovascular compromise and shock because the body does not have time to compensate for the decreased oxygen-carrying capacity. Compared with adults, children have a large physiologic reserve and can function quite well with chronically low Hb levels.

A patient with mild anemia may only feel slightly fatigued and reveal pallor at sites where capillary beds are visible through the mucosa (conjunctivae, palms, and nail beds). Clinically, anemia can be appreciated when the Hb concentration is below 8 to 9 g/dL, although the complexion of the child and the rapidity of onset may influence this value. In moderate anemia, the body begins to attempt to compensate for decreased oxygen delivery by increasing cardiac output; therefore, tachycardia and a systolic murmur may be present. A systolic flow murmur is often heard if the Hb level is below 8 g/dL. Symptoms at this time may include headache, excessive sleeping (especially in infants), poor feeding, and syncope. In severe anemia, the body's end-organ hypoxia increases, and the patient shows signs of decreased perfusion. Signs of severe anemia include tachypnea, altered mental status, and exertional dyspnea. Left untreated, anemia can progress to cardiovascular collapse.

A complete physical examination is important to establish the cause of anemia. Growth parameters should be obtained in all anemic patients. Failure to thrive suggests a more chronic anemia. Jaundice or darkened urine signifies a significant hemolytic process.

Hepatosplenomegaly is an important finding present in extramedullary hematopoiesis (in chronic hemolytic diseases such as thalassemia) or infiltrative disorders. Frontal bossing is another sign suggestive of extramedullary hematopoiesis.

The differential diagnosis of anemia is diverse. Physiologically, anemia can be divided into three categories: decreased or ineffective RBC production, premature RBC destruction, and blood loss. Causes of anemia can be further subdivided based on a morphologic approach using the reticulocyte index (see Diagnostic Approach) and the mean corpuscular volume (MCV) (Figure 50-1).

DIAGNOSTIC APPROACH

Through the combination of a thorough history, physical examination, and a few simple laboratory tests, the cause of anemia

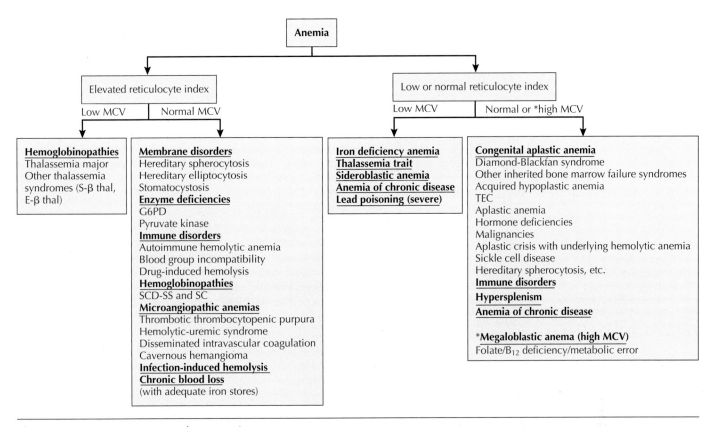

Figure 50-1 *Diagnostic approach to anemia.*

can usually be determined. The initial laboratory workup should include a CBC with differential and reticulocyte count. All three cell lines on the CBC need to be analyzed to determine whether the process causing the anemia is limited to erythroids or if other cells lines are affected.

Anemia is defined as a decrease in the Hb concentration more than 2 standard deviations below the mean for age (Table 50-2). The MCV and reticulocyte count are helpful measurements in

categorizing anemia. The MCV provides a quick, accurate, and readily available method of distinguishing the microcytic anemias (iron deficiency, thalassemia syndromes) from the normocytic (membrane disorders, enzyme deficiencies, AIHA, most hemoglobinopathies) or macrocytic (bone marrow or stem cell failure, disorders of vitamin B12, and folic acid absorption or metabolism) anemias. The MCV varies with age, necessitating the use of age-adjusted normal values (see Table 50-2).

Table 50-2 Normal Hematologic Values for Age			
Age	**Hb (g/dL) Mean (–2 SD)**	**HCT (%) Mean (–2 SD)**	**MCV (fL) Mean (–2 SD)**
Birth (cord blood)	16.5 (13.5)	51 (42)	108 (98)
1-3 d	18.5 (14.5)	56 (45)	108 (95)
2 wk	16.5 (12.5)	51 (39)	105 (86)
1 mo	14.0 (10)	43 (31)	104 (85)
2 mo	11.5 (9)	35 (28)	96 (77)
3-6 mo	11.5 (9.5)	35 (29)	91 (74)
6 mo-2 y	12.0 (10.5)	36 (33)	78 (70)
2-6 y	12.5 (11.5)	37 (34)	81 (75)
6-12 y	13.5 (11.5)	40 (35)	86 (77)
12-18 y			
Male	14.5 (13)	43 (37)	88 (78)
Female	14.0 (12)	41 (36)	90 (78)
18-49 years			
Male	15.5 (13.5)	47 (41)	90 (80)
Female	14.0 (12)	41 (36)	90 (80)

Hb, hemoglobin; HCT, hematocrit; MCV, mean corpuscular volume; SD, standard deviation.

Adapted from Orkin SH, et al., eds. *Nathan and Oski's Hematology of Infancy and Childhood*, ed 7. Philadelphia, Saunders Elsevier, 2009, p 1774.

Table 50-3 Diagnostic Tests for Evaluating Anemia

Diagnostic Test	Disease
DAT or Coombs test	AIHA
Hemoglobin electrophoresis	Sickle cell disease
	Thalassemia
RBC enzyme assays	G6PD deficiency
	PK deficiency
Osmotic fragility test	Hereditary spherocytosis
Iron studies	Iron-deficiency anemia
Folate, vitamin B12	Macrocytic or megaloblastic anemia
Bone marrow aspiration and biopsy	Myelodysplastic syndrome
	Aplastic anemia
	Malignancy
	Diamond-Blackfan anemia
ADAMTS13 activity and inhibitor level	TTP
Chromosomal breakage analysis	Fanconi's anemia

AIHA, autoimmune hemolytic anemia; DAT, direct antiglobulin; G6PD, glucose-6-phosphate dehydrogenase; PK, pyruvate kinase; RBC, red blood cell; TTP, thrombotic thrombocytopenic purpura.

The reticulocyte count should be performed and distinguishes anemias caused by impaired RBC production from those caused by increased RBC destruction. The reticulocyte count is expressed as a percent of total RBCs; it must be corrected for the degree of the anemia. A normal reticulocyte count is 1%. The easiest way to make this correction is to calculate the reticulocyte index (RI) by multiplying the reticulocyte count by the reported hematocrit divided by a normal hematocrit. For example, a reticulocyte count of 5% in a child with severe iron-deficiency anemia and a hematocrit of 7% is not elevated when corrected for the degree of anemia ($5\% \times 7\%/33\% = 1\%$).

After the cause of the anemia has been further categorized into broad disease categories, specific tests can be drawn. Table 50-3 lists specific diagnostic tests and their associated conditions.

MANAGEMENT AND THERAPY

Congenital Disorders

Therapy for patients with congenital RBC disorders is disease specific. In hereditary spherocytosis, splenectomy is curative but is associated with surgical and postsplenectomy infectious risks. There is also a possible increased risk for pulmonary hypertension after splenectomy. The procedure is reserved for severe cases and is usually deferred until at least 5 years of age because of the increased risk of infection with encapsulated organisms. Patients should be immunized against *Haemophilus influenzae*, *Streptococcus pneumoniae*, and *Neisseria meningitides* before surgery and require lifelong penicillin prophylaxis after surgery. Indications for splenectomy include severe anemia (Hb < 8 g/dL), poor growth, chronic fatigue, or recurrent hemolytic episodes requiring frequent RBC transfusions.

The best management strategy in G6PD deficiency is educating patients about avoidance of oxidative stressors that can trigger hemolysis. They should be instructed to avoid exposure to certain drugs, naphthalene (found in mothballs), and fava beans to prevent hemolytic crises. Management of an acute hemolytic crisis is supportive. Some patients may require an RBC transfusion if they develop severe symptomatic anemia.

For patients with β-thalassemia, the clinical phenotype ranges from transfusion dependence (thalassemia major) to a moderate anemia that does not necessitate chronic transfusions (thalassemia intermedia). The recommended treatment for β-thalassemia major involves regular blood transfusions every 2 to 5 weeks to maintain a nadir Hb of 9 to 10 g/dL. With regular blood transfusions, patients will develop iron overload, and if left untreated, it is fatal. At this time, patients with iron overload are treated with medications that bind iron known as chelators. The chelators currently in use in the United States include deferoxamine (Desferal), which is typically given as a 12-hour infusion intravenously or subcutaneously, and deferasirox (Exjade), an oral medication given once daily.

Therapy for patients with DBA includes an initial therapeutic regimen of chronic RBC transfusions followed by a corticosteroid trial. Forty percent of patients fail to respond to corticosteroid therapy. Those that do respond may remain steroid dependent. For an unknown reason, 20% of patients will go into remission. Allogenic bone marrow transplant is the only curative treatment.

Acquired Disorders

Therapy of patients with acquired RBC disorders involves correcting the underlying abnormality. In nutritional deficiencies, for example, treatment focuses on addressing the root cause and concurrently administering nutritional supplementation. The cause of iron deficiency needs to be determined for each patient. At the same time, the patient is given supplementation with 6 mg/kg/d of elemental iron divided two or three times per day. To fully replete the iron stores, the iron replacement should continue for 3 to 4 months until the CBC normalizes (including the MCV and RBC distribution width). With anemia of chronic disease, the treatment is focused on treating the underlying cause (i.e., oncologic process, rheumatoid arthritis).

AIHA can cause brisk, severe hemolysis and patients require close monitoring. Treatment of primary AIHA includes methylprednisone 1 to 2 mg/kg/d intravenously every 6 hours. After the Hb stabilizes, the patient can be switched to 1 to 2 mg/kg/d of oral prednisone. Steroids are then gradually tapered over a period of weeks to months. In cases of cardiovascular compromise, an RBC transfusion should be considered. However, because antibodies against RBCs cause AIHA, the patients' antibodies may also hemolyze the transfused blood. Extreme caution should be taken when transfusing these patients. Second-line therapy for AIHA includes intravenous immunoglobulin, and patients with refractory disease can be treated with exchange transfusion; plasma pheresis; or other immunomodulators, including rituximab, danazol, vincristine, or cyclophosphamide.

Treatment of patients with TEC or an aplastic crisis from parvovirus requires regular monitoring of CBCs until the anemia normalizes. Blood transfusion may be required if the patient is severely anemic with cardiovascular compromise. No other treatment is necessary, and patients undergo spontaneous resolution.

FUTURE DIRECTIONS

A new diagnostic test for hereditary spherocytosis is available. The test uses flow cytometry and is based on the fluorescence of RBCs after incubation with the dye eosin-5-malimide. The novel test has many advantages over the standard osmotic fragility test, including necessitating only a small amount of blood (100 microliters) and higher sensitivity and specificity (92% and 99%, respectively). Results of the flow cytometry test are available in 2 hours. Comparatively, the osmotic fragility test requires 3 mL of blood, and the sensitivity is only 80% (mild cases are not detected). Also, the specificity is lower in the osmotic fragility test because it can be falsely abnormal in other disease processes that result in spherocytes (e.g., AIHA).

Bone marrow transplant (BMT) is a treatment modality for patients with β-thalassemia major. BMT is reserved for only the most severe cases because of the risks and long-term side effects.

A novel treatment modality based on globin gene expression for β-thalassemia is currently in the experimental phase. Scientists have successfully manipulated globin gene expression in murine models but have not developed a specific targeting vector in humans yet. This potential target for gene therapy involves the insertion of normal β-globin gene into the patient's stem cells. If the treatment is developed successfully, it has the potential to cure β-thalassemia.

SUGGESTED READINGS

Brugnara, C, Oski FA, Nathan DG: Diagnostic approach to the anemic patient. In Orkin SH, Nathan DG, Ginsburg D, et al, editors: *Hematology of Infancy and Childhood*, Philadelphia, 2009, Saunders, pp 455-466.

Rund D, Rachmilewitz E: β-Thalassemia, *N Engl J Med* 353(11):1135-1145, 2005.

Segel GB: Anemia, *Pediatr Rev* 10(3):77-88, 1988.

Shah S, Vega R: Hereditary spherocytosis, *Pediatr Rev* 25(5);168-172, 2004.

Disorders of White Blood Cells

Daniel A. Weiser

51

White blood cells (WBCs), or leukocytes, are an integral part of the host immune system. Their microscopic appearance after Wright-staining categorizes them as either granulocytes (neutrophils, eosinophils, and basophils) or agranulocytes (monocytes, macrophages, and lymphocytes). Each WBC has a specific function within the immune system (Figure 51-1).

A complete blood count (CBC) and manual differential notes the total number of WBCs per microliter of sample as well as the percentages of each subset of WBC. Absolute counts for each WBC are more clinically meaningful than percentages. Reference ranges for the WBC differential vary by age. In general, newborns have high total WBC counts (≤30,000/μL). At about 1 week of age, an infant's total WBC decreases into the range of 5000 to 21,000/μL. Through the toddler and childhood years, the mean WBC count decreases slowly to an adult average of 7500/μL. Lymphocyte predominance is seen from 2 weeks to about 5 years of age. Then neutrophils are predominant, making up more than 50% of the differential. Monocytes, eosinophils, and basophils make up a very small percentage of the total WBC from the neonatal period through adulthood.

ETIOLOGY AND PATHOGENESIS

WBCs derive from hematopoietic progenitor cells in the bone marrow (Figure 51-2). Their maturation is induced by colony-stimulating factors.

This chapter focuses on congenital and acquired neutrophil disorders with a brief discussion regarding disorders of eosinophils, basophils, and monocytes. Disorders of lymphocytes, part of the body's acquired (adaptive) immunity, are discussed in the immunology section (see Chapter 21).

Neutrophils are part of the innate (natural) immune system. After they are released by the bone marrow, they remain in the circulation for 6 to 12 hours. They migrate to sites of infection and engulf, digest, and destroy microorganisms. A large portion of mature neutrophils reside in the bone marrow and along blood vessels in endothelial cells.

Neutropenia is defined as a decrease in the absolute neutrophil count (ANC) to less than 1500/μL. Neutropenia is considered severe if the ANC is less than 500/μL, moderate between 500/μL and 1000/μL, and mild between 1000/μL and 1500/μL. The risk of serious infection is inversely proportional to the ANC. Of note, the ANC is usually about 200 to 600/μL lower in African Americans compared with other races likely secondary to decreased neutrophil release from the bone marrow. This does not lead to a greater predisposition for infection.

CLINICAL PRESENTATION AND DIFFERENTIAL DIAGNOSIS
Congenital Disorders of Neutrophils

Because neutrophils play a key role in host defense, the primary signs and symptoms of neutropenia are related to an increased susceptibility to infection, particularly bacterial and fungal. Children with chronic neutropenia can develop cellulitis, perirectal or other deep tissue abscesses, oral ulcers, periodontal disease, pneumonia, and septicemia. Endogenous *Staphylococcus aureus* or gram negative organisms are frequently isolated. Clinical signs of infection, such as erythema and warmth, may be diminished secondary to a decreased neutrophil response.

There are multiple congenital neutropenias that are being further categorized as knowledge of the genetic basis of disease improves (Tables 51-1 and 51-2). These congenital disorders are exceedingly rare.

NEUTROPHIL FUNCTION DEFECTS

Complex physiologic processes are involved in neutrophil phagocytosis of microbes. An abnormality in any of the steps—adhesion, chemotaxis, opsonization, ingestion/phagocytosis, degranulation, and oxidative metabolism (bacterial killing)—results in inadequate neutrophil functioning. Susceptibility is to bacteria and fungi, with intact resistance to viral infections.

Although very rare in general, some neutrophil function defects are relatively more common (Table 51-3). Acquired defects of chemotaxis can also occur secondary to diabetes mellitus, metabolic storage diseases, malnutrition, immaturity, and burns.

Acquired Disorders of Neutrophils

Acquired neutropenia, which is much more common than congenital neutropenia, is the result of decreased WBC production secondary to suppression of bone marrow synthesis or antibodies directed against neutrophils.

INFECTION-ASSOCIATED NEUTROPENIA

Although infection often causes a transient reactive leukocytosis, many viruses cause neutropenia within the first couple of days of illness that can last up to 1 week. The cause of neutropenia from an infection is diverse, including decreased marrow production, depleted marrow reserves, increased neutrophil margination with decreased circulating neutrophils, antibody formation with increased peripheral destruction, or a combination of multiple factors. Viruses that can cause neutropenia include HIV, parvovirus B19, Epstein-Barr virus, cytomegalovirus, hepatitis A and B, influenza A and B, malaria, respiratory syncytial virus, and varicella.

AUTOIMMUNE NEUTROPENIA

Autoimmune neutropenia (AIN) can be primary or secondary to autoimmune diseases, drugs, infection, or immune dysregulation. Most cases of what was termed *benign neutropenia of childhood* are now believed to be primary AIN. Primary AIN is the most

Figure 51-1 Features of white blood cells in Wright-stained blood smears.

Features of Erythrocytes and Platelets in Wright-Stained Blood Smears

Cells	Diameter (µm)	Life span (days)	No. of cells/ L of blood	Shape and nucleus type	Cytoplasm	Functions
Erythrocyte (red blood cell) 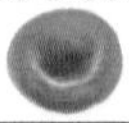	7–10	120	5×10^{12} in males; 4.5×10^{12} in females	Biconcave disc, anucleate	Pink because of acidophilia of hemoglobin; halo in center	Transports hemoglobin that binds O_2 and CO_2
Platelet (thrombocyte) 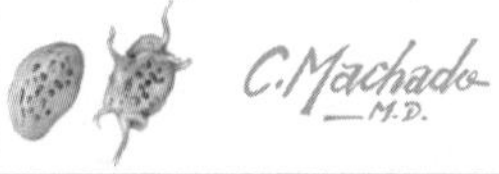	2–4	10	150 to 400×10^9	Oval biconvex disc, anucleate	Pale blue; central dark granulomere, peripheral less dense hyalomere	In hemostasis, promotes blood clotting; plugs endothelial damage

Features of Leukocytes in Wright-Stained Blood Smears (Total Number: 5–10 x 10^9/L Blood)

Cells	Diameter (µm)	Differential count (%)*	Nucleus	Cytoplasm	Functions
Granulocytes					
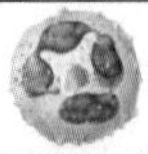 Neutrophil	9–12	60–70	Segmented, 3–5 lobes, densely stained	Pale, finely granular, evenly dispersed specific granules	Phagocytoses bacteria; increases in number in acute bacterial infections
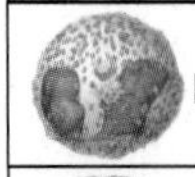 Eosinophil	12–15	1–4	Bilobed, clumped chromatin pattern, densely stained	Large homogeneous red granules that are coarse and highly refractile	Phagocytoses antigen-antibody complexes and parasites
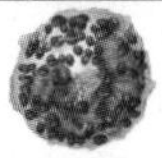 Basophil	10–14	0–1	Bilobed or segmented	Large blue specific granules that stain with basic dyes and often obscure nucleus	Involved in anticoagulation, increases vascular permeability
Agranulocytes					
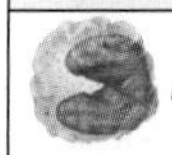 Monocytes	12–20	3–10	Indented, kidney shaped, lightly stained	Agranular, pale blue cytoplasm, with lysosomes	Is motile; gives rise to macrophages
Lymphocyte • Small • Medium to large	6–10 11–16	20–40	Small, round or slightly indented, darkly stained	Agranular, faintly basophilic, blue to gray	Acts in humoral (B cell) and cellular (T cell) immunity

*Note: Differential count (%) is based on adult values.

common cause of neutropenia in infancy and childhood and is usually found incidentally between the age of 2 months and 3 years. Affected infants and children may be asymptomatic or have recurrent mild infections, primarily of the upper respiratory tract or skin. It is rare to have more serious infection because the bone marrow is able to respond to stressors and increase granulocyte output two to three times. Because monocytosis precedes a brisk neutrophil response, it is not unusual to see an increased monocyte count in children with AIN. Antineutrophil IgG antibodies may also be identified. The prognosis is excellent with a self-limited course within 2 years in 95% of affected children. Secondary AIN will resolve when the underlying cause is treated.

ISOIMMUNE OR ALLOIMMUNE NEONATAL NEUTROPENIA

Within the first 2 weeks of life, neonates can develop neutropenia secondary to transplacental transfer of maternal antineutrophil IgG antibodies. This is similar to how Rh disease affects a newborn; however, isoimmune neonatal neutropenia is much more rare (one in 1000 neonates) and self-resolves within 4 to 6 months. The diagnosis is made by detecting antineutrophil alloantibodies in the maternal serum. Depending on the degree of neutropenia and the extent of other risk factors, neonates may present with infection as the first sign of this diagnosis. More often it is found incidentally.

DRUG-INDUCED NEUTROPENIA

Cytotoxic agents for the treatment of malignancies are known to cause severe neutropenia, anemia, and thrombocytopenia. Other more routine medications may be implicated in causing neutropenia (Table 51-4). Neutropenia is caused either by decreasing bone marrow synthesis or by evoking production of antineutrophil antibodies. Spontaneous resolution typically occurs after discontinuation of the offending drug.

OTHER CAUSES OF ACQUIRED NEUTROPENIA

Malignancies and marrow infiltrative processes do not usually cause an isolated neutropenia; multiple cell lines are more commonly affected (Table 51-5). Additionally, splenomegaly affects all cell lines because blood products get trapped in the enlarged spleen.

Leukocytosis

If a higher number of WBCs than expected are in the peripheral circulation, an underlying systemic process is likely. In the majority of children with leukocytosis, it is a reactive process to infection and subsides with resolution of the acute event. It can also occur in chronic inflammatory states such as autoimmune

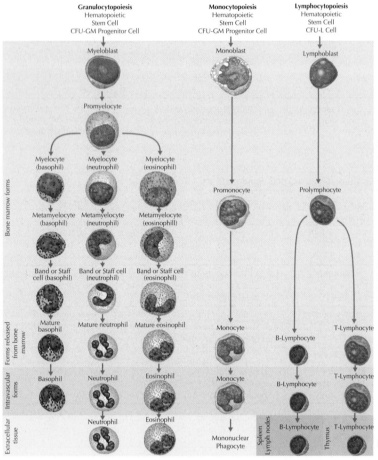

Granulocytopoiesis
Hematopoietic
Stem Cell
CFU-GM Progenitor Cell

Monocytopoiesis
Hematopoietic
Stem Cell
CFU-GM Progenitor Cell

Lymphocytopoiesis
Hematopoietic
Stem Cell
CFU-L Cell

Schematic showing stages of hematopoiesis. Although not all cells are included in each sequence, main cell types seen in bone marrow smears are shown in granulocytopoiesis (**left**), monocytopoiesis (**center**), lymphocytopoiesis (**right**). The various CFU cells that arise from the hematopoietic stem cell (not shown) closely resemble lymphocytes. Except for megakaryocytes, cells in erythroid and myeloid series as a rule get smaller during differentiation. Also, nuclear size declines, nuclear density increases, and special features related to cell lineage—such as hemoglobin production and nuclear extrusion in erythropoiesis, and specific granules (eosinophilic, basophilic, or neutrophilic) in granulocytopoiesis—appear. Various growth factors and cytokines mediate cell proliferation rate and survival and maturation of progenitor cells. Some of these are colony-stimulating factors, erythropoietin, thrombopoietin, interleukins (IL-1, IL-3, IL-6, IL-11), and stem cell factors.

Figure 51-2 *Stages of hematopoiesis.*

disease, rheumatologic disorders (systemic lupus erythematosus [SLE], juvenile idiopathic arthritis [JIA], inflammatory bowel disease [IBD], Kawasaki disease), and oncologic processes (leukemia, lymphomas, neuroblastoma). When the WBC is greater than 100k/μL, there should be a suspicion for a marrow infiltrative process such as leukemia. A history and physical examination may reveal lymphadenopathy or hepatosplenomegaly. A peripheral smear evaluation and manual differential count will note atypical lymphocytes (suggestive of a viral process) or blasts (premature WBCs suggestive of leukemia).

NEUTROPHILIA

An elevated neutrophil count can result from increased bone marrow production, increased movement of neutrophils out of the marrow and into the circulation, or possibly from decreased peripheral destruction if the spleen is not functioning. There are many causes of neutrophilia, some acute and some chronic in nature (Table 51-6).

MONOCYTOSIS

Monocytes develop much more rapidly than neutrophils in the bone marrow, and they give rise to macrophages. After bone marrow recovery from myelosuppressive chemotherapy,

monocytes are the first to reappear in the circulation; the reactive monocytosis is transient. An increased monocyte count is seen in particular infections such as tuberculosis, syphilis, typhoid, and brucellosis. Also, in chronic inflammatory states such as rheumatologic disorders (SLE, JIA), IBD, and Langerhans cell histiocytosis, a monocytosis can be present.

BASOPHILIA

Basophils are a nonspecific sign of a variety of disorders. Basophils are involved in immediate hypersensitivity diseases and may play a role in the defense against bacterial infections. An absolute value greater than 120 cells/μL is considered elevated, and this can occur in hypersensitivity reactions as well as chronic inflammatory states, particularly JIA, chronic sinusitis, IBD, and oncologic processes.

EOSINOPHILIA

Eosinophils have a role in both immunoenhancing and suppressive functions. They are very efficient in the destruction of invasive metazoan parasites, and they inactivate inflammatory mediators in immediate hypersensitivity reactions. Eosinophilia is characterized by the total eosinophil count. Mild eosinophilia, with an absolute count 600 to 1500/μL, is fairly common and

Table 51-1 Congenital Disorders of Neutrophil Development

Disorder	Clinical Manifestations	Defect	Inheritance Pattern	Severity of Neutropenia	Evaluation and Diagnosis	Treatment	Risk of Malignancy
Severe congenital neutropenia (Kostmann syndrome)	Life-threatening pyogenic infections often in infancy	Impaired myeloid differentiation caused by maturational arrest of neutrophil precursors	AR (AD rarely)	<200 since birth; associated mild anemia; occasional monocytosis and eosinophilia	Bone marrow demonstrates myeloid maturation arrest, 60%-80% have neutrophil ELA-2 mutations, less common *HAX1* mutations	GCSF	Increased risk of leukemia (AML) or myelodysplastic syndrome over time
Cyclic neutropenia	Cyclic fever, oral ulcers, gingivitis, periodontal disease, recurrent bacterial infections	Stem cell regulatory defect resulting in defective maturation	Sporadic or AD	<200 for 3-7 days every 3 weeks (range, 15- to 35-day cycle)	CBC two or three times a week for 6-8 wks to document cycles and nadir; ELA-2 mutation in 80%-90%	±GCSF	No increased risk of malignancy
Shwachman-Diamond syndrome	Triad of neutropenia, exocrine pancreas insufficiency, and skeletal abnormalities	May have defects in neutrophil mobility, migration, and chemotaxis in addition to neutropenia	AR	Chronic severe or intermittent; may be associated with anemia and thrombocytopenia	Neutropenia, low serum trypsinogen, elevated fecal fat excretion, metaphyseal dysostosis, rib cage abnormalities, short stature *SBDS* gene mutation in 90%	±GCSF, pancreatic enzyme replacement, yearly bone marrow	Increased risk for myelodysplastic syndrome or leukemia

AD, autosomal dominant; AML, acute myelogenous leukemia; AR,= autosomal recessive; CBC, complete blood count; ELA-2, elastase 2; GCSF, granulocyte colony-stimulating factor; SBDS = Shwachman-Bodian-Diamond syndrome gene, located on chromosome 7q11.

Table 51-2 Additional Congenital Disorders Associated with Neutropenia

Disorder	Clinical Manifestations
Cartilage-hair hypoplasia	Short limbs, dwarfism, abnormally fine hair
Myelokathexis with dysmyelopoiesis	Marrow retention of neutrophils, recurrent bronchopulmonary infections
Dyskeratosis congenita	Bone marrow failure syndrome; dystrophic changes in nails, skin (hyperpigmentation), and mucous membranes (leukoplakia)
Fanconi anemia	Bone marrow failure syndrome; GU and skeletal abnormalities, increased chromosome fragility
Organic acidemias (propionic, methylmalonic)	Initially well at birth, then toxic encephalopathy
Osteopetrosis	Defective bone turnover with resultant hematopoietic insufficiency and bone fragility
Reticular dysgenesis (congenital aleukocytosis)	Absent WBC, hypogammaglobulinemia, thymic hypoplasia, severe infection and death in infancy
Immunodeficiencies (severe combined immunodeficiency, common variable immunodeficiency, hyper-IgM)	Frequent infections, failure to thrive, hepatosplenomegaly
Glycogen storage disease type 1b (von Gierke disease) and other inborn errors of metabolism	Neutropenia and functional neutrophil defect, hepatosplenomegaly

GU, genitourinary; WBC, white blood cell.

usually transient. It most frequently results from allergies and resolves with control of the underlying disease process. Moderately severe eosinophilia is defined as an absolute count of 1500 to 5000/μL. Severe eosinophilia is greater than 5000/μL with the most common reason being visceral larva migrans (toxocariasis). The cause of eosinophilia is diverse; a history of fever, allergies, atopy, asthma, recent travel, diarrhea, environmental exposures, medication, or exposure to pets may help differentiate causes of eosinophilia (Figure 51-3).

EVALUATION AND MANAGEMENT

If isolated neutropenia is discovered incidentally on a routine screening CBC, a thorough history and physical examination should be completed. Recent fevers, upper respiratory infection symptoms, or diarrhea may point toward a preceding viral illness. If frequent infections are reported, a full understanding of the infection type and frequency is important to delineate. In the history, recent medication exposures should be reviewed. A diet history may elicit nutritional deficiencies as in vitamin B12 or folate. Family history of early unexplained deaths and parental blood counts can help to narrow down otherwise unrecognized inherited disorders. A comprehensive physical examination should identify phenotypic abnormalities that are associated with particular disorders. The clinician should carefully assess for hepatosplenomegaly or lymphadenopathy. If the child is otherwise healthy with normal examination results, a repeat CBC should be obtained in 2 to 3 weeks.

Neutropenia on three separate occasions over 8 weeks in an otherwise well child should prompt a more extensive workup. Discontinue drugs known to be associated with neutropenia. More specific testing should be guided by the patient's age, physical examination, and clinical presentation.

It is prudent to anticipate infection in patients with persistent severe neutropenia. Fever may be the first and only sign of a potentially life-threatening systemic infection. Fever is defined as a temperature greater than 101.5°F. Rectal thermometers

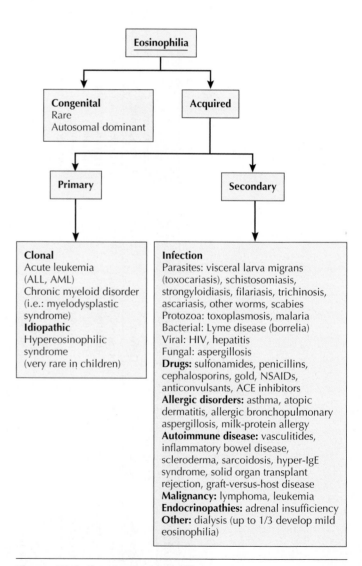

Figure 51-3 *Causes of eosinophilia.*

Table 51-3 Congenital Disorders of Neutrophil Function

Disorder	Clinical Manifestations	Functional Defect	Evaluation and Diagnosis	Frequency	Inheritance Pattern	Treatment	Prognosis
Leukocyte adhesion deficiency (types I, II, others)	Delayed separation of umbilical cord (≥3 wk), recurrent and severe bacterial and fungal infections without the accumulation of pus, poor wound healing, periodontal disease	Adhesion: neutrophils have diminished adhesion to surfaces and cannot migrate out of blood vessels	Neutrophilia ≤100k/μL, especially during infection; flow cytometry for deficiency of CD11/CD18 cell surface adhesive glycoproteins (for LAD I)	Very rare	AR	Prophylactic antibiotics	Depends on severity of deficiency, may die in infancy or have infrequent life-threatening infections
Hyper-immunoglobulin E syndrome (hyper-IgE, Job syndrome)	Severe eczema; bacterial infections, especially of the skin and lower respiratory tract; pneumatoceles; fungal infections	Chemotaxis	Increased IgE (>2500 IU/mL), eosinophilia; STAT3 (signal transduction) mutation analysis	Very rare	Sporadic, AD or less commonly AR	Supportive, prophylactic antibiotics	Good
Chediak-Higashi syndrome	Partial oculocutaneous albinism; peripheral and cranial neuropathies; neutropenia, recurrent pyogenic infections; accelerated HLH phase leads to death	Defects in granule morphogenesis, chemotaxis and degranulation; ineffective granulopoiesis	Giant granule formation in neutrophils and other granulocytes neutropenia, *CHS1* gene analysis	Very rare	AR	Prophylactic antibiotics, ascorbic acid; BMT if HLH	Few patients survive to the third decade of life
Myeloperoxidase deficiency	Usually clinically silent; rarely, disseminated candidiasis or fungal disease, usually in the setting of diabetes mellitus	Oxidative metabolism: H_2O_2-dependent killing not potentiated by myeloperoxidase	Flow cytometry for neutrophils with peroxidase activity; histochemical staining of neutrophils for peroxidase	One in 4000 (complete deficiency), one in 2000 (partial)	AR with variable expression	None if asymptomatic; aggressive treatment of fungal disease if they occur	Excellent
Chronic granulomatous disease	Recurrent purulent infections with fungal or bacterial catalase-positive organisms,* usually starting in infancy; chronic inflammatory granulomas	Oxidative metabolism: decreased or absent generation of superoxide (toxic to microbes) by NADPH oxidase	Nitroblue tetrazolium test; dihydro rhodamine fluorescence positive; genotyping for known mutations	One in 250,000	Primarily X-linked recessive rarely AR	Prophylactic antibiotics and antifungals, IFN-γ +/− BMT	Good prognosis with aggressive management of infection

*Catalase-positive organisms include *Staphylococcus aureus, Aspergillus* spp., *Escherichia coli, Klebsiella* spp., *Salmonella* species, *Serratia marcescens,* and *Burkholderia cepacia.* AD, autosomal dominant; AR, autosomal recessive; BMT = bone marrow transplantation; HLH, hemophagocytic lymphohistiocytosis; IFN, interferon; LAD, leukocyte adhesion deficiency; NADPH, nicotinamide adenine dinucleotide phosphate.

Table 51-4 Drugs Associated with Neutropenia*

Drug Class	Drugs
Antimicrobials	Trimethoprim–sulfamethoxazole, sulfonamides, macrolides, vancomycin, cephalosporins, semisynthetic penicillins (vancomycin), quinine, chloroquine, amphotericin B
Antiinflammatory drugs	NSAIDs (ibuprofen, others)
Psychotropic drugs	Clozapine, phenytoin
Gastrointestinal drugs	Histamine H2 receptor antagonists (ranitidine)
Antithyroid drugs	Methimazole, propylthiouracil
Cardiovascular	Antiarrhythmics, diuretics
Toxins	Benzene
Chemotherapeutic agents	Cytotoxic drugs

*This is a partial list only of the more commonly prescribed medications for children.

NSAID, nonsteroidal antiinflammatory drug.

Table 51-6 Causes of Neutrophilia

Infectious	Bacterial and viral
Rheumatologic	JIA, Kawasaki disease
Asplenia	Surgical or functional
Gastrointestinal	Liver failure, IBD
Endocrine	Diabetic ketoacidosis
Neutrophil function disorders	CGD, LAD (see Neutrophil Function Defects above)
Drugs	Corticosteroids (release neutrophils from marrow, slow egress from circulation into tissues, postpone apoptotic cell death), epinephrine (release of the marginating pool into circulation)
Stressors	Shock, trauma, emotional, burns, surgery, hemorrhage, hypoxia
Malignancy	Clonal expansion, especially if WBC >100,000/μL; leukemia, myeloproliferative disorders (note H&P, other cell lines, peripheral blasts)
Trisomy 21 (Down syndrome)	Defective proliferation and maturation of myeloid cells

CGD, chronic granulomatous disease; H&P, history and physical; IBD, inflammatory bowel disease; JIA, juvenile idiopathic arthritis; LAD, leukocyte adhesion deficiency; WBC, white blood cell.

should be avoided because of the lack of hygiene in the region. A blood culture and a CBC with differential should be drawn at the time of the fever. A urine culture should be added for infants and young children. Further infectious workup should be guided by the physical examination results. Fever with severe neutropenia (ANC < 500/μL) should be managed with empiric broad-spectrum antibiotics in a hospital setting for at least 24 hours. If a treatable organism is identified, antibiotic coverage can be narrowed. A well-appearing febrile patient with mild or moderate neutropenia can usually be managed as an outpatient with or without antibiotics depending on whether an infectious source has been identified.

Recombinant granulocyte colony-stimulating factor (GCSF) is readily available and often effective at increasing neutrophil counts and thereby decreasing infectious complications. GCSF is the standard treatment for patients with severe congenital neutropenia, for some patients with cyclic neutropenia, and for certain disorders if infectious complications are severe. Therapy should be tailored as necessary for specific WBC disorders as outlined in previous sections. Hematopoietic stem cell transplantation may be curative for some disorders.

Treatment of patients' neutrophil function disorders varies, although prophylactic antibiotics and prompt supportive care with fever is universal. Specifically, trimethoprim–sulfamethoxazole may enhance the bactericidal activity of

neutrophils, and interferon-γ decreases the frequency and severity of infections in chronic granulomatous disease. Patients with Chediak-Higashi syndrome may improve clinically when given ascorbic acid. Because the outcomes after bone marrow transplantation have improved, transplant may be a viable therapeutic option with the goal of reconstitution of normal neutrophil function.

FUTURE DIRECTIONS

Additional neutrophil function disorders continue to be described as a more elaborate understanding of the molecular basis for disease is elucidated. This will allow for improved diagnosis and targeted therapeutics. Increasingly, functional disorders of the hematopoietic system are being partially, or even fully, treated through hematopoietic stem cell transplantation.

Table 51-5 Other Causes of Acquired Neutropenia

Malignancies and bone marrow failure	Leukemia, lymphoma, preleukemic states, myelodysplastic syndromes, aplastic anemia
Nutritional deficiency	Vitamin B12, folate, copper or starvation
Other	Splenomegaly, complement activation (e.g., hemodialysis)

SUGGESTED READINGS

Kyono W, Coates TD: A practical approach to neutrophil disorders, *Pediatr Clin North Am* 49(5):929, 2002.

Lekstrom-Himes JA, Gallin JI: Immunodeficiency caused by defects in phagocytes, *N Engl J Med* 343(23):1703, 2002.

Schwartzberg LS: Neutropenia: etiology and pathogenesis, *Clin Cornerstone* 8(suppl 5):S5, 2006.

Segel GB, Halterman JS: Neutropenia in pediatric practice, *Pediatr Rev* 29:12-24, 2008.

Serwint JR, Dias MM, Chang H, et al: Outcomes of febrile children presumed to be immunocompetent who present with leukopenia or neutropenia to an ambulatory setting, *Clin Pediatr* 44(7):593, 2006.

Platelet Disorders

Jennifer Mangino

52

Platelets are small anucleate cell particles (5-7 μL in volume) that play a critical role in primary hemostasis. At the time of vascular injury, platelets rush to the site of vascular damage and adhere to the exposed collagen, forming a temporary platelet plug to prevent continued bleeding. The platelets are then activated and undergo changes in their shape and structure. These changes allow the platelets to bind to fibrinogen and aggregate with one another, thus propagating the platelet plug. Activation of platelets also causes secretion of the chemicals contained in the platelet storage granules. These chemicals recruit new platelets and contain many compounds needed to continue primary hemostasis and activate secondary hemostasis (Figure 52-1).

Platelets are made in the bone marrow via fragmentation of megakaryocytes. Formation of platelets is controlled by thrombopoietin (TPO), which is a compound that controls megakaryocyte growth and maturation. Platelets typically circulate for 7 to 10 days and are then removed by the reticuloendothelial system. A normal platelet count is 150,000 to 400,000/μL. Platelet disorders can involve a qualitative or quantitative defect, and they are either inherited or acquired.

ETIOLOGY AND PATHOGENESIS

Congenital Platelet Disorders

Congenital platelet disorders are individually very rare in the general population. They can have quantitative or qualitative abnormalities, and some disorders have both. Their mode of inheritance and their clinical significance vary. In general, children with congenital platelet disorders are more likely to have chronic bleeding symptoms that developed early in life. The following is a discussion of some of the important inherited platelet disorders.

GLANZMANN'S THROMBASTHENIA

Glanzmann's thrombasthenia is a rare autosomal recessive disorder of platelet function. It is the most common of the inherited platelet disorders. Patients with this disorder have an abnormality in the genes encoding either chain of the platelet αIIbβ3 integrin fibrinogen receptor. As a result, platelets cannot bind fibrinogen, resulting in clinically significant bleeding from infancy. Common types of bleeding include epistaxis, gastrointestinal hemorrhage, and menorrhagia. Carriers of this mutation have 50% normal fibrinogen receptors and generally do not have bleeding complications.

BERNARD-SOULIER SYNDROME

Bernard-Soulier syndrome is an autosomal recessive syndrome that occurs with a genetic mutation in the glycoprotein (GP) 1b/IX complex. The GP Ib/IX complex binds platelets to von Willebrand factor, a key step in the initial attachment of platelets to an injured vessel wall. Patients with Bernard-Soulier syndrome also have a variable degree of thrombocytopenia, making it both a qualitative and quantitative platelet abnormality. Heterozygotes for this condition are clinically normal but may have mild thrombocytopenia. Of note, children with 22q deletion syndromes can be heterozygotes for the Bernard-Soulier mutation given the proximity of the gene encoding the GP 1b/IX complex. They may have associated mild thrombocytopenia and minor platelet function abnormalities.

STORAGE POOL DEFECTS

Normal platelets contain granules that contain a number of biochemicals that are important for both primary and secondary hemostasis. Disorders related to abnormalities in granules are lumped together into a category of storage pool defects. These defects result in abnormalities of platelet function and have varying degrees of associated bleeding. There are a number of specific disorders in this category that are associated with other congenital anomalies. The most common disorders in this category are Hermansky-Pudlak syndrome (associated with albinism, vision problems, pulmonary fibrosis, and colitis) and Chediak-Higashi syndrome (associated with partial albinism and immune dysfunction).

THROMBOCYTOPENIA ABSENT RADII

Thrombocytopenia absent radii (TAR) is a disorder associated with thrombocytopenia and orthopedic abnormalities. Thirty percent of patients may also have cardiac abnormalities. The primary orthopedic problem is an abnormality or absence of both radii with maintenance of functional thumbs. This disorder is characterized by severe thrombocytopenia resulting from a decreased number of megakaryocytes in the bone marrow at birth. The thrombocytopenia improves as the children age and usually spontaneously resolves in the first year of life. Some patients with TAR may have an associated storage pool defect as well. The cause of this disorder is unknown.

CONGENITAL AMEGAKARYOCYTIC THROMBOCYTOPENIA

Congenital amegakaryocytic thrombocytopenia is an autosomal recessive disorder characterized by the absence of megakaryocytes in the bone marrow. This disorder results in severe thrombocytopenia at birth that persists throughout the lifetime of a child. This disorder often leads to aplastic anemia and can be fatal without bone marrow transplantation.

WISKOTT-ALDRICH

Wiskott-Aldrich is an X-linked disorder leading to a combination of thrombocytopenia, eczema, and immune deficiency. Often, the predominant feature of this disorder is a history of recurrent

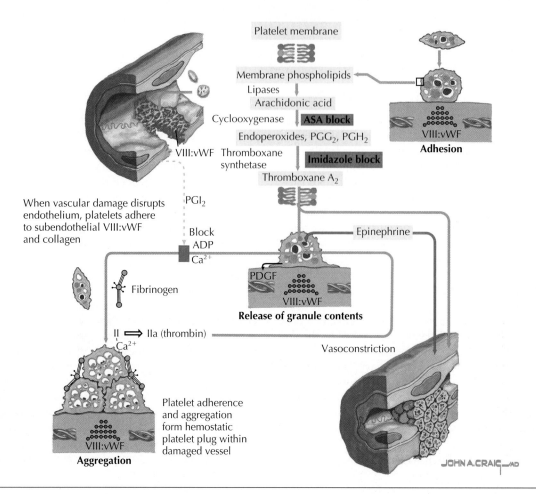

Figure 52-1 *Platelet adhesion, release, and aggregation.*

bacterial infections. The degree of thrombocytopenia varies with the extent of the genetic mutation. Of note, this disorder is associated with small platelets (microthrombocytes).

MACROTHROMBOCYTOPENIA DISORDERS

Several disorders characterized by macrothrombocytopenia are the result of various mutations in the cytoskeletal protein non-muscle myosin heavy chain IIA (MYH9). These disorders are characterized by thrombocytopenia with large platelets (macro-thrombocytes) and normal platelet function. May Hegglin anomaly is the most common, but other disorders in this spectrum include Sebastian, Epstein, and Fechtner syndromes. They may be associated with various other congenital anomalies, including sensorineural hearing loss, nephritis, or ocular abnormalities.

ESSENTIAL THROMBOCYTOSIS

Essential thrombocytosis is a very rare disorder characterized by an increase in the number of platelets, with platelet counts often above 1,000,000 to 2,000,000/μL. This disorder may be associated with other myeloproliferative disorders, and it is associated with a significantly increased risk of thrombosis.

ACQUIRED PLATELET DISORDERS

Acquired platelet disorders are far more common than congenital platelet disorders. The most common reason for acquired thrombocytopenia or an acquired platelet abnormality is drug exposure. Dozens of medications can cause thrombocytopenia or abnormalities in platelet function. These medications can act by inhibiting bone marrow production of platelets or activating or creating antibodies to platelets, or they can have a direct toxic effect on platelets. Refer to Table 52-1 for a list of some of the common medications resulting in thrombocytopenia and platelet function abnormalities. Heparin-induced thrombocytopenia (HIT) is a special case and is discussed again later this chapter.

In addition, there are many systemic disorders that are associated with thrombocytopenia by means of consumption, increased destruction or decreased production of platelets. Examples include disseminated intravascular coagulation, malaria, systemic lupus erythematosus, leukemia, lymphoma, thrombosis, viral infections, and HIV. Platelets can become sequestered in the spleen in syndromes associated with splenomegaly. Some systemic disorders, such as uremia, can cause abnormalities of platelet function as well. The following is a description of some acquired disorders of platelets.

Table 52-1 Common Medications Resulting in Thrombocytopenia or Platelet Function Abnormalities

Drugs Associated with Thrombocytopenia	Drugs Associated with Abnormal Platelet Function
Antibiotics • Linezolid • Penicillins • Quinidine • Rifampin • Sulfa-containing antibiotics (Bactrim) • Vancomycin Antiepileptics • Carbamazepine • Phenytoin • Valproate Chemotherapeutic agents GI medications • Cimetidine • Ranitidine	• Aspirin • NSAIDs (ibuprofen, ketorolac) • Clopidogrel and ticlopidine • Abciximab • Ethanol

GI, gastrointestinal; NSAID, nonsteroidal antiinflammatory drug.

Immune Thrombocytopenia

Immune thrombocytopenia (ITP) is an immune-mediated platelet disorder generated by immunoglobulin G (IgG) autoantibodies. It often presents acutely in childhood after a viral illness in an otherwise healthy child. IgG autoantibodies coat the surface of platelets and the platelets then undergo accelerated clearance through Fcγ receptors expressed on macrophages in the spleen and liver. In childhood, ITP is generally considered a benign self-limited disorder; 80% of patients spontaneously resolve within 6 months. However, a small percentage of patients (<20%) develop chronic ITP lasting longer than 12 months.

NEONATAL ALLOIMMUNE THROMBOCYTOPENIA

Neonatal alloimmune thrombocytopenia (NAIT) is associated with a mismatch between maternal and fetal platelets. The mother develops antibodies against an antigen on the surface of fetal platelets inherited from the father. The antibodies can cross the placenta and coat fetal platelets, forcing accelerated clearance in the spleen. This results in significant thrombocytopenia in the neonatal period. With the first pregnancy, the thrombocytopenia can be mild, but with subsequent pregnancies, it is severe and can lead to fetal intracranial hemorrhage. Human platelet antigen (HPA) 1a is the most common paternal–fetal antigen that results in the development of NAIT, causing 80% to 90% of the identified cases. The diagnosis of this disorder is confirmed by demonstration of maternal antibodies directed against a paternal platelet antigen.

THROMBOTIC THROMBOCYTOPENIC PURPURA

Thrombotic thrombocytopenic purpura (TTP) is a disorder characterized by a clinical pentad of fever, neurologic dysfunction, microangiopathic hemolytic anemia, renal insufficiency,

and thrombocytopenia. The thrombocytopenia seen in this disorder is secondary to platelet consumption in the development of thrombosis of the small vessels. TTP is associated with the presence of abnormally large von Willebrand multimers, which lead to increased activation of coagulation. It is now known that low levels of ADAMTS13, an enzyme responsible for cleaving large von Willebrand multimers, is at least partially responsible for this disorder. Low levels of ADAMTS13 can arise from an acquired IgG autoantibody or from a congenital deficiency.

HEPARIN-INDUCED THROMBOCYTOPENIA

HIT is a process in which exposure to heparin results in the development of moderate thrombocytopenia and arterial or venous thrombosis. This disorder is characterized by a mild to moderate thrombocytopenia (median, 50,000/μL) that typically develops within 5 to 10 days after heparin exposure but can occur within hours if the patient was previously exposed to heparin. The associated thrombocytopenia typically resolves within 1 to 2 weeks of stopping the drug. The mechanism of this disorder is related to the interaction of heparin and an antigen on the surface of platelets called platelet factor 4 (PF4). Heparin forms a complex with PF4, and in HIT, antibodies develop to the heparin–PF4 complex. These antibodies bind to the heparin–PF4 complex and cause platelet activation, resulting in undesired activation of platelets and resultant thrombosis.

CLINICAL PRESENTATION AND DIFFERENTIAL DIAGNOSIS

The clinical presentation of platelet disorders varies with the platelet count or the severity of the platelet function abnormality. The clinical picture of a patient with a platelet disorder is that of mucocutaneous bleeding. The patient may have epistaxis, easy bruising, petechiae, menorrhagia, or gingival bleeding. More significant mucocutaneous bleeding can be seen with a very low platelet count (<20,000/μL) or in disorders with severe platelet dysfunction. This may consist of gastrointestinal bleeding or hematuria. With extremely low platelet counts (<10,000/μL), there is a risk of spontaneous bleeding and an increased risk of intracranial hemorrhage. This is particularly of concern in NAIT (Figure 52-2). Some children may be asymptomatic but develop excessive bleeding with significant hemostatic challenges such as surgery, dental extractions, or trauma.

DIAGNOSTIC APPROACH

The diagnostic approach to a patient with a suspected platelet disorder starts with a thorough history and physical examination. In the history, one should pay special attention to any history of spontaneous bleeding, such as epistaxis, bleeding gums, or easy bruising. Pubertal girls should be questioned about their menses, specifically regarding the volume of bleeding and duration of menses. Parents should be questioned about prior hemostatic challenges such as circumcision, dental extractions, or surgical procedures. The past medical history may also provide clues about underlying medical diagnoses that can be associated with platelet abnormalities. A thorough medication

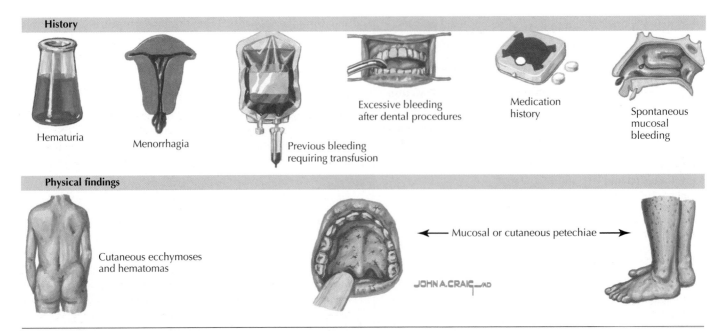

History

Hematuria

Menorrhagia

Previous bleeding requiring transfusion

Excessive bleeding after dental procedures

Medication history

Spontaneous mucosal bleeding

Physical findings

Cutaneous ecchymoses and hematomas

←— Mucosal or cutaneous petechiae —→

JOHN A. CRAIG—MD

Figure 52-2 *Clinical presentation of patients with bleeding disorders.*

history should be obtained, including herbal supplements, because many compounds have an effect on platelets. On physical examination, one should pay close attention to the skin examination, looking for bruises and petechiae. The mouth should be examined for the presence of wet purpura or gum bleeding. Congenital abnormalities such as albinism and radial defects should be noted because they can provide a clue to the diagnosis.

After the history and physical examination, a complete blood count should be obtained looking for thrombocytopenia. A blood smear should be examined, revealing differences in platelet size and the presence or absence of other hematologic abnormalities (Figure 52-3). If there is no thrombocytopenia present, formal platelet aggregation assays can help determine abnormalities in platelet function. A bleeding time is no longer recommended as a screening test for platelet disorders secondary to difficulty with standardization and unreliable results.

Platelet aggregation studies are laboratory tests in which compounds known to stimulate platelet aggregation are added to patient platelets, and the ability of platelets to aggregate in the presence of each compound is ascertained. These studies are particularly helpful if the diagnosis of a platelet function defect is under consideration. In Glanzmann's thrombasthenia, there are abnormalities in aggregation in the presence of all tested compounds, with the exception of ristocetin. Conversely, in Bernard-Soulier syndrome, platelets demonstrate poor aggregation in the presence of ristocetin, but they have normal aggregation when stimulated with epinephrine, collagen, or adenosine diphosphate.

ITP is a diagnosis of exclusion. Diagnostic tests, including antiplatelet antibodies, can be confirmatory, but these are only detected in approximately half of patients with ITP. In patients who have a classic presentation of ITP, a bone marrow evaluation is generally not necessary. Some providers perform bone

marrow aspirates on patients with suspected ITP to exclude leukemia before treatment with steroids.

MANAGEMENT AND THERAPY

The primary goal in the management of patients with platelet disorders is to prevent bleeding complications. Avoidance of significant trauma is integral in the management of these patients. In addition, preventive measures should be implemented before surgery and significant dental procedures.

In many of the congenital platelet disorders, judicious use of platelet transfusion may be required. However, transfusions should be used with caution in both Glanzmann's thrombasthenia and Bernard-Soulier syndrome because these patients can develop antibodies to normal transfused platelets and become refractory to platelet transfusions. DDAVP (desmopressin) has been effective in treating patients with bleeding associated with platelet function abnormalities and can be an alternative to platelet transfusions. In addition, antifibrinolytics such as aminocaproic acid can be used. There are small published case reports on the successful use of recombinant factor VIIa in patients with qualitative or quantitative platelet defects and severe bleeding. Recombinant factor VIIa works by increasing the thrombin generation on the surface of activated platelets. Patients with severe disorders of the bone marrow such as congenital amegakaryocytic thrombocytopenia require frequent platelet transfusions and bone marrow transplantation for definitive management.

In acquired platelet abnormalities secondary to an underlying disorder or medications, therapy is aimed at treating the underlying disorder or withdrawal of the offending agent. This is particularly true with HIT. If HIT is suspected, heparin should be discontinued immediately, and therapy with a direct thrombin inhibitor should be initiated.

In NAIT, infants are at risk for intracranial hemorrhage and spontaneous bleeding. In that instance, washed maternal platelets can be given to the infant. If maternal platelets are unavailable, either HPA-1a negative platelets or intravenous immunoglobulin (IVIG) can be used. In addition, if NAIT is suspected prenatally, the mother can be treated with immunosuppression before delivery to improve the infant's platelet count or fetal platelet transfusions can be performed. For acquired TTP, the treatment of choice is emergent plasmapheresis. For congenital TTP, infusions with fresh-frozen plasma are effective.

Controversy exists regarding the treatment of acute ITP. There is no evidence at this time that treatment alters the course of the disease. The sole purpose of treatment is to prevent significant bleeding complications and most importantly to prevent intracranial hemorrhage. Treatment is recommended if the patient has significant bleeding or if the platelet count is below 10,000/μL. In general, spontaneous bleeding is unlikely to occur in patients with platelet counts above 20,000/μL. Several therapies are available for the treatment of patients with acute ITP, including IVIG (1 g/kg), WinRho (50-75 μg/kg), or glucocorticoids (1 mg/kg twice a day). Treatment of patients with refractory or chronic ITP can include several other modalities from splenectomy to a variety of immune modulators, including rituximab, cyclosporine, vincristine, or cyclophosphamide.

FUTURE DIRECTIONS

Hematologists are continuing to research platelet disorders and possible therapies. The genetic components of many disorders are now known, and researchers are actively working on targeted genetic-based therapies for these disorders. A new class of medications was recently approved for the treatment of ITP that mimics the action of TPO. These medications are approved for use in adults, and clinical trials are opening in pediatrics for their use in a variety of the platelet disorders seen in childhood. In addition, advances in bone marrow transplantation continue to make them attractive options for children with severe platelet disorders such as congenital amegakaryocytic thrombocytopenia.

SUGGESTED READINGS

Aster RH, Bougie DW: Drug induced immune thrombocytopenia, *N Engl J Med* 357(6):580-587, 2007.

Cines DB, Bussel JB, Liebman HA, et al: The ITP syndrome: pathologic and clinical diversity, *Blood* 113(26):6511-6521, 2009.

Drachman JG: Inherited thrombocytopenia: when a low platelet count does not mean ITP, *Blood* 103(2):390-398, 2004.

Handin RI: Blood platelets and the vessel wall. In Nathan DG, Orkin SH, Ginsburg D, Look AT, editors: *Nathan and Oski's Hematology of Infancy and Childhood,* ed 6, Philadelphia, 2003, Saunders, pp 1457-1474.

Poncz M: Inherited platelet disorders. In Nathan DG, Orkin SH, Ginsburg D, Look AT, editors: *Nathan and Oski's Hematology of Infancy and Childhood,* ed 6, Philadelphia, 2003, Saunders, pp 1527-1546.

Warkentin T: Heparin induced thrombocytopenia. *Hematol Oncol Clin North Am* 21(4):589-607, 2007.

Wilson DB: Acquired platelet defects. In Nathan DG, Orkin SH, Ginsburg D, Look AT, editors: *Nathan and Oski's Hematology of Infancy and Childhood,* ed 6, Philadelphia, 2003, Saunders, pp 1597-1630.

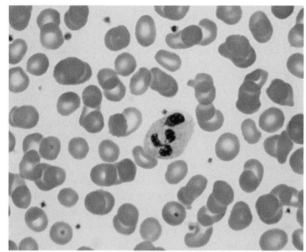

Normal*

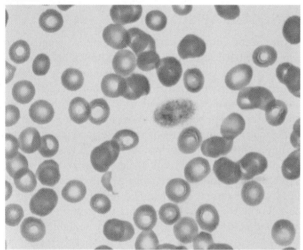

No platelets*

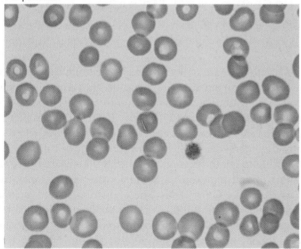

Giant platelet*

Pictures courtesy of Marybeth Helfrich

Figure 52-3 *Peripheral blood smears.*

Sickle Cell Disease

Connie M. Piccone

53

More than 100,000 Americans are affected with sickle cell disease (SCD), making it one of the most prevalent genetic disorders in the United States. The majority of affected individuals are of African or Mediterranean descent; this is related in part to the "natural selection" process because being a carrier of sickle hemoglobin (Hb) confers some resistance to malarial infection and a resultant survival advantage. The carrier rate among African Americans is approximately 8% (one in 12). Individuals with SCD can exhibit significant morbidity and mortality related to chronic hemolysis. Each year in the United States, an average of 75,000 hospitalizations are attributable to SCD, costing approximately $475 million. Neonatal screening, confirmatory diagnostic testing, family education, and routine comprehensive care of patients with SCD are imperative in reducing the morbidity and mortality of this lifelong disease.

ETIOLOGY AND PATHOGENESIS

SCD is a group of inherited hemoglobinopathies associated with hemolytic anemia and vaso-occlusive complications. All forms of SCD are inherited in an autosomal recessive fashion and are the result of mutations in the two β-globin genes. β-Globin is one of the major components of adult Hb and is part of a group of genes involved in oxygen transport. Two β-globin chains combine with two α-globin chains to form the predominant Hb found in human adults, HbA. In HbS, an amino acid substitution from glutamic acid to valine ultimately leads to the polymerization of HbS molecules, causing the "sickling" effect (Figure 53-1)

The most common form of SCD is homozygous SS. Other variants of SCD are the result of compound heterozygotes for HbS and other β-globin variants, including SC as well as Sβ+ thalassemia and Sβ0 thalassemia. All individuals who are homozygous or compound heterozygous for HbS exhibit some clinical manifestations of SCD. Symptoms usually appear by the first 6 months of life when fetal Hb dissipates, but there may be late presentations as well. There is considerable variability in clinical severity, which is related to genotype (Table 53-1). Patients with SS have the most severe clinical phenotype followed by individuals with Sβ0 thalassemia. Those with SC and Sβ+ thalassemia tend to have milder clinical phenotypes.

Whereas SCD was once seen as a disease in which morbidity and mortality were directly related to vascular occlusion by red blood cell (RBC) sickling alone, it is now evident that chronic hemolysis secondary to endothelial dysfunction and vasculopathy plays a significant role in morbidity. Researchers have found that the release of Hb and arginase from hemolyzed RBCs leads to nitric oxide (NO) bioavailability, thereby resulting in increased oxidative stress and accelerated intravascular hemolysis. SCD confers a state of NO resistance, and animal studies have provided evidence that a reduction in NO is associated with vasoconstriction, decreased blood flow, platelet activation, and end-organ injury.

CLINICAL PRESENTATION

SCD has a variable presentation in pediatric patients. Symptoms common to many patients include pallor and scleral icterus from the chronic hemolytic anemia, vaso-occlusive episodes, acute chest syndrome, splenic sequestration, and susceptibility to bacterial infections. Infection is the most common cause of mortality among children with SCD. Two infection prevention strategies—vaccination and penicillin prophylaxis—have significantly reduced mortality.

DIAGNOSTIC APPROACH

Currently in the United States, SCD testing is a standard component of newborn screening. Approximately 2000 infants with SCD are identified annually by national newborn screening programs. Patients with an abnormal newborn screen concerning for SCD should be referred to a pediatric hematologist. Confirmatory testing should be performed with Hb identification, molecular genetic testing (if available), and parental testing. Most importantly, when reviewing the results of a newborn screen, all patients with SS, Sβ0 thalassemia, and SC will have no HbA present, and patients with Sβ+ thalassemia will have some HbA, but the predominant Hb is HbS. In patients with sickle cell trait, the newborn screening will reveal FAS, in which the predominant Hbs are HbF and HbA (see Table 53-1).

MANAGEMENT AND THERAPY

Acute Complications

FEVER

Patients with SCD are at increased risk for certain bacterial infections secondary to functional asplenia, decreased opsonic activity in the serum, and poor antibody response to the polysaccharide component of the bacterial capsule. Bacterial sepsis remains one of the most common causes of death. Therefore, febrile illnesses are emergencies and require prompt medical evaluation and antibiotic administration. Immediate medical attention is required for all children with SCD who have temperatures greater than 38.4°C or 101°F. The evaluation should include a complete blood count (CBC), reticulocyte count, blood culture, physical examination, and pulse oximetry. Intravenous (IV) antibiotics should be given promptly and should have adequate coverage against *Streptococcus pneumoniae* and *Haemophilus influenza*; ceftriaxone is frequently used. A chest radiograph should be considered in patients younger than 3 years of age in whom an adequate lung examination may not be able to be obtained.

VASO-OCCLUSIVE EPISODES

Patients with acute pain require prompt evaluation and treatment. At initial presentation, it is important to determine the

Table 53-1 Sickle Hemoglobinopathies: Neonatal Screening and Diagnostic Tests

Genotype	Genotype % in the United States	Newborn Screening Results	Hemoglobin Range (g/dL) After 6 Months of Age	MVC After 6 Months of Age	Reticulocyte Range (%)
SS	65	FS	6-11	Normocytic	2-25
SC	25	FSC	9-12	Normocytic	1-13
Sβ⁺ thalassemia	8	FSA or FS*	9-12	Microcytic	1-7
Sβ⁰ thalassemia	2	FS	6-10	Microcytic	2-25

*The quantity of Hb A at birth can be insufficient for detection.
MCV, mean corpuscular volume.

cause of pain based on location and patient presentation because pain is not always related to SCD (Table 53-2). Assessment of pain should include age- and developmentally appropriate tools. Uncomplicated pain crises can be managed at home. Non-pharmacologic measures to help manage pain symptoms can be extremely helpful and include a heating pad or hot packs, massage, and play activities. Pharmacologic management of vaso-occlusive episodes (VOEs) includes a combination of non-steroidal antiinflammatory drugs (NSAIDs such as ibuprofen or ketorolac) and oral or IV analgesics (Tylenol, codeine, morphine, hydromorphone) (Table 53-3). It is important to adjust therapy according to the degree of pain (i.e., switching from oral to IV formulations) and to order medications to be given at scheduled intervals.

ACUTE CHEST SYNDROME

Acute chest syndrome (ACS) is a common complication in SCD and is defined by respiratory symptoms (i.e., cough, chest pain), fever, and evidence of a pulmonary infiltrate on chest radiography. Fever and cough are the most common presenting symptoms in patients with ACS. Radiographic findings are somewhat

variable and, in the absence of an infiltrate, patients should be treated presumptively for ACS if there is a strong clinical suspicion. Infiltrates may not appear on chest radiography. until 2 to 3 days after initial presentation. The cause of ACS is diverse and includes microbial infection, vaso-occlusion, fat embolism from ischemic bone marrow, and thromboembolism. In the 1970s, clinicians believed that most cases of ACS were caused by infection by *S. pneumoniae*, but more recent epidemiologic studies have revealed a change in ACS infectious epidemiology. *Mycoplasma* spp. and *Chlamydia pneumoniae* are also common bacterial causes of infection as well as respiratory viruses. The current antibiotic treatment for ACS should include coverage for *S. pneumoniae* and atypical microorganisms, for example, erythromycin and a cephalosporin. Patients may develop an

Table 53-2 Differential Diagnosis and Further Evaluation of Pain

Location of Pain	Other Conditions to Consider	Additional Studies to Consider
Head or face	• Hemorrhagic stroke • Sinusitis • Migraines • Meningitis	• MRI or MRA • CT • LP
Neck or throat	• Meningitis • Torticollis • Pharyngitis or tonsillitis	• LP • Throat culture
Chest	• Acute chest syndrome, pneumonia, RAD • Costochondritis • Cardiac • GER	• Chest radiography • ECG or echocardiography
Abdomen	• Appendicitis • Cholelithiasis or cholecystitis • Pancreatitis • Splenic sequestration • Urinary tract infection or pyelonephritis	• Abdominal radiography • Abdominal ultrasonography • Amylase or lipase • UA, ÷±culture
Limb or joint	• Osteomyelitis • Septic joint • Avascular necrosis • Painless limp may indicate stroke	• Plain radiography • Ultrasonography • MRI or MRA

CT, computed tomography; ECG, electrocardiography; GER, gastroesophageal reflux; LP, lumbar puncture; MRA, magnetic resonance angiography; MRI, magnetic resonance imaging; RAD, reactive airway disease; UA, urinalysis.
Adapted from Children's Hospital of Philadelphia Department of Hematology: *Guidelines for Patient Management*, July 1999.

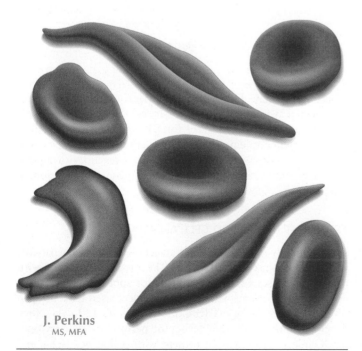

J. Perkins
MS, MFA

Figure 53-1 *Sickled red blood cells.*

Table 53-3 Guide to Common Pain Medications

Medication and Preparations	Route	Pediatric Dose	Adult Dose	Side Effects
Acetaminophen and NSAIDs				
Acetaminophen • Elixir: 160 mg/5 mL • Tablets: 325 mg • Chewable tablet: 80 mg	PO	10-15 mg/kg every 4-6 h	325-650 mg every 4-6 h or 1000 mg three or four times a day (not to exceed 4 g/d)	• Masking of fever • Liver toxicity (with prolonged use at high doses)
Ibuprofen • Suspension: 100 mg/5 mL • Tablets: 200 mg, 400 mg, 600 mg	PO	10 mg/kg every 6-8 h	400-800 mg every 6 h	• GI irritation • Masking of fever
Ketorolac • Parenteral	IM or IV	0.5 mg/kg/dose every 6-8 h; maximum, 30 mg/dose	0.5 mg/kg/dose every 6-8 h; maximum, 30 mg/dose	• Masking of fever • GI irritation • Renal and electrolyte abnormalities with prolonged use
Opioids (Agonists and Agonist–Antagonists)				

Codeine
• Solution:
  • Acetaminophen 120 mg
  • Codeine phosphate 12 mg/5 mL
• Tablet, as sulfate: 15 mg, 30 mg, 60 mg
	PO	0.5-1.0 mg/kg every 4 h (based on codeine)	15-30 mg every 4 h; maximum, 60 mg/dose	• Constipation
				• Nausea and vomiting

Morphine
• MS (immediate release):
  • Solution: 10 mg/5 mL
  • Tablets: 15 mg, 30 mg
• MS Contin (controlled release): 15-mg, 30-mg, 60-mg, 100-mg tablets
• Parenteral
	PO
	PO
	IV
		0.3 mg/kg every 3-4 h
		0.3-0.6 mg/kg every 8-12 h
		0.1-0.2 mg/kg every 3-4 h
			30 mg every 3-4 h
			15-30 mg every 8-12 h
			10 mg every 3-4 h
				• Pruritus
				• Nausea and vomiting
				• CNS depression
				• Respiratory depression
				• Constipation

Hydromorphone • Dilaudid: 2-mg, 4-mg tablets • Parenteral	PO IV	0.03-0.08 mg/kg every 3-6 h 0.015 mg/kg every 3-6 h	2-4 mg every 3-6 h 1 mg every 3-6 h	• Pruritus • Nausea and vomiting • CNS depression • Respiratory depression • Constipation
Nalbuphine • Nubain	IV	0.1 mg/kg every 3-6 h	10 mg every 3-6 h	• Pruritus • Nausea and vomiting • CNS depression • Respiratory depression

CNS, central nervous system; GI, gastrointestinal; IM, intramuscular; IV, intravenous; PO, orally.
Adapted from Children's Hospital of Philadelphia Department of Hematology: *Guidelines for Patient Management*, July 1999.

oxygen requirement, and close monitoring is essential to prevent significant morbidity, including respiratory failure necessitating intubation. Patients with more severe symptoms benefit from a simple blood transfusion to improve oxygen-carrying capacity and decrease sickle Hb levels.

SPLENIC SEQUESTRATION

Acute splenic sequestration is defined as a decrease in Hb in association with a rapidly enlarging spleen and evidence of increased bone marrow activity. Parental education helps establish early diagnosis, and prompt medical treatment decreases morbidity and mortality. Parents should be instructed on how to palpate the spleen and monitor for signs of splenomegaly and sequestration at home. Patients who require hospital admission should have an IV line placed with the administration of IV fluids. Blood should be sent for CBC, reticulocyte count, and type and screen. The spleen size should be documented and

monitored closely. The CBC and physical examination should be repeated at frequent intervals to assess the degree of sequestration and the potential need for RBC transfusion. Children who experience splenic sequestration are at risk for recurrent events. In children with recurrent events, prevention strategies should be considered, including either chronic transfusion or splenectomy.

TRANSIENT RED BLOOD CELL APLASIA

Approximately 70% to 100% of transient RBC aplasia in patients with SCD is caused by parvovirus B19 infection. Infection with parvovirus causes a reticulocytopenia for approximately 7 to 10 days. Because patients with SCD have a decreased RBC lifespan of 10 to 20 days (normal RBC life span is 90-120 days), they develop significant anemia during the period of reticulocytopenia. Clinically, patients can present with pallor, headache, and a marked decrease in their Hb level. The hallmark is a low reticulocyte count, indicating suppression of bone marrow activity. Blood transfusion is indicated in patients with significant anemia who are symptomatic.

Acute Stroke

Stroke is a major complication of SCD and occurs in approximately 11% of pediatric patients. The most common cause of stroke is obstruction of a distal intracranial internal carotid artery or proximal middle cerebral artery. The cause of stroke in this population is thought to be secondary to an arterial vasculopathy from progressive intimal hyperplasia. Signs and symptoms can include mild weakness to frank hemiparesis, visual and language disturbances, seizures, and altered mental status. If neurologic symptoms resolve in less than 24 hours and there is no evidence of brain ischemia, those events are termed *transient ischemic attacks*. If a patient presents with concern for an ischemic event, prompt evaluation and treatment are warranted. After initial stabilization, patients should undergo noncontrast computed tomography scan of the brain to rule out hemorrhage or other non-ischemic causes of symptoms followed by imaging with magnetic resonance imaging (MRI) and angiography (MRA). The treatment for patients with an acute stroke is RBC transfusion to decrease the percent HbS to less than 30%. If possible, exchange transfusion is preferred because it avoids the risk of hyperviscosity, which can lead to further cerebral injury.

Priapism

Priapism is defined as a sustained, painful penile erection. Related to vaso-occlusion, priapism occurs because there is an obstruction to the venous drainage of the penis. Prolonged priapism (an erection lasting more than 3 hours) is an emergency that requires prompt urologic consultation and evaluation. Treatment should include hydration and pain control. Prolonged episodes may require penile aspiration. Additional medications have also been used, including α-agonists (pseudoephedrine) and β-agonists (terbutaline). Recurrent episodes can lead to penile fibrosis and often impotence.

Routine Health Maintenance

IMMUNIZATIONS

Children with SCD should receive all routine childhood immunizations. In addition, patients should receive the 23-valent pneumococcal vaccine (Pneumovax) at age 2 years with a booster shot given at 5 years of age. They should also receive the influenza vaccine annually.

PENICILLIN PROPHYLAXIS

Penicillin prophylaxis for SCD was widely introduced after the PCN Prophylaxis Studies of the 1980s found a significantly reduced incidence of pneumococcal infections in individuals younger than 5 years of age. Prophylaxis should be started at 2 months of age with oral penicillin VK; children younger than 3 years of age should take 125 mg twice daily, and those 3 years and older should take 250 mg twice daily. Patients with a penicillin allergy can take erythromycin 10 mg/kg/dose twice a day.

Prophylaxis after the age of 5 years does not appear to significantly reduce the risk of pneumococcal infection compared with placebo. Continuation of penicillin prophylaxis after the age of 5 years is optional.

FOLIC ACID

Daily folic acid supplementation (1 mg/d) is recommended for patients with SCD secondary to increased RBC production and to prevent bone marrow aplasia from folate deficiency.

NUTRITION AND GROWTH

Children with SCD may have deficiencies in some vitamins and minerals, including fat-soluble vitamins and zinc. Additionally, patients have a delay in growth likely related to increased caloric requirements caused by chronic anemia. Families should be encouraged to adopt healthy eating habits, and patients should be monitored closely for growth and development. Nutritional supplements can be initiated if there are concerns about increasing growth delay. Patients can also take a daily multivitamin without iron.

STROKE SCREENING

As mentioned previously, stroke is a major complication of SCD. Patients with silent infarctions as well as overt stroke can experience significant neurocognitive impairment, making routine evaluation imperative. The use of screening transcranial Doppler (TCD) ultrasonography has lead to the early identification of vessel abnormalities and the identification of patients who are at high risk for stroke. Patients with SCD, type SS and Sβ⁰ thalassemia, should have a yearly TCD performed beginning at 2 years of age. Normal TCD rates are less than 170 cm/sec, patients with a conditional TCD (170-199 cm/sec) should be followed more closely, and those with an abnormal TCD (>200 cm/sec) should have an MRI or MRA of the brain performed and a chronic transfusion protocol initiated with the goal of maintaining the patient's trough HbS level at less than 30%.

EYE EXAMINATIONS

All SCD patients should have yearly ophthalmologic screening, including a dilated funduscopic exam, to monitor for vascular retinopathy, starting at age 5 years.

Chronic Issues

TRANSFUSION AND CHELATION THERAPY

Chronic RBC transfusion is a treatment modality in SCD used to treat and prevent disease-related complications, including stroke, recurrent VOE, and recurrent ACS. Prevention of neurologic complications is the most common reason for initiating a transfusion program. Transfusions help by decreasing the overall HbS percentage and increasing oxygen-carrying capacity. However, risks are associated with chronic transfusion, including alloimmunization (patients develop RBC antibodies) and iron overload. Because humans are unable to effectively excrete excess iron, it is necessary to use medications for iron chelation in patients with transfusional iron overload. The chelators currently in use include deferoxamine (Desferal), which is typically given as a 12-hour infusion IV or subcutaneously, and deferasirox (Exjade), an oral medication given once daily.

Excess iron deposits primarily in the heart and liver can lead to significant organ dysfunction and subsequent organ failure if not treated. MRI can be used to assess both cardiac and hepatic iron overload. Serum ferritin levels are also used to monitor iron overload, although ferritin measurements can be unreliable in patients with SCD because ferritin is an acute phase reactant and SCD is a chronic inflammatory state. Another option to minimize iron loading is erythrocytapheresis. Erythrocytapheresis (or RBC exchange) involves removing a patient's RBCs and replacing them with normal RBCs. With exchange transfusion, there is less overall iron loading. However, erythrocytapheresis requires more blood per procedure compared with a simple transfusion, thus exposing patients to more donor units.

HYDROXYUREA

Hydroxyurea is a drug used to increase fetal Hb levels, thereby increasing oxygen-carrying capacity, decreasing sickle Hb levels, and reducing many of the morbidities related to chronic hemolysis and hypoxia. Overall, it is a well-tolerated medication, but it can cause myelosuppression, so patients taking this drug are monitored closely.

AVASCULAR NECROSIS

Generally seen in patients with Hb SS, avascular necrosis (AVN, also known as osteonecrosis) is a painful destruction of bone related to sickle vasculopathy with thrombosis and joint ischemia. The femoral and humeral heads are most often involved. In pediatric patients, initial treatment is conservative and includes analgesics, NSAIDs, and physical therapy for weight-bearing recommendations. Joint-preserving surgical procedures can be used, including core decompression and osteotomy. No treatment has been found that can reverse or stop the progression of AVN. There is progressive flattening and eventual bony collapse of the femoral or humeral head. If the joint has collapsed, patients can have a joint replacement after the growth plate has closed.

FUTURE DIRECTIONS

Bone marrow transplantation (BMT) has been successful in multiple centers across the globe but has not become standard practice because of treatment-related complications and morbidities as well as disagreement on the timing of BMT in SCD patients. The first case report of BMT for SCD was published in 1984. Since that time, several groups have studied the efficacy of BMT in treating SCD in children with more severe complications, but there have not been any randomized controlled trials to provide clear evidence for the use of BMT in pediatric SCD. Newer BMT protocols using reduced-intensity conditioning may result in an increase in BMT referrals, but attempts at limiting side effects from conditioning may ultimately result in graft failure. In sum, the decision to recommend BMT for a pediatric SCD patient must be made carefully with input from the primary hematologist, the transplant team, and the family.

SUGGESTED READINGS

Ashley-Koch A, Yang Q, Olney RS: Sickle hemoglobin (Hb S) and sickle cell disease: a HuGE review, *Am J Epidemiol* 151(9):839-845, 2000.

Dunlop RJ, Bennett KCLB: Pain management for sickle cell disease, Cochrane Database Syst Rev (2):CD003350, 2006.

Johnson CS: The acute chest syndrome, *Hematol Oncol Clin North Am* 19:857-879, 2005.

Jones AP, et al: Hydroxyurea for sickle cell disease, Cochrane Database Syst Rev (2):CD002202, 2001.

Kwiatkowski JL, Cohen AR: Iron chelation therapy in sickle-cell disease and other transfusion-dependent anemias, *Hematol Oncol Clin North Am* 18:1355-1377, 2004.

Lee MT, Piomelli S, Granger S, et al; STOP Study Investigators: Stroke prevention trial in sickle cell anemia (STOP): extended follow-up and results, *Blood* 108(3), 2006: 847-852.

National Institute of Health, Division of Blood Diseases and Resources. The Management of Sickle Cell Disease. Available at http://www.nhlbi.nih.gov/health/prof/blood/sickle/sc_mngt.pdf.

Oringanje C, Nemecek E, Oniyangi O: Hematopoietic stem cell transplantation for children with sickle cell disease, Cochrane Database Syst Rev (1):CD007001, 2009.

Sickle Cell Disease Association of America: Available at http://www.sicklecelldisease.org/index.phtml.

Sickle Cell Kids: Available at http://www.sicklecellkids.org.

Wood KC, Hsu LL, Gladwin MT: Sickle cell disease vasculopathy: a state of nitric oxide resistance, *Free Radic Biol Med* 44(8):1506-1528, 2008.

Disorders of Thrombosis and Hemostasis

54

Alexis Teplick

The coagulation system is complex with intricately balanced interactions between the vascular endothelium, platelets, procoagulant, and anticoagulant proteins. With vascular injury, a cascade of interactions occurs between platelets and procoagulant proteins to initiate clot formation. After clot formation is initiated, anticoagulant proteins are activated to inhibit excessive clot formation. A dysregulation in this finely tuned system can lead to either a bleeding diathesis or a prothrombotic disorder.

EPIDEMIOLOGY

Congenital Bleeding Disorders

von Willebrand disease (vWD) is the most common congenital bleeding disorder, present in approximately 1% of the population. Hemophilia is the most common severe bleeding disorder and is the result of either a deficiency in factor VIII (hemophilia A) or IX (hemophilia B). The incidence of hemophilia is one in 5000 males, with 80% to 85% hemophilia A and 15% to 20% hemophilia B. There are no significant racial differences in the incidence of hemophilia.

Thrombosis

Advances in the treatment and support of critically ill children combined with an increasing awareness of thrombotic complications have likely resulted in an increase in the diagnosis of pediatric thromboembolic events. Although these events are increasing, they are still relatively rare compared with adults. This increase is most notable in comparing the rates from an older pediatric Canadian registry with an incidence of thromboembolic events of 5.3 in 10,000 hospitalizations, but a newer study from the United States reported a rate of 58 in 10,000 hospitalizations. There is a bimodal age distribution of thrombosis with peak rates in the neonatal and adolescent age groups.

ETIOLOGY AND PATHOGENESIS

Congenital Bleeding Disorders

vWD is a family of disorders caused by quantitative or qualitative defects of von Willebrand factor (vWF), a plasma protein that plays a role in both platelet adhesion and fibrin formation.

vWF is also a carrier protein for factor VIII; factor VIII unbound to vWF is rapidly degraded. vWD is classified into six types: 1, 2A, 2B, 2M, 2N, and 3. Table 54-1 provides a description and laboratory findings for all types of vWD.

Type 1 vWD is inherited in an autosomal dominant fashion and accounts for 70% to 80% of all vWD cases. It is

characterized by a partial quantitative defect resulting in decreased amounts of a functionally normal vWF protein. Type 3 is a complete quantitative defect with no vWF and subsequently decreased factor VIII levels. The type 2 variants are qualitative defects.

Hemophilia A is a deficiency of factor VIII, and hemophilia B is a deficiency of factor IX. Both types of hemophilia are X-linked recessive diseases. About 30% of cases of hemophilia represent new mutations. Clinical severity is classified by the patient's baseline factor level, severe less than 1%, moderate 1% to 5% and mild greater than 5%.

Acquired Bleeding Disorders

Children may develop bleeding disorders under various clinical conditions. The liver is responsible for the synthesis of most of the clotting factors. When synthetic liver dysfunction occurs, patients may develop abnormal coagulation profiles and clinical bleeding. Vitamin K plays a key role in the activation of coagulation proteins through the carboxylation of glutamate residues. Vitamin K deficiency can result from lack of exogenous vitamin K, as in an infant who is strictly breastfed or a child who is dependent on parenteral nutrition, or from infection or prolonged antibiotic administration. When vitamin K levels decline, the liver is unable to adequately synthesize functional factors II, VII, IX, and X, resulting in a bleeding propensity.

Disseminated Intravascular Coagulation

In disseminated intravascular coagulation (DIC), the normal physiology of coagulation is disturbed with resultant bleeding and thrombosis within the microvasculature. DIC is always secondary to a precipitating condition such as infection, tissue injury, malignancy, venom or toxin, or microangiopathic disorders. There is widespread deposition of intravascular fibrin leading to compromised organ function and capillary leak. Continued activation of this system leads to depletion of platelets and clotting factors, resulting in clinical bleeding (Figure 54-1).

Thrombosis

Deep venous thrombosis (DVT) is a consequence of Virchow's triad of venous stasis, endothelial injury, and a hypercoagulable state. More than 90% of children with DVT have an identifiable prothrombotic risk factor. The most common risk factor is the presence of a central venous catheter (CVC). More than 50% of DVTs in children and more than 80% in neonates are associated with a CVC. Venous stasis in children may be caused by a postoperative state, casting or splinting, or other causes of prolonged immobility. Endothelial injury may be caused by trauma,

Table 54-1 Classification of von Willebrand Disease

Type	Description	VW Antigen	VW Activity	Factor VIII Activity	Multimers
1	Partial quantitative deficiency	↓	↓	Nl to ↓	Normal
2A	Decreased high-molecular-weight multimers resulting in impaired vWF platelet binding	↓	↓↓	Nl to ↓	Abnormal
2B	Increased platelet and vWF binding	Nl to ↓	↓↓	Nl to ↓	Abnormal
2M	Decreased vWF and platelet binding	↓	↓↓	Nl to ↓	Normal
2N	Impaired vWF binding to factor VIII	Nl to ↓	Nl to ↓	↓↓	Normal
3	Complete quantitative deficiency	↓↓↓	↓↓↓	↓↓↓	Absent

↓, slightly decreased; ↓↓, moderately decreased; ↓↓↓, severely decreased; Nl, normal; vWF, von Willebrand factor.

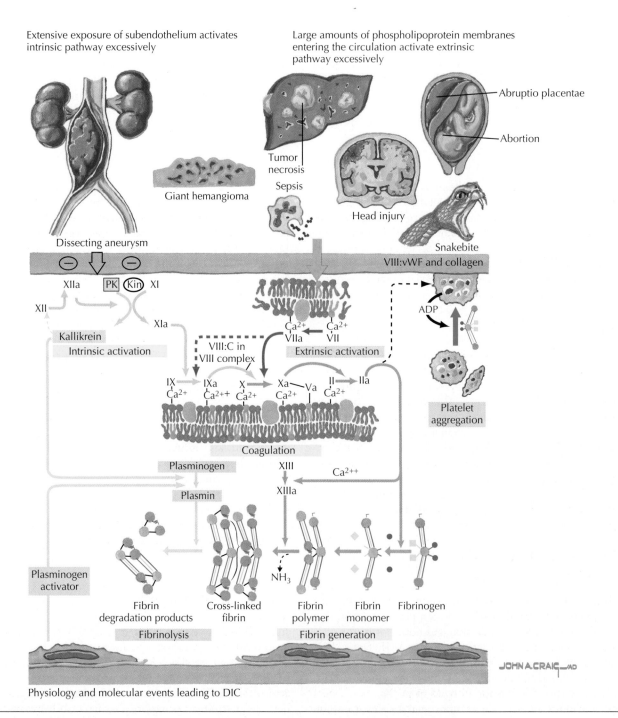

Figure 54-1 *Disseminated intravascular coagulation.*

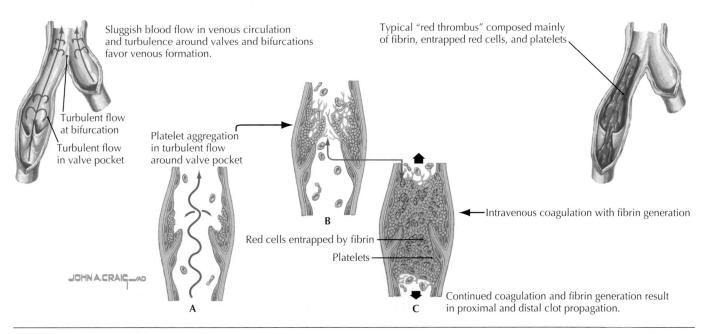

Sluggish blood flow in venous circulation and turbulence around valves and bifurcations favor venous formation.

Turbulent flow at bifurcation

Turbulent flow in valve pocket

Platelet aggregation in turbulent flow around valve pocket

JOHN A.CRAIG—AD

Typical "red thrombus" composed mainly of fibrin, entrapped red cells, and platelets

Intravenous coagulation with fibrin generation

Red cells entrapped by fibrin

Platelets

Continued coagulation and fibrin generation result in proximal and distal clot propagation.

A   B   C

Figure 54-2 *Venous thrombosis.*

infection, inflammation, or CVCs. Children may also have an inherited thrombophilia such as factor V Leiden or prothrombin gene mutations, deficiencies in the anticoagulant proteins including C, S, or antithrombin, hyperhomocysteinemia, or an elevated lipoprotein A. Acquired causes of thrombophilia include dehydration, antiphospholipid antibodies, malignancy, inflammatory states, anticoagulant deficiencies from consumption, or loss and exposure to certain medications such as estrogen-containing oral contraceptive pills or L-asparaginase (Figure 54-2).

CLINICAL PRESENTATION

Congenital Bleeding Disorders

Patients with vWD typically present with mucocutaneous bleeding, including epistaxis, gingival bleeding, abnormal bruising, or menorrhagia. Patients may also present with excessive postoperative bleeding.

The characteristic bleeding manifestations of hemophilia include palpable bruises, bleeding into joint spaces (hemarthroses), muscle hemorrhages, and excessive bleeding after surgery or trauma. The frequency and severity of bleeding correlate with the baseline measured factor activity. Whereas patients with severe hemophilia have spontaneous bleeding, patients with moderate hemophilia have bleeding with minimal trauma, and patients with mild hemophilia may only experience bleeding after a significant trauma or a surgical procedure.

In the newborn period, about 50% of boys with hemophilia have excessive bleeding with circumcision, and 3% to 4% have an intracranial hemorrhage. Muscle bleeds can also occur at the site of intramuscular immunization administration. Hemarthrosis is unusual in an infant and typically occurs after a child is ambulating. Patients with hemarthroses have pain, tenderness, warmth, swelling, and decreased range of motion of the affected joint. Muscle bleeds present with pain and swelling, and any

muscle can be affected. Intracranial hemorrhage is the most serious type of bleeding for patients with hemophilia with the highest mortality rate and can be the result of head trauma or spontaneous in patients with severe hemophilia (Figure 54-3).

Thrombosis

Presenting symptoms of an extremity DVT include swelling, erythema, or pain of the affected limb. Thrombosis of the jugular vein can present with neck pain, stiffness, or fullness. The clinical manifestation of cerebral sinus venous thrombosis is strongly influenced by the age of presentation, thrombosis location, and the presence of a venous infarction. Symptoms are diverse and nonspecific, including most commonly the triad of headache, emesis, and depressed mental status. Presenting signs and symptoms of pulmonary embolism (PE) may be mild to severe and may include cough, pleuritic chest pain, dyspnea, tachypnea, hypoxia, tachycardia, syncope, hemoptysis, and in the case of a massive PE, significant hemodynamic instability.

EVALUATION AND MANAGEMENT

Congenital Bleeding Disorder

In any patient that presents with findings concerning for a bleeding diathesis, it is appropriate to obtain a prothrombin time (PT), partial thromboplastin time (PTT), and a complete blood count (CBC). Hemophilia causes an isolated prolongation of the PTT; the same abnormality may be seen in patients with vWD, but the screening coagulation study results are frequently normal. Evaluation for vWD includes a vWF antigen, which indicates the quantity of vWF; a vWF activity, which represents the ability of vWF to cause platelet aggregation; and a factor VIII level. vWF levels, similar to factor VIII levels, may be elevated by illness or inflammation. As a result, vWF studies are

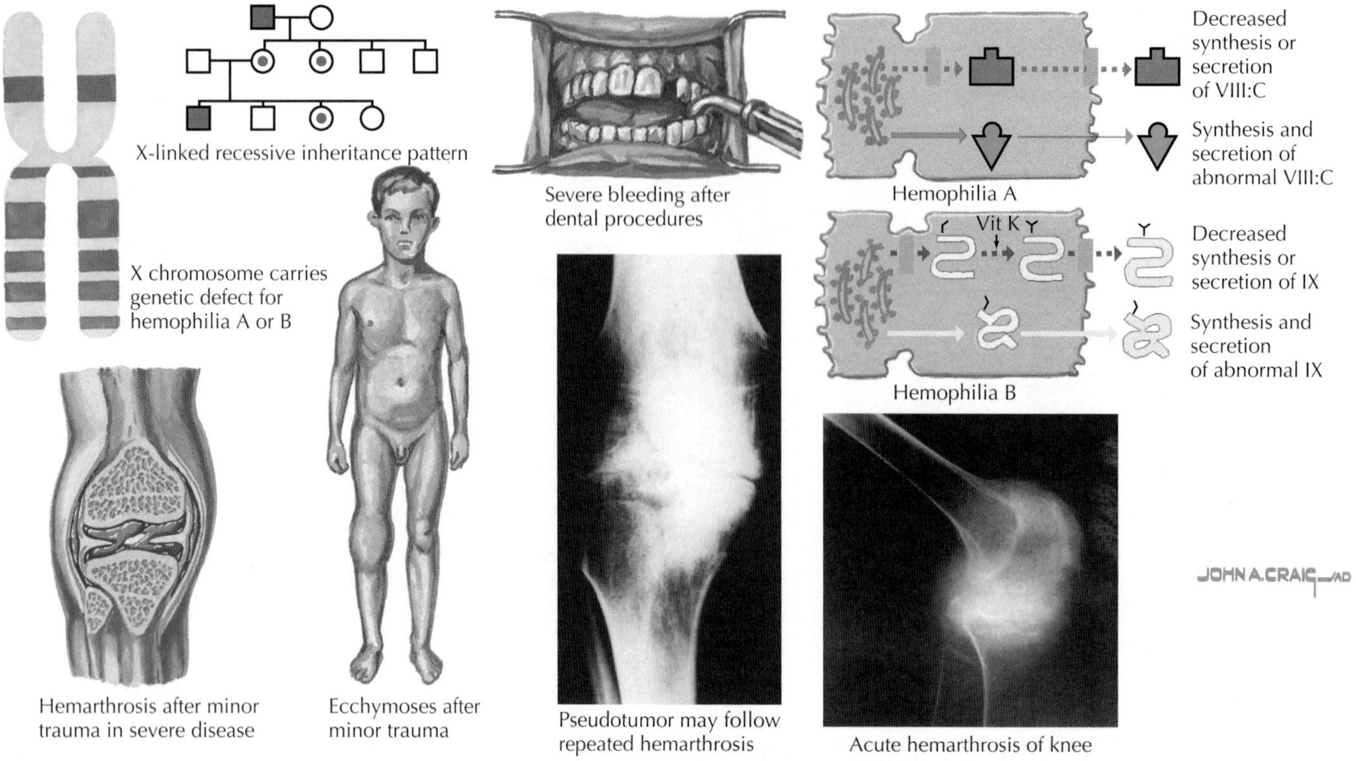

Figure 54-3 *Hemophilia A and B.*

routinely repeated to confirm the presence or absence of the disorder. A bleeding time is highly operator and patient dependent with unreliable results and is not recommended in children at this time.

Many types of vWD can be treated with DDAVP (desmopressin), which causes release of endogenous endothelial stores of vWF and factor VIII. DDAVP is ineffective in type 3 vWD and contraindicated in type 2B. DDAVP may be administered intranasally or intravenously. Both formulations have an antidiuretic effect, and total fluid should be limited to two-thirds maintenance for 24 hours after its administration to prevent hyponatremia and seizures. For significant bleeding or situations in which DDAVP cannot be used, a plasma-derived product containing vWF and factor VIII, such as Humate-P, can be used. In some anatomic areas, clot stabilization can be improved with the addition of antifibrinolytic therapy in the form of aminocaproic or tranexamic acid.

For pediatric patients with severe hemophilia prophylaxis, the routine replacement of factor to prevent bleeding and progressive joint damage is the standard of care. Treatment of bleeding episodes in patients with hemophilia begins with administration of the deficient factor. The target factor level depends on the severity of bleeding. There are several formulations of recombinant factor VIII available and only one formulation of recombinant factor IX. Various adjuvant therapies can also be used depending on the site of bleeding. For example, hemarthroses should be treated with factor replacement, immobilization, and ice. Oral bleeding in hemophilia may be managed with topical thrombin and antifibrinolytic therapy with factor administration if these initial measures are insufficient.

Patients with severe hemophilia may develop inhibitory antibodies against exogenous factor, leading to poor or no response to standard treatment. In some cases, a low titer inhibitor may be overcome with administration of higher doses of the deficient factor. However, some patients may be completely unresponsive to factor administration. In that case, bypass agents such as FEIBA (factor eight inhibitor bypass agent) or recombinant activated factor VII may be necessary.

Acquired Bleeding Disorders

Bleeding diatheses related to vitamin K deficiency and liver dysfunction are often discovered on screening coagulation profiles, although they may present with bleeding. For vitamin K deficiency, evaluation of coagulation factors may show a deficiency in factor II, VII, IX, and X. Factor V is often useful to differentiate between the two diagnoses because it is synthesized by the liver but is not vitamin K dependent. Treatment of vitamin K deficiency is most directly addressed by administration of oral, subcutaneous, or intravenous vitamin K. Coagulation factor deficiencies caused by liver dysfunction resolve when the underlying abnormality resolves. In the acute setting, bleeding from either cause may be treated with administration of fresh-frozen plasma (FFP).

Disseminated Intravascular Coagulation

Typical laboratory findings in DIC include thrombocytopenia, prolongation of the PT and PTT, and low fibrinogen. The fibrin degradation product elevation is quite sensitive but not

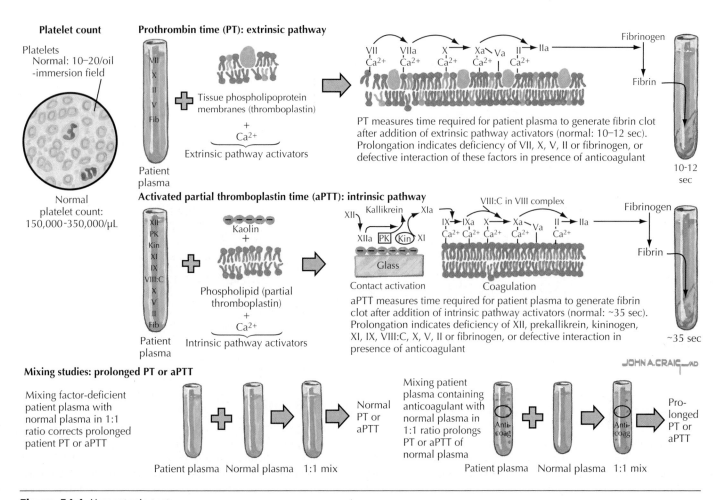

Figure 54-4 *Hemostasis tests.*

specific for DIC. Fibrinogen levels are expected to decrease but must be considered carefully; because it is an acute phase reactant, fibrinogen may initially maintain elevated or normal levels.

Treatment of patients with DIC must be directed at the underlying cause. In a patient who has clinical bleeding or severe laboratory derangements, administration of FFP and platelets may be helpful in maintaining hemostasis. At this time, multiple drugs, including activated protein C and antithrombin, were developed to correct the coagulopathy in DIC, but results have been disappointing.

Thrombosis

In a patient with a suspected DVT, imaging is the first diagnostic step. Although venography is the traditional gold standard, its invasiveness and technical difficulty have lead to the increased use of other modalities. Lower extremity, upper extremity, and jugular venous DVTs may all be visualized with Doppler ultrasonography. However, proximal extension of a lower extremity DVT into the inferior vena cava, intracranial extension of a jugular venous thrombosis, and subclavian vein thrombosis may not be appreciated with ultrasonography alone. For further evaluation of these thromboses or of other suspected DVTs, computed tomography (CT) or magnetic resonance venography is generally the modality of choice. PE may be evaluated with a

high-resolution or spiral CT or CT angiography. Ventilation/perfusion scans are used by some, but expertise with this modality is limited in many pediatric institutions.

Laboratory studies for evaluation of DVT and PE include a PT and PTT as well as a CBC (Figure 54-4). Renal function should be assessed. A D-dimer can be elevated in the presence of a DVT or PE but is not specific and can be elevated in other clinical settings and therefore is not diagnostic of the presence of thrombosis. A pregnancy test should be obtained in menstruating women. In many cases, it may be appropriate to evaluate a child for a predisposing thrombophilia, including factor V Leiden and prothrombin G20210 mutation analyses, protein C activity, protein S activity, antithrombin, homocysteine, lipoprotein(a) levels, dilute Russell Venom time, anticardiolipin, and anti-β2-glycoprotein antibodies.

When a DVT or PE is identified, anticoagulation is the definitive treatment but a decision must be made as to whether anticoagulation is appropriate, weighing the risk of bleeding versus the risk of clot propagation, embolization, or both. Acutely, therapy should be initiated with a continuous infusion of unfractionated heparin (UFH) or a subcutaneous administration of a low-molecular-weight heparin (LMWH) (Figure 54-5). Warfarin is an alternative anticoagulant that may be considered for maintenance therapy after adequate anticoagulation has been established with either heparin or a LMWH. The duration

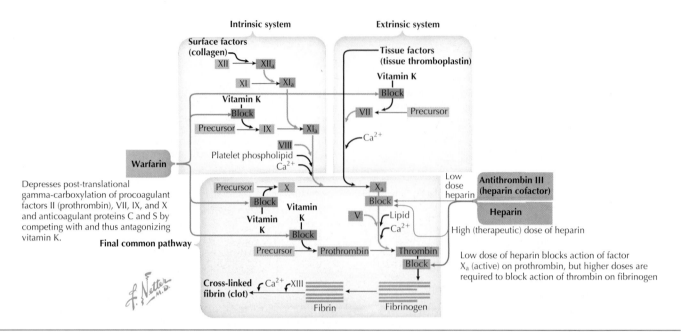

Figure 54-5 *Cascade of clotting factors and sites of action of heparin and warfarin.*

of anticoagulation depends on the clinical circumstances, size, site, and resolution of clot, as well as the presence of any thrombophilia.

Thrombolysis should be considered in patients who have a life- or limb-threatening thrombosis, such as an occlusive arterial clot with limb ischemia, sinovenous thrombosis unresponsive to anticoagulation with neurologic decompensation, or massive PE with hemodynamic instability. The most commonly used thrombolytic agents are tissue plasminogen activator and urokinase. Both agents act by catalyzing the conversion of plasminogen to plasmin, which then cleaves crosslinked fibrin. Lysis may be systemic, administered through an intravenous line, or directed, administered through a catheter positioned very close to the clot. Directed lysis may also use mechanical methods of clot disruption and removal. Thrombolysis carries a higher risk of bleeding than anticoagulation, and the risks and benefits must be weighed carefully. When a life- or limb-threatening thrombosis is present and thrombolysis is contraindicated or otherwise not possible, surgical thrombectomy may be considered.

Indications for the placement of an inferior vena cava filter include patients with an acute lower extremity DVT and a contraindication to anticoagulation or recurrent thrombosis despite adequate anticoagulation. A temporary filter is preferred because of the high risk of thrombosis below the filter.

FUTURE DIRECTIONS

Further study is necessary to elucidate the cause and treatment of inhibitors in patients with hemophilia. Gene therapy for hemophilia, in which normal copies of the factor VIII or IX gene are introduced back into the patient, is still in the early stages but has the potential to be curative in the future. Currently, there are limited studies regarding the treatment of thrombosis in children. Clinical decisions about anticoagulation versus thrombolysis, systemic versus directed thrombolysis, and duration of therapy are still based largely on expert opinion and experience from the adult literature. Studies will continue to elucidate these issues in the pediatric population.

SUGGESTED READINGS

Dunn AL, Abshire TC: Recent advances in the management of the child who has hemophilia, *Hematol Oncol Clin North Am* 18(6):1249-1276, viii, 2004.

Goldberg NA, Bernard TJ: Venous thromboembolism in children, *Pediatr Clin North Am* 55(2):305-322, 2008.

Levi M: Disseminated intravascular coagulation, *Crit Care Med* 35(9):2191-2195, 2007.

Robertson J, Lillicrap D, James PD: von Willebrand Disease, *Pediatr Clin North Am* 55:377-392, 2008.

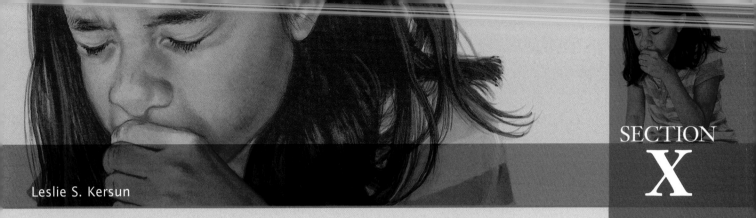

Leslie S. Kersun

Neoplastic Disorders

Leukemia

Abby Green and Susan R. Rheingold

55

Leukemia is the most common type of childhood cancer, accounting for more than 3000 new cases annually and 25% of all malignancies diagnosed in patients younger than 20 years in the United States. Subtypes and prevalence include acute lymphoblastic leukemia (ALL), 75%; acute myelogenous leukemia (AML), 20%; and chronic myelogenous leukemia (CML), less than 5% (Figure 55-1). Other types of chronic leukemia, including those of lymphocytic and myelomonocytic cell lineages, are extremely rare in childhood.

Cure rates of pediatric leukemia have improved drastically over the past 50 years as knowledge of genetic and molecular factors of the disease have increased, supportive care has improved, and treatment strategies have become more sophisticated. For pediatric patients, 80% to 85% of patients with ALL and 50% to 60% of patients with AML are cured of their disease.

ETIOLOGY AND PATHOGENESIS

ALL occurs more frequently in boys and Caucasian children. The incidence peaks at 2 to 5 years, as shown in Figure 55-2. AML affects boys and girls equally, and pediatric incidence peaks in the neonatal and late adolescent periods (see Figure 55-2). In the United States, Hispanic and African American children are diagnosed with AML slightly more often than Caucasian children.

Leukemic cells are derived from hematopoietic stem cells that acquire genetic alterations that affect their ability to mature or undergo apoptosis, leading to perpetual self-renewal. The etiology of most of these mutations is unknown; however, certain environmental exposures, familial factors, genetic syndromes, and infectious diseases have been investigated as predisposing agents in childhood leukemia.

Studies of twins, neonatal blood spots (Guthrie cards), and cord blood are beginning to provide insight into the development of acute leukemia. In twin studies, concordance for all leukemias in monozygotic pairs is 5% to 25%; 10% in ALL and approaching 100% in infant leukemia. The extraordinarily high twin concordance rate for infant leukemia is attributed to blood chimerism of monochorionic twins. It is thought that the leukemia cells are passed from one twin to the other via a shared blood supply. This chimerism also occurs through placental vascular anastomoses in approximately 8% of dichorionic twin pairs.

Upon review of Guthrie cards of children who later developed leukemia, genetic mutations unique to leukemic clones were found to be present at birth, suggesting some leukemia may originate in utero. Because not all children with these mutations at birth develop leukemia, the mutations are believed to be necessary but not sufficient to induce leukemogenesis. Clearly, a second mutation and probably multiple sequences of mutations are required. Based on twin concordance studies, these latter mutations most likely occur postnatally.

Prenatal and postnatal genetic insults resulting in leukemia can be extrapolated to nontwin patients. A survey of hundreds of cord blood samples revealed that 1% had a functional TEL-AML1 gene (a common chromosomal translocation in pre B-cell ALL). This rate is 100 times that of clinically diagnosed ALL in the pediatric population. This serves as additional evidence that the genetic abnormalities found in cord blood at birth are not sufficient alone to result in the development of ALL.

Several environmental factors are associated with pediatric leukemia. These include ionizing radiation and chemotherapeutic agents, such as topoisomerase II inhibitors and alkylating agents. Other suspected environmental exposures include hydrocarbons such as benzene and pesticides leading to AML. Children with inherited genetic syndromes, including trisomy 21, Fanconi anemia, ataxia-telangiectasia, Wiskott-Aldrich syndrome, and neurofibromatosis type I, have an increased risk of developing acute leukemia.

Infectious agents have been proposed as playing a role in the development of leukemia, especially ALL. The peak age of incidence correlates with the age of first exposure to many infections for children in developed countries. Additionally, pediatric leukemia is more common in industrial regions of developed countries than in developing countries. It is thought that the later onset of exposure to infectious agents seen in developed countries results in an abnormally rapid immune cell proliferation and dysregulation. This hypothesis is also supported by several studies that compared infectious exposures of children who did and did not attend daycare early in life. The results showed that children with early daycare attendance and earlier exposure to infectious agents were less likely to develop ALL.

GENETICS

Although little is known about the cause of initial mutations in the hematopoietic stem cell DNA of leukemia cells, the resultant genetic abnormalities are well studied. Leukemia is caused by multiple disruptions in cell DNA leading to (1) impaired maturation, (2) unregulated proliferation, and (3) lack of programmed cell death (apoptosis). In combination, this leads to the abnormal survival of mutated hematopoietic progenitor cells and unregulated growth of dysfunctional lymphoblasts or myeloblasts.

Some of the mutations are caused by chromosomal translocations resulting in fusion proteins that bring activated kinases and altered transcription factors together inappropriately. TEL-AML1 is the most commonly identified chromosomal translocation in pediatric ALL. TEL-AML1 t(8;21) is the product of the TEL gene responsible for recruiting progenitor stem cells into the bone marrow and the AML1 gene that plays a central role in hematopoietic cell differentiation. The Philadelphia chromosome is the product of a translocation of chromosomes 9 and 22, which is found in 95% of patients with CML and 2%

Acute lymphoblastic leukemia

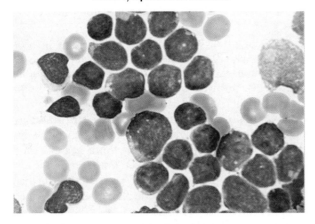

Acute myelogenous leukemia

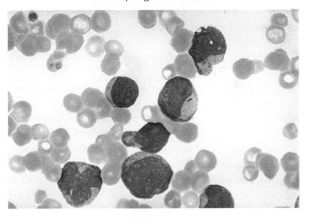

Chronic myelogenous leukemia

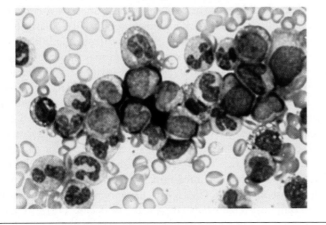

Figure 55-1 *Blood smears of leukemias.*

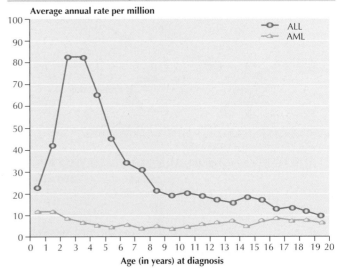

ALL and AML age-specific incidence rates, SEER*

Average annual rate per million

Age (in years) at diagnosis

Leukemia incidence rates by sex and race, SEER*		
Race/Ethnicity	**Male**	**Female**
All races	1.9 per 100,000 men	1.4 per 100,000 women
White	2.0 per 100,000 men	1.5 per 100,000 women
Black	1.1 per 100,000 men	0.8 per 100,000 women
Asian/Pacific Islander	1.6 per 100,000 men	1.3 per 100,000 women
American Indian/Alaska Native	1.3 per 100,000 men	
Hispanic	2.4 per 100,000 men	2.1 per 100,000 women

*All statistics in this report are based on SEER incidence statistics. Most can be found within:

Altekruse SF, Kosary CL, Krapcho M, et al. *SEER Cancer Statistics Review, 1975-2007,* National Cancer Institute. Bethesda, MD, http://seer.cancer.gov/csr/1975_2007/, based on Nov-ember 2009 SEER data submission, posted to the SEER web site, 2010.

Figure 55-2 *Incidence rates of acute lymphoblastic leukemia and acute myelogenous leukemia.*

of those with ALL. The translocation results in a fusion protein, BCR-ABL, which encodes a constitutively active tyrosine kinase protein. The tyrosine kinase activates proteins responsible for signaling within the cell cycle, therefore inducing uncontrolled cell proliferation, reducing apoptosis, and inhibiting DNA repair mechanisms (Figure 55-3). *MLL,* found on chromosome 11q23, partners with more than 40 genes and is found in childhood

AML, secondary (or therapy-induced) AML, and the majority of infant ALL. Because the *MLL* gene arrangement is associated with several types of leukemia, specifically secondary AML after prior topoisomerase II inhibitor exposure, investigators are evaluating environmental topoisomerase II exposures that might be responsible for in utero mutations resulting in infant leukemia.

The process of cytogenetic profiling involves evaluating leukemic blasts for both the number of chromosomes and specific translocations (see Figure 55-3). This information is used to classify leukemia subtypes and give prognostic information and is often part of treatment risk stratification algorithms. For example, in pre–B-cell ALL, hyperdiploidy (>50 chromosomes) is associated with a good prognosis. However, hypodiploidy (<45 chromosomes) signifies a poor prognosis. Patients with AML are considered to have good-risk disease if the leukemia cell contains t(8;21) and inv(16) mutations. Other genetic abnormalities such as monosomy 5 and 7 and abnormalities of 3q are considered unfavorable. As many as 40% of patients with AML have activating mutations within the *FLT3* gene,

Pathways affected by BCR-ABL

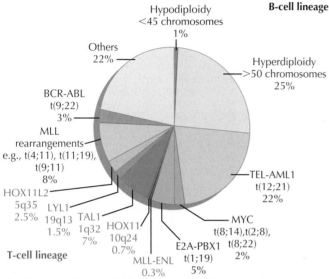

Many signal transduction pathways are influenced by the BCR-ABL tyrosine kinase. Interrupting these pathways results in uncontrolled cell proliferation, a halt in cell differentiation, and reduced apoptosis.

Estimated frequency of specific genotypes of ALL in children

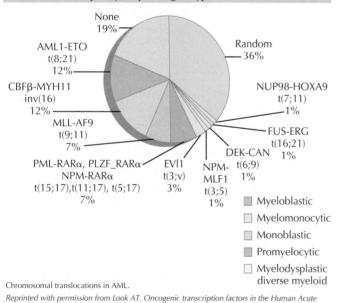

The genetic lesions that are exclusively seen in cases of T-cell lineage leukemias are indicated in purple. All other genetic subtypes are either exclusively or primarily seen in cases of B-cell lineage ALL.

Reprinted with permission from Pui CH, Relling MV, Downing JR. Acute lymphoblastic leukemia. N Engl J Med. 2004;350:1535-1548.

Estimated frequency of specific genotypes of AML in children

Chromosomal translocations in AML.

Reprinted with permission from Look AT. Oncogenic transcription factors in the Human Acute Leukemias. Science 1997;278:1059-1064.

Figure 55-3 *Genetics of acute lymphoblastic leukemia and acute myelogenous leukemia.*

which are known as internal tandem duplications (ITDs). Both increased number of ITDs and location within the *FLT3* gene are associated with poor clinical outcome.

High-resolution genetic analysis using single nucleotide polymorphism (SNP) array studies allow for more detailed profiling of additional genetic alterations. SNP arrays reveal mutations of genes involved in cell pathways such as lymphoid development, cell cycle regulation, apoptosis, and drug responsiveness. Clinically, this provides insight into the genotype and phenotype of leukemia and the underlying biology of the disease and can be associated with prognosis. SNP analysis can also follow the progression of genetic alterations during the disease course, which may predict response or resistance to therapy. SNP arrays have shown that genetic alterations in 60% of pre–B-cell ALL cases involve transcription factors that control B-cell differentiation. SNP analyses are increasingly important in providing clinical information about leukemia and have tremendous potential for discovering new molecular targets to treat specific leukemias.

CLINICAL PRESENTATION

Children with leukemia primarily present with symptoms of bone marrow failure. The leukemia cells overpopulate the marrow and prevent normal growth of other hematopoietic cells. Signs and symptoms of anemia include fatigue, headache, pallor, and tachycardia. Thrombocytopenia often presents with petechiae and easy bruising, and leukopenia results in infection and fevers. The crowding of the bone marrow can also cause bony pain, often mistaken for "growing pains" in school-aged children (Figure 55-4).

Other findings on physical examination are caused by leukemic infiltrate into normal tissues, such as the liver, spleen, lymph nodes, thymus, or testicles. The testicle is a common extramedullary site for ALL and may present as an enlargement of one or both testes. Leukemia cutis, or leukemic infiltration of the skin, has a varied presentation and may appear as single or multiple lesions commonly described as violaceous or hemorrhagic. Leukemia cutis most commonly presents in infant ALL and AML. Central nervous system (CNS) involvement at diagnosis is most often asymptomatic, but children with CNS disease may present with symptoms of increased intracranial pressure, visual disturbances, cranial nerve palsies, or gait disturbance. Other rare CNS effects not directly related to leukemic infiltration include intracranial hemorrhage and infarction. The presentation of CML can be very nonspecific and is often only suspected when a high white blood cell (WBC) count is seen on the complete blood count (CBC). Table 55-1 lists some of the life-threatening complications of leukemia at presentation and during therapy. Childhood leukemia presents similarly to many other common childhood illnesses (Table 55-2), and a bone marrow aspirate is necessary to make a definitive diagnosis.

EVALUATION

The initial laboratory evaluation should include a CBC with manual differential and basic metabolic panel including calcium

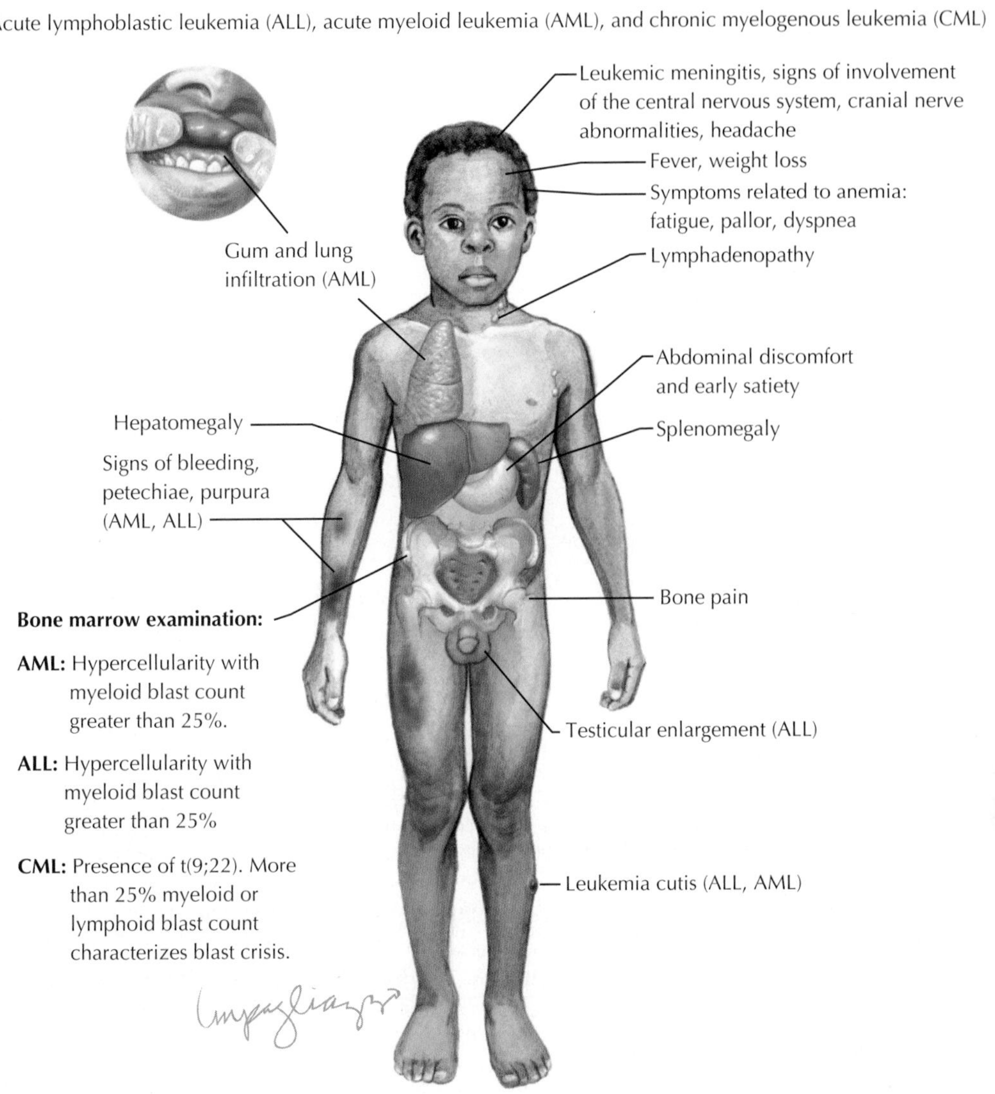

Acute lymphoblastic leukemia (ALL), acute myeloid leukemia (AML), and chronic myelogenous leukemia (CML)

Leukemic meningitis, signs of involvement of the central nervous system, cranial nerve abnormalities, headache

Fever, weight loss

Symptoms related to anemia: fatigue, pallor, dyspnea

Lymphadenopathy

Gum and lung infiltration (AML)

Abdominal discomfort and early satiety

Hepatomegaly

Splenomegaly

Signs of bleeding, petechiae, purpura (AML, ALL)

Bone pain

Bone marrow examination:

AML: Hypercellularity with myeloid blast count greater than 25%.

ALL: Hypercellularity with myeloid blast count greater than 25%

Testicular enlargement (ALL)

CML: Presence of t(9;22). More than 25% myeloid or lymphoid blast count characterizes blast crisis.

Leukemia cutis (ALL, AML)

Figure 55-4 *Clinical presentation of leukemia.*

and phosphorus, prothrombin time, partial thromboplastin time, fibrinogen, uric acid, and lactate dehydrogenase. Automated differentials are inadequate because myeloblasts are often identified as monocytes and lymphoblasts as atypical lymphocytes. Further laboratory testing may be necessary based on presenting signs and symptoms. Children with a suspected diagnosis of leukemia should be referred to a pediatric cancer center for stabilization, preparation for diagnostic procedures, and molecular testing.

Chest radiography should be performed before sedation or anesthesia is used to determine the presence of a mediastinal mass. A bone marrow aspirate and biopsy must be reviewed for morphology, immunohistochemistry, and cytogenetics (Figure 55-5). A lumbar puncture is also performed at diagnosis to determine the presence of leukemia within the CNS.

Morphologic review delineates the cell lineage and characteristics to classify the type of leukemia. Immunohistochemistry identifies specific cell surface cluster of differentiation (CD)

markers, which increases the accuracy of morphologic diagnosis. For example, B-cell precursor ALL blasts are known to express CD10, CD19, and CD20; AML blasts express CD13 and CD33. In some cases, morphology appears varied, and immunophenotyping may indicate a biphenotypic blast population with both lymphoid and myeloid blasts present. Identification of specific translocations and gene copy number alterations via karyotyping, fluorescence in situ hybridization, and SNP arrays indicate the cytogenetic profile of blast cells.

Specific molecular probes to known blast signatures have enabled monitoring of very small numbers of blast cells, or minimal residual disease (MRD), throughout therapy. Blasts may be detected at a level of 0.01%. This information is collected at regular intervals and used to tailor therapy or to predict relapse. MRD is a relatively new tool in leukemia therapy, and there is continued investigation into its clinical uses. The continued presence of MRD after the first 12 weeks of therapy is associated with a very poor prognosis.

Table 55-1 Life-threatening presentations of leukemia

Life-Threatening Presentation	Clinical Manifestations	Most Common Leukemia	Treatment
Infection or neutropenia	• Fever • Sepsis • Bacteremia • Typhlitis: necrotizing enterocolitis occurring in profoundly neutropenic patients	All types	• Blood cultures • Broad-spectrum antibiotics • Pressor support
Tumor lysis syndrome	• Rapid cell turnover leading to release of intracellular contents • Hyperuricemia, hyperkalemia, hyperphosphatemia, hypocalcemia • Renal failure	ALL • Elevated WBC at presentation • Burkitt leukemia • T-cell ALL	• Aggressive hydration • Alkalinize urine (bicarbonate-containing IV fluids) • Allopurinol/urate oxidase • Frequent monitoring of electrolytes and renal function
Hyperleukocytosis	• WBC > 100×10^3 • Hyperviscosity, sludging • CVA, renal insufficiency, pulmonary infarct	AML > ALL	• Exchange transfusion or leukapheresis • Treat leukemia rapidly
Hemorrhage or DIC	• CNS hemorrhage • Retinal hemorrhage • Thrombosis	APL (M3 AML)	• ATRA/chemotherapy • Blood product support
Airway compression or SVC syndrome	• Anterior mediastinal mass • Respiratory distress, cough, orthopnea • Headache, syncope • Facial swelling or plethora	T-cell ALL	• Chest radiography before sedation or anesthesia • Radiation therapy or steroids • Treat leukemia rapidly

ALL, acute lymphoblastic leukemia; AML, acute myelogenous leukemia; ATRA, all-trans retinoic acid; CNS, central nervous system; CVA, cerebrovascular accident; DIC, disseminated intravascular coagulation; IV, intravenous; SVC, superior vena cava.

Table 55-2 Presenting Signs and Symptoms of Common Childhood Illnesses that Mimic Leukemia

Disease	Anemia	Thrombocytopenia	Leukopenia	Leukocytosis	Fever	Hepatosplenomegaly	Bone Pain
Epstein-Barr virus	X		X	X	X	X	
Idiopathic thrombocytopenic purpura		X					
Juvenile inflammatory arthritis	X				X		X
Parvovirus	X		X		X		
Transient erythrocytopenia of childhood	X						
Aplastic anemia	X	X	X				
Pertussis				X	X		
Pneumococcus				X	X		

CLASSIFICATION

ALL is classified according to cell lineage as either B- or T-cell disease. B-cell disease is further categorized based on the level of differentiation of the B-cell involved (Table 55-3). Historically, the French-American-British (FAB) classification system divided ALL into three subtypes. Because this classification did not account for more sophisticated methods of immunophenotyping and cytogenetic profiling, it is no longer used. The FAB classification of AML is still in use and consists of subtypes M0 to M7 based on cell type and differentiation (Table 55-4).

Table 55-3 Acute Lymphoblastic Leukemia Subtypes and Frequency

Subtype	Frequency (%)
Early precursor B-cell	60-65
Precursor B-cell	20
Mature B-cell "Burkitt leukemia"	3
T-cell	15

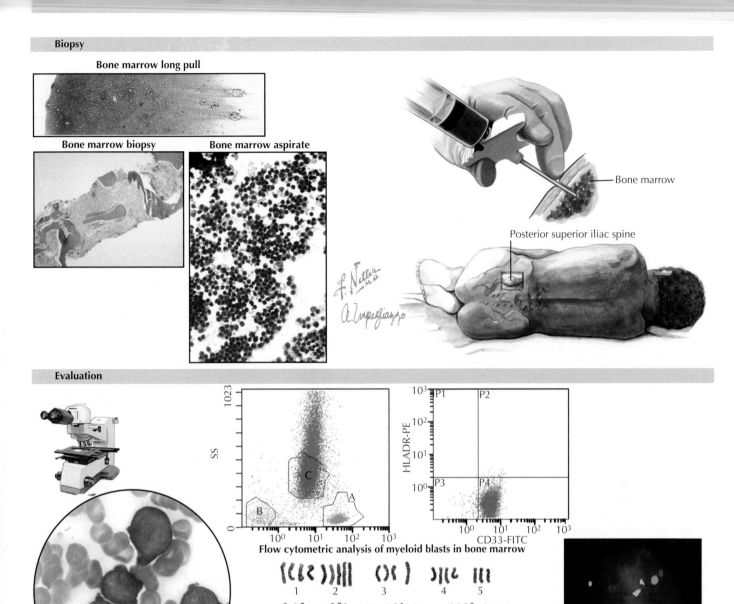

Biopsy

Bone marrow long pull

Bone marrow biopsy   Bone marrow aspirate

Bone marrow

Posterior superior iliac spine

Evaluation

Flow cytometric analysis of myeloid blasts in bone marrow

Positive myeloperoxidase staining in myeloid blasts

Conventional chromosome analysis showing 4 copies of many chromosomes

FISH results showing 3 copies of several chromosomes in ALL.

Figure 55-5 *Bone marrow biopsy.*

Subtype	Cell type	Details
M0	Undifferentiated stem cells	Very rare in children
M1	Immature myeloblasts	
M2	Slightly matured myeloblasts	Accounts for 25%-30% pediatric AML
M3	Promyelocytes (mature myeloblasts)	Also known as *acute promyelocytic leukemia*
M4	Immature monoblasts	Also known as *acute myelomonocytic leukemia*; most common in children younger than 2 years of age
M5	Monoblasts	Also known as *acute monocytic leukemia*; more common in children younger than 2 years of age
M6	Erythroblasts	Also known as *acute erythroblastic leukemia*; very rare in children
M7	Megakaryoblasts	Also known as *acute megakaryoblastic leukemia*

Table 55-4 Acute Myelogenous Leukemia Classification Based on Cell Type

AML, acute myelogenous leukemia.

CML classification is based on disease phase: chronic phase, accelerated phase, or blast crisis. Each phase requires specific monitoring and therapy. Most pediatric patients are diagnosed in the chronic phase, often resulting in mild symptoms. If untreated, the disease will progress to the accelerated phase. The accelerated phase is established based on one of the following parameters: thrombocytopenia, refractory thrombocytosis, increasing splenomegaly or leukocytosis, new cytogenetic abnormalities, or increasing blast load (10%-19%). The accelerated phase indicates progression of disease and impending blast crisis. Blast crisis occurs when there are more than 20% blasts in peripheral blood or bone marrow or when an extramedullary leukemic infiltrate develops.

MANAGEMENT AND PROGNOSIS

Acute Lymphoblastic Leukemia

As the survival rate of children with ALL improves, the goals of therapy include decreasing the toxicity of treatment for low-risk patients and escalating or targeting therapy for high-risk patients. Patients are considered high risk based on clinical characteristics, which are WBC greater than 50×10^3 or age older than 10 years at diagnosis. All others are defined as standard risk. Children younger than 1 year of age are considered to have infant ALL and undergo more intensive chemotherapy than their older counterparts. CNS or testicular involvement at diagnosis and slow early response to treatment are high-risk features, and intensified therapy is recommended for these groups. Molecular features, including immunophenotypic and cytogenetic profile, and MRD further define risk, prognosis, and need for treatment intensification.

ALL therapy in the United States generally consists of five phases: induction, consolidation, interim maintenance, delayed intensification, and maintenance, for a total duration of 2.5 to 3 years depending upon gender. ALL induction therapy has an excellent rate of remission (>99%) and a very low mortality rate from toxicity (<1%). Induction therapy is a 4-week phase and includes a steroid, vincristine, and asparaginase. Anthracycline therapy is added for high-risk patients. Methotrexate, given intrathecally, is used for CNS chemoprophylaxis in all patients with ALL. Cranial irradiation is added for high-risk patients and those with CNS involvement. Intensive outpatient chemotherapy continues for the first 6 to 8 months. The mainstay of ALL maintenance chemotherapy is low-dose oral 6-mercaptopurine and methotrexate as well as vincristine associated with a 5-day steroid pulses.

The 5-year survival rate for ALL is 80% to 85%. The prognosis depends on the factors that determine risk and the response to appropriate risk-stratified therapy.

Acute Myelogenous Leukemia

AML therapy also begins with induction but is much more intensive and often requires inpatient management. Eighty-five percent of patients achieve a remission at the end of induction. For those with favorable cytogenetics (t(8;21), inv(16)), chemotherapy is continued for five intensive cycles. Poor-risk patients (defined by unfavorable cytogenetics such as monosomy 5 or 7, high *FLT3* ITD ratio, or poor response to therapy) and

intermediate-risk patients with a human leukocyte antigen-matched related donor proceed to bone marrow transplant after three cycles of chemotherapy. Those without HLA-matched donors receive either several additional courses of chemotherapy or a bone marrow transplant from an unrelated donor.

The 5-year survival rate for AML is 50% to 60%. Prognosis largely depends on the ability to achieve remission and proceed to hematopoietic stem cell transplant with an appropriate donor.

Chronic Myelogenous Leukemia

Traditionally, children and adolescents with CML were treated with hydroxyurea for cytoreduction and best donor stem cell transplant. Now first-line therapy for chronic-phase CML is imatinib, a drug that inhibits the BCR-ABL tyrosine kinase, expressed in CML. Imatinib induces a complete molecular remission in more than 95% of CML patients, although the duration of remission in children is unknown. The only cure for patients in blast phase is chemotherapy and bone marrow transplantation. Imatinib combined with chemotherapy has also improved the outcome for *BCR-ABL*–positive ALL, which formerly had a dismal prognosis.

RELAPSE

Whereas patients with ALL have a 15% to 20% chance of relapse, 40% to 50% of patients with AML will relapse. The treatment and prognosis depend on the timing of relapse (early or late), site of relapse (bone marrow or extramedullary), and specific disease characteristics. Most children who relapse are given intensive reinduction chemotherapy to achieve remission and proceed to stem cell transplant. Isolated extramedullary relapse (CNS or testicular) may also require local radiation. Survival after relapse ranges from 10% in children who relapse during intensive therapy to 70% in children with isolated CNS or testicular relapse.

FUTURE DIRECTIONS

It is unlikely that classic cytotoxic therapy for treating acute leukemias can be intensified, especially in patients with AML. As we understand the molecular and genetic abnormalities that drive hematologic malignancies, we identify targets to kill these cells. Imatinib was the first targeted small molecule created to inhibit the abnormal BCR-ABL tyrosine kinase found in CML. Monoclonal antibodies are targeting the cell-specific proteins found on flow cytometry such as CD-33 (gentuzumab; Mylotarg) and CD-22 (epratuzumab), thereby avoiding generalized toxicity. *FLT3* inhibitors are being tested on infant MLL rearranged leukemias and AML. Oncologists are increasingly more successful at identifying high-risk patients who do not respond adequately to traditional chemotherapy. However, newer, targeted therapies still need to be identified in order to improve the cure rate for pediatric leukemia.

SUGGESTED READINGS

Bailey LC, Lange BJ, Rheingold SR, et al: Bone-marrow relapse in paediatric acute lymphoblastic leukaemia, *Lancet Oncol* 9(9):873-883, 2008.

Belson M, Kingsley B, Holmes A: Risk factors for acute leukemia in children: a review, *Environ Health Perspect* 115(1):138-145, 2007.

Campana D: Status of minimal residual disease testing in childhood haematological malignancies, *Br J Haematol* 143(4):481-489, 2008.

Gilham C, Peto J, Simpson J, et al: Day care in infancy and risk of childhood acute lymphoblastic leukaemia: findings from UK case-control study, *BMJ* 330(7503):1294, 2005.

Greaves MF, Maia AT, Wiemels JL, et al: Leukemia in twins: lessons in natural history, *Blood* 102(7):2321-2333, 2003.

Kantarjian H, Schiffer C, Jones D, et al: Monitoring the response and course of chronic myeloid leukemia in the modern era of BCR-ABL tyrosine kinase inhibitors: practical advice on the use and interpretation of monitoring methods, *Blood* 111:1774-1780, 2008.

Mullighan CG: Genomic analysis of acute leukemia, *Int J Lab Hematol* 31(4):384-397, 2009.

Pui CH, Robison LL, Look AT: Acute lymphoblastic leukaemia, *Lancet* 371(9617):1030-1043, 2008.

Pui CH, Relling MV, Downing JR: Acute lymphoblastic leukemia, *N Engl J Med* 350(15):1535-1548, 2004.

Pui CH, Schrappe M, Ribeiro RC, et al: Childhood and adolescent lymphoid and myeloid leukemia, *Hematol Am Soc Hematol Educ Program* Jan:118-145, 2004.

Rubnitz JE, Gibson B, Smith FO: Acute myeloid leukemia, *Pediatr Clinic of North Am* 55(1):21-51, 2008.

Smith MA, Ries LA, Gurney JG, et al: Leukemia. In Ries LAG, Smith MA, Gurney JG, et al, editors: *Cancer Incidence and Survival Among Children and Adolescents: United States SEER Program 1975-1995, NIH Pub. No. 99-4649.* Bethesda, MD, 1999, National Cancer Institute, SEER Program.

Lymphomas

Dana Sepe and Leslie Kersun

56

Lymphomas are malignant neoplasms of the lymphoid tissue and include Hodgkin's lymphoma (HL) and non-Hodgkin's lymphoma (NHL). They are the third most common type of pediatric cancer after leukemia and malignant brain tumors. In the United States, approximately 1700 children and adolescents younger than the age of 20 years are diagnosed with lymphomas each year. This is roughly 15% of the malignancies diagnosed in this age group. This chapter focuses on the presentation, diagnosis, evaluation, and management of children and adolescents with HL and NHL.

HODGKIN'S LYMPHOMA

ETIOLOGY AND PATHOGENESIS

HL is a B-cell malignancy that affects the reticuloendothelial and lymphatic systems. In addition, HL can affect other organ systems including the lungs, bone marrow, bone, liver, and rarely the central nervous system (CNS). The World Health Organization classification divides HL into classical HL (nodular sclerosis, lymphocyte rich, mixed cellularity, and lymphocyte depleted), which accounts for 90% of cases, and nodular lymphocyte predominant HL.

Previous epidemiologic studies suggest that the etiology of HL may be multifactorial and that environmental, genetic, and immunologic factors play a role in the development of the disease. Several studies have documented a link between HL and Epstein-Barr virus (EBV). The idea of this association was first proposed in 1966, and through modern molecular study techniques, it has been found that EBV DNA is expressed in the Hodgkin and Reed-Sternberg cells of 50% and 95% of the cases of HL in developed and developing countries, respectively. EBV is mostly associated with the mixed cellularity type of HL, shows a male predominance, and is more frequent in patients younger than 10 years of age.

Clustering of HL in families suggests a genetic predisposition to HL, with an increased incidence especially among same-sex siblings, monozygotic twins, and parent–child pairs. There is a three- to ninefold increased risk of HL among family members of patients affected by the disease, which leads to the hypothesis that at least a small proportion of cases are inherited.

CLINICAL PRESENTATION

The clinical presentation of HL can be varied but in most cases is asymptomatic. Approximately 70% to 80% of patients present with firm, rubbery, painless cervical lymphadenopathy. Often, patients will have been placed on antibiotics for presumed adenitis without improvement in the lymphadenopathy. Sixty percent of patients have mediastinal disease and may present with cough, chest pain, shortness of breath, orthopnea, or

superior vena cava (SVC) syndrome. However, patients can also have mediastinal involvement without any symptoms. It is therefore important to image this area for disease before any diagnostic procedures given the risk of sedation or anesthesia in this setting. Cytokine production by Hodgkin and Reed-Sternberg cells is believed to be responsible for many of the nonspecific systemic symptoms of HL commonly seen at diagnosis, including fatigue, weight loss, pruritus, urticaria, and anorexia.

Approximately 30% of patients present with at least one constitutional, or B, symptom. These include unexplained fevers of greater than 38°C for at least 3 days, unexplained weight loss of at least 10% within the preceding 6 months before diagnosis, and drenching night sweats. These symptoms are indicative of more advanced disease and have prognostic implications for the patient. The presence of B symptoms often places the patient in a higher risk group category for the purpose of determining appropriate treatment.

Physical examination of any patient suspected of having HL should include a thorough evaluation of all lymph node chains; the presence of hepatosplenomegaly; and signs of bone marrow involvement, including bruising, petechiae, and pallor.

The differential diagnosis for HL includes various infections, other malignancies, and other causes of lymphadenopathy (Table 56-1).

EVALUATION AND STAGING

Evaluation of HL should include a detailed history and physical examination, focusing specifically on the previously mentioned typical presenting signs and symptoms. Urgent signs and symptoms, such as cough, chest pain, orthopnea, bruising, and pallor should be evaluated promptly. Specific laboratory and radiographic tests and diagnostic procedures need to be performed to treat the patient and stage the disease. These include a complete blood count (CBC); erythrocyte sedimentation rate; comprehensive metabolic panel; chest radiograph; computed tomography (CT) scans of the neck, chest, abdomen, and pelvis; and a positron emission tomography (PET) scan to assess for disseminated disease. A bone marrow aspirate and biopsy is performed in certain cases.

Staging of pediatric HL is based on the Ann Arbor Classification and is outlined in Figure 56-1.

MANAGEMENT

Radiation therapy was the first curative modality for the treatment of HL. However, the high doses of radiation needed to cure HL as monotherapy resulted in side effects such as bone growth retardation, cardiac toxicity, and secondary malignancies in the radiation field. Therefore, response-based, low-dose, involved-field radiation is used as adjuvant treatment after chemotherapy.

Table 56-1 Differential Diagnosis of Hodgkin's and Non-Hodgkin's Lymphoma

	Hodgkin's Lymphoma	Non-Hodgkin's Lymphoma
Infections	Lymphadenitis	Lymphadenitis
	Cat scratch disease	Cat scratch disease
	Mononucleosis, EBV, CMV	Mononucleosis, EBV, CMV
	Brucellosis	Tuberculosis
	Tuberculosis	Toxoplasmosis
	Toxoplasmosis	Atypical mycobacterial infections
	Atypical mycobacterial infections	Appendicitis
Malignances	ALL	ALL
	Rhabdomyosarcoma	AML
	Germ cell tumors	Neuroblastoma
	Lymphoproliferative disorders	Rhabdomyosarcoma
		Wilms' tumor
		Lymphoproliferative disorders
Other	Bronchogenic cyst	Intussusception
	Lipoma	Sarcoidosis
	Teratoma	

ALL, acute lymphoblastic leukemia; AML, acute myelogenous leukemia; CMV, cytomegalovirus; EBV, Epstein-Barr virus.

Current treatment for pediatric HL is based on risk-adapted therapy and includes chemotherapy, radiation, or both. Two principles were critical for the development of chemotherapy treatment regimens for HL. First, multiple chemotherapeutic agents with different mechanisms of action are used to circumvent potential drug resistance. In addition, the treatment is structured to avoid combinations of medications with overlapping toxicities. Common agents used to treat HL include bleomycin, vinblastine/vincristine, etoposide, procarbazine, prednisone, methotrexate, doxorubicin, and cyclophosphamide. The combination and doses of medications depend on risk stratification. Table 56-2 depicts the current risk stratification system for The Children's Oncology Group; however, there may be small differences in this scheme for patients treated in other countries or cooperative groups.

HL has an excellent prognosis, with a 5-year overall survival (OS) for all patients (early stage or advanced disease) of approximately 90%. There is a subset of patients with disease recurrence who are subsequently cured because there are good salvage regimens for relapsed HL. Cure rates after relapse depend on the time from initial therapy, amount of initial therapy received (chemotherapy alone vs. chemotherapy and radiation therapy), and stage of relapsed disease. In particular, early relapses (<12 months from initial therapy) at more advanced stages with more initial therapy have a worse prognosis than later relapses with less initial therapy. Therapy for relapsed HL includes salvage chemotherapy, and depending on the aforementioned factors, can then be followed by high-dose chemotherapy and autologous stem cell transplant.

The general side effects of chemotherapy include nausea and vomiting, hair loss, mouth sores, and myelosuppression. However, each agent has specific acute and late toxicities that are important to carefully monitor during treatment and then follow for years after the completion of therapy. The late effects of therapy include pulmonary fibrosis (secondary to bleomycin exposure), cardiomyopathy (secondary to anthracycline therapy with doxorubicin, mediastinal radiation, or both) and infertility (secondary to alkylating agents like cyclophosphamide and procarbazine) and depend on the total cumulative dose of these medications. In addition, musculoskeletal and thyroid toxicity (secondary to radiation exposure) are of particular concern, with as many as 50% of survivors of HL experiencing hypothyroidism 10 years after treatment. Furthermore, approximately 30% of survivors of HL will develop a second malignant neoplasm (SMN) within 30 years after their initial treatment, with the most common SMNs being thyroid cancer, breast cancer, nonmelanomatous skin cancer, and NHL.

FUTURE DIRECTIONS

Future directions include evaluating the role of PET scan for diagnosis and follow-up of HL. In addition, in an attempt to decrease late effects of therapy while maintaining or improving upon the current excellent OS in HL, research and future studies are focusing on response-based therapy and targeted agents. Currently, targeted agents such as rituximab (anti-CD 20), bortezomib (NF-κB transcription factor inhibitor), SGN-30 (anti-CD 30), and SGN-35 (antibody–drug conjugate of tubulin inhibitor monomethyl auristatin E conjugated anti-CD30) are being studied.

Table 56-2 Risk Stratification of Patients with Hodgkin's Lymphoma

Risk Category	Stages
Low risk	IA, IIA; no bulk disease*
Intermediate risk	IA and IIA with bulk disease*
	All IB and IIB
	All IIIA and IVA
High risk	All IIIB and IVB

*Bulk disease is defined as a mediastinal mass greater than 33% of the chest width or any nodal aggregate that is larger than 6 cm.

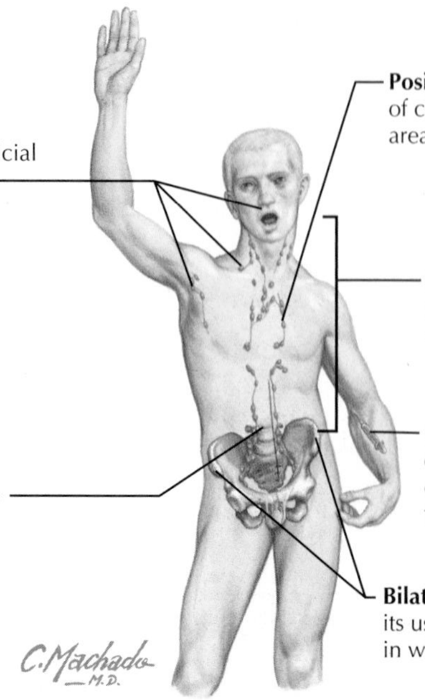

Physical examination including superficial lymph nodes and Waldeyer's ring

Positron emission tomography (PET) is the scan of choice to evaluate disease activity in involved areas.

Computed tomography (CT scan) with oral and intravenous contrast to evaluate chest/abdomen/pelvis and neck

Initial laboratory testing CBC with differential, erythrocyte sedimentation rate (ESR), electrolyte/chemistry panel, renal/liver function testing.

Lumbar puncture is used as part of the staging for patients with NHL.

Bilateral marrow aspiration/biopsy in most patients, its use is debated with early-stage, asymptomatic HL, in which it is rarely positive

C. Machado _M.D.

Ann Arbor Classification
Stage I
Involvement of a single lymph node region (I) or of a single extralymphatic organ or site (IE)
Stage II
Involvement of two or more lymph node regions on the same side of the diaphragm (II) or localized involvement of extralymphatic organ or site and of one or more lymph node regions on the same side of the diaphragm (IIE)
Stage III
Involvement of lymph node regions on both sides of the diaphragm (III), which may also be accompanied by localized involvement of extralymphatic organ or site (IIIE) or by involvement of the spleen (IIIS) or both (IIISE)
Stage IV
Diffuse or disseminated involvement of one or more extralymphatic organs or tissues with or without associated lymph node enlargement
Certain symptoms are commonly associated with lymphoma: * Night sweats   * Temperature > 38.5°C   * Weight loss > 10%   These are called "B" symptoms and are included in the stage designated to a patient. For instance, a patient with involved lymph nodes in the neck and under the arms only, and without any of the "B" symptoms, has stage IIA disease. The same patient with night sweats has stage IIB disease.

Figure 56-1 *Malignant lymphomas: staging.*

NON-HODGKIN'S LYMPHOMA

ETIOLOGY AND PATHOGENESIS

Pediatric NHLs are a diverse group of lymphoid neoplasms with varied pathology, cells of origin, natural history, and response to treatment. They arise from both mature and immature cells of both B- and T-cell origin. The four most common pathologic subtypes of pediatric NHL are Burkitt's lymphoma (BL), diffuse large B-cell lymphoma (DLBCL), anaplastic large cell lymphoma (ALCL), and lymphoblastic lymphomas (LL). There are rare and cutaneous types of pediatric NHL in addition to lymphoproliferative disorders that are not discussed in this chapter.

In developed countries, most individuals with NHL have no known cause. However, it is known that patients who are immunosuppressed, such as those with HIV or those who have undergone bone marrow transplantation, are at increased risk of developing NHL. In addition, patients who have been treated previously for HL are at higher risk of developing a secondary NHL. This appears to be an effect of the chemotherapy and radiotherapy of the HL treatment, as well as the immunosuppressive effects of the HL itself. In sub-Saharan Africa, there is a strong association between previous infection with malaria and EBV and the development of endemic BL.

CLINICAL PRESENTATION

Pediatric NHL usually presents acutely to subacutely, in contrast to many adult lymphomas, which are indolent. Constitutional symptoms are rare in NHL, with the exception of ALCL.

Table 56-3 Murphy Staging System of Non-Hodgkin's Lymphoma

Stage	Definition
I	A single tumor (extranodal) or single anatomic area (nodal), excluding mediastinum or abdomen
II	A single tumor (extranodal) with regional node involvement; or a primary GI tract tumor with or without associated mesenteric node involvement, grossly completely resected; or, on the same side of the diaphragm, two or more nodal areas or two single (extranodal) tumors with or without regional node involvement
III	All primary intrathoracic tumors (mediastinal, pleural, thymic); or all extensive primary intraabdominal disease that is unresectable; or all primary paraspinal or epidural tumors regardless of other sites; or on both sides of the diaphragm, two single tumors (extranodal) or two or more nodal areas
IV	Any of the above with initial CNS or bone marrow involvement (<25%)

CNS, central nervous system; GI, gastrointestinal.

Localized disease can manifest as lymphadenopathy or as a mass in any location. Patients with mediastinal involvement may complain of cough, chest pain, and dyspnea, and those with abdominal involvement may complain of constipation, abdominal pain, or distension. Focal bony pain or swelling may be present in patients with bone lymphoma and those with CNS involvement may develop altered mental status, meningismus, back pain, headache, or cranial nerve findings.

In general, patients with NHL look mild to moderately ill and can have pallor, dyspnea, cough, pain, and fever. Patients with a mediastinal mass can develop SVC syndrome and can have distended neck veins and plethora on physical examination. In addition, there are typical findings that can vary by subtype of NHL. For instance, BL tends to have a high growth fraction and can present as intussusception secondary to a rapidly growing abdominal mass. Nearly 75% of LL patients present with a mediastinal mass. Patients with ALCL sometimes present with painful skin lesions that may regress spontaneously, bone lesions, peripheral lymphadenopathy (especially inguinal), and hepatosplenomegaly.

The differential diagnosis of NHL can be found in Table 56-1.

EVALUATION AND STAGING

The evaluation for NHL is similar to that of HL and should include a CBC with differential as a preliminary screen for bone marrow involvement, as well as a comprehensive metabolic panel to look at renal and hepatic function. In particular, because BL can grow rapidly and there may be significant tumor burden at the time of initial presentation, tumor lysis can be of great concern. It is important to check an initial potassium, phosphorus, calcium, uric acid, blood urea nitrogen, and creatinine and to follow these levels closely before and during the initial treatment period. It is also standard practice to obtain a lumbar puncture with CSF differential to assess for CNS involvement and bilateral bone marrow aspirates and biopsies to evaluate spread into the marrow and differentiate certain types of NHL from leukemia. In addition, a radiographic evaluation is necessary for staging of the disease. This evaluation should include a neck, chest, abdomen, and pelvis CT scan and a PET CT.

In B-cell lymphomas, the primary presentation is not confined to a specific organ, nor is there a specific pattern of spread. Therefore, staging systems for NHL reflect tumor volume more than the degree of spread from the primary site. Several staging systems have been established for NHL. However, the Murphy staging system is the most widely accepted (Table 56-3).

MANAGEMENT

Patients with NHL are at risk for developing tumor lysis syndrome (TLS) both before and during the initial phases of chemotherapy because this can be a highly proliferative and bulky group of malignancies. TLS develops from the rapid turnover of malignant cells and the release of their contents, leading to hyperkalemia, hyperphosphatemia, and hyperuricemia. To prevent TLS, patients with NHL should be aggressively hydrated with alkalinized fluids containing sodium bicarbonate. These fluids should not contain potassium. If patients have evidence of renal insufficiency or oliguria at diagnosis, this balance of aggressive fluid management and potential need for dialysis should be discussed early with the nephrology team. In addition, patients should be placed on allopurinol to lower or prevent an increase in uric acid. Some patients in high-risk situations, including extreme elevations of uric acid or impaired renal function at time of presentation, may require the administration of rasburicase (a recombinant urate oxidase) to decrease their uric acid levels.

Current treatment for NHL includes combination chemotherapy, including medications directed at prevention of CNS recurrence. The backbone of therapy for pediatric NHL includes cyclophosphamide, methotrexate, and vincristine with the addition of various other agents depending on the subtype and staging of the disease. In addition, intrathecal chemotherapy is a crucial component of therapy and is given to patients with LL and those with a risk for CNS recurrence or CNS involvement at diagnosis.

The overall prognosis for NHL varies by stage at diagnosis and subtype. In patients with stage I and II mature B-cell NHL (BL and DLBCL) disease, there is a more than 90% disease-free survival (DFS) rate with chemotherapy alone. In patients with advanced disease (stage III or IV, bone marrow or CNS involvement), the OS is 80% to 90% with chemotherapy alone. With LL, neither the stage nor phenotype (T cell vs. B cell) seems to be a prognostic factor. DFS in LL is approximately 85%. However, in less favorable subgroups, such as BL with combined bone marrow and CNS involvement, primary mediastinal DLBCL, and in a certain subset of patients with systemic ALCL, the DFS ranges from 45% to 70%.

FUTURE DIRECTIONS

Great advancements have been made in the area of NHL research with current treatment leading to an overall DFS of greater than 80%. However, these therapies do not come without significant toxicity and late effects. Therefore, future directions in the field of NHL research include trying to better risk stratify patients such that low-risk patients can have a reduced-intensity treatment protocol. In addition, this would allow for high-risk patients to perhaps receive novel therapeutics earlier in their treatment course because salvage for relapsed or refractory NHL is difficult. Novel therapeutics would include biologically targeted agents, such as monoclonal antibodies and immunotherapy, which are currently under investigation. Finally, improved therapy targeting the CNS is undergoing investigation because patients with initial involvement of the CNS have a low OS compared with other groups.

SUGGESTED READINGS

Gross TG, Termuhlen AM: Pediatric non-Hodgkin's lymphoma, *Curr Oncol Rep* 9(6):459-465, 2007.

Olson MR, Donaldson SS: Treatment of pediatric Hodgkin lymphoma, *Curr Treat Options Oncol* 9:81-94, 2008.

Smith MA, Ries LA, Gurney JG, et al: Leukemia. In Ries LAG, Smith MA, Gurney JG, et al, editors: *Cancer Incidence and Survival Among Children and Adolescents: United States SEER Program 1975-1995, NIH Pub. No. 99-4649.* Bethesda, MD, 1999, National Cancer Institute, SEER Program.

Thomas RK, Re D, Zander T, Wolf J, Diehl V: Epidemiology and etiology of Hodgkin's lymphoma, *Ann Oncol* 13(suppl 4):147-152, 2002.

Weinstein HJ, Hudson MM, Link MP: *Pediatric Lymphomas.* Heidelberg, Germany, 2007, Springer.

Brain Tumors

57

Angela J. Sievert and Jane E. Minturn

*T*umors of the central nervous system (CNS) are the most common solid tumors of childhood and the primary source of cancer-related morbidity and mortality in this age group. Benign and malignant tumors may be equally life threatening because of an unfavorable location in the brain or spinal cord and the inability to safely achieve a surgical resection. Survival rates have improved significantly over the past 2 decades because of improvements in neuroimaging, neurosurgical techniques, radiation therapy, chemotherapy, and supportive care.

Nearly half of all childhood brain tumors arise infratentorially—in the brainstem, cerebellum, and fourth ventricle—and are classified according to histology. The most common malignant brain tumor is medulloblastoma, and the most common benign brain tumor is low-grade glioma. A discussion of the common pediatric tumors with emphasis on evaluation, management, and prognosis is outlined in this chapter.

ETIOLOGY AND PATHOGENESIS

Central nervous system tumors represent approximately 20% of all childhood cancers with 2.5 to 4 cases diagnosed per 100,000 children per year. There is a slight male predominance (male:female ratio, 1.29) at all ages younger than 20 years, and infratentorial location is more common in children 1 to 15 years of age.

The etiology of most childhood brain tumors is unknown. Specific genetic syndromes, such as neurofibromatosis (NF1 and NF2), tuberous sclerosis, and Li-Fraumeni and Turcot's syndromes, are associated with a higher incidence of tumors, but this group represents fewer than 10% of pediatric brain tumors. The only known environmental risk factor related to the development of brain tumors is exposure to ionizing radiation. Other exposures such as maternal diet during pregnancy, viral infections, cell phone use, and exposure to magnetic fields have been studied extensively with limited and conflicting data for an association with brain tumor risk.

Understanding the origin of brain tumors has been enhanced by the ability to detect specific molecular genetic alterations in tumor samples and the association of brain tumor development with inherited genetic disorders in which the gene defect is known. This has contributed to our understanding of the underlying biology of brain tumor initiation and progression and has led to the identification of therapeutic targets for drug development.

CLINICAL PRESENTATION

The presenting symptoms of a brain tumor are determined by tumor location rather than histology. Brain tumors may present with either generalized or localizing symptoms. Generalized symptoms are caused by obstruction of cerebrospinal fluid (CSF) with associated hydrocephalus and increased intracranial pressure (ICP). Increased ICP is more common with fourth ventricular or posterior fossa, pineal, suprasellar, and tectal tumors. Symptoms include headache (particularly in the morning), nausea, vomiting, and fatigue. On examination, paresis of upgaze, sixth cranial nerve palsies, and papilledema are often seen. In infants, macrocephaly, tense fontanelle, failure to thrive, developmental delay, and paresis of upgaze with downward eye deviation ("sun setting") are common. Posterior fossa tumors, such as cerebellar astrocytomas, often present with increased ICP (Figure 57-1).

Localizing symptoms depend on tumor location. Cerebellar tumors commonly present with ataxia and dysmetria. Brainstem tumors may cause cranial nerve deficits (diplopia, facial weakness, swallowing deficits), unsteadiness, and weakness (see Figure 57-1). Symptoms from hemispheric cortical tumors include seizures, hemiparesis, visual field deficits, and changes in behavior or school performance. Tumors in the suprasellar region often present with bitemporal visual field loss, decreased acuity, and hormonal dysfunction. Pineal region tumors frequently compress the tectal region of the brainstem and result in Parinaud's syndrome, characterized by paresis of upgaze, convergence nystagmus, pupils that respond better to accommodation than light (light-near dissociation), and eyelid retraction. Tumors of the spinal cord (primary or metastatic) may cause back pain, extremity weakness, sensory dysfunction, and bowel or bladder dysfunction. The most common presenting signs and symptoms are outlined in Table 57-1.

DIFFERENTIAL DIAGNOSIS

The clinical presentation can aid in localizing a brain tumor, and the anatomic location of a mass often narrows the differential diagnosis of the tumor type. Histologic confirmation is necessary in nearly all brain tumor cases with the exception of diffuse intrinsic brainstem (pontine) glioma, tectal glioma, and optic pathway gliomas in patients with NF1, in which neuroimaging alone can be sufficient for diagnosis. The differential diagnosis of brain tumors according to intracranial location is presented in Table 57-2.

EVALUATION AND MANAGEMENT

When a brain tumor is suspected, neuroimaging is the initial diagnostic test to obtain. Computed tomography (CT) is often the first imaging obtained because of its speed and availability and will detect nearly 95% of brain tumors. CT is useful as a rapid study to evaluate for hydrocephalus, hemorrhage, or the presence of calcifications in the tumor. However, because of its higher resolution, magnetic resonance imaging (MRI) with and without gadolinium is the established standard for diagnosis. Children with a brain tumor confirmed by MRI should be stabilized and referred to a tertiary hospital with experienced pediatric subspecialists in neurosurgery, neuro-oncology, and neuroradiology. The management of brain tumors depends on

Cystic astrocytoma of cerebellum

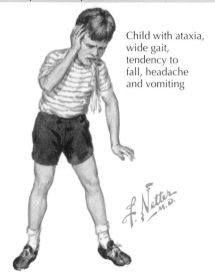

Child with ataxia, wide gait, tendency to fall, headache and vomiting

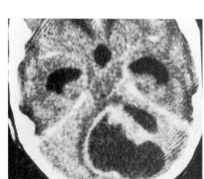

CT scan showing cystic tumor of cerebellum with nodule

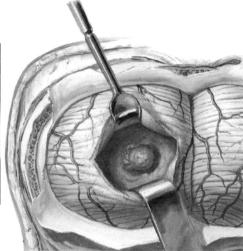

Cyst opened, revealing nodular tumor

Brain glioma

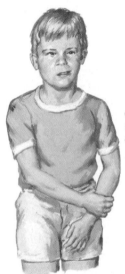

Child with sixth and seventh cranial nerve palsy on side of tumor and contralateral limb weakness

Glioma distorting brainstem and cranial nerves VI, VII, VIII

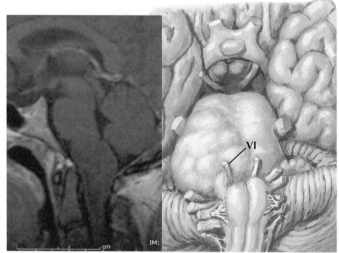

Sagittal MR T1-weighted image shows expansion of medulla to the pons

VI

Figure 57-1 *Clinical presentation of brain tumors.*

Table 57-1 Signs and Symptoms Associated with Intracranial Tumors
Headache
Vomiting
Seizure
Focal neurologic deficits (ataxia, diplopia, visual field cut, hemiparesis)
Triad of increased intracranial pressure (AM headaches, nausea, vomiting)
Meningismus
Neuroendocrine dysfunction

histology, tumor location and extent, and patient age but typically involves surgery, chemotherapy, and radiation therapy. Surgery for histology and to attempt maximal tumor debulking by an experienced pediatric neurosurgeon is required in most cases.

After surgery and histologic diagnosis, further studies are needed to stage the tumor. A postoperative MRI with and without gadolinium should be done within 24 to 48 hours after surgery to determine if residual tumor remains. The MRI must be repeated within this time frame so postoperative inflammatory changes are not confused for residual tumor or vice versa. For tumors with a high likelihood of spread via the CSF, complete multiplanar spine MRI and large-volume lumbar puncture for cytology should be performed. Medulloblastoma, the most

Table 57-2 Differential Diagnosis of Brain Tumors by Location

Location	Tumor
Cerebral hemisphere	Glioma
	Ependymoma
	PNET
Pineal	Germ cell tumor
	Glioma (tectal glioma)
	Pineoblastoma
	Pineocytoma
Cerebellum	Pilocytic astrocytoma
	Medulloblastoma
	Ependymoma
Brainstem	Glioma
Suprasellar	Craniopharyngioma
	Visual (optic) pathway glioma
	Germ cell tumor
	Pituitary tumor
Spinal Cord	Astrocytoma
	Ependymoma

PNET, primitive neuroectodermal tumor.

common malignant tumor in children, must be evaluated in this fashion (Figure 57-2). CSF and serum for the tumor markers α-fetoprotein and quantitative β-HCG should be sent if a germ cell tumor is diagnosed. Last, laboratory assessment of the hypothalamic–pituitary axis should be evaluated for any tumor involving the suprasellar region. Panhypopituitarism, including life-threatening diabetes insipidus, can be a relatively common postoperative complication in these children.

Treatment is tailored to specific tumor type and patient age. In general, regardless of tumor type, radiation therapy is avoided in infants and very young children because they are especially vulnerable to radiation-associated toxicities and neurocognitive deficits. Alternative therapies for this population include intensified chemotherapy followed by autologous stem cell transplant. For some brain tumors (e.g., low-grade gliomas), complete surgical resection may be the only therapy indicated. Common pediatric tumors with their relative incidences and prognoses are outlined in Table 57-3.

Most children with tumors of the CNS also require some form of supportive care in addition to tumor-directed therapy. This includes hormonal replacement for patients with neuroendocrine dysfunction; antiepileptic drugs for patients with seizure disorders; physical, occupational, and speech therapy;

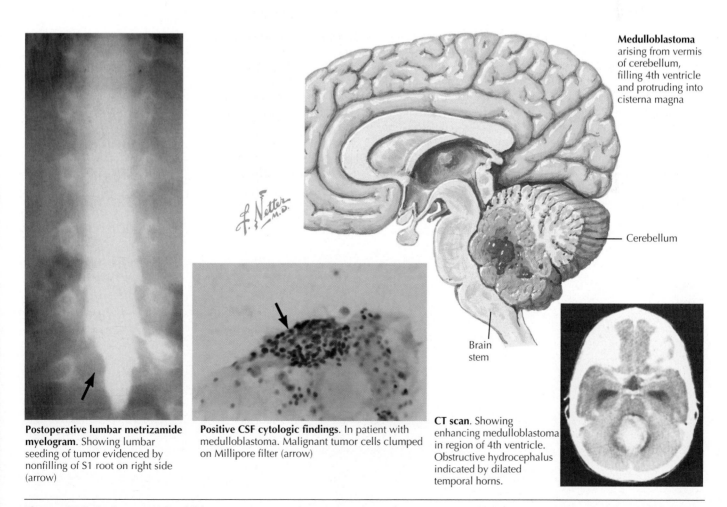

Medulloblastoma arising from vermis of cerebellum, filling 4th ventricle and protruding into cisterna magna

Cerebellum

Brain stem

Postoperative lumbar metrizamide myelogram. Showing lumbar seeding of tumor evidenced by nonfilling of S1 root on right side (arrow)

Positive CSF cytologic findings. In patient with medulloblastoma. Malignant tumor cells clumped on Millipore filter (arrow)

CT scan. Showing enhancing medulloblastoma in region of 4th ventricle. Obstructive hydrocephalus indicated by dilated temporal horns.

Figure 57-2 *Brain tumors in children.*

Table 57-3 Common Pediatric Brain Tumors: Incidences, and Prognoses

Tumor	Relative Incidence (%)	Prognosis (Overall Survival, 5 Years)
Low-grade glioma	35-50	90%-100% (pilocytic astrocytoma with complete resection) 60%-90% (other subtypes)
Medulloblastoma or PNET	16-20	85% overall (varies with age and stage) 20%-60% (infants) 33%-65% (supratentorial PNET)
Brainstem glioma	10-20	Median survival time, 9-13 mos (diffuse intrinsic pontine tumors) 80%-90% (localized tumors)
Ependymomas	8-10	67%-80% (complete resection + XRT) 22%-47% (incomplete resection + XRT)
Malignant glioma	10	25% (complete resection + XRT)
Germ cell tumors	4-7	Mature teratoma: 100% with complete resection Pure germinoma: >90% with surgery + radiation Nongerminomatous: 25%-55% with surgery + chemotherapy + XRT
Craniopharyngioma	3	95%
Aggressive infantile embryonal tumors (i.e., atypical teratoid rhabdoid tumor)	3	<10%-20%

PNET, primitive neuroectodermal tumor; XRT, radiation therapy.

and individualized educational planning for patients with learning challenges related to tumor or treatment.

FUTURE DIRECTIONS

Improvement in the long-term survival of children with brain tumors has come with a cost. Late effects of radiotherapy include neuropsychological and neurocognitive disorders (especially in young children who received large doses of radiation), endocrinologic disorders and growth delay, and the risk of secondary malignancies. The late effects of chemotherapy include prolonged bone marrow suppression, hearing loss, renal insufficiency, and risk of secondary malignancies such as leukemia. Individualized therapies targeted to specific patient populations, tumor types, and risk groups are being studied to minimize the risks of treatment-related toxicities while continuing to improve long-term survival.

SUGGESTED READINGS

Abdullah S, Qaddoumi I, Bouffet E: Advances in the management of pediatric central nervous system tumors, *Ann N Y Acad Sci* 1138:22-31, 2008.

Babcock MA, Kostova FV, Guha A, et al: Tumors of the central nervous system: clinical aspects, molecular mechanisms, unanswered questions, and future research directions, *J Child Neurol* 23:1103-1121, 2008.

Central Brain Tumor Registry of the United States: *Statistical Report: Primary Brain Tumors in the United States, 2000-2004.* Central Brain Tumor Registry of the United States, 2008.

Packer RJ, MacDonald T, Vezina G: Central nervous system tumors, *Pediatr Clin North Am* 55:121-145, 2008.

Neuroblastoma

58

Elizabeth M. Wallis and Nicholas Evageliou

Neuroblastoma is the most common extracranial solid tumor of childhood and accounts for 8% to 10% of all childhood cancers. The median age at diagnosis is 17 months, and the vast majority of neuroblastoma is diagnosed before age 10 years. The prognosis varies significantly and depends on age, tumor biology, and extent of disease at diagnosis. Whereas some disseminated tumors in infants may spontaneously regress, metastatic tumors diagnosed in slightly older children carry a long-term survival rate of around 40%. Although many children with neuroblastoma will need aggressive surgical resection and chemotherapy, some children can be safely observed over time. It is this dramatic heterogeneity of phenotypes that has prompted further evaluation of the implications of staging and treatment. Novel therapies are becoming increasingly important in treating refractory disease.

ETIOLOGY AND PATHOGENESIS

Neuroblastoma is characterized as a small, round, blue-cell tumor and arises from neural crest cells. The Shimada and Joshi staging system is based on the pathologic components of neuroblastoma. The important histologic components for classification are degree of neuroblast cell differentiation, mitosis-karyorrhexis index (MKI), and amount of stromal content. This combined with age at diagnosis divides patients into two categories: favorable and unfavorable histology.

Additionally, a number of genetic aberrations are important in classification and prognosis of neuroblastoma. The DNA content of tumor cells is characterized as near-diploid or hyper-diploid, the latter of which is associated with a more favorable outcome. Examples of other genetic abnormalities associated with prognosis include *MYCN* amplification, deletion of the short arm of chromosome 1p, and deletion of chromosome 11q. The most important of these, *MYCN* amplification, is associated with rapid tumor progression and poor prognosis, even in patients with otherwise lower stage disease. Neuroblastoma is most commonly an isolated diagnosis, but it has been associated with other neurocristopathies such as Hirschsprung's disease, congenital central hypoventilation syndrome (CCHS or Ondine's curse), and neurofibromatosis type 1. Additionally, a very small number of patients (1%-2%) present as part of a familial neuroblastoma syndrome. In this situation, the most common genetic abnormality is a germline mutation in the anaplastic lymphoma kinase (ALK) gene (Figure 58-1).

CLINICAL PRESENTATION

Neuroblastoma can arise anywhere along the sympathetic chain, and symptoms at the time of diagnosis depend on the location and extent of disease. Primary tumors most commonly occur in the abdomen (65%) and usually present as a painless abdominal mass. These patients may also present with vomiting, constipation, or symptoms of intestinal obstruction. Other common sites of primary tumors include the neck, chest, and paraspinal region. Tumors arising from the chest may be found incidentally on chest radiography, and cervical tumors may present as a Horner's syndrome or more rarely with superior vena cava syndrome (Figure 58-2).

Approximately half of patients have metastatic disease at the time of diagnosis. Infants with metastatic disease often present with massive hepatomegaly with or without respiratory compromise. Infants may also present with bluish, subcutaneous nodules, a hallmark of the disease in this population. Other symptoms of metastatic disease in any patient include anorexia, bone pain, irritability, fever, pallor, and hypertension (most often as a result of renal vascular compression). Periorbital ecchymosis and proptosis (from bony tumor infiltrate) are also characteristic of neuroblastoma. Rarely, children are symptomatic from tumor cell catecholamine release, resulting in flushing, sweating, headache, palpitations, and hypertension.

A small percentage of children (5%) present with symptoms of spinal cord compression. This oncologic emergency is associated with paraspinal neuroblastomas, and associated findings include lower extremity weakness, bowel and bladder dysfunction, back pain, and sensory loss. Neurologic function at the time of diagnosis has a strong association with long-term neurologic outcome (see Figure 58-2).

In addition, distinct paraneoplastic syndromes are associated with neuroblastoma. Secretion of vasoactive intestinal peptide by tumor cells results in intractable, watery diarrhea; hypokalemia; and poor growth. These tumors are often associated with favorable histology and good prognosis. The syndrome of opsoclonus–myoclonus is characterized by rapid, involuntary eye movements in all directions; irregular, frequent muscle jerking; and ataxia. These children usually also have a low-stage tumor with favorable biologic features. The presenting neurologic symptoms of opsoclonus–myoclonus and ataxia typically resolve after treatment; however, the majority of children have residual developmental delay.

The previously described clinical symptoms should be carefully evaluated in the physical examination. The abdominal examination should focus on the presence of a mass or hepatomegaly. Head and neck evaluation should include examination for proptosis, periorbital ecchymosis, and Horner's syndrome (ptosis, miosis, anhidrosis, and ipsilateral facial flushing). One should perform an examination of the cervical, supraclavicular, axillary, and inguinal areas for lymphadenopathy. It is essential to complete a careful neurologic examination because subtle findings can indicate an evolving paraspinal mass. Key neurologic findings include lower extremity weakness, hyperreflexia or diminished weakness, decreased rectal sphincter tone, bowel or bladder incontinence, and paraplegia.

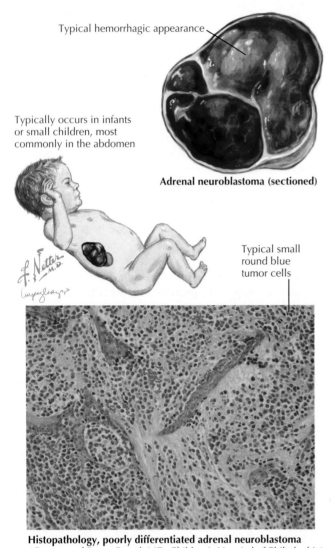

Typical hemorrhagic appearance

Typically occurs in infants or small children, most commonly in the abdomen

Adrenal neuroblastoma (sectioned)

Typical small round blue tumor cells

Histopathology, poorly differentiated adrenal neuroblastoma
(Courtesy of Bruce Pawel, MD, Children's Hospital of Philadephia)

Figure 58-1 *Overview of neuroblastoma.*

DIFFERENTIAL DIAGNOSIS

Because of its varied presentation, the differential diagnosis of a patient with suspected neuroblastoma is broad and should be based on specific signs and symptoms. The clinical presentation can be divided into categories: an abdominal mass or symptoms, a mass in another location, spinal cord compression, and nonspecific neurologic symptoms. Table 58-1 summarizes the differential diagnosis of neuroblastoma using these categories of presenting symptoms.

An abdominal mass is the most common physical examination finding in a patient with neuroblastoma. When evaluating an abdominal mass, it is important to determine whether it is secondary to an enlarged organ (hepatomegaly) or a discrete mass. Even though hepatomegaly may be mistaken for an abdominal mass, an enlarged liver can also be the result of an infection, storage disease, congenital hepatic fibrosis, or malignant infiltration. Splenomegaly may be attributable to leukemia or lymphoma, a hemolytic anemia, portal hypertension, or a storage disease.

There are many causes of spinal cord compression (see Table 58-1) in addition to neuroblastoma. However, in the case of spinal cord compression, the cause may not be immediately known, and steroid treatment can be initiated before a definitive diagnosis is made in select cases. In cases in which neurologic symptoms are rapidly progressing, immediate treatment is warranted to increase the prospect for preservation of neurologic function.

Opsoclonus–myoclonus occurs in 2% to 4% of children with neuroblastoma. It represents a specific syndrome characterized by rapid, irregular eye movements; ataxia; and myoclonus. Approximately 50% of children with this syndrome are found to have a primary neuroblastoma, and diagnostic workup should be undertaken to find a primary tumor in all children with these symptoms. The differential diagnosis is broad for any one of these symptoms; however, the constellation of symptoms significantly narrows the differential diagnosis.

EVALUATION

The initial workup for patients with suspected neuroblastoma includes laboratory and radiographic studies. The diagnosis is either made by tumor tissue biopsy or bone marrow biopsy consistent with neuroblastoma *combined with* increased urine catecholamines (homovanillic acid [HVA] and vanillylmandelic acid [VMA]). In a patient with suspected neuroblastoma, initial laboratory studies should include complete blood count, basic metabolic panel, hepatic function panel, lactate dehydrogenase, ferritin, and urine HVA and VMA. Radiologic evaluation should depend on primary tumor location, but often a variety of modalities are used to better delineate the diagnosis of neuroblastoma. Computed tomography imaging is best for tumors of the mediastinum, abdomen, and pelvis, but magnetic resonance imaging is superior for evaluation of paraspinal lesions and potential spinal cord compression.

Once neuroblastoma is the likely diagnosis, metaiodobenzylguanidine (MIBG) scan is important in finding a primary tumor as well as metastases. The MIBG isotope is concentrated in greater than 90% of neuroblastomas and is used in diagnosis as well as monitoring throughout therapy. Bilateral bone marrow biopsies and aspirates are also necessary to evaluate for the presence of metastatic disease even if tumor biopsy is used to make the initial diagnosis.

STAGING AND MANAGEMENT

Staging

The treatment approaches for neuroblastoma depend on a number of clinical and biologic characteristics of the tumor. Tumor risk assessment, as devised by the International neuroblastoma Risk Group, depends on tumor stage, age at diagnosis, and *MYCN* gene status. These factors along with other biologic variables (mainly genetic aberrations) and tumor histology are used to classify patients into low-, medium-, and high-risk categories. Tables 58-2 and 58-3 summarize tumor staging and risk stratification. Risk stratification (shown in a simplified form here) is essential in determining a treatment course and prognosis for patients with neuroblastomas.

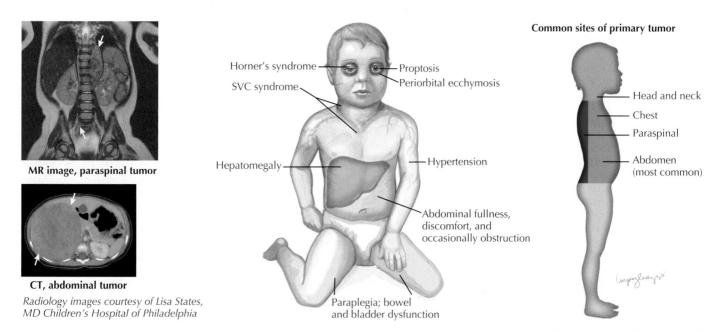

MR image, paraspinal tumor

CT, abdominal tumor

Radiology images courtesy of Lisa States, MD Children's Hospital of Philadelphia

Common sites of primary tumor

Horner's syndrome
Proptosis
Periorbital ecchymosis
SVC syndrome
Hepatomegaly
Hypertension
Abdominal fullness, discomfort, and occasionally obstruction
Paraplegia; bowel and bladder dysfunction

Head and neck
Chest
Paraspinal
Abdomen (most common)

Figure 58-2 *Summary of clinical presentation of neuroblastoma.*

Table 58-1 Differential Diagnosis of Neuroblastoma		
Abdominal Mass		
Intraabdominal mass	Neuroblastoma	Ovarian torsion
	Wilms tumor	Ovarian tumor
	Omphalocele	Teratoma
	Hernia	Lymphoma
	Pheochromocytoma	Hepatoblastoma
	Adrenal hemorrhage	Pancreatoblastoma
	Hemangioendothelioma	
Intestinal mass	Bezoar	Intussusception
	Volvulus	Abscess
	Megacolon	
Other intraabdominal pathologies	Pancreatic pseudocyst	Enlarged uterus
	Choledochal cyst	Constipation
	Hydrops of the gallbladder	Cystic kidney disease
Thoracic Mass		
Oncologic	Neuroblastoma	
	Lymphoma or leukemia	
	Germ cell tumor	
Non-oncologic	Congenital malformations	
	• Bronchogenic cyst	
	• Vascular malformations	
	Tuberculosis	
	Histoplasmosis	
	Pneumonia	
Spinal Cord Compression		
Oncologic	Sarcoma (most common)	
	Neuroblastoma	
	Leukemia	
	Lymphoma	

Table 58-2	International Neuroblastoma Staging System (Simplified)
1	Localized tumor with complete gross resection
2A	Localized tumor with incomplete resection and gross residual disease; ipsilateral lymph nodes without tumor cells
2B	Localized tumor with or without complete resection and ipsilateral lymph nodes positive for tumor cells
3	Unresectable tumor extending across the midline (directly or via nodal extension)
4	Any primary tumor with dissemination to distant lymph nodes, bone, bone marrow, liver, skin, or other organs (except 4S)
4S	Localized primary tumor (1, 2A, or 2B) in infants younger than 1 year old with dissemination limited to skin, liver, or bone marrow

Surgery

Surgery is a mainstay of therapy and is important in confirming the diagnosis as well as treating the disease. Gross total resection is the goal, provided the tumor can be safely removed without damaging vital organs. In patients with intermediate- and high-risk tumors, it may be necessary to attempt to reduce the tumor burden with chemotherapy before attempting resection. Surrounding lymph nodes are also sampled at the time of surgery.

Chemotherapy

A number of different chemotherapeutic regimens are used in patients with intermediate- and high-risk disease. The most common medications used for initial therapy include cisplatin, etoposide, doxorubicin, cyclophosphamide, topotecan, vincristine, and doxorubicin. In patients with high-risk tumors, five or six cycles of induction chemotherapy is undertaken before attempting surgical resection. Surgery of the primary site is followed by consolidation chemotherapy and then autologous stem cell transplantation. Patients with high-risk disease then receive radiation therapy and a maintenance phase of biologic and immunotherapy. Long-term, event-free survival for patients with high-risk tumors is 40% to 50%. Cooperative groups, including The Children's Oncology Group, continue to collaborate in evaluating novel chemotherapeutic regimens to improve long-term survival rates.

Radiation Therapy

The role of radiation therapy is evolving as novel chemotherapeutic and biologic treatments emerge, although there are still specific indications for its use. Radiation therapy is used in neonates with 4S disease who develop respiratory distress because of hepatosplenomegaly and in whom chemotherapy alone is not effective in resolving this symptom. Radiation therapy is also used for local control of the primary tumor in patients with high-risk disease. Pilot studies have investigated the use of total-body irradiation as part of the conditioning regimen for autologous stem cell transplant; however, this is not used as the standard of care. Additionally, radiation therapy plays an important role in palliative therapy for patients with end-stage disease.

Treatment of Paraneoplastic Syndromes

Opsoclonus–myoclonus is associated with immunoglobulin G (IgG) and IgM autoantibodies that bind neuronal cells, and up to 50% of cases of the syndrome are associated with neuroblastoma. In general, patients who present with this paraneoplastic syndrome have low-grade tumors that respond well to therapy. Initial treatment is designed to target the paraneoplastic syndrome and involves high-dose steroids, intravenous immunoglobulin, adrenocorticotropic hormone, and chemotherapy in some cases. With these treatments, many children have resolution of symptoms over time; however, 70% to 80% of children treated persist with some degree of developmental delay. Examples include delays in cognitive development, speech deficits, gross and fine motor skills, and behavioral disturbances.

FUTURE DIRECTIONS

Patients with high-risk disease, who are at significant risk for relapse, are now being treated with long-term biologic therapy to treat minimal residual disease (MRD). Currently, retinoids are the mainstay of this therapy (including 13-cis-retinoic acid), although the goal is to develop therapies that target the specific

Table 58-3 Risk Stratification (Simplified)		
Risk Group	**Stages Included**	**Treatment Summary**
Low risk	Stage 1 Stage 2 with >50% resected Stage 4S with favorable pathology and biology	Surgical resection only in most cases; if symptomatic (i.e., respiratory distress), may require chemotherapy Stage 4S without respiratory compromise may be treated with observation alone
Intermediate risk	Stage 3 and 4 <1.5 years with favorable biology Stage 3 >1.5 years with favorable pathology or biology	Chemotherapy Surgical resection
High risk	Stage 2 and 3 with unfavorable biology or pathology Stage 4 >1.5 years old Stage 4S with unfavorable biology	Induction chemotherapy before resection Surgical resection (as possible) with or without radiation therapy Consolidation with myeloablative therapy and autologous stem cell rescue Maintenance therapy for minimal residual disease

molecular characteristics of neuroblastoma. Other chemotherapeutics, including tyrosine kinase inhibitors, antiangiogenesis agents, and immunotherapies, are being used in novel ways to treat MRD as well as recurrent disease. Ongoing clinical trials are evaluating the efficacy of these therapies, and emphasis is also being placed on new molecular therapies that specifically target neuroblastoma.

The role of therapeutic MIBG is also being expanded for use in patients with refractory disease. This substance is selectively concentrated in neuroblastoma cells and was previously used only for diagnostic purposes. It can be used to transport bound radionucleotides to neuroblastoma cells, and therapeutic MIBG has demonstrated an excellent response rate in patients with refractory and relapsed disease. Even in the absence of tumor response, patients often have symptom relief. This is an expanding area of research and is being studied as an adjunct to current treatment strategies.

Although patients with low-risk disease have a generally favorable outcome, those with high-risk disease experience significant morbidity. The long-term, event-free survival for patients with high-risk disease is still approximately 40% to 50%. Patients who survive experience a number of long-term complications of treatment, including secondary malignancies later in life. As the specific molecular pathogenesis of neuroblastoma is better understood, the hope is to develop new therapies that target these factors. Novel approaches to treatment and combining molecular therapies with current chemotherapeutics will hopefully lead to more tailored treatment and better outcomes for patients.

SUGGESTED READINGS

Brodeur GM, Maris JM: Neuroblastoma. In Pizzo PA, Poplack DG, editors: *Principles and Practice of Pediatric Oncology*, ed 5, Philadelphia, 2006, JB Lippincott, pp 933-970.

Maris JM, Hogarty M, Bagatell R, et al: Neuroblastoma: a review, *Lancet* 369:2106-2120, 2007.

Matthay KK, Villablanca JG, Seeger RC, et al: Treatment of high-risk neuroblastoma with intensive chemotherapy, radiotherapy, autologous bone marrow transplantation, and 13-cis-retinoic acid. Children's Cancer Group, *N Engl J Med* 341:1165-1173, 1999.

Carly R. Varela and Kelly C. Goldsmith

*R*enal tumors account for 6% of all childhood cancers and are the sixth most common form of cancer in children. As with many pediatric cancers, there is no known environmental cause for childhood kidney tumors. Certain genetic syndromes are associated with a predisposition to developing renal neoplasms, specifically Wilms' tumor. The etiology of many renal tumors may be attributable to tumor-specific chromosomal abnormalities, discussed below. Although Wilms' tumor is one of the most curable tumors of childhood, other more rare pediatric renal tumors have a high mortality rate. Therefore, optimal management of the more rare renal tumors, such as tailoring therapy to tumor-specific genetic alterations to improve cure rates, is an active area of investigation.

ETIOLOGY AND PATHOGENESIS

Wilms' Tumor

Wilms' tumor accounts for the majority (85%) of pediatric renal tumors with 500 new cases per year in the United States (Figure 59-1). The more aggressive anaplastic histologic subtype of Wilms' makes up about 8% of all pediatric renal tumors. The mean age at presentation is 3 to 4 years for unilateral disease, and the majority of patients are younger than 10 years old at diagnosis. Patients with bilateral disease account for 5% of all Wilms' cases and present younger than those for unilateral disease at 2 to 2.5 years of age.

Wilms' tumor is an embryonic solid tumor derived from undifferentiated nephroblasts in the kidney. Thus, the persistence of embryonic renal tissue (nephrogenic rests) is often seen in kidneys resected for Wilms' tumor. The presence of multiple, diffuse nephrogenic rests is known as nephroblastomatosis, a premalignant condition prone to transforming into Wilms' tumor. Not all nephrogenic rests transform into Wilms' tumor; they may also regress or differentiate into mature kidney tissue. Therefore, children with diffuse nephroblastomatosis or a genetic predisposition for Wilms' are at highest risk of nephrogenic rests progressing to malignant Wilms' tumor.

Certain genetic syndromes are associated with the development of Wilms' tumor. Examples include overgrowth syndromes such as Beckwith-Wiedemann (organomegaly, neonatal hypoglycemia, macroglossia, and omphalocele; also associated with hepatoblastoma) and Perlman's (distinct facial features, macrosomia, genitourinary abnormalities and polyhydramnios), Denys-Drash (genital anomalies and nephropathy), and WAGR (**W**ilms' tumor, **a**niridia, **g**enitourinary anomalies, and mental **r**etardation) syndromes. These patients have germline genetic abnormalities, specifically at chromosome 11, that alter the genes responsible for growth and renal genesis.

The 11p locus has been shown to play an important role in Wilms' tumor pathogenesis. The *WT1* gene, thought to be a tumor suppressor gene, is located at 11p13. Deletions of this region are associated with WAGR syndrome, and mutations of this gene are associated with Denys-Drash syndrome. Loss of heterozygosity or loss of imprinting at the *WT2* gene, located at chromosome 11p15, has also been identified in patients with overgrowth syndromes such as Beckwith-Wiedemann and Perlman syndromes.

Specific genetic abnormalities that are exclusive to the tumor alone seem to be associated with a more aggressive form of Wilms' tumor. The combined loss of heterozygosity of chromosomes 16q and 1p in Wilms' tumors has been associated with a poorer prognosis in lower stage tumors. More recently, an X chromosome gene mutation, WTX, seen in one-third of sporadic Wilms' tumors, has been described.

Although most Wilms' tumors fall into the category of favorable histology, a subset of tumors can be categorized as diffusely "anaplastic," having irregular mitoses and hyperchromatic cells with large nuclei throughout, which carries a poorer prognosis. No specific genetic abnormalities have been determined thus far for this aggressive subtype of Wilms' tumor.

Rare Renal Tumors

Clear cell sarcoma of the kidney (CCSK) is the second most common malignant kidney tumor of childhood and accounts for about 2% to 4% of primary pediatric renal tumors. The majority of patients are younger than 5 years old at the time of diagnosis, and classic pathology shows nests of cells separated by septae. The majority of tumors also demonstrate variant patterns, which may resemble Wilms' tumor and make it difficult to differentiate CCSK from other renal tumors.

Rhabdoid tumor of the kidney (RTK) is a very aggressive renal tumor that is most often detected in infants but is not exclusive to infancy. RTK, like its central nervous system homologue, atypical teratoid rhabdoid tumor (ATRT) of the brain, carries a specific deletion of the *INI1* gene located at 22q11-2 that is a germline mutation in 20% of cases and can be used to confirm the diagnosis.

Renal cell carcinoma (RCC) is the most common form of adult renal cancer; however, pediatric RCC accounts for only 1% of all RCC and 5% to 6% of all pediatric renal tumors. Pediatric RCC seem to have a distinct tumor from adult RCC, with a genetic translocation involving chromosome Xp11. Interestingly, RCC has been described in a number of patients with a history of neuroblastoma. *Renal medullary carcinoma (RMC)*, a subset of RCC, is extremely rare and is seen almost exclusively in young adolescent patients with sickle cell trait; the etiology and rationale for the association is unclear. Patients with RMC generally present in the second to third decade of life with advanced disease and have a very poor prognosis.

Cystic nephroma, on the other hand, is a rare and benign tumor of the kidney that is associated with a very favorable prognosis after surgical resection alone.

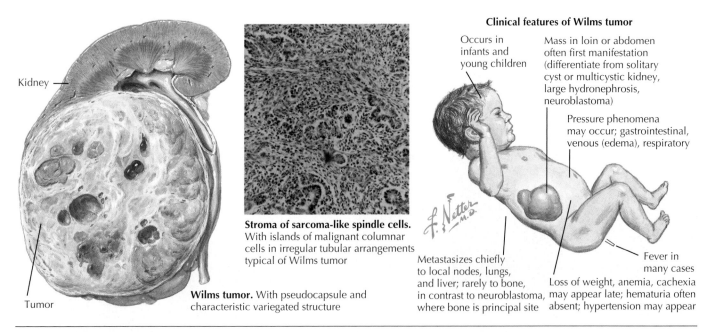

Clinical features of Wilms tumor

Occurs in infants and young children

Mass in loin or abdomen often first manifestation (differentiate from solitary cyst or multicystic kidney, large hydronephrosis, neuroblastoma)

Pressure phenomena may occur; gastrointestinal, venous (edema), respiratory

Kidney

Tumor

Stroma of sarcoma-like spindle cells. With islands of malignant columnar cells in irregular tubular arrangements typical of Wilms tumor

Wilms tumor. With pseudocapsule and characteristic variegated structure

Metastasizes chiefly to local nodes, lungs, and liver; rarely to bone, in contrast to neuroblastoma, where bone is principal site

Loss of weight, anemia, cachexia may appear late; hematuria often absent; hypertension may appear

Fever in many cases

Figure 59-1 *Nephroblastoma (Wilms' tumor).*

A kidney tumor noted on prenatal ultrasonography or in the first 6 months of life is almost always a *congenital mesoblastic nephroma (CMN)*. CMN occurs in one in 27,500 live births and is the most common benign renal tumor of infancy. Because of the differential diagnosis of an infant renal tumor including malignant Wilms' tumor and RTK, a nephrectomy is often performed to diagnose the lesion. The cellular variant of CMN is more aggressive with a 20% chance of local recurrence and shares the t(12;15)(p13;q26) gene fusion product ETV6-NTRK3 that is also found in infantile fibrosarcoma.

CLINICAL PRESENTATION

The clinical presentation for patients with a renal tumor often includes abdominal distension, hematuria, hypertension, and a palpable abdominal mass. Symptoms may also be generalized and include fevers, unintentional weight loss, or night sweats.

Wilms' Tumor

Patients with Wilms' tumor are often well appearing and asymptomatic and present only with a palpable abdominal mass. Often, patients come to medical attention after a caretaker feels an abdominal mass while bathing the toddler or a health care provider detects an abdominal mass on routine physical examination. Hypertension and hematuria may also be present because of tumor mass effects on the renal vessels. The most common site for metastatic disease is the lungs, which is often asymptomatic. Metastases may also involve regional or distant lymph nodes, liver, and rarely brain or bone. Patients with a propensity for bilateral disease may have synchronous tumors at the time of diagnosis or may present with unilateral disease and develop a contralateral tumor at a later time point (metachronous disease).

Rare Renal Tumors

CLEAR CELL SARCOMA OF THE KIDNEY

The majority of patients with CCSK are younger than 5 years old at the time of diagnosis, and the most common clinical presentation is a palpable abdominal mass. This tumor can spread to the lung, brain, and soft tissues and most commonly metastasizes to bone; hence, it is also known as the "bone metastasizing renal tumor of childhood."

RHABDOID TUMOR OF THE KIDNEY

Patients with RTK may present with hematuria, an abdominal mass, or signs of metastatic disease (including disease in the liver, lungs, brain, bone, and lymph nodes). Twenty percent of patients have a concomitant brain tumor (not necessarily metastatic) and may present with an altered neurologic examination.

RENAL CELL CARCINOMA

Pediatric patients with RCC are often older and more ill appearing than those with Wilms' tumor. The most common presenting symptoms include abdominal pain, fevers, and hematuria. Interestingly, adults do not often present with this classic triad of symptoms.

CONGENITAL MESOBLASTIC NEPHROMA

CMN may be detected on prenatal ultrasonography evaluation with associated polyhydramnios or can be identified by the presence of an asymptomatic palpable abdominal mass in infancy.

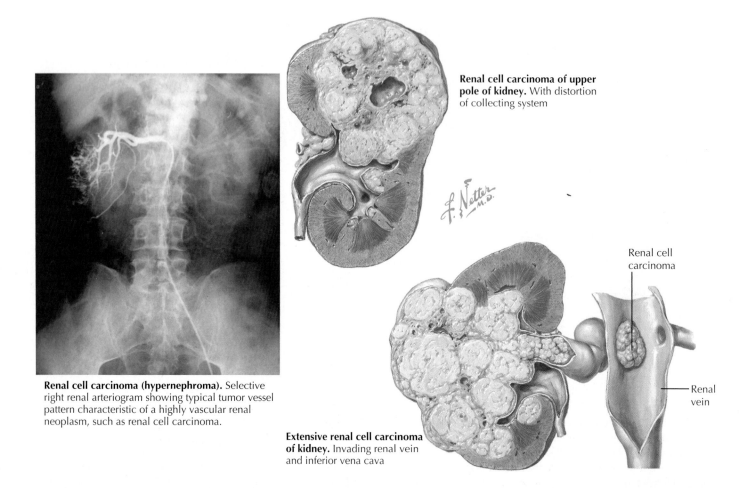

Renal cell carcinoma of upper pole of kidney. With distortion of collecting system

Renal cell carcinoma (hypernephroma). Selective right renal arteriogram showing typical tumor vessel pattern characteristic of a highly vascular renal neoplasm, such as renal cell carcinoma.

Renal cell carcinoma

Renal vein

Extensive renal cell carcinoma of kidney. Invading renal vein and inferior vena cava

Figure 59-2 *Malignant tumors of the kidney.*

EVALUATION AND MANAGEMENT

Evaluation of a child with any renal tumor begins with a detailed history and physical examination. It is imperative to evaluate on history and physical for anomalies that might suggest a Wilms' tumor predisposition syndrome, such as coarse facies (patients with *WT1* mutations), absence of intact iris (aniridia associated with WAGR), presence of undescended testicles or renal anomalies on radiologic examinations (i.e., horseshoe kidney may be seen in patients with WAGR and *WT1* mutations), developmental assessment, hemihypertrophy, large tongue, and ear pits or creases (as seen with Beckwith-Wiedemann syndrome). The presence of a predisposition syndrome will affect the diagnostic surgical procedure, recommended treatment, and posttreatment follow-up.

Laboratory evaluation should include a urinalysis; serum chemistry panel, including creatinine; and calcium because hypercalcemia is a paraneoplastic phenomenon found occasionally in RTK and CMN tumors. A complete blood count, lactate dehydrogenase, and uric acid may be helpful in differentiating kidney infiltration from leukemia, lymphoma, or the presence of bone marrow involvement from a more aggressive renal tumor.

Radiologic evaluation usually begins with abdominal ultrasonography to help determine the site of origin and whether the mass is cystic or solid. If a tumor arising from the kidney is identified, higher resolution imaging with computed tomography (CT) or magnetic resonance imaging (MRI) is recommended as well as imaging evaluation for metastatic disease (see for specific tumors below). Because of the propensity for Wilms' tumor and other more aggressive renal tumors to spread into the renal vessels and extend into the inferior vena cava (often into the right atrium, deemed "tumor thrombus"), it is essential to image the renal and large vessels with Doppler to assess extent of venous obstruction. Vascular invasion of tumor can affect the surgical approach, staging, and management decisions (Figure 59-2). The differential diagnosis for a patient with a renal mass is given in Box 59-1. One element of the differential diagnosis is shown in Figure 59-3 .

TUMOR-SPECIFIC EVALUATIONS AND MANAGEMENT

Wilms' Tumor

In addition to the dedicated renal imaging as described above, diagnostic evaluation for Wilms' tumor should include a CT scan of the chest to rule out metastasis.

Treatment for Wilms' tumor depends on the tumor stage and histology. The clinical stage of a Wilms' tumor is based on the amount of residual disease left behind after the diagnostic surgery (most often nephrectomy), whether lymph nodes are involved, and the absence or presence of metastatic disease. Surgery and chemotherapy are always part of the treatment, and patients may receive radiation to the abdomen and lungs based on the stage of the disease. Patients who have low-stage (I or II) favorable histology tumors are treated with nephrectomy followed by chemotherapy with vincristine and dactinomycin. Those with higher stage III (gross residual disease or nodal involvement) or IV (metastatic) disease receive the same surgery and chemotherapy as lower stage patients with the addition of doxorubicin and local abdominal (stage III) or metastatic site radiation. Based on data from International Society of Pediatric Oncology clinical trials for Wilms' tumor, newer study protocols are sparing lung radiation in stage IV patients whose lung metastases clear with 6 weeks of induction chemotherapy.

Anaplastic Wilms' tumor is associated with greater chemotherapy resistance, and despite the stage, it is more difficult to cure than the more common favorable histology variant. After upfront nephrectomy, chemotherapy for patients with anaplastic Wilms' tumor includes vincristine, cyclophosphamide, doxorubicin, and etoposide. Despite receiving more intensive chemotherapy as well as abdominal radiation, survival for patients with this variant remains poor.

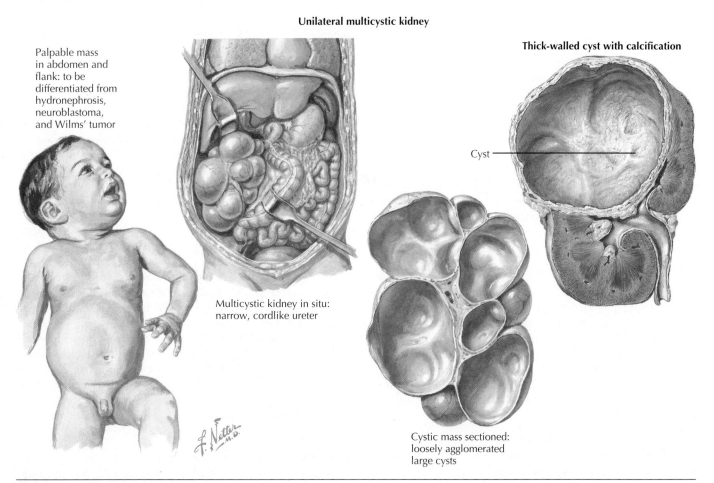

Unilateral multicystic kidney

Palpable mass in abdomen and flank: to be differentiated from hydronephrosis, neuroblastoma, and Wilms' tumor

Multicystic kidney in situ: narrow, cordlike ureter

Thick-walled cyst with calcification

Cyst

Cystic mass sectioned: loosely agglomerated large cysts

Figure 59-3 *Unilateral multicystic kidney.*

Treatment for bilateral Wilms' tumor differs from that of unilateral disease because bilateral nephrectomy is not a treatment option. Furthermore, patients with certain genetic syndromes who have unilateral disease are predisposed to renal failure genetically or from their potential to develop metachronous Wilms' tumors in the unaffected kidney. Therefore, the focus of management for this subset of patients is to preserve as much normal kidney tissue while still curing the patient of the cancer with local surgical resection, called *nephron-sparing surgery*. Most often, a urologist will perform this procedure because it requires intimate knowledge of renal anatomy. The goal is to obtain tumor-free margins while preserving renal parenchyma and function. Chemotherapy for patients with bilateral disease is based on the staging of the most involved kidney and is often given preoperatively to shrink the tumors to ensure adequate margins and maximal sparing of normal kidney tissue. Other patients for whom preoperative chemotherapy is recommended include patients with a solitary kidney; vascular extension of tumor into the inferior vena cava; and those with very large, unresectable tumors at diagnosis. Preoperative chemotherapy is a common therapeutic approach in Europe but remains controversial in American oncology study groups because patients are upstaged to receive abdominal radiation and doxorubicin if the tumor is not taken out before the initiation of chemotherapy.

Management of patients with Wilms' tumor predisposition syndromes or nephroblastomatosis is unique as well, both before and after development of a tumor. Screening for renal tumors in this unique group should begin early and continue until 7 to 8 years of age because this is the time period during which they are most likely to develop a tumor. Recommended screening includes renal ultrasonography every 3 months followed by CT scan if a mass is detected. Historically, there has been no standard therapy for these patients. Treatment with chemotherapy and nephron-sparing surgery when nephroblastomatosis is detected in the unaffected kidney has been described at a number of centers.

The prognosis for Wilms' tumor is excellent with overall survival greater than 90% for patients with non-metastatic, favorable histology disease. National Wilms' Tumor Study Group data also show that patients with stage IV (metastatic) favorable histology Wilms' tumor or favorable histology bilateral disease have a 10-year overall survival rate between 70 and 80%.

Rare Renal Tumors

CLEAR CELL SARCOMA OF THE KIDNEY

The diagnostic evaluation of a patient with CCSK should also include a bone scan for bony metastases. As with Wilms' tumor, surgery for CCSK is nephrectomy. Chemotherapy is more intensive and includes vincristine, cyclophosphamide, doxorubicin, and etoposide. Radiation therapy is used for patients with lymph node and bone involvement. With the exception of stage I disease, overall survival has slightly improved from less than 30% to 50% to 75% with the addition of doxorubicin to the chemotherapy regimen.

RHABDOID TUMOR OF THE KIDNEY

Because 20% of patients with RTK have an associated synchronous or metachronous brain tumor, imaging of the brain with CT or MRI is recommended at diagnosis. Brain tumor associations for RTK include primitive neuroectodermal tumor, medulloblastoma, or ATRT. The prognosis is poor despite multiagent chemotherapy and radiation. Survival correlates with stage, and there are very few survivors for those with high-stage disease.

RENAL CELL CARCINOMA

RCCs are more likely than Wilms' tumors to have calcifications on diagnostic imaging. Because this tumor can metastasize to the lung, liver, brain, bone, and regional lymph nodes, metastatic evaluation should include CT scans of the chest and abdomen and a bone scan. Brain imaging is indicated if neurologic abnormalities are detected on examination. RCC is notoriously resistant to chemotherapy. Therefore, the only cure is complete surgical resection, preferably by radical nephrectomy. Nephron-sparing surgery may be considered for patients with small tumors (≤4 cm). In adults, cure rates drastically decline if a patient's tumor size is greater than 4 cm in diameter despite complete resection. Interestingly, children with local lymph node involvement have a much better prognosis than their adult counterparts; however, both populations fare poorly if metastatic disease is present at diagnosis. Pediatric patients without distant metastases have a more favorable prognosis with an overall survival rate of 70% to 90%, and those with metastatic disease have less than 20% survival rate. Optimal treatment strategies for metastatic RCC are under investigation in adult and pediatric clinical trials and include nephrectomy and adjuvant therapy with immunomodulators (interleukin-2, interferon-α) as well as targeted therapy with tyrosine kinase inhibitors.

CONGENITAL MESOBLASTIC NEPHROMA

Although the prognosis for CMN is excellent, this tumor can be infiltrative and recur locally if not completely resected. Therefore, the treatment of choice is nephrectomy. Follow-up with an oncologist, including periodic ultrasonography for the first 3 years of life, is warranted for patients with CMN because there is the potential, albeit rare, for local recurrence or metastases. There is no role for chemotherapy or radiation in the treatment of these tumors.

FOLLOW-UP

Extensive follow up is required for all pediatric patients who have been treated for a malignant renal tumor. For the 5 years from diagnosis, evaluations at periodic intervals should include a detailed history and physical examination, imaging for metastases and local recurrence, and assessment of organ function based on prior therapy received. Patients with predisposition syndromes may warrant longer follow-up until 7 to 8 years of age. Most pediatric oncology centers have survivorship programs with clinical expertise in following patients for the long-term side effects of treatment.

FUTURE DIRECTIONS

Although the cure rate for patients with favorable histology Wilms' tumor has improved significantly over the past few decades, this does not hold true for children with anaplastic histology Wilms' tumor or with other less frequently seen malignant renal tumors. To improve patient survival and decrease treatment-related morbidity, goals of current and future renal tumor investigations include using response-based treatments, defining tumor biology to characterize high-risk patient subsets, and identifying tumor-targeted therapies for chemoresistant disease.

SUGGESTED READING

Argani P, Perlman EJ, Breslow NE, et al: Clear cell sarcoma of the kidney: a review of 351 cases from the National Wilms Tumor Study Group Pathology Center, *Am J Surg Pathol* 24:4-18, 2000.

Beckwith JB: Nephrogenic rests and the pathogenesis of Wilms tumor: developmental and clinical considerations, *Am J Med Genet* 79:268-273, 1998.

Bernstein L, Linet M, Smith MA, Olshan AF and the National Cancer Institute: Renal Tumors. Available at http://seer.cancer.gov/publications/childhood/renal.pdf.

Dome JS, Perlman EJ, Ritchey ML, et al: Renal tumors. In Pizzo PA, Poplack DG, editors: *Principles and Practice of Pediatric Oncology*, ed 5, Philadelphia, Lippincott, 2006, Williams & Wilkins, pp 905-932.

Geller JI, Dome JS: Local lymph node involvement does not predict poor outcome in pediatric renal cell carcinoma, *Cancer* 101:1575-1583, 2004.

Hartman DJ, MacLennan GT: Wilms tumor, *J Urol* 173:2147, 2005.

Huff V: Wilms tumor genetics: a new, UnX-pected twist to the story, *Cancer Cell* 11:105-107, 2007.

Kaste SC, Dome JS, Babyn PS, et al: Wilms tumor: prognostic factors, staging, therapy and late effects, *Pediatr Radiol* 38:2-17, 2008.

Lowe LH, Isuani BH, Heller RM, et al: Pediatric renal masses: Wilms tumor and beyond, *RadioGraphics* 20:1585-1603, 2000.

Perlman EJ, Faria P, Soares A, et al: Hyperplastic perilobar nephroblastomatosis: long-term survival of 52 patients, *Pediatr Blood Cancer* 46:203-221, 2006.

BONE TUMORS

Primary malignant bone tumors are the sixth most common group of malignant neoplasms in children and the third most common in adolescents and young adults. Together, malignant bone tumors account for about 6% of all childhood cancers. Osteosarcoma (OS) and the Ewing's sarcoma family of tumors (ESFT) are the most common primary bone neoplasms and together have an annual incidence of 8.7 per million in patients younger than 20 years of age. In total, approximately 650 to 700 children, adolescents, and young adults are diagnosed with malignant bone tumors in the United States per year.

OSTEOSARCOMA

Epidemiology and Pathogenesis

OS is the most common malignancy of bone in childhood, representing 15% of all primary bone tumors. The disease is somewhat more common in boys than girls (1.5:1), and the incidence is slightly higher in African Americans than in whites. The incidence is highest in patients between 10 and 20 years of age. OS is extremely rare in children younger than 5 years of age. Three percent of patients with OS have a germ line mutation in p53; many of these patients' families are affected by Li-Fraumeni syndrome. This is a familial cancer syndrome in which affected individuals have a risk of developing sarcomas, brain tumors, leukemia, breast cancer, and adrenal cortical carcinoma at a young age; this risk persists throughout patients' lifetimes. Patients who have had hereditary retinoblastoma are also at higher risk for the development of OS. OS is also associated with Rothmund-Thomson syndrome (skin rash, short stature, and skeletal abnormalities) and Paget's disease in patients older than 40 years of age.

The etiology of OS is unknown. Exposure to ionizing radiation, such as that used for treatment of previous malignancies, has been linked to secondary OS. There are no convincing data to support a link between other environmental or infectious exposures and OS.

Clinical Presentation

The most common clinical symptom at presentation is pain, often described as dull and aching, and typically of several months' duration. Other complaints include a palpable mass with or without swelling. Systemic complaints such as fevers, weight loss, and decreased appetite are rare. Eighty percent of OS occur in the extremities, and on examination, a mass (tender or nontender) may be noted (Figure 60-1). The examination may also reveal decreased range of motion or muscle atrophy. Regional lymphadenopathy is rare. The most common sites of disease include the distal femur, proximal tibia, and proximal humerus, although OS may occur in any bone. Involvement of

the axial skeleton can occur but is less common. Eighty percent of patients with OS have localized disease at the time of diagnosis. The lung is the most common site of detectable metastatic disease at diagnosis, although patients may present with multifocal bone disease without pulmonary involvement.

The differential diagnosis includes benign bone tumors, infections, and other malignant disorders. Benign tumors to be considered in the differential diagnosis include unicameral bone cysts, osteoblastomas, eosinophilic granulomas, giant cell tumors, aneurysmal bone cysts, osteochondromas, and fibrous dysplasia. Infections that may present in similar manner to OS include osteomyelitis and septic arthritis. Other malignancies must also be considered, including ESFT, chondrosarcoma, fibrosarcoma, leukemia, and metastatic lesions of other solid tumors.

Evaluation

Imaging studies are more helpful in making the diagnosis of OS than are laboratory tests. A plain radiograph will often reveal a lytic or blastic lesion of the bone with poorly defined borders (see Figure 60-1). Other findings include periosteal elevation adjacent to the primary lesion, a sunburst appearance, or a pathologic fracture. If OS is suspected, chest computed tomography (CT) and bone scan can be used to assess for pulmonary and bone metastases. Magnetic resonance imaging (MRI) should be performed to better evaluate the extent of the tumor and should include the joint above and below the involved area so that skip lesions are not missed (see Figure 60-1). In addition to delineating the intra- and extraosseous extent of the tumor, the MRI may provide information regarding tumor effects on critical neurovascular structures.

The diagnosis of OS can only be made by biopsy. Biopsies should be performed by an experienced orthopedic oncologist. The surgical approach at the time of biopsy may have an impact on the feasibility of future limb-sparing surgeries, which are necessary for local control of the tumor. In some situations, interventional radiologists are able to obtain the necessary biopsies with active participation by orthopedic oncologists. Involvement of the surgeon who will eventually perform the definitive surgical resection is preferable.

Under the microscope, OS classically appears to be composed of spindle cells associated with malignant osteoid (see Figure 60-1). The extent of osteoid production may vary among the osteoblastic, chondroblastic, fibroblastic, telangiectatic, and small cell subtypes; however, the presence of tumor osteoid is the key pathologic feature of this disease.

Management

Advances in chemotherapy over the past 30 years have resulted in higher overall survival rates and improved rates of limb salvage for patients with OS. Chemotherapy is used initially both to treat pulmonary micrometastases and to decrease the

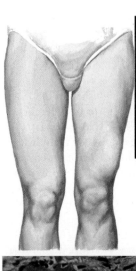

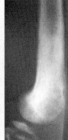

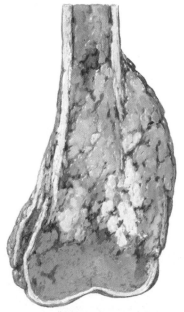

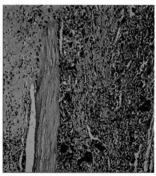

AP and lateral radiograph shows dense lesion and periosteal elevation

Mass on left distal femur palpable and tender but only slightly visible

Highly malignant stroma with cartilaginous and osteoid components (H and E stain)

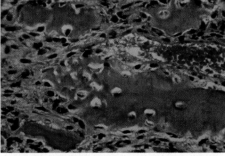

Tumor occupies entire metaphysis of distal femur and has extended into the soft tissues

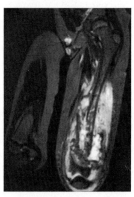

Masses of tumor cells with hyperchromatic nuclei interspersed with foci of malignant osteoid are typical histopathologic findings (H and E stain)

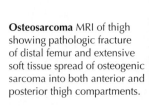

Osteosarcoma MRI of thigh showing pathologic fracture of distal femur and extensive soft tissue spread of osteogenic sarcoma into both anterior and posterior thigh compartments.

Figure 60-1 *Osteosarcoma.*

size of the primary tumor mass to facilitate surgical resection. Current treatment protocols for OS typically include preoperative (induction) and postoperative (adjuvant) chemotherapy. The total duration of treatment is approximately 8 to 12 months. Drugs that have been shown to be effective against OS include cisplatin, doxorubicin, and high-dose methotrexate. North American and European investigators are currently evaluating the role of ifosfamide and etoposide in OS therapy through an international clinical trial.

Complete surgical resection with wide margins is necessary for cure. Modern approaches to limb salvage surgery have resulted in local recurrence rates that are similar to those achieved with amputation. Limb salvage has therefore become the standard of care except when limb preservation would compromise disease control. Decision making with regard to approach to limb reconstruction is complex, particularly in patients who have not reached skeletal maturity. OS is not considered a radiosensitive tumor, although high-dose radiation may be considered for local control in rare cases in which tumor location precludes surgical resection. Surgery also remains the key therapeutic modality for macroscopic pulmonary metastases.

Prognosis

Most patients with localized OS involving an extremity can be cured. The 5-year survival rate for nonmetastatic OS is

approximately 60% to 70%. Patients with clinically detectable metastatic disease have a far worse prognosis; the overall survival rate for this patient group is approximately 25% to 30%. Among patients with localized disease at diagnosis, an inability to achieve a complete surgical resection of the tumor with negative margins is also associated with a poorer prognosis. Response to preoperative chemotherapy (i.e., degree of necrosis at the time of surgical resection) has also been shown to be an important prognostic factor for patients with localized disease because relapse-free survival rates are higher in patients with near-complete eradication of viable tumor compared with patients with a less extensive histologic response to therapy.

EWING'S SARCOMA FAMILY OF TUMORS

Epidemiology

ESFT is the second most common cancer of bone in children and adolescents, with an incidence of 2.1 per million children in the United States. Most patients are diagnosed during the second decade of life, although young adults may also be affected. Ewing's sarcoma (ES) of bone, Askin tumor (ES of the chest wall), extraosseous ES (arising from soft tissue), and peripheral neuroectodermal tumor make up the ESFT. ESFT is six times more common in white patients than in African Americans. It is slightly more common in males than in females.

ESFT does not appear to be associated with familial cancer syndromes, and the etiology of ESFT remains largely obscure.

Clinical Presentation

As in patients with OS, the most common presenting symptom of patients with ESFT of bone is pain. Before the diagnosis of the malignancy, bone pain may have been attributed to trauma or to athletic activities. As a result, the duration of symptoms before diagnosis may range from weeks to years. In addition to pain, patients may also complain of swelling or a palpable mass (Figure 60-2). Tender soft tissue masses may be palpable on examination. Fever and weight loss may be seen in patients with large tumors, but these symptoms are more common in the 25% of patients found to have metastatic disease at the time of diagnosis. Patients with tumors of the axial skeleton may present with neurologic symptoms, including paraplegia or bowel or bladder dysfunction, secondary to the paraspinal locations of these tumors.

The differential diagnosis in patients with ESFT and bony disease is similar to that of OS. It also includes benign bone tumors, infections, and other malignant disorders as discussed above. ESFT can only be definitively distinguished from OS and other bony lesions after a tumor biopsy; however, several characteristics might favor the diagnosis of ESFT. In contrast to OS, ESFT involves the axial skeleton more commonly than the long bones. Within the long bones, the diaphysis is the most common location for ESFT, but OS is more likely to arise in the metaphysis.

Evaluation

Radiography is typically the first imaging modality used to evaluate the primary site of disease (see Figure 60-2). Bony destruction with "onion skinning" of the periosteum may be seen. Tumor growth may lead to elevation of the periosteum and the formation of a triangular interface between the tumor and normal bone known as Codman's triangle. MRI of the primary site is critical in determining the extent and size of an ESFT involving bone, and the relevant bone or compartment should be imaged in its entirety.

Biopsies of suspected ESFT should be performed with the same care used for biopsies of other suspected bony malignancies. Because there may be extensive necrosis within a ESFT at the time of presentation, frozen sections are often necessary to confirm the presence of adequate diagnostic material within a biopsy sample. Importantly, biopsy samples should provide sufficient material for microscopy, immunohistochemical studies, and molecular diagnostic studies and should ideally be performed at a center that has a pathologist experienced in interpreting these diagnostic tests.

Under the microscope, ESFT appear to be composed of sheets of small, round, blue cells with scant cytoplasms (see Figure 60-2). The peripheral primitive neuroectodermal variant of ESFT may appear to contain aggregates of cells known as Homer-Wright rosettes. ESFT cells will frequently demonstrate membranous CD99 (cluster of differentiation molecule) positivity with immunohistochemical staining. CD99 staining is helpful in making the diagnosis of ESFT, but CD99 positivity can be seen in cells other than ESFT cells, including lymphoblasts. For this reason, molecular diagnostic studies are of critical importance in the ES tumor setting. In 95% of cases, a rearrangement involving the *EWS* (ES) gene is detected. Most occur via a t(11,22) translocation, which results in production of the EWS-FLI1 fusion protein. In approximately 10% of cases, other members of the ETS transcription factor family, including ERG, ETV1, or E1AF, are involved in gene rearrangements in ESFT. *EWS* rearrangements can be detected by reverse transcriptase polymerase chain reaction or by fluorescent in situ hybridization.

After confirmation of the diagnosis of ESFT, a staging evaluation must be performed. The most common sites of metastatic disease at diagnosis are lung, bone, and bone marrow. CT of the chest and bone scintography are used for detection of metastatic pulmonary and skeletal disease (see Figure 60-2). Bilateral bone marrow aspirates and biopsies are performed to detect marrow

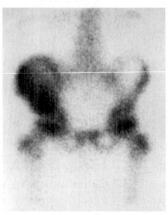
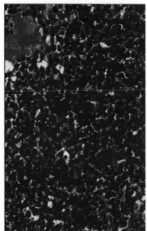

Tender bulge on proximal fibula with some inflammatory signs

Radiograph reveals mottled, destructive radiolucent lesion

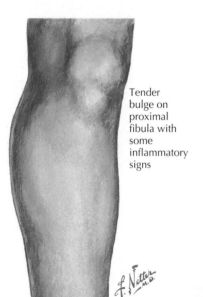
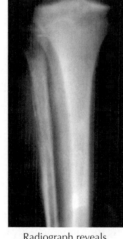

Bone scan shows lesion of mottled density involving anterior superior iliac spine

Section shows masses of small, round cells with uniformly sized hyperchromatic nuclei (H and E stain)

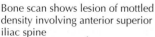

Figure 60-2 *Ewing's sarcoma.*

involvement. Functional imaging such as FDG (fluorodeoxy-D-glucose) positron emission tomography is being increasingly used in the staging and follow-up of patients with ESFT.

Management

The therapy of patients with ESFT involves multiple treatment modalities, including chemotherapy, surgery, and radiation therapy. Typically, treatment for ESFT begins with neoadjuvant (before surgery) chemotherapy to decrease tumor burden and to permit planning for definitive local control. Chemotherapeutic agents known to be active against ESFT include vincristine, doxorubicin, cyclophosphamide, ifosfamide, and etoposide. Treatment typically consists of alternating cycles of these agents on an every-2-week (compressed) schedule.

Local control can be achieved in ESFT with surgery, radiation therapy, or a combination of both. Surgical techniques similar to those used in OS may be used in ESFT, and complete surgical resection with resection margins clear of tumor is a critical goal in therapy. In contrast with OS, ESFT are responsive to radiation. Therefore, in cases that are not amenable to surgical resection, radiation can be used as the primary therapeutic modality for local control. Radiotherapy is also used after surgery if tumor is detected at the margins of resection. Adjuvant systemic chemotherapy is administered after local control. The total duration of ESFT therapy using modern intensive regimens is approximately 8 to 9 months.

Prognosis

The most important prognostic factor in ESFT is the extent of disease at diagnosis. Despite aggressive treatment regimens, fewer than one-third of patients with metastatic disease at diagnosis survive. However, for patients with localized disease, 5-year event-free survival rates near 80% have been reported. Age, site of disease, serum lactate dehydrogenase level, and histologic response to chemotherapy have also been identified as potential prognostic factors in newly diagnosed patients. Identification of prognostic factors in the relapse setting may also be useful because patients with localized, late recurrences appear to fare better than other patients.

FUTURE DIRECTIONS

The successful treatment of patients with localized OS and ESFT is a result of integrated, intensive multimodality care. Dramatic improvements in outcome have been achieved in the past 30 years, although late effects of the therapy delivered can have significant impact on survivors. The need to develop less toxic therapies for these patients is therefore pressing. In addition, the poor outcomes still observed in patients with metastatic bone tumors require the development of new approaches to the treatment of these diseases. Increased understanding of the basic biology of sarcomas will hopefully result in the development of rationally designed, targeted therapies for patients with bone tumors.

SUGGESTED READINGS

Bacci G, Bertoni F, Longhi A, et al: Neoadjuvant chemotherapy for high-grade central osteosarcoma of the extremity. Histologic response to preoperative chemotherapy correlates with histologic subtype of the tumor, *Cancer* 97(12):3068-3075, 2003.

Bernstein M, Kovar H, Paulussen M, et al: Ewing sarcoma family of tumors: Ewing sarcoma of bone and soft tissue and the peripheral primitive neuroectodermal tumors. In Pizzo PA, Poplack DG, editors: *Principles and Practice of Pediatric Oncology*, ed 5, Philadelphia, Lippincott, 2006, Williams & Wilkins, pp 1002-1032.

de Alava E, Gerald WL: Molecular biology of the Ewing's sarcoma/primitive neuroectodermal tumor family, *J Clin Oncol* 18(1):204-213, 2000.

Grier HE, Krailo MD, Tarbell NJ, et al: Addition of ifosfamide and etoposide to standard chemotherapy for Ewing's sarcoma and primitive neuroectodermal tumor of bone, *N Engl J Med* 348(8):694-701, 2003.

Gurney JG, Swensen AR, Bulterys M: Malignant bone tumors. In Ries LAG, Smith MA, Gurney JG, et al, editors: *Cancer Incidence and Survival Among Children and Adolescents: United States SEER Program 1975-1995*, NIH Pub. No 99-4649. Bethesda, MD, 1999, National Cancer Institute, SEER Program.

Link ML, Gebhardt MC, Meyers PA: Osteosarcoma. In Pizzo PA, Poplack DG, editors: *Principles and Practice of Pediatric Oncology*, ed 5, Philadelphia, Lippincott, 2006, Williams & Wilkins, pp 1074-1115.

Mirabello L, Troisi RJ Savage SA: Osteosarcoma incidence and survival rates from 1973 to 2004: data from the Surveillance, Epidemiology, and End Results Program, *Cancer* 115(7):1531-1543, 2009.

Disorders of the Renal and Urologic Systems

Hematuria and Proteinuria

Ryan M. Raffaelli and Madhura Pradhan

61

HEMATURIA

Hematuria is the medical term for the presence of blood in the urine and is a common pediatric problem. Gross hematuria is clearly visible. Whereas blood cells of a glomerular origin are usually present in brown, tea-colored, or cola-colored urine, blood from the lower urinary tract changes urine to pink or red. Microscopic hematuria is defined by the presence of five or more red blood cells (RBCs) per high-power field on at least three occasions over a 3-week period in a spun urine sample. Out of every 1000 children presenting to an emergency department, nearly 1.5 have gross hematuria; 1% to 2% of school-aged children have microscopic hematuria.

Several substances besides blood can cause discolored urine. Microhematuria is generally first detected on a dipstick test but should be confirmed by microscopic examination of the sediment of spun urine. Gross hematuria, without casts, should always be evaluated by renal ultrasound.

All children should have a screening urinalysis at school entry (age, 4-5 years) and during adolescence (age, 11-21 years). Serious conditions should be considered; however, most children with isolated microhematuria do not have a severe illness and do not require extensive investigation.

ETIOLOGY AND PATHOGENESIS

Table 61-1 and Box 61-1 provide a comprehensive differential diagnoses list for hematuria.

Hypercalciuria and Urolithiasis

Hypercalciuria can occur with low, normal, or high serum calcium levels. In eucalcemic patients, the most common cause is idiopathic; other causes include immobilization, Cushing's syndrome, distal renal tubular acidosis, and Bartter's syndrome. Disorders associated with hypercalcemia include hyperparathyroidism, vitamin D intoxication, hypophosphatasia, tumors, and immobilization bone resorption. Rare familial abnormalities of renal calcium channels are the cause of hypercalciuria with hypocalcemia. Hypercalciuria is the most common cause of stone disease.

Idiopathic hypercalciuria typically presents with asymptomatic microscopic hematuria. Stones can reveal their presence in a variety of ways to include dysuria, gross hematuria. and renal colic. Renal ultrasound or spiral computed tomography (CT) should be considered. Stones may be found incidentally after imaging is done for other reasons (e.g., radiographs for constipation). Radiographs can detect radiopaque stones but not those formed by uric acid.

The initial screening test for hypercalciuria is a urine calcium-to-creatinine ratio on a random urine sample. A ratio of greater than 0.2 in older children and adults is highly suggestive of hypercalciuria, with higher values in infants and young children.

Confirmation should be obtained by a 24-hour urine collection with an excretion of greater than 4 mg/kg/24 hours. Urine from this collection should be tested for cystine, citrate, oxalate, phosphorus, and uric acid excretion as well. The collection is difficult in younger children, however. Serum chemistries, including calcium, phosphorus, magnesium, uric acid, urine pH, and renal function, should also be obtained. A detailed family history for stone disease, diet history, and evaluation of medications and nutritional supplements should be sought. Recovery of a stone should be attempted for analysis. Stones caused by infection are rare in children.

Management of these patients is twofold (Figure 61-1). Pain management should be optimized. Surgical intervention or lithotripsy is indicated in cases of urinary obstruction or recurrent stones with superimposed urinary tract infections (UTIs). After the cause has been determined, therapy to prevent stone recurrence can be implemented; this includes increased fluid intake to ensure dilute hypotonic urine, dietary manipulation, and drug therapy in some cases.

Medications

Microscopic hematuria caused by drug exposure is not uncommon. Although some medications are commonly used in children, most are not. Gross hematuria associated with cyclophosphamide can be severe in some cases.

Glomerulonephritis

All forms of glomerulonephritis are discussed in Chapter 62.

Trauma

Traumatic injury to the urogenital tract is frequently seen with blunt force trauma and may be life threatening, depending on its severity. The presence of hematuria with minimal traumatic injury is highly suggestive of anatomic abnormalities of the kidney such as polycystic kidney disease.

Hematuria associated with renal trauma requires evaluation by CT scan, magnetic resonance imaging, or renal ultrasound. Urologic evaluation should be obtained before placement of a urethral or bladder catheter in cases of lower urinary tract trauma.

Most renal contusions or lacerations can be managed conservatively; however, significant lacerations of the kidney or injury to the collecting system or lower urinary tract may require emergent surgical intervention.

Malignancy

Wilms' tumor is the most common childhood malignancy of the kidney and is discussed further in Chapter 53. Microscopic hematuria is more commonly found than grossly bloody urine, but hematuria as the presenting sign of Wilms' tumor is rare.

Table 61-1 Distinguishing Features of Glomerular and Nonglomerular Hematuria

Feature	Glomerular	Nonglomerular
History		
Burning on micturition	No	Urethritis, cystitis
Systemic complaints	Edema, fever, pharyngitis, rash, arthralgias	Fever with UTIs; pain with calculi
Family history	Deafness in Alport syndrome, renal failure	Usually negative except with calculi
Physical Examination		
Hypertension	Often	Unlikely
Edema	Sometimes present	No
Abdominal mass	No	Wilms' tumor, polycystic kidneys
Rash, arthritis	SLE, HSP	No
Urine analysis		
Color	Brown, tea or cola colored	Bright red or pink
Proteinuria	Often	No
Dysmorphic RBCs	Yes	No
RBC casts	Yes	No
Crystals	No	May be informative

HSP, Henoch-Schönlein purpura; RBC, red blood cell; SLE, systemic lupus erythematosus; UTI, urinary tract infection.

Box 61-1 Differential Diagnosis of Hematuria

Non Glomerular Conditions
Urinary tract infections (see Chapter 93)
Bacterial, viral (adenovirus), tuberculosis
Structural abnormalities
   Congenital anomalies
   Polycystic kidneys
   Trauma
   Vascular anomalies: angiomyolipomas, arteriovenous malformations
   Tumors
Hematologic
   Sickle cell trait or disease
   Coagulopathies: von Willebrand disease, renal vein thrombosis
Hypercalciuria and nephrolithiasis
Exercise
Medications
Penicillins, polymyxin, sulfa-containing agents, anticonvulsants, Coumadin, aspirin, colchicine, cyclophosphamide, indomethacin, gold salts
Others
   Loin pain: hematuria syndrome
   Urethrorrhagia

Glomerular Conditions
IgA nephropathy
Alport syndrome
Benign familial hematuria
Acute poststreptococcal glomerulonephritis
Lupus nephritis
Membranoproliferative glomerulonephritis
Henoch-Schönlein purpura
Membranous nephropathy
Rapidly progressive glomerulonephritis

Hematologic Causes

Hematuria commonly occurs with sickle cell hemoglobinopathy. Affecting patients with either sickle cell disease or sickle cell trait, it is thought to be caused by sickling and sludging of RBCs in the renal medulla. Typically painless and occurring in adolescent boys, it can be precipitated by trauma, exercise, dehydration, or infection. Papillary necrosis is also seen with severe dehydration and renal infarction.

Hematuria is rarely the sole finding in a patient with a coagulopathy. However, coagulopathies should be investigated in patients without another source for painless, gross hematuria and a history of bruising/bleeding, or a family history of a bleeding diathesis.

Alport Syndrome

Alport syndrome is a hereditary nephritis associated with sensorineural hearing loss. Alport syndrome presents with persistent or recurrent microscopic or gross hematuria. It is further discussed in Chapter 62.

Benign Familial Hematuria

This disorder is defined by usually autosomal dominant transmission of persistent hematuria without proteinuria, hearing loss, or progressive renal disease.

This is a diagnosis of exclusion based on family history. Hematuria detected in the parents' or siblings' urine can support

the diagnosis that is only confirmed by renal biopsy. Biopsy shows thin basement membranes in most patients.

Loin Pain-Hematuria Syndrome

This syndrome is defined by recurrent episodes of pain in the lower abdomen with gross or microscopic hematuria usually occurring in women between 20 and 40 years of age, but it may occur in younger patients. The diagnosis is one of exclusion after investigating for other etiologies. There is often a psychological component. The usual management is pain control.

Urethrorrhagia

Painless terminal hematuria, or bloody spots in the underwear, occurring in boys between 4 and 17 years of age defines this process. Dysuria is present in 30%. Symptoms usually resolve in 2 weeks to 3 years in an average of 10 months. Complete resolution occurs in 92% overall. Treatment is watchful waiting after other causes of gross hematuria have been discounted. Cystoscopy should be avoided because urethral stricture may occur.

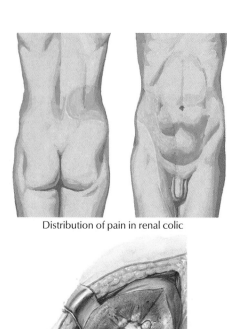

Distribution of pain in renal colic

Kidney split and widely laid open
for removal of multiple stones

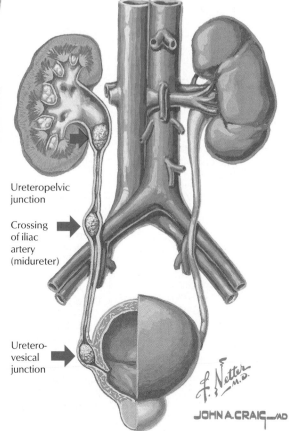

Ureteropelvic junction

Crossing of iliac artery (midureter)

Uretero-vesical junction

Common sites of obstruction

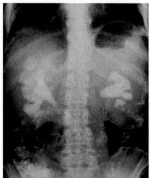

Staghorn calculus plus smaller stone

Bilateral staghorn calculi

Figure 61-1 *Kidney stones.*

CLINICAL PRESENTATION

History

A complete history is essential to guiding the diagnostic evaluation of hematuria.

- Previous episodes of gross hematuria or UTI
- Pattern of hematuria (initial, terminal)
- History of recent upper respiratory tract infections, sore throat, or impetigo
- Dysuria, frequency, voiding patterns, fever, weight loss, abdominal or flank pain, skin lesions
- Trauma or foreign body
- Drug, dietary, and vitamin or nutritional supplements
- Family history of renal disease including dialysis and transplant, hematuria, urolithiasis, sickle cell disease, coagulation disorders, hearing loss
- Travel to developing countries

Physical Examination

The examination of the patient should focus on the following:

- Blood pressure
- Edema
- Rash or purpura
- Arthritis
- Abdominal mass
- Ocular defects
- Genitourinary abnormalities

EVALUATION AND MANAGEMENT

The diagnostic evaluation of hematuria should be guided by findings on history and physical examination (Figure 61-2) and may include:

- Fresh urinalysis with microscopic examination of sediment for RBCs, crystals, and casts (Figure 61-3)
- Serum electrolytes: blood urea nitrogen, creatinine, calcium, phosphorus, uric acid
- Complete blood count with platelets
- Complement studies
- Antistreptolysin O or Streptozyme
- Antinuclear antibody
- Urine culture
- Urine Ca:Cr ratio or 24-hour urine Ca excretion
- Urinary excretion of cystine, oxalate, phosphorus, citrate, and urate

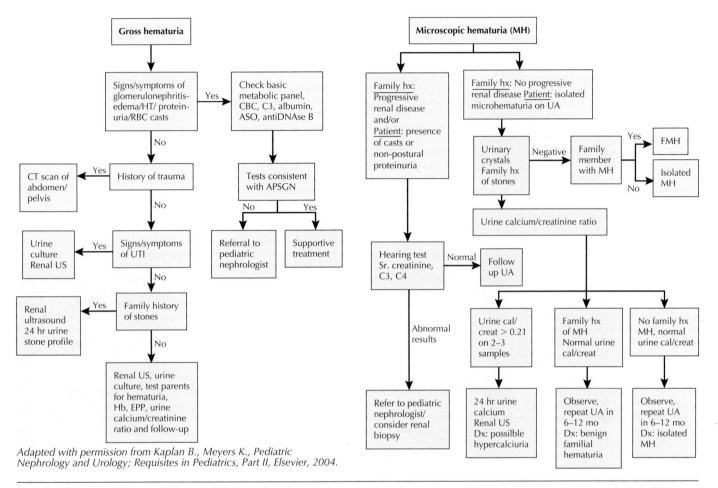

Adapted with permission from Kaplan B., Meyers K., Pediatric
Nephrology and Urology; Requisites in Pediatrics, Part II, Elsevier, 2004.

Figure 61-2 *Evaluation of the patient with hematuria: gross and microscopic.*

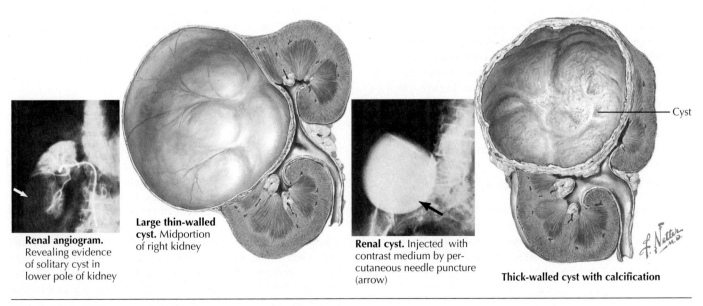

Renal angiogram. Revealing evidence of solitary cyst in lower pole of kidney

Large thin-walled cyst. Midportion of right kidney

Renal cyst. Injected with contrast medium by percutaneous needle puncture (arrow)

Thick-walled cyst with calcification

Cyst

Figure 61-3 *Solitary cysts of the kidney.*

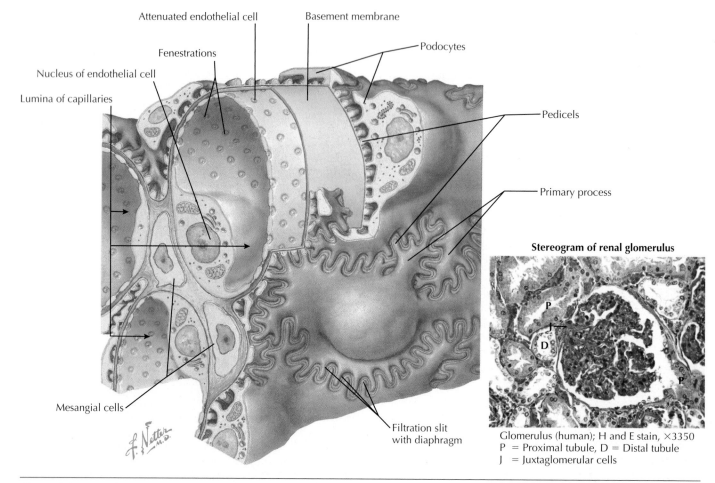

Figure 61-4 *Histology and fine structure of renal corpuscle.*

Diagnostic Modalities

Radiographic imaging is always indicated for evaluation of gross hematuria in the absence of RBC casts and proteinuria. Ultrasound evaluation of the kidneys and bladder should be part of the initial evaluation of hematuria unless the patient has isolated microhematuria. Magnetic resonance urography is useful for delineating the anatomic structure of the collecting systems as well as for defining functional obstructions. CT scans also provide valuable anatomic information. Additional studies such as nuclear scans, cystoscopy, angiography, or renal biopsy should be considered in consultation with a subspecialist.

TREATMENT OF HEMATURIA

The treatment of hematuria is driven by the underlying pathophysiology and is in large part conservative. Hematuria with concurrent proteinuria, hypertension, renal failure, trauma, or severe hemorrhage may indicate the need for more extensive investigation and therapy.

PROTEINURIA

Proteinuria, the presence of excessive protein in the urine, is a common finding in school-aged children. Up to 10% of children have proteinuria (30 mg/dL or higher on urine dipstick)

at some time. Its prevalence increases with age and peaks during adolescence. Although most proteinuria is transient or intermittent, it is the most common laboratory finding indicative of progressive renal disease. The challenge is to differentiate pathologic proteinuria from that of a physiologic nature. Normal urinary protein excretion in adults is less than 150 mg/d; in children, it is less than 4 mg/m²/h.

ETIOLOGY AND PATHOGENESIS

Benign Conditions

TRANSIENT PROTEINURIA

Transient proteinuria is unrelated to renal disease and resolves when the inciting factor disappears. It is rarely greater than 100 mg/dL on the dipstick. Febrile proteinuria usually appears with the onset of fever and resolves by 10 to 14 days. Proteinuria that occurs after exercise usually abates within 48 hours. Transient proteinuria seen with fever, exercise, and congestive heart failure is caused by hemodynamic alterations in renal blood flow that increases the passage of proteins across the glomerular basement membrane (Figure 61-4).

ORTHOSTATIC (POSTURAL) PROTEINURIA

Orthostatic proteinuria is elevated protein excretion that occurs only when the patient is upright. Although the exact mechanism is unclear, orthostatic proteinuria is most likely the result of excessive glomerular filtration of protein (see Figure 61-4). Orthostatic proteinuria is fairly common, accounting for 60% of all causes of childhood proteinuria. The prevalence is even higher among teenagers. Orthostatic proteinuria is an incidental finding. There are no specific clinical features (e.g., edema) and no known cause.

The diagnosis of orthostatic proteinuria can be made if urinary protein excretion is abnormal in samples obtained while the patient is upright but normal in samples obtained when the patient is recumbent. Total protein excretion should be less than 1 g/d. In some patients, orthostatic proteinuria is reproducible, but in others, it is intermittent. There are three approaches to evaluating orthostatic proteinuria:

1. **Dipstick analysis of first morning (recumbent) and daytime (upright) random urine samples.** Negative or trace protein in the first morning sample with a 30 mg/dL or greater protein in the daytime urine sample is suggestive of orthostatic proteinuria.
2. **Quantitative evaluation of proteinuria in a split collection.** Urine samples may be collected at timed intervals while the patient is recumbent as well as while ambulating and evaluated quantitatively for protein excretion. The timed urine samples should be collected by asking the child to void and discard the urine just before going to bed. The void should be collected into a container marked "recumbent" immediately upon arising. Then all the urine during the day, including the specimen voided just before going to bed, should be collected in a separate container labeled "ambulatory." In orthostatic proteinuria, the amount of protein in the ambulatory collection should be two to four times that of the recumbent collection.
3. **Calculation of the ratio of urine protein to urine creatinine.** The ratio of urine protein to urine creatinine is calculated on first morning and upright random urine samples. A normal ratio is less than 0.5 in children younger than 2 years of age and less than 0.2 in children older than 2 years; it is in the nephrotic range if it is greater than 2.

The prognosis for orthostatic proteinuria is thought to be very good.

PERSISTENT ASYMPTOMATIC ISOLATED PROTEINURIA

Persistent asymptomatic isolated proteinuria (PAIP) is defined as persistent proteinuria (>3 months) in an otherwise healthy child detected in more than 80% of the urine specimens tested, including recumbent samples. The prevalence in school-aged children is 6%. It is usually less than 1 g/d and is never associated with edema. Studies have reported divergent results with a significant number of patients having glomerulopathies such as focal sclerosis but others having normal histology or mild glomerular abnormalities. It is reasonable, in the absence of other findings, to consider a renal biopsy if proteinuria progresses to greater than 1 g/d or persists for more than 12 months. Children with PAIP form a heterogeneous group, and in the absence

of large prospective studies, the prognosis should be viewed with caution.

Pathologic Conditions
GLOMERULONEPHRITIS

Proteinuria occurs in most glomerular diseases. All forms of glomerulonephritis are discussed in Chapter 62.

NEPHROTIC SYNDROME

Nephrotic syndrome is defined by the presence of proteinuria, edema, hypercholesterolemia, and hypoalbuminemia. Nephrotic syndrome can be primary (isolated to the kidney) or secondary (part of a systemic disease, such as systemic lupus erythematosus). Nephrotic syndrome, including minimal change disease, focal and segmental glomerulosclerosis, and membranous nephropathy, is more fully discussed in Chapter 63.

TUBULAR DISEASES

Proteinuria caused by tubular disease can be from either congenital etiologies (dysplasia, polycystic kidney disease, Fanconi syndrome) or acquired ones (acute tubular necrosis, interstitial nephritis). Tubular proteinuria is usually less than 1 to 1.5 g/d.

CLINICAL PRESENTATION AND DETECTION

See Box 61-2 for a list of differential diagnoses. The clinical findings for patients with pathologic causes of proteinuria are discussed in Chapters 62 and 63.

Phase I Workup

The initial workup should begin with a complete history and physical examination. The physician should elicit history of recent infections (pharyngitis, impetigo), UTIs, oliguria or hematuria, and family history of renal disease. The physical examination should be focused on looking for hypertension (glomerulonephritis), edema (nephrotic syndrome), rash or arthritis (vasculitis), and short stature (chronic renal disease). Laboratory investigations in this phase should include a urine dipstick (ambulatory and recumbent), a urine analysis including microscopic examination, and a random urine protein-to-creatinine ratio.

Qualitative Protein Detection

The dipstick measures the concentration of protein in urine. A urine sample is considered positive for protein if it measures 1+ or greater when the specific gravity of urine is less than 1.015 or 2+ or greater when the specific gravity is greater than 1.015. A child is said to have persistent proteinuria if the dipstick is positive for protein on two of three random urine samples collected at least 1 week apart. The following can cause false-positive results on dipstick analysis: alkaline urine (pH >7.0), prolonged immersion, placing the strip directly in the urine stream, cleansing of the urethral orifice with quaternary ammonium compounds before collecting the sample, pyuria, and

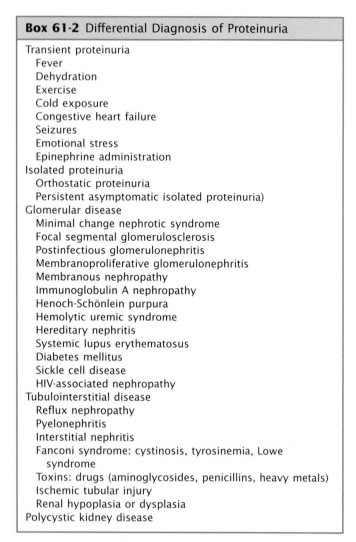

Box 61-2 Differential Diagnosis of Proteinuria

Transient proteinuria
  Fever
  Dehydration
  Exercise
  Cold exposure
  Congestive heart failure
  Seizures
  Emotional stress
  Epinephrine administration
Isolated proteinuria
  Orthostatic proteinuria
  Persistent asymptomatic isolated proteinuria)
Glomerular disease
  Minimal change nephrotic syndrome
  Focal segmental glomerulosclerosis
  Postinfectious glomerulonephritis
  Membranoproliferative glomerulonephritis
  Membranous nephropathy
  Immunoglobulin A nephropathy
  Henoch-Schönlein purpura
  Hemolytic uremic syndrome
  Hereditary nephritis
  Systemic lupus erythematosus
  Diabetes mellitus
  Sickle cell disease
  HIV-associated nephropathy
Tubulointerstitial disease
  Reflux nephropathy
  Pyelonephritis
  Interstitial nephritis
  Fanconi syndrome: cystinosis, tyrosinemia, Lowe
    syndrome
  Toxins: drugs (aminoglycosides, penicillins, heavy metals)
  Ischemic tubular injury
  Renal hypoplasia or dysplasia
Polycystic kidney disease

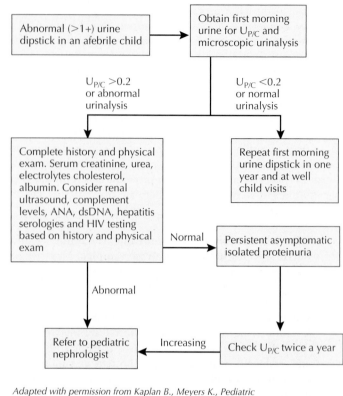

Adapted with permission from Kaplan B., Meyers K., Pediatric Nephrology and Urology; Requisites in Pediatrics, Part II, Elsevier, 2004.

Figure 61-5 *Suggested approach for the evaluation of proteinuria.*

bacteriuria. False-negative results can occur when the urine is too dilute (i.e., the specific gravity is <1.005) or when the patient excretes abnormal amounts of proteins other than albumin.

Quantitative Protein Detection

A timed urine collection for protein quantitation is essential to establish the degree of proteinuria. A 24-hour urine collection can be done by asking the child to void as soon as he or she wakes up and discarding the specimen; then every void should be collected for the next 24 hours, including the first void the next morning. In clinical practice, it is difficult to obtain timed urine collections in children. A random urine specimen can be analyzed for protein and creatinine concentration. Multiplying the random protein to creatinine ratio by 0.63 gives an estimated 24-hour total protein content in $g/m^2/d$.

EVALUATION AND MANAGEMENT

Phase II Workup

See Figure 61-5 for an evaluation algorithm. Split urine samples should be collected, and a 24-hour urinary protein level should be obtained.

Phase III Workup

If the initial workup suggests the presence of an underlying renal disease, a referral to a pediatric nephrologist should be made. A referral should be made in the following situations:

- Persistent fixed (i.e., nonorthostatic) proteinuria
- Family history of glomerulonephritis
- Systemic complaints (e.g., fever, rash, arthralgias)
- Hypertension
- Edema
- Cutaneous vasculitis or purpura
- Hematuria
- Abnormal renal function
- Abnormal renal ultrasound
- Increased parental anxiety

The nephrologist may perform a renal biopsy to define the etiology.

Most cases of proteinuria in children can be managed by a primary care physician at times in consultation with a pediatric nephrologist. Long-term follow-up is important because the prognoses in some of the conditions are not well defined.

FUTURE DIRECTIONS

Simple urinalysis is an easy way to ascertain proteinuria in the absence of clinical findings. It remains unclear if persistent proteinuria leads to glomerular damage, particularly focal sclerosis; however, angiotensin-converting enzyme inhibitors and angiotensin receptor blockers are proven to decrease protein excretion and may prevent chronic kidney damage in patients with seemingly "benign" forms of proteinuria.

SUGGESTED READINGS

Bergstein JM: A practical approach to proteinuria, *Pediatr Nephrol* 13:697-700, 1999.

Diven SC, Travis LB: A practical primary care approach to hematuria in children, *Pediatr Nephrol* 14:65-72, 2000.

Feld LG, Waz WR, Perez LM, et al: Hematuria: an integrated medical and surgical approach, *Pediatr Clin North Am* 44(5):1191-1210, 1997.

Hogg RJ, Portman RJ, Milliner D, et al: Evaluation and management of proteinuria and nephrotic syndrome in children: recommendations from a pediatric nephrology panel established at the National Kidney Foundation Conference on Proteinuria, Albuminuria, Risk, Assessment, Detection and Elimination (PARADE), *Pediatrics* 105:1242-1249, 2000.

Meyers KEC: Evaluation of hematuria in children, *Urol Clin of N Am* 31(3):559-573, 2004.

Yoshikawa N, Kitagawa K, Ohta K, et al: Asymptomatic constant isolated proteinuria in children, *J Pediatr* 119(3):375-379, 1991.

Glomerulonephritis

Matthew G. Sampson and Kevin E.C. Meyers

62

lomerulonephritis (GN) is a term used to describe an inflammatory insult to the kidney's glomeruli. A clinical pattern of hematuria, proteinuria, hypertension, red blood cell (RBC) casts, azotemia, oligoanuria, and edema occurs in various combinations. The inciting process varies from infectious to immunologic and from autoimmune to hereditary. Prompt recognition of GN is important because this disease can result in hypertensive emergency, hyperkalemia, heart failure, pulmonary edema, and renal failure. In addition, early diagnosis of GN permits prompt medical treatment of destructive subtypes that can cause long-term renal damage. Supportive care consists of strict attention to fluid and electrolyte management and blood pressure control. Certain types of GN require specific medical management to combat renal inflammation. An understanding of the diagnosis and management of GN ensures the best chance at reducing immediate morbidity and mortality as well as reducing the likelihood of progression to chronic kidney disease (CKD).

ETIOLOGY AND PATHOGENESIS

Most glomerulonephritides result from either circulating immune complex deposition within the glomerulus or in situ immune complex formation. This activates complement, as well as cellular and humoral pathways of inflammation. Within the glomerulus, there can be endothelial, epithelial, and mesangial hypercellularity, infiltration of leukocytes, thickening or duplication of the glomerular basement membrane, and necrosis (Figure 62-1). This results in loss of capillary integrity and obstruction of blood flow through the glomerular capillary loops. This capillary injury and obstruction of glomerular blood flow leads to the fluid overload, oligoanuric renal failure, hematuria, and RBC casts.

DIFFERENTIAL DIAGNOSIS

The two most common causes of GN in children are acute postinfectious GN (APIGN) and IgA nephropathy (IgAN). Other less common but important causes of GN include Henoch-Schönlein purpura (HSP), membranoproliferative GN (MPGN), rapidly progressive GN (RPGN), antineutrophilic cytoplasmic antibody– (ANCA-) positive vasculitis, systemic lupus erythematosus (SLE), and hemolytic-uremic syndrome (HUS).

Acute Postinfectious Glomerulonephritis

Acute poststreptococcal GN (APSGN) is the most common cause of APIGN in children and has a higher incidence in developing countries (Figure 62-2). APSGN is caused by nephritogenic forms of Lancefield group A streptococci. In most cases, there is clinical or laboratory evidence of antecedent streptococcal infection. APSGN must be confirmed or ruled out before looking for less common causes of post infectious GN (*Staphylococcus aureus, Streptococcus viridans*).

APSGN is characterized by sudden onset and variable presentation of hypertension, periorbital, lower extremity edema, oliguria, and painless gross hematuria. Urine microscopy reveals RBC casts. The glomerular damage in APSGN is immune mediated, with antigen–antibody reactions occurring in the circulation or in situ in glomeruli. These antigen–antibody reactions activate the alternative complement pathway cascade with reduction in the serum C3 concentration.

By light microscopy, findings in APSGN include glomerular enlargement, mesangial cell expansion and proliferation, and neutrophil exudation (see Figure 62-2). Electron microscopy (EM) reveals discrete subepithelial deposits.

IgA Nephropathy

IgA Nephropathy (IgAN) is an immune complex–mediated GN. Its course is highly variable and can range from asymptomatic microhematuria to recurrent episodes of gross hematuria to hypertension and acute and chronic renal failure. In Japan, of the children found by mass screening to have IgAN, 70% had asymptomatic microscopic hematuria. In these cases, IgAN is clinically silent. However, in up to 20% of patients who are referred to a pediatric nephrologist, IgAN will progress over decades to chronic renal failure.

The etiology of this disease is unknown. Although many children with IgAN present 1 to 2 days after the beginning of an upper respiratory infection, no infectious etiology has ever been identified. Most IgAN is sporadic, although an autosomal dominant form with incomplete penetrance has been found. Abnormally glycosylated IgA1 is found in the circulation and deposits in the skin and mesangium of the kidneys. The deposition of IgA in the mesangium causes activation of cytokines and growth factors, leading to mesangial expansion and extracellular matrix deposition.

Light microscopic findings show cellular and matrix expansion of the mesangium with deposition of IgA by immunofluorescence. Electron microscopy reveals electron dense deposits within the mesangium that may extend along capillary loops.

Henoch-Schönlein Purpura Nephritis

HSP nephritis is a small vessel vasculitis caused by IgA deposition within the glomeruli in the context of systemic HSP. Renal manifestations may present weeks after the onset of systemic HSP; rarely is it the first feature manifested in this syndrome. Prevalence of renal manifestations is subject to observer bias. Pediatric nephrology centers report that 50% of children with HSPN have hematuria and proteinuria, 8% have acute GN (AGN), 13% have nephrotic syndrome, and 29% have a mixed nephritic and nephrotic syndrome. Treatment of HSP nephritis is controversial because of a high rate of spontaneous remission and the lack of rigorous studies regarding treatment. Prognostic features are noted in Table 62-1.

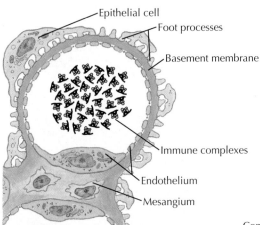
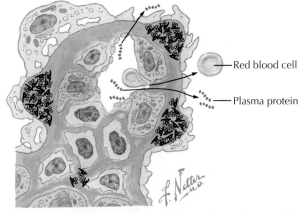

Epithelial cell
Foot processes
Basement membrane
Immune complexes
Endothelium
Mesangium

Red blood cell
Plasma protein

Circulating immune complexes, formed anywhere in the body, consisting of antigen, antibody, and complement components, arrive at glomerular capillaries in large amounts over a short period of time

Complexes penetrate endothelium and basement membrane of glomerular capillaries and form large isolated deposits (humps); foot processes fuse; mesangial and endothelial cells swell and proliferate, invading capillary lumen; fibrillar basement membrane–like material (mesangial matrix) is deposited between cells; increased porosity of capillary walls permits escape of plasma proteins and blood cells, causing proteinuria and hematuria

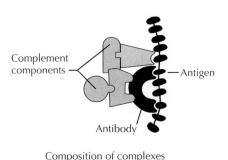

Complement components
Antigen
Antibody

Composition of complexes

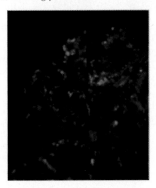

Immunofluorescent preparation, acute glomerulonephritis: irregular lumpy deposits of γ-globulin and complement, resembling experimental acute immune complex disease

Figure 62-1 *Hypothesis of pathogenesis of acute glomerular injury by circulating immune complexes (schematic).*

Rapidly Progressive Glomerulonephritis

Rapidly progressive glomerulonephritis (RPGN) may be idiopathic or secondary to Goodpasture's syndrome, HSP, Wegener's granulomatosis, SLE, APSGN, or IgAN. It is associated with rapidly deteriorating renal function. Glomerular crescents are present on biopsy. Patients with RPGN require renal biopsy to provide appropriate therapy.

Membranoproliferative Glomerulonephritis

Membranoproliferative glomerulonephritis (MPGN) is a form of GN with variable presentation, from asymptomatic proteinuria and hematuria to acute nephritis. MPGN requires prolonged therapy and can lead to CKD. It is an important differential diagnosis to consider in cases of presumed APSGN in which the serum C3 concentration does not revert to normal 6 to 8 weeks after the initial presentation.

Antineutrophilic Cytoplasmic Antibody–Positive Vasculitis/Pauci-Immune Glomerulonephritis

These are small vessel vasculitides (SVVs) that include Wegener's granulomatosis, microvascular polyangiitis, and Churg-Strauss syndrome. The pathogenesis involves antimyeloperoxidase and antiserinase 3 ANCAs (c-ANCA and p-ANCA). These patients may present with night sweats, fever, weight loss, cough, and hemoptysis. More than 50% present with a pulmonary–renal syndrome. The GN associated with SVV can be severe, with rapid progression to end-stage renal failure.

CLINICAL PRESENTATION

The clinical presentation of AGN is variable. Some children are asymptomatic and are found on screening, and others present to the emergency department with hypertensive emergency, edema, and acute renal failure. On history, the child's urine may be cola or iced tea colored; there usually is no associated dysuria. The child's face, abdomen, or legs may look swollen. One-third of patients will complain of cough, sore throat, fever, or headache. The most common physical examination findings are any combination of hypertension, edema, and gross hematuria. Nausea, vomiting, and abdominal pain are seen less often. Presentation with anuria, seizures, pulmonary edema, and symptoms of congestive heart failure occurs infrequently.

EVALUATION

Performing a directed patient history and physical examination focused toward the major causes of GN and targeted use of laboratory tests will help the practitioner with diagnosis.

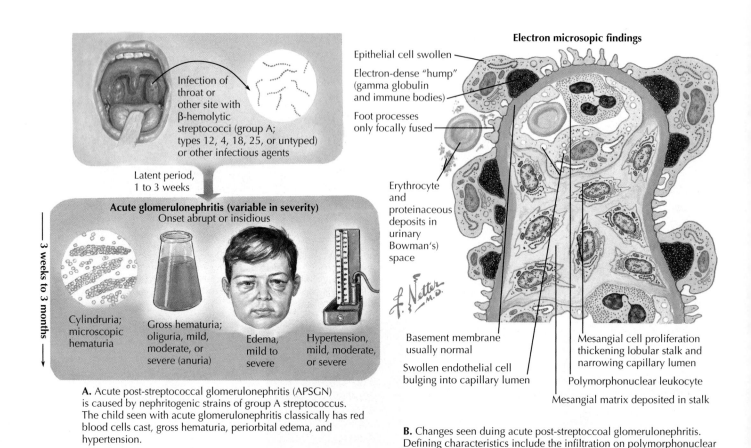

Figure 62-2 *Acute poststreptococcal glomerulonephritis.*

Recent Illnesses or Exposures

It is important to elicit the temporal relationship to any recent illnesses or exposures. ASPGN occurs after group A streptococcal infection of the throat (7-21 days later) or skin (14-28 days later). There may be a recent history of documented streptococcal pharyngitis or sore throat. Families may report that others in the family recently had sore throats but that the patient seemed unaffected. It is important to ask if there have been any skin infections (impetigo, infected bug bite, cellulitis) within the past month.

Table 62-1 Poor Prognostic Features of Selected Glomerulonephritides and Recommended Treatment

Disease	Poor Prognostic Features	First-Line Treatment
IgAN	Proteinuria >1 g/24 h, hypertension, azotemia, interstitial fibrosis, sclerotic glomeruli	If medical treatment,- corticosteroid ACEI
HSP	Presence of nephritic or nephrotic syndrome, renal failure, nephrotic-range ongoing proteinuria, interstitial fibrosis, sclerotic glomeruli	If medical treatment needed, corticosteroids, immunosuppressive agents
SLE	Diffuse proliferative GN (WHO Class IV), ↑ creatinine, persistent HTN, chronic anemia, nephrotic-range proteinuria	Corticosteroid therapy, cyclophosphamide, azathioprine, MMF
ANCA+ vasculitis or pauci-immune GN	Crescents on biopsy, frequent relapses	Corticosteroid therapy, azathioprine, MMF, cyclophosphamide
MPGN	Type II disease, nephrotic-range proteinuria	Corticosteroid therapy

ANCA, antineutrophilic cytoplasmic antibody; AZA, azathioprine; CCS, corticosteroids; GN, glomerulonephritis; HSP, Henoch-Schönlein purpura; HTN, hypertension; IgAN, IgA nephropathy; MMF, mycophenolate mofetil; MPGN, membranoproliferative glomerulonephritis; SLE, systemic lupus erythematosus; WHO, World Health Organization.

In IgA nephropathy, gross hematuria begins concurrently or 1 to 2 days after the start of an upper respiratory infection. A recent history of a visit to a zoo or farm or ingestion of undercooked hamburgers or unwashed fruits and vegetables might suggest HUS.

Other Symptoms and Review of Systems

Questions to ask in the review of symptoms include:

- Does the patient have abdominal pain or purpuric lesions that would suggest HSP nephritis?
- Is there a malar rash, pleuritic chest pain, neurologic changes, or other stigmata of SLE?
- Is there concomitant bloody diarrhea or a lobar pneumonia that would be seen in Shiga toxin or pneumococcal HUS, respectively?
- Is there any hemoptysis or sinusitis suggesting Wegener's granulomatosis or Goodpasture syndrome?
- Does the child have any hearing loss that would suggest a diagnosis of Alport's syndrome?
- Has the child fainted, felt dizzy, or had heart palpitations that could be indicative of arrhythmias caused by electrolyte imbalance?

Family History

In a child with suspected GN, it is also important to obtain a detailed family history, focusing on inherited forms of GN, especially Alport's syndrome (also known as hereditary nephritis). In all of these cases, it is important to construct a family tree because Alport's syndrome is usually X-linked. Questions to ask include:

- Has anyone else in the family ever had gross hematuria?
- Has anyone in the family been told that he or she has microscopic hematuria?
- Is there a history of renal failure, dialysis, or renal transplant in the family?

Physical Examination

In AGN, it is important to determine the degree of intravascular volume overload and to look for findings suggestive of the cause for the GN.

INTRAVASCULAR VOLUME STATUS

It is important to determine whether there is fluid overload that is compromising the child's cardiorespiratory status. Intravascular volume overload is suggested by weight gain in presence of elevated blood pressure; jugular venous distension; gallop rhythm; reduced oxygenation by pulse oximetry; increased work of breathing, rales, or crackles; hepatomegaly; and peripheral edema. The edema in AGN varies in severity. Hypertensive children may present with seizures, but headache and nonspecific behavioral changes are more common.

Table 62-2 Types of Glomerulonephritis with Possible Associated Physical Examination Findings

Disease	Notable Physical Examination Findings
ASPGN	Pharyngitis, healing or healed impetigo or ecthyma
IgAN	Coryza, congestion, pharyngitis, cough
HSP	Abdominal pain, palpable purpura
SLE	Malar or discoid rash, painless oral ulcers, neurologic changes, arthritis, serositis
ANCA positive: pauci-immune GN	Weight loss, fever, myalgias, sinusitis, hemoptysis (pulmonary–renal syndrome)
HUS: Shiga toxin positive	Bloody diarrhea
Pneumococcal	Lobar pneumonia

ANCA, antineutrophilic cytoplasmic antibody; APSGN, acute poststreptococcal glomerulonephritis; HSP, Henoch-Schönlein purpura; HUS, hemolytic-uremic syndrome; IgAN, IgA nephropathy; SLE, systemic lupus erythematosus.

OTHER PHYSICAL EXAMINATION FINDINGS

Physical examination findings that may indicate specific etiologies of AGN are detailed in Table 62-2.

Laboratory Evaluation

Laboratory evaluation is required to assess renal function and serum electrolyte concentrations, evaluate for the presence of GN, and determine the etiology of the glomerular inflammation. The presence of RBC casts should be determined in a fresh urine specimen examined by microscopy. The serum C3 concentration helps differentiate among the many causes of GN. A low serum C3 concentration is present in APSGN and MPGN. Patients with SLE may have low serum concentrations of C3 and C4. In those with IgAN, SVV, HUS, Alport syndrome, and HSP nephritis, the serum C3 concentration is normal. The serum C3 concentration should return to normal in 6 to 8 weeks in children with APSGN. If this does not occur and the patient remains symptomatic, then a biopsy should be considered to evaluate for MPGN. Studies used to differentiate among the glomerulonephritides are detailed in Table 62-3.

Imaging

Renal ultrasonography shows nonspecific echogenicity. Chest radiograph may show fluid overload or features of vasculitis.

Biopsy

The most definitive way to diagnose the cause and guide therapy of GN is with a percutaneous renal biopsy. Using a combination of light microscopy, immunofluorescence, and EM, the underlying GN type can be discerned.

Table 62-3 Laboratory Tests Important in Distinguishing Etiology of Glomerulonephritis

Disease	Laboratory Evaluation
APSGN	C3, ASOT, Streptozyme, rapid strep or throat culture
IgAN	Glycosylated IgA1, renal biopsy
SLE	C3, C4, ANA, anti-Smith, anti dsDNA, and renal biopsy
ANCA+ Vasculitis/ Pauci-Immune glomerulonephritis	ANCA titers, anti-PR3 Ab, anti-MPO Ab, and renal biopsy
HUS	Stool culture for *Escherichia coli* O157, stool Shiga toxin
MPGN	C3, C4, hepatitis panel (secondary causes of MPGN)
Alport's syndrome	Genetic test for mutations in type IV collagen gene COL4A5 and renal biopsy

ANCA, antineutrophil cytoplasmic antibody; ANA, antinuclear antibodies; APSGN, acute poststreptococcal glomerulonephritis; ASOT, antistreptolysin titer; C3/4, complement 3/4; HSP, Henoch-Schönlein purpura; HUS, hemolytic-uremic syndrome; IgAN, IgA nephropathy; MPGN, membranoproliferative glomerulonephritis; PR3, serine protease 3; MPO, myeloperoxidase; SLE, systemic lupus erythematosus.

MANAGEMENT

Management of fluid balance, control of hypertension, and correction of electrolyte abnormalities are the most acute components of the treatment of GN. After these have been addressed, use of other agents that may modify the course of disease are used. For patients with oliguria, fluid administration should be limited to insensible fluid losses plus replacement of urine output. Insensible losses can be estimated at one-third of daily maintenance requirements. Children who are volume overloaded can also be given intravenous furosemide. Over time, as the child's urine output improves, fluid intake can be liberalized. The combination of evaluation of daily weights and physical examination looking for signs of volume overload guides total daily fluid volume requirements. Hypertension associated with GN is caused by intravascular fluid retention with decreased glomerular filtration and by nitrous oxide–endothelin imbalance. Furosemide and calcium channel blockers should be used as initial therapy. Hyperkalemia can be life threatening, especially in the presence of acidosis, hemolysis, and anuria. The acute management of hyperkalemia focuses on the administration of calcium to stabilize the myocardium pari pasu with insulin or glucose and bicarbonate to shift potassium intracellularly. Kayexalate is used rectally to remove potassium from the body. Dialysis may be required to manage the hyperkalemia.

Therapies Targeting the Underlying Glomerulonephritis

The therapies described in this chapter are nonspecific and treat the homeostatic derangements directly attributable to the GN. Strategies in use that target the underlying glomerular inflammation include corticosteroids, cyclophosphamide, and plasmapheresis. Table 62-1 lists prognostic features for the different types of GN along with suggestions for first-line treatment.

FUTURE DIRECTIONS

Progress is being made in improving the evaluation and management of GN. Current studies focus on earlier detection of glomerular injury accompanied by directed therapy specific to each underlying cause of GN. Finally, research continues in understanding how to prevent, halt, or reverse the chronic renal damage caused by GN.

SUGGESTED READINGS

Kaplan BS, Meyers KEC: *Pediatric Nephrology and Urology; The Requisites in Pediatrics*, ed 1. Philadelphia, 2004, Elsevier, pp 131-162, 185-208.

National High Blood Pressure Education Program Working Group on High Blood Pressure in Children and Adolescents: The Fourth Report on the Diagnosis, Evaluation, and Treatment of High Blood Pressure in Children and Adolescents, *Pediatrics* 114:555-576, 2004.

Nephrotic Syndrome

63

Michelle Denburg and Shamir Tuchman

Nephrotic syndrome is defined by an association of the following four clinical and laboratory findings: (1) edema, (2) proteinuria, (3) hypoalbuminemia, and (4) hyperlipidemia. Nephrotic syndrome may be a manifestation of many underlying renal disease processes. Most often in children, however, the nephrotic syndrome is idiopathic, with an incidence of two to seven per 100,000 children younger than 16 years old. Idiopathic nephrotic syndrome can be broadly categorized based on the response to oral steroid treatment (steroid sensitive, steroid dependent, and steroid resistant). The majority of biopsy specimens comprise three underlying histologic lesions: minimal-change nephrotic syndrome (MCNS), focal segmental glomerulosclerosis (FSGS), and membranous nephropathy, the latter being rare in childhood. MCNS is the most common (60%-90% of cases), although there has been an apparent increase in the incidence of FSGS over the past several decades.

ETIOLOGY AND PATHOGENESIS

Although most often idiopathic, a variety of conditions and agents are associated with the nephrotic syndrome. These include (1) infections (e.g., HIV, hepatitis B and C, syphilis, toxoplasmosis, malaria), (2) drugs or toxins (e.g., nonsteroidal antiinflammatory drugs, lithium, ampicillin, penicillamine, heroin, mercury), (3) malignancy (lymphoma, leukemia), (4) allergens (e.g., certain foods and bee stings), and (5) obesity. Nephrotic syndrome may also be an associated feature of several glomerulonephritides, such as lupus nephritis, membranoproliferative glomerulonephritis (MPGN), and immunoglobulin A (IgA) nephropathy. With advances in molecular biology, there has been increasing discovery of genetic disorders resulting in steroid-resistant nephrotic syndrome (Table 63-1). The clinical course and histopathology depend on the underlying disease process or precipitating factors.

The frequent association of both the onset and relapse of "idiopathic" nephrotic syndrome with an antecedent upper respiratory tract infection or atopic event, as well as the response to immunosuppressive therapy, suggests that it is immunologically mediated. Multiple immunologic abnormalities and circulating factors that affect glomerular capillary permeability have been described, but the exact pathophysiology remains to be elucidated. The established familial occurrence (mostly in siblings) and similarity of the clinical course within families also implicate genetic factors.

Although the pathophysiologic mechanisms responsible for nephrotic syndrome clearly involve both environmental and genetic factors and differ based on the underlying diagnosis, the unifying pathology is damage to the glomerular filtration barrier either through injury to the glomerular basement membrane (GBM) or podocytes. On electron microscopy, there is effacement, retraction, and vacuolization of epithelial foot processes, and in the unique case of membranous nephropathy, there are immune complex deposits. Light microscopy may show no

abnormalities (minimal change), mesangial proliferation or matrix expansion, any of several morphologic variants of focal and segmental glomerulosclerosis (FSGS), or thickening of the GBM (membranous). Immunofluorescent staining results are typically negative in MCNS. There are characteristic patterns of staining in FSGS and membranous nephropathy as well as in the primary glomerulonephritides associated with nephrotic syndrome, such as lupus and MPGN (Figure 63-1). Although the histopathology is important, particularly if there is significant tubulointerstitial fibrosis and glomerulosclerosis, the response to steroid therapy is the most important predictor of clinical outcome.

CLINICAL PRESENTATION

Demographic Factors

The clinical and histopathologic distribution of nephrotic syndrome varies by age at onset and race. MCNS typically presents between 2 and 8 years of age (peak, 3 years). About 20% to 30% percent of nephrotic syndrome in adolescence is MCNS. FSGS occurs at a median of 6 years of age and is more common in adolescents than in younger children. MCNS is twofold more common in boys than girls until adolescence when both sexes are equally affected, and its incidence is higher in white and East Asian relative to black children. Steroid-resistant nephrotic syndrome is more common in black and Hispanic children. Genetic syndromes and congenital infections are considerably more common causes of nephrotic syndrome in infancy.

Edema

Edema is the main presenting feature, and its onset may be rapid or insidious. Edema is detectable when fluid accumulation is greater than 3% to 5% of body weight. Edema often presents in the periorbital region, is more pronounced in the morning, and is often misdiagnosed and treated as an allergic reaction or seasonal allergies. Edema may fluctuate with positional changes and activity, with lower extremity swelling being more noticeable over the course of the day. Edema develops in other dependent areas such as the sacral region and genitalia. Pleural effusions are generally asymptomatic but if large may cause respiratory compromise. Ascites may lead to umbilical or inguinal hernias as well as to more serious complications, such as spontaneous bacterial peritonitis (SBP). Bowel wall edema may produce diminished appetite; abdominal colic; and diarrhea, which, if chronic, can lead to a protein-losing enteropathy. Skin breakdown and infection can occur in the setting of severe edema (Figure 63-2).

Blood Pressure and Volume Status

Children with MCNS may have mild elevations in blood pressure, but significant hypertension is suggestive of another

Table 63-1 Genetic Causes of Steroid-Resistant Nephrotic Syndrome

Condition	Locus	Gene and Protein	Inheritance	Lesion	Additional Clinical Features
Finnish-type congenital nephrotic syndrome	19q	NPHS1 Nephrin	AR	Proximal tubular dilatation; Interstitial and periglomerular fibrosis; Glomerulosclerosis; Lymphocytic or plasma cell infiltration	Onset between birth and 3 months; Chronic renal failure; Failure to thrive; Recurrent infection; Renal vein thrombosis; Hypothyroidism; ↑ Maternal serum AFP and large placenta; Prematurity and SGA
Inherited SRNS	1q	NPHS2 Podocin	AR 20%–30% of sporadic SRNS	FSGS (some minimal change)	Early onset with rapid progression to ESRD
DMS; DMS in Denys-Drash syndrome	11p	WT-1 transcription factor	Sporadic or AR Germline mutation	Mesangial sclerosis; Collapsed tufts; Thickened GBM; Tubulointerstitial lesions	Onset between 3 and 6 months; Chronic renal failure; Hypertension; Ambiguous genitalia; Wilms' tumor
Frasier syndrome	11p	WT-1	AD	FSGS	ESRD in adolescence or early adulthood; Male pseudohermaphroditism • XY karyotype • Female external genitalia • Streak gonads; Gonadoblastoma
Pierson's syndrome	3p	LAMB2 Laminin β2 chain	AR	DMS	Neonatal onset; Microcoria
Galloway-Mowat syndrome	?	?	AR	DMS; FSGS; Minimal change	Onset <3 years of age; CNS abnormalities • Microcephaly • Wide sulci and abnormal gyri • Mental retardation • Seizures
Nail-Patella syndrome	9q	LMX1B transcription factor	AD	Abnormal GBM	<25% have renal involvement, <10% with renal failure; Dysplastic nails; Skeletal anomalies: absent or hypoplastic patellae, patellar dislocations, elbow abnormalities, iliac horns; Glaucoma
Dominant FSGS	19q 11q	ACTN4α-actinin-4 TRPC6	AD	FSGS	Later presentation and slower progression
Schimke immuno-osseous dysplasia	2q	SMARCAL1	AR	FSGS	Infantile and juvenile forms; Spondyloepiphyseal dysplasia; Short stature; T-cell deficiency

AD, autosomal dominant; AFP, α-fetoprotein; AR, autosomal recessive; CNS, central nervous system; DMS, diffuse mesangial sclerosis; ESRD, end-stage renal disease; FSGS, focal segmental glomerulosclerosis; SGA, small for gestational age; SRNS, steroid-resistant nephrotic syndrome.

underlying pathology, such as FSGS or glomerulonephritis with or without renal failure.

Careful assessment of volume status is critical. The child with anasarca may be profoundly intravascularly volume depleted. Tachycardia, orthostatic blood pressure changes, and hemoconcentration are indicative of hypovolemia. Children with nephrotic syndrome are at increased risk of cardiovascular collapse in the setting of ongoing volume loss (e.g., vomiting and diarrhea), particularly if compounded by adrenal insufficiency caused by long-term steroid administration. The acute management of hypovolemia in these patients consists of standard resuscitation with intravenous (IV) saline.

Urine

Nephrotic patients are often oliguric, and the urine appears concentrated and foamy. Nephrotic-range proteinuria is characterized by urine protein excretion greater than 40 mg/m^2/h on a 24-hour collection or a random urinary protein-to-creatinine ratio greater than 2. The specific gravity may be

Minimal disease

Foot processes fused

Epithelial cell

Basement membrane

Subendothelial "ßuff"

Glomerular capillary lumen

Endothelial cell

Mesangial cell

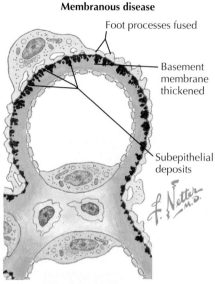

Electron microscopic findings. Only fusion of epithelial foot processes and some subendothelial "ßuff"

Membranous disease

Foot processes fused

Basement membrane thickened

Subepithelial deposits

f. Netter

Electron microscopic findings. Electron-dense deposits beneath epithelial cells, thickening of basement membrane, and fusion of foot processes

Proliferative disease

Epithelial cell proliferation

Foot processes fused

Endothlial cell proliferation

Mesangial cell proliferation

Basement membrane–like material

Fibrinoid

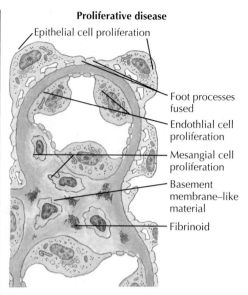

Electron microscopic findings. Epithelial, endothelial, and mesangial cell proliferation; little or no thickening of basement membrane, but variable amount of basement membrane–like material (mesangial matrix) deposited in mesangium; foot processes fused

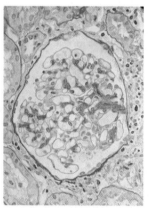

Light microscopic findings. Glomerulus appears normal; protein may be present in tubule lumina and lipoid droplets in tubule cells (PAS, ×250) ·

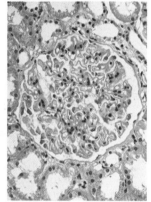

Light microscopic findings. Basement membrane thickened and eosinophilic; prominence but no numerical increase of epithelial, endothelial, and mesangial cells (H and E, ×250)

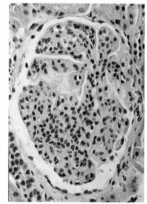

Light microscopic appearance. Cellular proliferation—epithelial, endothelial, and mesangial; very little, if any, basement membrane thickening (H and E, ×250)

Figure 63-1 *Pathology of the nephrotic syndrome.*

artificially high secondary to the proteinuria. Microscopic hematuria may be noted, but gross hematuria is rare.

Laboratory Findings

The laboratory abnormalities associated with nephrotic syndrome are listed in Box 63-1. Serum albumin is typically below 2.4 g/dL. Chronic hypoproteinemia produces transverse white bands in the nail beds, dull hair, and softening of ear cartilage.

Hyperlipidemia, particularly hypercholesterolemia but also hypertriglyceridemia, results from increased lipoprotein synthesis in the liver, attributed to low portal vein oncotic pressure and urinary loss of high-density lipoprotein and an unidentified regulatory substance. The associated hyponatremia (serum sodium, 120s-130 mEq/L) is typically not associated with central nervous system symptoms and is most likely caused by antidiuretic hormone–mediated free water retention but less commonly may be a sign of adrenal insufficiency. Blood urea

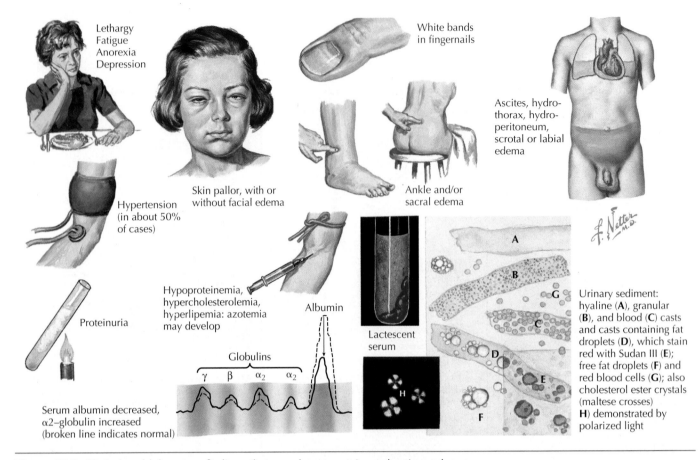

Figure 63-2 *Clinical and laboratory findings that may be present in nephrotic syndrome.*

nitrogen, serum creatinine, and hematocrit may be elevated secondary to intravascular volume depletion. Pseudohypocalcemia is caused by hypoalbuminemia. However, true hypocalcemia may result from loss of 25-hydroxyvitamin D–binding protein in the urine.

Complications

The two most important acute complications of nephrotic syndrome contributing to morbidity and mortality are infections and thromboembolic events. Common serious infections include pneumonia, SBP, and cellulitis. Several factors contribute to impaired immunity and infection: (1) defective opsonization

through complement loss, (2) changes in T-cell function and IgG concentrations, (3) edema, and (4) immunosuppressive treatment. Children with nephrotic syndrome are at higher risk for infection with encapsulated organisms, especially *Streptococcus pneumoniae*, as well as with gram-negative organisms, measles, and varicella.

The prothrombotic state of nephrotic syndrome is also multifactorial, resulting from a combination of disproportionate urinary loss of anticoagulant factors, increased production of clotting factors, thrombocytosis, increased platelet adhesion and aggregability, increased viscosity, and hyperlipidemia. This state may be exacerbated by diuretic and steroid therapy, venous catheters, and immobilization. Arterial sticks and catheters should be avoided because of the potential for arterial thrombosis and consequent ischemic injury to the extremity. Pulmonary embolus should be considered in a nephrotic patient with respiratory distress or pleuritic chest pain. Renal vein thrombosis should be suspected in the setting of acute azotemia, hypertension, flank pain, or gross hematuria.

Acute renal failure may develop in the setting of intravascular volume depletion, pyelonephritis, bilateral renal vein thrombosis, or medications associated with decreased renal perfusion (e.g., renin–angiotensin blockade and diuretics). Urinary loss of vitamin D–binding protein may lead to vitamin D deficiency and even secondary hyperparathyroidism. Hypothyroidism may result from loss of thyroid-binding globulin and thyroxine in the urine. Anemia may result from transferrin loss. Finally, trace

---

Box 63-1 Laboratory Findings in Nephrotic Syndrome

Hyperlipidemia (↑ cholesterol, ↑ triglycerides)
 Hyponatremia (serum sodium 120 to low 130 mEq/L)
 Azotemia (↑ BUN)
 ↓ Serum calcium (pseudohypocalcemia, true hypocalcemia)
 Hemoconcentration (↑ hemoglobin)
 Thrombocytosis
 ↑↑ ESR

BUN, blood urea nitrogen; ESR, erythrocyte sedimentation rate.

metal deficiencies (copper and zinc) may occur secondary to ceruloplasmin and albumin losses, respectively.

EVALUATION AND MANAGEMENT

Although idiopathic MCNS is most common in pediatric patients, careful attention should be focused on clinical characteristics that are inconsistent with MCNS and warrant a renal biopsy. These include (1) age younger than 12 months or older than 13 years at presentation; (2) extrarenal or constitutional symptoms, such as weight loss, recurrent fever, rash, or arthritis; (3) significant hypertension or pulmonary edema; (4) gross hematuria or the presence of red blood cell casts; and (5) renal failure. Glucocorticoid therapy without renal biopsy is indicated in the absence of such characteristics. Steroid resistance is an indication for renal biopsy. Careful history and physical examination should also identify patients with potential secondary causes of nephrotic syndrome, whether infectious, autoimmune, or malignant. Patients should be evaluated accordingly with serologies, complement levels, and computed tomography scans.

Supportive Therapy

Dietary restriction of sodium to less than 2 g/d decreases edema as well as the risk of steroid-induced hypertension. Dietary protein should neither be restricted nor enhanced. Children with nephrotic syndrome should consume the recommended daily allowance of protein. Administration of diuretics, such as furosemide and metolazone, with or without 25% IV albumin, may be used to treat symptomatic edema but should be used with caution to avoid acute volume overload or intravascular depletion. Empiric antibiotic coverage should be administered for suspected serious bacterial infections and peritoneal fluid sampled for cell count and culture to identify a causative organism.

Glucocorticoids

The standard treatment regimen at initial presentation is 4 to 6 weeks of prednisone 60 mg/m^2/d or 2 mg/kg of ideal body weight (maximum, 80 mg/d) followed by 4 to 6 weeks of 40 to 60 mg/m^2 on alternating days, after which the dose is gradually tapered. If there is concern about enteral absorption because of bowel wall edema, IV methylprednisolone may be used. Patients should have a PPD placed before starting therapy. The first morning urine sample should be monitored daily by urine dip. Remission is defined as at least 3 consecutive days of negative to trace urine protein. Approximately 95% of children with MCNS compared with 20% to 25% of those with FSGS go into remission after 8 weeks of prednisone. About 75% of children with MCNS are in remission by 2 weeks. Relapse is defined by 3 consecutive days of 2+ or greater urine protein. Approximately 80% of patients have at least one relapse, and 50% become frequent relapsers (i.e., two relapses in 6 months or three in 1 year). Steroid dependence is defined by a relapse while weaning or within 2 weeks of stopping steroid therapy. Steroid resistance is defined as lack of remission by 8 weeks of standard steroid therapy. Pulse IV methylprednisolone may produce remission in some steroid-resistant patients.

Other

Adjunctive therapies for steroid resistance (or steroid dependence with serious steroid side effects) include alkylating agents (e.g., cyclophosphamide), calcineurin inhibitors (e.g., cyclosporine, tacrolimus), and renin-angiotensin blockade (angiotensin-converting enzyme inhibitors, angiotensin receptor antagonists). Children and adolescents with progressive renal failure may require renal replacement therapy and a renal transplant. FSGS may recur after transplant in 30% to 50% of cases.

SUGGESTED READINGS

Avner ED, Harmon WE, Niaudet P, editors: *Pediatric Nephrology*, ed 5. Philadelphia, 2004, Lippincott Williams & Wilkins, pp 543-573.

Eddy AA, Symons JM: Nephrotic syndrome in childhood, *Lancet* 362:629-639, 2003.

Kaplan BS, Meyers KEC, editors: *Pediatric Nephrology and Urology: The Requisites in Pediatrics*. Philadelphia, 2004, Elsevier Mosby, pp 156-184.

Tryggvason K, Patrakka J, Wartiovaara J: Hereditary proteinuria syndromes and mechanisms of proteinuria, *N Engl J Med* 354:1387-1401, 2006.

Hemolytic-Uremic Syndromes

Christopher LaRosa and Kevin E. C. Meyers

64

Hemolytic-uremic syndromes (HUS) are clinical conditions characterized by acute kidney injury, thrombocytopenia, and microangiopathic hemolytic anemia with evidence of intravascular red blood cell (RBC) destruction demonstrated by fragmented cells (schistocytes) on blood smear. The kidney injury can manifest as hematuria, proteinuria, or azotemia, which can occur individually or in combination. HUS has clinical overlap with thrombotic thrombocytopenic purpura (TTP), a syndrome known to occur as a pentad that includes the HUS triad in addition to fever and neurologic abnormalities. TTP was first described by Moschcowitz in 1924 in a 16-year-old girl with fever, anemia, heart failure, and stroke; HUS was described by von Gasser in 1955 as a case series of five children with nonimmune (Coombs-negative) hemolytic anemia, thrombocytopenia, and small vessel renal thrombi. Generally, whereas neurologic features predominate in TTP, renal injury is a major component of HUS. The classification of these syndromes has become increasingly complex in view of the fact that multiple distinct underlying pathogenic mechanisms result in a similar disease phenotype. More precise etiologic definitions allows for a better understanding of associated clinical features and prognosis as well as rational treatment approaches.

ETIOLOGY AND PATHOGENESIS

Broadly defined, HUS and TTP are syndromes whose pathologic correlate is thrombotic microangiopathy (TMA). TMA describes the microvascular occlusion that occurs most frequently within capillaries and arterioles (Figure 64-1). It is seen histologically as thrombi, endothelial cell swelling, luminal narrowing, and fibrinoid necrosis of the vessel wall. TMA results from dysfunction of the endothelial cell–platelet interface and can originate from various underlying mechanisms, which form the basis for an etiologic classification. HUS can result from infectious causes, genetic causes, or medication-related causes or in association with secondary discrete pathologic entities. TTP results from a deficiency of von Willebrand factor-cleaving protease, (vWF-cp), which can be either acquired because of the presence of an autoantibody or congenital resulting from a mutation in the *ADAMTS13* gene.

The majority of childhood cases of HUS occur after a prodromal diarrheal illness. For this reason, it has been termed D+ or "typical" HUS, in contrast to the less common forms of HUS not associated with a diarrheal prodrome, known as D- or "atypical" HUS. A more precise classification for D+ HUS is Shiga toxin–associated HUS (Stx HUS), which is known to cause 90% of all HUS cases in children. As the name suggests, Stx HUS occurs as a result of Shiga toxin–producing organisms. The most common of these is Shiga toxin–producing *Escherichia coli* (STEC), also known as verocytotoxin-producing *E. coli*, so-called for their ability to lyse vero cells, a primate kidney cell line with epithelial characteristics. And of these, the most common serotype is O157:H7, which expresses somatic (O) antigen 157 and

flagellar (H) antigen 7. Stx HUS can occur at any age but primarily affects children younger than 5 years of age; the peak incidence is between the ages of 6 months and 4 years. It occurs both sporadically and in the form of epidemic outbreaks, most commonly during the summer and autumn months and largely in rural areas. The disease has an annual incidence of two to three per 100,000 children younger than 5 years of age in North America and Western Europe. The incidence decreases among older children. In countries such as Uruguay and Argentina, STEC infections are endemic and cause HUS in about 10.5 per 100,000 children per year.

The primary reservoir for STEC is cattle. Environmental sources of the infection include undercooked beef or poultry, deer jerky, unpasteurized milk or other dairy products, unpasteurized apple cider, fruits, vegetables, and contaminated municipal or swimming water. Additionally, STEC infection can be acquired as zoonoses from petting zoos, from human-to-human contact, or from urinary tract infection with the organism. Testing of stool may confirm Stx-producing organisms in up to two-thirds of cases, but the environmental source is rarely discovered in sporadic cases.

HUS not associated with enteropathic STEC (NStx) encompasses a disease group with heterogeneous etiologies. NStx HUS accounts for about 10% of all cases of HUS in children. Of this group, the most common cause is *Streptococcus pneumoniae*-associated HUS (pneumococcal HUS), accounting for about 40% of children with NStx HUS. Pneumococcal HUS has an estimated incidence of 0.4% to 0.6%, although the possibility that this underestimates the true incidence is noted by an overall lack of recognition of the disease.

Shiga Toxin–Associated Hemolytic-Uremic Syndrome

The most common causative organism of Stx-HUS is enterohemorrhagic *E. coli* (EHEC). Among the EHEC that cause HUS, serotype O157:H7 is predominant, accounting for 70% of cases in North America and Western Europe. There are several known STEC that are non-O157 strains (e.g., O111:H8, O103:H2, O121, O145, O26, and O113). *Shigella dysenteriae* type 1-associated HUS occurs more frequently in developing countries in Asia and Africa but rarely in industrialized countries. Other organisms such as *Aeromonas* spp. and *Citrobacter freundii* have been known to cause Stx HUS. *E. coli* O157:H7 infection can be confirmed by plating a stool sample on sorbitol-MacConkey agar. The O157:H7 strains cannot ferment sorbitol during an overnight incubation and appear as translucent colonies. The organism can be further confirmed by rapid assays that allow detection of Shiga toxin in the stool, including non-O157 serotypes. It is generally recommended to test stool samples by sorbitol-MacConkey agar as a first screening. The potential to detect the organism is higher in the first 6 days after onset of diarrhea.

Thrombocytopenia, hemolytic anemia,
and renal failure characterize HUS

Occlusive platelet
clumps in renal arteries
and capillaries

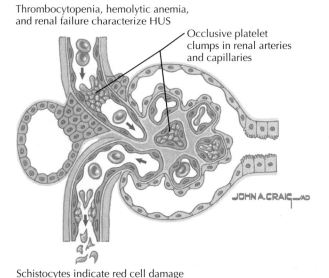

JOHN A. CRAIG—AD

Schistocytes indicate red cell damage
by occlusive platelet clumps and
microangiopathic hemolytic anemia

Proposed mechanisms in HUS

Damaged renal
endothelial cell

Precipitating factors:
gastroenteritis, pregnancy

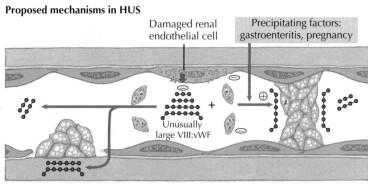

Unusually
large VIII:vWF

Platelet agglutination may be due to unusually large VIII:vWF polymers
in renal circulation followed by adsorption of the polymers onto exposed
subendothelial surfaces or, in the presence of cationic substances from
necrotic cells, onto platelets

Figure 64-1 *Thrombotic disorders: hemolytic-uremic syndrome.*

Shiga toxin is a potent exotoxin that functions as the virulence factor in STEC. All members of the Stx family share some degree of sequence homology, the protein products of which have common structures that include an enzymatically active A subunit linked to a pentameric B subunit (A_1B_5). The STEC can elaborate at least four plasmid-encoded Shiga-toxins: Stx1, Stx2, Stx2c, and Stx2d (Stx is used interchangeably with the term *VT*). Stx1 is nearly identical to the classic Shiga toxin, and Stx2 shares 60% homology with classic Shiga toxin. The Stx may be expressed individually or in combination with two or three different Shiga-toxins. The *Stx2* gene is carried by most *E. coli* O157:H7, and its expression individually causes more severe disease than Stx1 or the combination of Stx1 and Stx2.

Stx is responsible for the endothelial toxicity of HUS-causing STEC, giving rise to the pathologic hallmark of TMA. It is produced in the bowel and translocated into circulation, where it can localize to the glomeruli, gastrointestinal tract, pancreas, and various other host tissues by a mechanism that has yet to be fully understood. Central to enterocyte entry and subsequent toxemia, the Stx B subunit binds to a cell surface terminal carbohydrate moiety of the globotriaosylceramide receptor (Gb3). The Gb3 receptor is a key determinant for cell sensitivity to Stx, and along with enterocytes and other cell types is present on glomerular endothelial cells, thereby targeting the toxin to the renal microvasculature. In the intestine, binding of Stx to Gb3 commences a sequence of events beginning with receptor-mediated endocytosis. Stx can follow several different pathways: (1) it can be delivered intact to the intestinal submucosa and circulation via transcytosis; (2) it can induce direct cytotoxicity by trafficking to the cell endoplasmic reticulum via the Golgi apparatus in a process known as *retrograde transport*; or (3) it can, in lower concentrations, alter gene and protein expression of the cell without inducing cell death. Transcytosis of toxin to the intestinal microvascular circulation is thought to give rise to the characteristic intestinal lesion that has the clinical–pathologic

manifestation of bowel wall edema, thrombosis, and hemorrhage. Neutrophils localize to the intestinal mucosa during STEC infection, where they are thought to transport Stx to extraintestinal sites. They are known to bind Stx by a distinct receptor with a lower affinity than Gb3. The toxin is therefore not endocytosed, which allows it to be freely unloaded at various target sites (Figure 64-2).

The cytopathic effects of Stx result when the A subunit becomes enzymatically active within the host cell by proteolytic cleavage and in turn cleaves its target adenine residue (A4324) on the 28S rRNA of the 60S ribosomal subunit. This action blocks binding of the aminoacyl-tRNA to the subunit with resultant protein synthesis inhibition and cell death. Alternatively, subinhibitory concentrations of toxin are known to alter gene expression in the host cells. Stx has been found to increase expression of prothrombotic and inflammatory genes that affect the properties of endothelial cells. Various cell types undergo toxin-mediated increase in cytokine and chemokine production. For example, subinhibitory toxin concentrations cause endothelial cells to upregulate interleukin-8 (IL-8) and monocyte chemotactic protein-1 (MCP-1) as well as endothelin-1 and tissue factor. The effector functions of these molecules result in leukocyte migration or adhesion, vasoconstriction, and a procoagulant cellular milieu. Additionally, monocytes increase cytokine production of tumor necrosis factor-α and IL-1β, factors known to sensitize host cells to toxin via upregulation of Gb3.

A major virulence cofactor of pathogenic STEC is the ability of the organism to exploit the host enterocyte by secreting its own bacterial receptor into the cell such that it is expressed on its apical surface, in turn allowing firm attachment of the organism along the intestinal mucosal surface. This receptor incorporation occurs through a macromolecular complex called the type 3 secretion system, which results in cytoskeletal changes with associated loss of normal villous architecture, giving rise to a characteristic "attaching and effacing" lesion on the host cell.

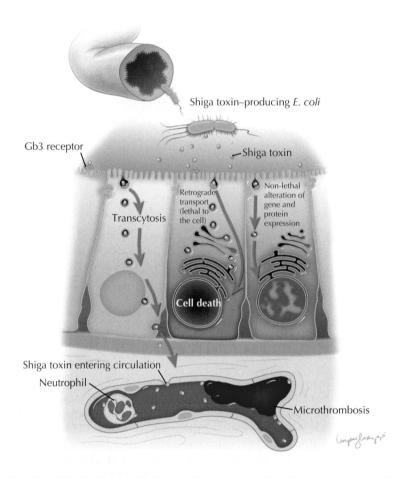

Figure 64-2 *Effects of Shiga toxin on enteric cells and endothelial cells.*

The genetic locus responsible for this process is found on what are known as pathogenicity islands of the bacterial chromosome. The genes encode the machinery of the type 3 secretion system as well as intimin, expressed on the bacterial cell surface, and the intimin receptor, which is translocated into the host cell for surface expression.

Pneumococcal Hemolytic-Uremic Syndrome

Infection with *S. pneumoniae* occurs in the form of bacteremia, pneumonia, empyema, and meningitis. Young children are particularly at risk. The prevalence of HUS associated with invasive pneumococcus peaks before age 2 years. The precise events leading to HUS in children with pneumococcal disease are unclear, but it is thought that the Thomson-Friedenreich (TF) antigen contributes to its pathogenesis. Human cells carry the TF antigen on their cell surfaces. The epitope is recognized by preformed circulating IgM antibody. However, this epitope is normally masked by neuraminic (sialic) acid from the cell glycocalyx. Neuraminidase, produced by various microbial pathogens, including pneumococcus, influenza A virus, and *Capnocytophaga canimorsus*, is released during infection and cleaves the *N*-acetyl-neuraminic acid from the surface of cells, thereby exposing the TF crypantigen. It is thought that exposure of the TF antigen on RBCs, platelets, and glomerular endothelium during the course of pneumococcal infection leads to a sequence of events that result in HUS. Although tempting to link the pathogenesis of pneumococcal HUS to recognition of exposed TF by anti-TF IgM antibody, this IgM is a cold antibody and as such is unlikely to cause RBC polyagglutination and hemolysis in vivo. Additionally, some children with invasive pneumococcal disease without HUS have evidence of TF antigen. Therefore, the mechanism of HUS in those with pneumococcal disease awaits further clarification.

Genetic Forms of Hemolytic-Uremic Syndrome

The genetic forms account for fewer than 3% of all HUS cases. They include mutations in various regulatory components of the complement cascade. Additionally, mutations causing a deficiency of specific proteins necessary for the intracellular metabolism of vitamin B12 are known to cause HUS. Forms of TTP also have a genetic basis associated with mutations in the *ADAMTS13* gene.

Complement component C3 was first noted in 1974 to be reduced in the serum of patients and relatives with inherited forms of NStx HUS. Low serum C3 can also occur with infection-related forms of HUS as a result of C3 consumption in the microvasculature. The low C3 in inherited HUS is

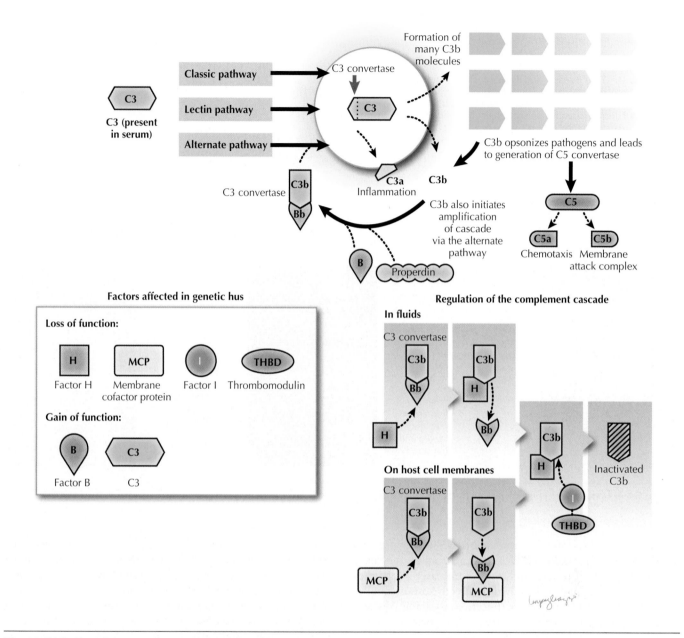

Figure 64-3 *Complement pathways and regulatory proteins.*

persistent and reflects abnormalities that give rise to hyperactivation of the complement cascade. The complement cascade is a key component of the innate immune system comprising groups of plasma and membrane-bound zymogen proteins that follow one of three activation pathways: classical, lectin, or alternative. These pathways converge with the generation of C3 convertase enzymes that convert C3 into C3a and C3b (see Figure 64-2). C3b is necessary for opsonization and generation of C5 convertase, which in turn is necessary for chemotaxis (C5a) and the generation of a membrane attack complex (C5b). This process is tightly regulated by specific regulatory proteins to prevent nonspecific destruction of host cells (Figure 64-3).

Mutations of at least four complement proteins are associated with NStx HUS. The mutations lead to deficiencies in complement factor H (fH), factor I (fI), or membrane cofactor protein (MCP), or they cause a gain in function of factor B. Factor H

mutations segregate to chromosome 1q32, known to be the locus for genes encoding the family of complement regulatory proteins. The mutations are seen in both autosomal dominant and autosomal recessive HUS. The 150 kDa fH is synthesized mainly in the liver and binds polyanionic sites on RBCs and vascular endothelium, thereby increasing its affinity for C3b. Factor H competes with factor B for binding to newly formed C3b, and when successful, it acts as a cofactor for factor I–mediated cleavage and degradation of C3b. It is thought that the polyanion-rich glomerular endothelium and basement membrane protect these components from complement attack. Clinical effects of fH deficiency are speculated to occur as a result of endothelial injury related to downstream effects of unregulated C3 convertase activity. Both homozygote and heterozygote fH deficiency persons can develop HUS. In homozygote persons, laboratory values generally reveal low serum C3,

Intravascular coagulation, hemolytic-uremic syndrome, and thrombotic microangiopathy

Common electron microscopic findings: Deposits (D) and mesangial cell cytoplasmic processes (M) in the subendothelial space; endothelium (E) swollen; both mesangial (MC) and endothelial cells (EN) contain many vacuoles and dilated rough endoplasmic reticulum; lumen (L) narrowed (may be slit-like); red blood cells (RC) may or may not be present; basement membrane (B) often wrinkled; epithelial foot processes (F) partly fused

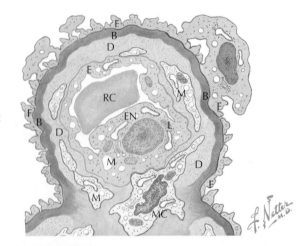

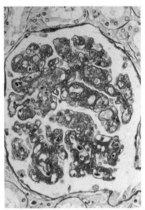

◀ Glomerulus showing thickening of capillary walls and partial capillary collapse (PAS stain, ×160)

▶ Fibrinogen deposition along capillary walls of glomerulus (immuno-fluorescent preparation, tagged anti-fibrinogen serum, ×100)

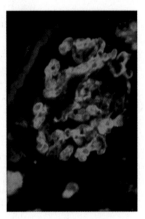

▶ **Small artery in kidney obstructed by fibrin thrombus.** (stained purple) (phosphotungstic acid, hematoxylin stain, ×100)

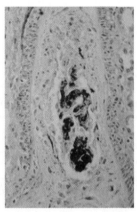

Figure 64-4 *Hemolytic-uremic syndrome (intravascular coagulation and thrombotic microangiopathy).*

fH, factor B, and CH50 concentrations. HUS usually presents in infancy or early childhood. Heterozygote carriers may have normal complement profiles and may present later in life after exposure to a trigger that directly or indirectly causes complement activation. These include infection, systemic disease, drugs, and pregnancy. There are isolated case reports of acquired NStx HUS in children with antibodies to fH.

Deficiency of MCP is implicated in HUS by virtue of its role as a transmembrane cofactor for factor I–mediated cleavage of C3b and C4b that deposits on the host cell surface. It is speculated that fH and MCP reinforce each other in the control of complement regulation on host cells. Factor I deficiency has been identified in small numbers of patients with NStx HUS. Similarly, a gain-of-function mutation has been identified in several families with NStx HUS and is thought to either increase formation or stabilize the alternative pathway C3 convertase (C3bBb).

Thrombotic Thrombocytopenic Purpura

Platelet adhesion and aggregation require the presence of vWF, which is produced by endothelial cells and platelets as large multimeric units. The vWF-cp is a liver-derived metalloproteinase that cleaves the multimers to vWF dimers. Inherited TTP results from autosomal recessive transmission of

mutations affecting the ADAMTS 13 gene on chromosome 9q34, which encodes vWF-cp. The result is enhanced platelet adhesion due to vWF multimers. In acquired TTP, this process occurs because of the presence of autoantibodies (or "inhibitors") to the vWF-cp. Antiplatelet agents ticlopidine and clopidogrel have been known to cause TTP with vWF metalloproteinase autoantibodies.

Secondary Hemolytic-Uremic Syndrome

HUS is known to occur secondarily in a variety of conditions, including autoimmune diseases such as systemic lupus erythematosus and antiphospholipid syndrome, HIV, adenocarcinomas, after hematopoietic stem cell transplantation, after solid organ transplantation; it may also be associated with pregnancy or use of medication. A complete discussion of these rare forms of HUS is beyond the scope of this chapter but can be found in a recent publication by Copelovitch and Kaplan.

Common Renal Pathology

The common "endotheliopathy" that results from various etiologic forms of HUS produces the histopathologic lesion of glomerular TMA (Figure 64-4). Thrombosis affects the glomerular capillaries and can extend proximally into the afferent arterioles, even rarely into interlobular arteries. Extensive thrombosis into the arteries may produce shrunken, ischemic glomeruli or cortical infarct, which can be responsible for severe hypertension. More commonly, the glomeruli have thickened capillary walls, luminal obstruction or thrombosis, and endothelial cell swelling. The glomeruli may appear large. In more severe cases of HUS, patchy cortical necrosis can be seen. Occasionally, necrosis can be more diffuse and affect the entire superficial cortex. It is important to note that whereas fibrin- and RBC-rich thrombi are seen in Stx and pneumococcal HUS, platelet thrombi are seen in TTP. In TTP, the platelet-dominant thrombi affect the heart, pancreas, kidney, adrenal glands, and central nervous system (CNS) in order of increasing severity. A renal biopsy is rarely necessary in the diagnosis of HUS or TTP.

CLINICAL PRESENTATION

There are several well-documented risk factors for the development of Stx-HUS—extremes of age (presumably from lack of antibody against Stx), the presence of Stx2, severe enteritis, fever during enteritis prodrome, leukocytosis, and female gender. Additionally, the use of antibiotics or antimotility agents is discouraged because they are thought to worsen disease.

The clinical spectrum of STEC infection ranges from possible asymptomatic infection to hemorrhagic colitis without HUS to postdiarrheal HUS. Generally, nonbloody diarrhea with abdominal pain, vomiting, and fever occurs 3 days after ingestion of STEC. In 90% of patients, bloody diarrhea then develops 1 to 3 days after these initial symptoms. At this time, leukocytosis may be present, and colonic edema and hemorrhage may be demonstrated as "thumbprinting" on barium enema study. The majority of patients with positive stool cultures for *E. coli* O157:H7 will have bloody diarrhea. HUS develops in about 15% of those patients, usually manifesting 6 days after the onset of diarrhea. In 85%, there is spontaneous symptomatic resolution without features of HUS. A clue to the diagnosis is a history of decreasing urine volume in a well-hydrated or volume-resuscitated child with diarrhea. Oligoanuria typically occurs 4 to 7 days after diarrheal onset followed by hematologic abnormalities. Similar to Stx disease, pneumococcal HUS typically develops 1 week after onset of symptoms.

Hematologic Features

The anemia of HUS results from microangiopathic or peroxidative injury. It manifests with hemoglobin generally lower than 8 g/dL and a blood smear with schistocytes, some appearing as helmet cells. As expected, intravascular hemolysis produces laboratory changes, including elevated lactate dehydrogenase, reticulocytosis, unconjugated hyperbilirubinemia, and decreased haptoglobin. The hemolysis in HUS is nonimmune, and Coombs' testing results are negative except in pneumococcal HUS, in which direct Coombs' testing results are positive because of exposed TF antigen on the cell surface of erythrocytes. In Stx HUS, hemolytic anemia requires RBC transfusion in up to 75% of patients and may recur in the first few weeks. Thrombocytopenia (usually <50,000/μL) may last up to 2 weeks. In most cases, there are no purpura or active bleeding, and coagulation study results are normal. Pneumococcal HUS

features longer durations of thrombocytopenia and greater requirement for blood product transfusions than Stx HUS. There is no correlation between severity of anemia or thrombocytopenia and renal injury.

Renal Features

The extent of acute kidney injury in HUS is variable and ranges from urinary abnormalities with mild renal insufficiency to oligo-anuric renal failure. Some patients have nonoliguric renal failure. The thrombotic glomerular injury in HUS generally causes a reduction in glomerular filtration rate (GFR) accompanied by an increased serum creatinine; biochemical abnormalities; and microscopic or macroscopic hematuria, occasionally with RBC casts. Hyperkalemia uncommonly occurs as a result of reduced GFR, hemolysis, and transcellular shifts from metabolic acidosis. In Stx HUS, this may be insidious in onset because of an initial hypokalemia resulting from gastrointestinal losses. Additionally, stool losses of bicarbonate and albumin (protein-losing enteropathy) may exacerbate metabolic acidosis and hypoalbuminemia. Reduced GFR with oliguria can lead to intravascular volume expansion, especially in the context of blood product transfusions. This may manifest as edema, hypertension, pulmonary venous congestion, and congestive heart failure.

Up to 50% of children with Stx HUS will require acute renal replacement therapy (RRT), but there is an overall favorable chance for renal recovery, and many experience a diuresis phase during recovery. Mortality in Stx HUS is about 3% to 5% and is particularly associated with CNS involvement. Chronic or late sequelae can occur in up to 25% of persons after the acute phase of Stx HUS. These include hypertension, proteinuria, and chronic renal insufficiency. An increased severity of acute illness, specifically a need for RRT, longer duration of oligoanuria, and the presence of CNS symptoms, are associated with worse outcomes. Recurrence of Stx HUS is rare, and posttransplant recurrence is not reported.

In contrast to Stx HUS, pneumococcal HUS results in a greater duration of oligoanuria, with 75% of children requiring RRT. The progression to end-stage renal failure (ESRF) is two to three times higher in pneumococcal HUS (10%), and overall mortality rates are higher (12%). Poor prognosis is especially seen in those with pneumococcal meningitis, in whom the development of HUS is associated with a disproportionately high rate of mortality.

Extrarenal Features

Stx HUS manifests with acute hemorrhagic colitis, which may be complicated by toxic megacolon, bowel wall necrosis, perforation, intussusception, or even frank gangrene of the colon. Hepatomegaly is common, and elevated transaminases can be present. Gallbladder hydrops can occur. The pancreas can be affected by Shiga toxin, causing pancreatitis or insulin-dependent diabetes mellitus secondary to islet cell necrosis and destruction.

Cardiopulmonary disease occurs in about 10% of patients. It may occur because of volume overload. Additionally cardiomyopathy, myocarditis, aneurysms, microthrombi, ischemia with troponin I elevation, pulmonary congestion, and respiratory failure with ARDS can occur in Stx-HUS.

CNS disease can present in about 25% in the form of reduced level of consciousness, tremors, twitching, irritability, seizures, stroke, and coma. Symptoms can result from accelerated hypertension related to volume overload, especially in association with blood product infusions. Hyponatremia and hypocalcemia may also contribute to CNS findings. Shiga toxin–mediated injury is thought to cause encephalopathy. CNS disease in Stx-HUS is associated with poor prognosis. Similarly, pneumococcal meningitis with associated HUS is associated with mortality, and CNS neuraminidase activity with TF antigen exposure is implicated in this finding.

DIFFERENTIAL DIAGNOSIS

HUS is marked by hemolytic anemia with fragmented erythrocytes on blood smear, a platelet count lower than $150 - \times 10^3/\mu L$, and acute renal injury. This may be difficult to distinguish from disseminated intravascular coagulation (DIC) that occurs in the context of a systemic inflammatory response to infection. DIC has clinical overlap with the HUS triad, and HUS can be misdiagnosed as DIC, especially in pneumococcal HUS. Distinguishing features include coagulation profiles: fibrinogen and prothrombin time and partial thromboplastin time are usually normal or slightly elevated in patients with HUS. Also in contrast to DIC, active bleeding is unusual in HUS. Definitive diagnosis can be made by renal biopsy showing TMA. However, biopsy is rarely necessary in HUS and is often precluded by thrombocytopenia.

MANAGEMENT

There are no targeted therapies for either Stx or pneumococcal HUS. Both conditions require supportive care with a high level of vigilance. Fluid status should be determined to ensure adequate perfusion without precipitating volume overload. Weight, urine volume, and blood pressure should be assessed frequently. About 50% of patients with Stx HUS develop oligoanuric renal failure and require dialysis. An increase in serum creatinine, elevated blood pressure, and decreasing urine output require prompt fluid restriction and planning for administration of dialysis. Dialysis indications are similar to those in other conditions: volume overload with hypertension or cardiopulmonary compromise, severe acidosis, or hyperkalemia. It is crucial to plan for and initiate dialysis early in the course of HUS because packed RBC transfusion is often required (80%) when hemoglobin drops to 6 to 7 g/dL or with evidence of cardiorespiratory compromise, and transfusion can precipitate hyperkalemia or accelerated hypertension in the setting of oligoanuria. Platelet transfusion should be avoided unless active hemorrhage occurs

or surgical interventions are required. An important consideration specific to pneumococcal HUS is the need to provide washed blood products if transfusion is required. This is because of the possible risk that preformed anti-TF antibodies are delivered with unwashed products.

In Stx HUS, antimotility agents delay gastrointestinal clearance of Stx and should be avoided, as should be antibiotics, some of which are known to promote release of Stx from STEC.

A number of therapies remain unproven in Stx HUS but continue to be used by some clinicians. Known ineffective therapies include plasma exchange or plasmapheresis, corticosteroids, anticoagulants, thrombolytics, antiplatelet agents, high-dose furosemide, intravenous immunoglobulin (IVIG), and oral toxin binders such as Synsorb Pk. Plasma exchange is also ineffective in pneumococcal HUS.

Plasma therapy is considered a first-line treatment to supply deficient proteins implicated in genetic forms of HUS (fH, fI) and TTP (vWF-cp). Plasma exchange allows removal of antibodies in acquired TTP and is thought to remove potentially injurious molecules in genetic forms of HUS. Inherited HUS has a relapsing or progressive course. Failure to induce remission with plasma therapy in inherited HUS generally results in progression to ESRF. Other therapies (steroids, IVIG) have been attempted without benefit. Renal transplantation is associated with high risk of recurrence in genetic HUS (50%). Graft failure is nearly inevitable in those with recurrence (>90%) and does not typically respond to plasma exchange. Combined liver–kidney transplants are recommended in high-risk patients to allow for correction of the genetic defect. Currently, monoclonal antibody therapy that blocks cleavage of C5 has been used successfully in patients with genetic HUS.

SUGGESTED READINGS

Constantinescu AR, Bitzan M, Weiss L, et al: Non-enteropathic hemolytic uremic syndrome: causes and short-term course, *Am J Kidney Dis* 43:976-982, 2004.

Copelovitch L, Kaplan BS: *Streptococcus pneumoniae*-associated hemolytic uremic syndrome, *Pediatr Nephrol* 23:1951-1956, 2008.

Copelovitch L, Kaplan BS: The thrombotic microangiopathies, *Pediatr Nephrol* 23:1761-1767, 2008.

Loirat C, Taylor CM: Hemolytic uremic syndrome. In Avner E, Harmon W, Niaudet P, editors: *Pediatric Nephrology*, ed 5, Philadelphia, Lippincott, 2004, Williams & Wilkins, pp 887-915.

Noris M, Remuzzi G: Hemolytic uremic syndrome, *J Am Soc Nephrol* 16:1035-1050, 2005.

Tarr PI, Gordon CA, Chandler WL: Shiga-toxin-producing *Escherichia coli* and haemolytic uraemic syndrome, *Lancet* 365:1073-1086, 2005.

Trachtman H, Kaplan B: Hemolytic uremic syndrome: Stx-HUS. In Kaplan B, Meyers K, editors: *Pediatric Nephrology and Urology: The Requisites*. Philadelphia, 2005, Elsevier Mosby, pp 203-208.

Acute and Chronic Renal Failure

65

Olivera Marsenic and H. Jorge Baluarte

ACUTE RENAL FAILURE

Acute kidney injury (AKI), previously referred to as acute renal failure (ARF), is defined as an abrupt reduction in kidney function measured by a rapid decline in glomerular filtration rate (GFR). AKI implies that an acute decline in kidney function is secondary to an injury that leads to functional or structural changes in the kidney. AKI is characterized by a disturbance of renal physiologic functions, including impairment of nitrogenous waste product excretion and inability to regulate water, electrolyte, and acid–base homeostasis. The precise incidence and prevalence of AKI in children is difficult to ascertain. The overall incidence of AKI appears to be rising because of advances in pediatric medical technology including bone marrow, hepatic, and cardiac transplantation, in surgery for congenital heart disease, and in the care of very low birth weight infants.

ETIOLOGY AND PATHOGENESIS

The causes of AKI can be related to any process that interferes with the structure or function of the renal vasculature, glomeruli, renal tubules, interstitium, or urinary tract. The causes of AKI can be categorized as prerenal, renal (intrinsic renal disorder), or postrenal.

Prerenal

AKI results from either volume depletion caused by bleeding, gastrointestinal (vomiting, diarrhea), urinary (diuretics, diabetes insipidus), cutaneous losses (burns) or decreased effective blood volume (heart failure, cardiac tamponade, hepatorenal syndrome, shock, sepsis). In this type of AKI, the kidneys are intrinsically normal, and AKI is reversible after renal blood flow is restored by correcting the underlying disturbance. However, prolonged prerenal injury results in intrinsic renal AKI.

Renal

AKI (intrinsic renal disease) is the result of disorders that involve the renal vascular, glomerular, or tubular–interstitial pathology. Acute tubular necrosis (ATN) results from ischemia caused by decreased renal perfusion or injury from tubular nephrotoxins (Figure 65-1). All causes of prerenal AKI can progress to ATN if renal perfusion is not restored or nephrotoxins are not withdrawn. Nephrotoxic AKI is mostly caused by toxic tubular injury by medications, including aminoglycosides, contrast agents, amphotericin B, chemotherapeutic agents (ifosfamide, cisplatin), and acyclovir. Toxic tubular injury can also be induced by the release of heme pigments, as it occurs from myoglobinuria caused by rhabdomyolysis and hemoglobinuria caused by intravascular hemolysis. Uric acid nephropathy and tumor lysis syndrome are causes of AKI in children with leukemia. During chemotherapy, a rapid breakdown of tumor cells causes increased release and subsequent excretion of uric acid, resulting in precipitation of uric acid crystals in the tubules and renal microvasculature. Hyperphosphatemia in tumor lysis syndrome results in precipitation of calcium phosphate crystals in the tubules. Acute interstitial nephritis most commonly results from hypersensitivity reactions to drugs, including penicillin analogs (e.g., methicillin), cimetidine, sulfonamides, rifampin, nonsteroidal antiinflammatory drugs, and proton pump inhibitors, but can also be idiopathic. Glomerulonephritis of any etiology (including those caused by vasculitis, systemic lupus erythematosus, or Goodpasture's syndrome) may present with AKI, with postinfectious glomerulonephritis being the most common cause of AKI in this group. Rapidly progressive glomerulonephritis presents as the most severe degree of any form of glomerulonephritis and presents with AKI. Vascular causes of AKI include cortical necrosis (mostly caused by hypoxic or ischemic injury in newborns), renal artery or vein thrombosis, and hemolytic-uremic syndrome (HUS).

Postrenal

AKI is caused by bilateral urinary tract obstruction unless there is a solitary kidney or caused by urethral obstruction. Examples of congenital disorders causing obstruction and AKI are posterior urethral valves (PUVs), bilateral ureteropelvic junction obstruction, and bilateral ureteroceles. Examples of acquired causes of obstruction and AKI are kidney stones and tumors.

CLINICAL PRESENTATION

A careful history and physical examination can frequently identify disease processes that underlie AKI and suggest an underlying diagnosis.

- A history of vomiting, diarrhea, hemorrhage, sepsis, or decreased oral intake resulting in hypovolemia associated with decreased urine output suggests AKI caused by prerenal disease or ATN. Physical examination findings that include tachycardia, dry mucous membranes, sunken eyes, orthostatic blood pressure changes, and decreased skin turgor suggest hypovolemia, resulting in AKI caused by prerenal disease or ATN.
- Nephrotic syndrome, heart failure, and liver failure causing prerenal AKI caused by a decrease in effective intravascular volume present with edema (see Chapter 63).
- In the hospital, history of hypotension (caused by sepsis or intraoperative events), administration of nephrotoxic agents or recent use of chemotherapy for leukemia may be responsible for AKI.
- History of use of medications that are known to cause a hypersensitivity reaction, together with a rash, fever, and arthralgias, suggests AKI caused by acute interstitial nephritis (see Chapter 62).

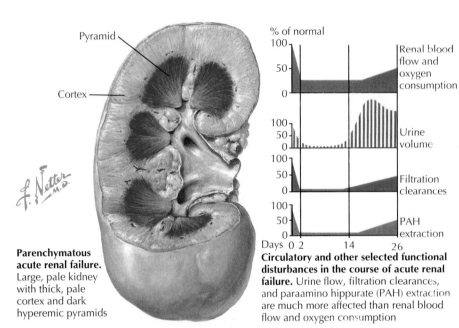

Pyramid

Cortex

% of normal

Renal blood flow and oxygen consumption

Urine volume

Filtration clearances

PAH extraction

Days 0 2   14   26

Parenchymatous acute renal failure. Large, pale kidney with thick, pale cortex and dark hyperemic pyramids

Circulatory and other selected functional disturbances in the course of acute renal failure. Urine flow, filtration clearances, and paraamino hippurate (PAH) extraction are much more affected than renal blood flow and oxygen consumption

Distal tubule   Glomerulus

Biopsy section. Glomerulus normal; distal convoluted tubules dilated, with flattened epithelium, "pretzel-like" distortion, and containing heme casts (H and E stain)

Figure 65-1 *Acute renal failure.*

- Clinical presentation that includes hypertension, edema, and gross hematuria is likely caused by AKI attributable to a glomerulonephritis. A history of pharyngitis or impetigo a few weeks before the onset of gross hematuria suggests postinfectious glomerulonephritis.
- History of bloody diarrhea and pallor and petechiae on physical examination are associated with HUS (see Chapter 64).
- Hemoptysis in the presence of renal impairment suggests a diagnosis of pulmonary–renal syndrome, such as Goodpasture's syndrome.
- Skin findings, such as purpura, malar rash, or petechiae or joint pain favor a diagnosis of vasculitis, such as systemic lupus erythematosus or Henoch-Schönlein purpura.
- Anuria or oliguria in a newborn suggests a congenital malformation (i.e., PUVs) or bilateral renal vein thrombosis.

EVALUATION AND DIAGNOSIS

In addition to a careful history and physical examination, the initial evaluation includes additional laboratory studies.

Serum Creatinine Concentration, Acute Kidney Injury Biomarkers, and Classification of Acute Kidney Injury

AKI is diagnosed by an increase in serum creatinine concentration, which strongly suggests a decrease in the GFR. However, it is accepted that the serum creatinine concentration is an insensitive and delayed measure of decreased kidney function after AKI. Biomarkers that allow recognition of the early stages of AKI have been identified. Clinical use of these markers may permit initiation of timely therapy. These biomarkers are serum neutrophil gelatinase-associated lipocalin (NGAL) and cystatin C, urinary NGAL, interlukin-18, and kidney injury molecule-1

(KIM-1). A standardized classification of AKI has recently been proposed in adults (RIFLE criteria) and adapted for children (pediatric [p] RIFLE criteria). pRIFLE stands for **r**isk for renal dysfunction, **i**njury to the kidney, **f**ailure of kidney function, **l**oss of kidney function, **e**nd-stage renal disease. These criteria better characterize AKI and reflect the course of AKI in children admitted to the intensive care unit (ICU).

Urinalysis

The urinalysis is the most important noninvasive test in the diagnostic evaluation because characteristic findings on microscopic examination of the urine sediment strongly suggest certain diagnoses. A normal or near-normal urinalysis result, characterized by few cells with little or no casts or proteinuria, suggests prerenal disease or urinary tract obstruction. Muddy brown granular casts and epithelial cell casts are highly suggestive of ATN. The finding of red blood cell (RBC) casts is diagnostic of glomerulonephritis, and heavy proteinuria is indicative of glomerular disease, both suggesting AKI caused by glomerulonephritis. The presence of many white blood cells (pyuria) suggests urinary tract infection, and white blood cells with granular or waxy casts and mild to moderate proteinuria suggest tubular or interstitial disease. Eosinophils in the urine suggest interstitial nephritis caused by a hypersensitivity reaction. Hematuria can be seen in glomerulonephritis and renal vein thrombosis and with renal calculi.

Urine Sodium Excretion

With AKI in children, measurement of the urine sodium concentration is helpful in distinguishing ATN (urine sodium >30-40 mEq/L) from prerenal AKI (urine sodium <10-20 mEq/L) in which the ability to conserve sodium and water is intact.

Fractional Excretion of Sodium

The fractional excretion of sodium (FENa) eliminates the effect of variations in urine volume on Na excretion in AKI, and it differentiates between prerenal AKI and ATN in children. FENa = [(UNa × PCr)/(PNa × UCr)] × 100, where UCr and PCr are the urine and serum creatinine concentrations, respectively, and UNa and PNa are the urine and serum sodium concentrations, respectively.

- A value less than 1% suggests prerenal disease (reabsorption of almost all of the filtered sodium represents an appropriate response to decreased renal perfusion).
- A value between 1% and 2% could be attributable to either disorder.
- A value greater than 2% indicates ATN.
- In newborns, the values for prerenal and ATN are less than 2.5% and greater than 2.5% to 3.5%, respectively, because of the decreased ability to reabsorb sodium.

Urine Osmolality

Loss of concentrating ability is an early and almost universal finding in ATN with the urine osmolality usually being below 350 mOsmol/kg. In contrast, a urine osmolality above 500 mOsmol/kg is highly suggestive of prerenal disease.

Urine Volume

The urine output is typically, but not always, low (oliguria) in prerenal AKI because of the combination of sodium and water avidity. AKI can present with decreased (oliguria), absent (anuria), normal, or increased (nonoliguric) urine output. Oliguria is defined as urine output less than 500 mL/24 h in older children, less than 0.5 mL/kg/h in younger children, and less than 1 mLkg/h in infants. Oliguria or anuria is likely to occur in AKI because of hypoxic or ischemic insults, HUS, glomerulonephritis or urinary tract obstruction. Nonoliguric AKI is associated with acute interstitial nephritis and nephrotoxic renal insults.

Serologic and Biochemical Abnormalities

In children with a clinical picture consistent with rapidly progressive glomerulonephritis (RPGN), antineutrophil cytoplasmic antibodies (ANCA), antinuclear antibodies (ANA), anti–glomerular basement membrane (GBM) antibodies, and complement levels are required to evaluate the etiology of the RPGN. Antistreptococcal antibody titers are necessary for diagnosis of acute poststreptococcal glomerulonephritis. Elevated serum levels of nephrotoxic medications (e.g., aminoglycosides) are associated with ATN. Markedly elevated uric acid levels are found in tumor lysis syndrome. Hyperkalemia, hyperphosphatemia occur in AKI because of their decreased renal excretion. Hypocalcemia in AKI can result secondary to hyperphosphatemia and decreased calcium absorption in the gastrointestinal tract because of inadequate renal production of 1,25-vitamin D. Acidosis seen in AKI results from decreased urinary excretion of hydrogen ions.

Box 65-1 General Management Principles of Acute Kidney Injury

- Maintenance of electrolyte and fluid balance
- Adequate nutritional support
- Avoidance of life-threatening complications
- Treatment of the underlying cause

Complete Blood Count

Microangiopathic hemolytic anemia associated with thrombocytopenia in the setting of AKI confirms the diagnosis of HUS. Severe hemolysis, whether drug induced or secondary to hemoglobinopathies, may also result in ATN caused by massive hemoglobinuria. Eosinophilia is associated with interstitial nephritis caused by a hypersensitivity reaction.

Renal Imaging

Renal ultrasonography should be performed in all children with AKI. It can document the presence of one or two kidneys, determine renal size (often enlarged in those with AKI) (see Figure 65-1), assess the renal parenchyma, and diagnose urinary tract obstruction or occlusion of the major renal vessels.

Renal Biopsy

A renal biopsy is done if diagnosis cannot be established by other noninvasive tests or if the initial presentation is suggestive of RPGN.

PREVENTION AND MANAGEMENT

The basic principles of the general management of AKI are shown in Box 65-1.

General measures to help prevent AKI include close monitoring of serum levels of nephrotoxic drugs, adequate fluid repletion in patients with hypovolemia, and aggressive hydration and alkalinization of the urine before chemotherapy. Unless contraindicated, a child with a history of fluid loss (vomiting and diarrhea), a physical examination consistent with hypovolemia (hypotension and tachycardia), or oliguria requires immediate intravenous (IV) fluid therapy in an attempt to restore renal function and perhaps prevent ischemic renal injury. Commonly used fluids are crystalloid solutions, such as normal saline (20 mL/kg) administered over 20 to 30 minutes, which may be repeated. If urine output does not increase and renal function fails to improve, invasive monitoring may be required to adequately assess the child's fluid status and help guide further therapy.

Hyperkalemia is a life-threatening complication of AKI that may result in fatal cardiac arrhythmia. Hyperkalemia is treated by shifting potassium from the intravascular to the intracellular space using IV glucose and insulin, β-agonists (albuterol inhalation), and bicarbonate and by using enteric exchange resins such as polystyrene sulfonate. IV infusion of calcium is used to stabilize cell membranes and decrease the risk of cardiac arrhythmias. Dialysis may be required to remove potassium.

Acid (H+) generated by diet and intermediary metabolism is excreted by the kidney, but in AKI, acid excretion is decreased, resulting in metabolic acidosis. Acidosis can be treated with IV or oral sodium bicarbonate or oral sodium citrate solutions.

Hyperphosphatemia and Hypocalcemia

Because the kidneys normally excrete a large amount of ingested phosphorus, hyperphosphatemia is common in AKI. Hyperphosphatemia is treated with dietary phosphorus restriction and with oral calcium carbonate (or other calcium compounds) that bind phosphorus and prevent gastrointestinal absorption of dietary phosphorus. Aluminum-containing compounds can be used for phosphate binding, but their use must be restricted to limit aluminum absorption. Hypocalcemia in AKI results from hyperphosphatemia and decreased production of 1,25-vitamin D. In the setting of acidosis, less calcium is bound to albumin, and more calcium is free in its ionized form. With the use of bicarbonate therapy for correction of acidosis or hyperkalemia, more calcium binds to albumin, and there is less free ionized calcium, which may cause symptomatic hypocalcemia with tetany. Therefore, if hypocalcemia is severe or bicarbonate therapy is necessary, IV calcium gluconate or calcium chloride should be given. Hypocalcemia may also be treated by oral administration of calcium carbonate or other calcium salts. Treatment of hypocalcaemia in the setting of severe hyperphosphatemia can result in metastatic calcifications because of a high Calcium × Phosphorus product.

Hypertension

Hypertension in AKI may be related to volume overload or alterations in vascular tone (i.e., renin mediated). If hypertension volume-mediated initial therapy with a loop diuretic can be attempted, fluid removal with dialysis or hemofiltration may be required. For severe hypertension, IV infusion therapy with nicardipine, labetalol, or sodium nitroprusside is indicated. Oral nifedipine, diltiazem, or clonidine can be used for initial control of acute less severe hypertension. After the blood pressure has been controlled, oral long-acting agents can be initiated. Angiotensin-converting enzyme inhibitors (ACEIs) and angiotensin receptor blockers (ARBs) should be used with caution in AKI because they reduce intraglomerular filtration pressure and retain potassium.

Nutrition

AKI can be associated with severe anorexia and subsequent malnutrition. Proper nutrition is essential in the management of children with AKI. If the gastrointestinal tract is intact and functional, enteral feedings with formula should be instituted in infants as soon as possible. Specialized formulations with attention to calcium, phosphorus, and potassium content should be used. In older children, a diet of high biologic value protein, low phosphorus, and low potassium foods can be used. At a minimum, daily maintenance calories should be provided, although calorie needs may be higher because of catabolism. Parenteral nutrition may be needed.

Box 65-2 Initiation of Renal Replacement Therapy

Signs and symptoms of uremia
- Pericarditis
- Neuropathy
- Change in mental status
  Azotemia
- BUN >80-100 mg/dL
- Rapid rate of increase of BUN
  Severe fluid overload state
- Hypertension
- Pulmonary edema
- Heart failure
  Severe electrolyte abnormalities (that are refractory to supportive medical therapy)
- Hyperkalemia
- Hypernatremia
- Hyponatremia
- Acidosis
  Need for intensive nutritional support in a child with
- Oliguria
- Anuria

BUN, blood urea nitrogen.

Renal Replacement Therapy

Renal replacement therapy in children with AKI should be initiated for the indications listed in Box 65-2.

Three dialysis modalities are available: peritoneal dialysis (PD), hemodialysis (HD), and continuous renal replacement therapy (CRRT). The choice of modality is influenced by the clinical presentation of the child, the availability of vascular access (necessary for HD), adequacy of the peritoneal membrane (necessary for PD), the presence or absence of multiorgan failure, and the overall goal of the dialysis (HD is most efficient in rapid correction of electrolyte and other solute abnormalities).

FUTURE DIRECTIONS

Biomarkers of AKI (cystatin C, NGAL, interleukin-18, KIM-1) and their ability to predict the duration and severity of AKI are under investigation. If these biomarkers prove to be sensitive for early detection of AKI, this will allow initiation of therapy in a timely manner, preventing further intrinsic renal disease.

Fenoldopam is a potent, short-acting, selective, dopamine-1 receptor agonist that decreases vascular resistance while increasing renal blood flow. Unlike dopamine, it was shown to decrease the incidence of AKI, the need for dialysis, ICU stays, and mortality. However, only limited experience in children is available at this time.

CHRONIC KIDNEY DISEASE

Chronic kidney disease (CKD) is a state of irreversible kidney damage or reduction of kidney function that can lead to a progressive decrease in kidney function. CKD more clearly defines renal dysfunction as a continuum rather than a discrete change in renal function. The term *CKD* replaces the clinical terms of

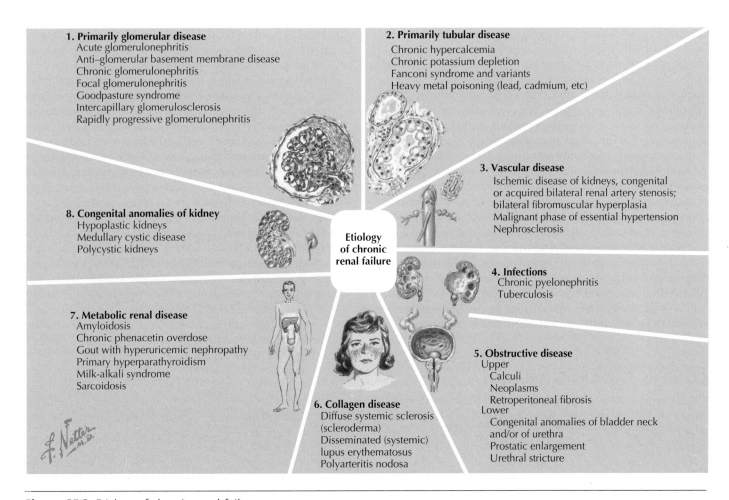

1. Primarily glomerular disease
Acute glomerulonephritis
Anti–glomerular basement membrane disease
Chronic glomerulonephritis
Focal glomerulonephritis
Goodpasture syndrome
Intercapillary glomerulosclerosis
Rapidly progressive glomerulonephritis

2. Primarily tubular disease
Chronic hypercalcemia
Chronic potassium depletion
Fanconi syndrome and variants
Heavy metal poisoning (lead, cadmium, etc)

3. Vascular disease
Ischemic disease of kidneys, congenital
or acquired bilateral renal artery stenosis;
bilateral fibromuscular hyperplasia
Malignant phase of essential hypertension
Nephrosclerosis

8. Congenital anomalies of kidney
Hypoplastic kidneys
Medullary cystic disease
Polycystic kidneys

Etiology
of chronic
renal failure

4. Infections
Chronic pyelonephritis
Tuberculosis

7. Metabolic renal disease
Amyloidosis
Chronic phenacetin overdose
Gout with hyperuricemic nephropathy
Primary hyperparathyroidism
Milk-alkali syndrome
Sarcoidosis

5. Obstructive disease
Upper
  Calculi
  Neoplasms
  Retroperitoneal fibrosis
Lower
  Congenital anomalies of bladder neck
  and/or of urethra
  Prostatic enlargement
  Urethral stricture

6. Collagen disease
Diffuse systemic sclerosis
(scleroderma)
Disseminated (systemic)
lupus erythematosus
Polyarteritis nodosa

Figure 65-2 *Etiology of chronic renal failure.*

chronic renal failure and *chronic renal insufficiency*. The National Kidney Foundation Kidney Disease Outcomes Quality Initiative (K/DOQI) has defined CKD as (1) the presence of markers of kidney damage for 3 months or longer, as defined by structural or functional abnormalities of the kidney with or without a decreased GFR, which is manifested by either pathologic abnormalities or other markers of kidney damage, including abnormalities in the blood, urine, or in imaging tests, or (2) GFR below 60 mL/min/1.73 m^2 for 3 months or longer with or without kidney damage. GFR is estimated by creatinine clearance.

The stages of CKD for children older than 2 years of age are based on estimated GFR (using the Schwartz equation) and are aimed at promoting early detection and treatment of CKD.

The annual incidence and prevalence of CKD, including its early stages, is reported as 12.1 per million children and adolescents younger than 20 years. The yearly incidence and prevalence in stages 4 and 5 is reported as 5.7 to 14.8 per million children in different countries. The variability in the worldwide incidence of CKD is thought to be affected by genetic and environmental factors, as well as the ability to detect CKD and provide care to children with significant renal impairment. In North America, the incidence of CKD is greater in African American than white children. The incidence and prevalence of CKD are greater in boys than girls because of the higher incidence of congenital anomalies of the kidney and urinary tract, including obstructive uropathy, renal dysplasia, renal hypoplasia, and prune belly syndrome, in boys.

ETIOLOGY AND PATHOGENESIS

Based on the registry of the North American Pediatric Renal Trials and Collaborative Studies, the causes of CKD are as follows: Congenital renal anomalies are present in 57% of cases (obstructive uropathy; renal aplasia, hypoplasia, or dysplasia; reflux nephropathy; and polycystic kidney disease), and glomerular disease is present in 17% of cases, with focal segmental glomerulosclerosis (FSGS) being the most common glomerular disorder (9% of all CKD cases; African American children are three times more likely to develop FSGS than white children). Other causes accounted for 25% of cases and included HUS, genetic disorders (e.g., cystinosis, oxalosis, hereditary nephritis), and interstitial nephritis. In large number of cases (18%), the primary disease is unknown because patients present in late stages of CKD. Unlike in adults, diabetic nephropathy and hypertension are rare causes of CKD in children (Figure 65-2).

After initial injury to the kidney, there is continued progression of renal disease and functional impairment, often leading to stage 5 CKD. This is a result of repeated and chronic insults to the renal parenchyma, leading to permanent damage or to the adaptive hyperfiltration response of the remaining nephrons in the kidney, which compensates for the loss of nephrons from the initial injury. Over time, the enhanced transglomerular ultrafiltration and glomerular pressure leads to glomerular damage and leakage of protein, resulting in interstitial inflammation and fibrosis. This long-term injury is characterized histologically by glomerulosclerosis, vascular sclerosis, and tubulointerstitial fibrosis and clinically by proteinuria and progressive renal insufficiency. The rate of progression of CKD is usually greatest during the two periods of rapid growth, infancy and puberty, when the sudden increase in body mass results in an increase in the filtration demands of the remaining nephrons. Other factors associated with acceleration of the progressive CKD include hypertension, obesity, dyslipidemia, proteinuria, anemia, intrarenal precipitation of calcium and phosphate, metabolic acidosis, and tubular interstitial disease. Some of these factors are modifiable, and timely therapeutic interventions may result in a reduced rate of deterioration of renal function.

CLINICAL PRESENTATION

Clinical presentation of CKD depends on the severity of renal disease and the underlying disorder. Stage 1 and 2 CKD are usually asymptomatic. As CKD progresses, patients become increasingly symptomatic. Signs and symptoms of CKD include different amounts of urine output (polyuria or oliguria), edema, hypertension, proteinuria, and hematuria. Glomerular diseases often present with hematuria, proteinuria, hypertension, and edema in the early stages of CKD. Polyuria may be an early presenting symptom as congenital anomalies of the kidney and urinary tract (e.g., obstructive uropathy); inherited disorders (e.g., nephronophthisis); and tubulointerstitial disorders caused by impairment in renal concentrating ability, which generally precedes a significant reduction in GFR. Poor growth is a common manifestation of CKD in children. More severe symptoms and signs of CKD begin to appear with stage 3 disease and worsen with stages 4 and 5.

Complications

A moderate to severe loss of GFR (stage 3-5 disease) is associated with a number of complications caused by impairment of many renal functions, resulting in disorders of fluid and electrolytes, acid–base homeostasis, metabolic bone disease, anemia, hypertension, dyslipidemia, endocrine abnormalities, and growth retardation.

- **Sodium and water balance.** Normal kidneys can adapt to a wide range of sodium and water intake, and these homeostatic mechanisms are usually maintained until the GFR decreases to advanced stages of CKD. Fluid abnormalities result in fluid retention and hypertension (particularly with glomerular diseases) or dehydration and hyponatremia (caused by polyuria with decreased renal-concentrating ability in nephronophthisis, congenital renal disorders, and obstructive uropathy).

- **Hyperkalemia** develops primarily because of decreased potassium excretion with reduced GFR as a result of decreased delivery of sodium to the distal tubule (type IV renal tubular acidosis [RTA]). Contributing factors to hyperkalemia include dietary potassium intake, increased tissue breakdown, metabolic acidosis, or hypoaldosteronism (administration of ACEIs or ARBs).

- **Metabolic acidosis** is a result of decreased ability of the kidney to excrete hydrogen ions (impaired ammoniogenesis), and in addition, there is reduction of titratable acid excretion and bicarbonate reabsorption.

- **Metabolic bone disease (renal osteodystrophy)**

- **Abnormalities in mineral metabolism and bone structure** are common findings in stage 3 CKD (Figure 65-3). There is retention of phosphate because of decreased GFR and decreased renal production of 1,25-dihydroxy vitamin D. This leads to decreased serum calcium levels and subsequent elevation of serum parathyroid hormone (PTH). This secondary hyperparathyroidism results in reabsorption of calcium from bone, leading to bone disease that presents with difficulty in walking, bone pain, skeletal deformities, and fractures.

- **Anemia** of CKD is initially normocytic and normochromic and is caused by reduced renal erythropoietin production. Iron deficiency, which is common, and vitamin B12 or folate deficiency may contribute to the anemia. Anemia results in progressive fatigue and weakness.

- **Hypertension** is caused by volume expansion or activation of the renin–angiotensin system. It can be present in the earliest stages of CKD. Cardiovascular abnormalities found in CKD include left ventricular hypertrophy (caused by hypertension) and evidence of early atherosclerosis (coronary artery calcification, increased aortic stiffness).

- **Dyslipidemia** results from abnormal lipid metabolism in CKD, causing an increase in triglyceride-rich lipoproteins and low high-density lipoproteins (HDL) cholesterol levels. This increases the risk of having cardiovascular disease.

- **Endocrine dysfunction** in CKD is reflected in disorders of growth hormone metabolism (end-organ resistance to growth hormone caused by increased levels of insulin growth factor binding proteins); thyroid function known as "sick euthyroid syndrome" (low total and free T4 and T3, normal thyroid-stimulating hormone and normal thyrotropin-releasing hormone); and reduced gonadal hormones, resulting in delayed puberty and anovulation.

- **Growth retardation** in CKD is caused by metabolic acidosis, decreased caloric intake, metabolic bone disease, and alterations in growth hormone metabolism.

- **Uremia** represents a constellation of symptoms and signs present in the final stage of CKD (Figure 65-4). These include anorexia, nausea, vomiting, growth retardation, platelet dysfunction (abnormal platelet adhesion and aggregation), pericardial disease (pericarditis and pericardial effusion), neurologic abnormalities (peripheral neuropathy, lethargy, seizures, coma, and death), and altered cognitive development (loss of concentration, poor school performance, and mental retardation).

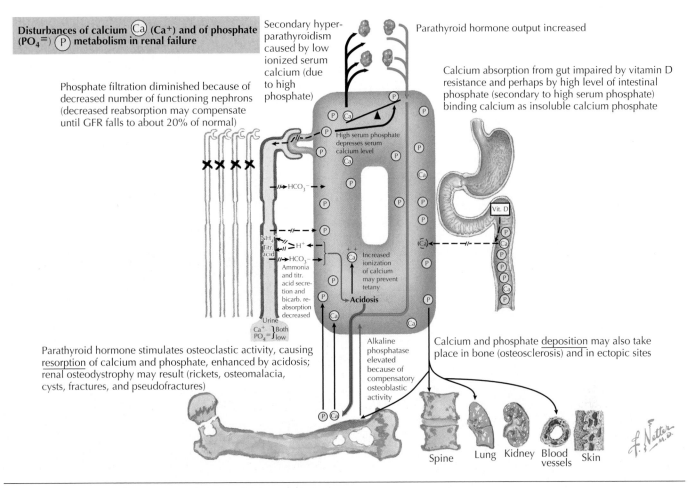

Figure 65-3 *Renal failure: calcium and phosphorus metabolism.*

EVALUATION

History

The history should include age at onset of symptoms, duration of symptoms, presence of uremic symptoms (weakness, fatigue, anorexia, vomiting), systemic diseases (fever, rash, arthralgias), specific renal disease, diagnosis of congenital anomaly of the kidney or urinary tract antenatally, and family history of renal disease or hypertension. The history is focused on signs of CKD and should include information about growth and development history; fluid and electrolyte abnormalities; elevated blood pressure; anemia; presence of polyuria, polydipsia, or enuresis; recurrent urinary tract infection; urologic abnormalities; bone abnormalities; and seizures.

Physical Examination

The examination should include measurement of growth parameters, blood pressure measurement, assessment for pallor, examination for any bone deformities, assessment for signs of hypervolemia (e.g., edema), and heart examination looking for pericardial rub (pericarditis) or diminished heart sounds (pericardial effusion).

Laboratory Testing

There is no single pattern of laboratory abnormalities that characterizes pediatric CKD, but some abnormalities are commonly present and are indicative of underlying chronic kidney dysfunction. Serum creatinine is the most commonly used test to estimate the GFR (creatinine clearance indirectly represents the GFR) using the Schwartz formula: GFR = kL/SCr, where k is a constant that varies with age and sex, L is length (cm), and SCr is serum creatinine in mg/dL (Table 65-1). The GFR is then used to determine the stage of CKD. Normal levels of GFR vary with age, gender, and body size (Table 65-2). GFR increases with maturation from infancy and approaches adult mean value by 2 years of age.

Electrolytes are tested to evaluate for hyperkalemia and metabolic acidosis. Serum calcium, phosphorus, and PTH level are needed to detect abnormalities in bone mineral metabolism. Lipid profile is needed to detect dyslipidemia. A complete blood count will detect anemia, and RBC indices will characterize the anemia and help eliminate other causes of anemia other than CKD, determining the iron profile (serum iron, total iron-binding capacity, percent transferrin saturation) and looking for possible blood losses (test for occult blood) is necessary.

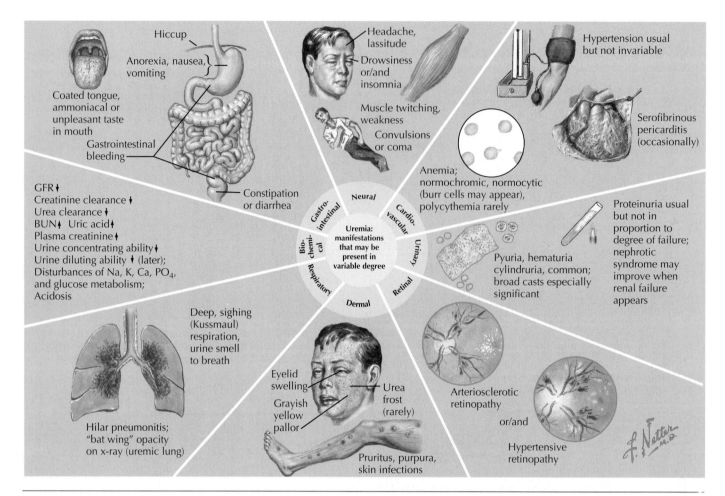

Figure 65-4 *Uremia.*

Urinalysis

Urinalysis as described for AKI can identify the underlying cause of both AKI and CKD. Proteinuria is an important biomarker associated with CKD because it may contribute to CKD progression.

Renal Ultrasonography

Renal ultrasonography is the most widely used imaging modality and is a noninvasive procedure. It assesses the renal size and

Table 65-1 Stages of Chronic Kidney Disease for Children Older Than 2 Years of Age

Stage	Glomerular Filtration Rate
1	Normal (≥90 mL/min/1.73 m²)
2	60-89 mL/min/1.73 m²
3	30-59 mL/min/1.73 m²
4	15-29 mL/min/1.73 m²
5	<15 mL/min/1.73 m² or ESRD

ESRD, end-stage renal disease.

Table 65-2 Normal Glomerular Filtration Rate Levels and the Schwartz Equation

Age (Gender)	Schwartz Equation (Serum Creatinine in mg/dL, Length in cm)	Mean GFR ± SD (mL/min/1.73m²)
1 wk (boys and girls)	GFR = 0.33*(Length/SCr) in preterm infants GFR = 0.45*(Length/SCr) in term infants	40.6 ± 14.8
2-8 wk (boys and girls)	GFR = 0.45*(Length/SCr)	65.8 ± 24.8
>8 wk (boys and girls)	GFR = 0.45*(Length/SCr)	95.7 ± 21.7
2-12 y (boys and girls)	GFR = 0.55*(Length/SCr)	133.0 ± 27.0
13-18 y (boys)	GFR = 0.70*(Length/SCr)	140.0 ± 30.0
13-18 y (girls)	GFR = 0.55*(Length/SCr)	126.0 ± 22.0

GFR, glomerular filtration rate; SCr, serum creatinine; SD, standard deviation.

structure. In CKD, the kidneys are usually smaller than normal, which indicates a loss of renal mass from an underlying renal disease, such as a congenital disorder (e.g., renal hypoplasia). It may also identify the cause of CKD such as detecting cystic kidney disease. Other imaging studies such as voiding cystourethrography, computed tomography, and magnetic resonance imaging are used in specific clinical settings.

Kidney Biopsy

Kidney biopsy provides diagnosis of the underlying renal disorder that caused CKD. The results also serve to guide therapy and provide information about disease severity, including whether the findings may be reversible, and about the degree of renal scarring.

MANAGEMENT

The general management of a patient with CKD includes the following components: treatment of reversible renal dysfunction (some renal function may be recovered if treatment is initiated early), prevention of progression of renal disease, treatment of complications, and identification of renal replacement therapy.

Slowing Progression

Slowing the progression of CKD is achieved by treating hypertension and decreasing proteinuria because these are known to accelerate the progression of CKD. ACEIs and ARBs are used in this regard. Additional intervention studies in adults with CKD such as dietary protein restriction, lipid-lowering therapy, and correction of anemia have shown inconclusive results. As far as the low protein restriction in children is concerned, the current consensus is to provide the age-appropriate recommended daily allowance of protein.

Management of Complications

Sodium and water retention occur as GFR becomes severely decreased in stages 4 and 5 CKD. This is treated with dietary sodium restriction and diuretics. Some children with obstructive uropathy or renal dysplasia have a poor urinary concentrating capacity and sodium wasting, making them prone to hypovolemia and hyponatremia.

- **Hyperkalemia** is treated with a low-potassium diet, loop diuretics, alkali therapy (sodium bicarbonate), and cation exchange resins (Kayexalate).
- **Metabolic** acidosis is corrected using sodium bicarbonate therapy with the goal of maintaining serum bicarbonate level at or above 22 mEq/L.
- **Bone metabolism and bone disease** of CKD are treated with dietary phosphate restriction, use of phosphate binding agents, and vitamin D replacement therapy.
- **Hypertension** is treated with weight reduction, exercise, dietary salt reduction, antihypertensive medications, and diuretics. Strict blood pressure control in all children with CKD is necessary, with a target blood pressure of less than

the 90th percentile for age, gender, and height and less than 120/80 mm Hg for adolescents with CKD.
- **Anemia** is treated with iron supplementation and erythropoietin replacement therapy. K/DOQI guidelines recommend a target hemoglobin between 11 and 12 g/dL.
- **Dyslipidemia** is managed with fibrates (i.e., gemfibrozil or fenofibrate) for elevated triglyceride level and with statin therapy (i.e., atorvastatin, simvastatin) for elevated low-density lipoprotein levels.
- **Nutrition** should be managed so that malnutrition of CKD (secondary to poor appetite, decreased intestinal absorption, and metabolic acidosis) is prevented. It is recommended that protein and caloric intake should be at least 100% of the recommended daily allowance for age. Nutritional support using nutritional supplements is often needed.

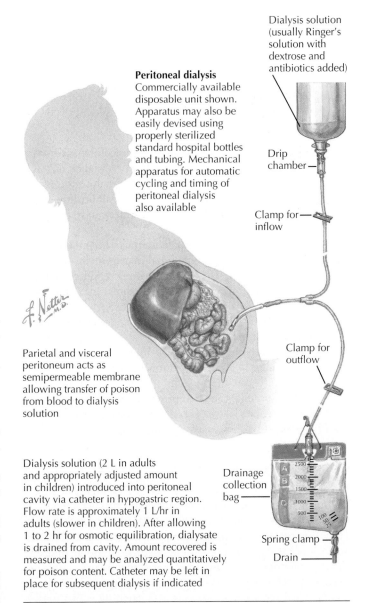

Peritoneal dialysis
Commercially available disposable unit shown. Apparatus may also be easily devised using properly sterilized standard hospital bottles and tubing. Mechanical apparatus for automatic cycling and timing of peritoneal dialysis also available

Dialysis solution (usually Ringer's solution with dextrose and antibiotics added)

Drip chamber

Clamp for inflow

Parietal and visceral peritoneum acts as semipermeable membrane allowing transfer of poison from blood to dialysis solution

Clamp for outflow

Dialysis solution (2 L in adults and appropriately adjusted amount in children) introduced into peritoneal cavity via catheter in hypogastric region. Flow rate is approximately 1 L/hr in adults (slower in children). After allowing 1 to 2 hr for osmotic equilibration, dialysate is drained from cavity. Amount recovered is measured and may be analyzed quantitatively for poison content. Catheter may be left in place for subsequent dialysis if indicated

Drainage collection bag

Spring clamp

Drain

Figure 65-5 *Peritoneal dialysis.*

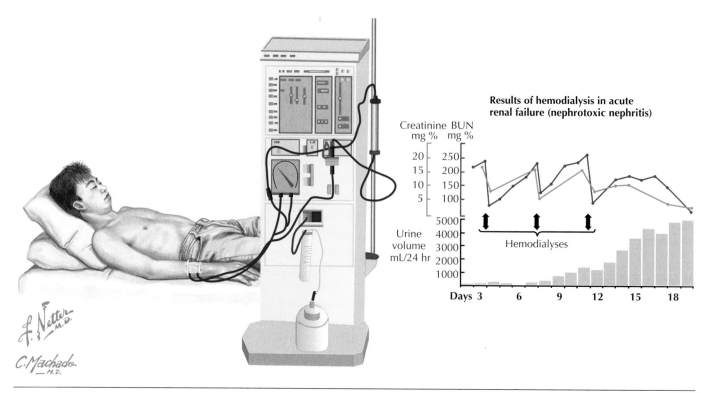

Figure 65-6 *Hemodialysis in progress.*

- **Growth retardation** is treated with recombinant human growth hormone (GH) therapy (GH resistance of CKD can be overcome using supraphysiologic doses of exogenous GH) and with management of malnutrition, renal osteodystrophy, acid–base abnormalities, and electrolyte disturbances.
- **Neurodevelopmental impairment** can be minimized by initiating dialysis and by optimal management of anemia and malnutrition. Infants and young children require frequent monitoring of head circumference and age-appropriate developmental evaluations. A more formal assessment is needed in older children, particularly if they have poor school performance.
- **Uremic bleeding** that occurs in uremia secondary to abnormalities in platelet adhesion and aggregation properties (mostly caused by reduced von Willebrand factor [vWF] in uremia) can be improved by using desmopressin, which increases levels of coagulation factor VIII and vWF by stimulating their release from storage sites.

Renal Replacement Therapy

Renal replacement therapy is achieved by PD, HD, and kidney transplantation. Renal replacement therapy is generally needed with GFR less than 15 mL/min/1.73 m² (stage 5 CKD). However, renal replacement therapy in children may be initiated sooner if there is poor calorie intake resulting in failure to thrive, symptomatic uremia (e.g., pericarditis), and significant delay in psychomotor or cognitive development. The choice among renal replacement options is dictated by family preference and technical, psychosocial and compliance issues.

- **PD** is more common in infants and younger children largely because of problems of vascular access in that age group (Figure 65-5). A PD catheter is surgically placed into the peritoneal space. PD fluid is pumped into the peritoneal space. Peritoneal membrane serves as a "filter" through which waste products and water are cleared from blood that circulates through blood vessels of the peritoneal membrane. Waste products and water are transferred to the PD fluid in the peritoneal space by processes of diffusion and osmosis. This fluid is then drained out of the peritoneal space. PD can be performed by parents at home, overnight with a cycling machine that allows the least disruption of home life, school, and work attendance.
- **HD** is more commonly used in older children (Figure 65-6). HD requires vascular access such as placement of an arteriovenous fistula, arteriovenous graft, or central venous catheter. Blood is pumped from the vascular access into the dialyzer, which contains an artificial membrane that serves as a filter through which waste products and water are cleared from the blood into the dialysis fluid by processes of diffusion, convection, and ultrafiltration. Dialysis fluid flows through the dialyzer countercurrent to the blood. HD is done in specialized HD centers using a HD machine and requires at least three weekly treatments that are each 3 to 5 hours long.
- **Renal transplantation** is performed using a deceased or living (related or unrelated) kidney donor. It can be performed in stage 4 or 5 CKD before dialysis begins (preemptive kidney transplantation). Renal transplantation is accepted as the optimal therapy of choice, which is based on the belief that successful transplantation not only

ameliorates uremic symptoms but also allows for significant improvement, and often correction of, delayed skeletal growth, sexual maturation, cognitive performance, and psychosocial functioning.

FUTURE DIRECTIONS

Currently, an ongoing prospective study, the Chronic Kidney Disease in Children Study (CKiD), is following children with CKD to identify risk factors for CKD progression and the impact of CKD on growth, cognition, and the risk of cardiovascular disease.

Recognition of the overestimation of GFR that regularly occurs when using the current estimating formulas has prompted studies on the development of newer and more accurate formulas as part of the multicenter CKiD study.

SUGGESTED READINGS

Akcan-Arikan A, Zappitelli M, Loftis LL, et al: Modified RIFLE criteria in critically ill children with acute kidney injury, *Kidney Int* 71(10):1028-1035, 2007.

Andreoli SP: Acute kidney injury in children, *Pediatr Nephrol* 24(2):253-163, 2009.

Andreoli SP: Management of acute kidney injury in children: a guide for pediatricians, *Paediatr Drugs* 10(6):379-390, 2008.

Benfield MR, Bunchman TE: Management of acute renal failure. In Avner ED, Harmon WE, Niaudet P, editors: *Pediatric Nephrology*. Philadelphia, Lippincott, 2004, Williams & Wilkins, pp 1253-1266.

Eddy AA: Progression in chronic kidney disease, *Adv Chronic Kidney Dis* 12:353, 2005.

Fine RN, Whyte DA, Boydstun II: Conservative management of chronic renal insufficiency. In Avner ED, Harmon WE, Niaudet P, editors: *Pediatric Nephrology*. Philadelphia, Lippincott, 2004, Williams & Wilkins, pp 1253-1266.

Greenbaum LA: Anemia in children with chronic kidney disease, *Adv Chronic Kidney Dis* 12(4):385-396, 2005.

Hadtstein C, Schaefer F: Hypertension in children with chronic kidney disease: pathophysiology and management, *Pediatr Nephrol* 23(3):363-371, 2008.

Nguyen MT, Devarajan P: Biomarkers for the early detection of acute kidney injury, *Pediatr Nephrol* 23(12):2151-2157, 2008.

Srivastava T, Warady BA: Overview of the management of chronic kidney disease in children, UpToDate 17.1, 2009.

Wesseling K, Bakkaloglu S, Salusky I: Chronic kidney disease mineral and bone disorder in children, *Pediatr Nephrol* 23(2):195-207, 2008.

Wong CS, Warady BA: Epidemiology, etiology, and course of chronic kidney disease in children. UpToDate 17.1, 2009.

Wong CS, Warady BA, Srivastava T: Clinical presentation and evaluation of chronic kidney disease in children. UpToDate 17.1, 2009.

Ulf H. Beier and Lawrence Copelovitch

This chapter reviews several common congenital and inherited anomalies of the kidney and urologic system. Congenital abnormalities are a frequent cause of renal failure in children, accounting for more than 30% of end-stage renal disease (ESRD). Congenital anomalies can be subdivided into three categories based on the stage of the primary abnormality in renal embryologic development (Figure 66-1). The first category refers to a failure to form a functional nephron, leading to renal parenchyma malformations, such as renal agenesis or cystic dysplasia. The second group of defects relates to a failure of the developing kidney to migrate to its appropriate destination. This may lead to renal ectopy (pelvic or thoracic kidneys) or fusion abnormalities, such as a horseshoe kidney. The third category describes defects of the urinary collecting system, such as double ureters or posterior urethral valves (PUVs). Here, changes of the renal parenchyma (hydronephrosis, dysplasia) are often secondary to obstructive uropathy or urinary reflux disease. Inherited conditions such as the polycystic kidney diseases (PKD) are the result of specific genetic mutations that may present with detectable renal abnormalities at birth or may not develop until later in life. The following sections detail common and exemplary conditions representative of these subcategories.

POLYCYSTIC KIDNEY DISEASE

PKDs are a group of genetically inherited conditions in which cyst formation and renal parenchymal replacement can occur at anytime from fetal life to adulthood. There are two major forms, autosomal dominant PKD (ADPKD) and autosomal recessive PKD (ARPKD) (Table 66-1). In addition, a number of rare pleiotropic disorders exist, which are loosely associated because of similar clinical and pathophysiologic features, including renal cystic and hepatobiliary disease (Table 66-2). All of these disorders share ciliary dysfunction as a common principle in their pathogenesis. PKD proteins have been localized to the cilia or basal body, and loss or abnormalities of cilia in the kidney are associated with cyst development (Figure 66-2).

Autosomal Recessive Polycystic Kidney Disease

ARPKD typically presents early in life and is commonly detected in utero by routine prenatal ultrasound. Severe cases may be associated with the Potter sequence (i.e., oligohydramnios with subsequent lung hypoplasia and characteristic limb and facial abnormalities resulting from decreased intraamniotic space). ARPKD is reported to have an incidence of one in 20,000. The phenotype can be quite variable. One-third of identified patients do not survive beyond the neonatal period mainly because of respiratory insufficiency. Of those who survive infancy,

approximately one-third will need chronic renal replacement therapy. In addition to the renal manifestations, cystic biliary dysgenesis is another hallmark of ARPKD. It can result in congenital hepatic fibrosis and may present later in childhood or adolescence, even in adults. Characteristically, patients presenting later in life have less severe renal disease and more prominent hepatic fibrosis. Hepatic fibrosis may lead to portal hypertension, gastrointestinal bleedings from esophageal varices, cholangitis, and hepatic failure. The gene identified with ARPKD is on the short arm of chromosome 6 and encodes fibrocystin (polyductin). Fibrocystin is expressed on the cilia of renal and bile duct epithelial cells and is thought to be critical in the maintenance of normal tubular architecture in the renal and biliary systems.

The diagnosis is established based on classical radiographic features. The classic sonographic appearances in newborns are large kidneys, increased echogenicity of the parenchyma, and loss of corticomedullary differentiation. There may be macrocysts that are less than 2 cm in diameter. The cysts are subcapsular extensions of radially oriented ectatic spaces. In addition to the sonographic findings, the diagnosis of ARPKD requires one or more of the following: (1) absence of renal cysts in both parents, (2) a previously affected sibling, (3) consanguinity, or (4) hepatic fibrosis.

Treatment is largely supportive. The primary prognostic determinant in the newborn period is the degree of lung hypoplasia. Renal failure and portal hypertension are treated with medications, dialysis, or transplant depending on an individual patient's symptoms. In childhood, the most common features are renal failure, electrolyte abnormalities, and hypertension. The hypertension is usually responsive to angiotensin-converting enzyme inhibitors. Hepatic fibrosis may cause portal hypertension with resulting esophageal varices, gastrointestinal bleedings, and hypersplenism with thrombocytopenia. Liver failure may in some cases require liver transplant. Cholelithiasis is common. Ascending cholangitis is a potentially life-threatening concern.

Autosomal Dominant Polycystic Kidney Disease

In contrast to ARPKD, ADPKD is usually diagnosed in adulthood, although it may be detected at any age, including prenatally. With an estimated incidence between one in 400 and one in 1000, it is one of the more common genetic disorders. There is a high degree of phenotypic variation, ranging from infants presenting in renal failure to asymptomatic elderly patients with adequate renal function. The disease may commonly lead to ESRD. In the United States, 4.4% of adult patients requiring renal replacement therapy have ADPKD. Morphologically, both kidneys show progressive bilateral development and

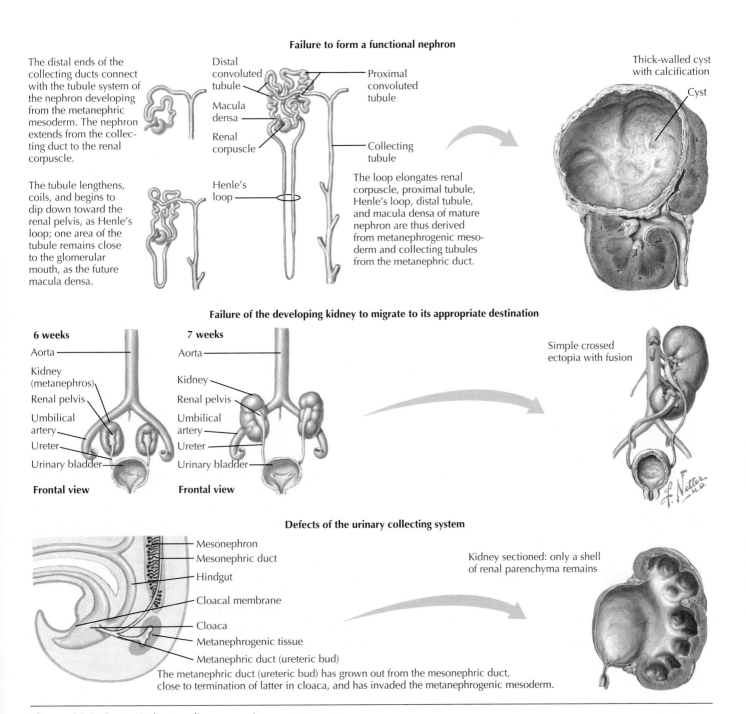

Failure to form a functional nephron

The distal ends of the collecting ducts connect with the tubule system of the nephron developing from the metanephric mesoderm. The nephron extends from the collecting duct to the renal corpuscle.

The tubule lengthens, coils, and begins to dip down toward the renal pelvis, as Henle's loop; one area of the tubule remains close to the glomerular mouth, as the future macula densa.

Distal convoluted tubule
Macula densa
Renal corpuscle
Henle's loop
Proximal convoluted tubule
Collecting tubule

The loop elongates renal corpuscle, proximal tubule, Henle's loop, distal tubule, and macula densa of mature nephron are thus derived from metanephrogenic meso-derm and collecting tubules from the metanephric duct.

Thick-walled cyst with calcification
Cyst

Failure of the developing kidney to migrate to its appropriate destination

6 weeks
Aorta
Kidney (metanephros)
Renal pelvis
Umbilical artery
Ureter
Urinary bladder
Frontal view

7 weeks
Aorta
Kidney
Renal pelvis
Umbilical artery
Ureter
Urinary bladder
Frontal view

Simple crossed ectopia with fusion

Defects of the urinary collecting system

Mesonephron
Mesonephric duct
Hindgut
Cloacal membrane
Cloaca
Metanephrogenic tissue
Metanephric duct (ureteric bud)

The metanephric duct (ureteric bud) has grown out from the mesonephric duct, close to termination of latter in cloaca, and has invaded the metanephrogenic mesoderm.

Kidney sectioned: only a shell of renal parenchyma remains

Figure 66-1 *Congenital anomalies categories.*

enlargement of focal cysts. ADPKD is a systemic disease, with cysts occurring in the liver, pancreas, and vasculature. In contrast to ARPKD, the liver disease is predominantly cystic, and hepatic failure is rare. Extrarenal manifestations of ADPKD are uncommon in children; however, intracranial aneurysms (intracranial saccular aneurysms, or "Berry aneurysms") and male fertility problems can occur in adulthood.

Two genes have been identified with ADPKD. The *PKD1* gene on chromosome 16p13.3 encodes polycystin 1 and accounts for 85% of all ADPKD cases. PKD2 on chromosome 4q13-q23 encodes for polycystin 2. Both affected proteins are involved with the ciliary apparatus. A small number of cases could

not be linked to either gene, suggesting the involvement of other genes.

Children with ADPKD may present with flank pain, hematuria, renal colic, urinary tract infections (UTIs), or hypertension, or they may be asymptomatic. ADPKD can be diagnosed by renal ultrasound, computed tomography, or magnetic resonance imaging. Multiple renal parenchymal cysts are generally visible and usually increase in size and number with age. The finding of a single cyst in a child may merit further observation. In general, the combination of a parent with ADPKD and more than one cyst in a child is considered diagnostic for ADPKD. Rarely, ADPKD may arise sporadically. Diagnosing ADPKD in

Table 66-1 Autosomal Recessive Polycystic Kidney Disease versus Autosomal Dominant Polycystic Kidney Disease

	Autosomal Recessive Polycystic Kidney Disease	Autosomal Dominant Polycystic Kidney Disease
Gene	Chromosome 6p21.2-p12	Chromosome 16p13.3, chromosome 4q13-q23
Protein	Fibrocystin	Polycystin 1, polycystin 2
Age of presentation	Commonly prenatally, childhood, adolescence	Highly variable
Renal cysts	Radial pattern	Anywhere in kidney, varying size
Extrarenal manifestations	Biliary obstruction, hepatic fibrosis with portal hypertension, liver failure	Liver cysts, pancreas cysts, vascular cysts ("Berry aneurysms")
Things in common	Renal cysts do not communicate. Disease may present at any age, including prenatally. Gene defect leads to malfunction of the ciliary body. The kidneys are usually enlarged. Usually bilateral disease (exception: early diagnosis ADPKD in childhood with positive family history)	

a presymptomatic, otherwise healthy child may not always be in the patient's best interest given the financial and psychosocial implications. Because of the complexities of these issues, pediatric practitioners should refer asymptomatic children to a pediatric nephrologist before undertaking any diagnostic investigations.

Analogous to ARPDK, the treatment of ADPKD is largely symptomatic. Notably, UTIs are relatively common in patients with ADPKD. A UTI in ADPKD may be difficult to diagnose because the infection may be contained within a cyst and may not provide diagnostic pyuria or bacteriuria. Conversely, a ruptured cyst may show hematuria and pyuria in the absence of a UTI. Furthermore, traditional first-line antibiotic agents for UTIs such as a cephalosporin or an aminoglycoside may be ineffective because of poor cyst penetration. A sulfonamide or quinolone is usually preferred. Screening for extrarenal manifestations, such as intracranial aneurysms, is not routinely recommended in children, and magnetic resonance angiography is

usually reserved for symptomatic patients and those with a strong family history of cerebrovascular disease.

HORSESHOE KIDNEY

Horseshoe kidney is the most prevalent fusion abnormality of the developing kidney. The fusion occurs commonly at the lower poles, and two separate excretory urinary systems are maintained (Figure 66-3) The incidence is reported between one in 400 and one in 1600. The isthmus may be located at or lateral to the midline (symmetric vs. asymmetric horseshoe kidney). It may contain actual parenchyma or a fibrous band. The kidneys arrest during their embryologic ascension toward the dorsolumbar position, usually between the fourth to ninth weeks of gestation. This is caused by the inferior mesenteric artery holding the isthmus and preventing further rostral migration. As a consequence, blood supply of the fused kidney is variable and may come from the iliac arteries or aorta or at

Table 66-2 Overview of the Ciliopathies*

Name	Eye Findings	Cerebellar and Brain Malformations	Gastrointestinal Malformations	Congenital Heart Disease	Osseous Changes
Senior Løken	Retinitis Pigmentosa, others				
Joubert	Coloboma, retinal degeneration	"Molar tooth sign," cerebellar vermis hypoplasia	Hepatic fibrosis		
Meckel Gruber		Occipital encephalocoele	Ductal proliferation, hepatic fibrosis		Postaxial polydactyly
Biedl Bardet	Retinitis pigmentosa	Anosmia	Hepatic fibrosis	Hypertrophic or dilated cardiomyopathy	Postaxial polydactyly
Jeune					Short upper limbs, asphyxiating thoracic dystrophy
Ellis–van Creveld				Multiple heart defects	Disproportionate dwarfism, postaxial polydactyly, ectodermal dysplasia, small chest
Alström	Retinal dystrophy	Sensorineural hearing loss	Obesity, hyperinsulinemia	Dilated cardiomyopathy	
Orofacialdigital					Facial, oral, and digital malformations

*All conditions are associated with cystic renal disease.

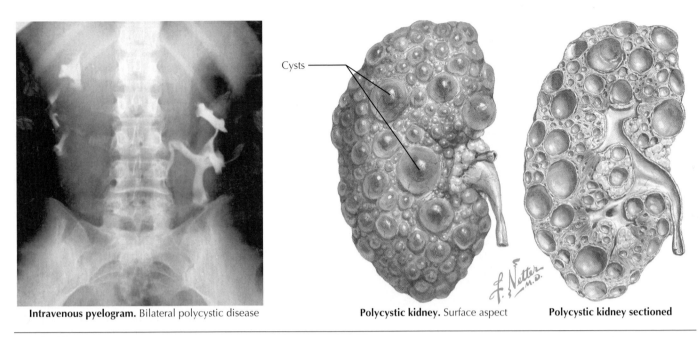

Cysts

Intravenous pyelogram. Bilateral polycystic disease   **Polycystic kidney.** Surface aspect   **Polycystic kidney sectioned**

Figure 66-2 *Renal cystic diseases.*

times, the hypogastric and middle sacral arteries. Horseshoe kidneys may occur in isolation or as part of a syndrome, such as Turner syndrome, trisomy 18, or less commonly trisomy 13 and 21. It is occasionally associated with other genitourinary findings, such as bicornuate or septate uterus in girls and hypospadias and undescended testis in boys. Most patients with horseshoe kidneys are asymptomatic and are diagnosed incidentally by ultrasonography. However, some patients may present with

pain, hematuria, obstruction, or UTIs. Hydronephrosis may be seen in up to 80% of children with horseshoe kidneys. The etiologies include vesicoureteral reflux (VUR), obstruction of the collecting system by external ureteric compression (from blood vessels, renal calculi), or ureteropelvic junction (UPJ) obstruction caused by a relatively high insertion of ureters. Twenty percent of patients have urolithiasis.

Patients with an isolated horseshoe kidney have a slightly increased risk of developing a Wilms tumor. The overall incidence of Wilms' tumor is 7.6 cases per million in children younger than 15 years and 14.9 per million (1.96 times higher) in children with horseshoe kidney. Because the risk still remains well less than 0.002%, screening for Wilms' tumor in patients with horseshoe kidney is not routinely done. The diagnostic evaluation of a horseshoe kidney is aimed at identifying VUR. These initial investigations include renal ultrasound and voiding cystourethrography (VCUG). The ultrasound may demonstrate the presence or absence of hydronephrosis. A voiding cystourethrogram should be done to exclude the possibility of reflux. A technetium 99m-labeled diethylenetriaminepentaacetic acid (DTPA) scan should be done if there is evidence of an obstruction on ultrasonography.

In most patients with a horseshoe kidney, no specific treatment is necessary. If VUR or obstructive uropathy has been identified, these patients should be referred to a pediatric urologist. Antibiotic prophylaxis and corrective surgery may be necessary.

UROLOGIC MALFORMATIONS

Double Ureter

Double ureters are part of a duplicated collecting system complex, defined as two pyelocaliceal systems within one renal unit. Both ureters may either drain separately or jointly over a single orifice into the bladder. Double ureters can be unilateral or bilateral and can be associated with a variety of congenital

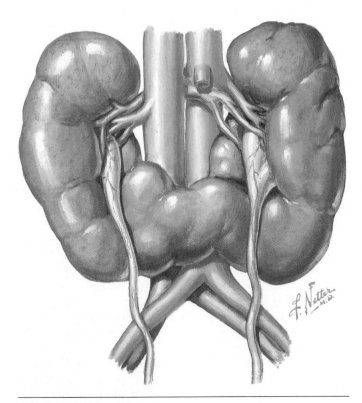

Figure 66-3 *Horseshoe kidney.*

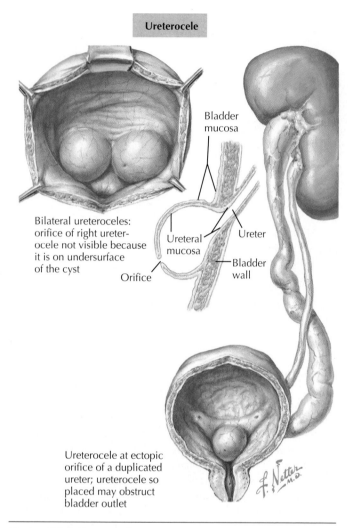

Ureterocele

Bladder mucosa

Bilateral ureteroceles: orifice of right ureterocele not visible because it is on undersurface of the cyst

Ureteral mucosa

Orifice

Ureter

Bladder wall

Ureterocele at ectopic orifice of a duplicated ureter; ureterocele so placed may obstruct bladder outlet

Figure 66-4 *Ureterocele.*

Table 66-3 Double Ureter: Associated Pathology	
Renal upper pole	Urinary obstruction from ectopic insertion of the ureter leading to upper pole hydronephrosis Ureterocele
Renal lower pole	Urinary reflux from maldevelopment of the ureter's valve mechanism

The diagnostic evaluation includes renal ultrasound and VCUG. The goal of imaging is to identify VUR, ureteroceles, and obstructive uropathy. If these are found, surgical correction may be indicated.

Ureteropelvic Junction Obstruction

UPJ obstruction is the most common cause of antenatally detected hydronephrosis. It is found in one of 500 live births on routine fetal ultrasound. UPJ obstruction is more commonly found in boys and more commonly on the left than on the right side. The UPJ diameter enlarges as a result of a partial restriction of urinary flow, resulting in hydronephrosis. The hydronephrosis may be progressive, arrest, or improve spontaneously, depending on both the reason for UPJ obstruction and the ability of the renal pelvis to expand and compensate for increased urinary pressure. Most patients are asymptomatic and found to have antenatal hydronephrosis on routine prenatal ultrasonography. Occasionally, newborns may present with abdominal masses or renal insufficiency if the obstruction is bilateral. The standard evaluation of a newborn with prenatal ultrasound findings suggestive of UPJ obstruction includes a confirmatory postnatal renal ultrasound. If the UPJ is persistent a VCUG to assess for urinary reflux disease should be considered. Urolithiasis and UTIs are possible complications of a UPJ obstruction. If patients are symptomatic, surgical intervention is frequently indicated. The surgical options include a reconstructive pyeloplasty or temporary nephrostomy tubes to alleviate pressure more acutely. If patients are managed by observation alone, antibiotic prophylaxis is usually not needed unless there is evidence of vesicoureteral reflux.

Posterior Urethral Valves

PUVs are the most common cause of lower urinary tract obstruction in male neonates (Figure 66-5). The reported incidence ranges from one in 8000 to one in 25,000 live births. The etiology of PUV is still disputed. Autopsy studies on stillborn fetuses with PUVs have found a congenital obstructing posterior urethral membrane (COPUM). It is possible that the valves classically seen on ultrasound and VCUG occur as a result of the perforation of the COPUM by an advancing Foley catheter.

The posterior urethra is formed by the cloacae and the urogenital sinus, and its lining contains transitional epithelium. The theory is that abnormal integration of the Wolffian ducts into the posterior urethra might lead to formation of the COPUM. PUV has a wide spectrum of clinical presentation largely depending on the initial degree of urethral obstruction. The associated morbidity is not limited to renal abnormalities and

genitourinary tract abnormalities. Most patients are asymptomatic, with double ureters being detected incidentally on imaging studies. Double ureters occur when two ureteral buds arise from the Wolffian duct. In cases of complete duplication, the lower renal unit typically drains into the normal ureteric insertion and the ureter of the upper renal unit drains ectopically in the bladder, urethra, or elsewhere. The ectopic ureter usually enters the bladder inferiorly and medially to the normal ureter. In girls, if the ectopic ureter inserts into the vagina, urethra, or uterus, urinary dribbling or incontinence may be the presenting sign. Most patients are asymptomatic. Symptoms usually occur in ureteric duplication if there is reflux into the ureter of the lower renal unit or if the ectopic upper renal unit ureter becomes obstructed (Figure 66-4). The typical complications observed with complete double ureter systems are summarized in Table 66-3. Recurrent UTIs can occur in obstructed or refluxing ureters. It is noteworthy that up to 80% of ureteroceles are associated with double ureters. In duplex kidneys, ureteroceles are usually an outgrowth of the ectopic ureter. Double ureters are common and noted to occur in 0.2% of live births. There is a 12% chance of a double ureter occurring in first-degree relatives of persons with this condition. Bilateral duplication is noted in 15% to 40% of individuals with complete duplication.

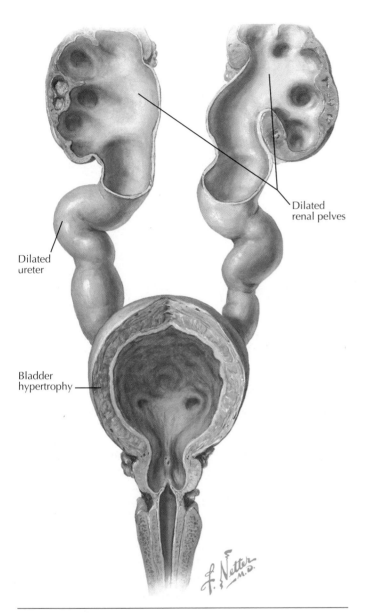

Dilated
renal pelves

Dilated
ureter

Bladder
hypertrophy

Figure 66-5 *Urethral congenital valve.*

may be related to impaired lung development in utero (Potter sequence), bladder wall thickening and dilatation, hydroureters, urinomas, and hydronephrosis. The obstructive uropathy may result in renal dysplasia, renal insufficiency, and end-stage renal disease. Up to 15% of patients who undergo renal transplantation in childhood have PUV as the underlying condition. The widespread use of prenatal ultrasound has resulted in most cases being diagnosed in the fetal or neonatal period. Some patients may be missed and present later in life. In those cases, a voiding history is of particular importance because patients with PUV usually have a diminished or abnormal urinary stream. Treatment consists of fulguration of the PUV by a urologist. Children commonly develop postobstructive diuresis and should be monitored carefully for electrolyte and volume instabilities. The prognosis depends on the degree of preserved renal function after the obstruction is relieved (see Figure 66-5).

SUGGESTED READINGS

Harris PC: 2008 Homer W. Smith Award: insights into the pathogenesis of polycystic kidney disease from gene discovery, *J Am Soc Nephrol* 20(6):1188-1198, 2009.

North American Pediatric Renal Trials and Collaborative Studies: NAPRTCS 2008 Annual Report. Available at https://web.emmes.com/study/ped/index.htm.

Neville H, Ritchey ML, Shamberger RC, et al: The occurrence of Wilms tumor in horseshoe kidneys: a report from the National Wilms Tumor Study Group (NWTSG), *J Pediatr Surg* 37(8):1134-1137, 2002.

Hildebrandt F, Attanasio M, Otto E: Nephronophthisis: disease mechanisms of a ciliopathy, *J Am Soc Nephrol* 20(1):23-35, 2009.

Krishnan A, de Souza A, Konijeti R, Baskin LS: The anatomy and embryology of posterior urethral valves, *J Urol* 175(4):1214-1220, 2006.

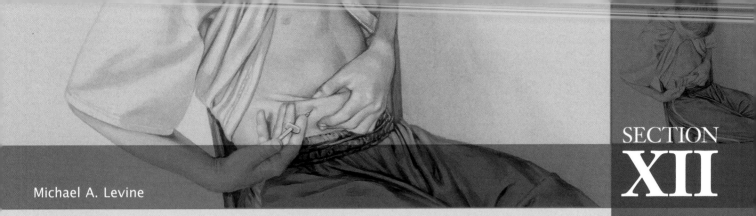

Michael A. Levine

SECTION
XII

Disorders of the Endocrine System

Puberty

Andrew C. Calabria and David R. Langdon

67

Puberty is the hormonally mediated transition between childhood and adulthood that facilitates development of secondary sexual characteristics, achievement of adult height, and reproductive maturity. Normal puberty requires interaction between the hypothalamus, pituitary, gonads, and internal sexual organs and the capacity to respond to the appropriate hormones. Disorders of puberty manifest as unusually early, late, or incomplete sexual development or abnormal growth. The initial clinical evaluation often depends on distinguishing early or late, but otherwise normal, sex hormone effects from conditions of excess or deficiency.

ETIOLOGY AND PATHOGENESIS

Hormonal Changes of Puberty

Pubertal onset is initiated by reactivation of hypothalamic gonadotropin-releasing hormone (GnRH) secretion (Figure 67-1). The hypothalamic–pituitary–gonadal (HPG) axis is active during fetal development and the first few months of life but is suppressed in infancy by neural input to the arcuate nucleus and remains so throughout childhood (juvenile pause). The transition from a quiescent state toward puberty involves gradually increasing, pulsatile release of GnRH by the hypothalamus, which leads to pituitary release of gonadotropins, first luteinizing hormone (LH) and then follicle-stimulating hormone (FSH). An increased amplitude and frequency of LH pulses during the night are the first detectable hormonal changes at the onset of puberty. Gonadotropins induce gonadal growth and maturation (gonadarche), marked by increasing production of sex steroids, mainly testosterone and estradiol. Apart from the increase in size of the testes, nearly all of the physical changes of puberty result from increasing levels of androgens and estrogens (Table 67-1).

Early androgenic physical changes commonly considered part of puberty in both boys and girls (pubic and axillary hair, body odor, acne) result from gradual mid-childhood maturation of the adrenal glands (adrenarche) and increasing secretion of adrenal androgens (DHEA [dehydroepiandrosterone], DHEA-S [dehydroepiandrosterone sulfate], and androstenedione). Adrenarche overlaps in timing with gonadarche, but the processes are separate and can occur independently.

Normal Pubertal Timing

The timing of the onset of puberty is determined by a variety of genetic factors and environmental influences in addition to gender. The heritability of pubertal timing has been estimated at 50% to 80% based on correlations within ethnic groups and families and between monozygotic twins. Recent genome-wide association studies have identified some of the genetic markers, particularly a height-related gene, LIN28B (6q21), that may affect the timing of menarche.

Much public attention has been paid recently to environmental factors, especially in the context of reports that children are entering puberty at earlier ages. Although several studies suggest that the age of pubertal onset has declined in recent decades, the decline is modest (menarche perhaps 3 months earlier than 30 years ago). Although many environmental factors have been identified as associated with earlier or later puberty, especially in girls, the magnitudes of effects are small and socially charged and can rarely be determined for an individual child. Much of the scientific attention has been directed at increased body mass and at environmental chemicals. Adiposity affects initiation of puberty, especially in girls, with larger body mass associated with earlier puberty and slender build associated with later puberty. Environmental hormones and endocrine-disrupting chemicals, such as polychlorinated biphenyls, organochlorine pesticides, and phthalates, can bind with sex steroid receptors and either mimic or inhibit the hormone effects. No assays for such agents are commercially available in clinical practice.

Although the age of onset may vary, the stages of puberty and their durations tend to be fairly constant (Figure 67-2). The most widely used system for describing the stages of puberty is the modified Tanner system (Figure 67-3), by which girls are assessed using the stage of breast development and pubic hair and boys by genitalia, pubic hair, and testicular volumes. The temptation to describe children with "unitary Tanner stages" should be resisted because it discourages recognition of important discordances that may indicate disease.

Girls tend to begin puberty earlier than boys. The first physical sign of female puberty is usually the appearance of breast buds (thelarche) at a mean age of 10.5 to 11 years. Pubic hair (pubarche) generally follows gonadarche by a few months but may precede it in 10% of girls. Menarche occurs approximately 2 years after thelarche. Pubertal growth acceleration coincides with thelarche for most girls and slows by menarche. Most girls are approaching adult height by 4 years after thelarche and 2 years after menarche.

In boys, the first sign of pubertal development is an increase in testicular volume to 4 mL, which occurs at a mean age of about 11.5 years. As in girls, pubarche usually follows but may precede gonadarche. Pubertal growth in boys accelerates more gradually, becoming noticeable in the second year, and reaches adult height about 6 years from the onset of puberty.

CLINICAL PRESENTATION

Two major clues to pathologic conditions are unusually early or late development and discordant development. Age thresholds for evaluation of early or late puberty are arbitrary and do not cleanly separate all disorders from "normal but unusually early or late" development. Evaluation for precocious puberty is usually recommended when secondary sex characteristics appear before the age of 8 years in girls or 9 years in boys. Evaluation

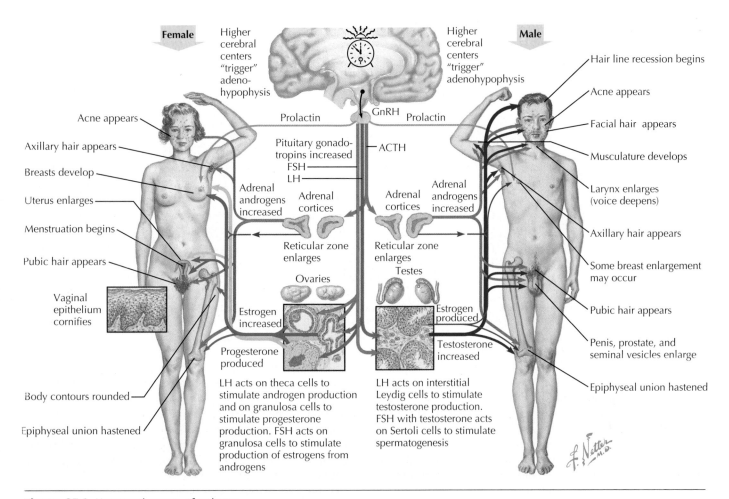

Figure 67-1 *Hormonal events of puberty.*

of a girl for delayed puberty is recommended when breast development has not begun by 13 years of age or when menarche has not occurred by 3 years after thelarche or by age 16 years. Evaluation of a delay in boys is warranted by lack of testicular enlargement by age 14 years.

Table 67-1 Physical Effects of Sex Hormones

Hormone Effect	Androgen Effects	Estrogen Effects
Early	Pubic hair development (stage 2-3) Acne Body odor	Breast development Growth acceleration
Moderate	Full pubic hair development Early axillary hair and facial hair (upper lip) Growth acceleration Penile enlargement	Uterine enlargement Endometrial thickening Vaginal mucosa dulls (pink) Physiologic leukorrhea
Advanced	Voice changes Increased muscle mass Broadening of shoulders Widening of jaw Full facial hair Growth acceleration	Menses Fat redistribution Pelvic widening

Recognition of discordant or interrupted development may suggest a need for evaluation even within the typical ages. Examples of discordance that may indicate specific disorders are stage 3 or 4 pubic hair in girls without breast development (perhaps congenital adrenal hyperplasia [CAH] in a tall 9-year-old girl or Turner's syndrome in a short 11-year-old girl), stage 3 or 4 pubic hair without testicular enlargement in boys (perhaps an LH receptor mutation), and advanced breast development without pubic hair in girls (perhaps androgen insensitivity).

DIFFERENTIAL DIAGNOSIS

Premature Sex Hormone Effects

Traditionally, early sex hormone effects have been classified as central, peripheral, or incomplete (Box 67-1). Central puberty reflects activation of the entire HPG axis, and the physical changes are typically those of normal puberty for a child of that sex. In contrast, peripheral sex hormone sources include adrenal and gonadal disorders, abdominal or pelvic tumors, or exogenous sex steroids. Physical changes reflect the predominant excess hormones (androgenic or estrogenic) and are often markedly discordant from normal pubertal development. *Incomplete puberty* describes early physical changes that do not have a pathologic source but do not progress to full development at the usual tempo.

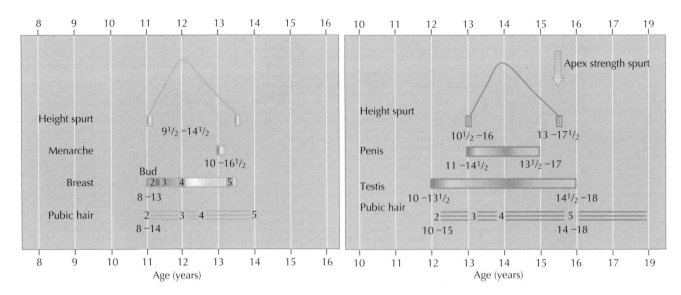

Adapted from Styne DM, Grumbach MM. Puberty: Ontogeny, Neuroendocrinology, Physiology, and Disorders. In Kronenberg H, Melmed S, Polonsky K, Larsen PR. Williams Textbook of Endocrinology, 11th Edition. Saunders, Elsevier, 2007.

Figure 67-2 *Relationship of pubertal milestones.*

Central precocious puberty, especially in girls, may be truly idiopathic and thus physically and hormonally normal in every respect except age of onset or may be attributable to any intracranial disorder that impairs the normal childhood suppression of the hypothalamus, such as central nervous system (CNS) tumors (astrocytomas, gliomas, germinomas); optic glioma; myelomeningocele; congenital anomalies (hamartomas); trauma; and damage from hypoxia, trauma, or radiation. Two rare forms of gonadotropin-dependent precocious central puberty have been described: (1) ectopic human chorionic gonadotropin (hCG) produced by a tumor, usually in the liver, can activate LH receptors in testes and induce what appears to be full puberty, but testicular size is not increased, and (2) prolonged, extreme elevation of thyroid-stimulating hormone (TSH) from primary hypothyroidism may induce precocious puberty through activation of gonadotropin receptors, presumably by partial structural homology.

Peripheral sex hormone effects, sometimes referred to as *precocious pseudopuberty* or *gonadotropin-independent puberty*, are less common and arise from acquired or congenital sex steroid excess by a process other than activation of the HPG axis. Endogenous estrogens may be produced by ovarian cysts or by gonadal or adrenal tumors. Genetic mutations resulting in autonomous activity of FSH receptors or the Gs protein that couples these receptors to activation of adenylyl cyclase can cause the ovaries to produce estrogen any time from infancy to late childhood. Activating mutations of Gs are typically associated with the clinical triad of McCune Albright syndrome (autonomous endocrine hyperfunction, fibrous dysplasia, and café au lait skin lesions) but may also occur in isolated ovarian cysts or testicular adenomas. Mutations that amplify aromatase activity can produce gynecomastia in males by increasing the fraction of testosterone converted to estradiol. CAH is the most common pathologic form of androgen excess in children of either sex. Most cases of CAH are caused by 21-hydroxylase deficiency and can be identified by elevated serum levels of

17-hydroxyprogesterone (see Chapter 70). Familial male-limited precocious puberty ("testotoxicosis") results from activating mutations of the LH receptor that cause constitutive Leydig cell hyperfunction and excessive testosterone production. Exogenous sources of estrogens or androgens should be sought but are rare. Examples include estrogen cream applied for labial adhesions or contact with a father's testosterone gel.

Incomplete or unsustained pubertal development is common, most often as isolated premature thelarche or adrenarche. Girls with premature thelarche typically display breast development during the first 2 years of life or after 6 years of age. Isolated premature thelarche is not accompanied by pubertal hormone levels, menarche, androgen effects, growth acceleration, advanced bone age, or compromised adult height. In older girls, premature thelarche can be an early stage of HPG axis maturation that only slowly progresses to central puberty. Isolated premature adrenarche is likewise not associated with progressive pubertal development. Children with premature adrenarche have signs of adrenal androgen production (pubic hair, acne, body odor) that progress slowly and do not accelerate growth or bone maturation. Premature adrenarche in girls may be associated with low birth weight (small for gestational age) with rapid catch-up growth and is a risk factor for later development of polycystic ovary syndrome and metabolic syndrome in adolescence.

Delayed Puberty (Box 67-2)

In most children, delayed puberty is constitutional (i.e., not a disease); in other cases, delayed puberty is related to a disorder of the HPG axis, systemic disease, or undernutrition. Constitutional delay of growth and puberty (CDGP) accounts for approximately 60% of cases of delayed puberty in boys and 30% in girls (see Chapter 73). A typical teenager with CDGP is a 14- or 15-year-old boy who presents after most of his peers have begun puberty and after several years of very slow growth. A

Breast development

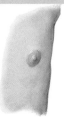
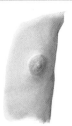
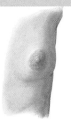
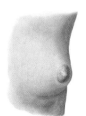
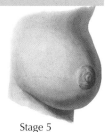

Stage 1
Elevation of papilla only

Stage 2
Breast bud: elevation of breast and papilla as a small mound and enlargement of areolar diameter

Stage 3
Additional enlargement of breast and areola with no separation of their contours

Stage 4
Areola and papilla project from surface of breast to form secondary mound

Stage 5
Mature stage with projection of papilla only with recession of the areola to the general contour of the breast

Female pubic hair development

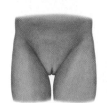
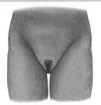
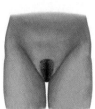
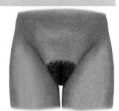

Stage 1
The vellus over the pubes is the same as that over the anterior abdominal wall

Stage 2
Sparse slightly pigmented, downy hair along the labia that is straight or only slightly curled

Stage 3
Hair spreads sparsely over the pubic region and is darker, coaser and curlier

Stage 4
Hair is adult type, but the area covered is smaller than in most adults, and there is no spread to the medial surface of the thighs

Stage 5
Hair is adult in quantity and type, distributed as an inverse triangle and spreads to the medial surface of the thighs but not up the midline anterior abdominal wall

F. Netter M.D. C. Machado M.D. K. Marzin

Male pubic hair and genital development

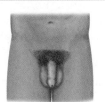
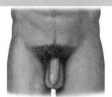

Stage 1
Penis, testes, and scrotum are the same size and proportion as in early childhood

The vellus hair over the pubic region is the same as that on the abdominal wall

Stage 2
Testes and scrotum enlarge and scrotal skin shows a change in texture and reddening

Sparse growth of straight or slightly curled pigmented hair appearing at the base of the penis

Stage 3
Penile growth in length more than width; further growth of the testes and scrotum

Hair is coarser, curlier, and darker; spread sparsely over the junction of the pubes

Stage 4
Further penile growth and development of the glans; further enlargement of testes and scrotum

Adult type hair, but area covered less than in most adults; no spread to the medial surface of the thighs

Stage 5
Genitalia are adult in size and shape

Adult in quantity and type of hair, distributed as an inverse triangle; spread is to the medial surface of the thighs

Figure 67-3 *Tanner staging system.*

family history of delayed puberty is often present. Male predominance of diagnosed CDGP partly reflects the greater psychosocial distress that teenage boys experience from shortness and sexual immaturity. Children with CDGP have hormone levels consistent with their stage of maturation and bone age, which reflects the degree of delay. They eventually undergo spontaneous pubertal development and usually achieve the target height predicted by midparental percentile.

Clues that delay may not be constitutional include prolonged delay, discordant development (e.g., pubic hair without breast development), recent growth failure, signs of undernutrition or systemic disease, or problems associated with pituitary or olfactory bulb (e.g., hyposmia) development. A practical approach to pathologic delay is based on identifying the site of the defect: systemic or nutritional, hypothalamic, pituitary, gonadal, or uterine or vaginal (see Box 67-2). Gonadotropins are among the most useful initial laboratory tests because sex steroid levels are apparent by body evidence, and current assays are poor at distinguishing early pubertal from prepubertal levels.

Systemic disease and undernutrition may either delay the onset of puberty or interrupt the progression. Most such conditions will be obvious, but inflammatory bowel disease, eating

---

Box 67-1 Differential Diagnosis of Precocious Puberty

Central precocious puberty
- Idiopathic (most frequent cause)
- Structural: tumors (optic glioma, astrocytoma, craniopharyngioma, neuroblastoma); congenital anomalies (hypothalamic hamartoma, hydrocephalus)
- Inflammatory or scarring: trauma, postsurgical, postirradiation, postchemotherapy, infection, abscess, infiltrative process
- Syndromes: Williams, Prader-Willi, neurofibromatosis type I, tuberous sclerosis
- Mimickers: hypothyroidism, hCG-secreting tumors (liver)
- Adoption from underdeveloped to developed region

Peripheral sex hormone effects
- Ovarian follicular cysts
- McCune-Albright syndrome
- Congenital adrenal hyperplasia
- Aromatase excess
- Male-limited precocious puberty (testotoxicosis)
- Tumors: gonadal, adrenal
- Exogenous sex steroids (estrogen creams, testosterone gels)

Incomplete pubertal development
- Premature thelarche
- Premature adrenarche
- Premature menarche

hCG, human chorionic gonadotropin.

Box 67-2 Differential Diagnosis of Delayed Puberty

Function Delay
- Constitutional delay of growth and puberty
- Systemic disease (inflammatory bowel disease, cystic fibrosis, eating disorders, chronic renal disease, AIDS, sickle cell disease, chronic lung disease, asthma)
- Excessive exercise
- Malnutrition
- Endocrinopathies (hypothyroidism, hyperprolactinemia, growth hormone deficiency, Cushing's syndrome, poorly controlled diabetes mellitus)

Hypothalamic or Pituitary

Primary
- Anatomic (septo-optic dysplasia, midline defects)
- Isolated gonadotropin deficiency (Kallman's syndrome)
- Multiple pituitary hormone deficiency (e.g., HESX1, LHX3, PROP1)
- Multisystem syndromes (e.g., Prader-Willi, Bardet-Biedl, CHARGE)

Secondary
- CNS tumors or infiltrative disease (craniopharyngioma, germinoma, gliomas, prolactinomas, astrocytomas, Langerhans cell histiocytosis), posttrauma, postradiation, post-CNS infection, hypophysitis

Gonadal
- Genetic: Turner's syndrome (girls), Klinefelter's syndrome (boys), gonadal dysgenesis
- Acquired: iatrogenic (radiation, chemotherapy, surgery), bilateral torsion, infection, autoimmune

Uterine or vaginal
- Anatomic defects (e.g., imperforate hymen, mullerian agenesis)
- Androgen insensitivity
- Biosynthetic defects (e.g., 5-α-reductase deficiency)

AIDS, acquired immune deficiency syndrome; CHARGE, coloboma of the eye, heart defects, atresia of the nasal choanae, retardation of growth or development, genital or urinary abnormalities, and ear abnormalities and deafness; CNS, central nervous system.

---

disorders, and endocrinopathies may be discovered during evaluation of pubertal delay. Gonadotropin levels in systemic disease may be low or pubertal.

Gonadotropin deficiency is often difficult to distinguish from constitutional delay in the absence of clues such as hyposmia or syndrome features. Permanent hypogonadotropic hypogonadism (HHG) can be congenital (primary) or acquired (secondary). One of the most common genetic forms of HHG in apparently healthy people is Kallmann's syndrome, in which isolated gonadotropin deficiency is associated with hyposmia. Most cases result from mutations of the KAL1 gene (located at Xp22.3) that encodes a protein, anosmin-1, necessary for early fetal migration of GnRH and olfactory neurons. Although classically X-linked, autosomal forms have also been identified that are associated with the KAL2 gene encoding FGFR1. Isolated gonadotropin deficiencies, possibly in combination with other pituitary hormone deficiencies, can also be caused by transcription factor gene mutations (PROP1, LHX3, and HESX1). Primary HHG can be associated with birth defects of the hypothalamus or pituitary (e.g., septo-optic dysplasia) or can be one of the features of multisystem syndromes such as Prader-Willi and Bardet-Biedl syndromes. Secondary causes of HHG include conditions that damage the hypothalamus or pituitary, such as tumors, trauma, or radiation. Tumors often associated with HHG include craniopharyngiomas, astrocytomas, gliomas, Langerhans cell histiocytosis, germinomas, and prolactinomas. When HHG is caused by congenital or acquired defects of the pituitary, other hormone deficiencies may be present, producing growth failure, polydipsia, or galactorrhea.

Primary hypogonadism (gonadal failure caused by defects of the gonads themselves) is easily confirmed by marked elevation of the gonadotropins (hypergonadotropic hypogonadism). Primary hypogonadism may be congenital or acquired and partial or complete. The most common congenital forms of primary hypogonadism result from abnormal numbers of sex chromosomes. Turner's syndrome occurs in about one in 2000 girls and Klinefelter's syndrome in about one in 500 to 1000 boys. These syndromes may often be difficult to recognize. Turner's syndrome should be suspected in short girls with pubarche but no thelarche. Girls lacking an X chromosome may have the full features of Turner's syndrome or may only display growth failure and lack of puberty. Gonadal dysgenesis caused by 45,X mosaicism or by a partially missing X chromosome, such as a deletion of Xq, is especially unlikely to be accompanied by the other features of Turner's syndrome. Pubertal development may be partial, even including some breast development. Most boys with Klinefelter's syndrome (47,XXY) have relatively normal pubertal development except for small, firm testes. Tall stature and social or academic problems are common. Sertoli cell function and spermatogenesis tend to be more deficient than testosterone effects in adolescence. Permanent bilateral gonadal failure can also be acquired and attributable to iatrogenic causes (radiation, chemotherapy, and surgery), bilateral torsion, and infectious or autoimmune processes.

EVALUATION AND MANAGEMENT

Precocious Puberty

The evaluation of a child with precocious sex hormone effects should include a history of duration, family timing, familial hyperandrogenic disorders, possible exposures to exogenous sex steroids, and growth pattern. Acceleration of growth within the past year may be strong evidence of central puberty. The physical examination should compile an inventory of androgen and estrogen effects; assessment of testicular size; and assessment of possible masses in the abdomen, pelvis, or testes; and the presence of neurocutaneous stigmata, CNS disease, high blood pressure, and Cushingoid features.

A bone age radiograph may help indicate whether sex hormone effects are systemic and suggests the possible duration of elevation. Blood tests should be chosen according to the features present. For predominantly androgen effects, the most useful initial tests include total testosterone, DHEA-S, 17-hydroxyprogesterone, and LH, but all should be measured using high-sensitivity assays that are designed for pediatric patients. Additional hormone measurements do not exclude any other conditions and often give false-positive results. For solely estrogen effects, the most useful screens include LH, FSH, and estradiol for girls and LH, FSH, hCG, and estradiol for boys. Abdominal or pelvic ultrasound may be useful if any of the steroid levels are elevated. When physical development is simply normal and concordant for the child's sex (e.g., breasts, pubic hair, and growth acceleration for girls; pubic hair, penile growth, and testicular enlargement for boys), the most useful tests are simply LH and FSH to document central puberty. Depending on age and the presence of clues to CNS abnormalities, the principal imaging decision is whether the probability of an intracranial abnormality is high enough to warrant cranial magnetic resonance imaging (MRI). In the absence of specific clues to CNS disease, the probability of an intracranial abnormality depends primarily on the age of onset of puberty and the sex of the child. An MRI abnormality is found in far fewer than 1% of girls with an onset of breast development after 7 years but is found in a far higher percentage of boys until onset exceeds 10 years of age.

Central precocious puberty can be suppressed with one of several GnRH analogs, most often monthly leuprolide injections or annual histrelin implants. Potential benefits of therapy are prevention of psychosocial distress and enhancement of remaining growth. However, the growth benefit is small in children older than the age of 6 years, and not all children need or will benefit from therapy. Treatment of peripheral sex hormone sources depends on the nature of the underlying disorder and can include adrenal suppression with glucocorticoids, surgical removal of tumors, or other measures to limit sex steroid secretion or block the effects. Incomplete forms of sexual precocity require no therapy but rather close monitoring to ensure lack of progression.

Delayed Puberty

Because of the variety of systemic conditions that may interfere with puberty, evaluation of children with delayed puberty requires a comprehensive history and examination. Inflammatory bowel disease and eating disorders are common causes of pubertal delay; thus, specific attention should be paid to abdominal symptoms and body attitudes. A prolonged period of markedly poor growth increases the likelihood of a systemic cause or intracranial pathology, as does bone age radiography that is consistent with chronological age. Screening laboratory tests should include a blood count, erythrocyte sedimentation rate, and general chemistries. Thyroid function tests, IGF-1, and IGF-BP3 are warranted if growth has been poor. Gonadotropins are usually prepubertal (i.e., low) in constitutional delay and HHG. They may be low or pubertal in systemic illness. However, a clear elevation of gonadotropins is a clear indicator of a primary gonadal defect, and a karyotype often confirms one of the forms of gonadal dysgenesis. The most difficult diagnostic distinction is between CDGP and HHG. No blood test reliably separates the two, and in the absence of a demonstrated gene abnormality, only increasing age, advancing bone age, and lack of response to brief courses of exogenous testosterone or estrogen shift the probability toward gonadotropin deficiency.

Treatment options depend on the underlying etiology. Suspected CGDP may be watched with reassurance. Alternatively, 4 to 6 months of low-dose testosterone or estrogen can relieve some of the social stress of delay by inducing the early physical changes of puberty. It may also hasten the onset of endogenous puberty. When endogenous puberty has not begun after two courses of low-dose supplementation, the likelihood of HHG is high, and more continual treatment at replacement doses can be resumed. When elevated gonadotropins indicate primary hypogonadism, replacement testosterone or estrogen can be provided continuously. The dose is gradually increased over several years to adult amounts. Progestin needs to be provided after 2 to 3 years of estrogen; an oral contraceptive is often used for the combination. If a chronic disease is identified, treatment of that process should be undertaken to allow spontaneous puberty to proceed.

SUGGESTED READINGS

Nathan BM, Palmert MR: Regulation and disorders of pubertal timing, *Endocrinol Metab Clin North Am* 34:617-641, 2005.

Ong KK, Elks CE, Li S, et al: Genetic variation in *LIN28B* is associated with the timing of puberty, *Nat Genet* 41:729-733, 2009.

Pescovitz OH, Walvoord EC: *When Puberty Is Precocious: Scientific and Clinical Aspects,* ed 1, Totowa, NJ, 2007, Humana Press.

Steinraber S: *The Falling Age of Puberty in U.S. Girls: What We Know, What We Need to Know,* ed 1, San Francisco, 2007, Breast Cancer Fund.

Tanner JM, Davies PS: Clinical longitudinal standards for height and height velocity for North American children, *J Pediatr* 107(3):317-329, 1985.

Thyroid Disease

68

Sara E. Pinney, Vaneeta Bamba, and Craig A. Alter

The follicular cells of the thyroid gland produce triiodothyronine (T3) and thyroxine (T4), thyroid hormones that have important roles in growth and development, as well as influential effects on metabolism, the central nervous system (CNS), and the cardiovascular system. This chapter reviews thyroid physiology, as well as the most common childhood thyroid disorders.

THYROID HORMONE PRODUCTION

Thyroid hormones are produced by the coupling of iodine molecules to the amino acid tyrosine (Figure 68-1). The principal secreted thyroid hormone is T4. The normal thyroid secretes only small amounts of T3, and most circulating T3 (≈70%-90%) is derived from peripheral deiodination of T4. Thyroid hormones circulate bound to carrier proteins, including thyroid-binding globulin (TBG), transthyretin (thyroxine-binding prealbumin), and albumin. Less than 1% of circulating T4 and T3 are unbound or "free."

Hypothalamic thyrotropin-releasing hormone (TRH) stimulates thyrotrope cells in the anterior pituitary to release thyroid-stimulating hormone (TSH), which stimulates production and release of thyroid hormone. When T4 levels are inadequate, a negative feedback loop activates the hypothalamic–pituitary axis and results in increased secretion of TSH, which then acts on the thyroid gland to stimulate increased hormone synthesis. When circulating levels of T4 and T3 are high, as in Graves' disease or overtreatment with exogenous T4, this negative feedback loop acts to reduce or suppress TSH secretion. Circulating levels of T4 are also influenced by peripheral conversion to either T3 or reverse T3 (rT3), an inactive form of thyroid hormone.

Circulating T4 and T3 enter cells by diffusion and carrier-mediated transport processes; inside the cell, T4 is then converted to T3. T3 is the most active thyroid hormone because it binds thyroid hormone receptors with approximately 10 times the affinity of T4. The T3–receptor complex is transported to the nucleus and regulates transcription of a variety of genes, ultimately leading to the synthesis of proteins that manifest thyroid hormone action in peripheral tissues. T4 is necessary for normal growth and development and is absolutely critical for brain development in utero as well as during the first 2 years of life.

CONGENITAL HYPOTHYROIDISM

Etiology and Pathogenesis

Congenital hypothyroidism (CH) is one of the most common causes of preventable mental retardation (Figure 68-2). Fortunately, early identification and rapid treatment lead to normal neurocognitive development. Although approximately 10% of cases of CH are transient and caused by factors such as iodine

exposure, prematurity, or maternal transfer of antithyroid antibodies, in most cases, hypothyroidism is permanent. Worldwide, iodine deficiency is the most common cause of CH. However, in areas of the world where iodine deficiency is uncommon, CH most commonly results from thyroid dysgenesis (≈75% of cases); thyroid dyshormonogenesis (≈10%), TSH deficiency (5%), and genetic defects in the TSH receptor are much less common. The incidence of CH is approximately one in 3000 to 4000 births. In most cases, CH is sporadic, but mutations in genes encoding transcription factors that are required for normal development of the thyroid gland are present in about 10% to 15% of cases. Circulating levels of TSH are elevated and thyroid hormone levels are low in those with CH.

A clinical picture that is similar to CH can occur in children who have genetic defects in the thyroid hormone receptor or in the MCT8 protein required to transport thyroid hormone into cells. Unlike CH, however, these patients have elevated serum levels of both TSH and thyroid hormones.

Clinical Presentation

Although there may be few obvious symptoms of CH in the first few weeks of life, a prolonged period of hypothyroidism during infancy can have profound neurocognitive consequences. Therefore, newborn screening (NBS) programs have been established in many countries to identify newborns with CH who require prompt treatment. Infants with untreated CH have an enlarged posterior fontanelle, prolonged jaundice, macroglossia, hoarse cry, distended abdomen, umbilical hernia, hypotonia, poor growth, weight gain, pericardial edema, or delayed development.

Long-term studies in adults with a history of CH indicate that when treatment is initiated before 2 months of age, there are only minor differences in intelligence, school achievement, and performance on neuropsychologic tests by comparison with control groups of classmates and siblings. Residual deficits in these patients may include visuospatial processing, selective memory, and sensorimotor defects. The prognosis for mental and neurologic performance in children with CH identified after 2 months of age is uncertain. Infants with CH who were not identified by the NBS but whose treatment was initiated between 2 and 3 months of age may manifest nonspecific developmental delays, including impaired arithmetic ability, speech, or fine motor coordination later in life. Long-term untreated CH can result in severe mental retardation and impaired growth.

Evaluation (Figure 68-3)

NBS for CH is based on collection of a blood sample from the newborn between 48 hours and 4 days of life. Earlier measurement may lead to erroneous results because of the normal physiologic surge in TSH that occurs soon after birth. NBS programs use blood spots collected on filter paper and use one of two

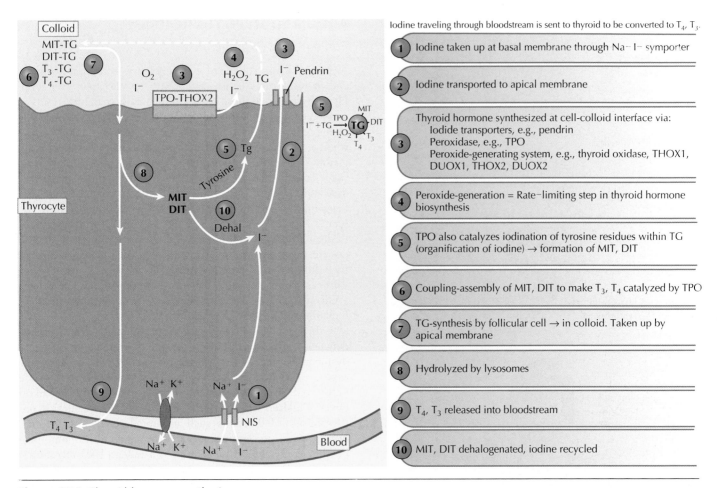

Figure 68-1 *Thyroid hormone synthesis.*

strategies to identify infants with CH: a primary TSH with backup T4 or a primary T4 with a backup TSH method. An abnormal result should be further evaluated immediately using serum-based assays for TSH and T4 or free T4. Premature or ill infants may have false-negative or false-positive results and should be retested by 7 days of age. Any infant with a TSH level above 40 mU/L with low T4 is considered to have primary hypothyroidism. In addition to T4 and TSH measurements, a thyroglobulin (TG) level may be helpful because elevation suggests dyshormonogenesis.

When there is history of maternal autoimmune thyroid disease, measurement of TSH–receptor binding antibodies in the infant or the mother may identify transient CH. Other diagnostic tests include thyroid ultrasonography and technetium or iodine (I-123) scans to identify functional thyroid tissue, as well as the perchlorate washout test to detect iodine organification defects that might indicate Pendred's syndrome. Treatment with levothyroxine (L-T4) should not be delayed to perform imaging.

Treatment

To avoid neurocognitive deficit, newborns with CH must be treated promptly with L-T4 and monitored closely by a pediatric endocrinologist. L-T4 is instituted at a dosage of 10 to 17 µg/kg/d initially, with a goal to normalize the serum T4 level within 2 weeks (fT4 >2 ng/dL) and serum TSH by 1 month of age. There are no suitable liquid preparations of L-T4, so tablets must be used. Tablets should be crushed and mixed with a few milliliters of formula, breast milk, or water. Soy-based formula, fiber, or iron may reduce absorption of L-T4 and should be given separately.

Serum levels of T4, T4 index or free T4, and TSH should be measured every 1 to 2 months during the first 6 months of life, every 3 to 4 months until 3 years of age, and then every 6 to 12 months until growth is complete. The half-life of T4 in the circulation is 1 week, so levels of TSH and T4 should be repeated 4 to 5 weeks after dose changes to ensure appropriate steady-state levels. An appropriately treated child will have serum T4 levels that are at or above the upper limit of normal with a serum TSH level of 1 to 2 mU/mL. The serum TSH level is not a reliable indicator of euthyroidism in children with pituitary or hypothalamic disorders, and in these patients, the T4 level should be maintained at the upper limit of the assay's normal range. Infants with suspected transient hypothyroidism should continue L-T4 therapy until at least age 2 years, when thyroid-dependent CNS myelinization is complete.

CONGENITAL HYPERTHYROIDISM

Neonatal hyperthyroidism is rare (one in 25,000), and most cases are caused by transplacental passage of maternal TSH-receptor stimulating immunoglobulins (TSIs). Although in

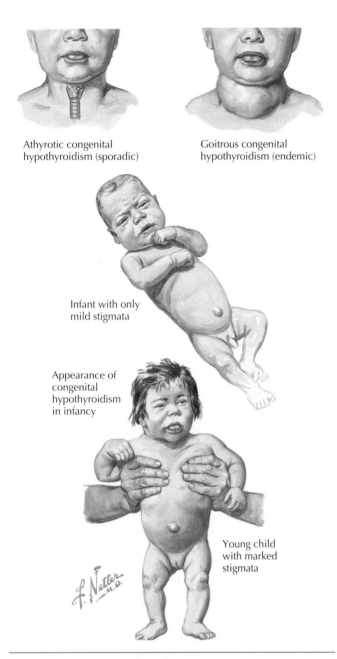

Athyrotic congenital
hypothyroidism (sporadic)

Goitrous congenital
hypothyroidism (endemic)

Infant with only
mild stigmata

Appearance of
congenital
hypothyroidism
in infancy

Young child
with marked
stigmata

Figure 68-2 *Congenital hypothyroidism.*

most cases the diagnosis of Graves' disease will be known during the pregnancy, in some cases, the mother may have only a remote history of treated Graves' disease. The fetus may develop a goiter and tachycardia, but clinical signs of thyrotoxicosis may be delayed if the mother is taking antithyroid medication. Symptoms of neonatal thyrotoxicosis include goiter, irritability, proptosis, tachycardia, hepatosplenomegaly, jaundice, and cardiac failure. Neonatal Graves' disease resolves spontaneously as maternal TSIs are degraded between 3 and 12 weeks of age. Treatment with methimazole is required until the maternal immunoglobulins are no longer present, and infants must be closely monitored to ensure normal levels of T4 and T3. In some cases, the presence of fetal hyperthyroidism leads to a permanent defect in TSH secretion with a consequent risk of hypothyroidism after maternal TSI has disappeared.

ACQUIRED HYPOTHYROIDISM

Etiology and Pathogenesis

Hypothyroidism is defined as a deficiency in thyroid hormone and in most cases is associated with an elevated TSH level. Hypothyroidism is more common in females than males and has an increased incidence in adolescents. The most common cause of hypothyroidism is chronic lymphocytic (Hashimoto's) thyroiditis, which results in autoimmune destruction of the thyroid gland. Goiter, caused by lymphocytic infiltration of thyroid tissue, and circulating antithyroid antibodies (antitissue peroxidase and anti-TG) are common but are not universally present. Hashimoto's thyroiditis is common in children who have the type 2 autoimmune polyglandular syndrome, which includes Addison's disease of the adrenal gland, pernicious anemia, celiac disease, type 1 diabetes mellitus, and juvenile rheumatoid arthritis. Children with chromosomal defects, such as trisomy 21, Turner's syndrome, 22q11 deletion syndrome, and Klinefelter's syndrome, have an increased incidence of autoimmune diseases, including autoimmune thyroid disease.

Other causes of hypothyroidism include chronic iodine deficiency, excessive iodine exposure, hypothalamic–pituitary dysfunction, acute infection, and medications. Excessive iodine exposure may lead to acute blockage of thyroid hormone release or thyroid hormone synthesis, known as the Wolff-Chaikoff effect. Children with CNS disease are at risk of central hypothyroidism. Medications such as amiodarone, antiepileptics, nitroprusside, and lithium can all affect thyroid hormone production or metabolism; dopamine can reduce TSH secretion.

Clinical Presentation (Figure 68-4)

Symptoms of hypothyroidism include dry skin, constipation, cold intolerance, and a decreased energy level. Severe thyroxine deficiency is associated with linear growth failure and delayed bone age, coarse hair, myxedema, galactorrhea, delayed or rarely precocious puberty, bradycardia, depressed reflexes, pallor, and hyperlipidemia. Carotenemia is more common in children than adults with hypothyroidism. Children with weight gain are often referred for evaluation of hypothyroidism. Although weight gain can occur in children with hypothyroidism, height is reduced, which is in contrast to exogenous obesity, in which height is often increased. On examination, the thyroid gland may be enlarged, asymmetric, and/or bosselated. In severe hypothyroidism, the gland may be atrophic. Reflexes are often slowed, the heart rate may be reduced, and the pulse pressure can be decreased. There is a family history of thyroid disease in 30% to 40% of patients.

Occasionally, patients with Hashimoto's thyroiditis present with elevations in T4 levels and suppressed TSH, mimicking Graves' disease, but without the eye symptoms. This is termed *Hashitoxicosis*, and it may occur because of excessive release of thyroid hormone from thyroid destruction. Patients with Hashimoto's thyroiditis can have TG antibodies or blocking TSH-receptor antibodies, both of which are known to destroy thyroid cells. TG antibodies are seen in Hashimoto's thyroiditis, and blocking TSH-receptor antibodies are seen in patients with atrophic thyroiditis. In addition, patients typically have thyroid peroxidase (TPO) antibodies, which are considered markers of inflammation. TPO antibodies also cause thyroid inflammation

Approach to a Newborn with Congenital Hypothyroidism

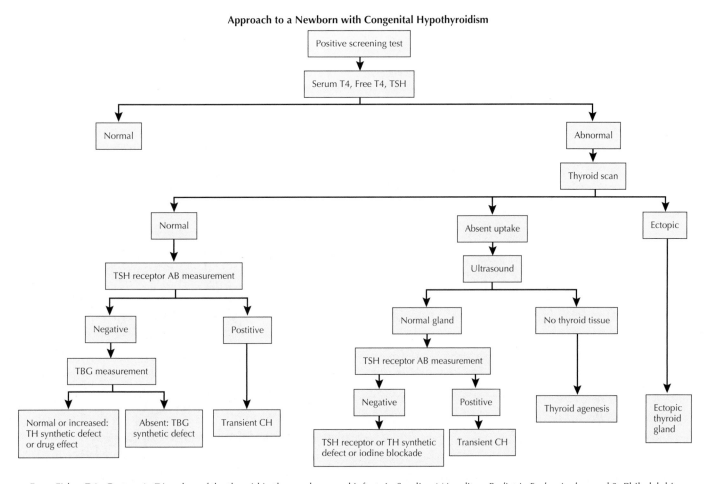

From Fisher DA, Gruters A: Disorders of the thyroid in the newborn and infant. In Sperling MA, editor: *Pediatric Endocrinology*, ed 3, Philadelphia, 2008, Sauders pp 198-226.

Figure 68-3 *Evaluation of congenital hypothyroidism.* AB, antibody; CH, congenital hypothyroidism; TBG, thyroid-binding globulin; TH, thyroid hormone; TSH, thyroid-stimulating hormone.

and thyroid disease to persist, interfering with the healing process. Patients with Hashitoxicosis can also have stimulating TSH-receptor antibodies, although their levels may not reach the high levels that cause hyperthyroidism in patients with Graves' disease.

In some ways, these patients can be described as having both Hashimoto's thyroiditis and Graves' disease because the antibodies associated with both diseases are often present. Thyroid uptake scans can differentiate between Hashitoxicosis with decreased uptake and true Graves' disease with increased uptake.

Evaluation

Typically, patients with hypothyroidism present with elevated TSH, low T4, and elevated TPO or TG antibodies. In the euthyroid state, TSH, T4, and T3 levels are in equilibrium. Decreased thyroid hormone production in hypothyroidism leads to negative feedback on the pituitary, with a concomitant increase in TSH levels. If the gland is unable to respond with an increase in T4 production, the TSH continues to increase, and there will be very low levels of T4, fT4, and T3.

Children with suspected hypothalamic or pituitary abnormalities should have yearly assessment of pituitary function,

including thyroid tests (T4, fT4, or both). Affected children have low fT4 levels; low-normal T4 levels; and normal, low, or mildly elevated TSH levels. In the case of central hypothyroidism, fT4 levels are monitored instead of TSH.

Children with slight elevations in TSH (<10 mIU/L) and normal T4 or fT4 levels, with or without antibodies, are considered to have subclinical hypothyroidism. In this scenario, treatment may be delayed unless the child has symptoms of hypothyroidism, a goiter, or increasing levels of TSH.

Treatment

Children with confirmed hypothyroidism should be treated with daily L-T4 with a therapeutic target of normalizing serum levels of T4 (or fT4) and achieving a TSH level of 1 to 2 mIU/L. When there is evidence of longstanding hypothyroidism, L-T4 may be started at a low dose and slowly increased to full replacement over several weeks. Serum levels of L-T4 and TSH should be measured 4 to 6 weeks after initiation of therapy or change of L-T4 dosage to ensure that the expected steady-state levels are achieved. In general, T4 and TSH levels should be tracked every 3 to 6 months as part of routine monitoring.

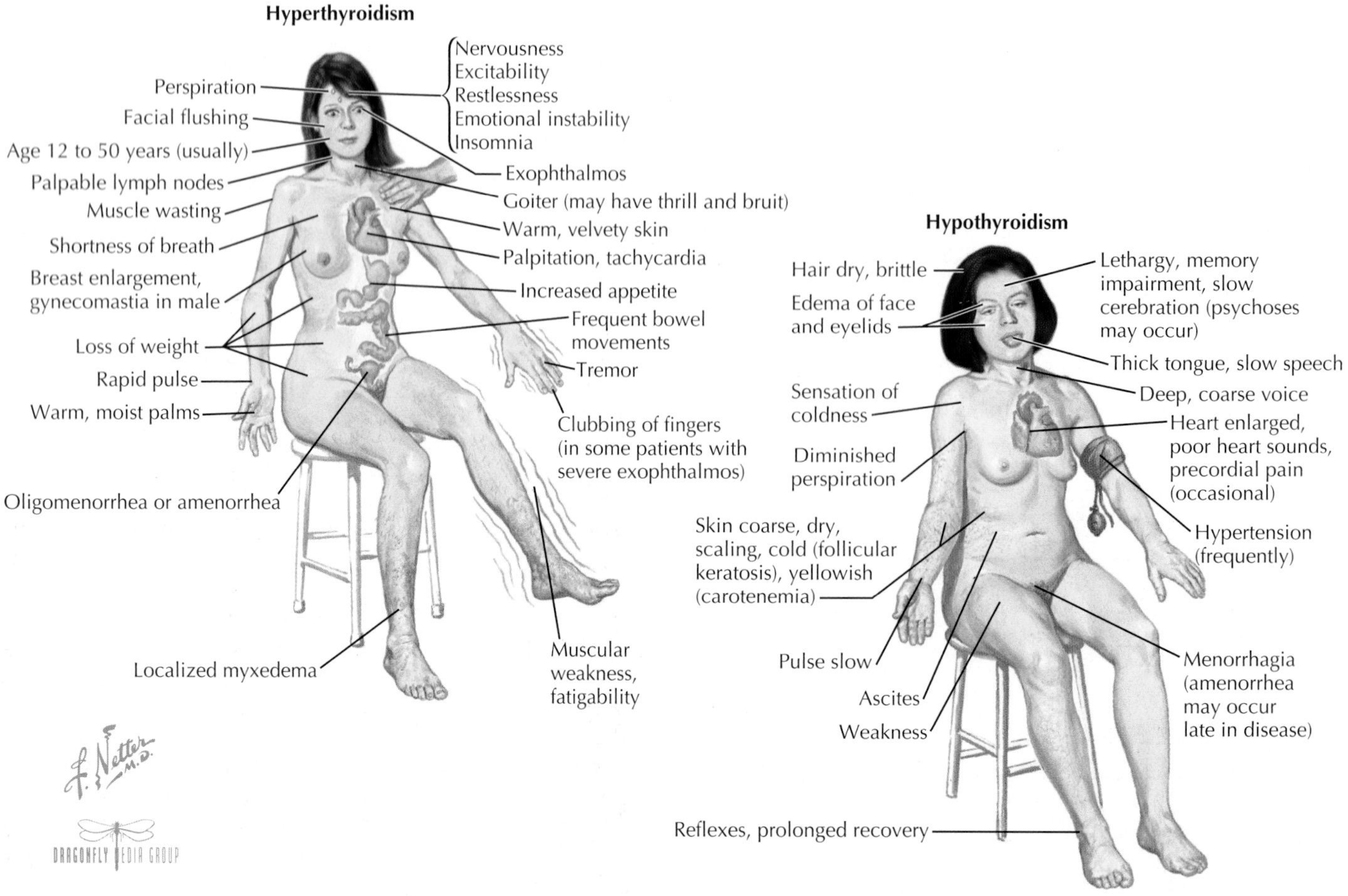

Figure 68-4 *Clinical features of hypothyroidism and hyperthyroidism.*

When used appropriately, L-T4 is a very safe medication, and the principal adverse effects are caused by overtreatment or undertreatment. In treatment of severe hypothyroidism, bone age may advance rapidly, which can impair ultimate height.

ACQUIRED HYPERTHYROIDISM

Etiology and Pathogenesis (Box 68-1)

Graves' disease accounts for over 90% of hyperthyroidism in children. Other less common etiologies include a hyperfunctioning toxic ("hot") nodule, transient hyperthyroidism as an early phase of chronic lymphocytic thyroiditis (Hashitoxicosis), and the hyperthyroid phase of subacute thyroiditis. Amiodarone, which contains 37% iodine by weight, causes hyperthyroidism

Box 68-1 Etiology of Hyperthyroidism
Graves' disease
Hashitoxicosis
Subacute or De Quervain's thyroiditis
Toxic adenoma
Thyroid cancer
Iodine-induced hyperthyroidism
TSH-producing pituitary adenoma
Thyrotoxicosis factitia (surreptitious levothyroxine)

TSH, thyroid-stimulating hormone.

in up to 12% of patients on long-term therapy. It has been suggested that amiodarone-induced myxedema predominates in areas in which the soil is iodide replete and that thyrotoxicosis occurs in areas of iodide deficiency.

Clinical Presentation (see Figure 68-4)

Children with hyperthyroidism often have hyperactivity with periods of fatigue and poor sleeping habits. Emotional lability, poor concentration, and a marked decrease in school performance are common. Children often come to medical attention because of cardiovascular complaints such as persistent tachycardia, palpitations, or syncopal episodes. Heat intolerance, weight loss, tremors, and diaphoresis are seen regularly. Although many children with hyperthyroidism indeed lose weight, paradoxical weight gain is common. Hyperthyroidism will also result in an increased appetite, and in some patients, an increased appetite and increased food intake may lead to weight gain despite the increase in metabolic rate that usually accompanies hyperthyroidism.

The eyes may reveal a "lid lag" or prominent eyes, with or without proptosis (exophthalmos) in which the eyes are pushed forward (may be asymmetric). In Graves' disease, the more severely hyperthyroid patients have the largest goiters (Figure 68-5). Mild polyuria may be seen. Frequent bowel movements, rather than diarrhea, are occasionally present.

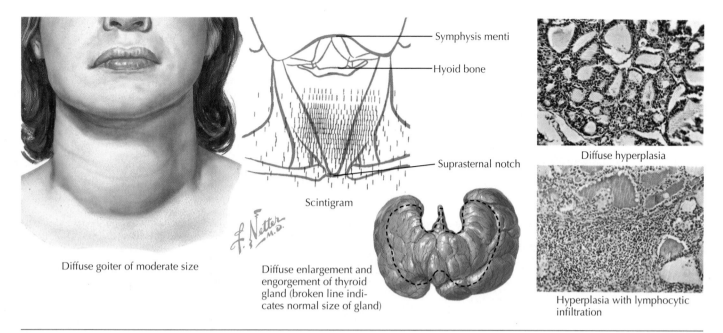

Diffuse goiter of moderate size

Symphysis menti

Hyoid bone

Suprasternal notch

Scintigram

Diffuse enlargement and engorgement of thyroid gland (broken line indicates normal size of gland)

Diffuse hyperplasia

Hyperplasia with lymphocytic infiltration

Figure 68-5 *Thyroid pathology in Graves' disease.*

Heart rate and blood pressure may be elevated with a widened pulse pressure. The degree of tachycardia parallels the severity of the hyperthyroidism. There may be normal to accelerated linear growth with concomitant weight loss. The skin is warm to the touch. The thyroid is smooth and diffusely enlarged, and there may be a palpable thrill or audible bruit caused by increased blood flow. Tremors and generalized restlessness are common. A change in mentation associated with hypertension and cardiovascular instability could indicate thyroid storm, which requires urgent hospitalization.

Subacute, or De Quervain's, thyroiditis is thought to be viral in origin and lasts weeks to months. In the first few months, hyperthyroidism may be seen because of leakage of thyroid hormone in a damaged gland. In time, hypothyroidism commonly develops.

Evaluation

After the diagnosis of hyperthyroidism has been established, it is important to establish the cause. Laboratory assessment of patients with hyperthyroidism should include measurement of total or free T4, T3, and TSH. In hyperthyroidism, TSH should be suppressed (<0.3 mIU/L on most assays). Because of intense stimulation of the gland by TSI, patients with Graves' disease typically have a disproportionately greater increase in T3 compared with T4. The degree of hyperthyroidism is related to the degree of elevation of fT4 and T3.

Thyroid TPO and TG antibodies can be present in both Graves' disease and chronic lymphocytic thyroiditis. Measuring TSI can be helpful when the diagnosis of Graves' disease is uncertain in a child with hyperthyroidism. An I-123 scan will show diffusely high uptake of iodine in patients with Graves' disease (see Figure 68-5) and patchy areas of uptake in those with chronic lymphocytic thyroiditis. The thyroid gland is hypervascular in Graves' disease, and this increased blood flow can be assessed by color-flow Doppler ultrasonography.

Treatment

Treatment of children with hyperthyroidism should be made in collaboration with a pediatric endocrinologist. Families should be informed of three treatment modalities: medication, radioactive iodine (I-131) ablation, and surgery. Most endocrinologists believe that initial treatment with antithyroid medication is indicated, especially because approximately 20% of children may go into a remission within 2 years of starting pharmacologic therapy.

The two antithyroid medications that are available in the United States are propylthiouracil (PTU) and methimazole. Both of these agents block synthesis of thyroid hormone, but only PTU can also prevent conversion of T4 to T3. The dosing of PTU is commonly two to three times per day compared with once or twice daily with methimazole. Methimazole has emerged as the preferred treatment based on recent reports that PTU usage, particularly in children, is associated with the occasional development of severe liver failure that often requires transplantation. Side effects from both medications occur in 5% to 14% of children and include skin rash, arthralgia, arthritis, lupus-like reaction, thrombocytopenia, and agranulocytosis. A β-blocker is used in patients with more severe cardiovascular signs.

Radioactive iodine ablation of the thyroid is an effective therapy for destroying the thyroid, although it does not ameliorate proptosis of the eyes. The destruction of the thyroid occurs 2 to 4 months after therapy with I-131. Surgery is used occasionally to treat children with Graves' disease, although complications include hypothyroidism, hypoparathyroidism, and damage to the laryngeal nerves.

Monitoring thyroid function frequently is particularly important in children with hyperthyroidism because of the fluctuating nature of the disease. Monthly laboratory assessments are common. An occasional complete blood count and chemistry panel, including hepatic function tests, may be useful to monitor for medication side effects.

FUTURE DIRECTIONS

Since 2008, reports of PTU use and subsequent fulminant hepatic failure in children treated for Graves' disease have led to a Food and Drug Administration black box warning regarding the use of PTU in the pediatric population. The antithyroid medication methimazole is still available to medically treat Graves' disease in children. It remains to be seen if the use of I-131 ablation or referral to surgery will become first-line therapies in the treatment of pediatric Graves' disease.

SUGGESTED READINGS

American Academy of Pediatrics, Rose SR, Section on Endocrinology and Committee on Genetics, American Thyroid Association, Brown RS, Public Health Committee, Lawson Wilkins Pediatric Endocrine Society,

Foley T, Kaplowitz PB, Kaye CI, et al: Update on newborn screening and therapy for congenital hypothyroidism, *Pediatrics* 117:2290-2303, 2006.

Fisher DA, Gruters A: Disorders of the thyroid in the newborn and infant. In Sperling MA, editor: *Pediatric Endocrinology*, ed 3, Philadelphia, 2008, Saunders, pp 198-226.

Gruters A, Krude H: Update on the management of congenital hypothyroidism, *Horm Res* 68(Suppl 5):107-111, 2007.

Kratzsch J, Pulzer F: Thyroid gland development and defects, *Best Pract Res Clin Endocrinol Metab* 22:57-75, 2008.

Ng SM, Anand D, Weundling AM: High versus low dose initial thyroid hormone replacement for congenital hypothyroidism. *Cochrane Database Syst Rev* (1):CD006972, 2009.

Osborn DA, Hunt R: Prophylactic postnatal thyroid hormones for prevention of morbidity and mortality in preterm infants. *Cochrane Database Sys Rev*(1):CD005948, 2007.

Disorders of Calcium and Bone Metabolism

69

Jill L. Brodsky and Michael A. Levine

Physiological concentrations of plasma calcium and phosphorus are necessary to ensure skeletal integrity and to maintain vital physiological processes, including muscle contraction, coagulation, energy metabolism, and neuronal excitation. Calcium and phosphorus homeostasis is regulated by both hormonal and nonhormonal factors, and increased appreciation of these complex interactions allows for a deeper understanding of the pathophysiology of the clinical disorders that occur when this delicate balance is disturbed.

REGULATION OF SERUM CALCIUM AND PHOSPHORUS

Most (99%) of the body's calcium exists as hydroxyapatite in bone, with the remaining 1% present in extracellular fluids. Serum calcium exists in three fractions: 50% to 55% is free (ionized) calcium; about 10% is complexed with low-molecular-weight anions; and 35% to 40% is bound to proteins, mainly albumin and, to a lesser extent, globulins. The calciotropic hormones calcitriol (the fully active form of vitamin D) and parathyroid hormone (PTH) act on their target organs, kidney, intestines, and bone to regulate mineral homeostasis (Figure 69-1). Phosphatonins such as FGF23 also play important regulatory roles in mineral metabolism and complement the actions of other calciotropic hormones; phosphatonins decrease renal phosphorus reabsorption while reducing synthesis of calcitriol and secretion of PTH.

The principal source of vitamin D is the skin. High-energy ultraviolet B light penetrates the epidermis and cleaves 7-dehydrocholesterol to produce previtamin-D_3. Previtamin D_3 then undergoes a thermally induced isomerization to vitamin D_3 (cholecalciferol) that takes 2 to 3 days to reach completion. Therefore, after a single sunlight exposure, cutaneous synthesis of vitamin D_3 continues for many hours. It is not possible to generate too much vitamin D_3 in the skin because prolonged sunlight exposure activates a mechanism that converts excess previtamin D_3 and vitamin D_3 to biologically inert products. Vitamin D can also be obtained from the diet, from plant sources as ergocalciferol (vitamin D_2), and from animal sources as cholecalciferol (vitamin D_3). Both of these forms of vitamin D are fat soluble and are absorbed from the small intestine into the lymphatics. About 50% of the vitamin D in chylomicrons is transferred to the plasma, where it circulates tightly bound to proteins, principally vitamin D–binding protein (DBP, also termed Gc protein).

Additional enzymatic steps are required to produce the fully active vitamin D metabolite calcitriol (also termed 1,25(OH)$_2$D$_3$). Dietary and endogenously produced vitamin D undergoes 25-hydroxylation in the liver by the cytochrome P450 enzyme CYP2R1 to form 25(OH)D. Subsequently, 25-(OH)D$_3$ is directed to the kidney, where it is either converted to 24,25-dihydroxyvitamin D$_3$ (an inactive derivative) or to 1,25-dihydroxyvitamin D$_3$ (calcitriol). Activation to calcitriol requires hydroxylation by a 1α-hydroxylase enzyme (CYP 27B1) that is tightly regulated and is the rate-limiting step in the bioactivation of vitamin D: PTH increases production of calcitriol by stimulating CYP27B1 activity, and FGF23 decreases CYP27B1 activity.

PTH is synthesized as a pre-prohormone by parathyroid cells and processed to a mature 84-amino acid peptide (intact or whole PTH) that is stored in secretory granules. Extracellular ionized calcium is the principal regulator of PTH release and interacts with G protein–coupled calcium-sensing receptors that are expressed on the cell membrane. Low or decreasing concentrations of ionized calcium stimulate secretion of stored PTH within seconds and subsequently increase synthesis of new hormone. PTH acts directly on bone and kidney and indirectly on the intestine to increase the extracellular calcium concentration. After release into circulation, PTH has a half-life of only 6 to 8 minutes and is degraded rapidly to inactive (or less active) fragments by endopeptidases in the liver and kidney. PTH binds to receptors on the surface of target cells that are coupled via guanine–nucleotide binding (G) proteins to activation of adenylyl cyclase and phospholipase C, which increase intracellular concentrations of the second messengers cyclic AMP, inositol triphosphate, and calcium.

Acutely, PTH acts on bone to activate osteoclastic bone resorption, which releases calcium (and phosphorus) into the circulation within minutes. Chronically elevated levels of PTH increase the number of osteoblasts and osteoclasts and stimulate bone remodeling, which over time leads to decreased bone mass and osteoporosis.

In the kidney, PTH increases distal tubular reabsorption of calcium and decreases proximal tubular and thick ascending limb reabsorption of sodium, calcium, phosphate, and bicarbonate. PTH (and hypophosphatemia) stimulates renal 25(OH)D-1α-hydroxylase, which increases synthesis of 1,25(OH)$_2$D$_3$ and promotes intestinal absorption of calcium.

Whereas most extracellular phosphate is located in bone mineral in the form of hydroxyapatite, intracellular phosphate is in nucleotides and nucleic acids, phosphoproteins, and phospholipids. Therefore, phosphate's important roles include maintenance of bone mineral, regulation of enzyme activity, and energy metabolism. Dietary phosphate is amply available and readily absorbed. Movement in and out of the bone mineral is regulated by PTH and 1,25(OH)$_2$D$_3$. In the kidney, PTH and phosphatonins (e.g., FGF23) inhibit phosphate transport by reducing membrane expression of Napi 2a and Napi 2c sodium-phosphate cotransporters in the proximal renal tubule cells.

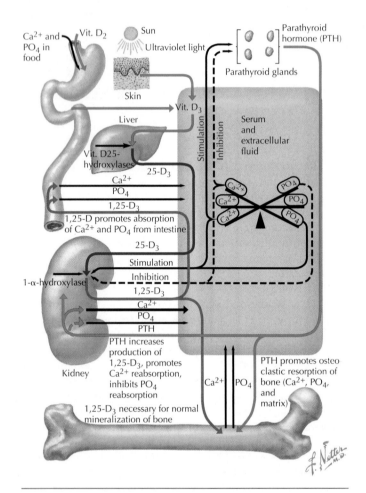

Figure 69-1 *Normal calcium and phosphate metabolism.*

DYNAMICS OF BONE HOMEOSTASIS

Skeletal development is a complex process sensitive to the hormonal, mechanical, and nutritional milieu of the bone. The shape and structure of bones are modified and renovated by two processes, modeling and remodeling. Remodeling is the major process in adults and does not result in a change of the bone shape. This process takes place in the basic bone multicellular units where bone resorption by osteoclasts is tightly coupled to bone formation by osteoblasts. Old or damaged bone is repaired by remodeling. By contrast, modeling occurs only during development and growth of the skeleton and facilitates new bone formation at a location different from the site of bone resorption. Growth in the diameter of the cortical shaft is the result of bone formation at the outer (periosteal) surface and bone resorption at the inner (endosteal) surface.

Bone modeling and remodeling are regulated by a variety of factors such as biomechanical loading, hormonal balance, acid–base status, and drug exposures (Figure 69-2). Bone adapts its strength in response to the magnitude and direction of the forces to which it is subjected. Mechanical forces on the skeleton arise primarily from muscle contraction. This capacity of bone to respond to mechanical loading with increased bone size and strength is greatest during growth, especially during puberty and adolescence. Increased production of estrogen and testosterone in addition to increased pulsatile secretion of growth

hormone are the hormonal hallmarks of puberty. These events act in an anabolic manner on bone to promote net bone formation.

In patients with comorbid conditions such as anorexia, uncontrolled hyperthyroidism, malabsorption, or inflammatory disorders requiring long-term use of glucocorticoids, multiple competing factors may tip the balance of bone homeostasis in favor of net bone resorption. Adequate intake and absorption of dietary calcium, vitamin D, and amino acids are necessary to promote bone acquisition in children. Adequate intake of calcium for children varies by age and is related to pubertal, pregnancy, and lactation status.

OSTEOMALACIA AND RICKETS

Osteomalacia is characterized by a defect in bone mineralization and occurs in both adults and children (Figure 69-3). By contrast, rickets represents a defect in mineralization of cartilage in the growth plate and therefore occurs only in children. Rickets and osteomalacia are classified as calcipenic or phosphopenic, depending on whether the defect in mineralization results from a primary deficiency of calcium and vitamin D or phosphorus. There are many forms of osteomalacia and rickets, both acquired and genetic, but the most common cause is nutritional deficiency of vitamin D. Other causes of vitamin D deficiency include chronic use of anticonvulsants, chronic kidney failure, hepatic disease, and malabsorption syndromes. Phosphopenic rickets can occur as a result of chronic use of medications that absorb phosphorus in the intestine or decreased renal phosphate reabsorption. The symptoms of osteomalacia may be subtle, with patients typically complaining of diffuse bone pain, proximal muscle weakness, and generalized fatigue. In children, rickets can cause growth failure and skeletal deformity. Over time, a waddling gait may result from the hip pain and thigh muscle atrophy. Biochemical abnormalities in patients with vitamin D deficiency include elevated serum levels of alkaline phosphatase and PTH, low serum phosphate, low or normal serum calcium, and low serum concentrations of 25(OH)D.

Nutritional Rickets

Nutritional rickets secondary to vitamin D deficiency is common throughout the world and reflects inadequate exposure to sunlight and poor intake of dietary vitamin D. Vitamin D deficiency is easily prevented, and the prevalence of this condition can be reduced by adequate nutritional intake of vitamin D or vitamin D–fortified foods (Figure 69-4). This form of rickets has a peak incidence between 3 and 18 months of age. Additional risk factors for vitamin D deficiency include dark skin, protracted exclusive breastfeeding, use of sunscreens or conservative clothing, fat malabsorption, use of anticonvulsants that induce hepatic P450 enzymes, marked prematurity, and lack of biliary secretions that may impair absorption of vitamin D and calcium. Mild to moderate vitamin D deficiency may be present for months before rickets is obvious on physical examination, and severe vitamin D deficiency may manifest as hypocalcemic seizures, growth failure, lethargy, irritability, and a predisposition to respiratory infections. Although relatively simple to prevent, vitamin D deficiency continues to be a significant problem

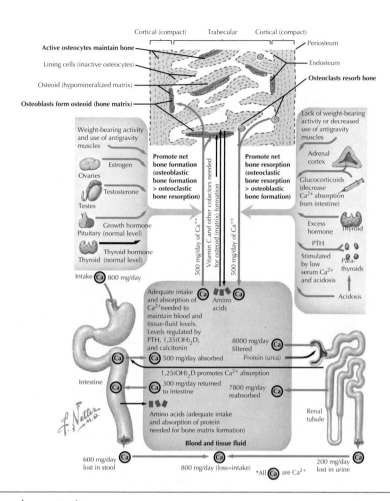

Figure 69-2 *Dynamics of bone homeostasis.*

worldwide, and vitamin D deficiency rickets continues to be a public health problem.

In 2008, the American Academy of Pediatrics issued revised guidelines regarding vitamin D supplementation in infants and children. The highlight of this revision was the recommendation that all infants and children, including adolescents, have a minimum daily intake of 400 IU of vitamin D_3 beginning the first few days of life and continuing through childhood. However, some patients may require more than 400 IU of vitamin D daily to maintain serum 25(OH)D levels that exceed 25 ng/mL, meeting the Institute of Medicine guideline for vitamin D sufficiency.

The treatment of vitamin D deficiency rickets requires supplementation with both vitamin D and calcium. In general, an older child or adult with vitamin D deficiency requires 300,000 to 500,000 IU of vitamin D to achieve normal vitamin D status, and a variety of therapeutic approaches can be used to achieve vitamin D replacement. Vitamin D may be prescribed as ergocalciferol or cholecalciferol (although cholecalciferol is preferred by many authorities) and administered orally on a once-daily or weekly schedule in low doses for several months. A daily dose of 2000 to 4000 IU is typically recommended, but daily doses of up to 10,000 IU appear to be safe. When compliance is a concern, it may be reasonable to replace vitamin D as "Stoss" therapy, a single one-time dose of 250,000 to 500,000 IU

administered, either orally or by injection. To achieve optimal mineralization of the skeleton during vitamin D therapy, it is recommended that patients also receive additional oral calcium.

Genetic defects that impair vitamin D activation (vitamin D–dependent rickets type 1) or responsiveness (vitamin D–dependent rickets type 2) can masquerade as vitamin D deficiency, but serum concentrations of 25(OH)D will be normal.

Hypophosphatemic Rickets

Hypophosphatemia most commonly occurs as a result of impaired renal reabsorption of phosphate. Renal hypophosphatemia can be acquired (e.g., tumors that secrete excessive FGF23) or genetic.

X-LINKED HYPOPHOSPHATEMIC RICKETS

This X-linked, dominant disorder is caused by mutations in the *PHEX* gene that encodes a specialized metalloprotease enzyme (Figure 69-5). X-linked hypophosphatemic rickets (XLHR) is the most common form of genetic rickets, with an estimated prevalence of one in 15,000. Loss-of-function mutations in *PHEX* are associated with reduced degradation and clearance of FGF23; in turn, elevated circulating levels of FGF23 reduce expression of renal sodium–phosphate cotransporters and

Childhood rickets

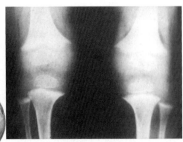

Impaired growth
Craniotabes
Frontal bossing
Dental defects
Chronic cough
Pigeon breast
(tunnel chest)
Kyphosis
Rachitic rosary
Harrison groove
Flaring of ribs
Enlarged ends of long bones
Enlarged abdomen
Coxa vara
Bowleg (genu varum)

Clinical findings (all or some present in variable degree)

Flaring of metaphyseal ends of tibia and femur. Growth plates thickened, irregular, cupped, and axially widened. Zones of provisional calcification fuzzy and indistinct. Bone cortices thinned and medullae rarefied

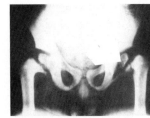

Coxa vara and slipped capital femoral epiphysis. Mottled areas of lucency and density in pelvic bones

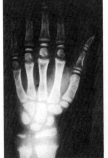

Radiograph of rachitic hand shows decreased bone density, irregular trabeculation, and thin cortices of metacarpals and proximal phalanges. Note increased axial width of epiphyseal line, especially in radius and ulna

Adult osteomalacia

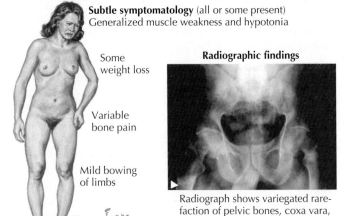

Subtle symptomatology (all or some present)
Generalized muscle weakness and hypotonia

Some weight loss

Variable bone pain

Mild bowing of limbs

Radiographic findings

Radiograph shows variegated rarefaction of pelvic bones, coxa vara, deepened acetabula, and subtrochanteric pseudofracture of right femur

Figure 69-3 *Childhood rickets and adult osteomalacia.*

inhibit 1-α-hydroxylase activity. Patients with XLHR have normal serum levels of 1,25(OH)$_2$D$_3$, which are inappropriate in the context of hypophosphatemia. In general, males and females are similarly affected.

Hypophosphatemia occurs within the first 6 months of life, but the first indication of XLHR is usually reduced growth rate and short stature that begins during the first year of life and is often associated with delayed standing or walking. Nevertheless, it is common for the diagnosis of XLHR to be delayed until age 3 to 5 years of age. Older children may have a history of short stature with delayed dentition or multiple dental abscesses. Widened joint spaces, flaring at the knees, and bowing of the weight-bearing long bones may become apparent in children by 1 year of age. Osteomalacia persists after closure of the growth plates, and bone pain, skeletal deformity, and advanced osteoarthritis are common complications in adult patients. Remarkably, patients do not have muscle weakness even though serum phosphorus levels are low.

Optimal treatment requires administration of both 1,25(OH)$_2$D3 (calcitriol) and neutral phosphate salts; the goal is not to normalize the serum phosphorus level but to facilitate skeletal mineralization and normalization of serum alkaline phosphatase. Treatment must be closely monitored because inappropriate dosages of calcitriol or phosphate can hinder improvement or lead to either secondary hyperparathyroidism or hypercalciuria. The use of human recombinant growth hormone therapy to enhance growth velocity after the rickets is under adequate control is still experimental. Despite aggressive treatment, many patients require osteotomies to improve lower extremity alignment.

AUTOSOMAL HYPOPHOSPHATEMIC RICKETS

The clinical and biochemical features of autosomal dominant (ADHR) and autosomal recessive (ARHR) hypophosphatemic rickets are very similar to those of XLHR. Some differences are worth noting, however. In contrast to XLDH rickets, ADHR shows incomplete penetrance, variable age at onset from childhood to adult, and often resolution during the second decade. Male-to-male transmission of hypophosphatemic rickets should alert the clinician to ADHR, which is caused by missense mutations within a specific region of the *FGF23* gene at 12p13 that appear to inhibit degradation of FGF23. Patients with ARHR have loss of function mutations in the *DMP1* or *ENPP1* genes that lead to overproduction of FGF23 by osteocytes. Thus, serum levels of FGF23 are elevated in both ADHR and ARHR (and XLHR) but owing to different mechanisms. Management of ADHR and ARHR is similar to that for XLHR, consisting of phosphate and calcitriol.

HEREDITARY HYPOPHOSPHATEMIC RICKETS WITH HYPERCALCIURIA

Hereditary hypophosphatemic rickets with hypercalciuria (HHRH) is an autosomal recessive form of hypophosphatemic rickets that can be distinguished from the previously discussed forms of hypophosphatemic rickets by the presence of hypercalciuria. Circulating levels of FGF23 are suppressed in patients with HHRH, which stimulates production of 1,25(OH)$_2$D$_3$.

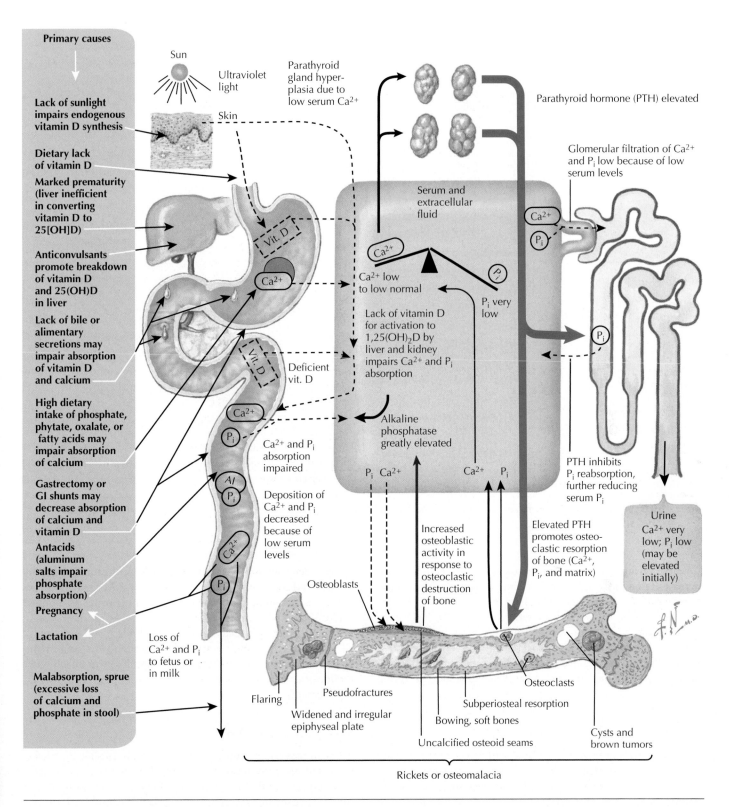

Figure 69-4 *Nutritional-deficiency rickets and osteomalacia.*

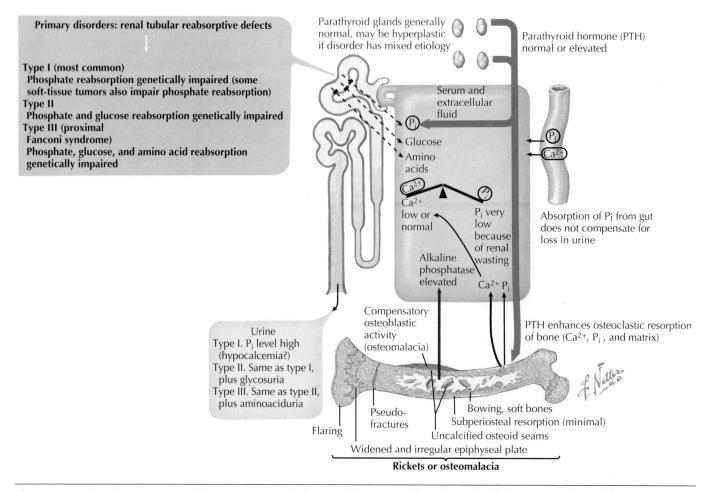

Figure 69-5 *Vitamin D–resistant rickets and osteomalacia caused by proximal renal tubular defects (hypophosphatemic rachitic syndromes).*

Elevated serum $1,25(OH)_2D_3$ decreases PTH secretion and increases bone resorption and intestinal absorption of calcium, thereby causing hypercalciuria and renal stone disease. HHRH is caused by loss of function mutations in the *SLC34A3* gene encoding the type 2c sodium–phosphate cotransporter (NaPi-IIc) that is expressed in the proximal tubule. Therefore, loss of NaPi-IIc protein reduces the tubular reabsorption of phosphorus directly, and hypophosphatemia stimulates secretion of FGF23.

FANCONI SYNDROME

Fanconi syndrome (FS) is associated with a variety of genetic defects (e.g., tyrosinemia) or can occur as a result of acute tubular necrosis, heavy metal and drug exposure, or protein malnutrition (Figure 69-6). Type 1 FS is the most common form and is the result of global tubular malfunction leading to urinary losses of bicarbonate, calciuria, phosphaturia, glycosuria, and proteinuria. Calcium losses in the urine cause secondary hyperparathyroidism; however, this increase in PTH cannot overcome the calcium and phosphate losses in the urine. Prolonged acidosis coupled with increased levels of PTH promoted bone resorption over time leads to rickets in children and osteomalacia in adults. Treatment consists of correcting any underlying primary disorder contributing to the development of FS, correction of acidosis, phosphate supplementation, and $1,25(OH)_2D_3$ replacement.

FUTURE DIRECTIONS

The complex balance of calcium and phosphorus homeostasis is regulated on many levels to ensure adequate bone mineralization. The recent discovery of FGF23 and a growing number of similar phosphatonins now adds greater complexity to our understanding of the control of mineral metabolism and provides additional targets for development of novel therapies.

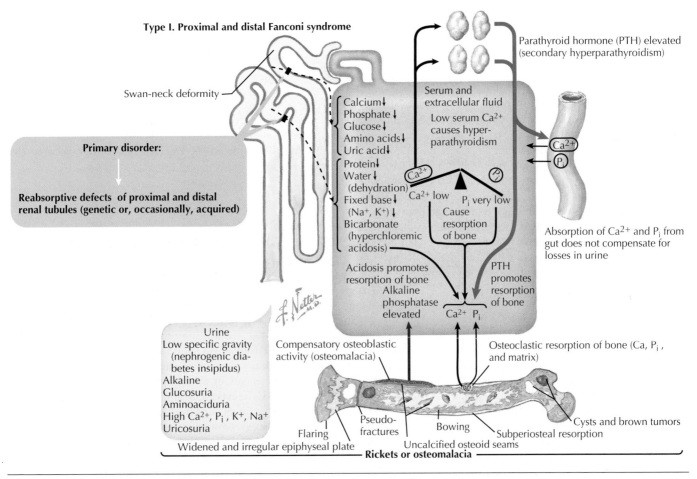

Figure 69-6 *Vitamin D–resistant rickets and osteomalacia caused by proximal and distal renal tubular defects.*

SUGGESTED READINGS

Consortium A: Autosomal dominant hypophosphatemic rickets is associated with mutations in FGF23, *Nat Genet* 26:345-348, 2000.

Goji K, Ozaki K, Sadewa AH, et al: Somatic and germline mosaicism for a mutation of the PHEX gene can lead to genetic transmission of X-linked hypophosphatemic rickets and mimics an autosomal dominant trait, *J Clin Endocrinol Metab* 91:365-370, 2006.

Holick MF: Vitamin D deficiency, *N Engl J Med* 357(3):266-281, 2007.

Institute of Medicine 2011 Dietary reference intakes for calcium and vitamin D. Washington, DC; The National Academies Press.

Lifshitz F. *Pediatric Endocrinology*, ed 5, New York, 2007, Informa Healthcare USA.

Misra M, Pacaud D, Petryk A, et al: on behalf of the Drug and Therapeutics Committee of the Lawson Wilkins Pediatric Endocrine Society. Vitamin D deficiency in children and its management: review of current knowledge and recommendations, *Pediatrics* 122(2):398-417, 2008.

Wagner C, Greer FR, American Academy of Pediatrics, Section on Breastfeeding Medicine and Committee on Nutrition: Prevention of rickets and vitamin D deficiency in infants, children, and adolescents, *Pediatrics* 122(5):1142-1152, 2008.

Wharton B, Bishop N: Rickets, *Lancet* 25:1389-1400, 2003.

Disorders of the Adrenal Gland

70

Roy J. Kim and Rachana Shah

The adrenal gland is really two separate organs: the adrenal medulla secretes epinephrine and norepinephrine, and the adrenal cortex secretes glucocorticosteroids, mineralocorticoids, and androgenic steroids. Glucocorticoids and mineralocorticoids are essential for maintaining metabolic homeostasis, particularly during times of stress; deficiency of these hormones can be life threatening if not recognized and treated. Conversely, excess of any of these hormones, although unusual, can lead to severe and permanent consequences. Accordingly, it is critically important to recognize disordered adrenal function and to institute treatment expediently. This chapter focuses on the physiology and pathology of the adrenal cortex.

ADRENAL GLAND PHYSIOLOGY

The adrenal cortex consists of three distinct zones, the glomerulosa, the fasciculata, and the reticularis. The fasciculata is the principal component of the hypothalamic–pituitary–adrenal axis. Glucocorticoid (cortisol) secretion from the fasciculata is regulated by adrenocorticotropic hormone (ACTH). ACTH is synthesized from pre-pro-opiomelanocortin (pre-POMC). The removal of the signal peptide during translation produces the 267 amino acid polypeptide POMC, which undergoes a series of posttranslational modifications to yield various polypeptide fragments with varying physiological activity. These fragments include the 39 amino acid polypeptide ACTH, as well as β-lipotropin, γ-lipotropin, melanocyte-stimulating hormone (α-MSH), and β-endorphin. POMC, ACTH and β-lipotropin are secreted from corticotropes in the anterior lobe of the pituitary gland in response to the hormone corticotropin-releasing hormone (CRH) released by the hypothalamus (Figure 70-1).

A reduction in circulating cortisol levels activates this axis, leading to increased secretion of ACTH; high levels of cortisol or exogenous steroids downregulate the axis and reduce secretion of adrenal cortisol. Aldosterone is produced in the zona glomerulosa under independent control through the renin–angiotensin system. Low blood pressure and intravascular volume contraction lead to renin release from the kidney, activating this system.

FUNCTIONS OF ADRENAL HORMONES

Cortisol plays important roles in cardiovascular stability (maintaining blood pressure by increasing the sensitivity of the vasculature to the vasoconstrictive effects of epinephrine and norepinephrine), metabolism (increasing gluconeogenesis to prevent hypoglycemia), and fluid and electrolyte balance (sodium retention and potassium excretion). It also inhibits bone formation and is a potent antiinflammatory agent (Figure 70-2).

Aldosterone acts on the distal tubules and collecting ducts of the kidney to increase conservation of sodium and water, secrete potassium, and increase blood pressure. Adrenal androgens produced in the zona reticularis play a role in pubarche and the development of secondary sexual characteristics (i.e., pubic hair) in both males and females during puberty (see Chapter 67).

ADRENAL INSUFFICIENCY

ETIOLOGY AND PATHOGENESIS

Primary Adrenal Insufficiency

Primary adrenal insufficiency is caused by congenital or acquired dysfunction of the adrenal cortex or the hormone-producing steroidogenic pathway (Table 70-1). The most common cause in the developed world is autoimmune adrenalitis, also known as Addison's disease. In developing countries, tuberculosis remains the most prominent cause. Destruction of the gland leads to deficiencies in all adrenal cortex hormones, but this process may be metasynchronous, and not all hormones are lacking in all patients. Enzyme defects can cause cortisol deficiency with an excess of precursor hormones. Loss of negative feedback from low cortisol levels leads to high ACTH in these disorders.

Secondary Adrenal Insufficiency

Secondary adrenal insufficiency reflects a defect in the pituitary or hypothalamic (central) regions that impair secretion of ACTH. Central adrenal insufficiency most commonly occurs in patients with congenital or acquired pituitary defects that arise as a consequence of surgery, trauma, radiation, hemorrhage, infiltrative disease, genetic mutation, or structural defect. Patients may have isolated ACTH deficiency or multihormonal deficiency (panhypopituitarism). Although the adrenal gland is essentially normal, lack of appropriate stimulation for hormone synthesis and release can lead to atrophy of the zona fasciculata. Mineralocorticoid secretion remains intact.

Iatrogenic Adrenal Insufficiency

Long-term use of glucocorticoid steroids is a common cause of central adrenal insufficiency. Daily administration of glucocorticoids in doses that exceed normal adrenal production can cause prolonged suppression of the hypothalamic–pituitary–adrenal axis and ultimately atrophy of the adrenal cortex. This occurs most commonly from oral administration of potent glucocorticoids but can also occur from inhaled glucocorticoids or even injection of depot steroids. Slow tapering of the daily dosage over weeks to months may be required before adrenal function recovers; however, until normal function is proven, the patient remains at risk for consequences of adrenal insufficiency during times of stress.

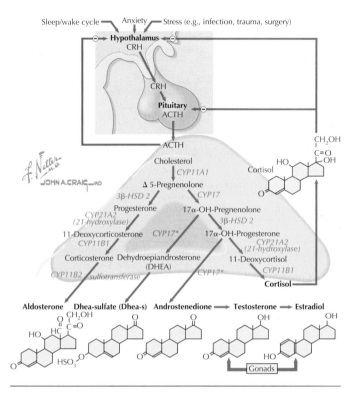

Figure 70-1 *Regulation of adrenal hormones.*

CLINICAL PRESENTATION

Chronic symptoms of adrenal insufficiency are vague and often unrecognized. Children experience fatigue, malaise, poor weight gain and growth, and anorexia. In primary adrenal insufficiency, pituitary secretion of ACTH is markedly increased and is often associated with hyperplasia of corticotrophic cells in the pituitary. Generalized hyperpigmentation of the skin and buccal mucosa may occur because of generation of α-MSH from ACTH (Figure 70-3).

Physical stress can trigger acute adrenal crisis, the most severe manifestations of which are a shocklike syndrome with tachycardia, hypotension, dehydration, and acute abdominal pain that is often mistaken for appendicitis. A distinguishing feature of shock caused by primary adrenal insufficiency is the presence of both hyponatremia and hyperkalemia; in central adrenal insufficiency, aldosterone continues to be produced, and therefore serum levels of potassium remain normal. Other laboratory findings include hypoglycemia, hypercalcemia, acidosis, eosinophilia, and elevated blood urea nitrogen and creatinine.

Many associated signs and symptoms are unique to the specific etiology of adrenal insufficiency. For example, patients may exhibit evidence of autoimmune disease (thyroiditis, vitiligo, type 1 diabetes) with Addison's disease; hypoparathyroidism and mucocutaneous candidiasis with autoimmune

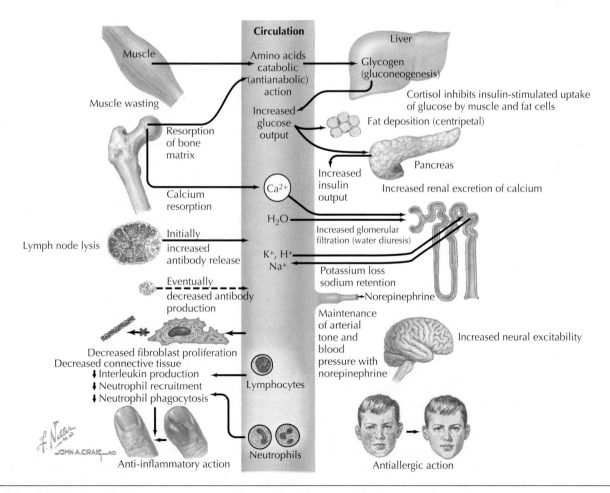

Figure 70-2 *Actions of cortisol.*

Table 70-1 Causes of Primary Adrenal Insufficiency

Cause	Associations or Pathogenesis	Diagnosis
Acquired		
Addison's disease	Other autoimmune disease	Adrenal antibodies
Autoimmune polyglandular syndrome	Type 1: hypoparathyroidism and mucocutaneous candidiasis	*AIRE* gene mutation in type 1
	Type 2: type 1 diabetes, thyroiditis, other autoimmune	
Infiltration or infection	TB, fungal, cancer, amyloidosis, sarcoid, hemochromatosis, CMV (HIV patients)	PPD, cultures, imaging, biopsy, ELISA or Western blot
Waterhouse-Friderichsen syndrome	Meningococcemia leading to adrenal hemorrhage	Cultures
Bilateral hemorrhage	Trauma, anticoagulants	Imaging
Medications: mitotane, ketoconazole	Destruction of gland, enzyme blockage	History
Congenital		
CAH	Autosomal recessive; mutation of 21-hydroxylase and others	Adrenal steroid profiles, genetic testing *CYP21*
Adrenoleukodystrophy; adrenomyeloneuropathy	X-linked; buildup of VLCFAs in adrenals and cerebral or spinal cord involvement; neuromuscular disease	Serum VLCFAs; *ALD* gene
X-linked congenital adrenal hypoplasia	Delayed puberty, contiguous gene mutations (Duchenne's muscular dystrophy, glycerol kinase)	*DAX1* gene testing
Triple A syndrome	Autosomal recessive; achalasia, alacrima, adrenal insufficiency	*AAAS* gene at 12q13
Other syndromes: IMAGE, Smith-Lemli-Opitz	Vary	Genetic testing
ACTH resistance	ACTH receptor or melanocortin 2 receptor accessory protein (MRAP) gene mutations	Genotyping of receptor or MRAP genes

ACTH, adrenocorticotropic hormone; CAH, congenital adrenal hyperplasia; CMV, cytomegalovirus; ELISA, enzyme-linked immunosorbent assay; HIV, human immunodeficiency virus; IMAGE, intrauterine growth restriction, metaphyseal dysplasia, adrenal hypoplasia congenita, genital abnormalities; PPD, purified protein derivative; TB, tuberculosis; VLCFA, very long chain fatty acid.

polyendocrinopathy syndromes; neuromuscular dysfunction with adrenoleukodystrophy; and weight loss, fever and pulmonary dysfunction with tuberculosis. In patients with central adrenal insufficiency, the presence of midline facial defects can suggest structural abnormalities of the pituitary, and poor growth or pubertal progression may reflect a more global disorder of the anterior pituitary gland.

EVALUATION AND MANAGEMENT

Laboratory Studies

In the setting of acute adrenal crisis, evaluation must be performed rapidly so as not to delay administration of life-saving glucocorticoid steroids. An elevated serum level of ACTH and low serum level of cortisol, along with the classic electrolyte abnormalities of hyponatremia and hyperkalemia, are diagnostic of primary adrenal insufficiency. An elevated plasma renin activity level and low aldosterone in the presence of hyponatremia or shock indicate concomitant mineralocorticoid deficiency. Because it takes considerable time to obtain the results of these specialized endocrine tests, it is prudent to draw blood for these hormones and to treat patients for suspected adrenal insufficiency until laboratory studies prove otherwise.

If the test results are equivocal or a patient does not have clinical signs of an acute crisis, it may be necessary to perform stimulation tests with ACTH or CRH. In general, the standard ACTH simulation test is performed with the 23-amino acid synthetic corticotropin (Cortrosyn, 15 µg/kg not to exceed 250 µg) to identify primary adrenal insufficiency, and low-dose

Cortrosyn testing (1 µg) is used to diagnose secondary adrenal insufficiency or recovery from adrenal suppression. Serum samples are collected at baseline and 60 minutes after stimulation for measurement of cortisol. CRH stimulation testing can be used to identify adrenal insufficiency caused by a pituitary lesion. Serum cortisol levels have a diurnal variation, with peak levels in the early morning; thus, the basal serum cortisol level at 8 AM is often checked as a screening test for adrenal insufficiency; a level greater than 12 µg/dL suggests normal cortisol production. In interpreting these tests, it is important to remember that the circadian rhythm for cortisol secretion is not established until a few months of life. After serum samples have been obtained, patients with suspected adrenal insufficiency should be treated without waiting for results.

Comprehensive analyses to determine the underlying cause of adrenal insufficiency should be pursued after treatment is initiated and the child is stabilized. Common tests include very long chain fatty acids (for adrenoleukodystrophy), adrenal antibodies (for Addison's disease), genetic testing, purified protein derivative (PPD) placement (for tuberculosis), and HIV testing (for AIDS). For secondary adrenal insufficiency, pituitary imaging and testing for other pituitary deficiencies (growth hormone, thyroid-stimulating hormone, and gonadotropins) is indicated.

Treatment and Prognosis

Treatment of adrenal insufficiency should be pursued in consultation with a pediatric endocrinologist and centers on appropriate replacement of cortisol and aldosterone, when necessary.

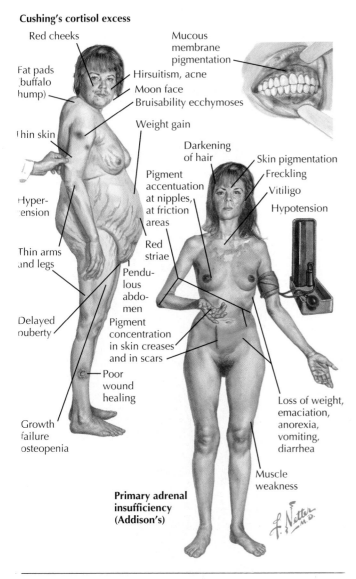

Cushing's cortisol excess

Red cheeks

Fat pads (buffalo hump)

Thin skin

Hypertension

Thin arms and legs

Delayed puberty

Growth failure osteopenia

Mucous membrane pigmentation

Hirsuitism, acne

Moon face

Bruisability ecchymoses

Weight gain

Darkening of hair

Pigment accentuation at nipples, at friction areas

Red striae

Pendulous abdomen

Pigment concentration in skin creases and in scars

Poor wound healing

Skin pigmentation

Freckling

Vitiligo

Hypotension

Loss of weight, emaciation, anorexia, vomiting, diarrhea

Muscle weakness

Primary adrenal insufficiency (Addison's)

Figure 70-3 *Signs and symptoms of primary adrenal insufficiency and Cushing's syndrome.*

maintenance dosage (i.e., 25 mg/m^2/d) can be given orally in three divided doses. In the event of vomiting, lethargy, or other conditions precluding oral intake, one recommendation is an intramuscular injection of hydrocortisone at a dose of 100 mg/m^2. In these cases, the child should be brought to the hospital for evaluation. In hospital settings, stress coverage for surgery or critical illness consists of 100 mg/m^2 of hydrocortisone intravenously or intramuscularly and then 100 mg/m^2/d intravenously divided every 6 hours until recovery, at which time maintenance doses can be resumed. For a child presenting in extremis with suspected adrenal insufficiency, baseline diagnostic laboratory studies should be obtained immediately and resuscitation initiated with isotonic fluids and glucocorticoid steroids.

CUSHING'S SYNDROME

ETIOLOGY AND PATHOGENESIS

Glucocorticoid excess caused by oversecretion of ACTH from a pituitary corticotrope adenoma is called Cushing's disease. *Cushing's syndrome* is a general term for glucocorticoid excess of any nonpituitary cause, including ectopic ACTH production, adrenal disease, and exogenous glucocorticoid use.

CLINICAL PRESENTATION

The signs and symptoms of Cushing's syndrome include weight gain, growth failure, fatigue, hypertension, glucose intolerance, and delayed puberty (see Figure 70-3). Osteopenia, acne, plethora, hirsutism, a dorsocervical fat pad ("buffalo hump"), and striae can occur. Hyperandrogenism and virilization can indicate an adrenal carcinoma.

A diagnosis of exogenous Cushing's syndrome may be obvious in a patient with a long history of glucocorticoid use. Exogenous obesity and monogenic or syndromic obesity must sometimes be differentiated from Cushing's disease.

EVALUATION AND MANAGEMENT

Documenting a loss of diurnal rhythm of cortisol secretion or excessive production of cortisol supports the diagnosis of Cushing's syndrome. This can be documented through a 24-hour urine collection and measurement of free cortisol (reference range, <40-50 µg/d), an 11 PM salivary cortisol determination (reference range, <4.2 nmol/L), or measurement of serum cortisol before 9 AM after administration of 1 mg of dexamethasone at 11 PM the evening before (reference range, <1.8 µg/dL). Abnormal results should be confirmed by repeating one or more of these tests. ACTH measurements should be performed, and a high dose dexamethasone test can be used to distinguish between ACTH-dependent and ACTH-independent Cushing's syndrome. Pituitary magnetic resonance imaging (MRI) with gadolinium can be used to visualize small adenomas. Adrenal masses can be identified using ultrasonography or abdominal computed tomography (CT). In some cases, ectopic secretion of ACTH can mimic a pituitary adenoma, and additional testing may be required. When an unequivocal pituitary tumor (>5 mm) is identified with MRI, further diagnostic evaluation may not be

Treatment is divided into maintenance (daily needs) and stress coverage (for times of illness or other physical stress). Maintenance doses of hydrocortisone are adjusted to provide 8 to 10 mg/m^2. Tablets should be used and can be crushed and mixed with liquids immediately before administration because commercial suspensions of hydrocortisone are unreliable. In secondary and iatrogenic adrenal insufficiency, the adrenal glands continue to be able to produce modest amounts of hormone; maintenance corticosteroids may not be needed. Symptoms such as abnormal fatigue and lethargy may suggest underdosing, and increased weight gain and decreased height velocity may suggest overdosage. Hydrocortisone is the preferred glucocorticoid because use of apparently equivalent doses of other more potent steroids is often associated with excessive steroid effects.

All patients with proven or assumed adrenal insufficiency should be instructed in the use of stress dose steroids for illness, injury, or other physical stress. Instructions for both oral and intramuscular stress dosing should be given and reviewed at regular intervals. During stress, such as a high fever, triple the needed depending on the clinical presentation. In such a case, referral to an experienced pituitary neurosurgeon is recommended. It is worth noting that at least 10% of the population have incidental tumors in the pituitary gland demonstrated on MRI. This means that at least 10% to 15% of patients with the ectopic ACTH syndrome also have an abnormal MRI of the pituitary gland. In patients in whom the diagnosis is not certain based on pituitary imaging, the single best test to confirm the presence or absence of an ACTH-secreting pituitary tumor is a procedure in which the inferior petrosal sinuses are catheterized with blood sampled for ACTH before and after the administration of CRH (which stimulates ACTH) and at 2, 5, and 10 minutes. This invasive study should be performed at a center with extensive experience in the procedure and has a diagnostic accuracy of 95% to 98%. Pituitary-dependent Cushing's disease is treated by transsphenoidal surgery. Adrenal adenomas and ACTH-independent micronodular or macronodular hyperplasia may be treated with surgery, but surgery and chemotherapy for adrenal carcinoma are not highly successful.

CONGENITAL ADRENAL HYPERPLASIA

ETIOLOGY AND PATHOGENESIS

Congenital adrenal hyperplasia (CAH) is a group of disorders characterized by defective adrenal steroid synthesis; accumulation of androgenic steroid intermediates; and variably, cortisol and mineralocorticoid deficiency. The most common form of CAH is caused by homozygous mutation of the *CYP21* gene that encodes 21-hydroxylase, the enzyme that catalyzes the conversion of 17-hydroxyprogesterone to 11-deoxycortisol and the conversion of progesterone to deoxycorticosterone (see Figure 70-1). The absence (or severe deficiency) of 21-hydroxylase results in a deficiency of cortisol and aldosterone.

CLINICAL PRESENTATION

Deficiency of 21-hydroxylase activity classically presents as a salt-wasting adrenal crisis during the second week of life; 46 XX females can have varying degrees of virilization with genital ambiguity (Figure 70-4). Affected children can also present later in childhood with premature development of pubic hair, penile enlargement in boys, or as infertility or a polycystic ovary syndrome– (PCOS-) like syndrome in women. Newborn screening programs now include measurement of 17-hydroxyprogesterone as a screen for 21-hydroxylase deficiency, as well as less common 11-hydroxylase deficiency. Both conditions are virilizing, but 21-hydroxylase deficiency is associated with salt wasting and low blood pressure, and 11-β-hydroxylase deficiency (*CYP11* gene) is associated with hypertension.

DIFFERENTIAL DIAGNOSIS

In infants presenting with shock, the differential diagnosis includes sepsis, primary adrenal insufficiency of other causes, cardiac or metabolic disease, and trauma. Newborns with ambiguous genitalia caused by CAH should have this distinguished from exposure in utero to sex hormones, androgenic enzyme inhibitors, gonadal steroid synthesis defects, or isolated

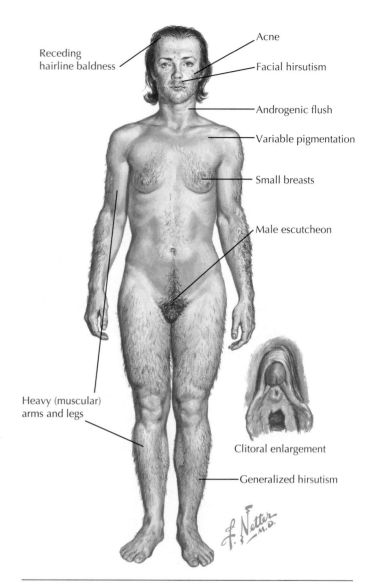

Figure 70-4 *Signs and symptoms of congenital adrenal hyperplasia in a female.*

or syndromic malformation of genitals from non-endocrine causes. CAH and late-onset CAH can present in childhood or later as virilization and precocious pubarche or precocious puberty and must be considered in the context of a differential diagnosis that includes virilizing tumors, particularly adrenal carcinoma, exogenous androgen exposure, PCOS, or other causes of infertility or menstrual irregularities.

EVALUATION AND MANAGEMENT

The diagnosis of CAH requires biochemical testing and may be confirmed through genetic analyses. As noted above, newborn screening programs throughout the United States enable early diagnosis of 21-hydroxylase deficiency and timely institution of hormone therapy to prevent life-threatening adrenal crisis. These screening programs assay levels of 17-hydroxyprogesterone in blood spots and use specific normal ranges that are adjusted for gestational age. Patients with abnormal newborn screen results should be referred to a pediatric endocrinologist immediately for confirmatory testing, including measurement of serum levels of adrenal steroid intermediates 17-hydroxyprogesterone, 17-hydroxypregnenolone, androstenedione, dehydroepiandrosterone, deoxycortisol, deoxycorticosterone, and testosterone. A high-dose ACTH stimulation test (see above) may be required in some cases to distinguish between less severe late-onset CAH, and genetic analysis of *CYP21* (or *CYP11*) should be considered to confirm the appropriate diagnosis. Abdominal imaging may be needed to rule out adrenal tumors as a source for androgen overproduction. The presence of hypertension can suggest 11-β-hydroxylase deficiency.

Adrenal crisis in patients with CAH requires urgent treatment, as described above, led by a pediatric endocrinologist. Long-term management of CAH requires treatment with glucocorticoids to prevent adrenal crisis and to reduce the overproduction of adrenal steroid intermediates. Suppression of excess adrenal androgens is critical to impede virilization, retard increased growth velocity, and prevent accelerated skeletal maturation that compromises final adult height. Glucocorticoid doses must be titrated carefully to reduce excessive secretion of adrenal androgens, but doses that are too high can suppress growth and cause Cushing's syndrome. Hydrocortisone is the preferred oral glucocorticoid because of its shorter half-life and lower growth-suppressing effect. Mineralocorticoid replacement with fludrocortisone prevents salt wasting and allows reduction in glucocorticoid dose.

FUTURE DIRECTIONS

Adrenal insufficiency, Cushing's syndrome, and CAH continue to be significant pediatric endocrine problems. Molecular diagnostics may permit earlier diagnosis of forms of adrenal insufficiency, CAH, and tumoral causes of Cushing's syndrome. Prenatal treatment of CAH is a possibility in families in which a known mutation is present. Because steroids remain a commonly used immunomodulating drug in children, their side effects should be monitored. The mechanisms by which glucocorticoids effect their biologic actions are still being investigated. A greater understanding of these pathways and how they vary in different target tissues may permit development of tissue-specific glucocorticoid analogues that, for example, suppress inflammation without also causing osteopenia or other features of Cushing's syndrome.

SUGGESTED READINGS

Clayton PE, Miller WL, Oberfield SE, et al: ESPE/ LWPES CAH Working Group: Consensus statement on 21-hydroxylase deficiency from the European Society for Paediatric Endocrinology and the Lawson Wilkins Pediatric Endocrine Society. Joint ESPE/LWPES CAH working group, *Horm Res* 58:188-195, 2002.

Shulman DI, Palmert MR, Kemp SF: Lawson Wilkins Drug and Therapeutics Committee: Adrenal insufficiency: still a cause of morbidity and death in childhood, *Pediatrics* 119(2):e484-e494, 2007.

Diabetes Mellitus

Alisa B. Schiffman, Kathryn M. Murphy, and Sheela N. Magge

71

Diabetes mellitus includes a variety of conditions that share in common hyperglycemia caused by a deficiency of insulin action. Diabetes can occur as a result of autoimmune destruction of insulin-producing pancreatic β-cells that causes absolute insulin deficiency (type 1 diabetes), insulin resistance in peripheral tissues with relative insulin deficiency (type 2 diabetes), genetic mutations in β-cell function (monogenic diabetes of the young [MODY] and neonatal diabetes), and other causes (Box 71-1). Although type 2 diabetes accounts for 90% to 95% of diabetes in the United States, type 1 diabetes is the most frequent form in children, occurring in about one in 1500 children by age 5 years and one in 350 children by age 18 years. Over the past 20 years, however, as a result of the obesity epidemic, type 2 diabetes has been increasing in prevalence in the pediatric population. This chapter focuses on type 1 diabetes, with relevant comparisons to type 2 diabetes in children.

ETIOLOGY AND PATHOGENESIS

Type 1 Diabetes Mellitus

Type 1 diabetes mellitus (T1DM) is the second most common chronic disease of childhood. It has two peaks in presentation, the first between 4 to 6 years of age and the second between 10 and 14 years (early puberty). Boys and girls are affected equally. T1DM most commonly affects whites of Northern European descent. T1DM is uncommon among blacks living in sub-Saharan Africa but is far more prevalent among U.S. black children of African descent.

T1DM can involve a genetic predisposition. Having a sibling with T1DM increases a person's lifelong risk by 3% to 6%, a parent increases the risk by 2% to 5%, and a monozygotic twin increases the risk by 30% to 50%. T1DM also occurs more frequently among individuals who have other autoimmune disorders, such as Addison's disease and Hashimoto's thyroiditis. These diseases are associated with increased frequency of certain human leukocyte antigens of the major histocompatibility complex (MHC). It is currently believed that T1DM is caused by a "two-hit phenomenon." An increased risk for T1DM is conferred via genes inherited in the MHC. Then, a second "hit" occurs after birth, activating the immune system and causing an immunologic attack on the pancreatic islets of Langerhans. Unfortunately, the nature of this second "hit" is not clear, and researchers have hypothesized that it may be caused by pregnancy-related and perinatal influences, viruses, vitamin D deficiency, or early ingestion of cow's milk and cereals.

Over a period of time, T cells infiltrate the islets and cause β-cell destruction with consequent insulin deficiency. However, clinical symptoms do not generally occur until insulin secretory capacity is reduced to approximately 30% of normal, although the exact percentage is controversial. Most patients with T1DM have circulating autoantibodies against a variety of islet cell proteins, including islet cells, glutamic acid decarboxylase (GAD65), protein tyrosine phosphatase-like protein (IA2), and insulin. These antibodies can be used to aid in diagnosis and as markers of risk. Of individuals who have the first three antibodies present, 50% will develop T1DM within 5 years.

Insulin is an anabolic hormone that stimulates glucose uptake and hepatic glycogen synthesis and inhibits hepatic gluconeogenesis and glycogenolysis. It also stimulates lipogenesis, amino acid uptake, and protein synthesis (see Chapter 4, Figure 4-1). The absence of insulin triggers a series of biochemical events that emulate a starvation state even when food intake is adequate and that result in hyperglycemia and ketoacidosis (Figures 71-1 and 4-2). Glucose uptake by peripheral tissues is reduced, and hepatic glycogenolysis and gluconeogenesis are stimulated by insulin deficiency, which produces hyperglycemia. Lipolysis, proteolysis, and fatty acid oxidation lead to the accumulation of ketone bodies (β-hydroxybutyrate and acetoacetate), which eventually leads to metabolic acidosis.

As the serum glucose increases above 180 mg/dL, the renal threshold for glucose reabsorption, glycosuria results. Glycosuria causes an osmotic diuresis, resulting in polyuria and compensatory polydipsia. Over time, hyperosmolarity and dehydration develop, and decreased tissue perfusion can elicit a mild lactic acidosis. Patients without free access to fluid, such as infants and those with developmental disorders, are especially at risk. The osmotic diuresis also leads to the loss of crucial electrolytes, such as sodium, potassium, phosphorus, magnesium, and calcium. Metabolic acidosis and dehydration also stimulate counterregulatory hormones, such as growth hormone, cortisol, and epinephrine, further antagonizing insulin action. The end result is a serious metabolic disorder termed *diabetic ketoacidosis* (DKA; see Chapter 4).

Type 2 Diabetes Mellitus

Although still rare in children and adolescents, type 2 diabetes mellitus (T2DM) has become more prevalent with the increase in pediatric obesity. T2DM results from a combination of genetic and environmental factors. Risk factors include obesity (particularly visceral adiposity), insulin resistance, race or ethnicity (Native Americans, African Americans, Hispanic, and Asian Americans are at greatest risk), family history (74%-100% have a first- or second-degree relative with T2DM), and physical inactivity. T2DM affects girls more often than boys, and children with T2DM often present during puberty, when there is a physiologic increase in insulin resistance.

Obesity increases insulin resistance, resulting in a compensatory hyperinsulinemia. Increased pancreatic insulin secretion cannot be sustained to meet demand, eventually resulting in a relative insulin deficiency and a loss of first-phase insulin secretion. The relative contributions of insulin resistance and the insulin secretory defect in T2DM are controversial.

Box 71-1 Diabetes Mellitus Types

Type 1 diabetes
- Immune mediated
- Idiopathic

Type 2 diabetes

Other types
- Genetic forms: β-cell defects
  - Monogenic diabetes of the young
  - Mitochondrial disease
- Genetic forms: insulin action defects
  - Donohue syndrome (formerly Leprechaunism)
  - Rabson Mendenhall syndrome
  - Type A insulin resistance
  - Lipoatrophic diabetes
- Exocrine pancreas defects
  - Cystic fibrosis
  - Pancreatitis
  - Hemochromatosis
  - Pancreatectomy
- Endocrinopathies
  - Cushing's syndrome
  - Pheochromocytoma
  - Hyperthyroidism
- Drug or chemical induced
  - Glucocorticoids
  - Diazoxide
  - Tacrolimus
  - β-Adrenergic agonists
  - Pentamidine
  - Nicotinic acid
  - Vacor
  - Dilantin
  - Thiazides
- Infections
  - Congenital rubella
  - Cytomegalovirus
- Uncommon forms of immune-mediated
  - "Stiff man" syndrome
  - Anti-insulin receptor antibodies
  - Other genetic syndromes associated with diabetes
  - Down's syndrome
  - Turner's syndrome
  - Klinefelter's syndrome
  - Prader-Willi syndrome
  - Friedreich's ataxia
  - Wolfram's syndrome
  - Myotonic dystrophy
  - Lawrence-Moon-Biedl syndrome
  - Alstrom's syndrome

Gestational diabetes

Adapted from American Diabetes Association: Diagnosis and classification of diabetes mellitus. Diabetes Care 34(suppl 1):62-69, 2011; and Botero D, Wolfsdorf JI: Diabetes mellitus in children and adolescents. Arch Med Res 2005;36:281-290.

CLINICAL PRESENTATION

The clinical presentation of diabetes varies from asymptomatic hyperglycemia to life-threatening severe DKA. The majority of children with diabetes present with symptoms such as polyuria, polydipsia, nocturia, polyphagia, weight loss, dehydration, abdominal pain, vomiting, or lethargy. A history of secondary enuresis is not uncommon. Hyperglycemia and fluid compartment shifts can also affect the lens of the eye, causing blurry vision. The breakdown of protein and fat stores results in weight loss. Ketonemia can cause abdominal pain and vomiting. Pancreatitis can occur. A family history of other autoimmune diseases, such as thyroiditis and celiac disease, may be present.

Complicating the presentation is the fact that patients with new-onset diabetes often present during an intercurrent illness, which may confound the classic presentation of diabetes. In addition, a number of other conditions should be considered in the differential diagnosis of diabetes (Table 71-1).

On physical examination, the respiratory status must be assessed first to determine the adequacy of the patient's airway. Patients in DKA can present with tachypnea and deep, labored respirations called *Kussmaul's respirations*. This breathing pattern occurs as respiratory compensation for the metabolic acidosis. It is important to evaluate a patient's hydration status (tachycardia; hypotension; poor skin turgor; dry mucous membranes; sunken eyes; and in infants, sunken fontanelles), perfusion status (cool skin, delayed capillary refill), and mental status. The degree of dehydration (e.g., 5%, 10%, 20%) should be estimated, keeping in mind that intravascular fluids are preserved at the expense of intracellular fluids, and the physical examination will underestimate the degree of dehydration. Any abnormal cardiac findings should prompt immediate evaluation because electrolyte abnormalities in DKA can cause life-threatening arrhythmias. It is essential to fully evaluate neurocognitive status, with particular emphasis on mental status, because of the risk of cerebral edema.

The physical examination can disclose additional significant findings, such as a fruity breath odor secondary to ketoacidosis, candidal infections (particularly in the genital area) resulting from hyperglycemia, and nasopharyngeal infection (rhinocerebral mucormycosis). Pubertal status should be noted. Patients should also be examined for evidence of other autoimmune disorders, such as thyroiditis (goiter) and Addison's disease (hyperpigmentation).

Type 2 Diabetes

The clinical presentation of T2DM in children can range from the incidental finding of glycosuria to severe acidosis or dehydration causing typical DKA. In addition to the signs described above for T1DM, children with T2DM often have specific characteristics that are related to insulin resistance, particularly obesity and acanthosis nigricans. In contrast to adults with T2DM, children with T2DM often have a shorter latency period of disease and commonly present with DKA. In addition, hyperglycemic hyperosmolar nonketotic coma (HHNK) is an extreme form of hyperosmolar dehydration seen more commonly in T2DM.

EVALUATION AND MANAGEMENT

Initial Evaluation

WELL-APPEARING CHILDREN

Initial biochemical evaluation of a patient suspected to have diabetes but not appearing ill should include a basic metabolic panel, including serum levels of electrolytes and glucose and urinalysis; a serum HbA1c can also be helpful. An oral glucose

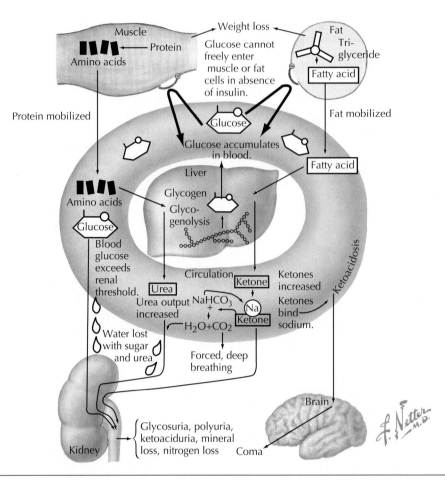

Figure 71-1 *Insulin deprivation.*

tolerance test is almost never necessary to diagnose T1DM but may be necessary for the early diagnosis of T2DM if the fasting blood glucose is not elevated. The American Diabetes Association (ADA) has established definitions for diabetes and increased risk for diabetes (prediabetes) (Box 71-2). Impaired glucose tolerance and impaired fasting glucose are both considered "prediabetes." These conditions are more relevant for T2DM and require close follow-up. In 2010, the ADA added Hba1c diagnostic criteria for diabetes and prediabetes as well.

Table 71-1 Differential Diagnosis

Symptom	Differential Diagnosis
Polyuria	Diabetes insipidus, urinary tract infection, psychogenic polydipsia
Polydipsia	Diabetes insipidus, psychogenic polydipsia
Glycosuria	Benign renal glycosuria
Weight loss	Anorexia nervosa, inflammatory bowel disease, celiac disease, infectious disease
Vomiting, abdominal pain	Gastroenteritis, inflammatory bowel disease, appendicitis, toxic ingestion, pancreatitis
Abnormal breathing	Pneumonia, asthma exacerbation
Hyperglycemia	Stress-induced hyperglycemia, medication-induced hyperglycemia

Box 71-2 American Diabetes Association Criteria

Criteria for diagnosis of diabetes:
1. Random blood glucose ≥200 mg/dL *and* symptoms of diabetes

or

2. Fasting plasma glucose ≥126 mg/dL*

or

3. 2-h glucose ≥200 mg/dL on an OGTT*

or

4. Hba1c ≥6.5% (must be performed using NGSP-certified method, standardized to DCCT assay)*

Criteria for diagnosis of prediabetes:
1. Fasting blood glucose: 100-125 mg/dL (impaired fasting glucose)

or

2. 2-h plasma glucose 140-199 mg/dL during a standard OGTT (impaired glucose tolerance)

or

3. Hba1c = 5.7–6.4%

DCTT, Diabetes Control and Complications Trial; NGSP, National Glycohemoglobin Standardization Program; OGTT, glucose tolerance test.
*In absence of obvious hyperglycemia, confirm by repeat testing.
Adapted from American Diabetes Association: Diagnosis and classification of diabetes mellitus. Diabetes Care 34(suppl):S62-S69, 2011; American Diabetes Association: Standards of medical care in diabetes—2011. Diabetes Care 34(suppl):S11-S61, 2011.

Table 71-2 Goals for Diabetes Control			
Age (y)	Pre-meal blood sugars (mg/dL)	Overnight blood sugars (mg/dL)	HbA1c (%)
0-6	100-180	110-200	<8.5
6-12	90-180	100-180	<8
Adolescents	90-130	90-150	<7.5

Adapted from American Diabetes Association: Standards of medical care in diabetes—2011. Diabetes Care 34(suppl):S11-S61, 2011.

ILL CHILDREN

For ill patients presenting with suspected diabetes, biochemical evaluation should include glucose, a comprehensive metabolic panel (including liver function tests), calcium, magnesium, phosphorus, venous or arterial (if respiratory compromise exists) blood gas, complete blood count (CBC) with differential, and urinalysis. In the case of potassium abnormalities, electrocardiography should be performed immediately. The serum sodium concentration is often low and is an unreliable measure of the degree of dehydration. This is partially because hyperglycemia causes osmotic movement of water into the extracellular space, thereby causing dilutional hyponatremia. Therefore, it is important to calculate the corrected sodium: for every 100 mg/dL of glucose over 100 mg/dL, the sodium concentration should be increased by 1.6 mEq/L [Measured sodium + ((Serum glucose − 100)/100) × 1.6].

DKA is common in patients with known T1DM, with a risk of about 1% to 10% per patient per year. In addition, about 25% of patients with new-onset diabetes present with DKA. DKA is present when a patient has marked hyperglycemia (glucose >300 mg/dL), ketonemia or ketonuria, and acidosis (pH<7.3 and bicarbonate <15 mEq/L). The details of evaluation and management of DKA are discussed in Chapter 4.

Children with new-onset diabetes and their families require intensive education with a multidisciplinary team of doctors, nurse practitioners, nutritionists, social workers, and case managers. When feasible, this is most effectively done while the child is still an inpatient. Additional screening laboratory tests should be performed to confirm the diagnosis of diabetes and screen for comorbidities. These tests include C-peptide, insulin (if not yet treated with insulin), HbA1c, diabetes autoimmune panel (see above), celiac screening antibodies, thyroid-stimulating hormone, thyroxine (T4), and antithyroid antibodies. In patients who fit the criteria for T2DM, liver function testing, fasting lipid panel, and urine microalbumin:creatinine ratio should also be obtained.

Post–Diabetic Ketoacidosis and Home Management

TYPE 1 DIABETES

Home management of children with diabetes involves careful balancing of insulin requirements with carbohydrate intake, exercise, and activity. Realistic blood glucose goals for children vary with age (Table 71-2). The risk of hypoglycemia in children who have hypoglycemia unawareness or lack the maturity to respond to the symptoms of hypoglycemia are limiting factors

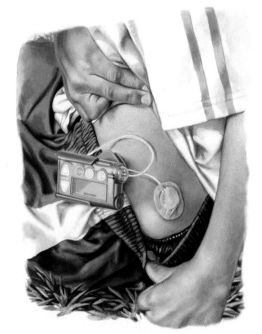

Insulin pump

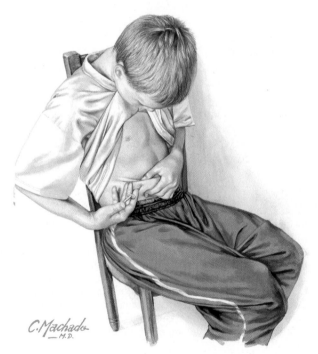

Multiple daily insulin injection

Figure 71-2 *Insulin delivery methods.*

in setting goals for intensive diabetes management in pediatric patients. Goals for intensive management should be set with the family, taking into consideration the abilities of the family and restrictions of age and social circumstances.

For their initial insulin regimen, children with diabetes are typically placed either on (1) a program of multiple daily injections (MDI) or (2) a basal and bolus program with injections or an insulin pump (see Figure 71-2). The MDI program generally consists of NPH (neutral protamine Hagedorn) insulin and a

Table 71-3 Types of Insulin

Type of Insulin and Brand Name	Onset	Peak	Duration
Short-Acting Insulin			
Humalog (lispro)	5-15 min	45-60 min	3-4 h
Novolog (aspart)	10-20 min	60-9 0 min	3-5 h
Short-Acting Insulin			
Regular	30-60 min	2 h	3-5 h
Intermediate-Acting Insulin			
NPH	2-4 h	4-6 h	12-16 h
Long-Acting Insulin			
Lantus (glargine) or Levemir (detemir)	1-2 h	no peak	20-24 h
Premixed Insulin			
Novolin or Humulin 70/30	30 min	2-4 h	14-24 h
Humalog 75/25	15 min	30 min-2.5 h	16-20 h

NPH, neutral protamine Hagedorn.

Table 71-4 Selecting Initial Total Daily Dose

Condition of Child	Insulin Dose (U/kg/day*)
DKA	0.8-1.0
Ketonuria or no DKA	0.5-0.7
Incidental	0.4-0.6

DKA, diabetic ketoacidosis.
*Adjust for age and puberty by adding up to 0.2 U/kg/d in pubertal children or subtracting 0.2 U/kg/d for preschool children.

form of short-acting insulin (Table 71-3). In a basal and bolus program, either an insulin pump or a combination of long-acting insulin (Lantus or Levemir) and short-acting insulin is used. Which regimen is initiated is decided in consultation with the patient and family, taking into careful consideration the family's schedule and lifestyle (Box 71-3).

Determination of the initial insulin total daily dose (TDD) depends on the patient's clinical presentation at diagnosis. In addition, within the first few weeks after diagnosis with T1DM, many patients have a decrease in their insulin requirements because of residual pancreatic β-cell function, referred to as the

"honeymoon period." This period can last from a few months up to 2 years. However, most children who are no longer making insulin need 0.7 to 1.0 U/kg/d. Children who present in DKA tend to require larger insulin doses than those children who present with mild hyperglycemia without acidosis (Table 71-4).

For children started on MDI or on a basal and bolus program of Lantus or Levemir, after the TDD has been established, the clinician must divide the TDD between long- and short-acting insulin (Table 71-5). Children who are started on an MDI program receive NPH before eating breakfast, dinner, and bedtime and short-acting insulin (Humalog or Novolog) before eating breakfast and dinner. Additional short-acting insulin can be given at lunch or bedtime to cover high blood glucose levels or to cover additional carbohydrates that are not planned into this coverage scheme (Table 71-6). Children on a basal and bolus program with Lantus or Levemir must receive short-acting insulin with *every* meal and snack to cover any hyperglycemia, as well as the carbohydrate load. Lantus or Levemir is typically given at dinner or bedtime and must be given as a separate injection and not mixed with the short-acting insulin. In younger children, the basal insulin may be split in half and given every 12 hours.

A postmeal dosing scheme can be used to cover carbohydrates in young children who have unpredictable eating patterns. The blood glucose level should be checked before the meal to calculate the need for a correction dose. After the meal, the insulin dose based on the grams of carbohydrate eaten is added to the correction dose to determine the total dose of short-acting insulin (see Table 71-6). The delayed onset of insulin action in this dosing scheme is not ideal but may be used temporarily to manage food issues in young children.

Dietary management for most children involves carbohydrate counting, which has replaced the older exchange system. The goal of dietary management is to provide a balanced diet while covering carbohydrate loads with insulin. A thorough dietary assessment should be conducted to determine overall caloric and nutrient requirements. A good rule of thumb to determine the amount of calories a child needs is 1000 calories

Box 71-3 Selecting an Initial Insulin Regimen

Consider Lantus or Levemir with meal time short-acting insulin (Novolog/Humalog) if:
- Infant or toddler with unpredictable eating habits *if* an adult is available to give daytime injections at school or daycare
- Child with schedule that needs maximum flexibility
- Child who plans to quickly transition to pump therapy
- *Do not consider* if an adult is not available to give daytime injections at school or daycare

Consider "split-mixed" dosing of NPH and short-acting insulin if:
- Lantus or Levemir is not an option
- Child or parents have needle phobia
- Family needs a simpler program because of multiple competing demands
- Family has a set daily schedule for meal or snack times
- Daycare or school is uncooperative with the requirement for lunchtime injection

Consider premixed insulin if:
- Type 2 patient
- Type 1 patient who requires a much simpler program because of competing demands or intellectual impairment
- Insulin program is likely to be temporary (e.g., steroid-induced hyperglycemia)
- Any patient with vision or learning limitations

Table 71-5 Splitting Basal and Bolus Doses

Time of Day	NPH Insulin	Lantus or Levemir	Premixed
Breakfast	50%		66%
Dinner	10%		34%
QHS	10%	40%–50%	0%
Short-acting insulin	30% (15% at breakfast and 15% at dinner)	50%–60% (use CHO counting)	0%

CHO, carbohydrate; NPH, neutral protamine Hagedorn; QHS, at bedtime

Table 71-6 Insulin:Carbohydrate Ratios and Correction Factors

Age	Insulin:CHO*	Correction
0-5	1 U/30 g	1 U/100-150 mg/dL
6-11	1 U/15 g	1 U/75 mg/dL
12+	1 U/8-10 g	1 U/50 mg/dL

CHO, carbohydrate.

*Insulin:CHO for children with no β-cell reserve ("non-honeymooning"). Children with some residual β-cell function require less insulin coverage for CHO.

+ (100 × Child's age in years [from 3-13 years]), with additional calories added for children with significant weight loss. Placing newly diagnosed children on a standard meal plan with a constant carbohydrate load allows the clinician to work with the family to determine individual insulin-to-carbohydrate ratios (Table 71-7). These ratios allow the family much more flexibility with meals and snacks, particularly when the child is on a basal and bolus program. Efforts should be made to customize the meal plan to the child's usual eating patterns before diagnosis. Tailoring the overall plan to lifestyle enhances the likelihood of long-term adherence.

Exercise and activity levels in children must be incorporated into decisions about carbohydrates and insulin dosing. Exercise has an overall effect of decreasing blood glucose that may be immediate or delayed (≤24 hours). Patients aware of the effect of exercise on their blood sugar can increase their carbohydrate intake or decrease their insulin dose in anticipation of a planned sports event to prevent hypoglycemia. In some children, the initial effect of strenuous exercise may be an increase in the blood glucose because of an adrenaline effect. Good record keeping is an essential tool in understanding the effects of exercise and responding to these trends.

Hypoglycemia (blood glucose <70 mg/dL) is a critical complication that must be anticipated in all children who are managed with intensive insulin regimens. Most children will experience two to four mild hypoglycemic events per week. The risk of hypoglycemia must be balanced with the child's ability to perceive and respond appropriately to low blood sugars. Mild hypoglycemia should be treated with 15 g of fast-acting carbohydrates. Treatment can be repeated in 10 minutes if the blood glucose remains below 80 mg/dL.

Families should be instructed in the use of a glucagon emergency kit to treat acute episodes of severe hypoglycemia by subcutaneous injection of glucagon. There are also commercially available over-the-counter products, including glucose gels and cake icing, that are useful aids for treating acute hypoglycemia orally when the child is in the care of someone who is not instructed in the use of glucagon (e.g., coaches, grandparents, scout leaders). A total of 15 g of gel or cake icing should be placed in the space between the gums and cheek where the product can be quickly absorbed through the buccal mucosa. Also available are glucose tablets (4 g of carbohydrate per tablet) that do not create the same temptation as candy and other foods. Medic Alert identification should be a standard expectation for all children with diabetes.

Educating families about ketone management ("sick day rules") is crucial to prevent progression to DKA and consequent hospitalization. Urine should be tested routinely for ketones if the blood glucose is 240 mg/dL or above or if the patient is sick (irrespective of the patient's blood glucose level). When ketones are present, additional short-acting insulin (10% of TDD) should be given every 2 to 3 hours. To prevent dehydration, patients should drink 1 oz of fluid for every year of age. If the patient's blood glucose is less than 200 mg/dL and additional insulin is given because of ketones, the patient should be encouraged to drink carbohydrate-containing fluids to prevent hypoglycemia. The most common reason for ketonuria after the initial diagnosis is an intercurrent illness. Other factors contributing to ketonuria are insulin omission and an insulin dose that is inadequate for the child's overall requirements (Figure 71-3).

Blood glucose levels should be measured before all meals and before bedtime snack; levels should also be checked at 2 AM when there are concerns about overnight safety. Information that should be recorded as families attempt to adjust insulin doses include:

- Blood glucose levels
- Insulin doses
- Carbohydrates (CHO): time and grams of CHO actually consumed
- Exercise: variations in overall activity level before that reading (e.g., 8-hour car ride, unexpected soccer practice)
- Any relevant factor that might explain variations in current reading (e.g., late or forgotten snack)

Accurate blood glucose documentation allows families to become proactive with day-to-day decision making about insulin, carbohydrates, and activity. For example, a child may require a lower NPH dose at dinner when there will be an evening soccer practice and a higher dose on days where the major evening activity will be homework. This level of insight can only be achieved through good record keeping and careful analysis.

It is important to verify the bolus insulin regimen before adjusting basal insulin. Consider adjusting the bolus insulin dose if the patient has recurrent postprandial hypoglycemia or hyperglycemia. Consider adjusting basal insulin if postprandial readings are in range but the patient has overall recurrent hyperglycemia or hypoglycemia that is not explained by variations in diet, exercise, or other factors. Adjust the dose of dinnertime (or bedtime) Lantus or Levemir to obtain fasting morning blood glucose levels that match the bedtime readings.

Table 71-7 Carbohydrate Counts by Age Groups

Age (y)	Meals (g)	Snacks (g)
1-3	30	15
4-5	30-45	15-20
6-8	45	15-20
9-11	60	15-20
12-14	75	30
15+ Girls	60	30
15+ Boys	90	45

8-year-old boy on NPH/Novolog insulin regimen has abdominal pain, diarrhea, hyperglycemia, and urine ketones. He is eating normally, with no vomiting.

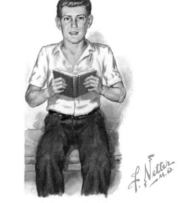

Current regimen:

	NPH (units)	Novolog (units)
Breakfast	15	5
Dinner	3	5
Bedtime	3	

Therefore, TDD=30 units, and patient's ketone dose is 10% for TDD or 3 units of Novolog every 2–3 hours.

Glucose log:

	10:00 am	12:00 pm	3:00 pm	5:30 pm (dinner)	8:00 pm	11:00 pm
Blood glucose:	497	392	458	227	147	107
Urine ketones:	Moderate	Moderate	Large	Moderate	Small	None
Intervention (units):	3 Novo	3 Novo	5 Novo	3 Novo	1 Novo	No insulin
+				**+**	**+**	
Home regimen (units):				5 Novo/3NPH	3NPH	

The patient received his usual insulin before breakfast but developed symptoms and ketones at 10 am. Because his urine ketones increased from moderate to large at 3:00 pm, his ketone dose was increased to 15% of TDD. At 8:00 pm, he had small ketones, so only 5% of TDD was given and three hours later his ketones had cleared. Note that his usual insulin dose was given in addition to his ketone dose, since he was eating normally.

Figure 71-3 *Ketone management example.*

TYPE 2 DIABETES MELLITUS

As in T1DM, the treatment goals in pediatric management of T2DM are aimed at normalizing blood glucose and avoiding hypoglycemia, with similar regimens to monitor blood glucose and ketones as in patients with T1DM.

An intensive management program must include lifestyle modification, with recommendations for improved nutrition and increased physical exercise when losing weight is necessary to improve insulin sensitivity. The American Academy of Pediatrics recommends at least 60 minutes of moderate to vigorous physical activity per day. Screen time (including sedentary activities such as television, computer use not related to school, video games, text messaging) should be less than 2 hours per day. The newer active video sports games and activities that require players to get up off the couch are preferred over more sedentary video games because these active games may increase energy expenditure as much as moderate-intensity exercise. Dietary changes should be made in consultation with a pediatric nutritionist. Simple steps to improve the diet include elimination of sugar-containing drinks (juice and soda), discouragement of skipping meals, avoidance of grazing on food throughout the day, controlling portion size, switching to low-fat foods, and increasing fiber intake through more fruits and vegetables.

Metformin is the only drug approved for the treatment of T2DM in children. Metformin improves insulin sensitivity, decreases hepatic glucose production, and facilitates weight loss. Common side effects include anorexia or nausea, bloating, gas, abdominal pain, and diarrhea. To avoid these problems,

metformin therapy should be initiated with a lower dose that can be increased gradually to achieve a target dose of 1000 mg by mouth twice daily given with food. Rare side effects include lactic acidosis and megaloblastic anemia, and families should be counseled about concerning signs and symptoms. Liver transaminases, CBC with differential, and pregnancy tests in young women should be checked at baseline and monitored while on treatment. Patients on metformin who require contrast for imaging studies should discontinue metformin for 48 hours before and after the study to decrease the risk of lactic acidosis.

Insulin therapy should be initiated for children with T2DM who present with a more severe clinical profile (e.g., HbA1c >8.5%). Lantus, Levemir, or a combination insulin preparation (e.g., Humulin 70/30 insulin) can be used, starting at 1 U/kg/d. Humulin 70/30 is a mixture of 70% Human Insulin Isophane Suspension and 30% Human Insulin Injection (rDNA origin). It is an intermediate-acting insulin combined with the more rapid onset of action of regular human insulin. The duration of activity may last up to 24 hours after injection. In the absence of acidosis, metformin can be started as well.

COMPLICATIONS AND COMORBIDITIES

Children with T1DM and T2DM are at risk for the same long-term complications that adults with diabetes face. General guidelines for screening and treating diabetic comorbidities and complications have been published by the ADA. Microvascular complications of diabetes include diabetic retinopathy, nephropathy, and neuropathy. Macrovascular concerns include coronary artery disease, stroke, and peripheral vascular disease. The Diabetes Control and Complications Trial showed that intensive glucose management reduces the risk of developing these conditions. HbA1c should be monitored every 3 months. Clinicians should consider baseline screening for complications within the first year of diagnosis to uncover any preexisting abnormalities. Annual screening should begin for nephropathy and retinopathy after the child is 10 years of age or has had diabetes for 3 to 5 years. The clinician should determine whether a family history of cardiovascular risk factors exists and should monitor the patient's blood pressure as part of routine care. Medical nutrition therapy (MNT) should be initiated for children with an elevated fasting low-density lipoprotein cholesterol level (≥100 mg/dL). If MNT fails, drug therapy may be necessary to minimize the risk of cardiovascular disease. Treatment with an angiotensin-converting enzyme inhibitor should also be considered for children with microalbuminuria or with persistently elevated blood pressure readings (>90th to 95th percentiles) who do not respond to lifestyle intervention.

Children with T1DM are also at higher risk for the development of other autoimmune disorders, particularly autoimmune thyroid disease and celiac disease. Consideration should be given to screening children at diagnosis and every 1 to 2 years.

Children with T2DM are often obese and are therefore at risk for the complications of obesity as well as diabetes (see Chapter 15). Polycystic ovarian syndrome (PCOS) and obstructive sleep apnea are important comorbidities of obesity and T2DM. PCOS should be considered in girls with irregular menses, hirsutism, or acne. Children with daytime somnolence, headaches, and snoring should be evaluated with a sleep study.

FUTURE DIRECTIONS

Since the discovery of insulin almost a century ago, the diagnosis and management of diabetes has evolved significantly. Diabetes was once thought to be an acute fatal disease and now has become a controllable chronic condition. Research and technology have transformed our understanding of the pathophysiology of diabetes and its complications and continue to provide improved approaches for successful management. Clinical trials are being performed using a variety of agents aimed at beta cell preservation in the newly diagnosed patient with T1DM. Since 2000, patients with long-standing diabetes have received islet cell transplants that offer limited success as a cure for diabetes. Insulin pumps offer children and adolescents flexibility in their daily activities, improving their quality of life. The use of continuous glucose sensors allows families to better understand glucose patterns over a 24-hour period that may not be picked up with routine blood glucose testing. In the near future, a closed-loop insulin delivery system (or "artificial pancreas") will become available. This system will combine a continuous glucose sensor and an insulin pump to titrate the insulin administered to the patient's blood glucose and has the potential to improve the quality of life and long-term outcomes in diabetic children tremendously.

The future of diabetes care is very promising; however, until a cure is found, patients with diabetes will continue to strive for optimal control of their diabetes to extend their lives and reduce the risk of complications.

SUGGESTED READINGS

American Diabetes Association: Diagnosis and classification of diabetes mellitus, *Diabetes Care* 34(suppl):S62-S69, 2011.

American Diabetes Association: Standards of medical care in diabetes—2011, *Diabetes Care* 34(suppl):S13-S61, 2011.

Botero D, Wolfsdorf JI: Diabetes mellitus in children and adolescents, *Arch Med Res* 36:281-290, 2005.

Diabetes Control and Complications Trial Research Group: The effect of intensive treatment of diabetics on the development and progression of long-term complications in insulin-dependent diabetes mellitus, *N Engl J Med* 329:977-986, 1993.

Diabetes Prevention Trial-Type 1 Diabetes Study Group: Effects of insulin in relatives of patients with type 1 diabetes mellitus, *N Engl J Med* 346:1685-1691, 2002.

Haller MJ, Atkinson MA, Schatz D: Type 1 diabetes mellitus: etiology, presentation and management, *Pediatr Clin North Am* 53:1553-1578, 2005.

Report of the Expert Committee on the Diagnosis and Classification of Diabetes Mellitus, *Diabetes Care* 26:3160-3167, 2003.

Hypoglycemia

Andrew A. Palladino and Diva D. DeLeón

72

Hypoglycemia is often the initial manifestation of a disorder of energy metabolism and regulation. The accurate diagnosis of the underlying condition facilitates institution of disease-specific therapy that can prevent long-term complications such as seizures, developmental delay, permanent brain damage, and even death. In children, the most common cause of persistent hypoglycemia is hyperinsulinism, a disorder affecting approximately 1 in 20,000 children in the United States.

ETIOLOGY AND PATHOGENESIS

In children, as in adults, blood glucose levels are maintained within a narrow range in the postabsorptive and fed state. Thus, normal fasting blood glucose levels should be above 70 mg/dL. A lower level of 50 mg/dL is recommended for diagnostic purposes only. The classic diagnostic triad of hypoglycemia, also known as "Whipple's triad," consists of a blood glucose level less than 50 mg/dL, symptoms of hypoglycemia, and resolution of symptoms with normalization of the blood glucose level.

To recognize the different causes of hypoglycemia, it is helpful to understand the fundamentals of energy homeostasis (Figure 72-1). In the fed state, as glucose levels increase, so do insulin levels. Insulin stimulates glucose uptake into cells for use as a source of energy and metabolic intermediate or for storage (see Chapter 4, Figure 4-1). Insulin has other effects that influence energy metabolism; in the liver, insulin inhibits glycogenolysis, gluconeogenesis, and ketogenesis. In the fasted state, insulin secretion is suppressed, allowing glycogenolysis and gluconeogenesis to commence, followed by fatty-acid oxidation, which leads to ketogenesis. In the absence of glucose, the brain uses ketones (e.g., β-hydroxybutyrate and acetoacetate) as energy sources. Insulin secretion from pancreatic β-islet cells is suppressed in the fasted state, and there is increased secretion of counterregulatory hormones that maintain blood glucose levels by stimulating glycogenolysis and gluconeogenesis, such as glucagon, cortisol, growth hormone, and epinephrine. Disorders that impair insulin regulation and counterregulatory hormone secretion, as well as storage or production of glucose, can result in hypoglycemia.

CLINICAL PRESENTATION

The symptoms of hypoglycemia can result from two different mechanisms. An adrenergic response (e.g., fight or flight) typically is triggered in response to a rapid decrease in blood glucose, as occurs with postprandial hypoglycemia (PPH). By contrast, the slower decline in blood glucose that occurs with fasting hypoglycemia may not trigger an obvious adrenergic response but can manifest as loss of consciousness caused by neuroglycopenia (Figure 72-2). In general, hypoglycemia in infants and children is fasting hypoglycemia. Hypoglycemia in neonates can present with irritability, shakiness, difficulty feeding, hypothermia, pallor, hypotonia, and seizures. In children, symptoms include sweatiness, unsteadiness, headache, hunger, nausea, weakness, tachycardia, change in mentation, and seizures. If symptoms suggestive of hypoglycemia are present, it is imperative, if possible, to send a blood specimen for a glucose level to the laboratory to confirm that hypoglycemia is at the root of the symptoms.

DIFFERENTIAL DIAGNOSIS

The differential diagnosis of hypoglycemia is expansive and includes not only disorders of carbohydrate metabolism but also disorders of fat oxidation, hormone deficiencies, and medication-induced hypoglycemia (Box 72-1). It is perhaps most useful to separate these disorders into those associated with hyperinsulinism and those associated with appropriately suppressed levels of insulin. Not included in this classification is transient neonatal hypoglycemia, typically seen within the first 6 hours of life, caused by immaturity of fasting mechanisms and poor glucose stores in premature infants and breastfed infants. In these cases, the hypoglycemia improves with feedings and typically resolves within the first day of life.

Hypoglycemia Secondary to Excessive and Inappropriate Insulin

INFANT OF A DIABETIC MOTHER

Infants of mothers with uncontrolled diabetes mellitus (DM) during pregnancy (regardless of type) are at risk of hypoglycemia because of transient hyperinsulinism. These infants are almost always large for gestational age. During gestation, the β cells of the fetal pancreas secrete high levels of insulin in response to chronic exposure to elevated glucose. After delivery, there is a sudden removal of the mother's elevated glucose supply, and hypoglycemia quickly occurs in the newborn, who continues to secrete increased levels of insulin. Hypoglycemia typically resolves in 1 to 2 days as the pancreatic islet cells reduce the insulin secretory rate. Infants exposed to oral hypoglycemic agents (e.g., sulfonylureas) can also develop hypoglycemia because of transient hyperinsulinism.

PROLONGED NEONATAL HYPOGLYCEMIA

When hypoglycemia persists beyond the first 2 or 3 days of life, one must consider the causes of persistent hypoglycemia. The most common cause of prolonged neonatal hypoglycemia is perinatal stress-induced hyperinsulinism (PSIH), a poorly understood, transient disorder that is characterized by dysregulated insulin secretion. PSIH occurs most commonly in neonates exposed to a perinatal stress, such as prematurity, asphyxia, intrauterine growth retardation (IUGR), or maternal toxemia. Newborns with PSIH have high glucose requirements, and during hypoglycemia, they show evidence of hyperinsulinism with insulin levels that are inappropriately detectable,

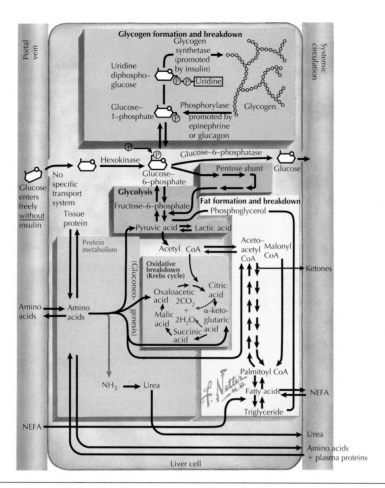

Figure 72-1 *Intermediary metabolism in the liver cell.*

suppressed levels of β-hydroxybutyrate and free fatty acids, and a robust glycemic response to glucagon (≥30 mg/dL increase in blood glucose levels after administration of glucagon). PSIH can last from weeks to months with a median age of resolution of 6 months.

PERMANENT HYPOGLYCEMIA (CONGENITAL HYPERINSULINISM)

The most common cause of persistent hypoglycemia in infants and children is congenital hyperinsulinism (CHI). In general, infants with CHI are large for gestational age and develop severe hypoglycemia shortly after birth. They require large amounts of intravenous (IV) glucose to maintain blood glucose above 70 mg/dL. During hypoglycemia (blood glucose <50 mg/dL), these infants have inappropriately normal or elevated serum insulin levels (although insulin levels may not be detected in all assays), suppressed free fatty acids and β-hydroxybutyrate, and a glycemic response to glucagon. Additional laboratory tests that may help distinguish specific forms of hyperinsulinism include ammonia (glutamate dehydrogenase hyperinsulinism), 3-hydroxy-butyrylcarnitine (short chain 3-hydroxacyl Co-A dehydrogenase hyperinsulinism), and abnormally processed transferrin (congenital disorders of glycosylation). Mutations in at least six genes have been associated with hyperinsulinism: the sulfonylurea receptor 1 (SUR-1), potassium inward rectifying channel (Kir6.2), glucokinase (GK), glutamate dehydrogenase (GDH), short-chain 3-hydroxyacyl-CoA dehydrogenase (SCHAD), and ectopic expression on the β-cell plasma membrane of *SLC16A1* (encodes monocarboxylate transporter 1 [MCT1]). Ectopic expression of MCT-1 on the plasma membrane of pancreatic β cells leads to exercise-induced hyperinsulinism.

The most common and severe form of CHI is caused by inactivating mutations of the adenosine triphosphate–sensitive potassium (K_{ATP}) channel, made up of SUR-1 and Kir6.2. Inactivating mutations in the K_{ATP} channel result in constitutive closure of the channel, allowing membrane depolarization and calcium influx into the β cell, resulting in constitutive insulin secretion from the β cell. In about half of cases, the baby has inherited a defective allele from each parent, resulting in diffuse hyperinsulinism. In the remaining cases, a loss of function mutation inherited from the father in combination with loss of heterozygosity with loss of tumor suppressor genes imprinted in the maternal allele results in focal hyperinsulinism.

INSULINOMA

An insulinoma must also be considered in children presenting with hypoglycemia that is consistent with hyperinsulinism. These patients typically present at an older age than children with CHI and with varying degrees of symptoms. Evaluation for

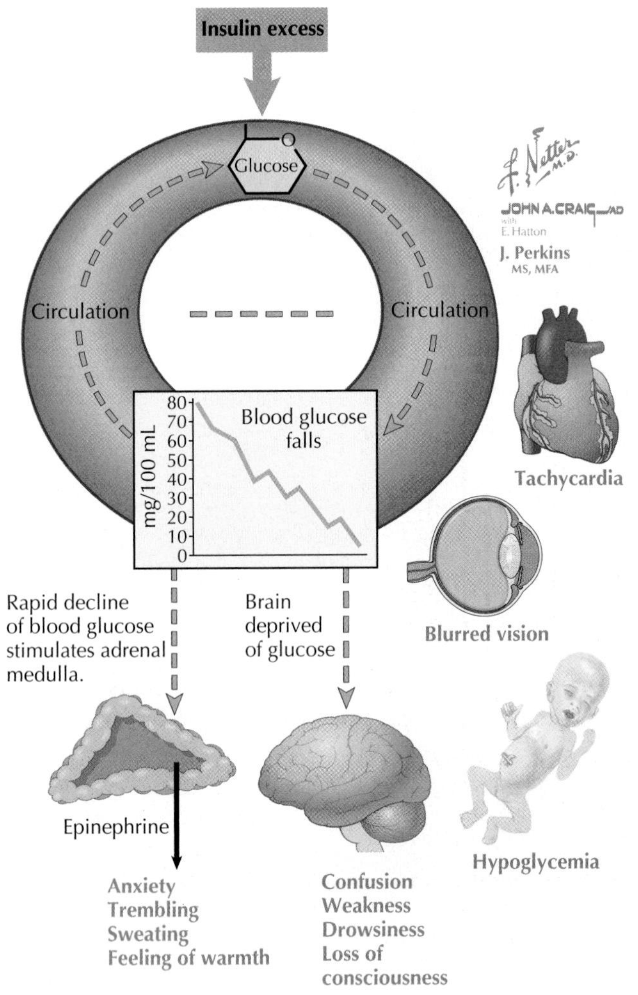

Figure 72-2 *Symptoms of hypoglycemia.*

Box 72-1 Differential Diagnosis of Hypoglycemia in Infants and Children

- Infant of a diabetic mother
- Prolonged neonatal hypoglycemia
  - Perinatal stress-induced hyperinsulinism
- Permanent hypoglycemia
  - Congenital hyperinsulinism
  - K_{ATP} channel hyperinsulinism
  - GDH hyperinsulinism
  - Glucokinase hyperinsulinism
  - SCHAD deficiency hyperinsulinism
  - Exercise-induced hyperinsulinism
- Insulinoma
- Other causes of hyperinsulinism
  - HN4-alpha mutations associated with familial monogenic diabetes
  - Factitious hyperinsulinism
  - Beckwith-Wiedemann syndrome
  - Anti-insulin and insulin receptor-stimulating antibodies
  - Congenital disorders of glycosylation
- PPH (dumping syndrome)
- Disorders of gluconeogenesis
  - GSD 1a
  - GSD 1b
  - F-1,6-Pase deficiency
  - Pyruvate carboxylase deficiency
- Disorders of glycogen storage
  - GSD 0
  - GSD 3
  - GSD 6
  - GSD 9
- Disorders of fatty acid oxidation
- Pituitary hormone deficiency
  - Panhypopituitarism
  - Isolated ACTH deficiency
  - Isolated growth hormone deficiency
- Primary adrenal insufficiency
- Medication-induced hypoglycemia
  - Sulfonylureas
  - Ethanol
  - β-Blockers
  - Salicylates
- Ketotic hypoglycemia

ATCH, adrenocorticotropic hormone; F-1,6-Pase, fructose-1,6-biphosphatase; GDH, glutamate dehydrogenase; GSD 0, glycogen synthase deficiency; GSD 1a, glucose-6-phosphatase deficiency; GSD 1b, glucose-6-phosphate translocase deficiency; GSD 3; debrancher enzyme deficiency; GSD 6, glycogen phosphorylase deficiency; GSD 9, phosphorylase kinase deficiency; K_{ATP}, adenosine triphosphate–sensitive potassium; PPH, postprandial hypoglycemia; SCHAD, short-chain 3-hydroxyacyl-CoA dehydrogenase.

---

an insulinoma requires a fasting test confirming the biochemical profile observed in conditions of excess insulin. Patients with insulinoma tend to have higher insulin-to-glucose ratios compared with healthy control subjects and an elevated proinsulin-to-insulin ratio. Imaging studies that can be useful in the diagnosis of an insulinoma include computed tomography, magnetic resonance imaging, and transesophageal ultrasonography. Complete surgical resection of the insulinoma is curative. A diagnosis of multiple endocrine neoplasia syndrome type 1 should be considered in patients with pancreatic islet cell tumors.

OTHER CAUSES OF HYPERINSULINISM

Factitious Hyperinsulinism

Surreptitious administration of insulin must always be suspected in patients with hypoglycemia consistent with hyperinsulinism. These patients may have increased insulin levels, as well as other markers of excessive insulin effects; however, they will have inappropriately low C-peptide levels relative to their insulin level. Administration of sulfonylurea drugs can cause a far more malicious form of factitious hyperinsulinism, as levels

of insulin and C-peptide will both be elevated. Therefore, a comprehensive toxicology screen should be performed in patients who are suspected of sulfonylurea abuse. Surreptitious insulin and sulfonylurea administration in neonates and children is almost always a result of Munchausen by proxy syndrome.

Beckwith-Wiedemann Syndrome

Beckwith-Wiedemann syndrome (BWS) is a clinically and genetically heterogeneous disorder characterized by macrosomia, macroglossia, hemihypertrophy, transverse creases of the ear lobes, hypoglycemia, and a predisposition to childhood tumors. Genetic testing for BWS is available, but approximately one-third of patients diagnosed with BWS do not have a known genetic mutation. Hypoglycemia occurs in up to 50% of patients with BWS, and it can vary from mild and transient to severe and persistent. The underlying mechanism of hyperinsulinism in these patients is unclear. Management of the hypoglycemia depends on the severity and includes the same treatment options as those for CHI. Most cases of hypoglycemia resolve spontaneously for reasons that are unknown.

Congenital Disorders of Glycosylation

Congenital disorders of glycosylation (formerly known as carbohydrate-deficient glycoprotein syndrome) are inherited metabolic diseases caused by defects in the biosynthesis or transfer of lipid-linked oligosaccharides to the nascent protein chain (type I) or compromised processing of protein-bound oligosaccharides (type II). Hypoglycemia with features of hyperinsulinism has been reported in cases of CDG-Ia and CDG-Ib and in a case of CDG-Id. The underlying mechanism behind the dysregulated insulin secretion in these conditions is unknown. Some patients have been successfully treated with diazoxide.

HYPOGLYCEMIA CAUSED BY NONHYPERINSULINEMIC STATES

A large number of disorders are associated with hypoglycemia with appropriately suppressed insulin levels. Accordingly, serum (and urine) levels of ketones are elevated in children with these conditions (except in cases caused by fatty acid oxidation [FAO] or defective ketone production), which distinguishes them from patients with hyperinsulinism.

Disorders of Gluconeogenesis

Glycogen storage disease (GSD) 1a (glucose-6-phosphatase deficiency) and GSD 1b (glucose-6-phosphate translocase deficiency), although typically classified as GSDs, are actually disorders affecting both gluconeogenesis and the release of stored glucose. Patients present with hypoglycemia, lactic acidosis, mild ketosis, hypertriglyceridemia, and massive hepatomegaly. Hypoglycemia occurs even after brief periods of fasting because patients are unable to access their glucose stores. A child with suspected or confirmed GSD 1 who is not tolerating oral feedings should be started on IV fluids containing dextrose. Long-term therapy for patients with GSD 1 includes frequent feedings, avoiding disaccharides containing fructose or galactose, and a regimen of uncooked cornstarch taken orally or via a gastrostomy tube every 4 to 6 hours.

Fructose-1,6-biphosphatase (F-1,6-Pase) deficiency and pyruvate carboxylase (PC) deficiency are disorders resulting in impaired gluconeogenesis. Both can present with hypoglycemia and lactic acidosis. Long-term treatment of F-1,6-Pase deficiency includes limited fasting (8-10 hours) and consuming a diet high in carbohydrates (excluding fructose), low in protein, and with a normal fat content. Continuous feedings via

nasogastric or gastrostomy tube is also a viable therapy. Treatment of PC deficiency is primarily symptomatic.

DISORDERS OF GLYCOGEN STORAGE

Patients with GSD 0 (glycogen synthase deficiency), GSD 3 (debrancher enzyme deficiency), GSD 6 (glycogen phosphorylase deficiency), and GSD 9 (phosphorylase kinase deficiency) may all present with fasting hypoglycemia, although not as severely as in those with GSD 1. GSD 0 presents as ketotic hypoglycemia and is the only GSD not associated with hepatomegaly. Children with GSD 0 have postprandial hyperglycemia with hyperlactatemia and hyperlipidemia. GSD 3 is characterized by fasting hypoglycemia without lactic acidosis and with hyperlipidemia, hepatomegaly, and short stature. GSD 6 and 9 both have hepatomegaly with hypoglycemia after prolonged fasting. Lactate levels are not increased in GSD 6 or 9. Treatment of GSD is regular administration of uncooked cornstarch and limiting fasting time.

DISORDERS OF FATTY ACID OXIDATION

Disorders in the pathway of FAO include defects in the carnitine cycle, β-oxidation, and the electron transport chain and in the synthesis or utilization of ketones. These patients can present with hypoketotic hypoglycemia with elevated free fatty acids. The best recognized of these disorders is medium-chain acyl-CoA dehydrogenase (MCAD) deficiency. Disorders of FAO can also affect liver, cardiac, and muscle function. Patients become symptomatic in the setting of illness or prolonged fasting. Because hypoglycemia can be a late manifestation of the disease, if a FAO disorder is suspected, treatment with IV dextrose should be initiated immediately. The diagnosis can usually be made based on metabolites observed in serum acylcarnitine or urine organic acid profiles. The primary treatment for disorders of fat oxidation is to avoid fasting.

PITUITARY HORMONE DEFICIENCY

Patients with neonatal panhypopituitarism can present with severe hypoglycemia caused by deficiencies of the counterregulatory hormones cortisol and growth hormone. The presentation can be similar to perinatal stress–induced hyperinsulinism, including suppressed ketones and fatty acids and a glycemic response to glucagon, presumably caused by the effect of elevated catecholamines. After the first year of life, children with panhypopituitarism manifest nonketotic hypoglycemia. Clues to this diagnosis include midline defects and a micropenis. Isolated growth hormone or adrenocorticotropic hormone (ACTH) deficiency can also present with hypoglycemia. If central adrenal insufficiency is suspected and the patient is stable, a corticotrophin-releasing hormone or low-dose ACTH stimulation test should be performed. If growth hormone deficiency is suspected, the patient should undergo a stimulation test with arginine and clonidine. If a patient has central adrenal insufficiency, growth hormone deficiency, or both, central hypothyroidism should also be considered and a free thyroxine (T4) level should be measured.

ADRENAL INSUFFICIENCY (ADDISON'S DISEASE)

Patients with primary adrenal insufficiency resulting in the loss of glucocorticoid production may present with hypoglycemia (see Chapter 70). Additionally, these patients can present with hyponatremia, hyperkalemia, and dehydration caused by a loss of mineralocorticoid production. Patients may also appear hyperpigmented secondary to the effects of excess ACTH. The diagnosis can be made by checking 8 AM cortisol and ACTH levels or by performing a high-dose ACTH stimulation test.

MEDICATION-INDUCED HYPOGLYCEMIA

In addition to sulfonylureas (see above), ethanol, β-blockers, and salicylates can all cause hypoglycemia. Ethanol diminishes the supply of nicotinamide adenine dinucleotide (NAD) in the liver, resulting in decreased gluconeogenesis. β-Blocking medications can lead to hypoglycemia because activation of β₂-adrenergic receptors normally stimulates glycogen breakdown and the release of glucagon from the pancreas. Salicylates may accelerate glucose utilization by interfering with gluconeogenesis and by augmenting insulin secretion.

POSTPRANDIAL HYPOGLYCEMIA (DUMPING SYNDROME)

PPH is extremely uncommon in children except in cases in which PPH (or late dumping syndrome) is caused as a consequence of Nissen or other fundoplication procedures. These children develop hyperglycemia shortly after a meal followed by hyperinsulinemia, and then a reactive hypoglycemia 2 to 3 hours after the feeding. Evaluation of a patient with suspected PPH consists of an oral glucose tolerance test or a mixed meal tolerance test. If the observed pattern is one of hyperglycemia followed by hypoglycemia, then PPH is the likely diagnosis. The cause of PPH is unclear, but it may involve rapid gastric emptying; overstimulation of enteroendocrine cells; and hypersecretion of glucagon-like peptide-1, an incretin hormone that stimulates insulin secretion. These patients are managed with feeding manipulations. Acarbose, an α-glucosidase inhibitor that slows down the absorption of carbohydrates, may be useful in older patients.

KETOTIC HYPOGLYCEMIA

Children with ketotic hypoglycemia have a shorter than expected fasting tolerance for their age and become appropriately ketotic at the time of hypoglycemia. The onset of symptoms may be as early as 6 months of age and typically occurs as infants begin to extend the intervals between meals. Patients with ketotic hypoglycemia do not require medical therapy but instead are instructed to avoid prolonged fasting, usually no more than 8 to 12 hours. During times of illness, their fasting tolerance is even shorter. If a child with ketotic hypoglycemia is not tolerating food or liquid by mouth, he or she should be taken to an emergency department to receive IV fluids containing dextrose. Ketotic hypoglycemia is a diagnosis of exclusion; its etiology is unknown, and it usually resolves by age 8 or 9 years.

EVALUATION AND MANAGEMENT

Glucose can be measured in whole blood or serum (i.e., plasma). In the past, blood glucose values were given in terms of whole blood, but most laboratories now measure and report serum glucose levels. By contrast, point-of-use glucometers typically measure and report whole blood glucose concentrations. Serum has a higher water content than blood cells and consequently contains more dissolved glucose than does whole blood. A calculated serum glucose level can be estimated from the whole-blood glucose by multiplying the blood glucose level by 1.15.

Additional caveats are worth noting. Blood samples that are not processed promptly can have erroneously low glucose levels owing to glycolysis by red and white blood cells (i.e., at room temperature, the decline of whole blood glucose can be 5-7 mg/dL/hr). In addition, hospital bedside glucose monitors and similar home glucose monitors are less precise than clinical laboratory methods and can be expected to have an error range of 10% to 15%. For practical reasons, the authors use the same threshold of 70 mg/dL if using plasma glucose or whole blood, but for diagnostic purposes, all measurements below 60 mg/dL should be verified with a plasma level in the clinical laboratory.

In severely symptomatic or clinically unstable patients with hypoglycemia, the first step should be administration of a 2 mL/kg bolus of 10% dextrose in water IV followed by a continuous infusion of 10% dextrose in an age-appropriate saline concentration at a glucose infusion rate of 6 to 8 mg/kg/min (Box 72-2). Whenever hypoglycemia is suspected in a clinically stable patient, the first step should be to send a "critical" blood sample to the laboratory to confirm hypoglycemia and to obtain the diagnostic tests necessary to establish the underlying cause of hypoglycemia (Box 72-3). If the patient is stable after the critical sample is sent, a glucagon stimulation test will help to refine the differential diagnosis (Figure 72-3).

The initial management, regardless of the etiology, is essentially always the same: dextrose-containing IV fluids. Long-term management of children with hypoglycemia depends on the cause of the hypoglycemia.

Treatment of Hyperinsulinism

The mainstay therapy for hyperinsulinism is diazoxide. Diazoxide suppresses insulin secretion by its action in the K_{ATP} channel. Because a functional K_{ATP} channel is required for diazoxide to exert an effect, most patients with K_{ATP} hyperinsulinism do not respond to diazoxide. A notable exception is a child with a dominant inhibitor mutation in a K_{ATP} gene, which causes a milder form of diffuse hyperinsulinism. The dosage of diazoxide is 5 to 15 mg/kg/day given orally and divided into two equal doses. The side effects of diazoxide include sodium and fluid retention and hypertrichosis. If it occurs, fluid retention can be managed with concomitant diuretic therapy.

Second-line medical therapy for infants unresponsive to diazoxide is octreotide. Octreotide is a long-acting somatostatin analog that inhibits insulin secretion distal to the K_{ATP} channel by inducing hyperpolarization of β cells, direct inhibition of voltage-dependent calcium channels, and more distal events in

Box 72-2 Treatment of Hypoglycemia

Emergency Treatment
- Dextrose bolus: 2 mL/kg of D10W
- Continuous infusion of D10 with NaCl with GIR*
  of 6-8 mg/kg/min

Specific Treatment
- Hyperinsulinism
  - Diazoxide: 5-15 mg/kg/day divided BID
  - Octreotide: 5-20 mcg/kg/day divided TID or QID or via
    continuous infusion
  - Glucagon: 1 mg IM or IV or 1 mg/d via continuous
    infusion
- Ketotic hypoglycemia
  - Limit fasting to 8-12 h
- Disorders of gluconeogenesis, glycogenolysis, and fatty
  acid oxidation
  - Limited fasting, frequent feedings, cornstarch (GSD)
- Adrenal insufficiency
  - Hydrocortisone:
    IV stress dose: 100 mg/m² once then 100 mg/m²/day
      divided every 4 hours
    Oral stress dose: 50 mg/m²/d divided every 8 hours
    Maintenance dose: 8-12 mg/m²/d divided TID
  - Growth hormone deficiency
    Growth hormone: 0.3 mg/kg/wk divided daily
- Postprandial hypoglycemia
  - Frequent smaller meals with low carbohydrate content
    or continuous feedings
  - Acarbose 12.5-50 mg before each meal

*GIR: $\dfrac{\text{IV rate (mL/h)} \times \text{Dextrose concentration (g/dL)}}{\text{Weight (kg)}} \times 6$

BID, twice a day; D10W, dextrose 10% in water; GIR, glucose
infusion rate; GSD, glycogen storage disease; QID, four times a day;
TID, three times a day.

Box 72-3 The Critical Sample and Glucagon
Stimulation Test

Blood and Urine Tests at the Time of Hypoglycemia
- Glucose
- Carbon dioxide
- Lactate
- β-Hydroxybutyrate
- Free fatty acids
- Insulin
- C-peptide
- Insulin-like growth factor binding protein-1
- Ammonia
- Acylcarnitine profile
- Free and total carnitine
- Growth hormone
- Cortisol
- Urine organic acids
- Urine ketones

Glucagon Stimulation Test
- Check blood glucose (time 0)
- Give 1 mg of glucagon IM or IV
- Check blood glucose every 10 min for 40 min
- If blood glucose does not increase by 20 mg/dL in
  20 min, rescue patient with dextrose
- Positive response: increase in blood glucose by 30 mg/dL
  by 40 min after glucagon administration

IM, intramuscular; IV, intravenous.

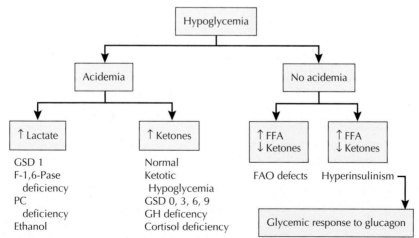

Results from the "critical" blood sample obtained at the time of hypoglycemia serve as the basis for distinguishing
four categories of disease: impairment of gluconeogenesis, normal and abnormal forms of ketotic hypoglycemia,
defects in fatty acid oxidation and ketogenesis, and impairment of lipolysis and ketogenesis. (GSD,
glycogen storage disease; F-1,6-Pase, fructose-1,6-biphosphatase; PC, pyruvate carboxylase; GH, growth hormone;
FFA, free fatty acids; FAO, fatty acid oxidation)

Figure 72-3 *Hypoglycemia diagnostic algorithm.*

the insulin secretory pathway. Octreotide is administered either subcutaneously every 6 to 8 hours or via continuous infusion at 5 to 20 µg/kg/d. The initial response to octreotide is good in most cases of hyperinsulinism, but tachyphylaxis develops after a few doses, rendering therapy inadequate for long-term use. Potential side effects of octreotide include nausea, diarrhea, gallstones, necrotizing enterocolitis, and suppression of growth hormone.

Glucagon can also be given as a continuous IV infusion of 1 mg/d to help maintain euglycemia in the hospital setting. Children with focal hyperinsulinism are excellent candidates for surgery if the lesion can be identified. Patients with diffuse hyperinsulinism require surgical resection of the pancreas to ameliorate or resolve the hypoglycemia if they do not respond to medical therapy (e.g., octreotide).

Gluconeogenesis, Glycogenolysis, and Fat Oxidation

The treatment of these children includes avoidance of prolonged fasting periods. In disorders of gluconeogenesis and GSDs, 1 to 2 g/kg of uncooked cornstarch is helpful in prolonging fasting tolerance.

Specific Hormonal Replacement

Patients with adrenal insufficiency should be treated with hydrocortisone (8-12 mg/m^2/d divided every 8 hours), plus a mineralocorticoid if they have primary adrenal insufficiency. If the patient is unstable, serum should be obtained and reserved for later measurement of cortisol and ACTH levels, and therapy with stress dose glucocorticoids should be initiated immediately: hydrocortisone (100 mg/m^2) as an IV bolus followed by hydrocortisone 100 mg/m^2/day divided every 4 hours for 24 hours or until the patient is stable. Infants with growth hormone deficiency should undergo pituitary imaging by magnetic resonance imaging and should be treated with replacement growth hormone (0.3 mg/kg/wk divided daily) to prevent future hypoglycemia.

FUTURE DIRECTIONS

In the past few years, significant advances in molecular genetics have contributed to our understanding of the most common causes of hypoglycemia in children. These advances should result in the development of specific, more effective therapies in the next few years that may improve the outcome in these children.

SUGGESTED READINGS

De León DD, Stanley CA: Mechanisms of disease: advances in diagnosis and treatment of hyperinsulinism in neonates, *Nat Clin Pract Endocrinol Metab* 3:57-68, 2007.

De León DD, Stanley CA, Sperling MA: Hypoglycemia in neonates and infants. In Sperling MA, editor: *Pediatric Endocrinology*, ed 3, Philadelphia, 2008, Saunders Elsevier.

Langdon DR, Stanley CA, Sperling MA: Hypoglycemia in the infant and child. In Sperling MA, editor: *Pediatric Endocrinology*, ed 3, Philadelphia, 2008, Saunders Elsevier.

Palladino AA, Bennett MJ, Stanley CA: Hyperinsulinism in infancy and childhood: when an insulin level is not always enough, *Clin Chem* 54:256-263, 2008.

Palladino AA, Stanley CA: A specialized team approach to diagnosis and medical versus surgical treatment of infants with congenital hyperinsulinism, *Semin Pediatric Surg* 20:32-37, 2011.

Stanley CA: Hypoglycemia in the neonate, *Pediatr Endocrinol Rev* 4(suppl):76-81, 2006.

Disorders of Growth

73

Dorit Koren and Adda Grimberg

Statural growth is an integral part of childhood development and normally occurs in a predictable pattern. Families often seek medical attention when a child does not seem to grow adequately, and the pediatrician's primary responsibility is to differentiate between normal variants of growth and abnormal patterns (i.e., between a healthy petite child and a child with an underlying systemic illness or other growth problem). Because early detection is important for diagnosing any underlying illness and intervening to maximize potential adult height, interval growth should be accurately assessed and plotted on a growth chart at each health maintenance visit. When judging a child's growth, it is useful to determine the sex-adjusted midparental height (genetic target height) by adding together the heights of the biological parents and adding 5 inches (13 cm) for a boy or subtracting 5 inches (13 cm) for a girl and then dividing by 2. This height, plus or minus approximately 4 inches, represents an estimate of the child's genetic height potential. Any deviations from normal growth patterns or the child's genetic height potential should be evaluated; the more the child's growth deviates from the usual pattern, the greater the chances of an underlying abnormality.

ETIOLOGY AND PATHOGENESIS

Normal Growth Patterns

Normal growth follows a predictable pattern. This pattern is depicted in widely used growth charts, which comprise sequential percentile curves showing the distribution of selected body measurements (usually length or height, weight, and weight for height or body mass index [BMI]) in children of a country. Growth is fastest during the fetal period; fetal size primarily relates to maternal health and nutrition. During infancy, the child's genetic factors come into play. Growth gradually slows, with average increase in length of 25 cm over the first year of life and 10 cm over the second year. In this period, infants often cross length percentiles (channelize) to a percentile more in line with their genetic potential. After the second birthday, growth proceeds at a slow, relatively constant velocity of 4 to 6 cm/y, and shifting percentile channels is *abnormal*. Childhood growth is slowest just before the onset of puberty and then accelerates during adolescence, resulting in the pubertal "growth spurt" (average growth velocity of 10 cm/y). At the end of puberty, growth ceases as the epiphyses (growth plates) fuse.

Longitudinal Growth and Mediating Factors

Longitudinal growth occurs via chondrocyte proliferation and subsequent endochondral ossification in the growth plates of long bones (and vertebrae). The growth plate is a cartilaginous zone located between the metaphysis and epiphysis (secondary ossification zone at the end of the bone). Growth is a complex process regulated by multiple factors, including nutrition, hormones, and growth factors that act either locally within the growth plate or systemically.

Growth hormone (GH) is the most important growth-regulating hormone; its pulsatile secretion from the anterior pituitary somatotrophs is regulated by two hypothalamic peptide hormones, GH-releasing hormone (GHRH) and somatostatin, which, respectively, stimulate and inhibit its release (Figure 73-1). Circulating GH is bound to GH-binding protein (GHBP), which corresponds to the extracellular domain of the GH receptor. Many, although not all, of GH's actions are mediated through insulin-like growth factor (IGF)-I (i.e., somatomedin-C). Serum IGF-I is produced principally in the liver in response to GH and circulates in the bloodstream bound to IGF-binding proteins (especially IGFBP-3) that control its bioavailability. IGF-I acts at target tissues by binding cell-surface IGF receptors and triggering multiple downstream effects that include cellular hypertrophy and proliferation. IGF-I and free fatty acids also inhibit GH secretion at the level of the pituitary and hypothalamus.

Other systemic hormones that affect growth include insulin (the principal growth-promoting hormone in utero), androgens and estrogens (which induce the pubertal growth spurt and, in the case of estrogens, epiphyseal fusion), thyroid hormone (which has a permissive effect on GH secretion and exerts direct action at the growth plates), and glucocorticoids (which inhibit growth both centrally and at the growth plate).

Abnormal Growth

Abnormalities in growth can be caused by systemic illness, psychosocial deprivation, malnutrition, or abnormalities in the secretion or action of any of the aforementioned hormones and growth factors. *Growth failure* is defined as height velocity that is less than expected for a child's age, sex, and pubertal stage or as the crossing downward of two or more major height percentiles (beyond 2 years of age). Growth failure always merits an evaluation. Normal height is a continuum; *short stature* is conventionally defined as a height that is below the child's genetic potential (as determined by parental heights) or more than 2 standard deviations (SDs) below the mean for age and sex. Thus, approximately 2.5% of a population will be classified as short, including some healthy children. Because the average adult height differs considerably among different ethnic groups, the actual height that corresponds to short stature differs from population to population.

CLINICAL PRESENTATION

The causes of short stature can be divided into three general categories: chronic disease (including undernutrition), familial short stature (FSS), and constitutional delay of growth and puberty (CDGP) (Figure 73-2). Endocrine diseases are rare

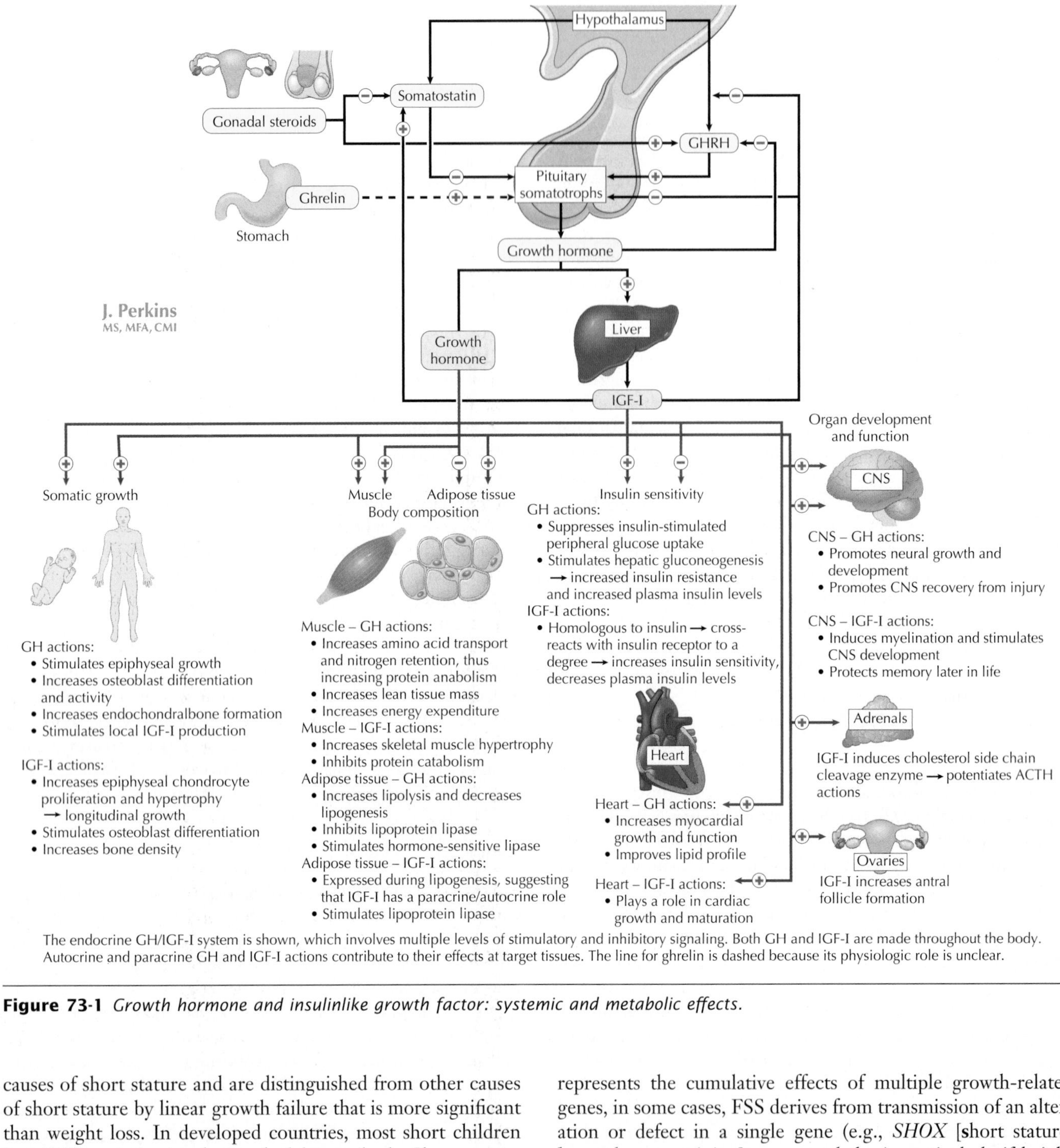

The endocrine GH/IGF-I system is shown, which involves multiple levels of stimulatory and inhibitory signaling. Both GH and IGF-I are made throughout the body. Autocrine and paracrine GH and IGF-I actions contribute to their effects at target tissues. The line for ghrelin is dashed because its physiologic role is unclear.

Figure 73-1 *Growth hormone and insulinlike growth factor: systemic and metabolic effects.*

causes of short stature and are distinguished from other causes of short stature by linear growth failure that is more significant than weight loss. In developed countries, most short children have FSS, constitutional growth delay, or both. Short stature and constitutional growth delay are diagnoses of exclusion. The following is a focused review of the clinical presentations of selected normal variants and causes of short stature; see Box 73-1 for a comprehensive list of growth disorders.

Familial Short Stature

FSS is the most common cause of short stature in otherwise well children. A child with FSS has a height that falls at the lower end of the population norm but that is consistent with the child's genetic potential. Although in most cases FSS

represents the cumulative effects of multiple growth-related genes, in some cases, FSS derives from transmission of an alteration or defect in a single gene (e.g., *SHOX* [**s**hort stature, **h**ome**o**b**ox**-containing] gene; see below), particularly if height is significantly below the third percentile. Both parents' heights are usually in the lower height percentiles, and the child's growth pattern and predicted adult height are *consistent* with that of his or her parents (and often siblings). The hallmark is a normal growth velocity, such that the child's growth curve is parallel to the standard population curve. In the absence of a family history of delayed puberty, the timing of puberty is usually average. The medical history, review of systems, and physical examination are typically unremarkable. The bone age is typically within the normal range, and laboratory workup results should be normal.

CDC 2000 Growth Curve: Boys ages 2–20 years

Tanner Height Velocity Curves for Boys

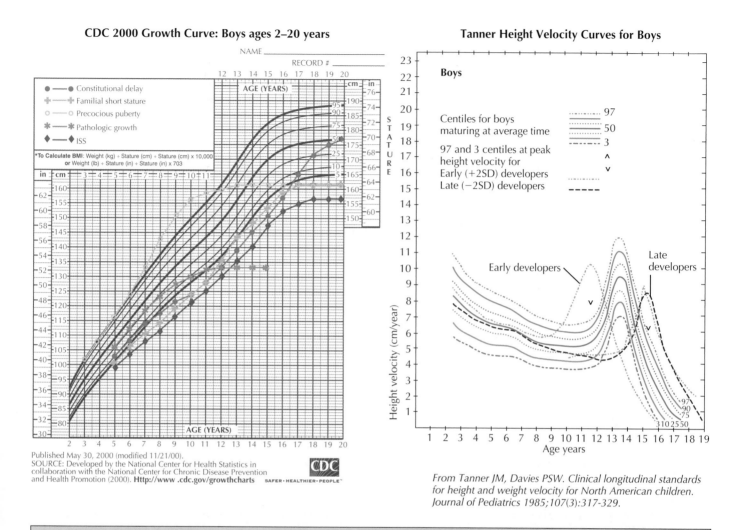

From Tanner JM, Davies PSW. Clinical longitudinal standards for height and weight velocity for North American children. Journal of Pediatrics 1985;107(3):317-329.

Genetics:	Nutrition:	Psychosocial:	Systemic illness:	Medications:	Endocrine:
· Turner syndrome	· Undernutrition	· Deprivation dwarfism	· HIV/AIDS	· Stimulants (for ADHD treatment)	· Hypothyroidism
· Down syndrome	· Eating disorders		· TB	· Glucocorticoids	· Growth hormone deficiency
· Noonan syndrome	· Celiac disease		· Cystic fibrosis	· Chemotherapy and/or radiation	· IGF deficiency
· SHOX haploinsufficiency	· IBD		· Cancer		· Puberty variants
· Skeletal dysplasias	· Other forms of malabsorption		· Congenital heart disease (esp. cyanotic)		· Endogenous gluco-corticoid excess
· Others	· GERD		· Renal disease		
	· Fe or Zinc deficiency		· Acidosis		
			· Chronic liver disease		

Figure 73-2 *Growth curves and disorders of growth. Illustrative growth patterns are shown, as well as multiple factors that may impact a child's growth. Many cases can be multifactorial.*

Constitutional Delay of Growth and Puberty

CDGP is the second most common cause of (transient) relative short stature in childhood. Children with CDGP usually have a normal birth length, begin crossing height percentiles by age 2 years, and settle in the lower percentiles, where they track until the onset of puberty in their peers, when they appear to drop further away from the growth curve. This growth pattern is associated with delayed puberty, which is defined as the absence of secondary sexual characteristics at an age beyond +2 SD for the population (see Chapter 67), that is, the absence of

thelarche (breast development) in girls older than age 13 years, no signs of puberty in boys older than age 14 years, or no menarche in girls by 4 years after thelarche or by age 16 years (primary amenorrhea). CDGP represents the late end of the spectrum of pubertal development. Because children with CDGP enter puberty (and thus accelerate their growth velocity) later than most of their peers, they develop a transient relative height and sexual maturation gap relative to their age-matched peers. However, children with CDGP continue to grow after their peers cease growth, and thus they eventually attain an adult height within the normal range. Family history often reveals

Box 73-1 Differential Diagnosis of Short Stature

I. Normal variants
  A. Familial Short Stature (excludes genetic problems inherited in an autosomal dominant fashion, which can also cause short stature in successive family generations)
  B. Constitutional delay of growth and puberty
  C. Idiopathic short stature
II. Abnormal causes
  A. Intrauterine growth retardation
  B. Bone disorders
    1. Osteochondrodysplasias: genetic abnormalities of cartilage, bone, or both; examples include:
      a. Achondroplasia and hypochondroplasia
      b. Achondrogenesis
      c. Mesomelic dysplasias
      d. Epiphyseal and metaphyseal dysplasias
    2. Osteogenesis imperfecta
  C. Chromosomal abnormalities
    1. Turner syndrome
    2. Trisomy 21
    3. Trisomies 8, 13, and 18
    4. 18q deletion
  D. Endocrine disorders
    1. Pituitary or hypothalamic dysfunction
      a. Idiopathic GH deficiency
      b. Structural abnormalities:
        • Associated with other midline defects (e.g., holoprosencephaly, septo-optic dysplasia)
        • Isolated hypothalamic or pituitary malformations (e.g., empty sella syndrome, ectopic neurohypophysis)
      c. Genetic causes:
        • Multiple pituitary hormone deficiencies: *HESX1* mutation, *PROP1* mutation, *POUF1* mutation
        • GHRH receptor mutation
        • GH gene (*GH1*) mutations
        • Growth hormone secretagogue receptor (GHSR) mutation
      d. Brain or hypothalamic tumors (e.g., germinomas, gliomas)
      e. Pituitary tumors (e.g., craniopharyngiomas, histiocytosis X)
      f. Surgical resection of the pituitary or pituitary stalk
      g. Trauma: generalized brain trauma or trauma specific to the hypothalamus, pituitary stalk, or anterior pituitary
      h. Inflammation of the pituitary or hypothalamus
      i. Irradiation of the brain or hypothalamus
    2. Primary insulin-like growth factor deficiency
      a. GH insensitivity (Laron syndrome)
      b. Post-GH receptor defects
    3. Hypothyroidism
    4. Glucocorticoid excess (Cushing syndrome)
    5. Diabetes mellitus (Mauriac syndrome)
    6. Pseudohypoparathyroidism
    7. Rickets
  E. Malnutrition
    1. Protein calorie (kwashiorkor)
    2. Generalized (marasmus)
    3. Anorexia nervosa
    4. Nutritional dwarfing and failure to thrive
    5. Micronutrient deficiencies (especially iron, zinc)
  F. Psychosocial (deprivation) dwarfism
  G. Nonendocrine chronic systemic diseases
    1. Malabsorptive disorders
      a. Celiac sprue
      b. Inflammatory bowel disease
      c. Short gut syndrome
    2. Renal disease
      a. Fanconi syndrome
      b. Renal tubular acidosis
      c. Uremia or chronic renal failure
    3. Cardiovascular disease
      a. Congenital (especially cyanotic)
      b. Congestive heart failure
    4. Pulmonary disease
      a. Cystic fibrosis
      b. Severe asthma
    5. Hepatic
      a. Chronic liver disease or liver failure
    6. Hematologic
      a. Profound anemia
      b. Thalassemia (especially if transfusion dependent)
      c. Hemosiderosis
    7. Oncologic
      a. Malignancy
      b. Secondary to treatment of oncologic process (chemotherapy or irradiation)
    8. Infectious
      a. AIDS or HIV infection (untreated)
      b. Tuberculosis
      c. Intestinal parasites
    9. Collagen vascular diseases
  H. Other genetic conditions
    1. Deletions of *SHOX* gene region of X or Y chromosomes
    2. Polymorphism: chromosome 12q11, 1q12, 2q36
    3. Russell-Silver syndrome
    4. Prader-Willi syndrome
    5. Noonan syndrome
    6. Others: Cornelia de Lange syndrome, insulin receptor gene mutations (Donohue syndrome), Rubinstein-Taybi syndrome, Aarskog syndrome, Bloom syndrome, Cochayne syndrome, progeria, Seckel syndrome
  I. Inborn errors of metabolism
    1. Glycogen storage diseases
    2. Galactosemia
    3. Mucopolysaccharidoses
    4. Glycoproteinoses
    5. Mucolipidoses
  J. Iatrogenic
    1. Chronic glucocorticoid exposure (e.g., in severe asthma, inflammatory conditions)
    Stimulant medications for ADHD

ADHD, attention deficit hyperactivity disorder; GH, growth hormone; GHRH, growth hormone–releasing hormone; GHSR, growth hormone secretagogue receptor.

relatives with similarly delayed puberty ("late blooming"). There are no other abnormalities present other than short stature and delayed puberty. A detailed history and physical examination and thorough review of the child's historical growth curve are essential steps to establishing this diagnosis; an isolated point on the growth curve at the time of the visit is insufficient. The differential diagnosis of CDGP includes Kallmann's syndrome and isolated gonadotropin deficiency; lack of anosmia can exclude the former, but only time or genetic analyses can help distinguish between CDGP and the latter. Bone age is significantly delayed, which provides reassurance that sufficient time for growth remains for the child to reach the predicted adult height. Any physical or biochemical abnormalities should suggest another diagnosis. When CDGP occurs superimposed on FSS, the child's short stature can appear severe; however, the child is still healthy, and his or her growth is still a normal variant.

Idiopathic Short Stature

Idiopathic short stature (ISS) refers to extreme short stature that does not have a diagnostic explanation after an ordinary growth evaluation. The U.S. Food and Drug Administration (FDA) set the threshold for ISS at a height more than 2.25 SD below the mean, roughly equal to the shortest 1.2% of the population. Although ISS may represent a statistical extreme, in some cases, specific genetic mutations may account for poor growth. For example, some 3% to 5% of children with ISS have deletions or mutations in the *SHOX* gene present on the short arms of the X and Y chromosomes (see below).

Intrauterine Growth Retardation and Small for Gestational Age

Intrauterine growth retardation (IUGR) results in a newborn who is small for gestational age (SGA); the most widely used definition for SGA is a birth weight less than 2.5 kg at a gestational age beyond 37 weeks or length or weight below the tenth percentile for gestational age. The SGA infant may have experienced IUGR caused by placental defects, infection (e.g., TORCH [**t**oxoplasmosis or *Toxoplasma gondii* infection, **o**ther infections, **r**ubella, **c**ytomegalovirus, and **h**erpes simplex virus]), or teratogens, but dysmorphic syndromes, chromosomal defects, and genetic mutations also account for prenatal growth impairment. Although most infants with SGA experience catch-up growth in the first 2 years of life, approximately 10% to 15% remain below the third height percentile. If history or physical examination in an SGA child suggests an intrinsic abnormality, an appropriate evaluation should be obtained (e.g., chromosomal analysis and genetics referral to evaluate possible syndromes or skeletal radiographs if the limbs are disproportionate).

Osteochondrodysplasias

The osteochondrodysplasias are a diverse group of genetic disorders whose common denominator is abnormality of cartilage, bone, or both. More than 100 different conditions falling under this heading have been identified. Most children with skeletal dysplasias grow slowly, and their growth is usually disproportionate because these disorders affect the limbs more than the torso. The ratio of upper-to-lower body segments is abnormal, but the sitting height may be only mildly reduced or normal. Moreover, based on the disorder, there may be disproportionate rates of growth between limb segments (rhizomelic affecting proximal limbs, mesomelic affecting distal limbs, or acromelic affecting the terminal parts of a limb). Osteochondrodysplasias are hereditary, so a careful family history should be obtained. However, many cases represent de novo mutations, so absence of a family history does not exclude the possibility. Careful measurement of body proportions should be taken; combined with radiographic evaluation, they can determine which bones are primarily involved (long bones, vertebrae, skull; epiphyses, metaphyses, or diaphyses).

Turner Syndrome (See Chapter 118, Figure 118-1)

Turner syndrome, a disorder in females associated with the partial or complete absence of one X chromosome, is relatively common (prevalence, one in 2500 live-born girls). As this variability suggests, girls with Turner syndrome may have a subtle or even normal phenotype. Short stature is the most common phenotypic manifestation in children and adults and is caused by loss of the *SHOX* gene. The *SHOX* gene is located on the short arm of each of the sex chromosomes in an area called the pseudoautosomal region. Genes in the pseudoautosomal regions do not undergo X inactivation, and healthy 46,XX and 46,XY individuals express two copies of these genes; thus, both copies of the *SHOX* gene are active and required for normal growth. *SHOX* encodes a transcription factor expressed in the growth plate that helps regulate chondrocyte differentiation and proliferation. Patients with Turner syndrome who lack the short arm of X (or one entire X chromosome) have only one functional copy of the *SHOX* gene. This condition, termed "*SHOX* haploinsufficiency," is responsible for the 20-cm difference in height between women with Turner syndrome and women of the referent population, as well as for several skeletal defects.

Turner syndrome may be recognized in infancy because of some characteristic features, particularly a webbed neck, lymphedema, or cardiac malformations. Beyond infancy, the two most common features are short stature and lack of puberty caused by primary ovarian failure. Skeletal abnormalities include relatively large hands and feet, a wide body, short neck, cubitus valgus (increased carrying angle with the elbows turned in and the forearms deviating away from body), genu valgum ("knock knees"), and shortened fourth metacarpals. Additional features may include ptosis, strabismus, low-set or deformed ears, micrognathia, a high-arched palate, dental abnormalities, a low posterior hairline, a shield chest, and hypoplastic areolae. Because of the phenotypic variability, Turner syndrome should be considered in any female with unexplained short stature, and a karyotype should be determined either by standard G-banding techniques or by comparative genomic hybridization.

Multiple-organ system abnormalities are associated with Turner syndrome, so a comprehensive evaluation is needed to screen for abnormalities of the aortic arch, descending aorta, kidneys, and pelvocaliceal collecting system; hearing loss; hip dysplasia (between infancy and age 4 years); scoliosis; and subtle neurocognitive deficits (especially involving visuospatial functions, although overall IQ is frequently normal). Women with Turner syndrome have an increased risk of potentially fatal aortic aneurysms and dissection and thus require lifelong monitoring.

Abnormalities of the Growth Hormone–Insulinlike Growth Factor Axis

Dysfunction may appear at any level of the GH–IGF axis, including the hypothalamus and higher brain centers (e.g., congenital malformations, trauma, inflammation, central nervous system [CNS] tumors), pituitary (e.g., structural defects, pituitary tumors, hypophysitis, idiopathic GH deficiency,) GH receptor (e.g., Laron syndrome or GH insensitivity), or postreceptor signaling defects (e.g., primary IGF-I deficiency and IGF insensitivity). Idiopathic GH deficiency (GHD) occurs in as many as one in 3500 U.S. children. Factors that raise suspicion for GHD include a history of prolonged neonatal jaundice; hypoglycemia; microphallus; traumatic delivery; craniofacial midline abnormalities (e.g., septo-optic dysplasia, holoprosencephaly, or a central maxillary incisor); family history of similar presentations; or a medical history of suprasellar tumor, CNS infection or infarction, cranial irradiation, or certain chemotherapies. Infants with congenital isolated GHD tend to have normal birth size; however, postnatal growth is overtly abnormal. Severe GHD in early childhood results in early growth failure and in slower muscular development, resulting in potentially delayed gross motor milestones, such as standing, walking, and jumping. Body composition (i.e., the relative amounts of bone, muscle, and fat) is affected in many children with severe deficiency, so that mild to moderate chubbiness is common (although GHD alone rarely causes severe obesity). Some severely GH-deficient children have recognizable, cherubic facial features characterized by maxillary hypoplasia and forehead prominence.

Other features of both congenital and acquired GHD include normal skeletal proportions, increased adiposity (especially truncal), poor lean body mass gain, delayed dentition, and delayed average age of pubertal onset. A child suspected of having GHD should be referred to a pediatric endocrinologist for diagnostic evaluation.

Poor Nutrition

Optimal statural growth requires optimal nutrition; malnutrition is the most common cause of poor growth globally (see Chapter 13). Total calorie and/or protein-calorie malnutrition suppresses hepatic IGF-I production, decreasing negative feedback to the hypothalamus and pituitary. This results in increased GH production and secretion and thus elevated basal and stimulated serum GH levels. Inadequate food intake and malabsorption are both important causes of malnutrition. Decreased nutrient intake can result from oropharyngeal malformations (e.g., Pierre Robin sequence, cleft lip or palate), abnormal oral-motor function (e.g., pervasive developmental delay), as well as loss of appetite caused by use of certain medications (e.g., stimulants for treatment of attention deficit hyperactivity disorder

or chemotherapeutic agents). Malabsorption can also cause malnutrition, and disorders such as celiac disease, inflammatory bowel disease, and cystic fibrosis can present as growth failure (see Chapter 111). Poor weight gain generally precedes the decrease, and eventual failure, of linear growth. Bone age and puberty are often delayed. Taking a detailed dietary history is essential to establishing this diagnosis. A 3-day diet log is a useful tool; this record can be analyzed for intake of total calories, macronutrients, and micronutrients. Laboratory evaluations should include all those involved in the evaluation for chronic illness.

Psychosocial Deprivation

Psychosocial growth failure, also known as psychosocial or deprivation dwarfism, is a disorder of growth associated with emotional deprivation, a pathologic environment, or both. It can affect children of all ages; failure to thrive is usually seen in infancy, but toddlers and older children often manifest bizarre behaviors surrounding food and eating and are frequently depressed. Delayed statural growth and puberty, growth arrest lines in long bones, and temporary widening of cranial sutures have been reported.

Chronic Systemic Illnesses

Many chronic illnesses are associated with short stature (see Box 73-1). General mechanisms include anorexia, nutrient malabsorption, chronic acidosis or hypoxemia, anemia, increased energy requirements, and medical therapy (e.g., glucocorticoids). In most children with short stature caused by chronic illness, weight tends to be depressed to a greater extent than height or there is a lag between the onset of weight deceleration and subsequent height deceleration. Bone age is usually delayed and approximates the height age. The growth curve typically shows a period of normal growth followed by growth deceleration or cessation consistent with the onset of illness.

Hypothyroidism

Growth failure is one of the most significant manifestations of hypothyroidism in children (see Chapter 68). Because most congenital hypothyroidism is detected with neonatal screening programs, most cases of hypothyroidism-associated growth failure are attributable to acquired hypothyroidism, most commonly from autoimmune Hashimoto (chronic lymphocytic) thyroiditis or from iodine deficiency. Growth retardation caused by acquired hypothyroidism can take several years to clearly manifest, but when it is clinically significant, it tends to be severe and progressive. Puberty is often delayed, but precocious puberty (still with a paradoxically delayed bone age) can be seen as well.

EVALUATION AND MANAGEMENT

Evaluation and therapy differ greatly depending on the cause of the short stature. The importance of a detailed history and thorough physical examination cannot be overemphasized because abnormalities of one or both often suggest the

Supine length

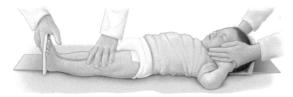

Two adults hold the child firmly in place, with the head against an inflexible board. The head is positioned in the Frankfurt plane (wherein the child's line of vision is straight up, perpendicular to the long axis of the trunk). The legs are held fully extended, and the ankles flexed perpendicularly with the feet flat against a moveable foot board.

Standing height

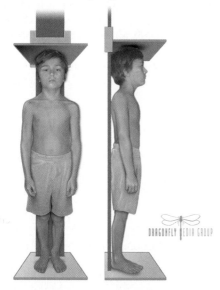

Using a wall-mounted stadiometer, the child's feet are placed together in parallel to each other, and heels, buttocks, thoracic spine, and back of head should all be up against the stadiometer's vertical axis. The child should be standing fully erect, knees straight, heels touching the ground, and head in the Frankfurt plane, as described above.

Figure 73-3 *Proper measurement techniques.*

diagnosis. The generalized method for further evaluation of normal and abnormal growth is described below.

Measurement Techniques and Growth Charts

Measurement of length or stature must be accurate and reproducible to correctly assess the degree of interval growth. Children younger than 2 years should be measured in a supine position, children older than 3 years of age should be measured standing, and children in between can be measured either way depending on their ability to stand erect for the duration of measurement. Whether supine or standing, proper measuring technique is crucial; both processes involve fixed measurement equipment and proper positioning (Figure 73-3). Recumbent lengths should be plotted on the length (ages birth-36 months)

growth charts and standing heights on the height (age 2-20 years) charts because a person's length usually exceeds his or her height. A child's current height and overall growth pattern should be interpreted within the context of standards typical for the local population. In the United States, most practitioners use the Centers for Disease Control and Prevention's growth charts, which are percentile curves that illustrate the distribution by age, in U.S. children, of length or height, weight, head circumference (for ages birth-3 years), and BMI (BMI = Weight (kg)/Height (m)^2). The data used to construct the updated 2000 growth charts were derived from cross-sectional population surveys rather than longitudinal studies following the same children over time. Thus, an individual's growth pattern may differ somewhat from the standardized pattern, especially during periods of rapid growth when timing is important (infancy and the pubertal growth spurt).

Specific Elements of the Physical Examination

When performing the physical examination, the practitioner should look for signs of underlying genetic abnormalities (e.g., dysmorphic features), midline defects suggesting possible hypothalamic or pituitary malformations (e.g., a central maxillary incisor), or systemic illness (e.g., papilledema, aphthous ulcers, rachitic rosary). The degree of dental maturation, which correlates with skeletal maturation (delayed dentition can imply delayed bone age), should also be assessed. Determining the child's pubertal status using the Tanner staging criteria is a critical part of the examination (see Chapter 67). Disproportionate growth can be ascertained via measurement of the upper-to-lower body segment ratio (upper segment length is the distance from top of the head to the top of the symphysis pubis, and lower segment length is the distance from the top of the pubic symphysis to the floor; normal ratios are 1.7:1 at birth, 1.3:1 at 3 years of age, and 1:1 by age 7 years) and arm span (distance between the tips of the middle digits with both arms fully extended; normally arm span is less than standing height before age 8 years, equal to height at ages 8-12 years, and greater than height after age 12 years).

Bone Age

A radiograph of the left hand and wrist is used to determine the child's bone age, which represents the maturation of the skeleton. The bone age is the only quantitative determination of somatic maturation, mirroring the tempo of growth and puberty and indicating the remaining growth potential. After the child is beyond infancy, an anteroposterior radiograph of the left hand and wrist is taken and compared with published standards (Greulich and Pyle or Tanner-Whitehouse); knee radiographs can be used at ages when hand and wrist films are not yet informative.

Diagnosis of Growth Hormone Deficiency

Because of the circadian rhythm of GH secretion, it is not useful to measure a random serum GH level. The evaluation of potential GHD involves measuring IGF-1 and its carrier protein,

Box 73-2 Pediatric Growth Hormone Indications

- Growth hormone deficiency
- Chronic renal insufficiency
- Turner syndrome
- AIDS wasting syndrome
- Prader-Willi syndrome
- SGA or IUGR
- Idiopathic short stature
- *SHOX* deficiency
- Noonan syndrome

IUGR, intrauterine growth retardation; SGA, small for gestational age; SHOX, short stature, homeobox containing.

IGFBP-3. Further evaluation may include provocative GH testing and is best deferred to a pediatric endocrinologist. All children with diagnosed GHD warrant magnetic resonance imaging of the brain with designated pituitary cuts to exclude an intracranial tumor or structural abnormality as the underlying cause.

Management

Management of abnormal growth depends on the underlying cause:

- **FSS** *is not a disease*, so treatment is not indicated. The patient and family should be reassured that the child is healthy, will likely enter puberty within the same time frame as his or her peers, and will likely reach a final height in keeping with family trends.
- **CDGP** *is a benign condition.* After excluding other causes of delayed puberty or abnormal growth, one can reassure the patient and family and monitor growth expectantly because spontaneous entry into puberty and attainment of family-appropriate adult height are anticipated. Because delayed puberty and consequent short stature in adolescence can have a significant social impact, it is also reasonable in severe or distressing cases to offer a short-term course of low-dose testosterone (for boys) or estrogen (for girls) to jump-start puberty. This intervention causes the adolescent to enter puberty earlier but does not increase the adult height. GH therapy is not indicated for treating CDGP.
- **Malnutrition and psychosocial:** refer to Chapters 13 and 14.
- **Hypothyroidism** is treated with daily replacement of levothyroxine, which often induces rapid catch-up growth (see Chapter 68).
- **Recombinant human (rh) GH therapy** should be managed by pediatric endocrinologists. Box 73-2 provides current FDA-approved GH indications for children. It is administered via nightly subcutaneous injections. Potential side effects include pseudotumor cerebri, slipped capital

femoral epiphysis, increased insulin resistance, increased size and number of nevi (but not increased risk of skin cancer), transient gynecomastia, and increased severity of scoliosis. Of note, current evidence supports a permissive role, but not a causal role, for both GH and IGF-I in causing cancer; thus, an active malignancy is a contraindication to treatment with GH.

FUTURE DIRECTIONS

In 2003, the FDA approved rhGH therapy for ISS (defined as height below −2.25 SD, abnormal growth velocity not expected to attain normal final height, and other causes of growth failure having been ruled out). This indication remains controversial because ISS is not a diagnosis (rather, it is a heterogeneous collection of short children), and treatment is both very expensive (estimated at $100,000 for an average gain of 1.9 inches) and often ineffective. The challenge for the future is to learn how to distinguish the various causes of ISS, determine which ones respond to rhGH, and thereby identify which children really warrant treatment.

SUGGESTED READINGS

AACE Growth Hormone Task Force: American Association of Clinical Endocrinologists: medical guidelines for clinical practice for growth hormone use in adults and children—2003 update, *Endocrine Pract* 9(1):64-76, 2003.

Centers for Disease Control and Prevention: CDC Growth Charts, United States. Available at http://www.cdc.gov/growthcharts.

Collett-Solbert PF, Petryk A, on behalf of the Members of the Drug and Therapeutics Committee of the Lawson Wilkins Pediatric Endocrine Society: Changes in Recombinant Human Growth Hormone (rhGH) Prescribing Information. Updated 2008. Available at http://www.lwpes.org/policyStatements/ChangesrhGHprescribing_information_31408.pdf.

Clayton PE: Management of the child born small for gestational age through to adulthood: a consensus statement of the International Societies of Pediatric Endocrinology and the Growth Hormone Research Society, *J Clin Endocrinol Metab* 92(3):804-810, 2007.

Greulich WW, Pyle SI: *Radiographic Atlas of Skeletal Development of the Hand and Wrist*, Stanford, 1959, Stanford University Press.

Grimberg A, Kutikov JK, Cucchiara AJ: Sex differences in patients referred for evaluation of poor growth, *J Pediatr* 146:212-216, 2005.

Growth Hormone Research Society: Consensus guidelines for the diagnosis and treatment of growth hormone (GH) deficiency in childhood and adolescence: summary statement of the GH Research Society, *J Clin Endocrinol Metab* 85(11):3990-3993, 2000.

Hall SS. Size Matters: *How Height Affects the Health, Happiness, and Success of Boys—And the Men They Become*, Boston, 2006, Houghton Mifflin.

Tanner JM, Goldstein H, Whitehouse RH: Standards for children's height at ages 2-9 years allowing for height of parents, *Arch Dis Child* 45:755-762, 1970.

Tanner JM, Whitehouse RH, Marshall WA, et al: Assessment of Skeletal Maturity and Prediction of Adult Height (TW2 Method), New York, 1975, Academic Press.

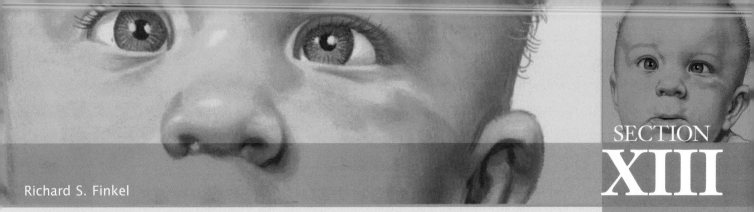

XIII

Richard S. Finkel

Disorders of the Nervous System

Seizures

Nicole Ryan

74

A seizure is a transient neurologic event caused by excessive or synchronous cortical neuronal activity in the brain. This can manifest as involuntary changes in body movement or function, sensation, awareness, or behavior. Seizures can be related to temporary conditions or associated with epilepsy, the syndrome of recurrent, unprovoked seizures.

Epilepsy is the most common serious neurologic condition, affecting 50 million people worldwide with prevalence in the United States of about 1%. Incidence rates vary by age with peaks both in early childhood and in adults older than the age of 65 years. Children with epilepsy are at higher risk for learning disorders and behavior problems.

ETIOLOGY AND PATHOGENESIS

Seizures can arise from many different sources (Figure 74-1). Primary seizures are thought to have a genetic or biochemical origin. Intracranial pathology, including tumor, vascular infarct or hemorrhage, arteriovenous malformation, trauma, infection, or congenital or developmental brain defects, can also result in seizure. They may also be provoked by electrolyte abnormalities (hypoglycemia, hypo or hypernatremia, hypocalcemia, hypomagnesemia), infection, anoxia, certain medications, drug intoxication or withdrawal, kidney or liver failure, and inborn errors of metabolism.

CLINICAL PRESENTATION

Seizure Classification

Classifying seizures is the most important first step toward appropriate diagnosis and treatment. Seizures are typically categorized as either partial or generalized. Whereas partial seizures begin in a focal area of the cerebral cortex, generalized seizures are characterized by onset simultaneously in both hemispheres and are usually associated with a loss of consciousness.

Partial seizures are further classified as either simple or complex. In simple partial seizures, consciousness is preserved, but in complex partial seizures, consciousness is impaired. Both types of partial seizures can spread to other cortical areas, resulting in a secondarily generalized seizure.

Symptoms of simple partial seizures are often determined by the cortical area involved. These symptoms may be motor, sensory, autonomic, or psychic in nature. For example, those arising from the motor cortex result in rhythmic movements of the contralateral face, arm, or leg. See Figure 74-2 for more examples.

A complex partial seizure typically begins with behavioral arrest and is followed by staring, automatisms, and postictal confusion. Occasionally, there is a preceding simple partial seizure or aura, warning of the oncoming seizure. Automatisms can include chewing, lip smacking, mumbling, or picking at clothes. Complex partial seizures typically last less than 3 minutes, and patients have no memory of the event. The postictal state can last from minutes to hours with symptoms of sleepiness, confusion, and headache, and a postictal ("Todd") hemiparesis, which typically lasts less than 1 day.

Generalized seizures are classified into six major categories: primary generalized tonic-clonic, tonic, clonic, myoclonic, atonic, and absence. The most commonly recognized type is the generalized tonic clonic seizure. These seizures are usually preceded by a cry followed by the sudden onset of tonic stiffening and convulsive movements. They are often associated with biting of the sides of the tongue and urinary incontinence.

Tonic seizures cause sudden stiffening of extensor muscles and are often associated with falls. Clonic seizures are characterized by rhythmic or semirhythmic muscle contractions, typically involving the upper extremities or the face. Myoclonic seizures consist of sudden, brief muscle contractions and may occur in clusters. Atonic seizures typically occur in patients with significant neurologic abnormalities. They are often referred to as *drop attacks* and result in sudden loss of muscle tone and collapse, frequently resulting in injury.

Absence seizures are brief episodes of impaired consciousness with no aura or postictal confusion. They typically last less than 20 seconds and are accompanied by few or no automatisms. Hyperventilation or photic stimulation often precipitates these seizures, which typically begin during childhood or adolescence, although they may persist into adulthood. In children, these seizures may initially go unnoticed and are often associated with decreased school performance or poor attention. The classic ictal electroencephalographic (EEG) correlate of absence seizures consists of 3-Hz generalized spike and slow-wave complexes (Figure 74-3).

FEBRILE SEIZURES

Febrile seizures are very common in childhood, affecting one in every 25 children between the ages of 6 months and 6 years. Children with recurrent febrile seizures are not considered to have epilepsy because the seizures are provoked by fever. Simple febrile seizures occur in neurologically normal children, are generalized, last less than 15 minutes, and do not occur more than once in a 24-hour period. Children with simple febrile seizures are at no greater risk for epilepsy than the general population. The risk is greater in children with complex febrile seizures (focal, prolonged, or multiple within 1 day) and in those with abnormal neurologic examination results or if they have a family history of epilepsy.

EPILEPSY SYNDROMES

Certain patterns of epilepsy in childhood have been further classified into syndromes (Figure 74-3). The diagnosis of these syndromes can further guide treatment choices and help to predict developmental outcome. The etiology may be

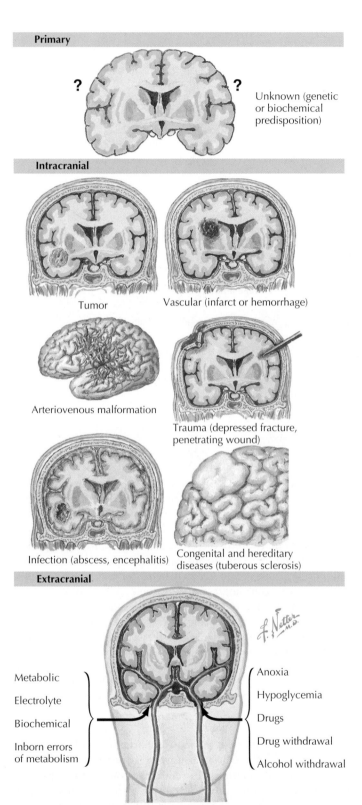

Figure 74-1 *Causes of seizures.*

flexor or extensor myoclonic jerks, which often occur in clusters upon waking or falling asleep. The cause of the syndrome may be symptomatic or cryptogenic. The typical age range is from 2 months to 2 years, but most children present in the first year of life. Although the spasms usually remit by age 2 years, often other seizure types emerge.

Lennox-Gastaut syndrome is a severe form of symptomatic generalized epilepsy. Seizures typically begin between 1 and 7 years of age and there are often premorbid developmental delays. Common seizure types include tonic, atonic, myoclonic, and atypical absence seizures. These patients are often refractory to treatment.

Benign rolandic epilepsy is the most common form of idiopathic focal epilepsy. The seizures usually occur upon awakening and involve unilateral facial sensory or motor symptoms, often with speech arrest, but without impairment of consciousness. The onset is typically between 3 and 14 years of age, and seizures usually resolve by the late teenage years. Treatment is often not necessary unless there is secondary generalization or seizures occur during the day.

Childhood absence epilepsy is a generalized idiopathic epilepsy syndrome affecting neurologically normal children between 4 and 10 years old. Absence seizures may be subtle and are often underrecognized. The EEG shows characteristic 3-Hz spike and wave discharges. The absence seizures occur multiple times a day and may be provoked in the pediatrician's office with hyperventilation.

Juvenile myoclonic epilepsy begins in the teenage years with myoclonic jerks; tonic-clonic seizures; and occasionally, absence seizures. The myoclonic jerks are typically bilateral and occur within the first few hours of waking. Patients will often describe dropping a toothbrush or silverware during breakfast. The EEG shows spike and wave complexes that may be precipitated by photic stimulation and sleep deprivation. It is an idiopathic generalized epilepsy that usually requires lifelong treatment.

STATUS EPILEPTICUS

A single seizure lasting at least 30 minutes or a cluster of seizures that occurs without a return to baseline mental status is defined as status epilepticus. This is a medical emergency because convulsive status epilepticus is associated with a 20% mortality rate. If convulsions have ceased but the patient continues to have a depressed mental status, an EEG must be performed to ensure that subclinical seizures are not ongoing.

DIFFERENTIAL DIAGNOSIS

Because the diagnosis of epilepsy is often based on clinical history and the presentation may be varied, epilepsy is commonly misdiagnosed. Conditions frequently misdiagnosed as seizures in children include psychogenic nonepileptic events, syncope, gastroesophageal reflux, stroke, tics or other movement disorders, benign myoclonus of infancy, migraine, breath-holding or shuddering spells, and parasomnia. At times, even normal childhood behavior, including temper tantrums, breath-holding, self-stimulation, and inattention, can be misinterpreted as seizures.

symptomatic (secondary to a known cause), idiopathic (presumed to be genetic), or cryptogenic (presumed to be symptomatic but with an unknown underlying abnormality).

West's syndrome is the clinical triad of infantile spasms, an interictal EEG pattern termed *hypsarrhythmia*, and developmental delay or deterioration. Infantile spasms are sudden, brief

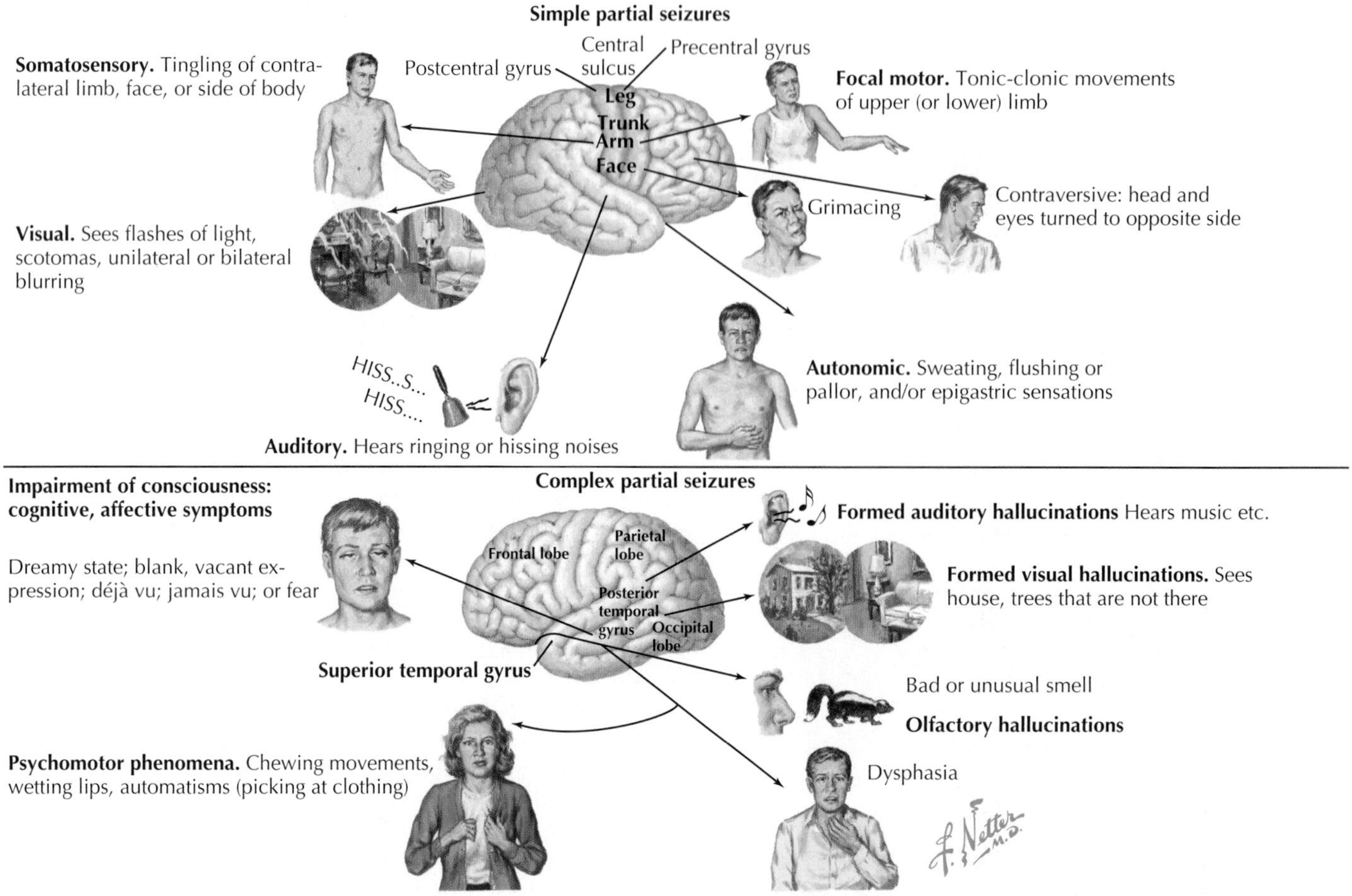

Simple partial seizures

Somatosensory. Tingling of contra-lateral limb, face, or side of body

Postcentral gyrus

Central sulcus

Precentral gyrus

Leg
Trunk
Arm
Face

Focal motor. Tonic-clonic movements of upper (or lower) limb

Grimacing

Contraversive: head and eyes turned to opposite side

Visual. Sees flashes of light, scotomas, unilateral or bilateral blurring

HISS..S...
HISS....

Autonomic. Sweating, flushing or pallor, and/or epigastric sensations

Auditory. Hears ringing or hissing noises

Complex partial seizures

Impairment of consciousness: cognitive, affective symptoms

Dreamy state; blank, vacant expression; déjà vu; jamais vu; or fear

Frontal lobe

Parietal lobe

Posterior temporal gyrus

Occipital lobe

Superior temporal gyrus

Formed auditory hallucinations Hears music etc.

Formed visual hallucinations. Sees house, trees that are not there

Bad or unusual smell
Olfactory hallucinations

Dysphasia

Psychomotor phenomena. Chewing movements, wetting lips, automatisms (picking at clothing)

Figure 74-2 *Partial seizures.*

EVALUATION

Routine blood tests should include a complete blood count and electrolytes (including glucose, calcium, and magnesium). Drug screening may be obtained when the history suggests an ingestion. Electrocardiography should be performed to evaluate for arrhythmia. If the child is younger than 1 year of age, an acute infection of the central nervous system is suspected, or there is status epilepticus, a lumbar puncture should be performed. In children younger than 2 years of age, a lumbar puncture should be strongly considered because symptoms of meningitis may be nonspecific.

EEG can support a clinical diagnosis of seizure and can help with the classification of seizure type. However, 50% of patients with epilepsy may have a normal interictal EEG. Certain techniques, such as hyperventilation and photic stimulation, may bring out abnormalities, particularly in certain epilepsy syndromes. Sometimes prolonged ambulatory or inpatient video EEG are required to capture an event and diagnosis of a seizure, differentiate from nonepileptic events, or clarify seizure type (Figure 74-4).

Structural imaging is important in the evaluation of seizure to determine whether a focal or diffuse abnormality exists. Magnetic resonance imaging (MRI) has higher sensitivity and specificity for identifying structural lesions than computed tomography (CT). These benefits outweigh the risk of sedation

required to perform MRI in young children. However, if MRI is unavailable or contraindicated (cardiac pacemaker or metal surgical implants), head CT may be performed.

Magnetoencephalography, functional MRI, and positron emission tomography are newer imaging modalities that may identify regions of abnormality not observed on standard MRIs. Research is ongoing to determine the usefulness of these techniques in surgical evaluation.

MANAGEMENT

Seizure First Aid

If a seizure is witnessed, the most important thing is to remain calm. Assess for adequate airway, breathing, and heart rate. Ensure that all objects or furniture that may cause harm are moved. Do not attempt to restrain or place anything into the mouth. Place the child recumbent and turned to the side to prevent aspiration if vomiting occurs.

It is not necessary to call an ambulance if the person is known to have epilepsy, if the seizure is shorter than 5 minutes long, and if the person is uninjured. Relatives and other caregivers often carry medicine such as rectal diazepam or buccal midazolam to rapidly end the seizure in a known epileptic patient. In a medical setting during or after a seizure, the blood sugar should be checked on an urgent basis.

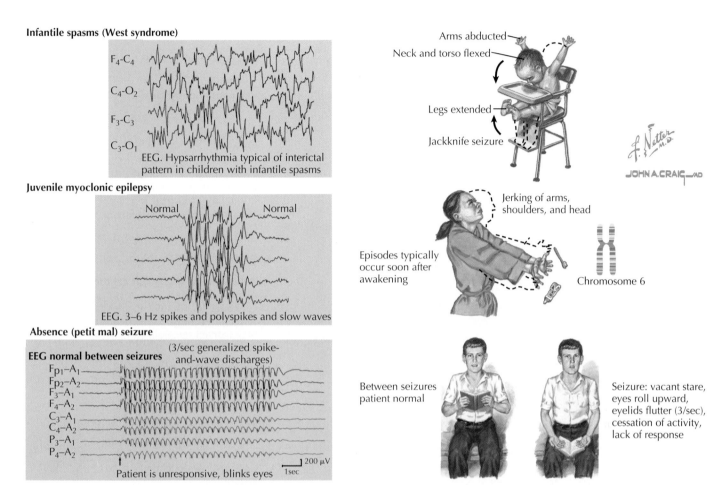

Infantile spasms (West syndrome)

F$_4$-C$_4$
C$_4$-O$_2$
F$_3$-C$_3$
C$_3$-O$_1$

EEG. Hypsarrhythmia typical of interictal pattern in children with infantile spasms

Juvenile myoclonic epilepsy

Normal   Normal

EEG. 3–6 Hz spikes and polyspikes and slow waves

Absence (petit mal) seizure

EEG normal between seizures   (3/sec generalized spike-and-wave discharges)

F$_{p1}$-A$_1$
F$_{p2}$-A$_2$
F$_3$-A$_1$
F$_4$-A$_2$
C$_3$-A$_1$
C$_4$-A$_2$
P$_3$-A$_1$
P$_4$-A$_2$

Patient is unresponsive, blinks eyes   200 µV   1sec

Arms abducted
Neck and torso flexed
Legs extended
Jackknife seizure

Jerking of arms, shoulders, and head

Episodes typically occur soon after awakening

Chromosome 6

Between seizures patient normal

Seizure: vacant stare, eyes roll upward, eyelids flutter (3/sec), cessation of activity, lack of response

Figure 74-3 *Epilepsy syndromes.*

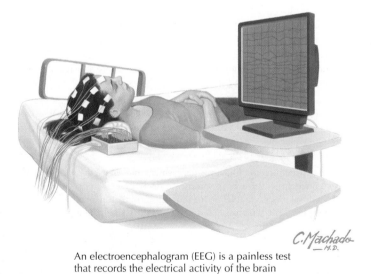

An electroencephalogram (EEG) is a painless test that records the electrical activity of the brain and helps identify abnormal activity.

Figure 74-4 *Epilepsy testing.*

ANTIEPILEPTIC MEDICATIONS

After a single unprovoked seizure, initiation of an antiepileptic drug (AED) is often not necessary. The probability of recurrence over the next 5 years after a single seizure has varied in research studies, ranging from 30% to 80%. If a second unprovoked seizure occurs, a diagnosis of epilepsy is made, and treatment is recommended.

AED choice is guided by seizure classification or the presence of an epilepsy syndrome. Common AEDs with usage and possible side effects are listed in Table 74-1.

ALTERNATIVE TREATMENTS

Unfortunately, 25% of patients with epilepsy have seizures that remain refractory to medication. Other treatment options do exist and include epilepsy surgery, the ketogenic diet, or the placement of a vagus nerve stimulator.

FUTURE DIRECTIONS

Several types of epilepsy have now been linked to specific genetic defects. Researchers continue to identify new genes and are hoping to also discover if genetic differences may play a role in

Table 74-1 Common Antiepileptic Drugs with Usage and Possible Side Effects

Drug	Usage	Use in Status Epilepticus	Possible Side Effects
Benzodiazepines • Diazepam • Lorazepam • Midazolam	Prolonged seizure (>5 minutes)	Yes; first line (rectal diazepam preparation)	Sedation Respiratory depression
Valproate	Broad spectrum JME CAE Infantile spasms	Yes	Weight gain Tremor Hair loss Pancreatitis Hepatic failure (especially children younger than age 2 years) Dose-related thrombocytopenia
Phenytoin	Partial seizures Status Epilepticus	Yes; first line (fosphenytoin IV preparation)	Gingival hyperplasia Hirsutism Allergic reactions
Phenobarbital	Broad spectrum Neonatal seizures	Yes	Psychomotor slowing Hyperactivity in younger children Allergic reactions
Carbamazepine	Partial seizures BRE	No	Leukopenia and aplastic anemia Allergic reactions May worsen generalized epilepsy
Oxcarbazepine	Partial seizures BRE	No	Hyponatremia Allergic reaction May worsen generalized epilepsy
Levetiracetam	Broad spectrum	Yes	Sedation Emotional lability Psychosis
Lamotrigine	Broad spectrum JME CAE	No	Allergic reaction May worsen myoclonic seizures
Topiramate	Broad spectrum Infantile spasms	No	Cognitive dysfunction Weight loss Kidney stones Hypohidrosis Metabolic acidosis Glaucoma (rare)
Zonisamide	Broad spectrum Infantile spasms	No	Similar to topiramate (little data in children)

BRE, benign rolandic epilepsy; CME, childhood absence epilepsy; IV, intravenous; JME, juvenile myoclonic epilepsy.

differential response to AEDs and identify those at risk for serious side effects. New imaging modalities may identify previously undiagnosed structural lesions. Medications with novel mechanisms of action are being introduced, and trials of deep brain stimulation may provide alternative options for refractory patients. The goal of rendering a patient seizure free and without treatment-related side effects remains elusive in approximately one-third of epilepsy patients and has obvious implications for that individual's ability to function fully and safely.

SUGGESTED READINGS

Hirtz D, Berg A, Bettis D, et al: Practice parameter: treatment of the child with a first unprovoked seizure: Report of the Quality Standards Subcommittee of the American Academy of Neurology and the Practice Committee of the Child Neurology Society, *Neurology* 60(2):166-175, 2003.

Riviello JJ Jr, Ashwal S, Hirtz D, et al: Practice parameter: diagnostic assessment of the child with status epilepticus (an evidence-based review): report of the Quality Standards Subcommittee of the American Academy of Neurology and the Practice Committee of the Child Neurology Society, *Neurology* 67(9):1542-1550, 2006.

Steering Committee on Quality Improvement and Management, Subcommittee on Febrile Seizures American Academy of Pediatrics: Febrile seizures: clinical practice guideline for the long-term management of the child with simple febrile seizures, *Pediatrics* 121(6):1281-1286, 2008.

Headache

Christina Lynch Szperka

75

Headache is a very common symptom in children. Epidemiologic studies estimate that approximately 20% of children have experienced a headache by the age of 5 years, jumping to 60% to 80% by school age. There are very little data about the prevalence of headaches of a specific cause other than migraine. Overall, its prevalence is in the single digits for children ages 7 to 10 years and increases to about 20% in teens. Young children with migraines are more commonly boys, but this pattern switches at the time of preadolescence.

ETIOLOGY AND PATHOGENESIS

The pathophysiology of headache is not fully understood. The blood vessels and meninges sense pain but refer it to the anterior or posterior scalp, explaining why pain from multiple etiologies and locations can feel similar.

The mechanism of migraine pain has been studied most extensively. Cortical spreading depression, which is associated with aura, is a rapid depolarization of neurons followed by prolonged hyperpolarization, which propagates as a wave through brain. This leads to release of ions, prostaglandins, and amino acids that irritate axon collateral nociceptors in the pia and dura mater. These nociceptors activate trigeminal and parasympathetic pain afferents in meningeal vessels, causing meningeal artery dilatation and activation of the trigeminal ganglion and then the trigeminal nucleus caudalis. The messages cross in the brainstem and continue to the ventroposterior thalamus, causing the sensation of pain (Figure 75-1).

CLINICAL PRESENTATION

Headaches have a wide variety of causes. Although many headaches are caused by primary headache syndromes, most commonly migraine and tension-type headache, an extensive history and physical examination must guide the differential diagnosis. Relevant elements of the history are listed in Table 75-1. The physical examination should include vital signs and general and neurological examinations, including visualization of the fundus. Table 75-2 outlines characteristics of many primary and secondary headaches, the recommended workup, and treatment where applicable.

EVALUATION AND MANAGEMENT

See Table 75-2 for workup based on specific to etiology. Indications for imaging are summarized here. Generally, magnetic resonance imaging (MRI) is preferred because it provides more detail, but CT is appropriate when looking for bony changes or bleeding or in emergent situations when MRI is not available. MR angiogram (MRA) and MR venogram (MRV) are sometimes important to obtain with MRI of the brain.

- Acute-onset, severe headache should be imaged emergently. The American Academy of Neurology Practice Parameter recommends imaging for any headache of less than 1 month's duration.
- Alteration of consciousness
- Symptoms or examination findings that suggest focal brain pathology (the brain and arteries should be imaged with MRI and MRA)
- Symptoms or examination findings that suggest increased intracranial pressure (ICP) (the brain and veins should be imaged with MRI and MRV)
- Comorbid seizures
- Change in headache quality, frequency, or severity
- Consider for any recurrent headache in which there is *no* family history of headache

Imaging is necessary before lumbar puncture if a patient has an abnormal physical examination result to ensure that it is safe to perform lumbar puncture (no signs of herniation nor significant edema). Indications for lumbar puncture (with opening pressure) include:

- Acute-onset, severe headache (looking for subarachnoid hemorrhage; the first and last tubes should be collected for a cell count to aid interpretation)
- Alteration of consciousness
- Symptoms or examination findings that suggest increased ICP
- Consider for symptoms or examination findings that suggest focal brain pathology when the differential diagnosis includes infectious or inflammatory pathology

Treatment

Treatment should be guided by the cause of the headache, and many of those are mentioned in Table 75-2. Most research in children has studied the use of medications for acute and preventive treatment of migraine.

ABORTIVE MEDICATIONS

These should be used at most two to three times per week to prevent medication overuse, which may transform headache from episodic to chronic. All abortive therapies should be given as soon as possible after symptom onset to maximize efficacy. Other than analgesics, studies of efficacy pertain to patients with migraine headache, and the intravenous (IV) therapies listed are generally for migraine except as noted above.

- **Analgesics:** remind patients of side effects; many of these are available over the counter.
  - Nonsteroidal antiinflammatory drugs (NSAIDs): contraindicated in renal disease or history of gastrointestinal (GI) bleeding
    - Ibuprofen
    - Naproxen
    - Ketorolac

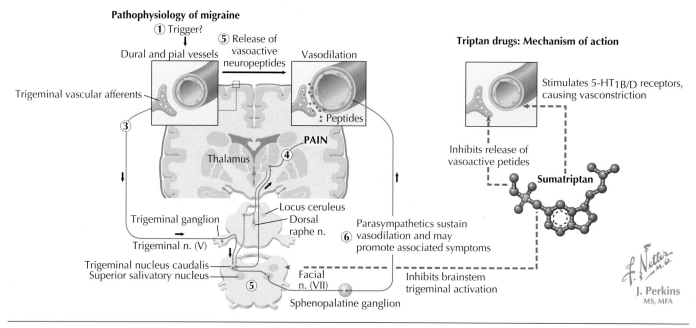

Figure 75-1 *Pathophysiology of migraine.*

- Acetaminophen: contraindicated in liver disease
- Except when other medications are contraindicated, opiates and preparations with caffeine should be avoided because they can be detrimental long term.
- **Triptans:** These are contraindicated in cardiovascular and liver disease, pregnancy, hemiplegic migraine, and patients with hypertension. Studies of triptans in teens with migraine have been limited by their extremely high response to placebo, making it difficult to prove statistical significance. Side effects include taste disturbance (for nasal sprays), burning (for injections), drowsiness, nausea or vomiting, dizziness, tingling, flushing, and infrequent chest tightness.
  - Sumatriptan (Imitrex): oral, subcutaneous, nasal effective in adolescents
  - Sumatriptan + naproxen (Treximet): no pediatric data
  - Rizatriptan (Maxalt): effective but no more than placebo
- Eletriptan (Relpax): effective but no more than placebo
- Zolmitriptan (Zomig): oral and nasal effective in adolescents
- Almotriptan (Axert): oral effective in adolescents
- Naratriptan (Amerge): no pediatric data
- Frovatriptan (Frova): pharmacokinetic data only in adolescents.
- **DHE (dihydroergotamine):** contraindicated in cardiovascular, renal, liver disease, pregnancy, hemiplegic migraine, and patients with hypertension or recent triptan use. Open-label case series of intravenous DHE in children have shown that it is effective for the treatment of status migrainosus.
  - Intranasal, subcutaneous, IV, intramuscular
  - Side effects include nausea or vomiting (can be prevented by premedication with an antiemetic), vasoconstriction.

Table 75-1 Headache History		
Description of the headache	Location and Radiation	Quality of pain
	Severity and school absence	Frequency and duration of attacks
	Pattern over time	Time of day and day of week
	Awaken patient from sleep	
Triggers and exacerbating factors	Stress at home and school	Food (MSG, caffeine, alcohol)
	Sleep changes	Valsalva maneuver, cough, sneeze
	Posture (recumbent, upright)	
Alleviating factors	Medication: clarify frequency and duration	Sleep
Associated symptoms	Nausea or vomiting	Photo- or phonophobia
	Weakness	Sensory changes
	Visual symptoms	Lacrimation or rhinorrhea
	Ptosis, pupillary changes	Pulsatile tinnitus
Other	Allergic symptoms	Snoring or teeth grinding
	Blurred vision	Family history

MSG, monosodium glutamate.

Table 75-2 Differential Diagnosis and Evaluation of Headaches by Cause

Headache Syndrome or Cause	Pertinent History	Pertinent Physical Examination Findings	Further Workup and Treatment
Primary Headaches			
Migraine			

Migraine without aura	• Unilateral frontotemporal or bilateral
	• Throbbing
	• Moderate to severe intensity
	• Aggravated by physical activity
	• Accompanied by nausea or vomiting or photophobia or phonophobia
	• 1–72 h when untreated
		Normal, may have photo- or phonophobia	• Image emergently if focal symptoms or signs
			• Non-urgent MRI if:
			  • Concern for secondary headache
			  • New onset, escalating, or changing quality
			  • Does not respond to medical therapy
			  • No family history

Migraine with aura	• Above + aura symptom for 5–60 min • Headache begins during the aura or within 60min • Aura is fully reversible visual or sensory symptoms (positive or negative) or speech disturbance (see Figure 75-2)	Normal; may fit aura	• Treat with analgesic, antiemetic, or triptan, and avoidance of triggers • Consider prophylaxis if >2 headache per month or disabling
Chronic migraine	• ≥15 or more days per month for ≥3 mo	Normal or may have photo- or phonophobia	Treat with prophylaxis
Status migrainosus	• Debilitating migraine lasting ≥72 h	Normal or may have photo- or phonophobia	• Treat with analgesic, antiemetic, or triptan • Consider IV fluids, antiemetic, ketorolac, valproic acid, DHE • IV steroids anecdotally efficacious; in adults, dexamethasone shown to decrease rebound headache
Familial hemiplegic migraine	• Migraine with aura, including motor weakness • Attacks can be triggered by mild head trauma • Positive family history; sometimes family history of cerebellar ataxia (same gene)	May include: • Focal weakness, sensory changes, or aphasia • Altered consciousness, fever, confusion	• MRI with diffusion to rule out focal lesion • Consider lumbar puncture (may have CSF pleocytosis during attack) • Consider genetic testing
Sporadic hemiplegic migraine	As above, no family history		
Basilar migraine	Migraine with aura symptoms from brainstem or both hemispheres (dysarthria, vertigo, tinnitus, hypacusis, diplopia, visual symptoms, ataxia, altered consciousness, bilateral)	May reflect aura symptoms	• Treat as above, avoiding triptans and DHE (may increase risk of stroke) • Consider prophylaxis
Retinal migraine	Monocular positive or negative visual phenomena	Visual field examination results may be abnormal	• Ophthalmologic examination to evaluate for optic neuropathy • MRI or MRA to evaluate for carotid plaque or dissection
Cyclic vomiting	• Intense nausea and vomiting lasting 1 h to 5 d; symptom-free between attacks • No GI/renal disease	Normal or may have findings of dehydration	

Abdominal migraine	• Abdominal pain lasting 1–72 hours:
	  • Midline, periumbilical, or poorly localized
	  • Dull or sore
	  • Moderate to severe
	• Accompanied by ≥2 of the following: anorexia, nausea, vomiting, pallor
	• No GI or renal disease
			• Rule out GI and other causes
			• May treat with abortive and preventive medications used for migraine

Benign paroxysmal vertigo of childhood	• Episodes of severe vertigo lasting minutes to hours • May be associated with nystagmus, vomiting, headache	Normal or may have nystagmus	Consider EEG to evaluate for seizure

continued

Table 75-2 Differential Diagnosis and Evaluation of Headaches by Cause—cont'd

Headache Syndrome or Cause	Pertinent History	Pertinent Physical Examination Findings	Further Workup and Treatment
Tension-Type Headache			
Episodic	• Bilateral • Pressing or squeezing • Mild to moderate intensity • Lasts minutes to days • May have photo- or phonophobia • May coexist with migraine	Normal or scalp may be tender	• Image if escalating or does not respond to long-term therapy • Adult studies support use of analgesics for acute management and amitriptyline for chronic headache • Other medications used for migraine, as well as psychological and complementary therapies may be helpful
Chronic	As above but ≥15 d per month for ≥3 mo		
Cluster Headache, Paroxysmal Hemicrania, Hemicrania Continua, Other Forms of Trigeminal Autonomic Cephalgia (Very Rare in Children)			
Secondary Headaches			
Headache Attributed to Non-Vascular Intracranial Disorder			
Posttraumatic headache	• No characteristic features • Severe head trauma with loss of consciousness more likely to cause demonstrable injury, but mild head trauma can cause headache as part of postconcussive syndrome	Look for signs of head trauma and focal neurologic findings	• Head imaging if examination results are abnormal; consider if duration <1 mo • Treat as the primary headache it resembles (migraine, tension type) • Consider magnesium supplementation; case series found low ionized magnesium in patients with posttraumatic headache
Intracranial neoplasm	• Headache worse in the morning • Progressive • Aggravated by physical activity, Valsalva maneuver, cough, sneeze, bending forward • Associated with nausea or vomiting	May have focal abnormality, papilledema, sixth nerve palsy, depressed mental status, abnormal gait	Head imaging
Hydrocephalus	• Headache worse in the morning • Aggravated by physical activity, Valsalva maneuver, cough, sneeze, bending forward • Associated with nausea or vomiting	May be associated with papilledema, sixth nerve palsy, depressed mental status, gait instability, increased head circumference	Head imaging
Idiopathic intracranial hypertension (pseudotumor cerebri)	• Daily, all-over aching headache aggravated by coughing or Valsalva maneuver • May be associated with tinnitus, transient visual obscurations, diplopia, constriction of visual field, enlarged blind spot • May be secondary to obesity, anemia, Lyme disease, lupus, medications (Retin A, tetracycline or minocycline, oral contraceptives)	• Papilledema; may have eye movement abnormalities • Lumbar puncture: increased opening pressure >250 mm H_2O in lateral decubitus position; patient should experience relief if pressure drained to 120–170 mm H_2O • CSF studies normal; if elevated protein or WBCs consider infectious or inflammatory causes (Lyme disease, lupus)	• MRI and MRV to exclude sinus venous thrombosis • Ophthalmologic examination with visual fields • Abnormal vision necessitates emergent therapy (lumbar puncture to drain fluid, acetazolamide ± steroids); otherwise treat underlying cause and start acetazolamide

Chiari type 1 malformation (cerebellar tonsils extend below foramen magnum into the cervical spinal canal)	• Occipital or posterior pain
	• Lasts hours to days
	• Worsens with cough or Valsalva maneuver
	• May have:
	  • Transient visual symptoms
	  • Dizziness, change in hearing, vertigo, nystagmus
	  • Other symptoms of brainstem, cerebellar, or cervical cord dysfunction, including spells of loss of consciousness
		Normal or may have:
		• Signs related to cervical cord, brainstem, lower cranial nerves, or ataxia or dysmetria
		• Signs of syrinx: abnormalities of sensation, strength, tone, reflexes
			• MRI of the brain
			• If present, MRI of the spinal cord to look for syrinx
			• Refer to neurosurgeon, although decompression may not cure headaches

Table 75-2 Differential Diagnosis and Evaluation of Headaches by Cause—cont'd

Headache Syndrome or Cause	Pertinent History	Pertinent Physical Examination Findings	Further Workup and Treatment
Intracranial hemorrhage (intraparenchymal, epidural, subdural)	• Acute onset; may be thunderclap headache • History of trauma suggests epidural or subdural • No history of trauma suggests intraparenchymal	Usually abnormal examination results, often with altered consciousness	Head CT; may require emergent surgery
Vascular malformation (aneurysm, AVM, cavernous angioma)	• New headache; may be thunderclap (suggests hemorrhage) • AVM can mimic migraine, but it is uncommon	May have painful third nerve palsy (points to posterior communicating artery aneurysm)	MRI and MRA or CTA
Sickle cell disease	• Increased incidence of migraine and tension-type headache in patients with sickle cell disease and possible association with pseudotumor cerebri • Headache can represent a pain crisis in scalp or face or symptom of stroke or moyamoya disease	Normal or may show focal signs of ischemia	• Head and vascular imaging; urgent if focal symptoms or signs • Treat as for primary headache, with precautions (e.g., acetazolamide can precipitate sickling)
Headache Attributed to Infection			
Systemic infection	Diffuse pain with symptoms of infection	Fever, signs of infection	• Guided by other symptoms or signs • Treat with analgesics
Intracranial infection	• Diffuse pain with nausea, photophobia, phonophobia • May develop chronic postmeningitis headache	May have focal findings, fever, meningismus, or altered mental status	• Head imaging if focal findings • CSF examination • Treat with antibiotics, analgesics
Headache Attributed to a Substance or Its Withdrawal			
Medication side effect	• Associated with many medications, especially hormonal contraceptives • Look for recent change in formulation (brand or generic) • Aseptic meningitis associated with ibuprofen, IVIG, penicillin, trimethoprim, and intrathecal injections	Normal, may have meningismus	• Consider changing medication or formulation • If meningismus, consider lumbar puncture
Medication overuse headache	Near-daily headache after overusing headache treatment (analgesic, ergot, triptan, opioid)	Normal	• Withdraw agent • Adult data show decreased withdrawal symptoms, less use of rescue meds when 6 day oral Prednisone taper was used during withdrawal
Headache Attributed to Disorder of Homeostasis			
Hypoxia or hypercapnia related to sleep apnea	• Bilateral headache almost daily upon awakening; resolves within 30 minutes • History of snoring	Enlarged tonsils, obese habitus may be present	Evaluate with overnight polysomnography
Psychiatric disease	• Rarely the direct cause • Comorbid anxiety and depression lead to increased rates of school absenteeism and lower rates of remission of chronic headaches	May have altered affect	Ask about mood and coping; refer for psychotherapy, biofeedback, psychiatry
Facial Pain			
Refractive error or eye misalignment	• Frontal or diffuse • Worse in afternoon or evening • History of blurred vision, eye strain, squinting	Decreased visual acuity, abnormal eye movements or alignment	Refer to optometrist or ophthalmologist

continued

Table 75-2 Differential Diagnosis and Evaluation of Headaches by Cause—cont'd

Headache Syndrome or Cause	Pertinent History	Pertinent Physical Examination Findings	Further Workup and Treatment
Rhinosinusitis	• Frontal headache accompanied by pain in face, ears, or teeth • May have halitosis, fatigue, cough, hyposmia or anosmia • Should remit within 7 days of treatment	Purulent nasal discharge, fever, tenderness to palpation of sinuses may be present	• Head imaging if diagnosis unclear • Treat with antibiotics, decongestants, nasal steroids • May be confused with tension, migraine, or medication overuse headache
Teeth or jaw abnormalities	• Frontal or diffuse headache • History of bruxism or pain precipitated by chewing or jaw movement	Noise or tenderness at TMJ with jaw movement, dental caries	• Refer to dentist or oral surgeon • Consider mouth guard, TCA, relaxation techniques for bruxism
Cervicogenic headache Occipital neuralgia	Pain referred from neck, perceived in head or face • Paroxysmal jabbing pain on the posterior scalp in the distribution of the occipital nerve • Primary headache syndromes (especially migraine) can also cause pain in a similar distribution	Tense or sore neck or back muscles Tenderness of posterior scalp	• Consider MRI of head and cervical spine to rule out posterior fossa lesion, C2 spinal nerve or joint problem, vascular imaging to rule out aneurysm • Treat cervicogenic with physical therapy • Treat with occipital nerve block; consider antiinflammatory or anticonvulsant medications

AVM, arteriovenous malformation; CSF, cerebrospinal fluid; CT, computed tomography; CTA, computed tomography angiography; DHE, dihydroergotamine; EEG, electroencephalography; GI, gastrointestinal; IV, intravenous; IVIG, intravenous immunoglobulin; MRA, magnetic resonance angiography; MRI, magnetic resonance imaging; MRV, magnetic resonance venography; TCA, tricyclic antidepressant; TMJ, temporomandibular joint; WBC, white blood cell.

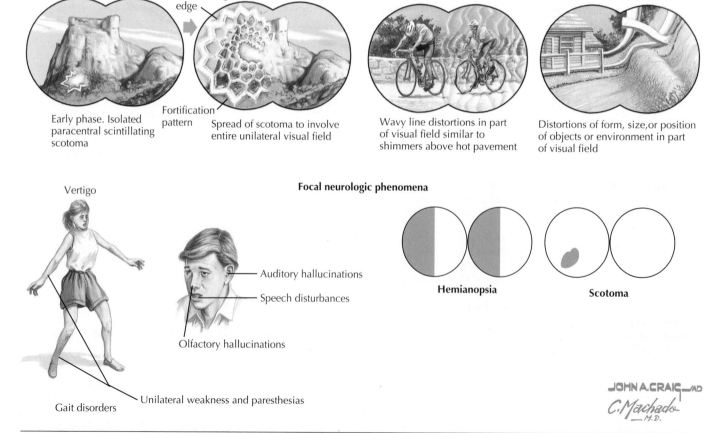

Figure 75-2 *Migraine prodromes.*

- **Antiemetics:** efficacious for migraine even in the absence of significant nausea. Side effects include dystonic reaction, which usually responds to diphenhydramine. Limited pediatric data.
  - Prochlorperazine (Compazine)
  - Metoclopramide (Reglan)
- **Steroids:** Limited data; a variety of doses are used. Use caution in patients with hypertension, renal disease, diabetes, active infections, and history of GI bleeding. Short-term side effects include increased appetite, weight gain, irritability or mood changes, insomnia, hyperglycemia.
  - Prednisone
  - Dexamethasone
- **Anticonvulsants:** see valproic acid below

PREVENTIVE MEDICATIONS

Very little data are available on children. The best evidence for migraine prophylaxis is with amitriptyline, topiramate, and valproic acid.

- **Antidepressants**
  - Amitriptyline
    - Side effects: sedation (advise taking 2–3 h before bed), dry eyes, dry mouth, urinary retention, constipation (patients should drink plenty of water), worsening of underlying prolonged QT (check electrocardiogram [ECG] before starting), weight gain
  - Other tricyclic antidepressants may have fewer side effects; these have not been studied in children
- **Antiepileptics**
  - Topiramate
    - Side effects: metabolic acidosis causing tingling (can treat with vitamin C or sodium bicarbonate supplementation), oligohidrosis or hyperthermia, weight loss, cognitive dulling and word-finding problems, uncommon kidney stones, blurred vision
  - Valproic acid
    - Oral for prophylaxis; can use IV to treat status migrainosus.
    - Side effects: hepatic and pancreatic dysfunction, anorexia or weight gain, teratogenic, tremor, hair loss, may be linked with polycystic ovarian syndrome
  - Gabapentin, lamotrigine, levetiracetam, zonisamide, carbamazepine are also used
- **NSAIDs:** contraindicated in renal disease or history of GI bleeding
  - Naproxen: see above; prophylactic use in menstrual or other predictable headache
  - Indomethacin: for hemicrania continua and paroxysmal hemicrania
- **Antiserotonergic**
  - Cyproheptadine (may also work as calcium channel blocker and is an antihistamine)
    - Side effects: sedation, appetite stimulation, weight gain
- **Antihypertensive**
  - Calcium channel blockers
    - Flunarizine has good evidence but is not available in the United States; consider verapamil
      - Side effects: sedation, weight gain, depression, constipation, arrhythmia (check ECG); contraindicated in patients with heart failure
  - β-Blockers (data thus far does not show clear efficacy)
    - Side effects: decreased exercise tolerance, hypotension or orthostasis, low energy, depression, vivid dreams, contraindicated in patients with asthma or existing depression
- **Acetazolamide:** limited pediatric data
  - Side effects: metabolic acidosis causing tingling (can treat with vitamin C or sodium bicarbonate supplementation), altered taste sensation, drowsiness, nausea, uncommon kidney stones
- **Nonpharmaceutical**
  - Riboflavin (vitamin B2): limited pediatric data; adult studies have been mixed
    - Side effects: turns urine bright yellow, diarrhea, polyuria
  - Magnesium: uncontrolled pediatric studies have been positive; one randomized, controlled trial (RCT) was equivocal
    - Side effects: diarrhea, GI upset
  - CoQ10: no RCT, open-label pediatric study in patients found to be deficient showed improvement in headache frequency and disability as level normalized
    - Side effects: stomach upset, procoagulant (may decrease efficacy of Coumadin)
  - Butterbur: no RCTs; uncontrolled study of children found decreased frequency of migraine
    - Side effects: burping, plant is toxic and can cause hepatic and pulmonary necrosis, cancer, and coagulopathy, so must use brand Petadolex, which is extracted without toxic alkaloids

NONPHARMACOLOGIC THERAPIES

These can be the mainstay of therapy or can complement medications.

- **Lifestyle changes and avoidance of triggers:** although these efforts are time consuming, they are very safe and can be quite effective. If patients find a lifestyle trigger, they often benefit from recognizing its predictability (Figure 75-3).
  - Sleep hygiene: sufficient sleep, consistent bedtime and wake-up time
  - Diet
    - Avoid fasting; eat regularly
    - Avoid dehydration; drink at least 72 oz/d of noncaffeinated fluids
    - There is poor evidence for some things thought of as common dietary triggers such as chocolate; the best evidence is for caffeine, alcohol or wine, and monosodium glutamate.
  - Exercise: believed to be preventive (not tested)
  - Stress: recognition of stressful life events at home and school, improvement of situation where possible, learning coping mechanisms (see below); stress letdown can also trigger headaches
  - Hormonal fluctuations: can be anticipated; may be appropriate to use prophylaxis for a few days around the time headache predicted

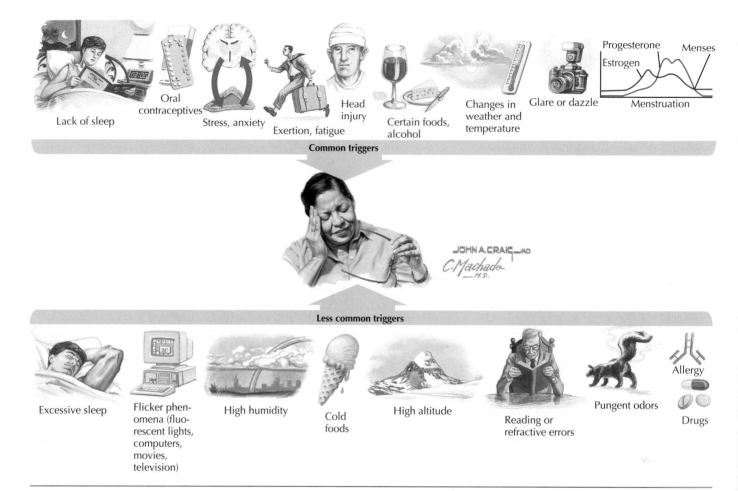

Figure 75-3 *Triggers of migraine.*

- Weather: can be anticipated; barometric changes are usually too frequent to use intermittent prophylaxis
- Odors: avoidance of smoke and perfumes
- **Psychological therapies**
  - Meta-analysis of studies of relaxation, cognitive behavioral therapy, and biofeedback in children concluded that there is good evidence that they are effective at reducing headaches
  - Biofeedback has been shown to be effective in children as young as 9 years of age
  - A listing of certified biofeedback practitioners is available at http://www.bcia.org
- **Acupuncture:** small pediatric trials, some uncontrolled, have shown a trend in reduction of headache frequency and severity for both migraine and tension-type headache

FUTURE DIRECTIONS

Most of the therapies used to treat pediatric headache are used off label, and there are limited supportive data. Furthermore, studies of pediatric headache are limited by the use of adult classification schemes, which do not entirely represent pediatric headaches. Moving forward, additional research should help to characterize the efficacy of current therapies and shed light on newer treatments such as nerve blocks and botulinum toxin that as of yet are used almost exclusively in adults.

SUGGESTED READINGS

Abend NS, Younkin D: Medical causes of headache in children, *Curr Pain Headache Rep* 11(5):401-407, 2007 Oct.

International Classification of Headache Disorders, ed 2, 2005. Available at http://ihs-classification.org/en/.

Lewis DL, Ashwal S, Dahl G, et al: Practice parameter: evaluation of children and adolescents with recurrent headaches: report of the Quality Standards Subcommittee of the American Academy of Neurology and Practice Committee of the Child Neurology Society, *Neurology* 59:490-498, 2002.

Winner P, Hershey AD, Li Z: Headaches in children. In Silberstein SS, Lipton RB, Dodick DW editors: *Wolff's Headache and Other Head Pain*, ed 8, New York, 2008, Oxford University Press, pp 665-690.

Neurocutaneous Disorders

76

Kathryn S. Taub

Neurocutaneous diseases encompass a group of diseases with neurologic manifestations and skin findings. More than 40 types have been described, and several have had a genetic mutation identified as the cause. The most common are tuberous sclerosis syndrome (TSC), von Hippel–Lindau (VHL) disease, neurofibromatosis 1 and 2 (NF-1 and -2), and Sturge-Weber syndrome (SWS).

TUBEROUS SCLEROSIS

TSC is a multisystemic disorder involving the eyes, heart, lung, kidney, brain, and skin (Figure 76-1). The prevalence of TSC is one in 6000 to 10,000 live births. TSC is caused by an autosomal dominant mutation in TSC 1 on chromosome 9q34 or TSC 2 gene on chromosome 16p13. TSC can result from inherited or de novo mutations. TSC 1 and 2 code for hamartin and tuberin, respectively, which form a protein complex involved in the regulation of cell growth. In TSC, there is loss of inhibition of Rheb (a rapamycin) by TSC 1–TSC 2 complex leading to uncontrolled cell growth of hamartomas in multiple organ systems. The diagnosis of TSC is based on clinical findings, and genetic testing is corroborative. The TSC Consensus Conference in 1998 revised the diagnostic criteria (Table 76-1); a patient must have two major features, or one major and two minor features. A patient with one major and one minor feature is diagnosed with probable TSC.

The skin lesions of TSC include hypopigmented macules ("ash leaf spots"), facial angiofibromas (adenoma sebaceum), shagreen patches, and ungual fibromas. Ash leaf spots, which are best seen with a Wood's lamp, occur in 90% of patients and appear during infancy. Facial angiofibromas first present in preschoolers on the nose and checks and become more prominent in adolescents extending down the nasolabial folds. These skin lesions may be treated with laser therapy. The shagreen patch is a fleshy, raised lesion often located on the lower back in teenagers. Ungual fibromas, a nodular lesion underneath the nail at the cuticle, also appear in teenagers.

Cardiac rhabdomyomas occur in 50% to 70% of infants with TSC. Fetal ultrasound often detects these benign tumors. The tumors may cause dysrhythmias, such as Wolff–Parkinson–White syndrome. Rhabdomyomas are often not treated and may remit spontaneously. However, an arrhythmia may require medical management, or cardiac outlet obstruction may require surgery.

Renal manifestations of TSC include renal cysts, angiolipomas, and renal cell carcinoma (RCC). The renal cysts are detected in infants and children. They may be asymptomatic or cause hypertension or renal failure. Angiolipomas occur in approximately 75% of TSC patients older than 10 years of age. They have abnormal vasculature that is at risk for bleeding, especially if the angiolipoma is larger than 3 or 4 cm. RCC is rare in TSC patients but may occur at a younger age than general population. Renal disease remains a significant cause of mortality in patients with TSC.

The neurologic manifestations of TSC include tubers, subependymal nodules, and giant cell tumors. Tubers are dysplastic cortical lesions resulting from disrupted proliferation, migration, and differentiation in early fetal life. Tubers are associated with the clinical triad of TSC—seizures, mental retardation, and behavior difficulties. Our appreciation of the significance of tuber count and its use in predicting prognosis has changed. It was once thought that increased tuber count correlated with a worse prognosis. However, the medical data supporting this correlation are quite limited. Current research suggests that the surrounding tissue of the tuber is epileptogenic and not the tuber itself. Subependymal nodules are hamartomas protruding from the ventricle walls. As they grow and calcify, they can obstruct the foramen of Monro, causing hydrocephalus. The symptoms and signs of hydrocephalus include lethargy, change in behavior, emesis, limited upgaze, headaches, and increased seizures. If a subependymal nodules grows to be larger than 1 cm, then it is considered a subependymal giant cell tumor. These are benign, but malignant transformation may occur. Subependymal giant cell tumors obstructing cerebrospinal fluid are surgically removed.

A total of 87% of TSC patients have retinal hamartomas, which are commonly asymptomatic. However, they may cause visual impairments, retinal detachment, or vitreous hemorrhage. The lungs in only adult-aged women may also be affected by TSC. Lymphangiomyomatosis cause shortness of breath, hemoptysis, or a pneumothorax.

Table 76-2 shows the tests and surveillance recommended for TSC.

The neurologic symptoms of TSC include epilepsy, behavior disturbances, and cognitive difficulties. Approximately 80% to 90% of patients have epilepsy. Infants with TSC are at risk for infantile spasms. The antiepileptic drug of choice for infantile spasms is vigabatrin. The goal of antiepileptic treatment is early seizure control to improve cognitive outcomes. Cognitive impairments range from mild learning disability to mental retardation. The neurobehavioral disturbances include autism and attention-deficit hyperactivity disorder.

VON HIPPEL–LINDAU DISEASE

VHL disease is a neurocutaneous disorder with benign and malignant tumors of the central nervous system (CNS), retina, ear, and pancreas. The prevalence is one in 39,000 live births. The inheritance pattern is autosomal dominant involving the VHL gene on chromosome 3p25, which codes for a tumor suppressor protein. The disease may also result from de novo mutations. According to the Massachusetts General Hospital Center for Cancer Risk Analysis and VHL Center, patients should be screened for VHL disease if they have a blood relative with VHL disease, have a VHL disease–associated tumor and a family history of VHL disease–associated tumors, or have two or more VHL disease–associated lesions. VHL disease–associated lesions include hemangioblastoma, clear cell renal carcinoma,

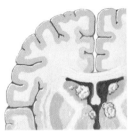

Tuber of cerebral cortex. Consisting of many astrocytes, scanty nerve cells, some abnormal sites

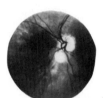

Multiple small tumors. Caudate nucleus and thalamus projecting into ventricles

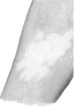

Tuber of ocular fundus

Depigmented skin area

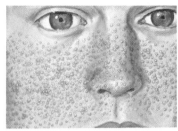

Adenoma sebaceum. Over both cheeks and bridge of nose

Sturge–Weber disease

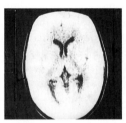

CT scan. Showing one of many calcified lesions in periventricular area

Multiple small angiomyolipomas or hamartomas in kidney

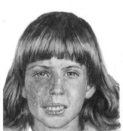

Rhabdomyomas of heart muscle

Facial nevus

CT scan. Showing calcifications and atrophy in temporoparietal area

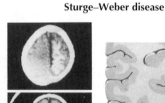

Calcific deposits and hypervascularity. In leptomeninges and gray matter of brain

X-ray film showing "railroad" calcification

Figure 76-1 *Tuberous sclerosis and Sturge-Weber disease.*

pheochromocytoma, middle ear endolymphatic sac tumor, epididymal papillary cystadenoma, pancreatic serous cystadenoma, and pancreatic neuroendocrine tumors (Figure 76-2). Individuals with clinical features listed in Box 76-1 should be screened for VHL.

Hemangioblastomas of the CNS are benign tumors with a rich capillary blood supply that develop most commonly in the second decade. They are the most common lesions in VHL disease. The CNS hemangioblastomas are located most commonly in the brainstem, spinal cord, and cerebellum. They do not metastasize but can apply pressure to adjacent structures and bleed. Treatment is observational, but surgical intervention is necessary with accelerated growth or symptomatic lesions.

Retinal angiomas are hemangioblastomas of the retina or optic nerve that develop during childhood. Complications

Table 76-1 Criteria for Tuberous Sclerosis Complex

Major Criteria	Minor Criteria
Facial angiofibromas or forehead plaque	Multiple randomly distributed dental enamel
Nontraumatic ungual or periungual fibroma	Hamartomatous rectal polyps
Hypomelanotic macules (>3)	Bone cysts
Shagreen patch (connective tissue nevus)	Cerebral white-matter "migration tracts"
Cortical tuber	Gingival fibromas
Subependymal nodule	Retinal achromic patch
Subependymal giant cell astrocytoma	Nonrenal hamartoma
Multiple retinal nodular hamartomas	"Confetti" skin lesions
Cardiac rhabdomyoma (single or multiple)	Multiple renal cysts
Lymphangiomyomatosis	
Renal angiomyolipoma	

From Roach ES, DiMario FJ, Kandt RS, et al. Tuberous Sclerosis Consensus Conference: recommendations for diagnostic evaluation. J Child Neurol 14:401-407, 1999.

Box 76-1 Screening for von Hippel–Lindau Disease

- Hemangioblastomas diagnosed before 30 years old
- >2 CNS hemangioblastomas
- Clear cell renal carcinoma diagnosed before 40 years old
- Bilateral or multiple pheochromocytomas
Family history of pheochromocytomas
- >1 pancreatic serous cystadenoma
- >1 pancreatic neuroendocrine tumor
- Multiple pancreatic cysts and any VHL disease–associated lesion
- Middle ear endolymphatic sac tumor
- Epididymal papillary cystadenoma
- Bilateral epididymal cysts

CNS, central nervous system; VHL, von Hippel–Landau.

Table 76-2 Tests and Surveillance Recommended for Tuberous Sclerosis Complex

Assessment	Initial Testing	Frequency of Testing
Brain imaging: MRI or CT scan	At diagnosis	Every 1–3 years
Renal ultrasound	At diagnosis	Every 1–3 years
Ophthalmic examination	At diagnosis	As indicated
Neurodevelopmental testing	At diagnosis	As indicated
EKG	At diagnosis	As indicated
ECHO	At diagnosis	As indicted
EEG	If seizures are present	As indicted
Chest CT	In adulthood (women only)	As indicated

CT, computed tomography; ECG, electrocardiography; ECHO, echocardiography; EEG, electroencephalography.

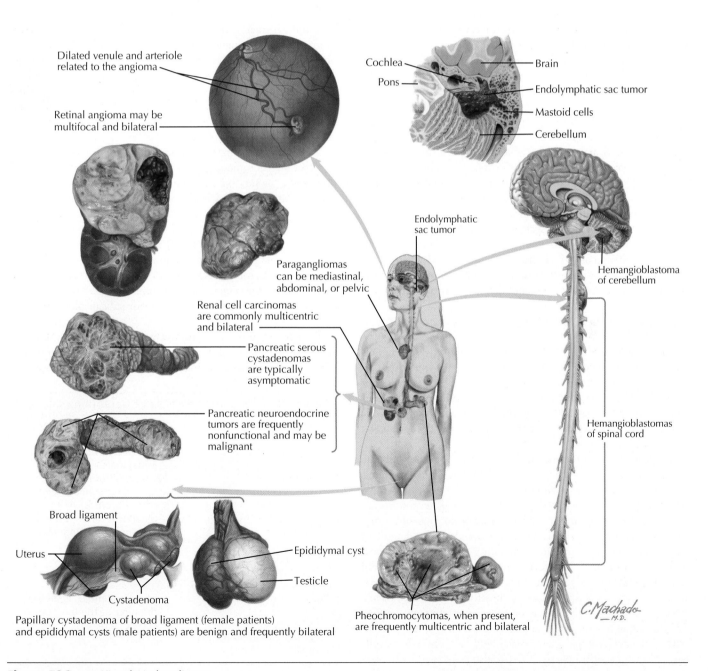

Figure 76-2 *von Hippel–Lindau disease.*

Table 76-3 Tests and Screening Recommended for von Hippel–Lindau Disease

Tumor Associated with von Hippel–Lindau Disease	Age Range for Screening	Tests or Screening Performed Yearly
Retinal hemangiomas	Infancy to adulthood	Eye examination
Pheochromocytomas	Infancy to adulthood	Plasma normetanephrine
	>11 years old to adulthood	Abdominal CT
Hemangioblastomas	>11 years old to adulthood	MRI with and without contrast of brain and spinal cord
Renal tumors and pancreatic tumors	>16 years to adulthood	Abdominal MRI or US
Endolymphatic sac tumors	At onset of symptoms or adulthood	ENT evaluation and MRI or CT or the internal auditory canal

CT, computed tomography; ENT, ear, nose, and throat; MRI, magnetic resonance imaging; US, ultrasound.
From Maher ER, Neumann HPH, Richard S. Hippel-Lindau disease: A clinical and scientific review. Eur J Human Genetics Mar 9, 2011, 1-7.

include hemorrhage leading to glaucoma, vision loss, or retinal detachment. Ophthalmic treatment for retinal lesions includes laser photocoagulation and cryotherapy.

There are many different tumors seen with VHL disease. Table 76-3 shows tests and screening recommended for VHL disease. RCC (clear cell type) is the highest mortality risk factor associated with VHL disease. It rarely develops before 20 years of age. Renal tumors greater than 3 cm are surgically excised. Patients present with hematuria, flank pain, or a palpable mass. Pheochromocytomas are associated with VHL in childhood. They are often asymptomatic with no clinical evidence of increased blood pressure. Endolymphatic sac tumors are papillary cystadenomas located within the posterior temporal bone. These lesions have an extensive vascular supply. Children present with hearing loss, vertigo, nystagmus, and facial muscle weakness. Treatment is surgical. Pancreatic lesions include cysts and serous cystadenomas, which are surgically excised when larger than 3 cm. VHL disease is also associated with asymptomatic papillary cystadenomas of the epididymis and broad ligament.

NEUROFIBROMATOSIS TYPE 1 AND 2

The inheritance pattern of neurofibromatosis type 1 (NF-1) is autosomal dominant. The disease is caused by a mutation in a tumor suppressor gene on chromosome 17, which encodes for neurofibromin. It is the most common neurocutaneous disorder (incidence of one per 3000 individuals). To make the diagnosis of NF-1, the patient must have at least two of the criteria shown in Table 76-4.

Neurofibromas are benign Schwann cell tumors of the peripheral nervous system. The subcutaneous and cutaneous neurofibromas may be asymptomatic, cause cosmetic deformity, or cause pruritus or pain (Figure 76-3). Spinal neurofibromas cause sensory and motor deficits. Plexiform neurofibromas involve multiple nerve fascicles and grow along the length of the nerve. They may invade surrounding tissue (muscle, bone, and internal organs). Plexiform neurofibromas cause pain and neurologic deficits. They may transform into spindle cell sarcomas or malignant peripheral nerve sheath tumors, which have a poor prognosis. Optic gliomas occur in approximately 15% to 25% of patients with NF-1 during childhood. Patients present with visual acuity impairment, visual field loss, optic disc swelling, strabismus, or proptosis. NF-1 is also associated with moyamoya disease (vascular abnormality within the brain), cardiac

malformations, and renal arterial stenosis. NF-1 patients may have mild behavior and cognitive difficulties. Treatment management involves analgesics for the pain associated with neurofibromas, symptomatic neurofibroma resections by soft tissue surgeons and neurosurgeons, yearly evaluations for scoliosis, annual ophthalmologic examinations for optic pathway gliomas, magnetic resonance imaging (MRI) surveillance scans for diagnosed gliomas, hypertension management, and orthopedic surgery for bone deformities.

The inheritance pattern of neurofibromatosis type 2 (NF-2) is autosomal dominant. It results from a mutation in a tumor suppressor gene on chromosome 22, which codes for neurofibromin-2. NF-2 is diagnosed if a patient has at least one of the following:

- Bilateral cranial nerve VIII masses, such as acoustic neuromas or vestibular schwannomas; *or*
- Family history of NF-2 in a first-degree relative and two of the following: neurofibroma, meningioma, glioma, schwannoma, or juvenile posterior subcapsular cataract.

Patients often present with deafness or tinnitus. Others have facial numbness, facial weakness, headaches, vertigo, or ataxia. They may also have café-au-lait lesions similar to NF-1. A

Table 76-4 Diagnostic Criteria of Neurofibromatosis-1

Café-au-lait spots	≥6 lesions that are >5 mm in prepubertal individuals and >15 mm in postpubertal individuals
Neurofibromas	≥2 neurofibromas of any type (including subcutaneous neurofibromas) or 1 plexiform neurofibroma
Freckling	In the axillary or inguinal region
Optic glioma, melanocytic iris hamartomas (also known as Lisch Nodules)	≥2
Bony lesion	Such as sphenoid dysplasia, thinning of the long bone cortex, scoliosis
First-degree family history of NF-1	

NF, neurofibromatosis.

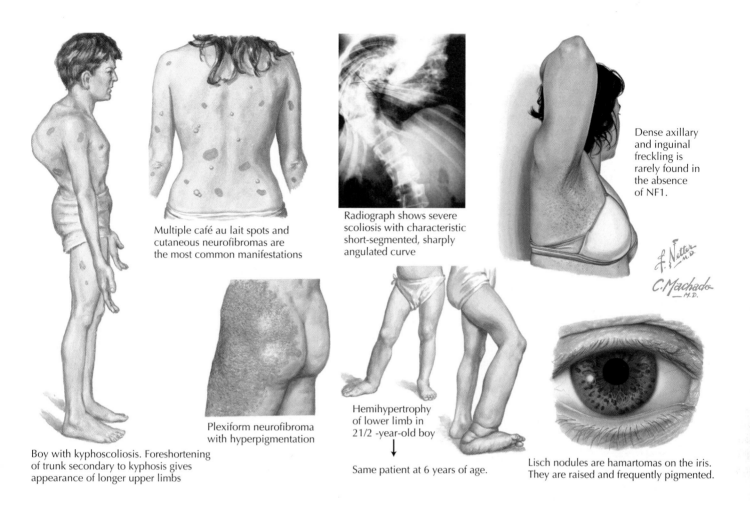

Multiple café au lait spots and cutaneous neurofibromas are the most common manifestations

Radiograph shows severe scoliosis with characteristic short-segmented, sharply angulated curve

Dense axillary and inguinal freckling is rarely found in the absence of NF1.

Plexiform neurofibroma with hyperpigmentation

Hemihypertrophy of lower limb in 2 1/2 -year-old boy

↓

Same patient at 6 years of age.

Boy with kyphoscoliosis. Foreshortening of trunk secondary to kyphosis gives appearance of longer upper limbs

Lisch nodules are hamartomas on the iris. They are raised and frequently pigmented.

Figure 76-3 *Neurofibromatosis type 1.*

workup for NF-2 involves an MRI with contrast of the internal auditory canal and brain. Genetic testing is available. A hearing test should also be performed.

STURGE-WEBER SYNDROME

SWS is a congenital disorder with an unknown cause. It is characterized by skin angiomas known as port-wine stains and leptomeningeal angiomas. The port-wine stain often involves the V1 and V2 distribution of the trigeminal nerve. The majority of children with facial port-wine stains do not have SWS, especially if they are limited to the midline of the forehead ("stork bite" birth mark). However, involvement of the upper and lower eyelid has a greater association with leptomeningeal angiomas than involvement of the upper eyelid alone. Port-wine stains may also involve the trunk and extremities. These lesions are present at birth and become hyperpigmented and larger with age. Leptomeningeal angiomas occur ipsilateral to the facial angiomas. Venous angiomas form in the pia mater and cause venous congestion leading to parenchymal hypoxia, hemispheric atrophy, and parenchymal calcifications. MRI of the brain is the study of choice to diagnose leptomeningeal angiomas. However, it should be noted that MRI findings may not be apparent at birth, so if a child is stable, the MRI should be done after 1 year

of age. However, an MRI in infancy is recommended if seizures, ocular findings, or hemiparesis is present.

The clinical presentation of SWS involves seizures (mostly symptomatic partial seizures), port-wine stains, vision loss caused by glaucoma or other vascular abnormalities of the eye, a visual field cut caused by leptomeningeal angiomas and parenchymal calcifications, and mental retardation. Children may also have strokelike episodes secondary to thrombosis within the leptomeningeal angioma or hypoxia. Hemiparesis and limb atrophy on the contralateral side of the leptomeningeal angioma often develop with the onset of seizures. Patients are also at risk for hydrocephalus secondary to venous congestion. Treatment involves laser therapy of the port-wine stains, antiepileptics for seizures, ophthalmic surgery or medical management of glaucoma, physical therapy for hemiparesis, and special educational programs for mental retardation. Occasionally, surgical treatment of refractory epilepsy is necessary. Management of recurrent strokes is problematic and no clear consensus has been reached.

SUGGESTED READINGS

Butman JA, Linehan WM, Lonser RR: Neurologic manifestations of von Hippel-Lindau disease, *JAMA* 300(11):1334-1342, 2008.

Comi A: Topical review: pathophysiology of Sturge-Weber syndrome, *J Child Neurol* 18;509-516, 2003.

Crino PB, Nathanson KL, Henske EP: Medical progress: the tuberous sclerosis complex, *N Engl J Med* 355(13):345-1356, 2006.

Ferner RE: Neurofibromatosis type 1 and neurofibromatosis type 2: a twenty-first century perspective, *Lancet Neurol* 6:340-351, 2007.

Listernick R, Ferner RE, Liu GT, et al: Optic pathway gliomas in neurofibromatosis-1: controversies and recommendations, *Ann Neurol* 61:189-198, 2007.

Lonser RR, Glenn GM, Walther M, et al: von Hippel-Lindau disease, *Lancet* 361(9374):2059-2067, 2003.

Maher ER, Neumann HPH, Richard S: Hippel-Lindau disease: A clinical and scientific review, *Eur J Human Genetics* 1-7, Mar 9, 2011.

Roach ES, DiMario FJ, Kandt RS, et al: Tuberous Sclerosis Consensus Conference: recommendations for diagnostic evaluation, *J Child Neurol* 14:401-407, 1999.

Roach ES, Sparagana SP: Diagnosis of tuberous sclerosis complex, *J Child Neurol* 19(9):643-649, 2004.

Thomas-Sohi KA, Vaslow DF, Maria BL: Sturge-Weber syndrome: a review, *Pediatr Neurol* 30(5):303-310, 2004.

Umeoka S, Koyama T, Miki Y, et al: Pictorial review of tuberous sclerosis in various organs, *RadioGraphic* 28(7):e32, 2008.

Williams VC, Lucas J, Badcock MA, et al: Neurofibromatosis type 1 revisited, *Pediatrics* 123:124-133, 2009.

Cerebral Palsy

77

Courtney J. Wusthoff

Cerebral palsy (CP) is an "umbrella diagnosis" describing a group of chronic syndromes of nonprogressive motor and postural dysfunction caused by brain lesions occurring early in development. Although the disorder does not involve degeneration over time, the features may change over the course of a lifetime. This may relate to expected changes across neurodevelopment, evolving musculoskeletal contractures, or changes in symptoms related to comorbidities. CP has an estimated prevalence of about two to three per 1000, with an overall 30-year life expectancy of 90%.

ETIOLOGY AND PATHOGENESIS

CP can arise from many different causes and is often multifactorial. The majority of children with CP have brain lesions arising prenatally or in the perinatal period. Approximately 15% of causes occur in the neonatal period or early in childhood. There is no consensus for an upper age limit when brain injury would no longer cause symptoms classified as CP. Although research groups sometimes set a maximum age of brain injury ranging from 2 to 5 years, such cutoffs are less important in clinical practice.

The most important prenatal and perinatal risk factors associated with CP are prematurity and low birth weight. About half of new cases of CP occur in children born weighing less than 1000 g. Intracranial hemorrhage, intrauterine growth retardation, and placental pathology are associated with higher rates of CP. Increasingly, infection (including maternal chorioamnionitis) and stroke have been recognized as contributors. Multiple pregnancy increases the risk for CP, with higher risk conferred with each multiple. Less common factors include congenital abnormalities, such as brain malformation and genetic disorders. In the past, many cases of CP were attributed to birth asphyxia. Although perinatal hypoxia or ischemia may be present in up to 15% of children with later CP, it is now thought that only a small number of cases are attributable to this alone. In fact, other pathologies are identified in more than 95% of cases of CP.

Causes of CP occurring after birth include infection, neonatal stroke, hypoxic brain injury, traumatic brain injury, and kernicterus. Infection may cause CP either through sepsis leading to secondary brain hypoperfusion or through direct central nervous system (CNS) infection. Kernicterus is the sequelae of severe hyperbilirubinemia; this typically causes a choreoathetoid movement disorder in conjunction with gaze abnormalities and hearing impairment.

CLINICAL PRESENTATION

Some children with CP have recognized risk factors (e.g., prematurity and low birth weight) leading to early neurologic and developmental screening. In these children, follow-up visits or early intervention evaluations should include serial assessments of tone and motor development. In the first few months, early signs may include low tone or decreased movements in affected limbs (Figure 77-1). However, not all such clinical presentations progress to CP. Although severe CP may be evident in the first months of life, it is generally difficult to make a definitive diagnosis before 1 year of age. Some clinicians advise not giving the diagnosis to a child younger than 2 years of age. This is because many children identified as having tone or motor abnormalities before 12 months of age will be free of symptoms by school age. Caution is necessary to avoid overdiagnosis in infancy.

In children without recognized risk factors, CP most often presents as delayed motor development. In the first year, this may manifest as difficulty with use of an affected limb. Some children are identified when "toe walking" becomes obvious as toddlers. Delay in reaching gross and fine motor milestones or early asymmetry in limb posture or use should prompt consideration of CP in the differential diagnosis.

In all children with CP, a careful history must confirm a nonprogressive course. The pregnancy and birth history are particularly important in eliciting possible etiologies. If the child was born prematurely or received intensive care as a neonate, specific details should be obtained. Reports of any prior neuroimaging should be obtained. The clinician should assess for other factors causing functional impairment that may mimic motor dysfunction, such as musculoskeletal or sensory difficulties. Current medications must be inventoried, particularly any sedating medications that might affect tone or motor activity at the time of examination. A developmental history is useful in recognizing the trajectory of development, as well as whether nonmotor delays coexist. A family history of neurologic disease should raise suspicion for the possibility of a genetic or metabolic process.

It can be helpful to classify CP by the type and distribution of motor impairment. There is no universally recognized set of categories, and some providers may subtype CP by more specific features, severity, and etiology (when known). Overlap may occur, with at least 10% of cases considered "mixed" CP. Nonetheless, the history and physical examination allow the clinician to classify CP into the broad categories described here.

Spastic Cerebral Palsy

Spastic CP is the most common type, comprising about 70% of cases. It may be further subdivided according to the pattern of limb involvement. Spastic diplegia primarily involves the lower limbs and may be symmetric or asymmetric (see Figure 77-1). Parents often give a history of "tiptoeing" even when walking holding on to furniture. Spastic hemiparesis involves the upper and lower limb on one side, usually with the upper extremity more affected than the lower (see Figure 77-1). Parents may report early handedness (before 2 years) or that the child did not support his or her weight as well on the affected side when crawling. Spastic quadriparesis evenly involves all four limbs (see Figure 77-1).

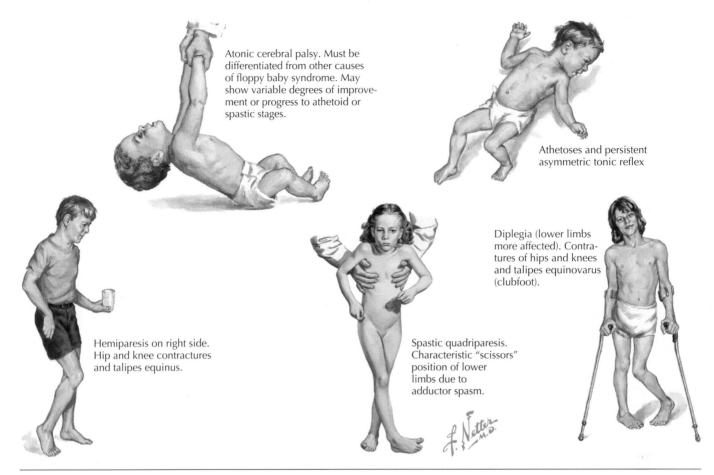

Figure 77-1 *Cerebral palsy.*

In the clinical history, patients with spastic CP are more likely to have been at risk for a cortical brain injury. Certain types of spastic CP are more highly associated with certain risks for brain injury. Children with spastic diplegia have likely had injury to both cerebral hemispheres; this most often is periventricular leukomalacia related to premature birth. Children with spastic hemiparesis more likely had unilateral injury, such as prenatal or perinatal stroke. Risk factors for stroke, such as a family history of hypercoagulability, should be assessed. Children with spastic quadriparesis may be the most severely affected. Global brain injury has often occurred, and there is a higher rate of associated cognitive impairment, epilepsy, and other disabilities.

Spastic CP is characterized on physical examination by signs of an upper motor neuron syndrome, indicating a CNS process. On observation, the clinician may see a characteristic pattern in spastic limbs (Figure 77-2). Affected upper extremities have a tendency toward flexion at the elbow and wrist, with pronation of the forearm and fingers kept closed or fisted. Affected hips are adducted and are "scissored" in extreme cases. There is partial flexion at the knees and plantarflexion at the ankles. Torticollis and truncal hyperextension or twisting may also be present. After inspection, the clinician may perform passive range of motion, revealing increased tone in the affected limb. Typical of spasticity is "velocity dependence," meaning resistance increases with more rapid passive movement. In some cases, a

spastic "catch" may be elicited in a limb with passive joint extension in which the increase in tone is momentarily reduced. Tone may also be increased in states of stress or excitement and decreased in sleep. In long-standing or severe cases, range of motion may be limited by secondary joint contractures, which typically evolve later in infancy or childhood. Strength may be intact, although this varies, and an element of weakness and motor fatigue is common. Reflex testing reveals hyperreflexia. This is the result of a hyperexcitable stretch reflex and in extreme forms presents as clonus. Extensor plantar responses (i.e., Babinski's sign) may be present on the affected side. Children with spastic CP may experience difficulties with fine motor movements (e.g., sequential finger movements) or in isolated effortful movements. In mild cases, this may appear as "clumsiness" with easy fatigability. Observation of gait is helpful both in recognizing the pattern of involvement and in assessing functional impairment.

Dyskinetic Cerebral Palsy

Dyskinetic CP comprises about 15% of CP. Involuntary movements interfering with voluntary motor function are characteristic. Dyskinetic CP may be further divided by primary movement type into choreoathetoid CP and dystonic CP (Figure 77-3). Choreoathetoid movements have a smooth, fluctuating dancelike quality (chorea) and a writhing or wriggling quality

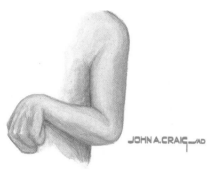

JOHN A. CRAIG—AD

Spastic paresis of upper extremity
with predominance of flexor tone

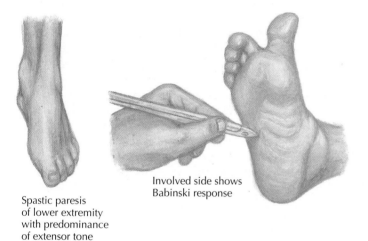

Spastic paresis
of lower extremity
with predominance
of extensor tone

Involved side shows
Babinski response

Figure 77-2 *Characteristic pattern in spastic limbs.*

(athetosis) in the distal extremities. Dystonia is abnormal sustained movement or posturing in a repetitive, patterned fashion. Although dystonias are also quite common in spastic CP, dystonic CP refers to the case in which dystonia is the primary feature. Even in retrospect, dyskinetic CP may not be noticed

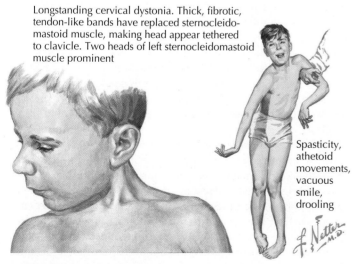

Longstanding cervical dystonia. Thick, fibrotic, tendon-like bands have replaced sternocleidomastoid muscle, making head appear tethered to clavicle. Two heads of left sternocleidomastoid muscle prominent

Spasticity, athetoid movements, vacuous smile, drooling

Figure 77-3 *Dyskinetic cerebral palsy.*

until after age 2 or 3 years because infants without CP have some degree of choreoathetoid movement. The movement disorder in dyskinetic CP reflects injury to the basal ganglia. Clinical history should explore risk factors for such injury, including hyperbilirubinemia or hypoxic ischemic injury at term or postnatally. Children with dyskinetic CP are often described as having "fluctuating tone." This reflects involuntary, often sustained muscle contraction that may be mistaken for intermittent spasticity. The physical examination should include observation of involuntary movements, recognizing that multiple movement types may be present. Sustained posture (e.g., extension of the arms) or distraction may elicit involuntary movements. Serial assessments of tone may be necessary to characterize whether spasticity is also present.

Ataxic Cerebral Palsy

Ataxic CP comprises about 5% of cases. Slow, jerky, uncoordinated movements characterize ataxic CP. Ataxia may be apparent in gait, titubation, or speech. In some cases, it may be elicited by complex motor tasks, such as rapid alternating hand movements or tandem gait. For some children, there is an associated global hypotonia. Ataxic CP may only be diagnosed after other causes of incoordination have been ruled out, such as weakness, movement disorder, and spasticity. Ataxic CP is often diagnosed later than the other subtypes because of the subtlety of symptoms in toddlers. This possibility should be kept in mind when considering "benign hypotonia" in infants.

DIFFERENTIAL DIAGNOSIS

The differential diagnosis of CP includes neurodegenerative disorders, spinal cord lesions, and neuromuscular disease. The history and physical examination typically exclude these possibilities. Alternate diagnoses are suggested by a progressive course of impairment, developmental regression or loss of milestones, peripheral hypotonia and weakness, or a family history of neurologic impairment. When dystonic symptoms present in isolation, particularly in the absence of neuroimaging abnormalities or CP risk factors, dopa-responsive dystonia should be considered. This genetic movement disorder usually presents between ages 6 and 16 years, and patients respond very well to low-dose L-dopa/carbidopa administration.

EVALUATION AND MANAGEMENT

CP is a clinical diagnosis; investigations may clarify the etiology. Neuroimaging is indicated for all children with CP who have not had prior studies (i.e., in the neonatal period). Magnetic resonance imaging (MRI) is the preferred method, revealing abnormalities in 68% to 100% of children with CP. In conjunction with clinical history, MRI can help determine the cause of the brain lesion causing CP. The severity and pattern of lesions on MRI may also be helpful in guiding the prognosis.

Metabolic and genetic testing is not indicated for all children with CP but should be considered if the history or examination is suggestive. Examples include dysmorphic features, a family history suggesting a genetic etiology, or characteristic

Table 77-1 Conditions Commonly Associated with Cerebral Palsy

System	Condition (Prevalence Among Children with Cerebral Palsy)
Neurodevelopmental	Speech or language disorder (38%-59%)
	Seizures (25-45%)
	Cognitive impairment (25%-75%)
Sensory	Strabismus or refractive error (50%)
	Vision impairment (10%-39%)
	Hearing impairment (4%-15%)
Nutrition	Malnutrition
	Excess adipose tissue
Gastrointestinal	Constipation (74%)
	Swallowing dysfunction (60%)
	Reflux (32%)
Respiratory	Aspiration (41%)
Orthopedic	Osteopenia
	Hip subluxation
	Scoliosis
Genitourinary	Voiding dysfunction (30%)

abnormalities on neuroimaging to suggest a metabolic cause. In cases of hemiplegia or when neuroimaging is consistent with stroke, a prothrombotic screening may be considered. Electroencephalography is only recommended if there are features of the history suggestive of seizure.

The American Academy of Neurology and the Child Neurology Society suggest screening for common comorbidities as part of the initial assessment of children with CP. Indeed, 50% to 75% of children with CP have another disability. As part of the initial assessment, screening for mental retardation, vision and hearing impairment, speech and language disorders, and disorders of oromotor function is advised. Importantly, although such screening for comorbidities is necessary, care should be taken not to assume that there is related cognitive impairment, especially in children with spastic diplegia.

Initial and follow-up visits should include screens for other conditions commonly associated with CP (Table 77-1). The pediatrician should identify these conditions and refer the patient for further evaluation and management when appropriate. Although CP itself is not curable, many commonly associated conditions are highly amenable to treatment and may impact quality of life even more than the motor impairment itself. Furthermore, mortality in CP is almost always caused by secondary difficulties, such as aspiration.

Because CP affects multiple domains of function and has many comorbidities, special attention should be paid to the integration of care. Ideally, a multidisciplinary team coordinates the many aspects of a child's care. An awareness of the psychosocial needs of the family is particularly important. This includes caregiver education, identification of educational needs, facilitation of accommodations, procurement and maintenance of adaptive devices, referral to appropriate community groups or resources (e.g., United Cerebral Palsy, WE MOVE), and discussions of respite care, when appropriate.

In managing the motor dysfunction of CP, many options exist. Unfortunately, there is a paucity of evidence to support specific treatments in children. The brain lesion causing CP is not correctable. Treatment instead targets specific symptoms affecting function or quality of life.

Oromotor Dysfunction

Oromotor dysfunction can affect communication, nutritional intake, and control of secretions. Speech therapy is used to facilitate communication and to help with oromotor training. Occupational therapy may facilitate oral nutritional intake. In some cases, a gastrostomy may provide a safer, more efficient means of providing medications and nutrition to the child.

Drooling is a very common problem for children with CP. Therapies can train and reinforce improved swallowing of saliva for some children. Oral medications may also be used to decrease saliva production. These are largely anticholinergics, including glycopyrrolate, hydroxyzine, and scopolamine. Injection of botulinum toxin into the salivary gland may also decrease saliva production. There are conflicting data regarding the comparative efficacy of oral medication versus botulinum toxin injection. In refractory cases, partial surgical resection may also be performed. However, this can cause irreversible symptoms of dry mouth and affect dentition, so should be used only after other therapies have failed. There is an increased risk of dental issues when such oromotor concerns are present.

Spasticity

A cornerstone of symptomatic treatment for CP is spasticity management. Improving spasticity can facilitate motor function. This would be the case, for instance, when improved ankle flexion facilitates ambulation for a child with spastic diplegia. In other cases, spasticity management is needed to facilitate caregiving. An example is a child with spastic quadriparesis whose positioning, dressing, and changing become much easier as limb flexion and adduction decrease. Finally, improvements in spasticity may postpone or preclude later orthopedic procedures and joint contractures.

The first step in spasticity management is detailed assessment of the involved muscle groups and the degree of spasticity in each. The modified Ashworth Scale is a grading from 0 (no increased tone) to 4 (rigid) that quantifies the subjective assessment. A quantitative record of spasticity may help track subtle responses to treatment that are gradual over time. The functional impairment the patient and family identify should guide the targets of spasticity management. If spasticity is present but causes no functional limitation, treatment need not be as aggressive.

When spasticity is focal, limited to a few muscle groups, injectable botulinum toxin can be particularly helpful. Botulinum toxin blocks neuromuscular transmission and thus relieves spasticity by partially weakening the targeted muscle. Evidence has supported its efficacy in quantitative measures of spasticity, particularly in the lower extremities, although there is conflicting evidence regarding longer term functional impact. Injections must be repeated every 3 to 8 months and should be done in conjunction with physical therapy (PT), which has a synergistic benefit. A more permanent effect is seen with phenol or ethanol injection, which causes chemodenervation of the targeted muscle.

For global spasticity, oral medications may be used. These include benzodiazepines, baclofen, tizanidine, and dantrolene. Benzodiazepines are systemic sedatives acting on GABA (γ-aminobutyric acid) in the CNS. Diazepam is among the most commonly used. Baclofen likewise works through GABA pathways but through a different mechanism. Tizanidine is an α-adrenergic medication that has been used widely but has no published evidence supporting its use in children. In each of these medications, sedation is a common adverse effect. Children with truncal low tone or drooling may also have a worsening of these symptoms. Frequently, adverse effects limit oral medications' usefulness for treatment of spasticity and argues for slow titration. Dantrolene acts directly upon muscle and thus does not have associated sedation. However, a potentially fatal hepatotoxicity has been associated with dantrolene, thus limiting its use. When baclofen is effective but associated sedation is limiting, intrathecal baclofen is an option. Intrathecal baclofen may be infused into the cerebrospinal fluid through a surgically placed pump and catheter terminating in the T10 region of the spinal cord. A single test dose infused through a standard lumbar puncture is performed initially to demonstrate benefit. Although this avoids cognitive sedation, pump-related difficulties may occur in 20% to 50% of children.

In some cases, surgical options target spasticity. This includes selective dorsal rhizotomy (SDR). SDR is partial transection of the dorsal lumbosacral spinal roots, interrupting sensory input to selected levels of the spinal cord, which in turn diminishes the motor output at that level. This is most useful for children with spasticity in the lower extremities who are old enough to have achieved a stable gait. Tendon release is another common surgical intervention, which decreases the mechanical tension across a joint that contributes to spasticity.

Finally, PT and occupation therapy (OT) are established components of spasticity management programs despite uncertainty as to the best regimen. PT focuses primarily upon lower limb motor impairment and ambulation issues, and OT addresses mainly upper limb and fine motor concerns. In many cases, a trained professional initiates this therapy and teaches parents exercises to continue at home. These customized regimens seek to build strength, maintain range of motion, reduce excessive muscle tone, and improve motor function. Caregivers should understand that medication and surgical interventions are to be used in conjunction with physical therapy, not as substitutes. Speech therapy (ST) is used to address oromotor and speech-related issues, as previously described.

Persuant to a U.S. federal law, all states are required to have an "early intervention" program for at-risk infants and children from birth to 3 years old, with screening and delivery of PT, OT, ST services usually in the home setting. At age 3 years, a transition to a local school-based system occurs. Physicians need to be aware of these services and promote them for patients with CP and other developmental disorders.

Dyskinesias

The movement disorder of dyskinetic CP is particularly difficult to treat. In some cases, chorea responds to chronic benzodiazepine administration, although again this is limited by sedation. Haloperidol has been used with success in some cases, but rigorous evidence for use in children with CP is lacking. Likewise, valproic acid use has been reported, but data regarding use in children outside of epilepsy are lacking.

For dyskinetic CP with dystonia as the primary feature, trihexyphenidyl will provide some relief, but not for all children. Injectable botulinum toxin is an option for focal symptoms, such as cervical dystonia. Intrathecal baclofen may also provide some benefit in patients with combined spastic and dyskinetic (primarily dystonic) CP.

Alternative and Complementary Therapies

It is helpful to become familiar with alternative and complementary therapies families may explore. Examples include conductive education, hyperbaric oxygen, and stem cell infusion. Unfortunately, over the past 25 years, there have been fewer than a dozen randomized controlled trials of alternative or complementary treatments for children with CP. Some have had limited evidence of benefit in case series or select populations but not enough to support an overall benefit. As such, treatments must be considered individually for physiologic plausibility, potential benefits, potential harms, and the cost and energy required.

Pain

Musculoskeletal aches from limited joint mobility are not unusual among children with CP. Painful muscle spasms occur when abrupt spastic contractions occur, usually in the severe spastic diplegic, quadriplegic, and dystonic forms of CP. These spasms often respond to the pharmacologic interventions mentioned above, especially benzodiazepines and intrathecal baclofen (if frequent).

PROGNOSIS

At the time of diagnosis and throughout the care of children with CP, caregivers often hope for prognosis of future functional impairment. It is difficult to say if or when a particular child will sit, walk, or speak. However, some features may help guide expectations. The most helpful for each particular child is the trajectory of motor development. For example, children who walk independently by 24 months are more likely to walk and climb stairs without limitation by adolescence, although their speed and coordination may be impaired. Few children who do not sit independently by 24 months will walk independently. Conversely, children who do not walk independently by 9 years of age are very unlikely to walk later in life. The Gross Motor Function Classification System is a formalized description of the trajectories of different "levels" of CP and may be useful in prognostication. Survival is related to the degree of disability. Overall life expectancy among high-functioning adults is essentially the same as the general population. However, children with CP who are immobile and without oral feeding abilities may have an average life expectancy as short as 10 years, according to Wood. This is primarily attributable to aspiration pneumonia and undernutrition.

FUTURE DIRECTIONS

Recent research has greatly enhanced understanding of the risk factors for CP. Future work will seek to clarify the distinct pathophysiologies and unifying features of these disorders. In particular, the influence of genetics on CP is an area of study rapidly expanding. An emphasis upon emerging strategies in neuroprotection may offer interventions to decrease subsequent CP in high-risk neonates. For symptom management, more research is needed to provide evidence for which interventions are most effective in children. Particularly, more data are needed to clarify which therapy regimens may be most beneficial for different children.

SUGGESTED READINGS

Ashwal S, Russman BS, Blasco PA, et al: Practice parameter: diagnostic assessment of the child with cerebral palsy: report of the Quality Standards Subcommittee of the American Academy of Neurology and the Practice Committee of the Child Neurology Society, *Neurology* 62(6):851-863, 2004.

Cooley WC: Providing a primary care medical home for children and youth with cerebral palsy, *Pediatrics* 114(4):1106-1113, 2004.

Tilton A: Management of spasticity in children with cerebral palsy, *Semin Pediatr Neurol* 16(2):82-89, 2009.

Wood E: The child with cerebral palsy: diagnosis and beyond, *Semin Pediatr Neurol* 13(4):286-296, 2006.

Demyelinating Diseases

78

Amy T. Waldman

emyelinating diseases are acquired autoimmune disorders affecting the central nervous system (CNS) in children and adolescents. Presenting with acute neurologic symptoms, these disorders are often difficult to distinguish from each other because of considerable overlap in the clinical presentation, paraclinical tests (e.g., cerebrospinal fluid [CSF] analysis), and neuroimaging features. Although some disorders, such as acute disseminated encephalomyelitis (ADEM), can be self-limited with a generally favorable prognosis, other demyelinating diseases, including multiple sclerosis (MS) and neuromyelitis optica (NMO), are chronic relapsing conditions that are potentially disabling.

ETIOLOGY AND PATHOGENESIS

The pathogenesis of demyelinating diseases is quite complex and incompletely understood. Autoimmune mechanisms are thought to have a fundamental role in the pathogenesis of these disorders, possibly initiated by an environmental trigger in a genetically susceptible individual. Previously, these disorders were thought to be primarily driven by a T-cell–mediated process; however, B-cells, macrophages, and microglia have now also been identified to have a role. Environmental factors, such as Epstein-Barr virus (EBV) and human herpes virus-6, have also been implicated in the pathogenesis of MS. Twin studies of adults with MS have revealed a 30% concordance rate among identical twins; multiple genes are probably involved. Although demyelination is a key feature of these disorders, there is axonal injury and neuronal loss as well, particularly in MS and relapsing disease, and this neuronal aspect may be the primary cause of chronic morbidity.

CLINICAL PRESENTATION AND DIFFERENTIAL DIAGNOSIS

Acute Disseminated Encephalomyelitis

Historically, ADEM was defined by the development of neurologic symptoms after a vaccination or a viral or bacterial infection. In 2007, an International Pediatric MS Study Group (IPMSSG) proposed working definitions for demyelinating disorders in children. ADEM is currently defined as a first demyelinating or inflammatory event in which the child is polysymptomatic and encephalopathic. Encephalopathy can be mild (e.g., confusion or irritability) but must be present to distinguish ADEM from a clinically isolated syndrome (described below). Although a preceding illness or infection is identifiable in approximately 75% of children (with an average latency between the febrile illness and neurologic symptoms of 7-14 days), such an event is not required for the diagnosis. Magnetic resonance imaging (MRI) of the brain typically reveals multiple large (>1-2 cm) asymmetric lesions affecting the supra- and infratentorial white matter that are easily visualized using T2-weighted and fluid-attenuated inversion recovery (FLAIR) sequences. Symmetric gray matter involvement of the thalami and basal ganglia and confluent spinal cord lesions have also been described in ADEM. CSF analysis may demonstrate an elevated white blood cell (WBC) count or protein or the presence of oligoclonal bands, although the latter is more frequent in MS. The presence of encephalopathy, a preceding illness or vaccination, large asymmetric white matter lesions on MRI, symmetric gray matter involvement, and CSF WBC greater than 50 cells/mm are highly suggestive of ADEM rather than a first attack of MS. The clinical and radiographic involvement may fluctuate for the first 3 months. Thereafter, relapses may occur in the same (recurrent ADEM) or a different (multiphasic) CNS site but must meet the diagnostic criteria for ADEM described above to differentiate these conditions from MS.

Clinically Isolated Syndrome

The IPMSSG defined a clinically isolated syndrome (CIS) as a first demyelinating event that may be monofocal or multifocal in the absence of encephalopathy (with the exception of a brainstem lesion, which may result in altered mental status, lethargy, or coma). Whereas the name suggests a single event, these disorders may represent the initial presentation of MS.

OPTIC NEURITIS

Optic neuritis is characterized by acute or subacute visual loss, altered color vision, periorbital pain that is exacerbated by eye movements, and visual field defects. The neuro-ophthalmologic examination may reveal a relative afferent pupillary defect (in unilateral cases) or optic disc edema (Figure 78-1). MRI of the orbits often reveals T2/FLAIR abnormality in the optic nerve or chiasm with or without enhancement using gadolinium. Visual recovery from idiopathic optic neuritis is excellent for most children, especially in the absence of alternate diagnoses such as NMO.

TRANSVERSE MYELITIS

Transverse myelitis (TM) is characterized by acute bilateral sensory, motor, or autonomic dysfunction localizable to the spinal cord. The distribution is typically asymmetric; however, this is not required for the diagnosis. Neurologic symptoms present rapidly, within hours to days, often beginning with sensory symptoms. Weakness, urinary dysfunction, and pain frequently occur depending on the extent and location of disease. In 2002, the Transverse Myelitis Consortium Working Group proposed diagnostic criteria for TM. According to these guidelines, inflammation in the spinal cord must be demonstrated by CSF analysis (pleocytosis or elevated immunoglobulin G [IgG] index) or MRI (gadolinium enhancement), which helps

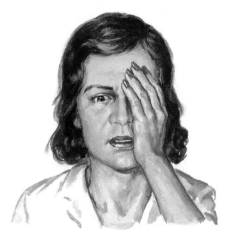
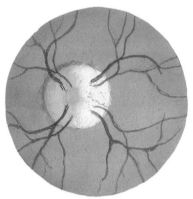
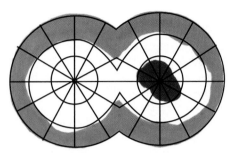

Sudden unilateral blindness, self-limited (usually 2 to 3 weeks). Patient covering one eye, suddenly realizes other eye is partially or totally blind.

Temporal pallor in optic disc, caused by delayed recovery of temporal side of optic (II) nerve

Visual fields reveal central scotoma due to acute optic neuritis

Figure 78-1 *Ocular manifestations of multiple sclerosis.*

differentiate noninflammatory causes of spinal cord disease (including previous radiation, anterior spinal artery thrombosis, tumor, syrinx, and compressive myelopathy) from idiopathic TM. However, these criteria have not been validated in children, and normal CSF profiles have been reported. If inflammation is not detected in the CSF or on MRI, the Working Group recommends a repeat spinal tap or MRI 2 to 7 days after symptom onset to further look for signs of inflammation. In addition, idiopathic TM should be distinguished from symptomatic TM caused by CNS infections (e.g., Lyme disease, HIV, human T-lymphotropic virus-1, syphilis, *Mycoplasma*, herpes simplex virus types 1 and 2 [HSV-1 and HSV-2], HHV-6, varicella zoster virus, EBV, cytomegalovirus, and enteroviruses) or systemic diseases (e.g., connective tissue disorders such as systemic lupus erythematosus, Sjögren's disease, sarcoidosis, or antiphospholipid antibody). Other than the presence of gadolinium enhancement, there are no proposed diagnostic criteria for the size or extent of the lesion upon neuroimaging of the spine. Nevertheless, whereas TM is often associated with longitudinally extensive lesions (greater than three or more vertebral segments), discrete lesions are more common in the initial presentation of MS. At the time of the development of TM, the presence of T2 or FLAIR abnormalities on an MRI of the brain is suggestive of a first attack of MS. The prognosis for full recovery is less favorable than for the other demyelinating diseases because some children may have residual disability in ambulation, sensation, or bladder function.

Multiple Sclerosis

MS is a chronic demyelinating inflammatory disorder characterized by the dissemination of neurologic signs and symptoms in time and space in both children and adults. The development of a neurologic symptom lasting more than 24 hours is referred to as an "attack" or "flare." Children most often present with paresthesias or optic neuritis. Motor dysfunction, ataxia, cranial nerve palsies, vestibular symptoms, and other neurologic

symptoms also occur. As described above, a first demyelinating event is called a CIS. The evolution of disease over time affecting multiple areas of the CNS distinguishes MS from a truly monophasic CIS. Using the 2005 Revisions to the McDonald Criteria established for adults, dissemination in time is defined clinically as the separation of symptom onset by 30 days or by the appearance of a new T2 or FLAIR lesion (compared with a reference scan) in the brain or spinal cord on MRI imaging performed at least 30 days after the onset of the initial attack (Figure 78-2). Alternatively, the detection of gadolinium enhancement on a repeat MRI scan performed at least 3 months after the onset of the initial clinical event at a different site (not corresponding to the initial clinical symptoms) also meets criteria for dissemination in time. The IPMSSG suggested that in children a time frame of 3 months be used for both the appearance of a new T2 or FLAIR lesion or gadolinium-enhancing lesion. Dissemination in space is defined by objective clinical evidence of two or more lesions (i.e., two or more abnormalities found on neurologic examination either transiently or permanently). MRI and lumbar puncture can also be performed to document dissemination in space. According to the McDonald criteria and IPMSSG, dissemination in space is fulfilled by three of the following four features: (1) at least one gadolinium-enhancing brain or spinal cord lesion or nine T2 hyperintense lesions in the brain or spinal cord in the absence of a gadolinium-enhancing lesion, (2) at least three periventricular lesions, (3) at least one juxtacortical lesion, or (4) at least one infratentorial or spinal cord lesion. Children are less likely than adults to fulfill these criteria. Therefore, dissemination in space can also be demonstrated in a patient with an MRI showing two or more lesions (one of which must be in the brain) consistent with MS and the presence of oligoclonal bands or an increased IgG index in the CSF. These criteria have not been validated in children but are supported by the IPMSSG and used in clinical practice. Most children have relapsing-remitting MS; primary progressive MS and progressive relapsing MS are rare. Although there are limited data, the natural history of pediatric MS suggests a

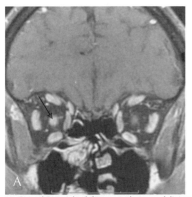

(A) Coronal T1-weighted, fat-saturated, post–gadolinium-enhanced image shows enhancement and enlargement of the right optic nerve (*arrow*).

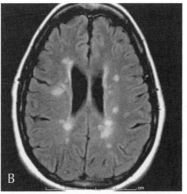

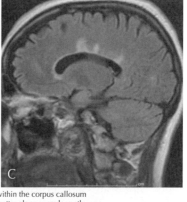

(B and C) Axial and sagittal FLAIR images with increased T2 signal within the corpus callosum and paraventricular white matter with extension into central white matter along vascular pathways

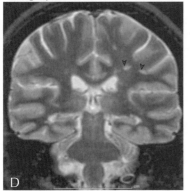

Also illustrated in **D**, coronal T2, where the typical oval lesions are oriented along vascular pathways, typical of "Dawson fingers" (*arrowheads*).

Reprint with permission from Misulis K, Heat T. Netter's Concise Neurology, page 303. Saunders, Elseiver 2007.

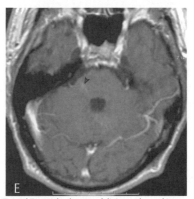

(E) Axial T1-weighted post–gadolinium-enhanced image shows enhancement of T2 bright lesion shown in other sequences in the right cerebellar penduncle. The enhancement suggests disease activity.

(F) Sagittal T2-weighted image shows T2 bright lesion in posterior cord at C2-3.

Figure 78-2 *Imaging of multiple sclerosis.*

slower progression of disease than in adults; however, children develop secondary progressive MS at younger ages than adults.

Neuromyelitis Optica

NMO is a chronic, relapsing demyelinating disease of the CNS affecting the optic nerves and spinal cord either concurrently or sequentially (with attacks separated by months). The symptoms can be significant with complete vision loss and quadriplegia or paraplegia depending on the location and extent of spinal cord involvement. Clinical criteria for the diagnosis include the presence of optic neuritis and acute myelitis. In addition, children must have a longitudinally extensive lesion extending over three or more vertebral segments on spinal MRI or have a positive NMO-IgG antibody. This IgG autoantibody binds selectively to the aquaporin-4 water channel, a component of a protein complex found in the foot processes of astrocytes at the blood–brain barrier, causing complement activation and disrupting glutamate transport. The NMO–IgG antibody is also detected in other autoimmune diseases causing demyelination in the optic nerves, brain, and spinal cord, including Sjögren's disease. Other autoimmune markers, such as antinuclear antibody, may also be elevated even in the absence of further evidence of another autoimmune process. Although the disease is defined by lesions elsewhere in the CNS, brain lesions in the

hypothalamus, brainstem, or diffuse cerebral white matter have been described in children with typical features of NMO. CSF analysis, although not required for the diagnosis, may reveal a pleocytosis (≥50 WBC) or positive CSF NMO-IgG, although serum is preferred for the detection of the autoantibody.

EVALUATION AND MANAGEMENT

The evaluation of a child with suspected demyelinating disease varies slightly based on the suspected disorder. Most physicians use neuroimaging (MRI of the brain and cervical or thoracic spine), a lumbar puncture, neurophysiologic testing (visual evoked potentials, somatosensory evoked potentials, and brainstem auditory evoked potentials) to detect evidence of inflammation and blood work to exclude other nutritional, metabolic, and inflammatory conditions. A referral to a pediatric neuro-ophthalmologist may be helpful in symptomatic and asymptomatic patients to characterize the extent of disease, including subclinical involvement of a seemingly unaffected eye. For children with suspected MS, the IPMSSG recommends at least the following tests: complete blood count with differential, erythrocyte sedimentation rate, and antinuclear antibody. Abnormalities in these tests are not typical of demyelinating disorders. Further genetic, infectious, inflammatory, or metabolic tests depend on the clinical presentation.

Acute Therapy

Corticosteroids are used to decrease inflammation associated with demyelinating attacks. Intravenous (IV) methylprednisolone (15-30 mg/kg/d; maximum, 1 g) is given for 3 to 5 days followed by an oral corticosteroid taper (range, 2 weeks–3 months) depending on the clinical presentation and physician judgment. Relapses of all demyelinating disease may occur with corticosteroid tapers. In general, IV corticosteroids do not alter the long-term prognosis but may hasten recovery as demonstrated in the Optic Neuritis Treatment Trial (ONTT). The ONTT was a randomized clinical trial (RCT) performed in adults with acute optic neuritis. Some patients in the ONTT received oral corticosteroids without preceding IV corticosteroids. These patients had an increased recurrence rate; therefore, oral corticosteroids alone are not recommended in the management of acute optic neuritis. Second-line therapies include IV immunoglobulin (IVIG) and plasma exchange. There have been no clinical trials performed in children to evaluate the efficacy of corticosteroids, IVIG, plasma exchange, or any other therapy in acute demyelinating attacks.

Special Considerations

MULTIPLE SCLEROSIS

There are disease-modifying therapies (DMTs) that are used in adults with MS to alter the course of disease by decreasing the severity and number of relapses and reducing the number of new lesions on MRI. However, there have been no RCTs of these drugs in children; therefore, these medications are not approved by the Food and Drug Administration for younger than age 18 years. Small cohort studies have reported safety and efficacy data in children who are offered these DMTs, including intramuscular or subcutaneous interferon β-1a, subcutaneous interferon β-1b, or subcutaneous glatiramer acetate. Flulike symptoms may occur with the interferons; these symptoms may be prevented with acetaminophen or ibuprofen before the injection. Subcutaneous injections may cause local irritation. The role of natalizumab therapy in children with MS is unclear at this time, partly because of the risk of progressive multifocal leukoencephalopathy identified in adults treated with this drug.

NEUROMYELITIS OPTICA

NMO is perhaps more aggressive than other demyelinating diseases and does not respond to the immunomodulatory medications used to treat MS, making the distinction between the two important for therapeutic considerations. Similar to MS, no RCTs have been performed in children, although a small cohort study has proposed immunosuppressive agents, such as rituximab, azathioprine, or mycophenolate mofetil, may be effective.

TRANSVERSE MYELITIS

Prompt evaluation and treatment with IV methylprednisolone may result in greater recovery. Supportive care, such as mechanical intubation, may be required for cervical involvement. Relapses can occur, raising clinical suspicion for MS or NMO.

FUTURE DIRECTIONS

There is greater recognition of pediatric demyelinating disorders. Validation of the definitions set forth by the IPMSSG and others will allow for better understanding of the spectrum of these disorders in children. Additional clinical trial data about the safety and efficacy of the immunomodulatory and immunosuppressive medications in children are needed to decrease disability, especially in relapsing diseases such as MS and NMO.

SUGGESTED READINGS

Beak RW, Cleary PA, Anderson MM Jr, et al: A randomized, controlled trial of corticosteroids in the treatment of acute optic neuritis, *N Engl J Med* 326:581-588, 1992.

Hahn JS, Pohl D, Rensel M, et al: Differential diagnosis and evaluation in pediatric multiple sclerosis, *Neurology* 68(suppl 2):S13-S22, 2007.

Krupp LB, Banwell B, Tenembaum S, for the International Pediatric MS Study Group: Consensus definitions proposed for pediatric multiple sclerosis and related disorders, *Neurology* 68(suppl 2):S7-S12, 2007.

Lotze TE, Northrop JL, Hutton GJ, et al: Spectrum of pediatric neuromyelitis optica, *Pediatrics* 122:e1039-e1047, 2008.

Pohl D, Waubant E, Banwell B, et al for the International Pediatric MS Study Group: Treatment of pediatric multiple sclerosis and variants, *Neurology* 68(suppl 2):S54-S65, 2007.

Polman CH, Reingold SC, Edan G, et al: Diagnostic criteria for multiple sclerosis: 2005 revisions to the "McDonald Criteria." *Ann Neurol* 58:840-846, 2005.

Tenembaum S, Chamoles N, Fejerman N: Acute disseminated encephalomyelitis: a long-term follow-up study of 84 pediatric patients, *Neurology* 59:1224-1231, 2002.

Transverse Myelitis Consortium Working Group: Proposed diagnostic criteria and nosology of acute transverse myelitis, *Neurology* 59:499-505, 2002.

Stroke

79

David R. Bearden and Lauren A. Beslow

S troke refers to acute vascular events involving the brain or brainstem. Childhood stroke occurs at a rate approximating that of childhood brain tumors. It is among the top 10 causes of death in children and is a significant cause of morbidity among survivors. Pediatric stroke can be subdivided into perinatal stroke, occurring from 28 weeks of gestation to 1 month of age, and childhood stroke, occurring from 1 month to 18 years. Important subtypes of stroke include arterial ischemic stroke (AIS), watershed infarction, intracerebral hemorrhage (ICH), and cerebral sinus venous thrombosis (CSVT). AIS is usually defined as an acute neurologic deficit of any duration consistent with focal brain ischemia conforming to an arterial distribution. Transient ischemic attacks (TIAs) are defined as focal deficits in a vascular territory lasting less than 24 hours, with some authors including the caveat that there must be no magnetic resonance imaging (MRI) evidence of infarction (Figure 79-1).

ETIOLOGY AND PATHOGENESIS

Estimates of the incidence of stroke in children range from two to 13 per 100,000 children per year. As opposed to adults in which ICH accounts for about 15% of stroke, ICH accounts for about half of pediatric stroke. The incidence of perinatal stroke is approximately one per 4000 live births, with 80% of these secondary to AIS. One-quarter of all strokes in children take place during the perinatal period. The incidence of cerebral venous sinus thrombosis is approximately 0.3 to 0.7 per 100,000 per year, with almost half of these occurring in the perinatal period. Strokes are more common in boys than in girls, with 55% to 60% of all childhood strokes occurring in boys. In the United States, strokes are more common among African American children, even when controlling for the presence of sickle cell disease (SCD).

Unlike adults, in whom hypertension, diabetes, and atherosclerosis predominate as risk factors for ischemic stroke, children presenting with AIS have much more varied etiologies. Approximately 50% of children presenting with stroke have an obvious underlying cause at the time of presentation, with arteriopathy, congenital heart disease, and sickle cell anemia representing some of the most common causes. In an additional 20% to 40%, an underlying cause can be found with further investigation. Somewhere between 10% and 30% are cryptogenic. Factors associated with pediatric AIS include inherited or acquired prothrombotic states, cardiac disease, arteriopathies or vasculopathies, trauma, and infections (Box 79-1). In older teenagers, traditional risk factors for adults, such as hypertension, diabetes, high cholesterol, and smoking, may also play a role. Cocaine or sympathomimetic medications are additional risk factors. Watershed strokes can be seen after cardiac arrest or other causes of shock, near drowning, and cardiac surgery.

ICH in children is also etiologically distinct from ICH in adults. Unlike adults, in whom hypertension and amyloid angiopathy are the most common causes, childhood ICH is most commonly caused by ruptured vascular malformations (e.g., arteriovenous malformations, cavernomas, and aneurysms), hematologic abnormalities, and brain tumors (Box 79-2 and Figure 79-2).

The major risk factors for CSVT include dehydration, head and neck infections, hypercoagulable states, malignancies, congenital heart disease, inflammatory bowel disease, oral contraceptives, and the use of certain chemotherapeutics.

AIS occurs when occlusion of an artery with a thrombus or embolus prevents blood flow to the region supplied by that artery. In watershed infarctions, global or near-global hypoperfusion preferentially damages areas on the border of two different vascular territories. The end result is a complex chain of events in cerebral neurons and support cells in which lack of oxygen and glucose leads to mitochondrial dysfunction, ion pump failure, calcium influx, and glutamate-induced neurotoxicity, eventually producing cell necrosis or apoptosis. The extent of ischemic damage to the region is determined by oxygen demand, collateral blood flow, and time to reperfusion. After an acute ischemic insult, there is a core area of infarction in which cells have sustained irreversible injury. This core is surrounded by an area with reversible ischemia known as the *ischemic penumbra*. If no further improvement of blood flow takes place or if additional insults occur, the tissue within the penumbra will eventually infarct over a period of hours to days, potentially causing additional neurologic impairment. In TIAs perfusion is restored before infarction can take place, and neuronal dysfunction induced by ischemia is reversed.

In ICH, blood extravasates into the brain parenchyma (intraparenchymal hemorrhage) into the ventricles (intraventricular hemorrhage), or into the subarachnoid space (subarachnoid hemorrhage). Intraparenchymal hemorrhage causes neuronal damage through a combination of mechanical damage and chemical irritation. Secondary ischemic stroke can occur as well because of mechanical deformation of cerebral vasculature by mass effect, vasospasm, and altered pressure dynamics leading to decreased cerebral perfusion pressure. Intraventricular hemorrhage can lead to hydrocephalus.

In CSVT, obstruction of venous blood by clot formation alters blood flow dynamics and overall venous drainage is decreased. Increased cerebral venous pressure causes resistance to cerebral perfusion and can cause venous infarction or hemorrhage. All contribute to increasing intracranial pressure (ICP).

CLINICAL PRESENTATION

The clinical presentation of a child with stroke depends on the location, type, and size of the stroke and the age and developmental stage of the child. The diagnosis is often missed or delayed in children because of a low index of suspicion on the part of care providers. In addition, children are much more likely than adults to present with headaches, seizures, or altered mental status as the first sign of stroke. Any child with acute

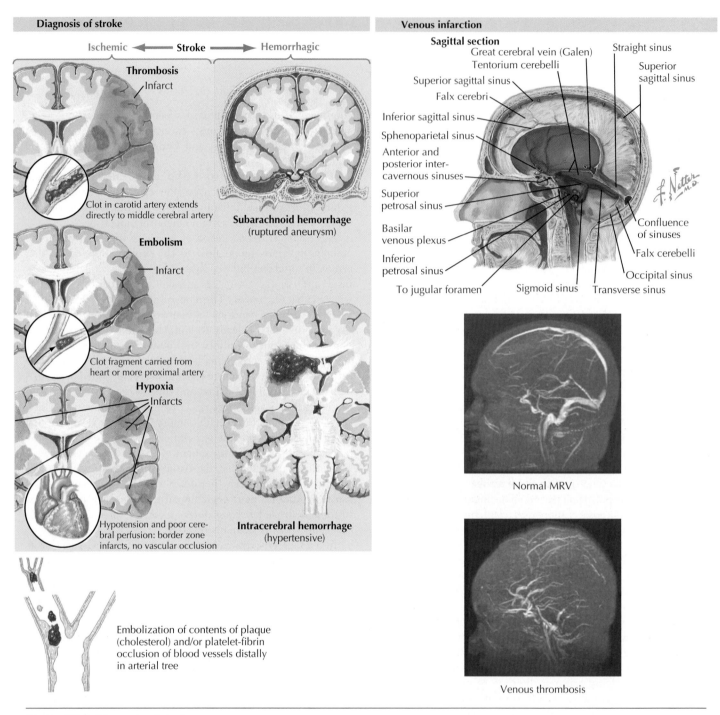

Figure 79-1 *Diagnosis of stroke.*

onset of a focal neurologic deficit should be investigated for possible stroke, but other situations that should be investigated for possible stroke include seizures in the newborn, seizures in a child of any age occurring after cardiac surgery, and changes in mental status associated with headache.

Approximately 75% percent of AIS in children occurs in the anterior circulation coming from the internal carotid arteries. Older children with ischemic strokes most commonly present with acute hemiparesis, hemisensory loss, or aphasia but may also present with isolated seizures or hemichorea. Children with posterior circulation strokes affecting the vertebrobasilar distributions may present with ataxia, vertigo, visual field cut, or brainstem signs. Children with watershed strokes can present with proximal greater than distal weakness.

Intraparenchymal hemorrhage classically presents with focal neurologic signs or seizures accompanied by severe headache, emesis, and loss of consciousness but may be impossible to distinguish from AIS based on clinical features alone because presentations vary (see Figure 79-2). Children with CSVT may present acutely with headaches, emesis, seizures, altered mental status, or focal neurologic signs but can also present more insidiously with symptoms of increased ICP such as chronic headache, blurry vision, or diplopia secondary to sixth cranial nerve palsies.

Box 79-1 Etiologies of Pediatric Arterial Ischemic Stroke

Arteriopathy
- Focal cerebral arteriopathy of childhood
- Postvaricella arteriopathy
- Moyamoya disease and syndrome
- Cervicocephalic dissection of carotid or vertebral artery
- Fibromuscular dysplasia
- Congenital vascular anomalies
- Radiation-induced arteriopathy
- HIV-related arteriopathy
- Arteriopathy secondary to meningitis or encephalitis
- Primary or secondary CNS vasculitis

Hematologic
- Sickle cell disease
- Inherited or acquired prothrombotic disorders (see Evaluation section)
- Disseminated intravascular coagulation
- Hemolytic uremic syndrome
- Thrombotic thrombocytopenic purpura
- Hypercoagulable state caused by malignancy

Cardiac
- Congenital heart disease
- Valvular heart disease
- Intracardiac septal defect permitting passage of peripheral embolus
- Intracardiac tumors: atrial myxoma, fibroelastoma, or rhabdomyoma

- Cardiomyopathy
- Arrhythmia
- Cardiac surgery or cardiac catheterization
- Extracorporeal membrane oxygenation related

Infectious
- Arteriopathy secondary to meningitis or encephalitis
- Postvaricella vasculopathy
- HIV-related arteriopathy
- Endocarditis
- Syphilis

Rheumatologic
- Primary or secondary CNS vasculitis
- Antiphospholipid syndrome

Metabolic
- Fabry disease
- Homocystinuria
- Mitochondrial disorders (e.g., MELAS)
- CADASIL
- Organic and amino acidurias

Other
- Traumatic vascular disorders
- Drug abuse, especially cocaine and amphetamines
- Inherited connective tissue disorders (e.g., Marfan's syndrome, Ehlers-Danlos syndrome)
- Migraine

CADASIL, cerebral autosomal dominant arteriopathy with subcortical infarcts and leukoencephalopathy; CNS, central nervous system; MELAS, mitochondrial encephalopathy with lactic acidosis and strokelike episodes.

DIFFERENTIAL DIAGNOSIS

The most common mimics of stroke in children are complicated migraine and postictal Todd's paralysis. Other considerations are hypoglycemia and other metabolic derangements, syncope, cerebral mass lesions such as brain tumor or abscess, demyelinating diseases, and functional disorders. Clues to the diagnosis of complicated migraine include a strong personal or family history of migraine, headache appearing after the onset of neurologic symptoms, and the presence of positive visual phenomena such as scintillating scotoma. Clues to the diagnosis of Todd's paralysis include a history of convulsions, characteristic aura occurring before the onset of symptoms, and nonvascular distribution of weakness. It is crucial to recognize that diagnoses such as complicated migraine are diagnoses of exclusion.

Box 79-2 Etiologies of Pediatric Intracerebral Hemorrhage

- Vascular malformations
- Coagulopathy
- Thrombocytopenia
- Hypertension
- Malignancy
- Mycotic aneurysms
- Hemorrhagic encephalitis or meningitis
- Ischemic stroke with hemorrhagic transformation
- CVST with hemorrhage

EVALUATION

The initial evaluation of a child with suspected stroke should focus on confirming the diagnosis and ruling out common stroke mimics. The initial history and physical examination should assess the child's ability to maintain a natural airway and adequate perfusion. Initial testing should include a complete blood count, electrolytes, blood glucose, prothrombin time, international normalized ratio, partial thromboplastin time, toxicology screen, and electrocardiography (ECG). Brain imaging should be obtained as soon as is possible. In most cases, unless MRI can be performed immediately, head computed tomography (HCT) should be performed first. HCT is fast and widely available and allows for the quick assessment of hemorrhage or mass lesions. In AIS, HCT results may be normal early in symptom evolution, but subtle findings of AIS, such as hyperdense middle cerebral artery (MCA) sign or blurring of the gray-white matter border can sometimes be seen. However, MRI is usually required to confirm the diagnosis of AIS. The most sensitive MRI sequence for detecting acute ischemic stroke is diffusion-weighted imaging with apparent diffusion coefficient; abnormalities on these sequences usually last 7 to 10 days from the acute stroke (Figure 79-3).

Additional testing should attempt to identify the etiology of the stroke (Box 79-3). Imaging of the vessels of the head and neck with MR angiography (MRA) or computed tomography angiography (CTA) should be performed to look for arterial dissection (Figure 79-4) or other arteriopathy. In certain cases, conventional catheter angiography may be necessary.

In children with ICH, MRA, CTA, or conventional angiography should be performed to evaluate for vascular

Pathology	CT scan	Pupils	Eye movements	Motor and sensory deficits	Other
Caudate nucleus (blood in ventricle)		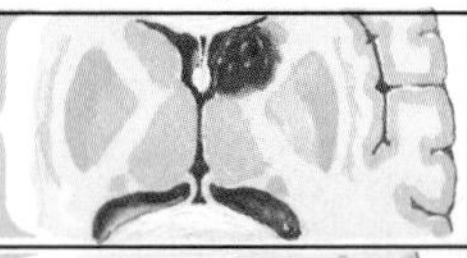 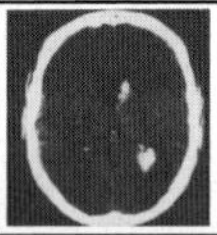 Sometimes ipsilaterally constricted	Conjugate deviation to side of lesion; slight ptosis	Contralateral hemiparesis, often transient	Headache, confusion
Putamen (small hemorrhage)		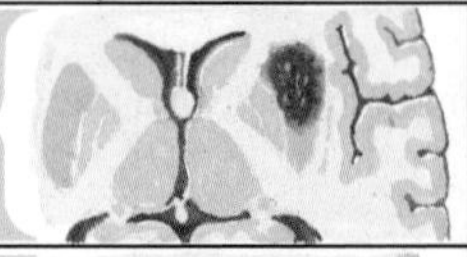 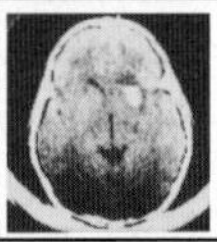 Normal	Conjugate deviation to side of lesion	Contralateral hemiparesis and hemisensory loss	Aphasia (if lesion on left side)
Putamen (large hemorrhage)		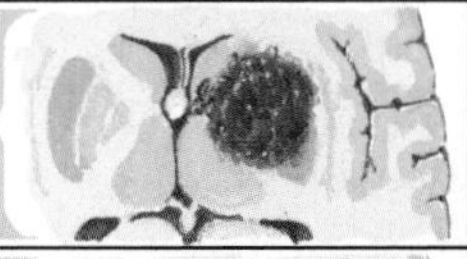 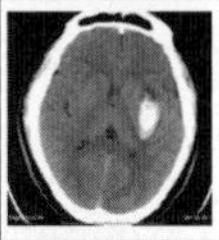 In presence of herniation, pupil dialated on side of lesion	Conjugate deviation to side of lesion	Contralateral hemiparesis and hemisensory loss	Decreased consciousness
Thalamus		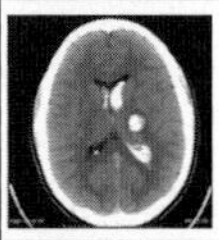 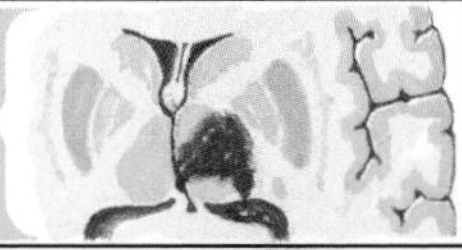 Constricted, poorly reactive to light bilaterally	Both lids retracted; eyes positioned downward and medially; cannot look upward	Slight contralateral hemiparesis, but greater hemisensory loss	Aphasia (if lesion on left side)
Occipital lobar white matter		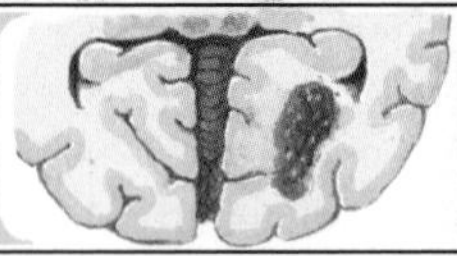 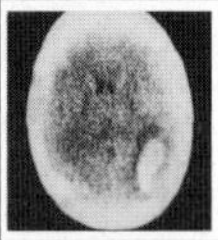 Normal	Normal	Mild, transient hemiparesis	Contralateral hemianopsia
Pons		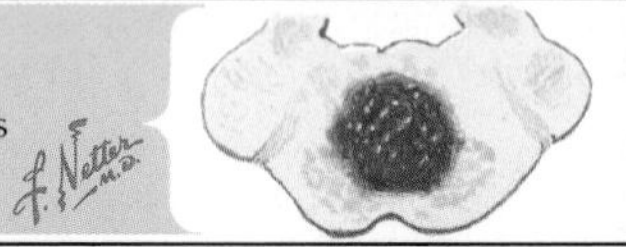 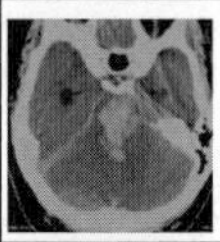 Constricted, reactive to light	No horizontal movements; vertical movements preserved	Quadriplegia	Coma
Cerebellum		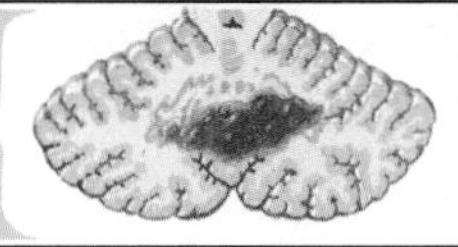 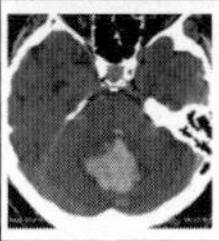 Slight constriction on side of lesion	Slight deviation to opposite side; movements toward side of lesion impaired, or sixth cranial nerve palsy	Ipsilateral limb ataxia no hemiparesis	Gait ataxia, vomiting

Figure 79-2 *Intracerebral hemorrhage: clinical manifestations related to site.*

malformations. If such a lesion is suspected but is not found in the acute setting, arterial imaging may need to be repeated at intervals because overlying hemorrhage may obscure the detection of vascular malformations. In children with suspected or confirmed CSVT, MR venography is the modality of choice to evaluate the dural sinuses for clot and residual blood flow.

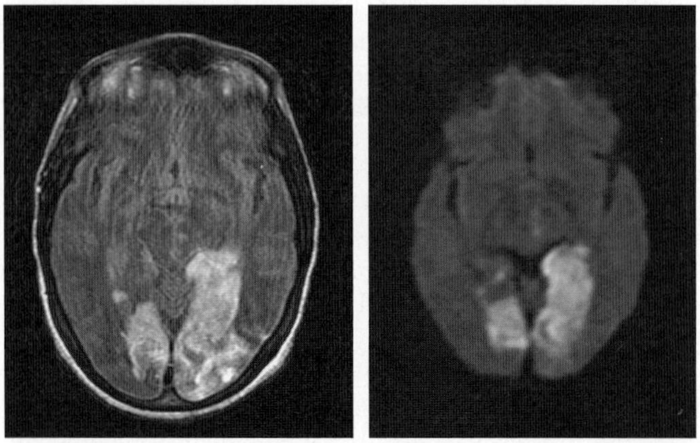

In children with either AIS or CSVT, an evaluation for prothrombotic states should be performed. Hematology should be consulted regarding the most up-to-date recommendations, but currently testing includes protein C and S activity, factor V Leiden mutation, antithrombin III level, antiphospholipid

Cerebral infarction: Bilateral posterior cerebral artery infarction affecting both occipital lobes. Left panel shows the FLAIR image, which is most sensitive for pathology. Right panel shows the diffusion weighted imaging (DWI) which is sensitive for acute or subacute infarction.

Figure 79-3 *Diagnostic tests for infarction.*

Box 79-3 Suggested Evaluation after the Hyperacute Period

Arterial ischemic stroke
- Brain, cervical, and intracranial arterial imaging (ideally MRI and MRA)
- Echocardiography with evaluation for right-to-left shunting
- Prothrombotic states (see text for laboratory tests to consider)
- Additional tests as indicated by patient history or examination

Intracerebral hemorrhage
- Brain, intracranial arterial imaging (ideally MRI and MRA)
- Bleeding diathesis if no vascular cause is determined or suspected

Cerebral sinus venous thrombosis
- Brain, intracranial venography (ideally MRI and MRV)
- Prothrombotic states (see text for laboratory tests to consider)
- Additional tests as indicated by patient history or examination

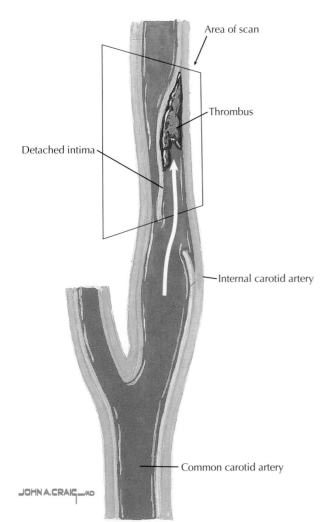

Intimal tear allows blood flow to dissect beneath intimal layer, detaching it from arterial wall. Large dissection may occlude vessel lumen.

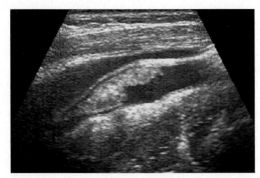

Carotid dissection: Ultrasound of the carotid artery with clot formed between layers of the artery.

Figure 79-4 *Arterial dissection.*

antibodies (anticardiolipin antibodies, β2 glycoprotein, diluted Russell's viper venom time), prothrombin gene mutation, lipoprotein (a), and homocysteine. In the appropriate clinical setting, testing for infectious causes of vasculopathy, including varicella, HIV, and syphilis, is appropriate. Evaluation of the heart for cardiac sources of thrombi should be performed in all children with AIS. Transthoracic echocardiography is usually the initial cardiac imaging modality, but if there is a strong suspicion for a cardiac source, transesophageal echocardiography should be considered, even when the transthoracic test results are normal. A "bubble study" (agitated saline contrast) during the ECG is used to detect any abnormal arterial–venous connections. More extensive testing may be appropriate if the initial evaluation does not demonstrate a clear cause or if an underlying metabolic, infectious, or inflammatory disease is suspected.

MANAGEMENT

The phrase "time is brain" has been used in adult stroke to emphasize that a stroke is a "brain attack" that should be recognized and treated emergently. Unfortunately, treatment of childhood stroke is often delayed by more than 24 hours because parents and physicians often do not recognize childhood stroke immediately. The goal of therapy in acute ischemic stroke is to save as much of the penumbra as possible by restoring perfusion, minimizing demand, and avoiding additional insults such as hyperglycemia. Thrombolytics have not been studied in children younger than 18 years of age, so therapy is primarily supportive.

An overview of initial therapy is summarized in Figure 79-5. In the acute setting, the child should lie supine with the head of the bed flat and isotonic intravenous fluids given to maximize perfusion. Hypertension is an adaptive response to ischemia, and thus outside of extreme hypertension, blood pressure should not be aggressively reduced. In most cases, aspirin should be given after hemorrhage has been excluded with neuroimaging; however, in many centers, anticoagulation with a heparinoid is started after hemorrhage is excluded. In certain cases of AIS such as arterial dissection, cardioembolism, or a known prothrombotic disorder, anticoagulation should strongly be considered (see Figure 79-5). Fever and seizures should be treated to minimize additional metabolic demands, and normoglycemia should be maintained. After the neonatal period, dextrose-free fluids are preferred to minimize the risk of hyperglycemia.

After the child has been stabilized, attention should be directed at identifying the cause of the stroke and minimizing risk factors for recurrence. Speech, physical, and occupational therapy and other rehabilitation services should be involved early in the child's hospitalization course so a recovery plan can be initiated in a timely manner.

In the acute management of patients with ICH and CSVT, the head of the bed should be elevated to at least 30 degrees to promote venous drainage and thereby lower ICP. The management of ICH is sometimes surgical, and prompt consultation with a neurosurgeon is advised. The need for acute lowering of ICP should be continuously reassessed. In CSVT, anticoagulation should be strongly considered, even in the presence of associated hemorrhage. In neonatal CSVT, the data for anticoagulation is less clear, and the approach should be highly individualized.

Special Considerations

PERINATAL ARTERIAL ISCHEMIC STROKE

The perinatal period is the most common period in childhood for ischemic strokes, and the stroke rate in neonates

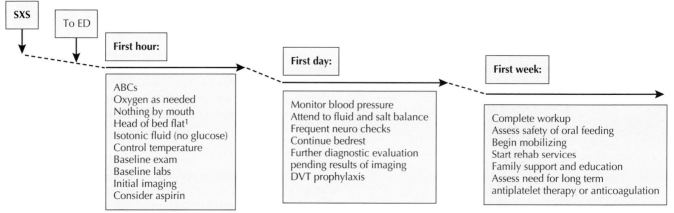

¹Head of bed flat if ischemic stroke, elevate 30° if ICH or CSVT

SXS-symptoms; ED-emergency department; ABCs-airway, breathing, circulation; Baseline exam-vital signs, brief general examination, auscultation of heart and neck, neurologic examination excluding walking; Baseline labs-electrolytes, complete blood count with platelets, prothrombin time/international normalized ratio, partial thromboplastin time, electrocardiogram, toxicology screen; Initial imaging-non-contrast head computed tomography; DVR-deep vein thrombosis; ICh-intracerebral hemorrhage; CSVT-cerebral sinus venous thrombosis

Adapted from Ichord RN, unpublished.

Figure 79-5 *Acute management of a child with suspected acute stroke.*

approaches that in the elderly. The most common presentation of perinatal stroke is seizure during the first few days of life, but perinatal stroke may present only with lethargy or poor feeding or may be completely asymptomatic. Many infants who have perinatal stroke are only diagnosed later in childhood upon evaluation of early hand preference, developmental delay, or emerging hemiparesis.

The pathophysiology of perinatal ischemic stroke is incompletely understood but is thought to be secondary to intrinsic hypercoagulability, dehydration, and shifts from the fetal to the mature circulation that lead to clot formation. The majority of strokes are in the anterior circulation, and there is a predilection for the MCA territory. There is a moderate preponderance of left-sided stroke in the perinatal period, presumably secondary to altered flow dynamics from the ductus arteriosus. Watershed infarcts are common, both in the classic distribution between the MCA and anterior cerebral artery territories and in a watershed area unique to the perinatal period between the territory of the long circumferential and paramedian penetrating branches of the basilar artery. This leads to a linear-shaped infarction affecting structures in the brainstem governing feeding and respiratory drive and thus can present solely with unexplained apnea or poor feeding.

Risk factors for perinatal stroke include complications during pregnancy or delivery, congenital heart disease, and thrombophilias in both the infant and the mother. However, in about 50% of cases of perinatal stroke, no specific cause can be identified. Evaluation of the neonate with suspected stroke should include the same elements as that of the older child, although infectious causes and maternal prothrombotic states should also be investigated. The placenta should be evaluated for pathology when possible. Management of a neonate with suspected stroke is different from that of an older child in that hypotonic and dextrose-containing fluids are acceptable. In addition, aspirin is rarely used. The prognosis depends on the extent and location of the injury, with complete MCA territory strokes and bilateral

basal ganglia infarction portending a poor prognosis in almost all cases. Cerebral palsy is a common sequela, occurring in 30% to 50% of survivors of perinatal stroke. Because most perinatal stroke is secondary to factors unique to the perinatal period, recurrence is rare.

SICKLE CELL DISEASE

Children with SCD are at increased risk for stroke both secondary to sludging from sickling and from early arteriopathy. Stroke is an important cause of morbidity and mortality among patients with SCD, in one study accounting for 12% of all SCD-related deaths. The cumulative risk of stroke for children with SCD increases with age, with more than 20% showing MRI evidence of stroke by age 20 years. Even in children with so-called "silent" infarctions, MRI evidence of ischemia is associated with cognitive deficits and learning and behavior problems. Stroke risk for children with SCD can be predicted by increased blood flow velocity on transcranial Doppler ultrasonography (TCD), with high-risk children having an annual stroke risk of up to 10% per year. Thus, children with SCD should be followed with annual TCD. Children with increased risk of stroke by TCD should have MRI and MRA and should usually be placed on chronic transfusion therapy because this has been demonstrated to reduce the risk of a first stroke by up to 90% in a clinical trial. In the setting of acute stroke, aspirin may be less helpful than in other causes of stroke, and exchange transfusion should be considered.

FOCAL CEREBRAL ARTERIOPATHY OF CHILDHOOD

Focal cerebral arteriopathy of childhood (FCA) is a recent term that describes a focal stenosis in a cerebral artery. FCA excludes dissection, moyamoya, sickle cell arteriopathy, postvaricella arteriopathy, radiation-induced arteriopathy, and vasculitis. A frequent distribution of FCA is unilateral focal or segmental stenosis of the distal carotid artery or its branches that leads to AIS or TIA in previously healthy children. Lenticulostriate branches of the MCA are preferentially affected, often leading to strokes in the basal ganglia or internal capsule. FCA is likely a heterogeneous arteriopathy because some stenoses may continue to progress for several months during which additional strokes may occur; in other children, the stenotic vessel may improve but may never completely normalize. Postvaricella angiopathy can cause a very similar arteriopathy in children who have had varicella infection within the preceding year, leading many to believe that at least some cases of FCA are caused by other viruses.

MOYAMOYA DISEASE AND SYNDROME

Moyamoya disease is a noninflammatory vasculopathy in which gradual occlusion of one or both internal carotid arteries leads to the formation of fragile collaterals that give a characteristic "puff of smoke" appearance on angiography. Idiopathic moyamoya disease is more common among children of Japanese descent and classically presents with ischemic strokes in the first decade of life and intracranial hemorrhages thereafter. However, multiple other syndromes can also be associated with moyamoya vessels, including SCD, trisomy 21, Williams syndrome, neurofibromatosis type 1, and Alagille syndrome. In most patients, a revascularization procedure should be considered; however, the benefit of revascularization procedures is less clear in patients with sickle cell anemia.

ARTERIAL DISSECTION

Arterial dissection is a common cause of arteriopathy in children and can affect the carotid or vertebral arteries in the neck as well as the intracranial vessels. Arterial dissection is caused by a tear along the inner wall of an artery. A small pouch called a "false lumen" can form in which blood can pool. Strokes can occur if a "pseudoaneurysm" forms, which can impede blood flow or even rupture; if clot forms in the false lumen and extends distally; or if clot forms in the false lumen and then embolizes distally. Dissection can occur after minor or major trauma but can sometimes occur spontaneously, especially in patients with connective tissue disorders. Dedicated arterial imaging of the head and neck is required to make a diagnosis of dissection.

VASCULITIS

Central nervous system (CNS) vasculitis is an inflammatory arteriopathy of the brain and meninges and is a rare cause of childhood stroke. It is primary when the process is isolated to the CNS and is not explained by another condition. Vasculitis is secondary when it is the result of another process such as rheumatologic diseases such as lupus, infection such as meningitis, or drugs such as amphetamines. Large-, medium-, or small-caliber vessels can be affected. Conventional catheter angiography and sometimes brain and meningeal biopsy are required to confirm the diagnosis. Treatment depends on the underlying cause, but systemic immunosuppression may be necessary.

METABOLIC STROKE

Unlike AIS, which is caused by hypoperfusion, metabolic strokes are usually caused by inherited defects in metabolic pathways that lead to an inability to compensate for metabolic stresses. In the setting of metabolic stress, neuronal energy production is unable to keep up with metabolic demand, leading to a final common pathway of cell death. Metabolic strokes or strokelike episodes are most commonly associated with mitochondrial disease such as MELAS (mitochondrial encephalopathy with lactic acidosis and strokelike episodes). However, they can be seen in a variety of metabolic diseases in which energy production is impaired, including organic and amino acidurias, disorders of fatty acid oxidation, and carnitine transport disorders. Clues to the diagnosis of metabolic stroke include a history of developmental regression, decompensation in the setting of acute illness, recurrent episodes in the absence of any vascular or hematologic pathology, unexplained acidosis, and nonvascular distribution of infarct. MRI findings suggestive of metabolic stroke include bilateral basal ganglia or bilateral occipital lobe infarcts. Further evaluation of a child with suspected metabolic stroke should include urine organic acids, serum amino acids, an acylcarnitine profile, lactate, pyruvate, and ammonia. MR spectroscopy (MRS) can also be very helpful, with lactate peaks over the basal ganglia suggestive of metabolic stroke. However, an MRS can be delayed because lactate might be elevated in the setting of any acute infarction. Management of a child with metabolic stroke depends on the underlying disease, but the emphasis should be on minimizing metabolic stress. Conventional measures to decrease thrombus formation or increase cerebral perfusion are unlikely to be effective because the origin of the "stroke" is not thrombus but is instead neuronal energy failure.

CONCLUSIONS AND FUTURE DIRECTIONS

Stroke is a common cause of morbidity and mortality in children. Childhood stroke includes AIS, ICH, and CSVT. The outcome of stroke in children varies from severe deficits to complete recovery and may depend in part on timely recognition and treatment. The future of this field rests on collaborative trials to evaluate acute therapies such as thrombolytics in AIS and therapies to enhance recovery of function such as transcranial magnetic stimulation. In addition, efforts to improve the classification of childhood AIS and to identify predictors of outcome in childhood ICH are underway.

SUGGESTED READINGS

Adams RJ, McKie VC, Hsu L, et al: Prevention of a first stroke by transfusions in children with sickle cell anemia and abnormal results on transcranial Doppler ultrasonography, N Engl J Med 339:5-11. 1998.

Amlie-Lefond C, Bernard TJ, Sebire G, et al: Predictors of cerebral arteriopathy in children with arterial ischemic stroke: results of the international pediatric stroke study, Circulation 119:1417-1423, 2009.

deVeber G, Andrew M, Adams C, et al: Cerebral sinovenous thrombosis in children, N Engl J Med 345:417-423, 2001.

Elbers J, Benseler SM: Central nervous system vasculitis in children, Curr Opin Rheumatol 20:47-54, 2008.

Fullerton HJ, Johnston SC, Smith WS: Arterial dissection and stroke in children, *Neurology* 57:1155-1160, 2001.

Fullerton HJ, Wu YW, Zhao S, et al: Risk of stroke in children: ethnic and gender disparities, *Neurology* 61:189-194, 2003.

Hutchison JS, Ichord R, Guerguerian AM, et al: Cerebrovascular disorders, *Semin Pediatr Neurol* 11:139-146, 2004.

Jordan LC: Stroke in childhood, *Neurologist* 12:94-102, 2006.

Jordan LC, Hillis AE: Hemorrhagic stroke in children, *Pediatr Neurol* 36:73-80, 2007.

Lynch JK: Cerebrovascular disorders in children, *Curr Neurol Neurosci Rep* 4:129-138, 2004.

Lynch JK, Han CJ: Pediatric stroke: what do we know and what do we need to know? *Semin Neurol* 25:410-423, 2005.

Kirton A, deVeber G: Therapeutic approaches and advances in pediatric stroke, *NeuroRx* 3:133-142, 2006.

Nelson KB, Lynch JK: Stroke in newborn infants, *Lancet Neurol* 3:150-158, 2004.

Roach ES, Golomb MR, Adams R, et al: Management of stroke in infants and children: a scientific statement from a Special Writing Group of the American Heart Association Stroke Council and the Council on Cardiovascular Disease in the Young, *Stroke* 39:2644-2691, 2008.

Shellhaas RA, Smith SE, O'Toole E, et al: Mimics of childhood stroke: characteristics of a prospective cohort, *Pediatrics* 118:704-709, 2006.

Scott RM, Smith ER: Moyamoya disease and moyamoya syndrome, *N Engl J Med* 360:1226-1237, 2009.

Zimmer JA, Garg BP, Williams LS, et al: Age-related variation in presenting signs of childhood arterial ischemic stroke, *Pediatr Neurol* 37:171-175, 2007.

Spinal Cord Disorders

Saba Ahmad

80

Disorders of the spinal cord are exceedingly diverse. They range in etiology from congenital malformation to neurodegenerative, inflammatory, infectious, ischemic, and traumatic. The spinal cord functions as the primary communication between the brain and the body. Disorders of the spinal cord, termed myelopathies, typically conform to neuroanatomic pathways and vascular territories, resulting in classic neurologic syndromes. Acute myelopathies require urgent attention. Profound physical disability may result.

ETIOLOGY AND PATHOGENESIS

According to the Centers for Disease Control and Prevention, spina bifida, the most common neural tube defect, occurs at a rate of two in 10,000 live births and results in varying degrees of disability from clinically normal to paraplegia. Traumatic spinal cord injury occurs at a rate of about 40 cases per million people per year and annually costs $9.7 billion in health care costs. Of these cases, it is estimated that up to half occur in adolescence and young adulthood. To diagnose and treat the disorders of the spinal cord, an understanding of its anatomy and how to examine for dysfunction of the spinal cord is imperative. The spinal cord is divided into four sections: cervical, thoracic, lumbar, and sacral (C, T, L, and S). It terminates at vertebral body level L2–L3 in infants, and in grown children and adults, it terminates at level L1–L2, where the cauda equina, the collection of nerves exiting the cord, begins. The spinal cord itself is sectioned in to a central H-shaped region of gray matter and surrounding white matter tracts (Figure 80-1).

The anterior horn of the gray matter contains motor nuclei, which receive information from the descending motor tracts. The axons of the motor neurons leave the ventral horn via the ventral root and synapse at the neuromuscular junction. The dorsal horn of the gray matter processes sensory information. It contains afferents from muscle spindles that participate in spinal cord reflexes. It also contains second-order neurons that mediate the various sensory inputs from the body.

There are three major white matter tracts of clinical importance when assessing myelopathy. The major descending tract is the lateral corticospinal tract (located posterolaterally within the cord). This tract contains the upper motor neurons originating from the primary motor cortex. The descending fibers cross at the cervicomedullary junction and descend, innervating the side of the body opposite the cortex. Within the tract, fibers that carry information to the upper extremities are located medially, and fibers that control the lower extremity movement are located laterally. The dorsal columns contain ascending proprioceptive and vibratory information and decussate in the medulla. These fibers are arranged so that information from the upper body is carried most laterally, in the fasciculus cuneatus, and that from the lower half is most medially, in the fasciculus gracilis. The spinothalamic tract (located anterolaterally in the cord) carries pain, temperature, and crude touch sensory information. These tracts decussate within a few levels of entering the spinal cord; therefore, they contain primarily contralateral sensory information. Within the spinothalamic tract, upper body information is carried medially, and lower body information is carried laterally.

The vascular anatomy of the spinal cord is divided into anterior and posterior circulations, arising from the vertebral arteries in the neck. The anterior spinal artery supplies the anterior two-thirds of the spinal cord. The two posterior spinal arteries primarily supply the posterior columns.

CLINICAL PRESENTATION AND DIFFERENTIAL DIAGNOSIS

The clinical examination is extremely helpful in localizing lesions within the spinal cord and can help determine the pathophysiology of spinal cord disease depending on the pattern of deficits. When examining a patient with suspected spinal cord disease, a thorough history and neurologic examination are essential to localizing the problem and generating a differential diagnosis. Cranial nerve examination can be helpful in distinguishing pure spinal cord disease from disease that involves the brainstem as well. It is important to perform a detailed motor, coordination, and reflex examination, including muscle bulk tone and strength, to determine patterns of weakness and elicit upper and lower motor neuron signs. Upper motor neuron signs include weakness, hypertrophy, spasticity, hyperreflexia, clonus, and a positive Babinski's sign. Lower motor neuron signs include weakness, flaccidity, atrophy, fasciculations, and hyporeflexia. Tenderness along the spine can help with localization, and a sensory examination should detail the pattern of reported sensory loss and always include sensory level elicited by determining pinprick sensation and light touch along both sides of the spinal cord. Assessment of rectal tone and bowel and bladder function is critical. Respiratory function should be evaluated with vital capacity and negative inspiratory force. Importantly, an acute spinal cord lesion can present with signs of "spinal shock," which includes reduced tone (or flaccidity in the extreme situation), hyporeflexia distal to the lesion, and reduced rectal sphincter tone. Only later will the upper motor neuron signs evolve. The sensory examination takes on greater emphasis toward localizing a spinal cord lesion in the acute setting.

There are common patterns of motor and sensory involvement depending on the localization of disease within the spinal cord. Table 80-1 describes the features of some typical patterns or spinal cord disease and their common causes (Figure 80-2).

The time course of the presentation can suggest the cause. Whereas traumatic injury such as transection or ischemic injury is usually sudden in onset, symptoms of spinal cord contusion develop over hours. Epidural abscesses, hematomas, transverse myelitis, and infectious myelopathy can have an acute to subacute course, which progress over hours to days. Tumors usually are very gradual in progression, over days to months, and

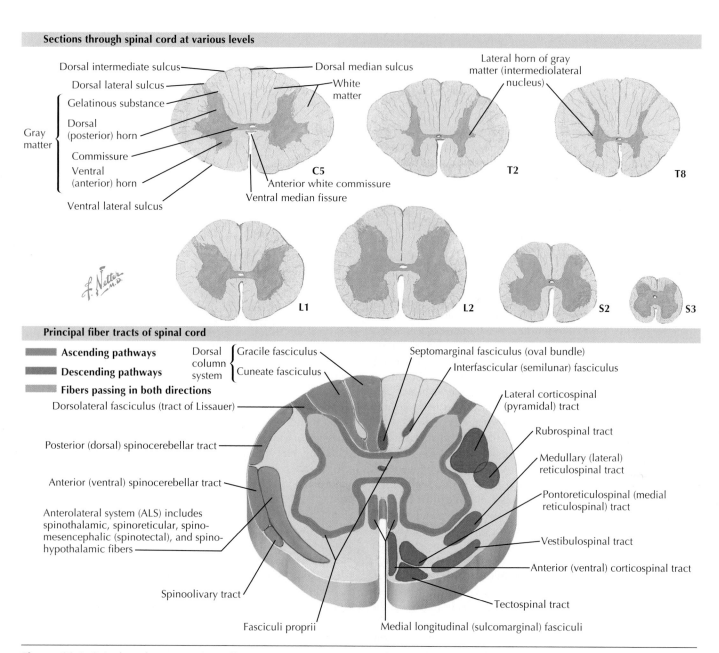

Figure 80-1 *Spinal cord cross-sections: fiber tracts.*

neurodegenerative conditions typically change over months to years.

EVALUATION AND MANAGEMENT

Evaluation of spinal cord disease typically depends on clinical presentation. In a trauma patient, assessment of the patient's airway, breathing, and circulation should take precedence. A transection above C3 can be rapidly fatal because it can involve the cessation of respiration. The cervical spine should be immobilized in a collar to prevent or minimize damage.

In all patients who present with an acute or subacute spinal cord process, urgent or emergent imaging is indicated. Typically, magnetic resonance imaging (MRI) is done with and without contrast of the suspected area, including diffusion-weighted imaging if the clinical history is suspicious for

ischemia. MRI evaluation is always preferable to computed tomography for imaging the spinal cord.

If the injury is traumatic, there is some evidence in the adult literature that supports the use of steroids also in the emergent setting. In blunt traumatic spinal cord injury, one steroid has been the most extensively studied: methylprednisolone sodium succinate. This medication, when administered within 8 hours of injury, has been shown to improve neurologic outcome up to 1 year postinjury. The regimen used in the Second National Acute Spinal Cord Injury Study (NASCIS II) was a bolus of 30 mg/kg administered over 15 minutes with a maintenance infusion of 5.4 mg/kg/h infused for 23 hours. In the Third National Acute Spinal Cord Injury Study (NASCIS III), this regimen was administered if the patient presented within 3 hours, and if the patient presented with 3 to 8 hours, the methyl-prednisolone infusion was continued for a total of 47 hours. In

Table 80-1 Features of Typical Patterns or Spinal Cord Disease and Common Causes

Localization	Common Pattern of Weakness and Sensory Loss	Common Causes in Pediatric Patients
Cervical spinal cord	Neck pain Lower motor neuron signs in the upper extremities at the level of the lesion Upper motor neuron signs in the lower extremities Sensory level: all sensory modalities Bowel or bladder involvement	Trauma Epidural hematoma or abscess Tumors Transverse myelitis (infectious and demyelinating)
Thoracic or lumbar spinal cord	Back pain Spared upper extremities Upper motor neuron signs in the lower extremities Sensory level: all sensory modalities Bowel or bladder involvement	Trauma Epidural hematoma or abscess Tumors Transverse myelitis
Ventral cord syndrome	Lower motor neuron signs at the level of the lesion +/− Upper motor neuron signs below the level of the lesion Sensory level to pain or temperature Spared vibration or proprioception	Infarction Trauma Tumor Radiation myelopathy
Dorsal cord syndrome	Decreased proprioception or vibration Preserved pin or light touch sensation +/− Upper motor neuron signs below the lesion	Trauma Infarction Epidural hematoma or abscess Tumors Tabes dorsalis Friedreich's ataxia Vitamin B12 deficiency HIV/AIDS myelopathy
Central cord syndrome	Suspended sensory level to pain or temperature at the level of the lesion Spared vibration or proprioception Lower motor neuron signs at the level of the lesion	Syrinx Intramedullary tumors
Brown-Séquard syndrome (hemi-cord syndrome)	Ipsilateral upper motor neuron signs below the level of the lesion Ipsilateral impaired vibration or proprioception below the level of the lesion Contralateral loss of temperature or pain below the level of the lesion Spared bowel and bladder function	Trauma Transverse myelitis (infectious and demyelinating)
Pure motor spinal cord syndrome	Upper or lower motor neuron signs, no sensory involvement	Viral myelitis (polio, Coxsackie, enterovirus 17, West Nile virus, Japanese encephalitis) Spinal muscular atrophy Hereditary spastic paraplegia
Cauda equina syndrome	Asymmetric multiradicular leg pain and sensory loss (all modalities) Lower motor neuron signs in lower extremities Bladder dysfunction	Epidural hematoma or abscess Tumors
Conus medullaris syndrome	Bladder or bowel dysfunction Saddle anesthesia	Trauma Epidural hematoma or abscess Tumors

this study, there was improvement in the functional mobility scores, which was not statistically significant at 6 months. There was also increased morbidity in the group that received the 47-hour infusion, with these patients having a higher incidence of severe sepsis and pneumonia. These data did not include pediatric patients younger than 13 years old; therefore, the use of steroids in this setting should be determined on an individual basis, with the involvement of the neurosurgeon. Steroids should not be used in the setting of penetrating traumatic injury.

For other causes of spinal cord injury, treatment depends on the etiology. In the nontraumatic setting, obtaining MR imaging, is crucial to establishing the diagnosis. If the clinical course or imaging suggests an abscess as the cause, early empiric antibiotic administration that treats *Staphylococcus aureus* infection is

important to prevent extension of the infection and further cord damage. With any compressive lesions, early decompressive neurosurgical intervention can minimize the damage to the spinal cord and may benefit functional recovery. When cord compression is caused by cancer, the use of dexamethasone may reduce swelling and compression of the spinal cord. In the adult literature, the dosage of dexamethasone was given as a 20 mg IV bolus followed by 10 mg IV every 6 hours. These data did not include pediatric patients and should be considered on an individual basis in conjunction with an oncologist and a neurosurgeon.

Because the etiology of transverse myelitis is so diverse, from demyelinating and inflammatory or autoimmune disease to infections to nutritional and metabolic derangements, the

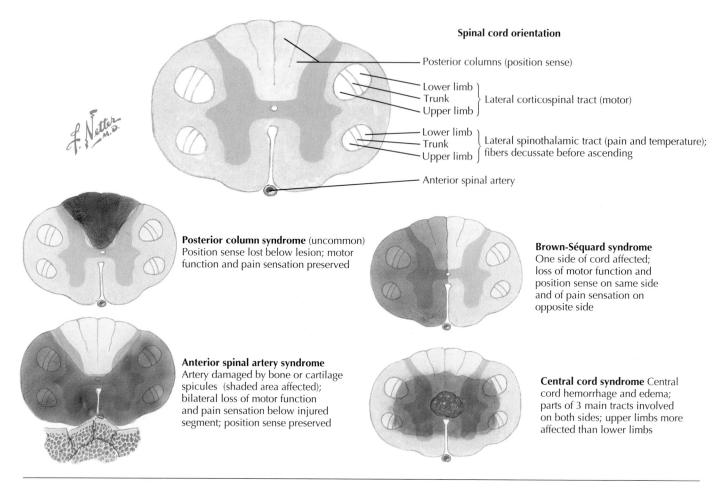

Spinal cord orientation

Posterior columns (position sense)

Lower limb ⎫
Trunk ⎬ Lateral corticospinal tract (motor)
Upper limb ⎭

Lower limb ⎫
Trunk ⎬ Lateral spinothalamic tract (pain and temperature);
Upper limb ⎭ fibers decussate before ascending

Anterior spinal artery

Posterior column syndrome (uncommon)
Position sense lost below lesion; motor
function and pain sensation preserved

Brown-Séquard syndrome
One side of cord affected;
loss of motor function and
position sense on same side
and of pain sensation on
opposite side

Anterior spinal artery syndrome
Artery damaged by bone or cartilage
spicules (shaded area affected);
bilateral loss of motor function
and pain sensation below injured
segment; position sense preserved

Central cord syndrome Central
cord hemorrhage and edema;
parts of 3 main tracts involved
on both sides; upper limbs more
affected than lower limbs

Figure 80-2 *Cervical spine injury: incomplete spinal cord syndromes.*

evaluation of these patients is similarly broad. The evaluation for transverse myelitis should include an MRI of the brain to look for lesions above the foramen magnum that would suggest multiple sclerosis (see Chapter 78). It should also include serum tests such as inflammatory markers, vitamin levels (such as B12, folate, vitamin D, and copper), a rheumatologic evaluation (including autoantibody seen in systemic lupus erythematosus, Sjögren's syndrome, sarcoidosis, and other autoimmune disease), as well as serum infectious evaluation as indicated (Lyme disease, Mycoplasma, HIV, Epstein-Barr virus, cytomegalovirus). If there are risk factors, the patient should have evaluation for tuberculosis. Finally, cerebrospinal analysis including cell count, glucose, protein, culture, cytology, oligoclonal bands, myelin basic protein, immunoglobulin G, and viral polymerase chain reaction tests (enterovirus, herpesviruses) as indicated are important for determining diagnosis and treatment. For viral myelitis, treatment is typically supportive.

In the setting of spinal cord infarction, treatment is typically supportive. Minimizing risk factors, such as hypercoagulability, and evaluating for the source of ischemia, such as an embolism, vasculitis, or venous thrombophlebitis, are important to reduce the chances of further ischemic events. In adult populations in which spinal cord infarction is more common, particularly after aortic surgeries, there is some evidence that suggests lumbar drain placement to augment spinal perfusion pressure improves

functional outcome. This has not been studied in pediatric patients.

FUTURE DIRECTIONS

Spinal cord diseases, although uncommon in children, are often very disabling conditions. At this point in time, there is only one treatment option that has been used extensively in traumatic spinal cord injury with evidence of benefit. Steroids have also been used with some success in inflammatory conditions, but this medication is not without its consequences, and it is far from curative.

Currently, there are two major approaches actively being studied focusing on improving functional outcome in spinal cord disease. The first is neuroprotection, which attempts to reduce the tissue loss by mediating secondary intracellular cascades that cause neuronal tissue damage. These neuroprotective agents being studied include mediators of excitotoxicity such as pregabalin and mediators of lipid metabolism. The second strategy involves promoting regeneration of axons, such as stem cell transplant and growth factors, to improve functional outcomes. These strategies seem promising to help treat a multitude of conditions that have a very high financial cost to the health care system and immeasurable physical and emotional cost to the patient.

SUGGESTED READINGS

Bracken, MB: Steroids for acute spinal cord injury. Cochrane Database Syst Rev 2:CD001046, 2002.

Bracken MB, Holford TR: Neurological and functional status 1 year after acute spinal cord injury: estimates of functional recovery in National Acute Spinal Cord Injury Study II from results modeled in National Acute Spinal Cord Injury Study III, *J Neurosurg* 96(3 suppl):259-266, 2002.

Defresne P, Hollenberg H, Husson B, et al: Acute transverse myelitis in children: clinical course and prognostic factors, *J Child Neurol* 18(6):401-406, 2003.

Hall ED, Springer JE: Neuroprotection and acute spinal cord injury: a reappraisal, *NeuroRx* 1(1):80-100, 2004.

Kaplin AI, Krishnan C, Deshpande DM, et al: Diagnosis and management of acute myelopathies, *Neurologist* 11(1):2-18, 2005.

Lammertse D, Dungan D, Dreisbach J, et al; National Institute on Disability and Rehabilitation: Neuroimaging in traumatic spinal cord injury: an evidence-based review for clinical practice and research, *J Spinal Cord Med* 30(3):205-214, 2007.

Wagner R, Jagoda A: Spinal cord syndromes, *Emerg Med Clin North Am* 15(3):699-711, 1997.

Neuromuscular Disorders

81

Jennifer L. McGuire

Neuromuscular disorders include a highly variable group of diseases that affect the peripheral nervous and muscular systems on any level of the neuraxis. Pathology ranges from disorders affecting the spinal motor neuron to the muscles by way of the peripheral nerves (Figure 81-1). In this chapter, several of the more common pediatric neuromuscular disorders are reviewed and classified based on their level of involvement in the neuraxis.

ANTERIOR HORN CELL

Spinal Muscular Atrophy

The spinal muscular atrophies encompass a heterogeneous group of genetically based disorders, all of which involve a progressive degeneration of the anterior horn cells in the spinal cord and motor nuclei in the lower brain stem. The term *spinal muscular atrophy* (SMA) refers to the most common form, described here, but other rare forms have similar terminology (e.g., X-lined SMA). Together, they are the leading genetic cause of infant deaths, occurring in about one in 10,000 live births, with a carrier frequency of about one in 40.

ETIOLOGY AND PATHOGENESIS

SMA is caused by an autosomal recessive mutation in the survival of motor neuron 1 (SMN1) gene on chromosome 5q13. The gene product, SMN protein, plays an important role in RNA processing and is expressed in all cells but seems to be of particular importance in motor neurons. In humans, a near-identical homocopy, the *SMN2* gene, rescues an otherwise lethal disorder, and the number of copies of *SMN2* is inversely related to severity of the phenotype.

CLINICAL PRESENTATION

SMA is subclassified into four types based on age of onset and the maximal level of motor skills achieved. SMA type 1 (or Werdnig-Hoffmann disease) is the most common and severe of these disorders, accounting for approximately 60% of cases. SMA type 1 presents in the early infancy period (0–6 months) with generalized hypotonia, proximal and symmetric flaccid muscle weakness (initially lower more than upper limbs), and absent deep tendon reflexes. This frequently comes to the attention of the pediatrician with gross motor milestone delay and may present subacutely or more indolently. Most infants also have tongue fasciculations, and some have postural tremor of the fingers or joint contractures. Diaphragmatic sparing with intercostal muscle involvement results in paradoxical breathing and the classic bell-shaped torso (Figure 81-2). Importantly, these infants are alert and interactive with normal cognitive development and no sensory loss or impairment of eye movements. Systemic complications of SMA include pneumonia, scoliosis, poor weight gain, sleep difficulties, and joint contractures. These infants never achieve independent sitting. Most individuals' expected life span is less than 2 years without invasive ventilatory and nutritional support.

SMA type 2 refers to infants who present usually between 6 and 18 months of age and achieve independent sitting but not ambulation and rely upon power wheelchairs for mobility. SMA type 3 presents after 18 months of age, and these children achieve community ambulation, but about half lose this ability by age 10 years. SMA type 4 presents in the adult years and tends to be slowly progressive.

The differential diagnosis includes other disorders causing acute weakness, including poliomyelitis and infantile botulism. In addition, the general differential diagnosis for hypotonia and more chronic weakness in an infant should be considered (Table 81-1).

EVALUATION AND MANAGEMENT

SMA type 1 diagnosis is suspected in individuals with an appropriate clinical history and is confirmed with molecular genetic testing for homozygous deletion of the *SMN1* gene. Electromyography (EMG) and nerve conduction studies (NCS) confirm a motor neuron process but is not necessary when the clinical presentation is strongly suggestive of SMA. Muscle biopsy is no longer performed as a diagnostic test. Genetic counseling and carrier testing is important after the diagnosis has been established.

There is no cure for SMA. The level of supportive care provided for SMA type 1 includes an ethical dimension, given the progressive nature of the disorder, with many parents electing to pursue a palliative course at home. Nonetheless, with aggressive management of dysphagia, malnutrition, and respiratory insufficiency, the lifespan can be extended considerably, often for several years. This entails early placement of a gastrostomy tube for supplemental feedings and early initiation of bilevel positive airway pressure (BiPAP), cough assist, and using a pump to suction oral secretions. Similar but less intensive nutritional and pulmonary support for patients with type 2 SMA, along with close attention to evolving scoliosis and joint contractures, has enabled these children to live into the third decade and beyond, often attending college, gaining employment, and forming interpersonal relationships. Children with type 3 SMA need mainly orthopedic and physical therapy support.

FUTURE DIRECTIONS

Much of the research into SMA is now focused on the molecular genetic mechanism of the disease. Several clinical drug trials based on encouraging preclinical data have been conducted on neuroprotection (riluzole), histone diacetylase (HDAC) inhibition (valproic acid), and regulators of *SMN2* expression (hydroxyurea and sodium phenylbutyrate). None, however, has

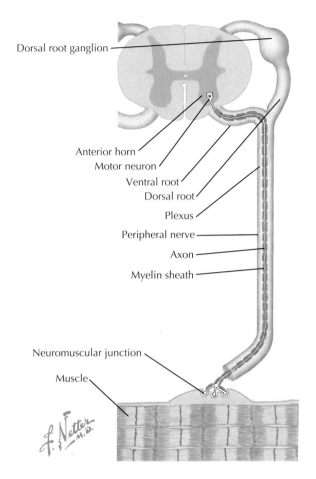

Motor neuron
Primary motor neuron diseases
  Amyotrophic lateral sclerosis
  Spinal muscular atrophy
    Type 1: Werdnig-Hoffmann disease
    Type 2: Intermediate form
    Type 3: Kugelberg-Welander
  Progressive muscular atrophy
  Poliomyelitis
  Tetanus

Dorsal root ganglion
  Herpes zoster
  Friedreich ataxia
  Hereditary sensory neuropathy

Spinal nerve (dorsal and ventral roots)
  Disk extrusion or herniation
  Tumor

Plexus
  Erb's palsy
  Tumor
  Trauma
  Idiopathic plexopathy
  Diabetic plexopathy

Peripheral nerve
  Metabolic, toxic, nutritional, idiopathic neuropathies
  Arteritis
  Hereditary neuropathies
  Infectious, postinfectious, inflammatory neuropathies (Guillain-Barré syndrome)
  Entrapment and compression syndromes
  Trauma

Neuromuscular junction
  Myasthenia gravis
  Lambert-Eaton syndrome
  Botulism

Muscle
  Duchenne muscular dystrophy
  Myotonic dystrophy
  Limb-girdle muscular dystrophy
  Congenital myopathies
  Polymyositis/dermatomyositis
  Potassium-related myopathies
  Endocrine dysfunction myopathies
  Enzymatic myopathies
  Rhabdomyolysis

Figure 81-1 *Classification of neuromuscular disorders by level in the neuraxis.*

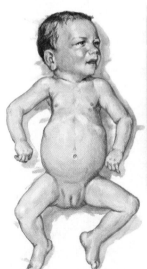

Infant with typical bell-shaped thorax, frog-leg posture, and "jug-handle" position of upper limbs

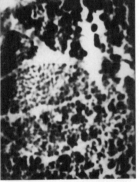

Muscle biopsy specimen showing groups of small atrophic muscle fibers and areas of normal or enlarged fibers (group atrophy) (trichrome stain).

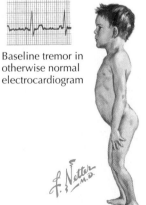

Baseline tremor in otherwise normal electrocardiogram

Boy with much milder, late-onset form of disease (Kugelberg-Welander disease). Marked lordosis and eversion of feet

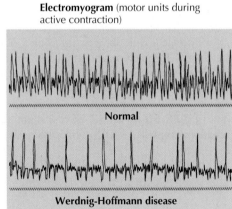

Electromyogram (motor units during active contraction)

Normal

Werdnig-Hoffmann disease

Figure 81-2 *Werdnig-Hoffmann disease.*

Table 81-1 Differential Diagnosis of the Floppy Baby, Infant, and Child

Localization	Diagnoses (Examples)
Brain/Systemic	Chromosomal (Turner's syndrome, trisomy 21, Prader-Willi syndrome)
	Benign congenital hypotonia
	Infection (sepsis, meningitis, encephalitis, TORCH infections, tick paralysis)
	Metabolic (electrolyte abnormalities, hypothyroidism, hepatic encephalopathy, mitochondrial and peroxisomal disorders, amino and organic acidemias)
	Toxins (alcohol, narcotics, heavy metal poisoning, organophosphates, anticholinergics)
	Neonatal encephalopathy
	Trauma
Spinal cord	Hypoxic-ischemic myelopathy
	Compression
	Syringomyelia
Anterior horn cell	Spinal muscular atrophy
	Infection (polio, Coxsackie)
	Cytochrome C oxidase deficiency
Peripheral nerve	Demyelinating (Guillain-Barré syndrome, hereditary motor-sensory neuropathy type I, congenital hypomyelinating neuropathy)
	Axonal (familial dysautonomia, hereditary motor-sensory neuropathy type II, infantile neuronal degeneration)
Neuromuscular junction	Infection (botulism)
	Myasthenia gravis
Muscle	Myopathies and congenital muscular dystrophies
	Metabolic (acid maltase deficiency, hypo- or hyperthyroid myopathy, carnitine deficiency)
	Muscular dystrophies
	Inflammatory (dermatomyositis, polymyositis)
	Mitochondrial myopathies

TORCH, toxoplasmosis or *Toxoplasma gondii*, other infections, rubella, cytomegalovirus, and herpes simplex virus.

demonstrated clinical efficacy as yet. The use of novel oligo-nucleotides and small molecule drugs that increase *SMN2* expression are currently in development, and stem cell and gene correction strategies are being considered.

PERIPHERAL NERVE

Guillain-Barré Syndrome

The name Guillain-Barré syndrome (GBS) encompasses a variety of acute immune-mediated polyneuropathies. It is the most common cause of acute flaccid paralysis in infants and children in the postpolio era, with an annual incidence of 0.38 to 0.91 pediatric cases per 100,000 children. A total of 50% to 82% of pediatric cases have an antecedent respiratory or gastro-intestinal (GI) infection associated with a variety of organisms, but most commonly *Campylobacter jejuni* (≤30% of cases). GBS has also been reported after use of several different vaccines, including influenza and rabies. There are multiple different types of GBS. Here, we will discuss acute demyelinating poly-radiculoneuropathy (AIDP), which accounts for 85% to 90% of GBS cases.

ETIOLOGY AND PATHOGENESIS

Pathologically, the two primary changes seen in GBS are acute inflammatory demyelinating polyradiculoneuropathy and acute axonal degeneration, both of which are thought to be caused by cross-reacting antibodies to the various gangliosides expressed in peripheral and cranial nerves. *Campylobacter* infections can result in molecular mimicry with the GM1 ganglioside, such that patients with *C. jejuni* infections are at 100-fold higher risk of developing GBS than the general population (Figure 81-3).

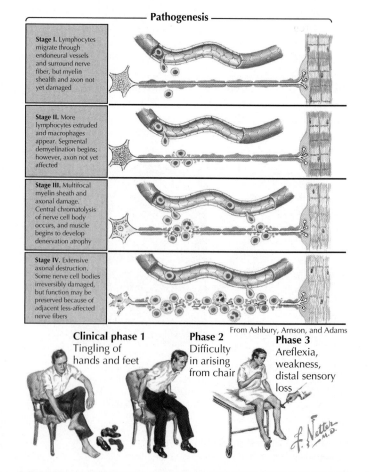

Figure 81-3 *Guillain-Barré pathophysiology.*

CLINICAL PRESENTATION

AIDP presents 2 to 4 weeks after a respiratory or GI illness with paresthesias of the extremities and a symmetric, length-dependent weakness (beginning distally in the lower limbs) with areflexia that may ascend over hours to days. About 50% of children have autonomic dysfunction as well, including cardiac dysrhythmias, blood pressure fluctuations, or bladder dysfunction.

The differential diagnosis of GBS should include other causes of peripheral neuropathy (including toxic neuropathy, critical care neuropathy, or tic paralysis), diseases of the neuromuscular junction, or spinal cord pathology.

EVALUATION AND MANAGEMENT

A child with suspected GBS should be evaluated with lumbar puncture, which classically shows albuminocytologic dissociation (high protein without pleocytosis) in the cerebrospinal fluid (CSF). The CSF may be normal within the first week of symptom onset, though, and in a child with clinical GBS and a normal CSF profile, treatment should still be initiated. EMG and NCS demonstrate multifocal demyelination or axonal degeneration. Magnetic resonance imaging of the spine should be considered in children with atypical presentation to rule out external compressive myelopathy and often demonstrates enhancing nerve roots after gadolinium administration.

In the appropriate clinical context, treatment for GBS should be initiated based on history and examination with supportive studies when able. First, children should have forced vital capacity (FVC) and negative inspiratory force (NIF) followed regularly and cardiorespiratory instability closely monitored with cardiac monitor and pulse oximeter. Hypertension may need medication to control. About 15% to 20% of children with GBS require assisted ventilation for respiratory failure sometime during their course. If the child is immobile in bed, sequential compression devices should be used, as well as consideration of prophylactic subcutaneous heparin. In children with stable or improving weakness without respiratory distress, supportive care may be enough.

In children with rapidly worsening weakness, worsening respiratory status, significant bulbar weakness, or inability to walk, more aggressive therapy should be initiated with intravenous immunoglobulin (IVIG) or plasmapheresis. Corticosteroids are not effective in AIDP.

Children with GBS typically have a shorter course with more complete recovery (in ≈85%) compared with adults. The best indicator of prognosis is based on EMG or NCS and the degree of axonal damage involved in a given case. Children who have had GBS should not receive live vaccinations for 1 year after their clinical symptoms. Recurrence is uncommon.

NEUROMUSCULAR JUNCTION

Myasthenia Gravis

Myasthenia gravis (MG) is the most common disorder of neuromuscular transmission in the United States with a prevalence of about 12.5 cases per 100,000 people. Approximately 11% to 24% of patients with MG have symptom onset in childhood or adolescence. Childhood forms of myasthenia include congenital myasthenic syndromes, neonatal MG, and juvenile MG (JMG). Congenital myasthenic syndromes are caused by genetic defects in presynaptic, synaptic basal lamina, and postsynaptic components of the neuromuscular junction. Transient neonatal MG occurs in 10% to 20% of infants born to myasthenic mothers, most of whom have active clinical disease. This is a transient disease mediated by passive transfer of maternal antibodies across the placenta that self-resolves when those antibodies are destroyed, typically in the first 2 months of life. This topic review focuses on the most common form of myasthenia, JMG, which is the childhood onset of autoimmune MG seen in adults.

ETIOLOGY AND PATHOGENESIS

MG is caused by an antibody-mediated response attacking the nicotinic acetylcholine receptor on the postsynaptic motor endplate of the neuromuscular junction (Figure 81-4). Two specific antibodies are thought to be responsible for most MG. The first is an antibody directed against the acetylcholine receptor (anti-Ach-R Ab), which is positive in 56% of prepubertal children with JMG and 82% of children with peripubertal onset. Of the adult patients that test negative for anti-Ach-R Ab, 40% to 70% have antibodies that bind to the extracellular domain of muscle specific kinase (anti-MuSK Ab). The prevalence of anti-MuSK Ab is unclear in children.

Because of this dysfunction at the neuromuscular junction, patients with MG are particularly sensitive to nondepolarizing neuromuscular blocking drugs (e.g., vecuronium), aminoglycoside antibiotics, phenytoin, magnesium and β-blockers. If a patient presents with a sudden flare of uncertain etiology, his or her medication list should be checked for possible offending drugs.

CLINICAL PRESENTATION

JMG typically presents after 10 years of age (although cases have been reported in children younger than 1 year old) and is characterized by fatigable weakness of ocular, facial, bulbar, respiratory, and extremity striated muscles. Most patients present with ocular symptoms, but others can present with generalized fatigue, swallowing dysfunction, slurred speech, acute respiratory failure, or difficulty chewing. Differential diagnosis of MG includes is broad and includes a similar list as that of GBS.

EVALUATION AND MANAGEMENT

A clinical diagnosis of myasthenia is suspected based on the presentation above. Physical examination findings specific to MG include the hallmark of fatigable weakness (test for eyelid droop with sustained upward gaze, the curtain sign, Cogan's eyelid twitch), and frequently a preferential involvement of proximal limb muscles. Neck flexion and extension strength may correlate with respiratory muscle strength.

The edrophonium (Tensilon) test is useful in establishing the diagnosis when there is definite weakness that can be objectively assessed for change. This test should be done in a child in a controlled setting with a cardiac monitor and with atropine available if a bradycardic response evolves. Diagnosis is made

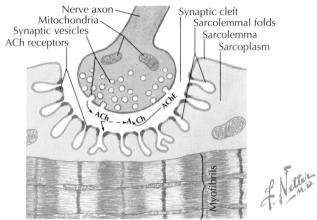

Normal neuromuscular junction
Synaptic vesicles containing acetylcholine (ACh) form in nerve terminal. In response to nerve impulse, vesicles discharge ACh into synaptic cleft. ACh binds to receptor sites on muscle sarcolemma to initiate muscle contraction. Acetylcholinesterase (AChE) hydrolyzes ACh, thus limiting effect and duration of its action.

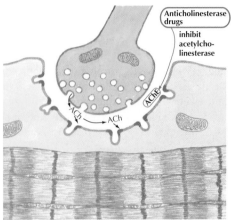

Myasthenia gravis
Marked reduction in number and length of subneural sarcolemmal folds indicates that underlying defect lies in neuromuscular junction. Anticholinesterase drugs increase effectiveness and duration of ACh action by slowing its destruction by AChE.

Figure 81-4 *Myasthenia gravis pathophysiology.*

serologically, looking for anti-Ach-R antibodies and or anti-MuSK antibodies in the serum. Conventional NCS with slow repetitive stimulation of nerves in affected limbs shows a classic decremental response of the compound muscle action potential. Single-fiber EMG shows increased jitter and blocking of motor unit generation.

Most children with JMG who require maintenance therapy are treated with anticholinesterase agents (e.g., pyridostigmine) with or without a variety of immunosuppressive agents. Oral corticosteroids may control symptoms and reduce the incidence of disease generalization at 2 years in patients with pure ocular MG. Other steroid-sparing immunosuppressive agents used in JMG treatment include azathioprine, cyclosporine, mycophenolate, and cyclophosphamide. Plasmapheresis or IVIG may be used as a chronic, intermittent therapy in patients with refractory disease. IVIG is sometimes preferred as first-line chronic therapy over corticosteroid mediation in growing children. As with adults, thymectomy has been demonstrated to be beneficial for generalized disease but is not typically used for purely ocular myasthenia.

For myasthenic crisis, FVC, NIF, and clinical examination should be followed closely. Overuse of anticholinergic medication in a patient on pyridostigmine therapy needs to be considered as a cause. Plasmapheresis and IVIG are also used in crisis.

FUTURE DIRECTIONS

Most research in MG is currently trying to better understand the disease, what exactly causes the autoimmune response, and attempts to better define the relationship between the thymus gland and MG.

Infantile Botulism

Infantile botulism is a rare but potentially life-threatening toxin-mediated neuroparalytic disorder. The offending toxins are produced by *Clostridium botulinum*, a gram-positive, spore-forming, anaerobic organism found in soil, marine animals, and bird intestines. *C. botulinum* toxins irreversibly block presynaptic cholinergic transmission, resulting in smooth muscle and skeletal muscle weakness and autonomic dysfunction. Approximately two per 100,000 live births, or 70 to 100 total cases occur annually throughout the United States, affecting infants from birth to 12 months of age. Infantile botulism is most prevalent in Pennsylvania, Utah, and California, presumably related to favorable soil conditions there.

ETIOLOGY AND PATHOGENESIS

Botulinum spores reside primarily in soil and are disrupted by local construction or agricultural cultivation. Less commonly, they may be found in contaminated wild honey or home-canned foods. Infection occurs when spores are ingested and germinate in the intestines, which leads to bacterial colonization and toxin release. Infants may be more susceptible to infection than adults because of immaturity and age-related changes in the competitive bowel flora, which allows extensive colonization.

CLINICAL PRESENTATION

Affected infants incubate their botulinum spores for 3 to 30 days and then present with a progressive clinical picture of neuromuscular blockade, nadiring at 1 to 2 weeks. Infants initially demonstrate poor feeding and constipation followed by a subacute progression of descending bulbar and extremity hypotonia and weakness (Figure 81-5). Cranial nerve dysfunction manifests early as pupillary paralysis, ptosis, diminished extraocular movements, facial diplegia, and a weak suck and gag. Autonomic dysfunction presents with decreased salivation and tearing, widely fluctuant heart rate and blood pressure, and flushed skin. Decreased extremity movement and areflexia are later signs followed by flaccid paralysis and respiratory failure in 50% to 70%.

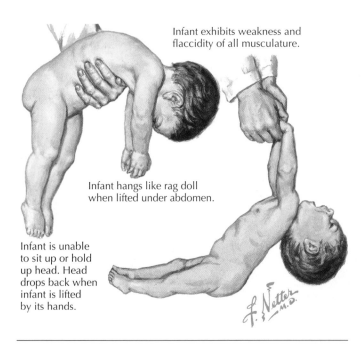

Infant exhibits weakness and flaccidity of all musculature.

Infant hangs like rag doll when lifted under abdomen.

Infant is unable to sit up or hold up head. Head drops back when infant is lifted by its hands.

Figure 81-5 *The floppy baby.*

Without treatment, the total duration of illness is approximately 1 to 2 months.

The differential diagnosis is that of the hypotonic infant (see Table 81-1). In clinical practice, SMA type 1 and metabolic disorders are the most frequent mimics of infantile botulism.

EVALUATION AND MANAGEMENT

Infantile botulism should be suspected in any infant with weak suck, ptosis, inactivity, and constipation, particularly in an endemic area. The gold standard of diagnosis is isolation of *C. botulinum* spores from stool and is confirmed by the identification of botulinum toxin in stool samples. However, collection of stool may be difficult because of the accompanying constipation, and anaerobic stool cultures may take up to 6 days to grow, resulting in a significant delay in treatment if all cases were confirmed before initiation. Electrophysiologic testing may be helpful in the diagnosis of infantile botulism, but findings of abnormal incremental response with repetitive nerve stimulation and short-duration, low-amplitude motor unit potentials on EMG are not pathognomonic and are not always present in very early disease.

For any case of suspected infantile botulism, the California Department of Health Services, Infant Botulism Treatment and Prevention Program should be contacted (http://www.infantbotulism.org/ or 24-hour telephone number, 510-231-7600), and the infant should be immediately treated empirically with intravenous botulism immune globulin (or "babyBIG") while the prolonged confirmatory testing described above is pending. Prompt babyBIG therapy has been shown to decrease the mean duration of hospital stay from 5.7 to 2.6 weeks, decrease the duration of mechanical ventilation from 4.4 to 1.8 weeks, and decrease hospital costs by $89,000 (in 2004 United States dollars). Management of patients with infantile botulism is otherwise supportive. Aminoglycoside antibiotics should be avoided because they can potentiate the effects of the toxin. With appropriate treatment, the case fatality rate is under 2%, and full recovery is expected.

FUTURE DIRECTIONS

Research directed at development of a variety botulism vaccines is currently underway, and in clinical trials, some vaccines are already available to adults at risk, particularly those in the military to counteract the risk of bioterrorism with botulinum toxin.

MUSCLE

Duchenne Muscular Dystrophy

Muscular dystrophies (MDs) are progressive, genetically based, disorders of the skeletal muscle. Dystrophinopathies are a subset of MD caused by a mutation in the dystrophin gene, which is located in the Xp21 region, and encodes for the 427-kD subsarcolemmal protein dystrophin. The most common and severe of the dystrophinopathies is Duchenne's muscular dystrophy (DMD), which is caused by complete absence of dystrophin. Becker's muscular dystrophy (BMD) is a less severe allelic form, in which there is a reduction in the dystrophin protein.

ETIOLOGY AND PATHOGENESIS

The dystrophin gene is the largest human gene isolated to date, spanning 2.5 million base pairs, and including 79 exons, which make up 0.6% of the gene. In approximately 60% of DMD patients, a deletion of one or more exons is found. Other causes are exon duplication, small insertions, or deletions or single-base pair changes, which may result in a premature stop codon. These mutations all result in stunted and abnormal RNA, which rapidly decays and leads to the production of a small amount of truncated and nonfunctional proteins. Identifying the type of mutation is now important for both genetic counseling and because newer treatments focus on the type of mutation (see below).

DMD occurs in about one per 3500 live male births and is transmitted in an X-linked recessive mechanism; however, about 30% of cases are spontaneous new mutations. Most patients are therefore boys; however, girls may also rarely manifest some DMD symptoms because of uneven lyonization or Turner's syndrome. The severity of disease is frequently related to the effect of the deletion on the disruption of the protein transcription reading frame.

CLINICAL PRESENTATION

Patients with DMD classically present around the age of 3 years old with gross motor delay, excessive falling, and gait abnormalities. Calf hypertrophy and neck flexion weakness are evident by 3 to 4 years of age. Hip girdle muscles are typically affected sooner than shoulder girdle muscles, causing the classic Trendelenburg (or waddling) gait and the Gowers' sign (Figure 81-6). As the disease progresses, weakness spreads distally. Joint contractures can develop and further worsen gait. Untreated, DMD follows a fairly predictable progressive course. Untreated,

Gower's maneuver

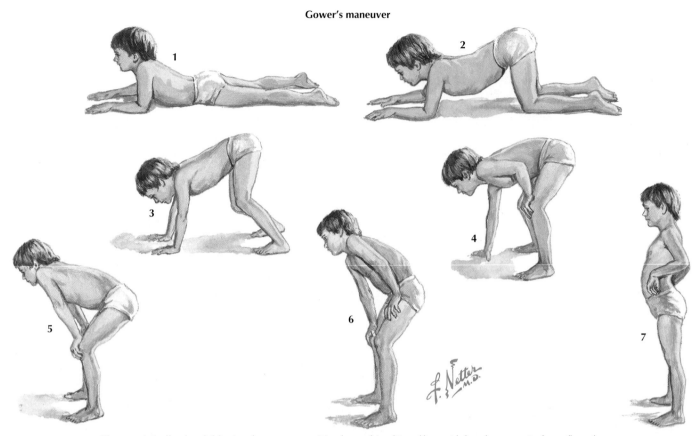

Characteristically, the child arises from prone position by pushing himself up with hands successively on floor, knees, and thighs, because of weakness in gluteal and spine muscles. He stands in lordic posture.

Figure 81-6 *Duchenne's muscular dystrophy.*

children lose the ability to walk (typically by 10 years of age and always by 13 years of age), then develop kyphoscoliosis, and finally develop cardiac and respiratory involvement and failure in the later second decade of life. The differential diagnosis includes other myopathies (see Table 81-1), dystrophies, and SMA type 3.

EVALUATION AND MANAGEMENT

Creatine kinase (CK) is elevated in affected children, from 10,000 to 30,000 IU (reference range, <250 IU). EMG may be helpful in distinguishing a myopathic process from a neurogenic disorder if this is in question. Definitive confirmation of a dystrophinopathy is made with molecular genetic testing; the diagnosis of DMD versus BMD remains a clinical one. Muscle biopsy is infrequently needed for diagnosis, but dystrophin protein expression can be identified by specific monoclonal antibody tagged immunostains or quantified with Western Blot analysis.

Glucocorticosteroids (prednisone or deflazacort) are the only medications with demonstrated benefit for DMD. They improve strength and motor function in the short term and prolong the time to reach nonambulatory status. They also postpone significant scoliosis, deterioration in pulmonary function, and possibly the evolution of cardiomyopathy. Thus, morbidity has been reduced and mortality extended since steroid use has been widely adopted and better pulmonary, cardiac, and orthopedic management implemented.

The remainder of the management is multidisciplinary. Pulmonary manifestations of DMD largely result from weakness of intercostal and diaphragmatic muscles, although it is also complicated by scoliosis. Monitoring of pulmonary function is important to pursue regularly by the early teen years, with annual spirometry and cough force, and if the patient is symptomatic for nocturnal hypoventilation, with a sleep study. Treatment includes implementing a cough-assist device and BiPAP, regular immunizations, and prompt attention to respiratory infections. Cardiac manifestations include dilated cardiomyopathy and regional wall motion abnormalities in areas of fibrosis (on echocardiography), arrhythmias, and chronic heart failure. Echocardiographic abnormalities are uncommon in the first decade but are seen in all boys with DMD by the late teens. Monitoring with regular electrocardiography and echocardiography is recommended every 2 years up to age 10 years and then annually. Treatment of heart failure is usually with an angiotensin-converting enzyme inhibitor, such as lisinopril, and a β-blocker is sometimes added.

With improved supportive care, the mean age of mortality has extended from 17 years to the mid-twenties, and some patients now survive into the fourth decade. Recent clinical care guidelines for DMD have been published (see Suggested Readings). Death is still usually from cardiomyopathy.

Boys with DMD overall have an intelligence quotient (IQ) curve shifted to the left, with one study identifying the mean as 83. DMD patients are also more prone to dysthymic disorder and major depressive disorder than their nonaffected peers.

There are several specific drug considerations in caring for DMD patients. In particular, they should not receive anticholinergic drugs or ganglionic blocking agents given the risk of decreased muscle tone. They may also be more susceptible to malignant hyperthermia, which care providers should be aware of before administration of general anesthesia. Cardiotoxic drugs should not be used.

FUTURE DIRECTIONS

Novel research into DMD is focusing on strategies to bypass the dystrophin mutation. Clinical trials are currently exploring two approaches: ribosomal read-through of premature stop codons, in the approximately 13% of DMD patients with this type mutation, by a small molecule drug named PTC124 (ataluren) and exon skipping, using oligonucleotides, now being tested for a subset of patients with deletions. In addition, pharmacologic therapies to ameliorate disease are targeting fibrosis, inflammation, and other downstream secondary pathways.

SUGGESTED READINGS

Arnon SS, Schechter R, Maslanka SE, et al: Human botulism immune globulin for the treatment of infant botulism, *N Engl J Med* 354:462-471, 2006.

Barras BT, Korf BR, Urion DK: Dystrophinopathies. Last updated March 2008. Available at http://www.ncbi.nlm.nih.gov/bookshelf/br.fcgi?book=gene&part=dbmd.

Bushby K, Finkel R, Birnkrant D, et al: The diagnosis and management of Duchenne muscular dystrophy–part 1. Diagnosis, and pharmacological and psychosocial management, *Lancet Neurol* 9:77-93, 2010.

Bushby K, Finkel R, Birnkrant D, et al: The diagnosis and management of Duchenne muscular dystrophy–part 2. Implementation of multidisciplinary care, *Lancet Neurol* 9:177-189, 2010.

Chiang LM, Darras BT, Kang PB: Juvenile myasthenia gravis, *Muscle Nerve* 39:423-431, 2009.

Domingo RM, Haller JS, Gruenthal M: Infant botulism: two recent cases and literature review, *J Child Neurol* 23:1336-1345, 2008.

Hughes RA, Swan AV, Raphael JC, et al: Immunotherapy for Guillain-Barré syndrome: a systematic review, *Brain* 130:2245-2257, 2007.

The Infant Botulism Treatment and Prevention Program: Available at http://www.infantbotulism.org/09.

Lunn MR, Wang CH: Spinal muscular atrophy, *Lancet* 371:2120-2133, 2008.

The Myasthenia Gravis Foundation of America: Available at http://www.myasthenia.org.

Rabie M, Nevo Y: Childhood acute and chronic immune-mediated polyradiculneuropathies, *Eur J Paediatr Neurol* 13:209-218, 2009.

Ryan MM: Guillain-Barré syndrome in childhood, *J Paediatr Child Health* 41:237-241, 2005.

Wang, CH, Finkel RS, Bertini ES, et al: Consensus statement for standard of care in spinal muscular atrophy, *J Child Neurol* 22(8):1027-1049, 2007.

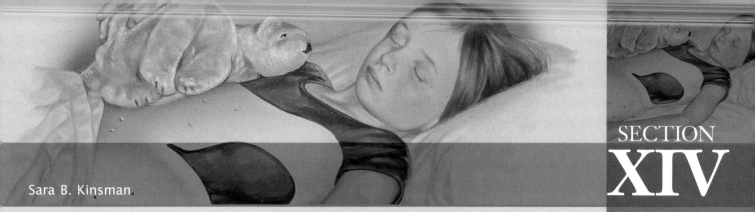

Sara B. Kinsman.

SECTION XIV

Adolescent Medicine

Substance Abuse

82

Daniel B. Horton and Sara B. Kinsman

Adolescence marks a time of transition from childhood to young adult life. As part of this process, a majority of U.S. adolescents will initiate health risks, including cigarette smoking, drinking alcohol, and experimenting with illicit substances. Although the majority of adolescents will avoid significant harm, immediate health risks associated with the use of alcohol and other substances include an increased likelihood of involvement in a motor vehicle crash, violence against others, self-harm, an unwanted sexual encounter, or an unprotected sexual encounter. The substance associated with the highest risk of death during adolescence is alcohol. Every year an estimated 5000 adolescents younger than 21 years of age die from underage drinking. Among college students, approximately 700,000 students are assaulted by other students who have been drinking, and about 100,000 students are victims of alcohol-related sexual assault or date rape.

The long-term risks associated with adolescent substance use include alcohol dependency and nicotine addiction, which together account for greater than half of all adult morbidity and mortality in the United States. Early alcohol use, independent of other risks, strongly predicts the development of alcohol dependence. Almost half of adults with alcohol dependence were found to be dependent before they had reached 21 years of age. The majority of adult smokers (80%-90%) started smoking before 18 years of age, and most regret having become addicted to nicotine. Pediatricians play a critically important role in identifying adolescents at increased risk for self-harm or addiction and offering appropriate interventions to reduce immediate and long-term risks.

EPIDEMIOLOGY AND PATHOGENESIS

Patterns of drug initiation and drug use vary by age, gender, race, ethnicity, and substance availability in an adolescent's community. Monitoring the Future Study (MTFS) is a nationally representative study that follows trends in adolescent drug use and attitudes. As adolescents mature, they report higher rates of substance use (Figure 82-1). Notably, alcohol is the most commonly reported substance used by adolescents followed by cigarette use and marijuana use. Use of other illicit drugs substances, although less common, poses risks resulting from acute impairments in judgment or long-term addiction. More recent surveys have highlighted the increased availability and recreational use of prescription drugs such as hydrocodone bitartrate (Vicodin), oxycodone (Percocet), and methylphenidate hydrochloride (Ritalin). Although illicit substances can signify an increased risk for an individual adolescent, pediatricians need to routinely discuss alcohol-related issues given that 43% of 12th graders; 29% of 10th graders; and 16% percent of 8th graders reported using alcohol based on 2008 MTFS data. Although adolescents drink less frequently than adults, when consuming alcohol, teens tend to drink more at one time compared with adults. Remarkably, from the same survey, 25% of 12th graders, 16% of 10th

graders, and 8% of 8th graders report having consuming five or more drinks on at least one occasion.

Pediatricians will find that a substantial proportion of their adolescent patients will report trying substances, yet of these teens, only a minority will abuse a substance or become physiologically dependent (Figure 82-2). Progression from experimentation to abuse or physiologic dependence results from the complex interplay of numerous biopsychosocial risks and protective factors, including adolescent physical, emotional, and cognitive development, and environmental factors, including peers' and family's attitudes and behaviors, genetic predisposition, and mental health stressors.

Recent research elucidates how maturation of the prefrontal cortex impacts risks associated with substance use. Initially, the adolescent brain learns to feel intense emotions with limited self-control followed later by the maturation of regulatory systems, which temper these emotions and allow the adolescent to assess immediate and long-term risks. This developmental sequence helps to explain why younger adolescents may experience excessively positive emotions associated with a substance and less moderation of behavior, resulting in risk of immediate harm and long-term dependence. Adolescents who physically mature earlier are at increased risk because they may have the opportunity to socialize with older adolescents and be exposed to a wider variety of substances. Learning what substances are commonly available and used by adolescents in a particular school or community can be extremely helpful in screening for particular substance use. Although availability and social cues from peers are strongly correlated with continued substance use, the highest predictor of long-term substance use or abuse is the adolescent's family's substance use patterns. This may be due to ongoing behavioral stimuli or a genetic predisposition; both mechanisms have been implicated in alcohol dependency and nicotine addiction.

Mental health issues and past traumas can increase the risk that an adolescent will begin using substances on a regular basis to elevate mood, dull anxiety, or avoid feelings altogether. Adolescents with depression, anxiety, attention-deficit/hyperactivity disorder, and conduct disorders are at significantly increased risk for using substances to manage symptoms related to these disorders (Figure 82-3). A history of having experienced childhood physical or emotional abuse, past or ongoing family conflict, inadequate parental supervision, isolation from school, poor academic achievement, and sexual or gender identity concerns can increase the risk that an adolescent may begin to use and experience harm from substances.

EVALUATION AND CLINICAL PRESENTATION

Screening Adolescents for Substance Use

Substance use and its disorders often emerge through the screening of otherwise well-appearing adolescents. For this

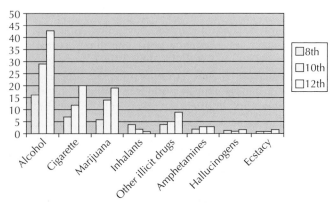

Based on the Monitoring the Future Study (2008), more adolescents use alcohol than any other substance, followed by cigarettes and marijuana. Use of most substances increases with age, except for inhalants, which are more commonly used in early adolescence. In this figure, "other illicit drugs" include illegal drugs other than marijuana, as well as substances such as amphetamines and sedatives used recreationally, not under a doctor's care. *Adapted from Johnston, LD, O'Malley, PM, Bachman, JG, & Schulenberg, JE. (2008). Monitoring the Future national results on adolescent drug use: Overview of key findings, 2007 (NIH Publication No. 08-6418). Bethesda, MD: National Institute on Drug Abuse.*

Figure 82-1 *Thirty-day reported substance use by grade.*

reason, all adolescent patients should be screened for risks associated with substance use at each visit. A complete family history includes questions related to mood disorders, history of suicide or suicide attempts, and substance use by siblings, parents, aunts, uncles, and grandparents. A complete review of systems

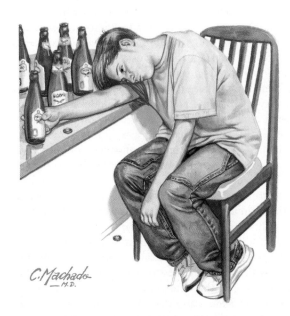

Disordered substance use in adolescents may be associated with poor school performance, accidental injury, violence towards self or others, and isolation and social alienation. Substance dependence (addiction) suggests compulsive, uncontrolled use accompanied by tolerance, withdrawal symptoms, and negative consequences.

Figure 82-2 *Substance dependence (addiction).*

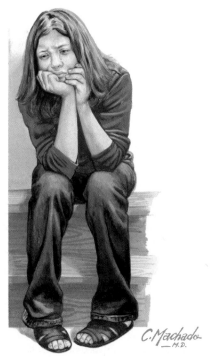

Mood disorders such as depression may lead affected adolescents to use substances to help with their mood symptoms. Some of these individuals ultimately develop concomitant substance use disorders. Conversely, substance use can also trigger or worsen an underlying psychiatric condition, leading to an increased risk of adverse outcomes including suicide.

Figure 82-3 *Mood disorders.*

is an important nonthreatening way that a pediatrician may be alerted of a problem related to substance use. For example, an adolescent who reveals weight loss, insomnia, and the symptom of a fast racing heart beat may be experiencing overuse of highly caffeinated beverages, diet pills, or other amphetamines. An adolescent who admits to mood changes, including poor concentration, lack of motivation, and irritability may be struggling with depression, daily marijuana use, or both.

Substance use screening can be included as one portion of a broader psychosocial screening tool. When asking teens about the social aspects of their lives, it is important for pediatricians to remember that most adolescents report wanting to speak to their pediatricians about these health issues. When the pediatrician assures adolescent patients that discussions related to the social aspects of their lives are confidential—with the important caveat that the pediatrician must tell their adolescent patients that the pediatrician will need to get help from other trusted adults if the adolescent has experienced physical or sexual harm or is planning to harm themselves or someone else—most adolescents are quite forthcoming and appreciate the opportunity to speak with their pediatrician about how substance use fits into and impacts their life. When using screening tools such as "SSHADESS," the pediatrician may ask about *s*trengths, *s*chool, *h*ome, *a*ctivities, *d*rugs, *e*motion/depression, *s*exuality, and *s*afety. When asking about *d*rugs, questions about the commonly available substances in the adolescent's peer group may help to contextualize the adolescent's use and avoid a sense of confrontation.

Next the pediatrician should ask directly about the adolescent's use of alcohol, cigarettes and other tobacco products, marijuana and other drugs including use of club drugs, prescription drugs, over-the-counter medications, and inhalants. Furthermore, pediatricians may ask adolescents how they feel about their drug use. Specifically, if relevant, the pediatrician should learn about past attempts to decrease use and current level readiness to reducing use.

Acute visits with an adolescent patient may also prompt concern for substance use. Recurrent asthma exacerbations or exacerbations that are refractory to treatment may be related to ongoing cigarette or cannabis use. A seizure in an otherwise well-controlled adolescent with epilepsy may indicate use of substances that reduce the seizure threshold. An adolescent presenting with a sexually transmitted infection (STI), including HIV, or unwanted pregnancy may have had unwanted or unprotected sexual intercourse related to substance use.

Physical Examination Finding Related to Substance Use

Although the interview is the best tool that pediatricians can use to screen for substance use in the practice setting, the physical examination may sometimes raise concern for substance use that was not revealed during the interview. Vital signs can give important clues to ongoing intoxication or withdrawal. The constellation of tachycardia, hypertension, or hyperthermia may correlate to use of stimulants or withdrawal from a chronically used depressant. Constricted pupils can be associated with either narcotics or stimulant withdrawal, and dilated pupils may suggest stimulant use or narcotic withdrawal. Nystagmus may indicate use of depressants or 1-(1-phenylcyclohexyl)piperidine or phencyclidine (PCP). Conjunctival injection can result from the recent use of alcohol, cannabis, or inhalants, and nasal mucosa may be irritated or ulcerated by intranasal drug use. An adolescent with sharp midepigastric pain may have pancreatitis related to alcohol use, and recurrent abscesses may be associated with injection steroid or drug use.

MANAGEMENT

After an adolescent has been identified as using a substance, the pediatrician should assess the need for an emergency evaluation, referral for specialized substance abuse treatment, referral for outpatient psychiatric consultation and counseling, or an office-based intervention.

Adolescents with acute intoxication or a significant change in mental status, including somnolence, confusion, agitation, aggression, paranoia, or hallucination, and those who appear to pose a safety risk to themselves or others will need immediate medical and psychiatric evaluation in an emergency department, including laboratory testing for substance use. Laboratory assessment of substance abuse consists primarily of urine and serum toxicology, which is often reserved for the emergency setting. Adolescents should be informed of the limits of laboratory testing, including the possibility of false-positive test results, when pediatricians are asking their consent for this testing. A pediatrician may forego an adolescent's consent for laboratory screening when the patient does not have decision-making

capacity (e.g., significantly altered mental status). Positive test results should be confirmed by secondary analysis, usually mass spectrometry or gas chromatography. The clinical scenario will guide additional testing, including blood alcohol concentration, rapid glucose, electrolytes, creatinine, hepatic function panel, pancreatic enzymes, pregnancy and STI testing.

Indications for inpatient management of patients with substance abuse or dependence include severe, acute, or life-threatening presentations; drug dependence that requires specialized care to prevent withdrawal; psychiatric comorbidities that prohibit safe, reliable treatment as an outpatient; or the failure of outpatient management. Inpatient options include hospitalization on medical or psychiatric wards as well as residential treatment facilities for longer term care.

For patients not requiring immediate referrals, the pediatrician should assess by discussing the degree to which the substance use is the main concern or exploring if there are symptoms of other mental health issues that require referral for specialized mental health care. Adolescents who are using substances to manage severe depression will benefit from an evaluation and therapy with a child psychiatrist. While supporting adolescents and respecting their confidentiality, pediatricians can help adolescents to share their concerns with caring adults who can facilitate referral to this mental health professional. Referral for outpatient family-based therapy programs can be effective in treating adolescents with substance use disorders, particularly when familial stress and substance use contribute to the adolescent's substance use.

For adolescents who have experimented with substances or are thinking about trying a new substance, pediatricians can provide important and accurate information regarding the immediate and long-term risks. Pediatricians who are aware of the commonly used substances in an adolescent community can begin an ongoing dialogue before an adolescent is likely to be exposed to the substance so that risks associated with initial experimentation and later use are easily discussed.

Different intervention models have been proposed to manage different types of substance use. One model for talking to an adolescent regarding smoking use is based on the U.S. Department of Health and Human Services Clinical Practice Guideline; Treating Tobacco Use and Dependence. These intervention models have proven to be effective in decreasing tobacco use among adults and may be of promise among youth, although adequate studies are not conclusive. These guidelines recommend that primary care providers follow the "five As." First, the provider should (1) *a*sk every patient at *every* visit about their tobacco use, (2) the provider should *a*dvise patients that the best thing they could do for their health would be to quit smoking, (3) the provider then can *a*ssess patients' interest and willingness to quit smoking at this time, (4) if the patient is interested in quitting, the provider can *a*ssist the patient in quitting, and (5) the provider should always *a*rrange for a follow-up to further discuss substance use and cessation.

Pediatricians caring for adolescents report that they often find themselves at a loss about what to do if an adolescent reports that he or she does not wish to stop smoking or using other substances. In this case, the U.S. Department of Health and Human Services Clinical Practice Guidelines recommend that the provider follows the "five Rs"—(1) the provider can ask if cessation would even be *r*elevant or meaningful for the patient, (2) the provider may ask the patient if he or she associates any *r*isks related to smoking and any potential *r*ewards associated with quitting, (3) for example, an adolescent may believe that by buying cigarettes, he or she *r*isks not being able to save to go to the prom, and a *r*eward of quitting would be increased savings, (4) by helping the patient identify *r*oadblocks to quitting, such as how to deal with being around friends and family who smoke, the pediatrician can start a dialogue about ways to overcome some of these challenges, and (5) *r*epetition and follow-up are key for increasing motivation to decrease or stop substance use. A more specialized technique, motivational interviewing, may also have promise with adolescents who smoke and are not yet ready to commit to quitting. This technique focuses on expressing empathy, enhancing awareness of discrepancies between desires and behavior, accepting resistance, and supporting self-efficacy. Studies focusing on adolescent alcohol use have not yet definitely described effective office-based interventions, although pediatricians working in coordination with family and schools may promote a comprehensive community-wide intervention that decreases alcohol use among adolescents.

FUTURE DIRECTIONS

Future research will continue to help pediatricians become more effective in screening for and managing substance use by adolescent patients. Interventions using in-office motivational counselors, online programs, and brief, repetitive counseling sessions may help to increase the effectiveness of pediatricians in reducing substance use and improving the immediate and long-term health of adolescents.

SUGGESTED READINGS

Agency for Healthcare Research and Quality: Treating Tobacco Use and Dependence: 2008 Update, a Public Health Service-sponsored Clinical Practice Guideline, Available at http://www.ncbi.nlm.nih.gov/books/bv.fcgi?rid=hstat2.chapter.28163.

Centers for Disease Control and Prevention: Youth Risk Behavior Surveillance, Available at http://www.cdc.gov/HealthyYouth/yrbs/index.htm.

Kulig JW, the American Academy of Pediatrics Committee on Substance Abuse: Tobacco, alcohol, and other drugs: the role of the pediatrician in prevention, identification, and management of substance abuse, *Pediatrics* 115(3):816-821, 2005.

National Institute on Alcohol Abuse and Alcoholism: Available at http://www.niaaa.nih.gov.

National Institute on Drug Abuse: Available at http://www.nida.nih.gov.

Office of National Drug Control Policy: Listing of Drug Street Names, Available at http://www.whitehousedrugpolicy.gov/streetterms/default.asp.

Regents of the University of Michigan: Monitoring the Future, Available at http://www.monitoringthefuture.org.

Steinberg L: Cognitive and affective development in adolescence, *Trends Cognitive Sci* 9(2):69-74, 2005.

Substance Abuse and Mental Health Services Administration: Available at http://www.samhsa.gov.

Toumbourou JW, Stockwell T, Neighbors C, et al: Interventions to reduce harm associated with adolescent substance use, *Lancet* 369:1391-1401, 2007.

Menstrual Disorders

83

Kamillah Wood and Sara B. Kinsman

Menstrual irregularity is one of the most common concerns that pediatricians address with their adolescent female patients. Being prepared to provide anticipatory guidance regarding the normal menstrual cycle will help ensure that adolescent females do not experience complications associated with dysfunctional uterine bleeding such as changes in lifestyle, anemia, hospitalization, and transfusions. When adolescent females and their caretakers are taught the risks of excessive menstrual flow, they may be more likely to call a pediatrician before an adolescent has developed a significant anemia. Teaching patients to keep a calendar of their menstrual cycles can help adolescent females to actively care for their own health and begin to communicate effectively with their providers about a number of related health topics, including dysmenorrhea, nutritional needs, and reproductive health needs.

Dysfunctional uterine bleeding (DUB) is menstrual bleeding that is not consistent with the expected timing or flow for average menstrual cycle. The normal menstrual cycle occurs every 28 days with a normal range from 21 to 35 days. Menstrual bleeding typically lasts 4 days with a normal range of 2 to 7 days. Typical blood loss is expected to be 30 mL of blood per cycle with the upper limit of normal being 80 mL per cycle. The average age for menarche in the United States is currently 12.3 years. Although anovulation is common in the first 12 to 24 months after menarche affecting approximately 50% of cycles, excessively frequent menses or high volumes of menstrual flow need to be managed carefully to avoid significant blood loss. Specifically, pediatricians can teach adolescent females and their caretakers that excess blood loss may result from when menstrual flow soaks more than six full pads or tampons per day, lasts for greater than 7 days, and occurs more frequently than every 21 days.

EITOLOGY AND PATHOGENESIS

The most common cause of DUB in young women is anovulation. A normal menstrual cycle starts on the first day of menstruation and begins with the follicular phase. During this phase, a developing ovarian follicle synthesizes estrogen, which promotes endometrial growth and proliferation. As estrogen levels continue to increase, estrogen provides positive feedback centrally to the pituitary gland, causing a surge in luteinizing hormone (LH) excretion. This results in release of the ovum from the follicle. The follicle forms the corpus luteum and the beginning of the luteal phase. Estrogen levels decrease, and the corpus luteum begins to produce progesterone. The progesterone promotes stabilization of the endometrial mucosa as well as glandular changes within the endometrial wall to provide an environment for implantation of a fertilized ovum. Without implantation, the corpus luteum cannot maintain production of progesterone, leading to sloughing of the endometrial lining or menstruation approximately 14 days after ovulation.

Anovulatory cycles result when the increase in estrogen during the follicular stage does not result in a surge of LH and therefore ovulation cannot occur. Because the endometrium is mainly exposed to estrogen without progesterone, it can become highly thickened, resulting in heavy, prolonged, or unsynchronized sloughing of the lining (Figure 83-1).

CLINICAL PRESENTATION

The pediatrician should take a detailed history, including questions regarding the degree and pattern of vaginal bleeding. Asking these questions of the adolescent with the caretaker present can be helpful. Sometimes a dialogue between the adolescent and her caretaker may facilitate a fuller understanding of her bleeding pattern. Questions should include the age of menarche, the duration and amount of bleeding associated with the first few menses, the duration of menstruation subsequently, frequency, the color of menstruation, the presence of clots in the menstrual discharge, the number of pads or tampons used daily, and any need to change pads or tampons during the night. The presence of dysmenorrhea will also be helpful. Despite careful history taking, most adolescent and adult females cannot accurately account for the total amount of blood loss; however, aspects of this history will still inform the pediatrician's laboratory evaluation.

In a confidential setting, the pediatricians should ask the adolescent directly about her sexual history, including consensual and nonconsensual sexual intercourse, history of sexually transmitted diseases, use of hormonal contraceptive methods or intrauterine devices (IUDs), and history of pregnancies or abortions. Questions of physical or sexual abuse are important, although adolescent females may need to be reminded that pediatricians are mandated reporters and will need to ensure the adolescent's safety by reporting history of abuse to other helping adults.

The review of systems can assess for the presence of other etiologies that could cause DUB. The report of weight changes, oral lesions, or dental decay may raise concern for an eating disorder; visual changes, headaches, and galactorrhea may raise concern for a prolactinoma; acne, hirsutism, acanthosis nigricans, and obesity may raise concern for polycystic ovarian syndrome (PCOS); and nosebleeds, bruising, or petechiae may raise concern for bleeding dyscrasias.

The family history should include information regarding the history of heavy or prolonged menses, chronic anemia, bleeding disorders, PCOS, and endocrine disorders such as thyroid disease.

The pediatrician will also be interested in medication use, even those that a caretaker may not be aware of such as an oral contraceptive pill (OCP), IUD, or excessive aspirin use.

For the general physical examination, close attention to vital signs may reveal tachycardia or have orthostatic hypotension associated with severe anemia. In addition, the pediatrician should document visual field testing; thyroid enlargement; the

Hypothalamic regulation of pituitary gonadotropin production and release

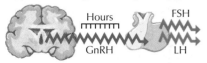

Pulsed release of GnRH by hypothalamus
(1 pulse /1–2 hr) permits anterior pituitary
production and release of FSH and LH (normal)

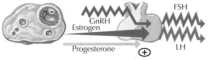

Continuous, excessive, absent, or more frequent
GnRH release inhibits FSH and LH production
and release (downloading)

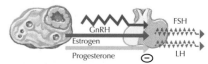

Decreased pulsed release of GnRH
decreases LH secretion but increases
SH secretion (slow-pulsing model)

Ovarian feedback modulation of pituitary gonadotropin production and release

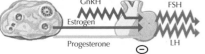

Pulsed GnRH and low estrogen and
progesterone levels result in increased levels of
pulsed LH and FSH (negative feedback)

Pulsed GnRH, rapidly increasing levels
of estrogen, and small amounts of progesterone
result in high pulsed LH and moderately
increased pulsed FSH levels (positive feedback)

Pulsed GnRH and high levels of
estrogen and progesterone result
in decreased LH and FSH levels
(negative feedback)

Correlation of serum gonadotrophic and ovarian hormone levels and feedback mechanisms

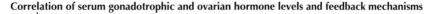
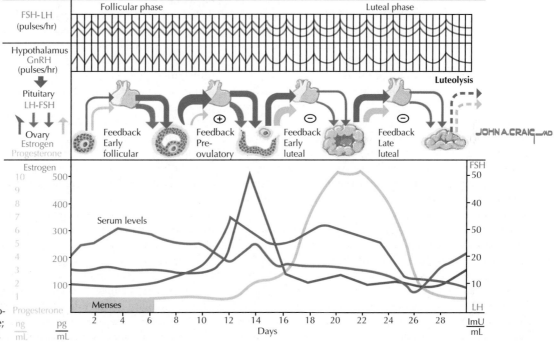

FSH, follicle-stimulating
hormone; GnRH, gonado-
tropin-releasing hormone;
LH, luteinizing hormone.

Figure 83-1 *Neuroendocrine regulation of menstrual cycle.*

presence or absence of galactorrhea; signs of androgen excess; and signs of extramenstrual bleeding, including bruising and petechiae.

The external genital examination can identify pubertal Tanner staging, clitoromegaly, and heavy ongoing vaginal bleeding that may be due to trauma or malodorous discharge that may be associated with a retained foreign body or anatomic abnormality. For young and nonsexually experienced adolescents, a pelvic examination may not be indicated or possible in the pediatrician's office. If no significant concern for acute vaginal tear, foreign body, or anatomic etiology is present, the pelvic examination can be deferred.

For adolescents who are sexually active, direct observation of the source of bleeding from the vaginal mucosa or cervix may be helpful. Cervical testing for gonorrhea and chlamydia can be

obtained. With a bimanual examination, the clinician can also assess the degree to which the adolescent is experiencing cervical motion tenderness, uterine tenderness, or pelvic fullness.

Laboratory evaluation should begin with a urine pregnancy test and complete blood count and differential. If there is a concern for a coagulopathy, prothrombin time, partial thromboplastin time, and a von Willebrand panel are indicated before starting hormonal treatment. Consultation with a hematologist may facilitate a comprehensive assessment of bleeding disorders. Endocrine evaluation, including thyroid-stimulating hormone, serum prolactin, free testosterone, FSH, LH, and estradiol can be helpful.

Ultrasonography is useful in adolescents who cannot undergo a full speculum examination and is indicated for adolescents who are pregnant or for whom an anatomic abnormality is suspected.

Pelvic ultrasonography will be more sensitive than most pediatricians' examination to exclude an anatomic abnormality.

DIFFERENTIAL DIAGNOSIS

The most common cause of DUB in adolescents during the 2 years after menarche is anovulatory cycles, but before making this diagnosis, other causes of DUB must be excluded. Foremost, pregnancy, ectopic pregnancy, and pregnancy-related complications must be excluded. Threatened, spontaneous, or incomplete abortions can cause DUB.

Blood dyscrasias are also a major cause of DUB. In one study, almost 20% of patients with complications of DUB had von Willebrand disease. Adolescents with these disorders frequently report excessive or prolonged menstrual bleeding starting at the time of menarche. Other bleeding disorders, including leukemias or lymphomas, may present with changes in uterine bleeding.

Infections with *Neisseria gonorrhoeae* and *Chlamydia trachomatis* may cause an inflammation of the endometrium or endometritis, resulting in prolonged menstrual bleeding and cervical friability. In developing countries, endometrial infiltration with tuberculosis is an important cause of DUB.

Endocrinopathies, including hypothyroidism and hyperthyroidism, prolactinomas, late-onset 21-hydroxylase deficiency, Cushing's disease, Addison's disease, and PCOS, can result in DUB. Disorders that affect the hypothalamic–pituitary–ovarian axis, including bulimia nervosa, are also a consideration.

Medications that impact the ovulatory cycle, such as tricyclic antidepressants, valproic acid, and antipsychotics, may be causative. Other medications that affect coagulation, such as aspirin-containing compounds, can exacerbate bleeding.

Trauma to the vagina or cervix, retained foreign body, and vascular or anatomic lesions must be included in the differential diagnosis. Congenital anatomic abnormalities may be considered when the patient reports having regular, red-colored menstrual bleeding followed by brown or prune-colored discharge between cycles. This is caused by the normal uterus emptying in a cyclic pattern while the obstructed uterus or vagina empties into a fistula slowly over a period of time. A foul smell may accompany this intermenstrual discharge because of infection with anaerobic bacteria (Figure 83-2).

TREATMENT

The treatment for DUB is determined by the severity of symptoms, the underlying etiology, and complicating comorbidities. A treatment plan should be developed that stops active bleeding and prevents recurrence.

In adolescents with DUB that is not associated with significant anemia, the best approach is to provide anticipatory guidance regarding normal parameters, asking patients to keep a menstrual calendar, and periodic visits to check hemoglobin if bleeding exceeds normal expectations. A diet high in iron or adding a multivitamin with iron may be initiated as a preventive measure against anemia.

Combined hormonal contraception, such as an OCP that includes estrogen and progesterone, can be used to treat an adolescent with DUB that affects the adolescent's daily activities or results in anemia. The rationale for using OCPs is that the estrogen component will help to stop blood loss at the actively bleeding sites within the endometrium. Estrogen also increases platelet aggregation and levels of fibrinogen, as well as factors V and IX. The progesterone component adds stabilization to the endometrium and decreases the risk of endometrial sloughing. If an adolescent has an underlying condition that does not allow for use of estrogen (i.e., a clotting disorder), therapy with progesterone only can be substituted. However, progesterone only therapy is considered less effective. An OCP with 30 μg of ethinyl estradiol is generally recommended in the combined therapy.

An adolescent with DUB and mild anemia who is not actively bleeding may be started on OCPs once daily. When active bleeding is present, the pediatrician may prescribe one pill every 6 hours until 24 hours after menses stops followed by a slow taper (i.e., one pill three times a day for 3 days, one pill twice daily for 2 days, and then one pill daily). The estrogen component of the pill may cause nausea, so an antiemetic medication may be prescribed. Bleeding usually subsides within the first 48 hours of treatment; however, if bleeding persists beyond this time frame, a higher dose of OCP may be indicated, and reevaluation of the cause of the DUB should be considered. If bleeding occurs during the hormonal taper, the medication dose should be readjusted to control bleeding. To ensure that the adolescent has time to replete iron stores, continuous hormonal therapy should be maintained for several weeks (8-12 weeks) without use of the placebo OCP. The patient and the caretaker need to be aware that the first withdrawal bleed after using OCP may be unusually heavy. OCPs can be continued for 6 months or more to give the adolescent female time to mature and increase the likelihood that her neuroendocrine system will be able to synchronize ovulatory menstrual cycles. In addition, if an adolescent is sexually active, she may choose to stay on an OCP for a longer period.

Significant anemia (hemoglobin <8 g/dL) with hemodynamic instability merits inpatient admission. Although an OCP can be used in the acute setting with dosages of estrogen at 30 μg every 4 hours, conjugated intravenous estrogen doses of 25 mg every 4 to 6 hours will usually stop the bleeding within 24 hours. If bleeding does not subside, gynecologic consultation should occur to assess the need for dilatation and curettage. Blood transfusion is indicated for adolescents who have severe anemia and are hemodynamically unstable.

Treatment of DUB related to other chronic conditions will require treatment specific to the underlying cause.

CONCLUSION

The pediatrician plays an important role in educating adolescent females about normative menstrual cycles and the risks associated with excess bleeding. Learning how to quickly assess DUB in the office will reduce the need for increased levels of care for a problem that can easily and comfortably be managed in the office setting. An added positive experience for pediatricians and adolescent patients is the benefit of beginning a dialogue about general and reproductive health needs.

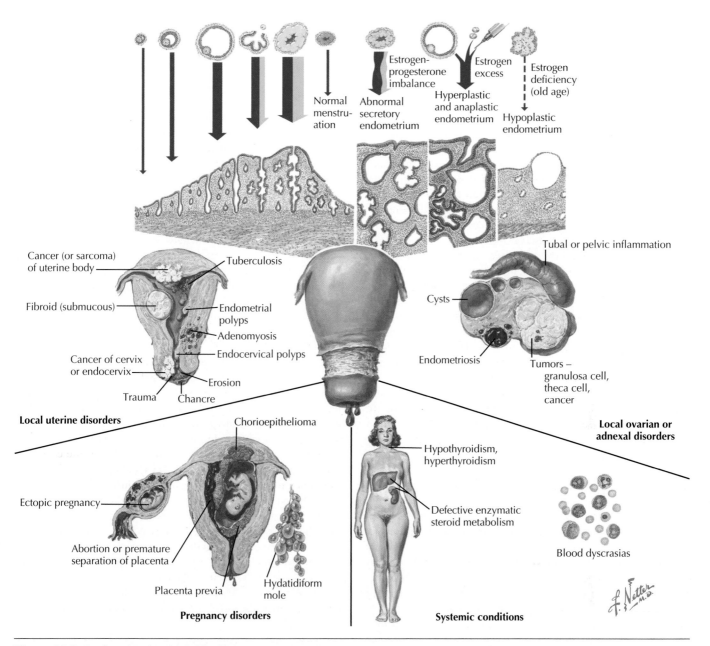

Figure 83-2 *Dysfunctional uterine bleeding.*

SUGGESTED READINGS

El-Hemaidi I, Gharaibeh A, Shehata H: Menorrhagia and bleeding disorders, *Curr Opin Obstet Gynecol* 19(6):513-520, 2007.

Emans SJ: Dysfunctional uterine bleeding. In Emans SJ, Laufer MR, Goldstein DP, editors: *Pediatric and Adolescent Gynecology*, ed 5, Philadelphia, Lippincott, 2005, Williams & Wilkins, pp 270-286.

Lavin C: Dysfunctional uterine bleeding in adolescents, *Curr Opin Pediatr* 8(4):328-332, 1996.

Lazovic G, Radivojec U, Milicevic S, et al: The most frequent hormone dysfunctions in juvenile bleeding, *Int J Fertil Womens Med* 52(1):35-40, 2007.

Messinis IE: From menarche to regular menstruation: endocrinological background, *Ann N Y Acad Sci* 1092:49-56, 2006.

Rimza ME: Dysfunctional uterine bleeding, *Pediatr Rev* 23:227-232, 2002.

Toth M, Patton DL, Esquenazi B, et al: Association between *Chlamydia trachomatis* and abnormal bleeding, *Am J Reprod Immunol* 57(5):361-366, 2007.

Polycystic Ovarian Syndrome

84

Oana Tomescu and Sara B. Kinsman

*P*olycystic ovarian syndrome (PCOS), the most common endocrinopathy affecting women, frequently presents during adolescence. PCOS is characterized by anovulatory menstrual dysfunction, hyperandrogenism, obesity, and metabolic disturbances including insulin-resistance and dyslipidemia. Pediatricians who learn to identify and manage PCOS can help address their adolescent patients' immediate health concerns and reduce the likelihood of later sequelae, including endometrial hyperplasia and cardiovascular disease.

In 1935, Stein and Leventhal first described a syndrome characterized by enlarged ovaries, hirsutism, and chronic anovulation. Since that time, diagnostic guidelines have evolved. In 2009, the Androgen Excess and PCOS (AE-PCOS) Society Task Force published the following diagnostic guidelines for PCOS: (1) hyperandrogenism (clinical, biochemical, or both), (2) ovarian dysfunction (oligoanovulation, polycystic ovaries, or both), and (3) the exclusion of related disorders. Additionally, these new guidelines stress the importance of screening women with PCOS for metabolic syndrome. Metabolic syndrome includes a set of biological risks, including abdominal obesity, elevated serum triglycerides, and insulin resistance, that significantly increase the likelihood that an individual will develop cardiovascular disease.

ETIOLOGY AND PATHOGENESIS

PCOS is thought to result from an interaction involving multiple genetic loci and environmental factors that disrupt several metabolic pathways. Resulting androgen excess can present as hyperandrogenism (Figure 84-1). One androgen pathway involved in PCOS is altered luteinizing hormone (LH) function, which can lead to increased androgen production by ovarian theca cells. This finding is especially common in thin or normal weight women with PCOS. Another potential pathway that leads to elevated androgens involves insulin resistance and compensatory hyperinsulinemia. Elevated insulin levels can also stimulate androgen production by ovarian theca cells while simultaneously inhibiting liver synthesis of sex hormone–binding globulin (SHBG), which in turn results in an increased fraction of bioavailable or free testosterone.

CLINICAL PRESENTATION

PCOS typically presents during adolescence with one or more of these symptoms: menstrual irregularities, androgen excess including hirsutism, acne that is resistant to treatment, male pattern hair loss, and obesity. Menstrual dysfunction may present as primary amenorrhea, oligomenorrhea, secondary amenorrhea, or dysfunctional uterine bleeding. Eighty percent of women with PCOS present with menstrual irregularity; however, 20% experience "regular" anovulatory vaginal bleeding. One of the factors that can delay diagnosis of PCOS during early adolescence is the high frequency of developmental anovulation ($\approx$50% of cycles) during the 2 years after menarche. Although irregular menses is common during this stage of development, this is not accompanied by clinical or biochemical evidence of androgen excess.

Clinical signs of hyperandrogenism may include hirsutism, acne and androgenic alopecia (thinning of the crown hair with preservation of the anterior hairline). Hirsutism affects approximately 70% of women with PCOS. Significant virilization, such as severe hirsutism, clitoromegaly, or bitemporal hair recession, is rarely seen with PCOS. Obesity is present in approximately 50% of women with PCOS. Insulin resistance and dyslipidemia are also very common. One center noted that 25% of their adolescent females with PCOS had metabolic syndrome.

DIFFERENTIAL DIAGNOSIS

PCOS is the most common diagnosis for adolescent females presenting with androgen excess, although other causes must be excluded, including androgen-secreting neoplasms (ASNs), nonclassic congenital adrenal hyperplasia (NC-CAH), other endocrinopathies, and exposure to drugs. Androgen-secreting neoplasms (ASNs) should be considered when there is rapidly progressive onset of hyperandrogenism and significant virilization. Nonclassic ("late-onset") CAH (NC-CAH) is the second most common cause of androgen excess during adolescence and typically results from a mild deficiency of 21-hydroxylase. Much rarer etiologies of androgen excess include mild deficiencies of 3-β-hydroxysteroid dehydrogenase and 11-β-hydroxylase. Other endocrine disorders that can disrupt the menstrual cycle but rarely present with hyperandrogenism include thyroid disease, hyperprolactinemia, Cushing's syndrome, and premature ovarian failure. Drugs, including anabolic steroids and valproic acid, may also result in symptoms of androgen excess.

SCREENING AND EVALUATION

Testosterone is abnormally elevated in approximately 70% of patients with PCOS. The most sensitive test for PCOS is plasma free testosterone or calculated free testosterone. Mild elevation in dehydroepiandrosterone sulfate (DHEA-S) or androstenedione can account for the androgen excess in 10% of patients with PCOS; importantly, significantly elevated levels of DHEA-S or androstenedione suggest a virilizing adrenal disorder. Elevated levels of 17-hydroxyprogesterone may suggest the diagnosis of NC-CAH. Obtaining thyroid-stimulating hormone, free thyroxine, prolactin, LH, follicle-stimulating hormone, random serum cortisol, and estradiol levels will help to exclude other endocrinopathies.

An ultrasound to evaluate for the presence of polycystic ovaries may be helpful, although lack of polycystic ovaries if other criteria are present will not change management. Although 80% of adult women with PCOS have polycystic ovaries, only 20% of women with polycystic ovaries meet criteria for PCOS.

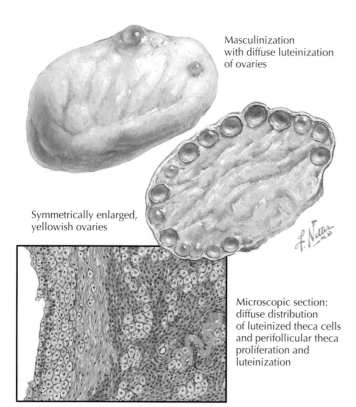

Masculinization with diffuse luteinization of ovaries

Symmetrically enlarged, yellowish ovaries

Microscopic section: diffuse distribution of luteinized theca cells and perifollicular theca proliferation and luteinization

Figure 84-1 *Polycystic ovarian disease.*

Because polycystic ovaries typically do not develop until 2 or more years after menarche, ultrasound findings may be normal in younger adolescents with PCOS.

After the diagnosis of PCOS has been confirmed, many experts suggest that each patient should be screened for dyslipidemias and insulin resistance with an oral glucose tolerance test, even if fasting blood sugar and insulin levels are normal.

MANAGEMENT

The management of PCOS should focus on the clinical concerns of the patient (e.g., menstrual irregularity, hirsutism, or acne) and the long-term consequences of PCOS, such as endometrial hyperplasia and cardiovascular disease risk factors.

To treat menstrual irregularity, prescribing a combined oral contraceptive pill is the first-line treatment. Adolescent females who have contraindications to combined oral contraceptive pills can schedule regular withdrawal bleeds using a progestin such as medroxyprogesterone. For concerns related to androgen excess, OCPs are also the first-line treatment. A pill containing 30 to 35 µg ethinyl estradiol combined with a progestin with minimal androgenicity (norgestimate, desogestrel, or drospirenone) will help improve acne and stop progression of hirsutism. To further manage hirsutism, an antiandrogen such as spironolactone can be added. Eflornithine HCl Cream (Vaniqa) or mechanical hair removal may be used by some adolescent females to reduce unwanted facial hair. For obese patients with PCOS, assisting the patient to exercise and achieve modest weight loss (≈5% of total body weight) can result in restored menstrual cycles. Metformin may be considered to suppress appetite, enhance weight loss, and reduce insulin level. Adolescents should be assured that when they plan to get pregnant, their physician will recommend treatment, possibly including metformin to enhance fertility.

CONCLUSION

PCOS should be considered in any adolescent female who presents with menstrual irregularity, symptoms of androgen excess including hirsutism, persistent or severe acne, or male pattern balding and obesity. A full diagnostic evaluation can exclude other etiologies of androgen excess and allow the pediatrician to start treatment. Effective strategies to manage symptoms and reduce long-term health risks can significantly improve the immediate and long-term well-being of adolescents with PCOS.

SUGGESTED READINGS

Center for Young Women's Health at Boston Children's Hospital: Polycystic Ovary Syndrome (PCOS): A Guide for Teens, Available at http://www.youngwomenshealth.org/pcosinfo.html.

Pfeifer SM, Kives S: Polycystic ovarian syndrome in the adolescent, *Obstet Clin North Am* 36:129-152, 2009.

Eating Disorders

85

Levon H. Utidjian and Sara B. Kinsman

*P*ediatricians are well positioned to screen their preadolescent and adolescent patients routinely for eating disorders. With increased awareness, pediatricians can often effectively decrease the progression of disordered eating and manage potentially harmful consequences of significant weight loss, including electrolyte abnormalities, risk of osteoporosis, and chronic patterns of disordered eating. During adolescence, many teens become self-conscious and report food restriction or increased exercising to achieve a thinner appearance. For most adolescents, these are short-term behavioral changes that do not negatively impact long-term health, but for adolescents at risk for an eating disorder, these common behaviors may result in significant long-term medical and emotional sequelae.

ETIOLOGY AND PATHOGENESIS

In the United States, it is estimated that the lifetime prevalence of anorexia nervosa is 0.5% and 1% to 3% for bulimia nervosa. Ten percent of all eating disorder patients are males. The current *Diagnostic and Statistical Manual of Mental Disorders* (DSM-IV) outlines the criteria for the diagnosis of anorexia nervous and bulimia nervosa as summarized in Box 85-1. Although a main feature of the diagnosis of anorexia nervosa is a body weight that is below 85% of that expected for age and height, for younger patients, the diagnosis can be made without weight loss from previous visits if the patient fails to make the expected weight gains of normal growth. The DSM-IV criteria for bulimia nervosa require recurrent episodes of regular binge eating with inappropriate compensatory behaviors to avoid weight gain. Eating disorder not otherwise specified encompasses eating disorders that do not meet full DSM-IV criteria for either anorexia or bulimia nervosa. Some reports show that more than 50% of adolescents with eating disorders fall into this category; these patients still require appropriate treatment because they have the same underlying eating behaviors and can develop the same life-threatening complications.

CLINICAL PRESENTATION

Pediatricians may be alerted to the early stages of an eating disorder during their evaluations at the patient's routine and acute visits. Weight loss or failure to gain weight may be an initial finding. Vital signs may also reveal bradycardia, a lower blood pressure, or hypothermia compared with previous visits. A patient with anorexia nervosa may present with thinning of scalp hair, lanugo or fine hair growth on the extremities, dry skin, acrocyanosis, and bruising or calluses related to overexercising. Bulimia nervosa may be considered if the pediatrician notes scarring or abrasions in the back of the mouth, parotid gland hypertrophy, dental enamel erosions, or calluses on the dorsum of the fingers known as Russell's sign, which result from self-induced vomiting. Some of the symptoms of patients with bulimia nervosa are summarized in Figure 85-1.

If a pediatrician becomes concerned that a patient may be at risk for an eating disorder, screening for known risk factors may be helpful. Although patients and even their parents or guardians may not be fully able to report the degree of restriction or purging during the early stages of weight loss, reports of changing eating patterns, such as giving up favorite foods or eating away from family members, may be useful information. In addition to changing eating patterns, pediatricians should screen for known risk factors, including history of dieting, childhood or family concerns regarding weight gain, participation in competitive sports that focus on maintaining a specific weight such as gymnastics or wrestling, or participation in sports that can result in lower body fat stores such as cross-country running or swimming. Social history will shed light on other psychiatric diagnosis that could increase the risk of an eating disorder, including obsessive-compulsive symptoms associated with anorexia nervosa and substance use or alcohol misuse associated with bulimia. Difficulties in family communication, ability to manage conflict, or marital tension may also be risk factors.

The family history may be notable for a first-degree relative with an eating disorder as studies have found that adolescents whose first-degree relatives have eating disorders are 6 to 10 times more likely to develop an eating disorder.

DIFFERENTIAL DIAGNOSIS

The differential diagnosis of eating disorders includes other medical and psychiatric conditions that can account for the symptoms of weight loss or, in the case of bulimia, chronic vomiting or electrolyte abnormalities (Box 85-2). These diagnoses need to be excluded by history or laboratory evaluation because the resulting malnutrition associated with these chronic conditions can look very much like an eating disorder.

Laboratory evaluation will also help to assess the degree to which an adolescent is affected by the disorder. Laboratory evaluation includes a complete blood count, erythrocyte sedimentation rate, electrolytes, calcium, magnesium, phosphorus, serum glucose, blood urea nitrogen, creatinine, and urinalysis. If the patient has amenorrhea, pregnancy should be ruled out; in addition, thyroid function tests, serum prolactin, follicle-stimulating hormone level, luteinizing hormone level, and estradiol can be obtained. A morning screening serum cortisol and adrenocorticotrophic hormone level will help to exclude Addison's disease, which has been reported to present similarly to anorexia nervosa. An electrocardiogram (ECG) should be obtained to assess any changes that may result from electrolyte shifts and to document the degree of bradycardia. Patients with long-standing amenorrhea may benefit from a bone densitometry study.

MANAGEMENT

Adolescents with eating disorders are best cared for by an interdisciplinary treatment team, including a pediatrician or medical gain. Expected rates of weight gain depend on the patient's percent ideal body weight. Outpatient treatment for an adolescent who is medically stable typically aims to increase weight at 1 to 2 lb per week. During the period of initial weight gain, the medical provider may prescribe multivitamins and additional calcium. Clinicians vary in their comfort in providing short-term promotility agents and osmotic laxatives to enhance gut motility and minimize the symptoms of constipation.

The nutritionist will educate patients regarding balanced nutrition, assist patients in making specific dietary choices, and help patients to gain weight following a controlled plan.

Ensuring that the patient receives care from a mental health provider with experience in treating eating disorders in adolescent patients is essential for long-term healing. Effective treatment strategies include cognitive behavioral approaches, interpersonal psychotherapies, and family-based therapies, including the Maudsley method.

Pharmacotherapy for anorexia nervosa has not demonstrated significant efficacy, but comorbid disorders such as obsessive-compulsive disorder may benefit from treatment. Antidepressants such as selective serotonin reuptake inhibitors can reduce binge-eating and purging behaviors and reduce relapse rates in bulimia nervosa.

Inpatient hospitalization or psychiatric residential treatment may be required for severely affected adolescents who are dehydrated, have significant bradycardia, demonstrate risk for arrhythmia on ECG (i.e., a prolonged QTc), have electrolyte abnormalities, are poorly motivated for recovery, or express suicidality. A major complication of the treatment of anorexia nervosa or any patient who is severely malnourished is refeeding syndrome. This occurs when rapidly refeeding leads to hypophosphatemia, which can affect multiple organ systems, producing cardiac, neurologic, neuromuscular, pulmonary, and hematologic complications, and may present as confusion, coma, convulsions and death. Thus, refeeding must be performed carefully with close monitoring and potential supplementation of phosphate, as well as other electrolytes.

PROGNOSIS

Almost half of patients with anorexia nervosa recover without long-term sequelae. An estimated 25% of patients improve but remain symptomatic, and approximately another 25% of patients may have chronic symptoms of anorexia nervosa. Long-term mortality may be as high as 10% and usually results from malnutrition, suicide, or other physiologic complications. The majority of adolescents with bulimia recover with effective treatment. Patients with a history of high frequency of pretreatment vomiting, longer duration of symptoms before initiation of treatment, and substance abuse are at increased risk for developing relapsing bulimic behaviors.

CONCLUSION

In the past decade, pediatricians have been challenged to balance messages related to the risks of obesity with prevention messages related to the risks of unhealthy dieting to achieve thinness. Having regular visits with children and adolescents allows pediatricians to observe weight trends and health behavior

clinician, a nutritionist, and a mental health provider. Having a system of communication that allows for the three providers to update one another regarding progress and concerns will greatly improve coordination of the team's care plan.

The pediatrician should monitor weight gain; vital sign stability, including bradycardia; electrolyte abnormalities that may result from dehydration, refeeding, or purging; and long-term concerns, including amenorrhea and osteopenia. The pediatrician should schedule weekly visits to assess vital signs and weight

Box 85-2 Eating Disorder Differential Diagnosis

- Endocrine: diabetes mellitus, thyroid disease, hypopituitarism, Addison's disease
- Gastrointestinal: inflammatory bowel disease, malabsorption, celiac disease
- Infectious: chronic, occult infections
- Oncologic: central nervous system tumor
- Psychiatric: major depression, obsessive-compulsive disorder, substance abuse

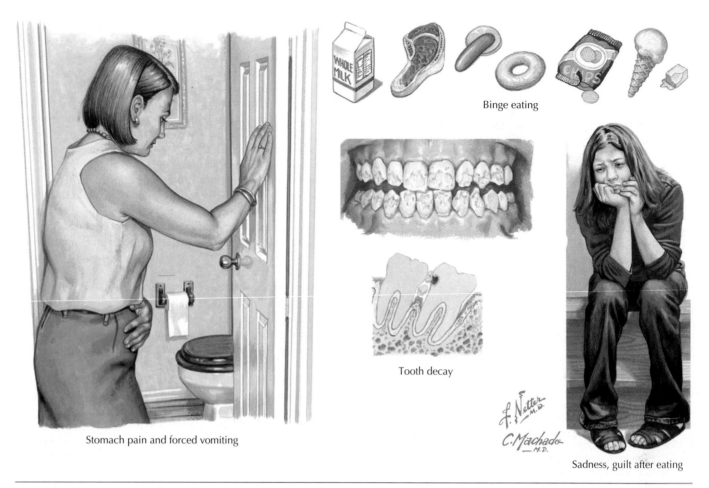

Binge eating

Tooth decay

Stomach pain and forced vomiting

Sadness, guilt after eating

Figure 85-1 *Signs and symptoms of bulimia nervosa.*

patterns over the course of the patient's development. Being attuned to the adolescent's concerns related to his or her body, screening for risk factors associated with an eating disorder, and addressing potential eating disorders early will help to minimize the long-term risks associated with an eating disorder. Developing an interdisciplinary team to address patients who have eating disorders is essential in ensuring recovery. Advocating for access to effective care if the patient requires hospitalization or long-term care may be time consuming for the pediatrician but is extremely important. With the support of informed and effective pediatricians, adolescents at risk for an eating disorder will have a much better chance of avoiding

significant risks and developing safe and healthy eating and exercise patterns for life.

SUGGESTED READINGS

American Academy of Pediatrics Committee on Adolescence: Identifying and treating eating disorders, *Pediatrics* 111(1):204-211, 2003.

American Psychiatric Association: *Diagnostic and Statistical Manual of Mental Disorders*, ed 4, text revision. Washington, DC, 2000, American Psychiatric Association.

American Psychiatric Association: *Practice Guideline for the Treatment of Patients with Eating Disorders*, ed 3, Washington DC, 2006, American Psychiatric Association.

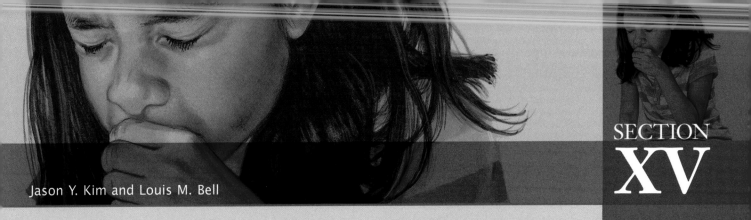

Jason Y. Kim and Louis M. Bell

SECTION
XV

Infectious Disease

Fever of Unknown Origin

86

Elizabeth E. Foglia

Fever is one of the most common signs that prompt parents to seek medical attention for their children, accounting for up to 15% of office visits to pediatricians. Although most pediatric febrile illnesses have an easily identifiable source, a small percentage of children have prolonged fevers with no clear etiology. In children, fever of unknown origin (FUO) has classically been defined as a 2-week history of daily fevers >38.3°C with no identifiable etiology after a thorough physical examination and an initial screening diagnostic evaluation have been performed.

DIFFERENTIAL DIAGNOSIS

The differential diagnosis for FUO can be broadly divided into the following categories: infection, collagen vascular or autoimmune, and malignancy. A number of case series have followed children who were evaluated for FUO to determine the underlying etiology of fever in these patients (Table 86-1). Many of these reports are decades old and may not comprise the underlying infectious etiologies of FUO because of the advancement of clinical microbiologic laboratory and diagnostic imaging modalities, as well as the emergence of novel pathogens. Nonetheless, these studies are informative in that the most commonly identified etiologies for FUO have remained stable through time.

Infection

Infections comprise the majority of identifiable causes of FUO in children, accounting for up to 50% of all final diagnoses. In most cases, the underlying diagnosis reflects an unusual presentation of a common illness rather than a typical presentation of an uncommon entity.

BACTERIAL INFECTIONS

Identification of bacterial sources of FUO is important because early diagnosis can lead to prompt initiation of antimicrobial therapy and fewer long-term consequences. The most common bacterial infections causing FUO in children are upper and lower respiratory tract infections (including otitis media, sinusitis, and pneumonia), urinary tract infections (UTIs), and osteomyelitis. Although the history and physical examination often point to these diagnoses, many of these infections may present with isolated fever. In particular, UTI should be considered in all patients with FUO because physical examination findings are not reliable in patients with UTIs, and in younger, nonverbal children, the history may not suggest UTI.

Soft tissue infections of the head and neck (including tonsillopharyngitis, peritonsillar abscess, and cervical adenitis) can also lead to prolonged fevers, although localizing symptoms usually prompt earlier diagnosis of these entities. Endocarditis is an important cause of FUO in patients with congenital or acquired heart disease; this entity can also occur in patients without an underlying structural heart anomaly, particularly in the case of infections with *Staphylococcus aureus*. Although isolated prolonged fever rarely occurs in bacterial meningitis, it should be considered in the differential diagnosis of all febrile patients. The incidence of occult bacteremia has decreased in recent years after the introduction of *Streptococcus pneumoniae* and *Haemophilus influenzae* type B vaccines. Still, it should be considered in the case of isolated fevers, particularly in young children who are not fully immunized or who have not received vaccinations.

Bartonellosis, or cat scratch disease, is an increasingly identified etiology of FUO in children and should especially be considered in patients with marked regional adenopathy or a history of exposure to cats or kittens. Enteric infections, such as salmonellosis and yersiniosis, have also been identified as sources of FUO; a history of gastrointestinal (GI) complaints is suggestive in these cases. Returned travelers or recent immigrants may present with typhoid (*Salmonella typhi* or *Salmonella paratyphi*) or typhoidal rickettsial infections. Both pulmonary and extrapulmonary tuberculosis (TB) must be included in the differential diagnosis in every patient with FUO because isolated prolonged fever is often the only presenting sign. Zoonotic infections are less common, but still identifiable, causes of FUO. Among these are tularemia, brucellosis, and Q fever, and they should be considered with the appropriate exposures. Ehrlichiosis, anaplasmosis, and Rocky Mountain spotted fever are tickborne infections and may present with prolonged fever; the incidence of these infections varies greatly with geography and season.

VIRAL INFECTIONS

Viral infections are frequent causes of FUO in children. Although these infections are generally self-limited, their identification can help avoid further testing and imaging in patients in whom a diagnosis has not been established. Epstein-Barr virus (EBV) remains one of the most common causes of FUO in children. Other systemic viral infections responsible for FUO include systemic cytomegalovirus (CMV), enterovirus, and adenovirus. Viruses in the herpes family, particularly human herpesvirus-six (HHV-6), are commonly found in children and may present with prolonged isolated fever. Newer molecular techniques for identification of parvovirus have demonstrated its prevalence in children with fever. Finally, HIV is a possible source of FUO, both acutely and chronically, in association with opportunistic infections (see Chapter 95).

OTHER INFECTIONS

In patients with an appropriate travel history, malaria is a potential source of FUO in children. Similarly, fungal infections, such as blastomycosis and histomycosis, may present with prolonged fever in children who live in or have traveled to endemic regions.

Table 86-1 Underlying Diagnosis in Fever of Unknown Origin in 545 Patients from Compiled Case Reports

Diagnosis	Total (*n*)	Established Diagnoses (%)
Infectious	**262**	**62**
Epstein-Barr virus	26	6
Viral syndrome	22	5
Urinary tract infection	22	5
Pneumonia	19	4
Osteomyelitis	18	4
Viral meningitis or encephalitis	17	4
Bacterial meningitis	14	3
Pharyngitis or tonsillitis	14	3
Viral upper respiratory infection	12	3
Streptococcosis	9	2
Otitis media	8	2
Bartonellosis	8	2
Bacterial enteritis	7	2
Viral gastroenteritis	7	2
Sinusitis	6	1
Subacute bacterial endocarditis	5	1
Tuberculosis	5	1
Rickettsial infection	5	1
Cytomegalovirus	5	1
Tularemia	4	1
Other Infections	29	7
Collagen Vascular or Autoimmune	**65**	**15**
Juvenile idiopathic arthritis	28	7
Inflammatory bowel disease	11	3
Rheumatic fever	7	2
Other collagen vascular	19	4
Malignancy	**27**	**6**
Leukemia	14	3
Lymphoma	4	1
Other malignancy	9	2
Other	**65**	**17**
Drug reaction	8	2
Factitious fever	6	1
Miscellaneous	51	14
Total established diagnoses	**426**	**78**
Diagnosis unknown	**119**	**22**

Collagen Vascular and Autoimmune Disorders

Fever may be a major presenting symptom in many noninfectious inflammatory conditions. Among these, the acute onset of fever occurs most commonly in systemic juvenile idiopathic arthritis and Kawasaki's disease (KD) (see Chapters 26 and 28). The incidence of KD varies greatly with geography. In the United States, the average incidence ranges between 3.1 and 8.9 cases per 100,000 children per year. Apart from being the more common noninfectious inflammatory causes of fever among children, these disorders are important because they require early recognition and treatment to prevent long-term complications.

Systemic lupus erythematosus (SLE) accounts for a subset of patients with FUO, although this entity does not usually present with isolated fever but rather with multiorgan involvement.

Apart from KD, other vasculitides may present with fever in addition to other organ involvement. Juvenile Behçet's disease in children older than age 1 year may include fever as a symptom, and polyarteritis nodosa should be considered in older children with fever and muscle and skin involvement. Remaining identified vasculitides are either very rare in children or are unlikely to present with isolated fever, such as Henoch-Schönlein purpura (see Chapter 28).

Recurrent intermittent fevers may occur as part of a periodic fever syndrome. The most commonly encountered of these is periodic fever, aphthous stomatitis, pharyngitis, and cervical adenitis disease (PFAPA). The syndrome is rarely associated with fevers that last longer than 1 week. The hereditary fever disorders are far less common but are potential etiologies of recurrent fevers in children. One hereditary fever syndrome that may present with prolonged fever is tumor necrosis factor receptor–associated periodic syndrome (TRAPS). In young children and especially infants with persistent or recurrent fevers, an underlying immunodeficiency should be considered (see Chapter 21).

Inflammatory bowel disease (IBD), particularly Crohn's disease, has become an important diagnostic consideration in children with FUO. Because this entity may be difficult to diagnose at an early age, patients may present with a history of prolonged isolated fever and growth failure with or without intestinal manifestations (see Chapter 110).

Malignancy

Malignancy remains an important diagnostic consideration for children with FUO, and early identification of oncologic processes allows for earlier initiation of directed therapy. In most cases, children with neoplastic processes present with other systemic symptoms or local findings, but it is possible that isolated fever is the only presenting sign. The oncologic processes most likely to present with fever depend on the age of the patient. The most common malignancies to present with isolated fever include leukemia, lymphoma, neuroblastoma, neoplasms of the bone, and Wilms' tumor. Additionally, central nervous system (CNS) malignancies and metastases to the CNS may present with FUO if the thermoregulatory system of the hypothalamus is involved.

Miscellaneous

Other conditions are included in the differential diagnoses for FUO in children. Drug fevers are frequently overlooked as potential causes of FUO in children. Although a history of new medications is often elicited, chronic medications are commonly responsible for drug fevers, especially in drugs that are known to be sensitizing. Sulfa-containing drugs, antiseizure medications, antiarrhythmics, sleep medications, and narcotics are known causes of drug fevers.

Derangements of the thermoregulatory system may lead to prolonged fevers and present as FUO. In addition to malignancy, other noninfectious inflammatory entities that affect the CNS may lead to FUO in children, as can dysautonomia.

Finally, factitious fever is a diagnosis of exclusion and may enter the differential diagnosis only after a thorough investigation has been performed. In children, Munchausen by proxy syndrome is also a cause of factitious fevers. Hospitalization of the patient for close observation and measurement of body temperature can be instructive in the case that a concern exists for factitious fevers.

APPROACH TO THE PATIENT

In a well-appearing child who continues to thrive, the evaluation for FUO may be performed in the outpatient setting. A thorough history will offer many clues to the potential etiology of FUO and will help guide the appropriate diagnostic workup. The major exception to this is an infant younger than 90 days old with fever. Because fever is a less common but more concerning presenting sign in this population, these patients warrant an immediate laboratory evaluation to assess for serious bacterial infections (see Chapter 105).

Table 86-2 Localizing Symptoms in Patients with Fever of Unknown Origin

Organ System	Symptoms
Central nervous system	Headache
	Neck stiffness
	Lethargy or irritability
	Personality or cognitive changes
Respiratory	Nasal congestion or rhinorrhea
	Sinus pain
	Otalgia
	Cough
	Dyspnea
	Chest pain
	Hemoptysis
Ocular	Painful or dry eyes
	Ocular discharge
Oral	Oral ulcers
Gastrointestinal	Abdominal pain
	Abdominal distension
	Changes in appetite
	Vomiting
	Diarrhea
	Hematochezia
Genitourinary	Dysuria, frequency, urgency
	Back pain
	Urethral ulcers or discharge
Musculoskeletal	Extremity or joint swelling or pain
	Limp or limited extremity use

History

A careful fever history is of extreme importance. Although many parents initially report a history of daily fever for 2 weeks or more, it is important to distinguish one prolonged febrile episode from many serial illnesses. The height and pattern of fever should also be recorded.

The child's overall state of health should be described, including activity level and appetite. A history of any localizing or coexisting symptoms should be elicited because they may help target the investigation (Table 86-2). The patient's age and any underlying conditions may offer clues to the diagnosis and help to organize the differential diagnosis. A thorough medication history should be recorded, particularly when considering drug fever. A detailed family history should explore for family members with a history of rheumatologic conditions, malignancy, or IBD.

The social history should include any exposure to ill contacts. Risk factors for TB exposure should be determined. A detailed travel history is important because tropical or exotic infections should be considered. Zoonotic exposures, including contact with livestock, cats, rodents, and reptiles, should be investigated. A dietary history should include consumption of unpasteurized dairy products.

Physical Examination

The physical examination has the highest yield when the child is comfortable in the presence of his or her parents. The child's overall state of health should be noted, including a lethargic or wasted appearance, level of activity, hydration status, and the presence of irritability or inconsolability. Growth percentiles should be charted; stunted growth may point to a more chronic underlying disease process. If a rash is present, it is important to understand the history and evolution of the lesions. Oral lesions may coexist with a rash or occur independently.

The respiratory tract is a common source of infection in children. Vital signs will indicate tachypnea or hypoxia. The overall work of breathing should be noted. An examination of the upper respiratory tract may reveal cough, middle ear effusions, sinus tenderness, rhinorrhea, or stridor. Likewise, auscultation of the lower respiratory tract is important for identification of rales, rhonchi, wheezing, or decreased aeration.

The cardiovascular examination should include auscultation for murmurs and examination of the skin and extremities for signs of endocarditis, such as petechiae, Janeway's lesions, Osler's nodes, and splinter hemorrhages. These stigmata are often absent in younger children. The abdominal examination may reveal hepatosplenomegaly, localizing tenderness, or palpable masses. Suprapubic tenderness and costovertebral tenderness should be elicited. A rectal examination with guaiac smear for occult blood should be performed, particularly if a concern exists for IBD. Potential findings on the genitourinary examination include ulcerations or discharge.

An ophthalmologic examination should be performed; this may reveal uveitis, Roth spots, or signs of infection. The presence of adenopathy should be noted, as well as any tenderness or signs of adenitis. The musculoskeletal examination may help localize the source of fever. Any point tenderness, refusal to bear weight, or limited use of an extremity may suggest an underlying osteomyelitis or malignancy. The patient should be witnessed walking or bearing weight, if developmentally appropriate. All joints should be examined for effusions or arthritis. Muscle tenderness or weakness may suggest myositis. Any positive findings from the physical examination should be used to focus the diagnostic evaluation.

Diagnostic Testing

As the sensitivity and availability of laboratory tests and imaging modalities advance, the identifiable underlying causes of FUO in children continue to evolve (Fig. 86-1). Specifically, viral pathogens and fastidious bacteria that were formally difficult to isolate in culture are more easily detected with polymerase chain reaction (PCR) testing. Additionally, improvements in computed tomography (CT) and ultrasonography for imaging the abdominal cavity have virtually eliminated the need for exploratory laparotomy as a final resort in diagnosis in FUO. Finally, newer techniques in positron emission tomography (PET) scanning allow for identification of regions with increased metabolic activity, making it possible to find potential sources of FUO even in the absence of localizing clinical signs. Still, the diagnostic workup should proceed in a stepwise fashion, using the history and physical examination to guide the testing modalities selected for each patient.

SCREENING EVALUATION

An initial screening laboratory evaluation is appropriate and may be performed in the outpatient setting (Box 86-1). A

Box 86-1 Initial Diagnostic Evaluation in Patients with Fever of Unknown Origin

- Complete blood count and differential
- Complete metabolic panel
- C-reactive protein
- Erythrocyte sedimentation rate
- Urinalysis
- Urine culture
- Blood culture
- Purified protein derivative tuberculin skin test
- Chest radiography

---

complete blood count with differential may be very revealing. An elevated white blood cell count is a nonspecific sign of inflammation, but the degree of elevation is informative. The types of cells that are prominent in the differential count may point toward the source of inflammation. In addition, some infections are associated with leucopenia as well. Microcytic anemia can occur in the setting of chronic disease. Thrombocytosis is a nonspecific marker of inflammation because platelets are acute phase reactants. The suppression of cell lines may point to a rheumatologic or hematologic or neoplastic process. Inflammatory markers, such as C-reactive protein and erythrocyte sedimentation rate are not specific if elevated, but they give an overall impression of level of inflammation. Baseline inflammatory markers are useful in tracking the course of illness. Urinalysis, urine culture, and blood culture should be obtained in all patients. A complete metabolic profile may demonstrate transaminitis or indicate impaired kidney function. Chest radiography is part of the initial evaluation of all patients and may identify parenchymal disease, pulmonary nodules, hilar adenopathy, or cardiomegaly. A purified protein derivative tuberculin skin test should be done on all patients, regardless of known risk factors for infection with TB.

LABORATORY TESTING

Further laboratory testing should be directed by the history and physical and screening evaluation using less invasive testing preferentially. This workup may continue in the outpatient setting initially. Hospitalization is indicated in ill-appearing children and in patients who have had weeks of prolonged fever with no identifiable source after an extensive outpatient investigation.

Common infections should be considered first given the relatively high likelihood of these processes causing FUO; testing for these infections should be performed early in the diagnostic evaluation. Serologic testing for EBV and *Bartonella henselae* (if there is a kitten exposure) should be performed. Common systemic viral infections should also be considered early. PCR testing is available for many viral pathogens and can be performed from many sources, including blood, urine, stool, respiratory secretions, and cerebrospinal fluid. Increasing the number of sources of body fluids or tissue samples that are sent for PCR testing raises the likelihood of identifying a given pathogen. PCR testing for enterovirus, adenovirus, CMV, parvovirus, and HHV-6 should be performed early in the evaluation for FUO.

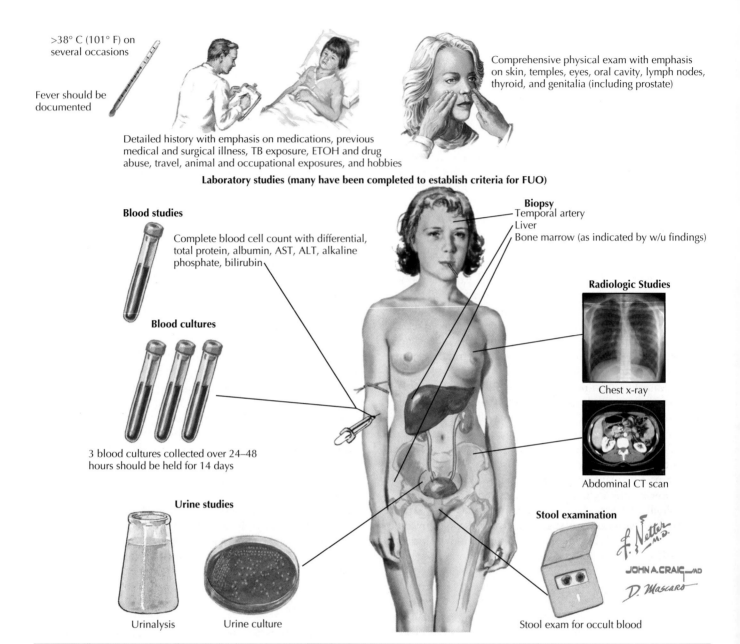

>38° C (101° F) on several occasions

Fever should be documented

Detailed history with emphasis on medications, previous medical and surgical illness, TB exposure, ETOH and drug abuse, travel, animal and occupational exposures, and hobbies

Comprehensive physical exam with emphasis on skin, temples, eyes, oral cavity, lymph nodes, thyroid, and genitalia (including prostate)

Laboratory studies (many have been completed to establish criteria for FUO)

Blood studies

Complete blood cell count with differential, total protein, albumin, AST, ALT, alkaline phosphate, bilirubin

Blood cultures

3 blood cultures collected over 24–48 hours should be held for 14 days

Urine studies

Urinalysis   Urine culture

Biopsy
Temporal artery
Liver
Bone marrow (as indicated by w/u findings)

Radiologic Studies

Chest x-ray

Abdominal CT scan

Stool examination

Stool exam for occult blood

Figure 86-1 *Diagnostic considerations in fever of unknown origin.*

The stool should be cultured if GI symptoms are present. Serial large-volume blood cultures should be obtained if endocarditis is a concern. A low threshold should exist for performing for lumbar puncture in patients who are ill appearing, have meningeal signs, or a history of symptoms involving the CNS. HIV antibodies should be obtained if risk factors exist for HIV, such as sexual activity or intravenous drug use. Specific testing for zoonotic or geographically specific infections should not be performed universally but only in cases as indicated by history.

Although antineutrophil antibodies are a poor screening test for all rheumatologic conditions, this test should be obtained if a concern for SLE exists. Because other collagen vascular conditions are made on a clinical basis, additional laboratory testing should not be used in a "shotgun" approach to rule out rheumatologic and autoimmune conditions (see Chapter 26).

DIAGNOSTIC IMAGING

Imaging studies augment the diagnostic tools available in the evaluation of FUO. The potential benefit of imaging studies should always be weighed against the degree of radiation exposure to the patient. Plain radiographs are appropriate in the initial evaluation of localized limb pain. Contrast imaging of the GI tract is appropriate. Ultrasound technology has the benefit of being fast and painless, and it does not include radiation. The uses of ultrasound include initial abdominal imaging to identify fluid collections, masses, or lesions. Ultrasound is also useful for assessing joint fluid collections as well as superficial fluid collections or masses in the soft tissues. Echocardiography should be obtained in patients with a concern for endocarditis.

Cross-sectional imaging such as CT and magnetic resonance imaging (MRI) provide superior anatomic detail. CT can be performed quickly and can provide anatomic detail for large sections of the body at once. The major disadvantage of CT imaging is the high radiation exposure to the patient. MRI is highly sensitive for detailing anatomic lesions, and it does not involve radiation. However, MRI takes longer to perform, and young children often require sedation to maintain one position during the entire scanning process.

CT is the imaging modality of choice for sinusitis. CT of the head can identify structural abnormalities, such as ventriculomegaly, tumors, or abscesses. MRI of the brain is more sensitive for identifying small lesions and inflammatory processes in the brain parenchyma. CT scanning is also useful for imaging the chest, abdomen, and pelvis for masses, fluid collections, lesions, or adenopathy. CT of the abdomen with oral contrast can also assess the GI tract for bowel wall thickening, fistulae, or other signs of IBD. MRI is especially useful in the assessment of localized bony tenderness to rule out osteomyelitis.

Nuclear medicine studies, such as bone scans and PET scans, may be used when no localizing signs are present. This technology uses tagged tracers that are introduced to the body on a biologically active molecule, such as a glucose analogue. Full-body imaging is then performed to identify regions of tracer uptake that indicate increased metabolic activity. These regions often correlate with infectious or malignant processes. Bone scans may be used if limb pain or limp is present but no focal tenderness is identifiable to localize for MRI scanning or to survey the entire body for occult osteomyelitis. PET scanning may be used to identify regions within the entire body with increased cellular activity. Although these studies may help initially localize regions of interest, they provide no anatomic detail. They are therefore often used in conjunction with CT.

INVASIVE TESTING

Invasive testing may be necessary in the diagnostic evaluation of FUO. Bone marrow biopsy is indicated when a concern for hematologic neoplasm exists. Biopsy of other suspicious masses or lesions is also often necessary to obtain tissue for pathology. Endoscopy is often used in patients for whom IBD is a serious concern. These tests should be performed conservatively and in conjunction with expert consultation.

CONCLUSION

In up to 40% of cases, the underlying etiology for FUO is never determined. Many of these patients' fevers will spontaneously resolve with no diagnosis ever established. It is important to eliminate treatable and potentially life-threatening conditions from the differential diagnosis, but it is not essential that a final diagnosis be established for all patients with FUO. The identifiable etiologies of FUO will continue to evolve in the future in concert with the advancement of diagnostic testing.

SUGGESTED READINGS

Bleeker-Rovers C, van der Meer J, Oyen W: Fever of unknown origin, *Semin Nucl Med* 39:81-87, 2009.

Cunha B: Fever of unknown origin: clinical overview of classic and current concepts, *Infect Dis Clin North Am* 21:867-915, 2007.

Feigin RD, Shearer WT: Fever of unknown origin in children, *Curr Prob Pediatr* 6:3-64, 1976.

Hofer M, Mahlaoui N, Prieur A-M: A child with a systemic febrile illness: differential diagnosis and management, *Best Pract Res Clin Rheumatol* 20:627-640, 2006.

Jacobs R, Schutze G: *Bartonella henselae* as a cause of prolonged fever and fever of unknown origin in children, *Clin Infect Dis* 26:80-84, 1998.

Lohr JA, Hendley JO: Prolonged fever of unknown origin: a record of experiences with 54 childhood patients, *Clin Pediatr* 16:768-773, 1977.

McCarthy P: Fever, *Pediatr Rev* 19:401-408, 1998.

McClung HJ: Prolonged fever of unknown origin in children, *Am J Dis Child* 124:544-550, 1972.

Pizzo PA, Lovejoy FH, Smith DH: Prolonged fever in children: review of 100 cases, *Pediatrics* 55:468-473, 1975.

Infections of the Head and Neck

Jessica L. Hills

87

CERVICAL LYMPHADENITIS

Cervical lymph node enlargement is a common problem in children and adolescents. Almost all children have small palpable cervical lymph nodes. Cervical lymphadenopathy is defined by lymph nodes measuring more than 1 cm in diameter. Lymphadenitis refers specifically to inflammation of lymph nodes and is characterized by enlarged and tender nodes with warmth or erythema of the overlying skin.

ETIOLOGY AND PATHOGENESIS

The cervical lymphatic system consists of a collection of both superficial and deep lymph nodes that protect the head, neck, nasopharynx, and oropharynx against infection (Figure 87-1). Lymph nodes can enlarge by either proliferation of normal cells intrinsic to the node such as lymphocytes or infiltration by cells extrinsic to the node such as neutrophils or malignant cells. The most common cause of cervical lymphadenopathy in children is reactive intranodal hyperplasia secondary to infection. The majority of lymphatics of the head and neck drain to the submandibular lymph nodes and the anterior and posterior cervical lymph node chains. Consequently, these nodes are involved in most children with cervical lymphadenitis.

Many different organisms have been implicated in cervical lymphadenitis (Box 87-1). The most common cause of cervical lymphadenitis is viruses that infect the upper respiratory tract, including adenovirus, respiratory syncytial virus, influenza, and parainfluenza. When bacterial in origin, cervical lymphadenitis may be a primary process or result from direct extension of a local infection such as pharyngitis or dental abscess. In the case of acutely inflamed and enlarged unilateral nodes, aspirates reveal infection by *Staphylococcus aureus* or *Streptococcus pyogenes* (group A β-hemolytic streptococci [GABHS]) in the majority of cases. Recent studies of suppurative lymphadenitis show the predominance of *S. aureus* and the increased prevalence of community-acquired methicillin-resistant *S. aureus* (CA-MRSA). More indolent causes of cervical lymphadenitis include *Bartonella henselae*, mycobacterial infections, and *Toxoplasma gondii*. The age of a child plays a role in predicting the infectious etiology of cervical lymphadenitis (Table 87-1).

CLINICAL PRESENTATION AND DIFFERENTIAL DIAGNOSIS

The presentation of cervical lymphadenitis can be divided into three broad categories: (1) acute bilateral, (2) acute unilateral, and (3) subacute or chronic. The most common causes of acute bilateral cervical lymphadenitis are viral upper respiratory tract infections followed by pharyngitis caused by GABHS. In general, the lymph nodes are small, soft, and mobile without associated erythema, warmth, or significant tenderness. Additional clinical features such as gingivostomatitis in herpes simplex virus or

pharyngoconjunctival fever caused by adenovirus may help to identify the causative virus. Viral causes of generalized lymphadenopathy, such as Epstein-Barr virus (EBV) and cytomegalovirus (CMV), can cause acute bilateral cervical lymphadenitis associated with infectious mononucleosis. In both cases, posterior cervical lymph node enlargement is most prominent followed by anterior cervical nodes.

Acute unilateral cervical lymphadenitis is caused by *S. aureus* and *S. pyogenes* in the majority of cases. The onset may be associated with an upper respiratory tract infection, pharyngitis, or periodontal disease, and associated fever is common. Typically, the onset is acute with development of large, tender, erythematous, and warm lymph nodes that may become fluctuant over a few days (Figure 87-2). In addition, a cellulitis–adenitis syndrome caused by group B streptococcus in infants between 3 and 7 weeks of age is associated with irritability, fever, and unilateral facial or submandibular swelling with erythema and tenderness.

The most common causes of subacute or chronic lymphadenitis are mycobacterial infections, cat scratch disease, and toxoplasmosis. Lymph node enlargement is typically gradual in onset and progresses over weeks to months. The most common presentation of nontuberculous *mycobacterium* (NTM) disease in children is cervical lymphadenitis. The lymph nodes are large and indurated but nontender, and the overlying skin often becomes violaceous and thin (see Figure 87-2). Untreated lymphadenitis caused by NTM may resolve, but often it progresses to lymph node necrosis followed by fluctuance and spontaneous drainage. Cervical lymphadenitis caused by *Mycobacterium tuberculosis* has a similar presentation, but there are clinical and epidemiologic differences. NTM is uncommon in children older than 5 years of age compared with tuberculosis, which can occur at any age. With NTM, involvement is usually unilateral and associated with a normal chest radiograph and a normal or minimally indurated purified protein derivative (PPD). In contrast, children with tuberculous cervical lymphadenitis are more likely to have bilateral lymph node involvement, systemic symptoms, an abnormal chest radiograph, and an abnormal PPD result.

Cat-scratch disease, caused by *B. henselae*, most commonly affects the axilla and cervical regions. Most patients have a history of recent contact with cats or kittens. Clinical manifestations begin with a papule or pustule that develops at the inoculation site a few days to weeks after a bite or scratch followed by lymphadenitis proximal to the site. Lymphadenitis is tender and erythematous and often associated with fever. Lymphadenitis typically persists for several weeks to months and may suppurate. Acquired *Toxoplasma* infection, when symptomatic, generally presents as cervical lymphadenopathy and fatigue without fever. Lymphadenitis most frequently involves a solitary node in the head and neck region without systemic symptoms. Lymphadenitis secondary to toxoplasmosis tends to be nonsuppurative and may persist for many months. In addition, viral etiologies

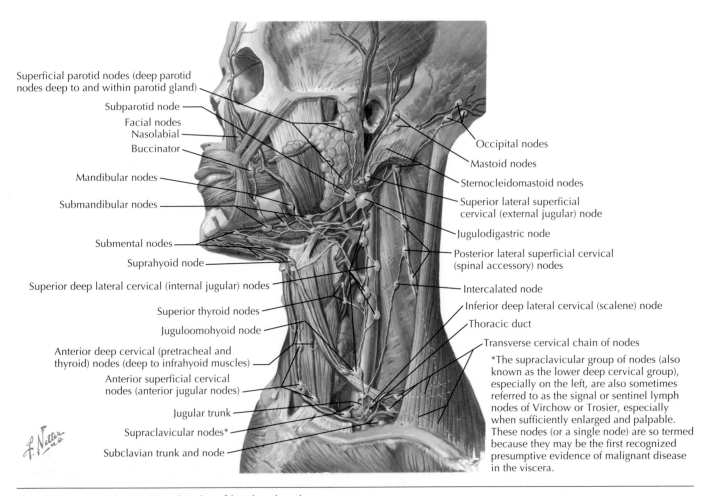

Superficial parotid nodes (deep parotid nodes deep to and within parotid gland)

Subparotid node

Facial nodes
Nasolabial
Buccinator

Mandibular nodes

Submandibular nodes

Submental nodes

Suprahyoid node

Superior deep lateral cervical (internal jugular) nodes

Superior thyroid nodes

Juguloomohyoid node

Anterior deep cervical (pretracheal and thyroid) nodes (deep to infrahyoid muscles)

Anterior superficial cervical nodes (anterior jugular nodes)

Jugular trunk

Supraclavicular nodes*

Subclavian trunk and node

Occipital nodes

Mastoid nodes

Sternocleidomastoid nodes

Superior lateral superficial cervical (external jugular) node

Jugulodigastric node

Posterior lateral superficial cervical (spinal accessory) nodes

Intercalated node

Inferior deep lateral cervical (scalene) node

Thoracic duct

Transverse cervical chain of nodes

*The supraclavicular group of nodes (also known as the lower deep cervical group), especially on the left, are also sometimes referred to as the signal or sentinel lymph nodes of Virchow or Trosier, especially when sufficiently enlarged and palpable. These nodes (or a single node) are so termed because they may be the first recognized presumptive evidence of malignant disease in the viscera.

Figure 87-1 *Lymph vessels and nodes of head and neck.*

such as EBV, CMV, and HIV can cause bilateral subacute cervical lymphadenitis.

Noninfectious causes of lymphadenitis in children are less common but should always be considered in the differential diagnosis. Congenital cysts such as branchial cleft cysts, cystic hygromas, and thyroglossal duct cysts can mimic lymphadenitis, especially when infected. Malignancies such as lymphoma, leukemia, neuroblastoma, and rhabdomyosarcoma can present as cervical lymphadenopathy. Malignancy should be considered in

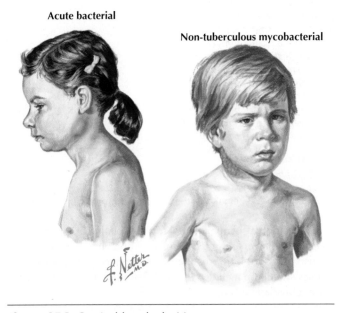

Acute bacterial

Non-tuberculous mycobacterial

Figure 87-2 *Cervical lymphadenitis.*

Table 87-1 Etiology of Cervical Lymphadenitis by Age Group

Age	Etiology
Infants	*Staphylococcus aureus*
	Group B streptococcus
Children age 1-4 y	*S. aureus*
	Group A streptococcus
	Nontuberculous *mycobacterium*
	Bartonella henselae
School-age children and adolescents	*S. aureus*
	Group A streptococcus
	Anaerobes
	B. henselae
	Toxoplasma gondii

Box 87-1 Infectious Etiologies of Cervical Lymphadenitis

Viruses
- Adenovirus
- Coronavirus
- Coxsackievirus
- Cytomegalovirus
- Enteroviruses
- Epstein-Barr virus
- Herpes simplex virus
- Human herpesvirus 6
- HIV
- Influenza
- Mumps
- Parainfluenza
- Parvovirus B19
- Respiratory syncytial virus
- Rhinovirus
- Rubella
- Varicella

Fungi
- *Aspergillus fumigatus*
- *Candida albicans*
- *Coccidioides immitis*
- *Histoplasma capsulatum*

Bacteria
- Anaerobes
- *Actinomyces israelii*
- Atypical mycobacterium
- *Bacillus anthracis*
- *Bartonella henselae*
- *Brucella* spp.
- *Corynebacterium diphtheriae*
- *Francisella tularensis*
- *Haemophilus* spp.
- *Leptospira interrogans*
- *Mycobacterium tuberculosis*
- *Mycoplasma pneumoniae*
- Nontuberculous mycobacterium
- *Nocardia* spp.
- *Pasteurella multocida*
- *Salmonella typhi*
- *Staphylococcus aureus*
- *Streptococcus pyogenes* (GABHS)
- *Streptococcus agalactiae* (GBS)
- *Yersinia pestis*

Protozoa
- *Toxoplasma gondii*

GABHS, group A β-hemolytic streptococci; GBS, group B streptococci.

Box 87-2 Noninfectious Etiologies of Cervical Lymphadenopathy

Congenital Cysts
- Branchial cleft cysts
- Cystic hygromas
- Thyroglossal duct cysts

Malignancies
- Lymphoma
- Leukemia
- Neuroblastoma
- Rhabdomyosarcoma

Miscellaneous
- Castleman's disease
- Collagen vascular disease
- Kawasaki's disease
- Kikuchi-Fujimoto disease (histiocytic necrotizing lymphadenitis)
- Kimura's disease
- PFAPA
- Rosai-Dorfman disease (sinus histiocytosis with massive lymphadenopathy)
- Sarcoidosis

PFAPA, periodic fever, aphthous stomatitis, pharyngitis, and cervical adenitis.

---

cases of indolent lymphadenopathy, especially with a history of weight loss, fevers, night sweats, or lymphadenitis that is unresponsive to antibiotic treatment. Other causes of cervical neck masses should be included in the differential diagnosis of cervical lymphadenitis (Box 87-2).

EVALUATION AND MANAGEMENT

Lymphadenitis is a clinical diagnosis based on physical examination findings of enlarged and inflamed palpable lymph nodes. The evaluation and management of cervical lymphadenitis is directed by a thorough history and physical examination. Patients with acute small, bilateral nodes with minimal tenderness along with symptoms of fever or respiratory tract infection most likely have a viral syndrome and can be managed conservatively with observation and supportive care. If GABHS pharyngitis is suspected, a rapid streptococcal antigen test or throat culture should be performed. In patients with acute large, unilateral, erythematous, and tender nodes associated with fever, bacterial infection is most likely. Antimicrobial therapy should be directed at *S. pyogenes* and *S. aureus* with cephalexin being a reasonable choice. Because of the continuing rise of CA-MRSA in many areas, clindamycin is also an appropriate first-line option. In older children and adolescents, anaerobic bacteria should be suspected in cases of cervical lymphadenitis associated with gingival infections or dental abscesses. In these cases, amoxicillin–clavulanate or clindamycin provide anaerobic coverage in addition to gram-positive coverage. Cervical lymphadenitis can be managed on an outpatient basis for most children who are well-appearing, well-hydrated, and have no evidence of abscess. Hospital admission for intravenous (IV) antibiotics should be considered in infants, ill-appearing children, children who have fluctuant nodes or associated cellulitis, and patients who have failed outpatient treatment. IV antibiotic choices include cefazolin, oxacillin, and ampicillin-sulbactam. In regions with a high prevalence of CA-MRSA, clindamycin or vancomycin provides adequate coverage. The total treatment course should be 10 to 14 days. If there is no response to antibiotic treatment within 48 to 72 hours or clinical worsening, the next steps include evaluation for abscess formation. Ultrasound is useful to detect the presence and extent of an abscess if lymph node fluctuance is not obvious by examination. Surgeons may request a computed tomography (CT) scan before performing an incision and drainage to obtain more detailed imaging of adjacent and deep

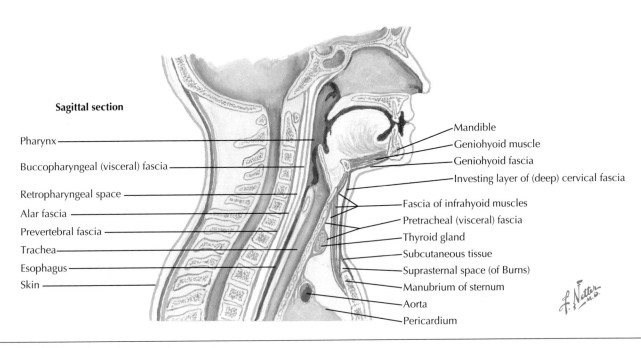

Sagittal section

Pharynx

Buccopharyngeal (visceral) fascia

Retropharyngeal space

Alar fascia

Prevertebral fascia

Trachea

Esophagus

Skin

Mandible

Geniohyoid muscle

Geniohyoid fascia

Investing layer of (deep) cervical fascia

Fascia of infrahyoid muscles

Pretracheal (visceral) fascia

Thyroid gland

Subcutaneous tissue

Suprasternal space (of Burns)

Manubrium of sternum

Aorta

Pericardium

Figure 87-3 *Major fascial spaces of the neck.*

structures that may not be seen on ultrasound. However, ultrasound offers the advantage of avoiding radiation exposure. Aspirated or drained material from a suppurative node should be sent for Gram stain and both aerobic and anaerobic bacterial culture. Acid-fast stain and culture for mycobacterium and fungi should be considered with the appropriate clinical picture.

In cases of subacute or chronic lymphadenitis, evaluation for tuberculosis, NTM, HIV, EBV, CMV, cat scratch disease, and toxoplasmosis should be considered based on history and physical examination findings. A PPD can be helpful in distinguishing tuberculous from NTM lymphadenitis. Serologic testing is available for *B. henselae*, *T. gondii*, EBV, and CMV. Polymerase chain reaction is the preferred diagnostic test for HIV. Toxoplasmosis and cat scratch disease are typically self-limited infections that do not require treatment. For patients with systemic disease secondary to *B. henselae*, treatment with azithromycin is an option. However, the role of antimicrobial therapy in cat scratch disease remains controversial. With NTM lymphadenitis, excisional biopsy of the node can provide a definitive diagnosis and is the preferred treatment. If surgery is not feasible because of the location of involved nodes, clarithromycin or azithromycin with ethambutol or rifampin should be considered. When the etiology of cervical lymphadenitis remains unclear after negative infectious workup results, patients should be monitored closely for systemic signs of disease. An excisional biopsy may be necessary to establish the diagnosis in cases of persistent lymphadenitis that do not respond to appropriate antibiotic treatment or when nodes are nontender and fixed to adjacent tissue suggestive of malignancy.

DEEP NECK INFECTIONS

Multiple layers of cervical fascia encase the contents of the neck, creating three clinically important spaces: the peritonsillar area,

retropharyngeal space, and parapharyngeal space (Figure 87-3). Peritonsillar, retropharyngeal, and parapharyngeal infections are among a group of potentially life-threatening deep neck infections in children that can present significant diagnostic challenges. All of these infections have the potential to progress from cellulitis to organized phlegmon (pre-abscess stage) and then to mature abscess. The initial step in the evaluation of a child with a potential deep neck space infection is rapid assessment for upper airway obstruction and need for emergent airway management. Therefore, prompt diagnosis of these conditions is essential for successful treatment and prevention of complications.

ETIOLOGY AND PATHOGENESIS

Despite the widespread use of antibiotics for the treatment of tonsillitis and pharyngitis, peritonsillar abscess remains the most common deep infection of the head and neck. It occurs most frequently in older school-age children and adolescents. The peritonsillar space lies between the palantine tonsil and the superior pharyngeal constrictor muscle. Peritonsillar abscess is defined as a collection of pus between the tonsillar capsule, superior constrictor muscle, and palatopharyngeus muscle. It typically occurs in the superior pole of the tonsil. Peritonsillar abscess is generally preceded by tonsillitis or pharyngitis. When it occurs without preceding infection, a possible mechanism involves Weber's glands, a group of salivary glands located superior to the tonsil. These glands clear the tonsillar area of debris, and if they become obstructed, an abscess can develop.

The retropharyngeal space is bordered posteriorly by the prevertebral fascia and anteriorly by the pretracheal fascia. Its superior border is the base of the skull, it extends inferiorly to the posterior mediastinum, and it communicates with the parapharyngeal space laterally. The retropharyngeal space contains two chains of lymph nodes that drain the nasopharynx, adenoids, and paranasal sinuses. Suppurative infection of these lymph nodes can result in abscess formation. Accordingly, retropharyngeal infections in children tend to be preceded by upper respiratory tract infections such as pharyngitis, tonsillitis, sinusitis, and cervical lymphadenitis. Retropharyngeal abscess occurs most commonly in preschool-age children. The reduced incidence of retropharyngeal infections in older children has been attributed to atrophy of these lymph nodes with age. In older children and adolescents, retropharyngeal abscess is more likely to result from trauma to the posterior pharynx, foreign body, or dental abscess.

The parapharyngeal (lateral pharyngeal) space is located in the lateral aspect of the neck. Structurally, it can be thought of as an inverted cone, with its base at the skull and apex at the hyoid bone. It can be further subdivided into an anterior and posterior compartment. The anterior compartment is near the tonsillar fossa and contains lymph nodes, connective tissue, and muscle. The posterior compartment consists of the carotid sheath, which protects the carotid artery, internal jugular vein, vagus nerve, cervical sympathetic trunk, and the ninth to twelfth cranial nerves. Sources of infection of the parapharyngeal space include pharyngitis, tonsillitis, parotitis, otitis media, mastoiditis, and dental infections. Parapharyngeal space infections most often arise via contiguous spread from a peritonsillar or retropharyngeal abscess.

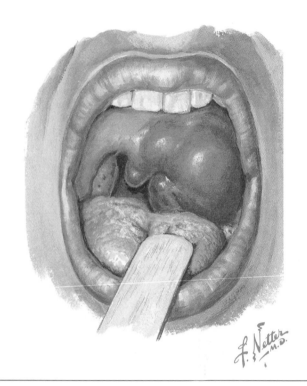

Figure 87-4 *Peritonsillar abscess (quinsy).*

CLINICAL PRESENTATION AND DIFFERENTIAL DIAGNOSIS

Patients with peritonsillar or retropharyngeal abscess present with fever, severe sore throat, neck pain, odynophagia, and decreased oral intake. Throat pain is more severe on the affected side and is often referred to the ipsilateral ear. Other associated findings include trismus, cervical lymphadenopathy, and pooling of saliva or drooling. With peritonsillar abscess, the physical examination usually reveals a patient with a partially opened mouth speaking in a muffled or "hot potato" voice. The oropharynx is erythematous with fullness or bulging of the superior pole of the tonsil. The uvula and tonsil may be deviated to the opposite side by the abscess (Figure 87-4). With retropharyngeal abscess, the physical examination may reveal neck swelling or torticollis. Bulging of the posterior pharyngeal wall lateral to the midline is suggestive of retropharyngeal abscess but is not consistently present. If left untreated, a peritonsillar or retropharyngeal abscess can spread through the deep tissues and produce complications such as airway compromise, mediastinitis, thrombophlebitis, and aspiration pneumonia if rupture occurs.

The clinical manifestations of parapharyngeal infections can be subtle and depend on whether the anterior or posterior compartment is involved. Infections of either compartment can be associated with systemic toxicity, fever, cervical lymphadenopathy, and parotid gland swelling. The key clinical features of parapharyngeal abscess in the anterior compartment include odynophagia, trismus, and pain involving the ipsilateral side of the neck and jaw. On physical examination, there is induration and swelling below the angle of the mandible and medial displacement of the lateral pharyngeal wall and posterior tonsillar pillar. If swelling occurs in the area of the larynx or epiglottis, stridor and respiratory distress may be present. Posterior compartment involvement produces signs of sepsis with minimal trismus or pain. Swelling of the pharyngeal wall can be missed on oropharyngeal examination when it is deep to the palatopharyngeal arch. In these cases, the development of neurologic or vascular complications secondary to involvement of structures in the posterior compartment may lead to the diagnosis. Abscess in the posterior compartment may result in unilateral tongue paresis, vocal cord dysfunction, facial nerve weakness, Horner's syndrome, hemorrhage from carotid artery erosion, or internal jugular vein thrombosis (Lemierre's syndrome). In addition, intracranial complications such as meningitis, brain abscess, and thrombosis of the cavernous sinus may occur.

It can be difficult to differentiate between the early findings of peritonsillar, retropharyngeal, and parapharyngeal infections. Therefore, these diagnoses should all be considered in the differential diagnosis of deep neck infections. Patients with retropharyngeal or parapharyngeal abscesses may be misdiagnosed with meningitis because of neck pain and stiffness. Other diagnostic considerations include epiglottitis secondary to the signs of drooling and respiratory distress and laryngotracheobronchitis if the patient presents with stridor. The differential diagnosis of peritonsillar abscess includes severe tonsillopharyngitis and peritonsillar cellulitis. The lack of trismus and fluctuance in tonsillopharyngitis help to distinguish it from a peritonsillar abscess. It can be difficult to distinguish peritonsillar cellulitis from peritonsillar abscess clinically; however, with peritonsillar cellulitis, the uvula usually remains in the midline, and there is a lack of purulent material during a needle aspiration. A list of other differential diagnoses appears in Box 87-3.

Box 87-3 Differential Diagnosis of Deep Neck Infections

- Caustic burns of the posterior pharynx
- Cervical lymphadenitis
- Cervical osteomyelitis
- Cystic hygroma
- Epiglottis
- Foreign body
- Hemangioma
- Laryngotracheobronchitis
- Meningitis
- Penetrating pharyngeal trauma
- Retromolar abscess
- Tonsillopharyngitis

EVALUATION AND MANAGEMENT

Laboratory evaluation is not necessary to make the diagnosis of deep neck infections, but it may help to assess the degree of illness and response to therapy. Leukocytosis with neutrophil predominance and elevated inflammatory markers are common, but these abnormalities are nonspecific. Associated bacteremia is uncommon, but a blood culture should be considered in an ill-appearing patient. Routine GABHS antigen test or throat culture should be done, keeping in mind the possibility of a carrier state with a positive result.

The diagnosis of peritonsillar abscess can usually be made clinically and is confirmed by a collection of pus at the time of drainage. A lateral neck radiograph may be obtained initially to exclude epiglottis and retropharyngeal abscess. In the case of retropharyngeal and parapharyngeal abscess, definitive diagnosis is established with radiographic studies. A lateral soft tissue radiograph of the neck may show widened prevertebral soft tissues and the presence of air-fluid levels within the retropharyngeal space. When retropharyngeal infection is present, the prevertebral soft tissue measures more than half the width of the adjacent vertebral body. The prevertebral space can appear falsely widened during neck flexion or with crying. Therefore, proper technique including imaging during inspiration and with the neck fully extended is essential. The most useful imaging modality for deep neck infections is a CT scan, which can define the source and extent of infection and determine whether there is abscess formation verses cellulitis or phlegmon. Magnetic resonance imaging (MRI) is another imaging option and avoids the irradiation that accompanies CT scan. However, sedation is typically required for young children, and the risk of sedating a child with potential airway compromise must be considered.

Aggressive monitoring and management of the airway is the most urgent and critical aspect of care for deep neck infections followed by appropriate antibiotic treatment and surgical drainage when necessary. There is a trend toward conservative early medical management with IV antibiotics for 24 to 48 hours when imaging is consistent with phlegmon, fluid collections are small, and there is no airway compromise. If there is worsening of clinical status or a suboptimal response to appropriate antibiotics, incision and drainage are necessary. Mature abscesses require surgical drainage. In the case of peritonsillar abscess, drainage is performed by either needle aspiration or incision and drainage.

Peritonsillar, retropharyngeal, and parapharyngeal abscesses tend to be polymicrobial in nature, consisting of both aerobic and anaerobic organisms. Empiric therapy should include coverage for *S. pyogenes*; non–group A streptococcus; *S. aureus*; and respiratory anaerobes such as *Prevotella*, *Bacteroides*, and *Peptostreptococcus* spp. Treatment failure with penicillin monotherapy because of the emergence of β-lactamase production among oral anaerobes has changed the preferred treatment to broader spectrum antibiotics. In areas where *S. aureus* remains susceptible to methicillin, ampicillin–sulbactam is appropriate. In areas with increased prevalence of CA-MRSA, antibiotic choices include clindamycin and vancomycin. IV therapy should be continued until the patient is afebrile with improvement in symptoms and resolution of any airway compromise. Oral therapy should be continued to complete a 14-day course. Appropriate oral regimens include amoxicillin–clavulanate, clindamycin, or linezolid. The use of steroids remains controversial, and there is not a clear role for them in the treatment of deep neck infections.

PERIORBITAL AND ORBITAL CELLULITIS

Periorbital cellulitis, also referred to as preseptal cellulitis, involves infection or inflammation of the eyelid and its subcutaneous tissues that are anterior to the orbital septum. Orbital cellulitis, also referred to as postseptal cellulitis, involves infection of the fat and muscle within the bony orbit that are posterior to the orbital septum. Orbital cellulitis occurs less frequently than periorbital cellulitis but can result in much more serious sequelae. Therefore, it is extremely important to distinguish between these two infections.

ETIOLOGY AND PATHOGENESIS

The anatomy of the eye and its contiguous structures play an important role in the pathogenesis of periorbital and orbital cellulitis. The orbital septum is a fibrous tissue that extends from the periosteum of the superior and inferior orbital rims and reflects into the upper and lower eyelids. The orbital septum protects the periorbital area from the paranasal sinuses and provides a barrier to the spread of infection from the periorbital area into the orbit. Periorbital cellulitis most commonly arises from secondary bacterial infection of soft tissue injuries to the face or eyelids such as lacerations or insect bites or from spread of local infection such as conjunctivitis, dacryocystitis, or hordeolum. Periorbital cellulitis can also develop secondary to hematogenous spread of nasopharyngeal pathogens to the periorbital tissues. In addition, periorbital swelling can occur with acute sinusitis as a result of inflammatory edema because of poor venous drainage.

In contrast to the periorbital area, the orbit is surrounded by the paranasal sinuses. Many of the bony walls of the sinuses are thin and porous and allow spread of infection into the orbit. Orbital cellulitis most commonly results from extension of sinusitis with the ethmoid sinuses involved most frequently (Figure 87-5). Pathogens may also gain access to the orbit through direct trauma from a fracture or foreign body. In addition, spread of infection from adjacent structures can occur,

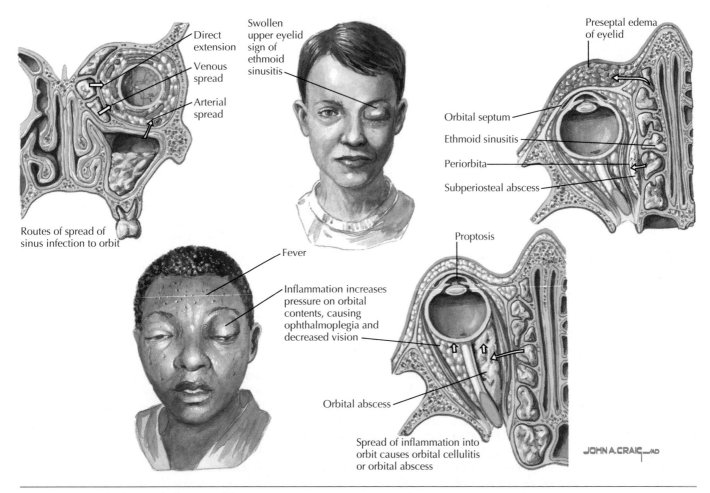

Figure 87-5 *Orbital spread of sinus infection.*

such as an odontogenic infection extending into the maxillary sinus and subsequently into the orbit. Infection can also travel through the valveless venous system that drains the orbit and sinuses. These veins drain into the cavernous sinus, which can allow hematogenous spread of sinus infections into the orbit and result in complications such as thrombosis of the cavernous sinus, compression of the optic nerve, meningitis, or intracranial abscess.

CLINICAL PRESENTATION AND DIFFERENTIAL DIAGNOSIS

Periorbital and orbital cellulitis are both characterized by unilateral eyelid erythema, edema, induration, and tenderness. Only orbital cellulitis is associated with proptosis, impairment of extraocular movements, pain with extraocular movements, chemosis, or decreased visual acuity. The presence of fever or toxic appearance is variable, but both are more common with orbital cellulitis. Tearing may occur, but significant conjunctival injection and purulent drainage are not common unless there is associated conjunctivitis. Because the majority of patients with orbital cellulitis have concomitant sinusitis, a history of a recent upper respiratory tract infection or symptoms of sinusitis such as headache or sinus tenderness may be present (see Chapter

33). The clinician should inquire about recent trauma, insect bites, and skin or eye infections.

Several noninfectious conditions can present with eyelid swelling and should be considered in the differential diagnosis of periorbital and orbital cellulitis. Allergic reactions may cause acute eyelid swelling but typically are pruritic and bilateral and do not exhibit tenderness. Blunt trauma can cause unilateral periorbital swelling, ecchymosis, and tenderness to the eyelid. Historical information will help to differentiate trauma from infection. Hypoalbuminemia can cause eyelid swelling secondary to edema, but periorbital swelling tends to be bilateral, nontender, and without erythema. Other causes of periorbital swelling include chemical irritation, chalazion, dacryocystitis, and conjunctivitis. The differential diagnosis of orbital cellulitis also includes conditions that cause orbital inflammation. Orbital pseudotumor, an autoimmune inflammation of the orbital tissues, presents with eyelid swelling, pain, and decreased extraocular movements. These patients are typically afebrile, and CT scan reveals an intraorbital mass and no evidence of sinusitis. Intraocular tumors such as retinoblastoma and rhabdomyosarcoma usually cause gradual onset of proptosis without evidence of inflammation. Other conditions that may present similarly to orbital cellulitis include a subperiosteal hematoma and a ruptured dermoid cyst.

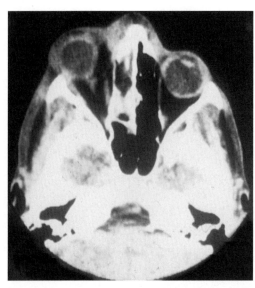

CT scan of orbital cellulitis.

Figure 87-6 *Orbital cellulitis.*

EVALUATION AND MANAGEMENT

Most cases of periorbital cellulitis can be diagnosed clinically. A CT scan should be performed in any patient with suspected orbital cellulitis to evaluate the extent of infection in the orbit, detect coexisting sinus disease, and identify an orbital or subperiosteal abscess (Figure 87-6). Leukocytosis with neutrophil predominance is often present in patients with periorbital and orbital cellulitis, so obtaining a complete blood count does not necessarily help to differentiate between the two diagnoses. Inflammatory markers are usually elevated, but these tests are neither sensitive nor specific. Blood cultures are typically negative but worth considering in an ill-appearing patient. Drainage aspirates of sinuses or abscesses associated with orbital cellulitis should be sent for culture when surgery is indicated.

Most cases of periorbital cellulitis can be safely managed on an outpatient basis with oral antibiotics and close follow-up. Hospitalization and IV antibiotics should be considered in patients who are younger than 1 year old, toxic appearing, cannot tolerate oral antibiotics, or failed outpatient management. All patients with suspected orbital cellulitis require hospitalization for IV antibiotics and close observation for progression of symptoms by ophthalmology. If CT scan demonstrates sinus disease as a likely etiology, an otolaryngologist should be consulted because surgical drainage may be necessary. If there is no improvement after 24 to 48 hours of IV antibiotics or if there is worsening of clinical status at any time, repeat imaging to assess for abscess formation may be necessary to determine if surgery is required.

Antibiotic choices should be aimed at the most likely pathogens. For periorbital cellulitis secondary to trauma or adjacent soft tissue infection, antibiotic therapy should be targeted at *S. aureus* and *S. pyogenes*. Amoxicillin–clavulanate is an appropriate oral antibiotic. Because of the continuing rise of CA-MRSA in many areas, clindamycin is an alternative. Children who are hospitalized should receive IV ampicillin–sulbactam or clindamycin. The duration of treatment should be a total of 10 to 14 days. For orbital cellulitis, antibiotic therapy should be aimed at respiratory pathogens originating from the paranasal sinuses, including *Streptococcus pneumoniae*, nontypable *Haemophilus influenzae*, *Moraxella catarrhalis*, and anaerobes in addition to *S. aureus* and *S. pyogenes*. Ampicillin–sulbactam is an appropriate choice with a high dose of ampicillin to cover resistant *S. pneumoniae*. Clindamycin can be added to ampicillin–sulbactam for CA-MRSA coverage. A third-generation cephalosporin with clindamycin added for broader CA-MRSA and anaerobic coverage is another reasonable option. The total duration of antibiotic treatment is 14 to 21 days. For children who are admitted to the hospital, discharge criteria include resolving clinical symptoms with improved ophthalmologic examination, afebrile for 24 hours, and able to tolerate oral antibiotics.

FUTURE DIRECTIONS

With the continuing rise of CA-MRSA and potential development of other resistant bacterial strains, empirical antibiotic therapy for infections of the head and neck will continue to be challenging. The trend toward more conservative management of head and neck infections with a trial of IV antibiotics before attempting incision and drainage places additional significance on initial antibiotic choices. In addition, more randomized, controlled studies are necessary to delineate if there is a role for steroids in the treatment of deep neck infections. Furthermore, as awareness continues to increase regarding radiation exposure via imaging with CT scan, the use of other imaging modalities such as ultrasound and MRI to diagnose infections of the head and neck and follow progression will likely increase.

SUGGESTED READINGS

Cervical Lymphadenitis

Friedman AM: Evaluation and management of lymphadenopathy in children, *Pediatr Rev* 29:53-59, 2008.

Leung AK, Davies HD: Cervical lymphadenitis: etiology, diagnosis, and management, *Curr Infect Dis Rep* 11:183-189, 2009.

Nield LS, Kamat D: Lymphadenopathy in children: when and how to evaluate, *Clin Pediatr* 43:25-33, 2004.

Peters TR, Edwards KM: Cervical lymphadenopathy and adenitis, *Pediatr Rev* 21:399-404, 2000.

Deep Neck Infections

Basel A, Salleen HB, Hagr A, et al: Retropharyngeal abscess in children: 10-year study, *J Otolaryngol* 33:352-355, 2004.

Brooks I: Microbiology and management of peritonsillar, retropharyngeal, and parapharyngeal abscesses, *J Oral Maxillofac Surg* 62:1545-1550, 2004.

Craig FW, Schunk JE: Retropharyngeal abscess in children: clinical presentation, utility of imaging, and current management, *Pediatrics* 111:1394-1398, 2003.

Johnson RF, Stewart MG, Wright CC: An evidence-based review of the treatment of peritonsillar abscess, *Otolaryngol Head Neck Surg* 128:332-343, 2003.

Rafei K, Lichenstein R: Airway infectious disease emergencies, *Pediatr Clin North Am* 53:215-242, 2006.

Periorbital and Orbital Cellulitis

Givner LB: Periorbital versus orbital cellulitis, *Pediatr Infect Dis J* 21:1157-1158, 2002.

McKinley SH, Yen MT, Miller AM, et al: Microbiology of pediatric orbital cellulitis, *Am J Ophthalmol* 144:497-501, 2007.

Nageswaran S, Woods, CR, Benjamin DK, et al: Orbital cellulitis in children, *Pediatr Infect Dis J* 25:695-699, 2006.

Wald ER: Periorbital and orbital infections, *Infect Dis Clin North Am* 21:393-408, 2007.

Osteomyelitis and Other Bone and Joint Infections

88

Ann Chahroudi

OSTEOMYELITIS

Osteomyelitis is inflammation of bone caused by bacterial or, less often, fungal infection. Osteomyelitis is categorized both by the mechanism of pathogen transmission to the bone (hematogenous, direct extension) and by the clinical presentation (acute, subacute, or chronic). In children, hematogenous spread of bacteria to the bone is the most common mode of transmission (Figure 88-1). Less often, osteomyelitis is the result of contiguous spread from a soft tissue infection or direct inoculation by penetration, such as after trauma or surgery. Vascular insufficiency is a rare cause of osteomyelitis in children. Eighty-five percent of cases of osteomyelitis occur in children younger than 16 years of age (50% in children younger than 5 years of age), with a male-to-female ratio of 2:1, except within the first year of life, when both genders are affected equally. Long bones (femur, tibia, humerus, in that order of frequency) followed by bones of the hands and feet and pelvis are the most common sites involved (see Figure 88-1). Approximately 5% of patients have multiple foci.

ETIOLOGY

Isolation of a bacterial source of osteomyelitis occurs in 50% to 80% of patients when both blood and bone are cultured. The bacteria responsible for osteomyelitis in children vary by age and underlying condition (see Figure 88-1). *Staphylococcus aureus* is the most common pathogen in any age group (70%-90% of cases), with community-acquired methicillin-resistant *S. aureus* (CA-MRSA) becoming more prevalent in recent years. In infants younger than 2 months of age, group B streptococci and gram-negative enteric bacteria are seen in addition to *S. aureus*. In children younger than 5 years of age, *S. aureus*, *Streptococcus pyogenes*, *Streptococcus pneumoniae*, and *Kingella kingae* are leading causes of osteomyelitis. Children older than 5 years of age are most commonly infected by *S. aureus* or *S. pyogenes*. *Neisseria gonorrhoeae* may be the etiologic agent in sexually active adolescents.

Approximately 10% of cases of acute hematogenous osteomyelitis are caused by *S. pyogenes*, a pathogen that tends to cause higher fever and white blood cell (WBC) count than *S. aureus*. An upper respiratory tract infection often precedes osteomyelitis with *K. kingae*, and this organism has been associated with outbreaks at daycare centers. Joint involvement is more common with *S. pneumoniae* than with *S. aureus* and *S. pyogenes*, perhaps because children with osteomyelitis caused by *S. pneumoniae* tend to be younger.

After introduction of the *Haemophilus influenzae* type b (Hib) conjugate vaccine, the frequency of osteomyelitis caused by this organism has significantly decreased. *Actinomyces* spp. have been isolated in facial and cervical osteomyelitis. Mixed flora, including *Pseudomonas* spp., *S. aureus*, and anaerobes, are seen in osteomyelitis that occurs after a puncture wound to the foot through sneakers. *Salmonella* spp. are an important cause of osteomyelitis in patients with sickle cell disease. *Mycobacterium tuberculosis* causes skeletal lesions in 1% of children with tuberculosis, typically manifested by lower thoracic vertebral osteomyelitis (Pott's disease).

PATHOGENESIS

The pathogenesis of acute hematogenous osteomyelitis is dictated by the anatomy of growing bone in young children. The rich vascular supply of the metaphysis and its sluggish flow allow deposition of bacteria that enter via the nutrient artery (Figure 88-2). An absence of macrophages in the metaphyseal capillary loops allows bacterial replication, inducing an inflammatory response that may lead to abscess formation, infarction of bone, and necrosis. Acute hematogenous osteomyelitis is preceded by minor trauma to the site of infection in one-third of cases; resultant small hematomas may make the underlying metaphysis more favorable for bacterial deposition.

Transphyseal vessels in children younger than 18 months of age can lead to spread of the infection from the metaphysis into the epiphysis and joint space, causing a secondary septic arthritis. The growth plate, after it has formed, serves as a barrier to extension of infection into the epiphysis and joint. The hip or shoulder joint can be involved at any age because the metaphyses of the proximal humeri and femurs are located within their respective joints.

CLINICAL PRESENTATION

Patients with acute hematogenous osteomyelitis describe localized bone pain that worsens over a brief period of time; the majority of these patients present to medical attention within 2 weeks of symptom onset. Pain precludes use of an affected extremity (pseudoparalysis). Fever is often present. Less common associated signs include malaise, anorexia, and vomiting. On physical examination of a patient with acute hematogenous osteomyelitis, swelling, erythema, warmth, and point tenderness that is out of proportion to the soft tissue findings may be present over the affected bone.

Ten percent of hematogenous osteomyelitis is categorized as subacute based on a slower progression of mild to moderate pain over the site of infection and the absence of systemic symptoms. Chronic osteomyelitis is characterized by waxing and waning pain and swelling that does not respond to prolonged antibiotics.

The clinical presentation of pelvic osteomyelitis includes pain in the hip, buttock, groin, lower back, or abdomen; gait abnormality; and, in some cases, fever. There is point tenderness over the affected bone and pain with manipulation of the hip.

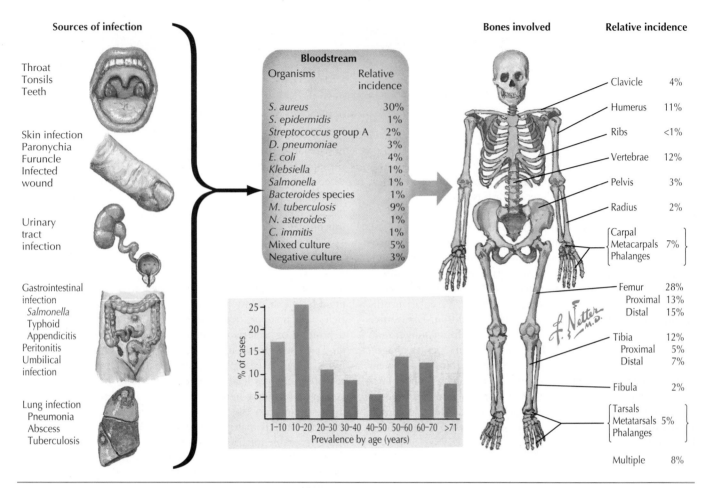

Figure 88-1 *Etiology and prevalence of hematogenous osteomyelitis.*

Distinguishing pelvic osteomyelitis and septic arthritis of the hip can be difficult, although range of motion of the hip joint is typically preserved in pelvic osteomyelitis.

Vertebral osteomyelitis can present with back, abdominal, chest, or leg pain; low grade–fever; and tenderness over the affected vertebrae. Fewer than 25% of patients demonstrate neurologic abnormalities. Symptoms can be subtle and slowly progressive, making diagnosis difficult. Vertebral osteomyelitis can be similar in presentation to diskitis but tends to affect older children and adolescents.

Chronic recurrent multifocal osteomyelitis is a distinct auto-inflammatory disorder that is characterized by episodes of pain, swelling, and low-grade fever that recur over several years, radiographic findings of multiple lesions that have the appearance of osteomyelitis, an inability to isolate an infectious etiology, and a lack of clinical response to antimicrobial therapy. Girls are more commonly affected than boys, with symptom onset around 10 years of age.

DIAGNOSIS

The diagnosis of osteomyelitis is made by a high index of clinical suspicion in the setting of confirmatory laboratory and imaging studies. Blood and bone cultures should be obtained before initiation of antibiotic therapy, if possible. If a joint is involved,

synovial fluid cultures may aid in the microbiologic diagnosis. The peripheral white blood cell count and platelets may be normal or elevated. The erythrocyte sedimentation rate (ESR) and C-reactive protein (CRP) are elevated in the majority of cases. The CRP typically peaks 48 hours after treatment initiation and returns to normal in 1 week. The ESR typically peaks 3 to 5 days after treatment initiation and may take 3 weeks to return to normal.

Plain radiographs show soft tissue swelling within 3 days of symptom onset; osteolytic lesions and periosteal elevation are apparent after 10 to 20 days; and after 1 month of symptoms, sclerosis of bone can be seen. Technetium-99 bone scanning has a sensitivity of 80% to 100% for osteomyelitis and can be helpful early on when plain films are normal and can identify multiple sites of infection, when present. Because the radionuclide bone scan can be falsely negative in 5% to 20% of children in the first few days of illness, magnetic resonance imaging (MRI) may be performed. MRI has a sensitivity of 92% to 100% for osteomyelitis and is effective in distinguishing soft tissue infection (e.g., cellulitis) from osteomyelitis. Pelvic and vertebral osteomyelitis are best imaged by MRI. Additionally, chronic osteomyelitis may have a different appearance from acute osteomyelitis on MRI (Figure 88-3).

The differential diagnosis of localized bone pain in children includes trauma, fracture, malignancy, and bone infarction. The

Terminal branches of metaphyseal arteries form loops at growth plate and enter irregular afferent venous sinusoids. Blood flow slowed and turbulent, predisposing to bacterial seeding. In addition, lining cells have little or no phagocytic activity. Area is catch basin for bacteria, and abscess may form.

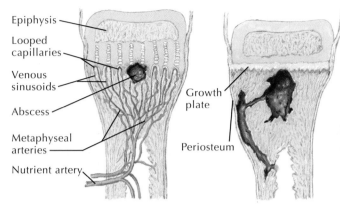

Abscess, limited by growth plate, spreads transversely along Volkmann canals and elevates periosteum; extends subperiosteally and may invade shaft. In infants under 1 year of age, some metaphyseal arterial branches pass through growth plate, and infection may invade epiphysis and joint.

As abscess spreads, segment of devitalized bone (sequestrum) remains within it. Elevated periosteum may also lay down bone to form encasing shell (involucrum). Occasionally, abscess is walled off by fibrosis and bone sclerosis to form Brodie abscess.

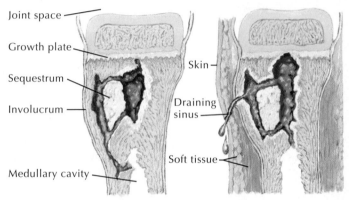

Infectious process may erode periosteum and form sinus through soft tissues and skin to drain externally. Process influenced by virulence of organism, resistance of host, administration of antibiotics, and fibrotic and sclerotic responses.

Figure 88-2 *Pathogenesis of hematogenous osteomyelitis.*

differential diagnosis of multifocal bone lesions includes leukemia, neuroblastoma, and histiocytosis X.

TREATMENT AND PROGNOSIS

Treatment of osteomyelitis depends on the selection of appropriate antibiotic therapy and surgical intervention when indicated. Empiric parenteral antibiotics should be started while cultures are pending, the choice depending on the patient's age and underlying medical condition, while ensuring coverage against *S. aureus* as well as adequate bone penetration. Antibiotic therapy is then modified based on culture results. Good outcomes are reported when conversion from parenteral to oral antibiotics is made in patients who are afebrile, demonstrating clinical improvement, and have a normalizing CRP. Intravenous (IV) therapy by means of a central venous catheter may be used to complete treatment at home for a patient in whom adherence to oral therapy is in question, but the risk of catheter complications increases with prolonged use. The total duration of therapy ranges from 4 to 6 weeks depending on the organism and clinical scenario.

Indications for surgery in a patient with osteomyelitis include (1) prolonged fever, pain, erythema, and swelling; (2) persistent bacteremia despite appropriate antibiotic therapy; (3) imaging results consistent with soft tissue or subperiosteal abscess;

(4) the presence of necrotic bone; or (5) development of a sinus tract.

Complications of osteomyelitis include secondary septic arthritis and subsequent joint destruction, epiphyseal injury leading to impaired bone growth, development of chronic osteomyelitis, and pathologic fractures. The recurrence rate is approximately 2% to 5%. Poorer outcomes are seen with younger patients, a delayed diagnosis, and shorter durations of antibiotic therapy.

SEPTIC ARTHRITIS

Septic or pyogenic arthritis is a bacterial infection of the joint space, most commonly affecting the joints of the lower extremities (knees, hips, ankles). A single joint is affected in more than 90% of cases. The greatest incidence of disease is in children younger than 3 years of age, with a male-to-female ratio of 2:1.

ETIOLOGY

Isolation of a bacterial organism from blood or synovial fluid of patients with septic arthritis occurs in 65% to 75% of cases. In general, the same pathogens cause septic arthritis as those

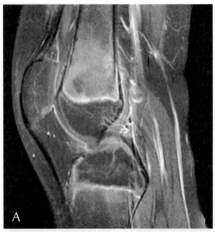

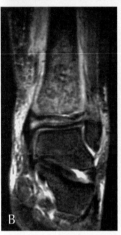
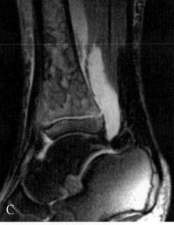

(A) Lateral T2-weighted MRI of distal femur with early acute osteomyelitis. 10-year-old female with progressive pain in left knee region and difficulty walking. Plain radiographs normal. MRI showed signal changes of distal femur metaphyseal region consistent with osteomyelitis.

AP (B) and lateral (C) of T2-weighted MRI of the distal tibia with late acute osteomyelitis. Note the inflammatory changes in the distal tibia metaphysis, the signal changes beneath the elevated periosteum, and the large posterior abscess from pus breaking through the periosteum.

Figure 88-3 *Magnetic resonance imaging findings in early and late acute osteomyelitis.*

that cause acute hematogenous osteomyelitis, including special clinical scenarios, such as hemoglobinopathies. In addition, pauciarticular arthritis of the large joints can be a complication of *Borrelia burgdorferi* infection in endemic areas.

Since the introduction of the conjugate Hib vaccine, infection with *H. influenzae* has become rare. Similarly, it is expected that a decrease in the cases of septic arthritis caused by the serotypes of *S. pneumoniae* contained within the heptavalent pneumococcal vaccine introduced in 2000 will be seen because an overall reduction in invasive pneumococcal disease has been shown.

PATHOGENESIS

Similar to acute osteomyelitis, hematogenous spread of bacteria to the vascular synovium is the most common cause of septic arthritis in children (Figure 88-4). The precise mechanism by which the presence of bacteria leads to joint destruction is unknown, but the resultant inflammatory response causes activation of host leukocytes, cytokine secretion, and chondrolysis.

Degradation of the joint begins as early as 8 hours after infection and can lead to irreversible synovial fibrosis and bony ankylosis.

Contiguous spread of bacteria into the joint space from rupture of a nearby focus of osteomyelitis occurs in approximately 10% of cases. Metaphyseal bone infection in children younger than 18 months of age can migrate through the growth plate to the epiphysis and then into the joint space by means of transphyseal blood vessels. The intracapsular location of the proximal metaphyses of the femur and humerus permits direct spread into the hip and shoulder joints, respectively.

Less frequently, septic arthritis develops as a consequence of direct penetrating injury or joint manipulation (such as intraarticular injections or prosthetic joint surgery).

CLINICAL PRESENTATION

Septic arthritis is characterized by the acute onset of joint pain with systemic symptoms including fever and irritability. An older child may limp or refuse to walk, and an infant may demonstrate increasing irritability with passive movement of the joint. If the infection is in the upper extremity, the patient may refuse to use the affected joint.

On physical examination, there may be swelling, erythema, and warmth over the affected joint. Most helpful for diagnosis is the presence of severe limitation in movement of the affected joint and pain with manipulation, so-called micromotion tenderness. Infection of the hip may cause referred pain to the knee or thigh, and signs of external inflammation may be absent. Patients with septic arthritis of the hip classically keep the hip and knee flexed with the hip abducted and externally rotated, a position that alleviates the most pain.

DIAGNOSIS

Rapid diagnosis of septic arthritis is crucial in preventing further joint destruction. Any child with fever, acute onset of pain, and limited range of motion on examination should be promptly evaluated. For microbiologic diagnosis, both blood and synovial fluid should be obtained for Gram stain and culture. Synovial fluid can be used to distinguish septic from other causes of arthritis: typically with a bacterial etiology, the fluid is cloudy, the WBC count is greater than 50,000/mm³, and polymorphonuclear cells predominate. Lyme arthritis can have a similar synovial fluid composition, so appropriate serologic testing is conducted as dictated by region. Measuring the levels of glucose and protein in the synovial fluid is generally not helpful. When *N. gonorrhoeae* is suspected in an adolescent patient, cultures of skin lesions and the throat, rectum, and cervix or urethra should also be sent.

Upon examination of the peripheral blood, the ESR is typically greater than 20 mm/h, and the CRP and peripheral WBC count are often elevated. CRP peaks by day 2 or 3 of treatment and normalizes in 7 to 9 days; ESR peaks by day 7 of treatment and normalizes in 3 to 4 weeks.

Plain radiographs in septic arthritis may be negative early on, but joint space widening and capsular distension can be seen (Figure 88-5); erosion of subchondral bone is evident 2 to 4 weeks into infection. Other pathologies such as fracture,

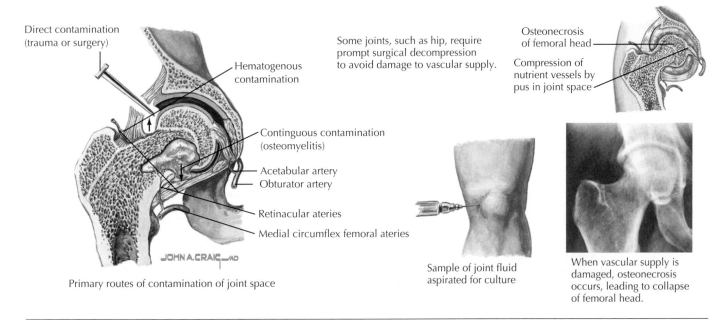

Direct contamination (trauma or surgery)

Hematogenous contamination

Some joints, such as hip, require prompt surgical decompression to avoid damage to vascular supply.

Osteonecrosis of femoral head

Compression of nutrient vessels by pus in joint space

Continuous contamination (osteomyelitis)

Acetabular artery
Obturator artery
Retinacular ateries
Medial circumflex femoral ateries

JOHN A. CRAIG—AD

Primary routes of contamination of joint space

Sample of joint fluid aspirated for culture

When vascular supply is damaged, osteonecrosis occurs, leading to collapse of femoral head.

Figure 88-4 *Septic arthritis.*

osteomyelitis, and malignancy can be identified on the plain radiograph. With septic arthritis of the hip, plain films may again be negative, but the characteristic finding early on is swelling of the hip capsule and lateral displacement of the gluteal fat planes; later, there is upward and lateral displacement of the femoral head. Ultrasound of the hip can be performed to detect fluid in the joint and to guide arthrocentesis. Bone scan, CT scan, and MRI are typically not performed for diagnosis of septic arthritis, but can be useful for evaluating deep joints, such as the sacroiliac joint and identifying osteomyelitis.

The differential diagnosis of septic arthritis includes transient (toxic) synovitis, viral arthritis, tuberculous arthritis, fungal arthritis, reactive arthritis, Reiter's syndrome, juvenile idiopathic arthritis, rheumatic fever, trauma, malignancy, Legg-Calvé-Perthes disease, and a slipped capital femoral epiphysis (Table 88-1).

TREATMENT AND PROGNOSIS

Treatment of septic arthritis is aimed at joint decompression and sterilization for the prevention of serious sequelae. Arthrocentesis is performed both to obtain fluid for diagnosis and to decompress the joint. Repeated joint aspiration may be needed after reaccumulation of fluid. Prompt surgical drainage is warranted for septic arthritic of the hip or shoulder to prevent vascular compromise and ischemic necrosis of the femoral or humoral head, respectively.

Empiric IV antibiotic therapy should be started pending culture results even in patients with negative synovial fluid Gram stain results when the combination of clinical, laboratory, and imaging studies is suggestive of septic arthritis. Initial antibiotic choice depends on the patient's age, clinical status, and local antibiotic resistance profiles.

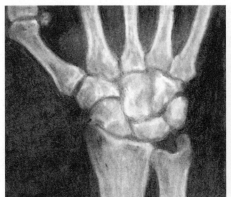
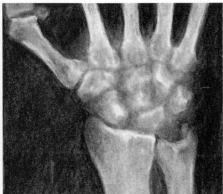
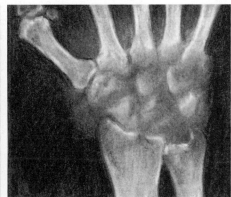

Rapid progression of wrist involvement within 4 weeks, from almost normal (left) to advanced destruction of articular cartilages and severe osteoporosis (right)

Figure 88-5 *Septic arthritis: imaging.*

Table 88-1 Differential Diagnosis of Septic Arthritis

Condition	Differential Diagnosis from Septic Arthritis
Appendicitis	Possible psoas muscle irritation that may result in flexion of the right hip, abdominal tenderness
Bursitis	No joint effusion, swelling in the area of affected bursa
Cellulitis	No joint effusion, marked erythema of skin
Gout	Intense pain, great toe common involvement, crystals seen on joint aspiration
Hemarthrosis	History of trauma, bloody fluid on aspiration
Juvenile rheumatoid arthritis	Gradual onset of symptoms, morning stiffness, better joint motion
Lyme disease	Indolent onset, boggy synovium
Osteomyelitis	No joint effusion, better range of motion
Rheumatic fever	Less effusion, arthralgia
Reactive arthritis	Less pain and effusion; joint fluid white blood cell count, 10,000 to 20,000 per mm^3
Transient synovitis	Hip involvement only, no systemic symptoms, better range of motion, may require aspiration to be differentiated from septic arthritis

Reprinted with permission from Greene W: Netter's Orthopaedics. Philadelphia, Saunders, Elsevier, 2006, p 157.

The duration of antibiotic therapy is dictated by the pathogen involved, site of infection, and clinical response, as evidenced by symptoms and levels of inflammatory markers. Emerging data suggest that shorter courses (10 days) of oral antibiotics after brief IV administration may be equivalent in terms of clinical outcome to a more traditional longer course (30 days) of therapy.

Septic arthritis leads to residual joint problems in 10% to 25% of patients. These problems include abnormal bone growth, chronic joint dislocation, joint instability, and limited range of motion. Risk factors for complications include age younger than 6 months, delay of more than 4 days in diagnosis (and thus treatment), infection of adjacent bone, infection of the hip or shoulder, and infection with *S. aureus* or gram-negative organisms.

DISKITIS

Diskitis is characterized by inflammation of intervertebral disk spaces and vertebral body end plates, primarily involving the lumbar or lower thoracic spine. The exact incidence and etiology of diskitis are unknown, but it typically affects children younger than 6 years of age, likely because of the rich blood supply to the intervertebral disk that involutes later in life. Inflammation is thought to result from low-grade bacterial or viral infection of the disk space, although trauma may also play a role. Blood and disk space culture results from patients with diskitis tend to be negative, but *S. aureus* (most commonly), *K. kingae*, and other bacterial organisms have been isolated.

The most common presenting symptoms are the gradual onset of a limp, leg pain, or refusal to walk as well as progressive back pain and, less frequently, abdominal pain. Low-grade fever may be present. On physical examination, the patient may be irritable with hip flexion and complain of pain with palpation of the lower back. Laboratory tests reveal an elevated ESR rate and normal or slightly elevated peripheral WBC count. Plain radiographs of the spine demonstrate characteristic disk space narrowing and irregularity of the vertebral end plates 2 to 6 weeks after symptom onset.

Diskitis is treated with bedrest, spine immobilization, and antibiotics (with empiric antistaphylococcal coverage) for patients who do not demonstrate a prompt response to immobilization.

SUGGESTED READINGS

Gutierrez K: Bone and joint infections in children, *Pediatr Clin North Am* 52(3):779-784, 2005.

Kaplan SL: Osteomyelitis in children, *Infect Dis Clin North Am* 19(4):787-797, 2005.

Peltola H, Pääkkönen M, Kallio P, Kallio MJ, Osteomyelitis-Septic Arthritis (OM-SA) Study Group: Prospective, randomized trial of 10 days versus 30 days of antimicrobial treatment, including a short-term course of parenteral therapy, for childhood septic arthritis, *Clin Infect Dis* 48:1201-1210, 2009.

Poehling KA, Talbot TR, Griffin MR, et al: Invasive pneumococcal disease among infants before and after introduction of pneumococcal conjugate vaccine, *JAMA* 295:1668-1674, 2006.

Zaoutis T, Localio AR, Leckerman K, et al: Prolonged intravenous therapy versus early transition to oral antimicrobial therapy for acute osteomyelitis in children, *Pediatrics* 123(2):636-642, 2009.

Sexually Transmitted Infections

89

Kristen A. Feemster

Sexually transmitted infections (STIs) present a significant source of morbidity among adolescents, especially young women. According to 2007 surveillance data, adolescents represent 25% of the sexually active population but account for 50% of new STIs. The high incidence of STIs is associated with greater susceptibility of the adolescent female reproductive tract, poor access to STI prevention services, inconsistent use of barrier prophylaxis, and high prevalence among sexual partners.

STIs present with a wide range of symptoms and physical findings. Moreover, many infections are asymptomatic. Thus, regular screening among sexually active adolescents is highly recommended.

This chapter focuses on the most common clinical syndromes among adolescents: vaginitis, urethritis, cervicitis, human papillomavirus (HPV) infection, herpes genitalis, chlamydia, gonorrhea, and syphilis.

VAGINITIS

Vaginitis is one of the most common symptoms among adolescent females. It typically presents as increased or malodorous vaginal discharge and vulvovaginal erythema or edema. Although this can be caused by chemical or physical irritation, infectious causes include *Trichomonas vaginalis*, bacterial vaginosis (caused by *Gardnerella vaginalis*, genital *Mycoplasmas*, anaerobic bacteria) and *Candida* spp. In postpubertal women, normal vaginal flora is dominated by lactobacilli, which decrease the pH within the vaginal canal and prevent colonization by pathogens. However, any change to the genital environment can alter this balance and result in infection. Except *T. vaginalis* vaginitis, infectious vaginitis is not an STI. However, vaginitis is frequently diagnosed as part of the evaluation for STIs. The signs, symptoms, diagnostic criteria, and treatments for each infection are shown in Table 89-1.

URETHRITIS AND CERVICITIS

EPIDEMIOLOGY AND PATHOPHYSIOLOGY

Urethritis and cervicitis are most often caused by *Neisseria gonorrhoeae* and *Chlamydia trachomatis*. Gonorrhea and chlamydia are the most common reportable diseases in the United States, with approximately 360,000 cases of gonorrhea and 1.1 million cases of chlamydia reported in 2007. Adolescents are overrepresented: 50% of gonorrhea cases occur in individuals 15 to 24 years of age, and chlamydia infection among 15- to 19-year-old young women is 10 times the national average (3004 cases vs. 370 cases per 100,000 population). The transmission rate for each pathogen is much higher from males to females. Transmission occurs by oral, vaginal, or anal sexual contact. Each organism may be transmitted vertically to a newborn via passage through an infected birth canal.

N. gonorrhoeae is a gram-negative, oxidase-positive diplococcus, with 70 different strains. Its virulence is associated with the presence of pili and an outer membrane protein that increase adhesion of gonococci to tissues. *C. trachomatis* circulates as an elementary body. At epithelial cell attachment, it is ingested and then transforms into a reticulate body. It then reproduces within the infected cell, producing several elementary bodies, which are released. *C. trachomatis* also has a predilection for columnar epithelial cells, which are prevalent in the adolescent ectocervix.

CLINICAL PRESENTATION

The clinical presentations of urethritis and cervicitis and their associated infections are detailed in Table 89-2 and Figure 89-1.

Pelvic Inflammatory Disease

Pelvic inflammatory disease (PID) is an important complication of cervicitis, most commonly caused by *N. gonorrhoeae* and *C. trachomatis*. Other vaginal and enteric pathogens may be involved, including *Bacteroides* spp., *Ureaplasma urealyticum,* and *Mycoplasma hominis*. Gonococcus, *C. trachomatis*, and other organisms may ascend into the uterus and fallopian tubes. Infected material in the fallopian tubes may result in tubo-ovarian abscess, and overflow may lead to peritonitis or perihepatitis. The risk of PID is associated with young age at first intercourse, multiple partners, vaginal douching, and use of intrauterine devices.

The presenting symptoms of patients with PID are described in Table 89-2. Some patients may have subclinical infection that is not diagnosed until evaluation for infertility reveals fallopian tube scarring. On examination, patients usually have lower abdominal tenderness. Pelvic examination may reveal cervical discharge; an inflamed cervix; cervical, adnexal, or uterine tenderness; or an adnexal mass. Timely diagnosis of PID is important to prevent infertility. Because the signs and symptoms of infection are not specific, the Centers for Disease Control and Prevention developed criteria to guide diagnosis and empiric treatment (Table 89-3). Fulfillment of minimal criteria indicates presumptive treatment.

Other Manifestations of Gonococcal and Chlamydial Infection

Nongenitourinary manifestations of gonococcal and chlamydial infection include pharyngitis, conjunctivitis, and disseminated infection. Gonococcal pharyngitis should be considered for exudative pharyngitis in a sexually active adolescent. Disseminated gonococcal infection often manifests as arthritis, tenosynovitis,

Table 89-1 Infectious Causes of Vaginitis

	Signs and Symptoms	Diagnosis	Treatment
Trichomonas vaginalis 50% of women are asymptomatic 90% of men are symptomatic	Pruritus, dysuria Frothy cream or green-colored discharge Dyspareunia, postcoital bleeding Strawberry cervix, vulvovaginal edema, erythema Urethritis (men)	Wet mount: trichomonads Vaginal pH >4.5 Culture (sensitive but expensive) Rapid test (OSOM Trichomonas Rapid Test* or Affirm nucleic acid probe†)	Metronidazole, tinidazole
Bacterial vaginosis	Most common cause of abnormal vaginal discharge: grayish white with fishy odor, adherent to vaginal walls 50% of patients are asymptomatic No vulvovaginal erythema or edema	Three of the following four criteria • Homogenous, white discharge on vaginal walls • Presence of clue cells on wet prep • Vaginal pH >4.5 • Positive "whiff test" result (fishy odor after adding 10% KOH) Gram stain to look for replacement of lactobacilli with coccobacilli	Metronidazole oral or topical gel Clindamycin oral or topical gel
Vulvovaginal candidiasis *Candida* spp. are part of commensal vaginal flora Infection is associated with diabetes; pregnancy; and oral contraceptive, steroid, antibiotic use	Burning and pruritus Vulvar edema and erythema Thick "cottage cheese–like" discharge with no odor Dysuria or dyspareunia May have satellite lesions on thighs and in skin folds	Pseudohyphae on wet mount Vaginal pH <4.5	Butoconazole 2% cream Clotrimazole 1% cream or vaginal tablets Miconazole 2% cream or vaginal suppository Nystatin vaginal tablets Oral regimen: fluconazole

KOH, potassium hydroxide.
*Genzyme Corp., Cambridge, Mass.
†BD, Franklin Lakes, NJ.

Table 89-2 Signs and Symptoms of Urethritis, Cervicitis, and Associated Syndromes in Men and Women

	Men	Women
Urethritis	Dysuria Purulent urethral discharge	Dysuria Urinary frequency Urethral exudate Suprapubic pain
Epididymitis develops in 10%-30% of untreated men	Urethral discharge or dysuria Scrotal pain, swelling, erythema Inguinal or flank pain Pain or swelling of epididymis or spermatic cord	
Endocervicitis		Increased vaginal discharge Dyspareunia Cervical erythema, edema, friability
Endometritis or salpingitis (PID) Develops in 10%-20% of acute urogenital infection		Abdominal pain Intermenstrual bleeding Menorrhagia Dyspareunia Cervical motion tenderness
Anorectal gonorrhea	Proctitis or anal discharge Rectal bleeding Anorectal pain Tenesmus or constipation	Usually asymptomatic Purulent exudate Erythema or edema of rectal mucosa
Perihepatitis (Fitz-Hugh-Curtis syndrome) Usually associated with salpingitis	Rarely occurs in men	RUQ abdominal pain Fever Nausea or vomiting

PID, pelvic inflammatory disease; RUQ, right upper quadrant.

Cervicitis

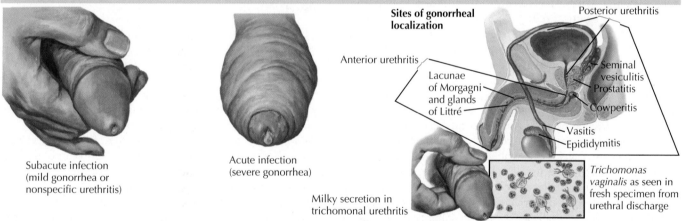

Primary sites of infection
1. Urethra and Skene's gland
2. Bartholin's gland
3. Cervix and cervical glands

Subsequent sites of infection
4. Fallopian tubes (salpingitis)
5. Emergence from tubal ostium (tubo-ovarian abscess and peritonitis)
6. Lymphatic spread to broad ligaments and surrounding tissues (frozen pelvis)

Urethritis

Subacute infection
(mild gonorrhea or
nonspecific urethritis)

Acute infection
(severe gonorrhea)

Milky secretion in
trichomonal urethritis

Sites of gonorrheal
localization

Posterior urethritis

Anterior urethritis

Lacunae
of Morgagni
and glands
of Littré

Seminal
vesiculitis
Prostatitis
Cowperitis
Vasitis
Epididymitis

*Trichomonas
vaginalis* as seen in
fresh specimen from
urethral discharge

Infected cervical glands

Appearance of cervix
in acute infection

Gonorrheal infection
(Gram stain)

Non-specific infection
(Gram stain)

Figure 89-1 *Cervicitis and urethritis.*

Table 89-3 Signs and Symptoms of Pelvic Inflammatory Disease

Minimal Criteria	Additional Criteria	Definitive Criteria
Uterine or adnexal tenderness *or* Cervical motion tenderness	Temperature >38.3°C Abnormal cervical or vaginal discharge WBCs on microscopic evaluation of vaginal discharge Elevated ESR and CRP Laboratory documentation of gonorrhea or chlamydial infection	Evidence of endometritis from endometrial biopsy Transvaginal sonography showing thickened fluid-filled tubes, free pelvic fluid, or tubo-ovarian complex Laparoscopic abnormalities

CRP, C-reactive protein; ESR, erythrocyte sedimentation rate; WBC, white blood cell.

Table 89-4 Treatment Recommendations for Urethritis, Cervicitis, and Pelvic Inflammatory Disease*

	Treatment	Special Considerations
Nongonococcal urethritis or cervicitis	Azithromycin Doxycycline Erythromycin Ofloxacin Levofloxacin	Patients should abstain from sexual intercourse for 7 days from starting treatment. Partners should be notified and treated.
Gonococcal urethritis or cervicitis	Ceftriaxone *or* Cefixime Spectinomycin Cefoxitin IM + Probenecid PO	*Fluoroquinolones are no longer recommended for treatment because of resistance.* Unless chlamydia is definitely ruled out (i.e., by use of NAAT), include coverage for chlamydia.
Pelvic inflammatory disease	Parenteral regimen Cefotetan *or* cefoxitin *plus* Doxycycline PO or IV for 14 d *Plus* clindamycin or metronidazole if TOA Outpatient regimen Ceftriaxone IM *or* Cefoxitin IM + probenecid PO *plus* doxycycline PO for 14 d ± metronidazole	IV antibiotics until 24 h after improvement; then continue PO doxycycline to complete 14-d course. As above, patients should abstain from sexual intercourse for 7 days from initiation of treatment. Partners should be evaluated and treated.
Epididymitis	Ceftriaxone IM *plus* Doxycycline PO	

IM, intramuscular; IV, intravenous; NAAT, nucleic acid amplification test; PO, oral; TOA, tubo-ovarian abscess.
*Additional alternate regimens for special populations or for those with allergies are available at www.cdc.gov/std/treatment.

and dermatitis. Chlamydia is associated with Reiter's syndrome (urethritis, spondylitis, uveitis). Both chlamydia and gonorrhea can also cause neonatal infection (see Chapter 105).

EVALUATION AND MANAGEMENT

Gonorrhea can be diagnosed by gram stain and culture from urethral and endocervical swabs. Chlamydia, as an intracellular organism, is difficult to grow in culture and has therefore been more difficult to diagnose. Newer and more rapid diagnostic methods include nucleic acid amplification techniques that have greatly increased the ease and sensitivity of testing. They can be performed on urine samples in addition to urethral or endocervical swabs. The other bacterial causes of urethritis—cervicitis and PID—are not generally isolated from cultures.

Patients with gonorrhea or chlamydia are at risk for co-infection. Therefore, treatment guidelines recommend covering for both pathogens when treating urethritis, cervicitis, or PID (Table 89-4). This is critical in PID, in which cervical culture results are often negative. Recommendations for PID also include anaerobic coverage because of the polymicrobial nature of the infection.

ANOGENITAL LESIONS

The most common causes of anogenital lesions in adolescents include herpes genitalis, HPV, and syphilis. The differential diagnosis should also include chancroid caused by *Haemophilus ducreyi*. Although only 23 cases of chancroid were reported in the United States in 2007, it is prevalent in certain regions and groups. In general, painful ulcerative lesions are associated with herpes genitalis and chancroid. Painless ulcers are associated with syphilis, and HPV causes painless anogenital growths.

SYPHILIS

Syphilis is a systemic infection caused by the spirochete *Treponema palladium*. The agent is usually transmitted via sexual contact but can also be transmitted in utero, through blood transfusions, or through direct contact with infectious lesions. After the organism enters the body, infection spreads through the blood and lymphatic systems, infiltrating cells and causing granuloma formation and endarteritis. If left untreated, the infection is chronic and can be transmitted for up to 4 years.

The overall incidence of syphilis has significantly declined since the 1970s, and in contrast to other STIs, the incidence of syphilis is lower among adolescents compared with other age groups. Most new cases occur among 20- to 30-year-old young adults. However, recent outbreaks of syphilis have occurred among adolescents who participate in commercial sex trades or illicit drug use.

The protean clinical manifestations of syphilis depend on the stage of infection, as shown in Table 89-5 and Figure 89-2.

Diagnosis

The diagnosis of syphilis should always be considered in the presence of any ulcerative anogenital or oral lesion. Breasts and fingers can also be affected. Because primary infection can present with either a small lesion or asymptomatically, regular screening for syphilis is recommended for sexually active adolescents and pregnant women.

Diagnosis uses screening nontreponemal antibody tests (rapid plasma reagin [RPR] and Venereal Disease Research Laboratory [VDRL]) and confirmatory specific treponemal antibody tests (fluorescent treponemal antibody absorption [FTA-ABS]). The RPR is a qualitative test that requires confirmation by the FTA-ABS. The VDRL is a quantitative test used to monitor

Table 89-5 Clinical Manifestations of Syphilis

	Timing	Clinical Manifestations
Primary syphilis	9-90 days after exposure	1- to 2-cm *painless* chancre or ulcerative lesion on external genitalia Typically single lesion but can have multiple Heals in 3-6 wk
Secondary syphilis	6-8 wk (after exposure) 4-10 wk (after chancre)	Generalized macular, papular, or papulosquamous rash of trunk and extremities, including palms and soles Any type of rash can appear Rash is bilateral and symmetric, follows line of cleavage, and can involve mucous membranes General or regional painless lymphadenopathy Flulike syndrome with malaise, sore throat, fever, and so on Rash lasts few weeks to 12 months
Latent syphilis	Early (within first year) vs. late (after first year)	No clinical signs or symptoms of syphilis Persistently positive serologic test results (VDRL and FTA-ABS) Negative syphilis test results from CSF
Late syphilis	2-10 years after infection	Gummas (hypersensitivity reaction) Cardiovascular syphilis *Has not* been reported in adolescents
Neurosyphilis	Within 2 years	Asymptomatic: CSF pleocytosis, increased protein, and positive CSF VDRL results Acute meningitis with cranial nerve palsies Meningovascular syphilis: local infarction resulting in headache, memory loss, hemiparesis, Argyll-Robertson pupils, tabes dorsalis; *Rare* in adolescents

CSF, cerebrospinal fluid; FTA-ABS, fluorescent treponemal antibody absorption test; VDRL, Venereal Disease Research Laboratory.

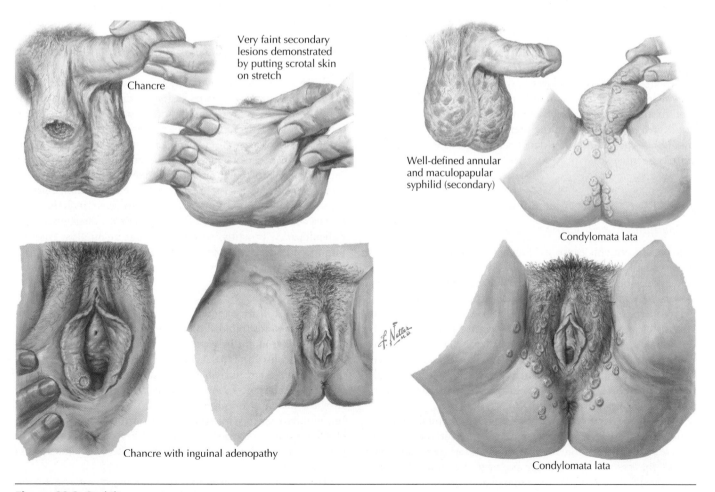

Chancre

Very faint secondary lesions demonstrated by putting scrotal skin on stretch

Well-defined annular and maculopapular syphilid (secondary)

Condylomata lata

Chancre with inguinal adenopathy

Condylomata lata

Figure 89-2 *Syphilis.*

Table 89-6 Treatment of Syphilis

Primary or secondary syphilis	Benzathine penicillin G IM Other preparations of penicillin are not appropriate for treatment.	In the setting of penicillin allergy, doxycycline or tetracycline can be used.
Early latent syphilis	Benzathine penicillin G	Alternate: doxycycline
Late latent or tertiary syphilis	Benzathine penicillin G	LP should be performed to look for neurosyphilis
Neurosyphilis	Aqueous crystalline penicillin G *or* Procaine penicillin + probenecid	LP should be repeated every 6 months until pleocytosis has resolved

IM, intramuscular; LP, lumbar puncture.

treatment. The treponemal-specific antibody test also yields antibody titers, but levels do not change in response to treatment; the FTA-ABS result will remain positive for life. The sensitivity of these tests depends on the timing after infection: they are most sensitive 4 weeks after infection but before the onset of late syphilis. There is also a high likelihood of false-positive results, particularly for the nontreponemal tests. False-positive results can occur with viral, spirochetal, mycoplasmal, other bacterial infections, and autoimmune vasculitides. Although screening test results are confirmed with the FTA-ABS, definitive diagnosis is made through dark-field examination of transudate from lesions or through direct fluorescent antibody.

Treatment

The mainstay of treatment for syphilis is penicillin. Although other regimens are available to treat primary and secondary syphilis for patients who are allergic to penicillin, their efficacy has not been well demonstrated. The treatment regimens are shown in Table 89-6. Follow-up should include repeat non-treponemal quantitative antibodies (VDRL) at 6, 12, and 24 months after completion of therapy. If initially high titers have not decreased fourfold or if the titers have increased, treatment should be repeated. Further detail is available at www.cdc.gov/std/treatment.

HERPES GENITALIS

Epidemiology and Pathophysiology

The most common cause of anogenital ulcerative lesions is herpes simplex virus (HSV). HSV has two serotypes: HSV 1 is primarily associated with herpes labialis, and HSV2 is primarily associated with herpes genitalis (although ≤50% of primary genital herpes lesions are caused by HSV-1). Overall, herpes is responsible for 90% of anogenital ulcerative lesions, and it is the second most prevalent STI across all age strata. The prevalence is highest among young adults ages 20 to 29 years but has been increasing among adolescents. Overall, 20% of individuals in the United States are HSV-2 positive, and 6% of adolescents ages 12 to 19 years are positive.

The virus is transmitted through genital–genital or oral–genital sexual contact. Viral shedding is highest in the presence of lesions, but asymptomatic shedding also occurs, especially within the first 3 months after primary infection. Shedding occurs in salivary, cervical, and seminal secretions. After infection, the virus replicates in skin or mucosal cells and then spreads via sensory nerves. After primary infection in herpes genitalis, the virus becomes latent, remaining in sacral dorsal root ganglia until reactivation. During reactivation, the virus spreads along peripheral sensory nerves back to skin or mucosal surfaces, resulting in recrudescence of skin lesions. Recurrence occurs in 70% to 90% of individuals with HSV-2.

Clinical Presentation

Primary infection usually begins with a burning sensation in the genital area followed by the development of small (1-2 mm) vesicular lesions with an erythematous base that erode and become ulcers. The distribution of lesions can be extensive, involving the labia, vagina, perineum, cervix, and penis (Figure 89-3). The lesions are almost always painful. In primary infection, regional tender lymphadenopathy, fever, and malaise occur. Patients may also have dysuria, urinary retention, or dyspareunia. Lesions typically last from 4 to 15 days before crusting, and systemic symptoms usually peak in the first 3 to 4 days and then resolve.

Recurrent episodes are usually less severe and involve fewer lesions. Overall, the episodes last approximately 1 week compared with 3 weeks for primary infection, and the virus sheds for 2 to 7 days. There may be paresthesias or pain in the anogenital region before the appearance of ulcers but mild systemic symptoms can occur. The likelihood and frequency of recurrence varies; recurrences are more frequent in the first year after infection. Although herpes results in chronic infection, episodes are usually self-limited. Complications can occur, including secondary bacterial infection of lesions, labial adhesions, sacral radiculopathy, proctitis, encephalitis, and meningitis. Another important complication is neonatal herpes (see Chapter 105).

Diagnosis and Management

If the clinical history and appearance of lesions suggest herpes genitalis, the most rapid and inexpensive test is a Tzanck smear of scrapings from the base of the lesions, looking for multinucleated giant cells. It has a sensitivity of only 30% to 80%. Other diagnostic tests are available; the historic gold standard is viral culture, which is most sensitive when samples are obtained from vesicles, pustules, or ulcers. HSV can grow in 1 to 7 days. Immunofluorescence microscopy, DNA probes, and polymerase chain reaction are highly sensitive and specific assays. HSV type-specific serologic tests exist but may be falsely negative in early infection.

Treatment will not clear infection but may decrease the duration of symptoms and viral shedding in both primary and

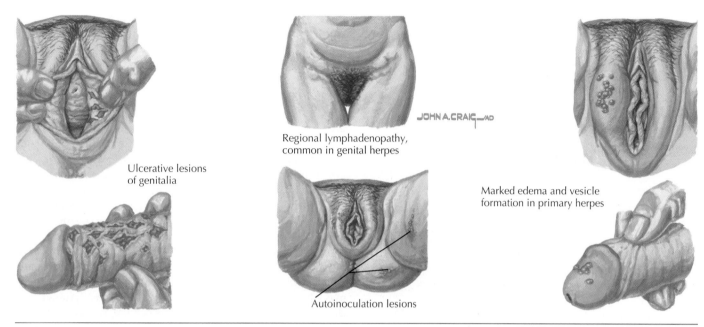

Ulcerative lesions
of genitalia

Regional lymphadenopathy,
common in genital herpes

Marked edema and vesicle
formation in primary herpes

Autoinoculation lesions

Figure 89-3 *Lesions of herpes simplex.*

recurrent infection. To be effective, episodic treatment should begin within 1 day of lesion appearance. In severe infection, patients require intravenous acyclovir, 5 to 10 mg/kg every 8 hours for 2 to 7 days until improved followed by oral therapy to complete a 10-day course. Topical therapy has not been shown to be effective for herpes genitalis. Long-term suppressive antiviral therapy can also be given to decrease the frequency of recurrences. See Table 89-7 for treatment of HSV infections.

HUMAN PAPILLOMAVIRUS

HPV is the most common STI in the United States, affecting at least 80% of women and men at some point during their lives. Similar to other STIs, adolescent and young adult women are most likely to be affected. In the United States, a recent study found that 25% of 14- to 19-year-old individuals and 45% of 20- to 24-year-old individuals were infected with at least one type of HPV. HPV is usually acquired shortly after sexual initiation, and the number of partners is the most important risk factor for HPV infection.

Epidemiology and Pathophysiology

HPV is a double-stranded DNA virus of which there are 130 known genotypes. Approximately 40 of these genotypes infect the anogenital region and are divided into low- and high-risk types based on their association with clinical disease. Although most HPV infections are asymptomatic and self-resolve, infection with low-risk types can cause anogenital warts, and high-risk types can cause precancerous anogenital lesions (i.e., cervical dysplasia) and anogenital cancers. Low-risk types 6 and 11 cause approximately 90% of anogenital warts. High-risk types 16 and 18 cause approximately 50% of high-grade cervical dysplasia and 70% of cervical cancers. Generally, HPV is thought to cause all cervical cancers.

Transmission of HPV is primarily through sexual contact; however, genital lesions can also be caused by autoinoculation from skin warts. There is also evidence that HPV types that cause skin warts are transmissible via fomites, although such evidence does not exist for genital HPV types. HPV infect rapidly dividing basal epithelial cells that predominate in the cervical transformation zone and genital areas during sexual intercourse (Figure 89-4).

Clinical Presentation

Four different types of genital warts can develop: condyloma acuminata, papular warts, keratotic warts, and flat-topped warts (Figure 89-5). The lesions are usually pinkish, red, gray, or white and are usually painless. They can, however, sometimes be associated with burning, itching, or bleeding.

Table 89-7 Treatment of Herpes Simplex Virus		
Primary Infection	**Suppressive Therapy**	**Episodic Therapy**
Acyclovir: 400 mg TID *or* 200 mg five times a day for 7-10 d Famciclovir: 250 mg TID for 7-10 d Valacyclovir: 1 g PO BID for 7-10 d	Acyclovir: 400 mg BID Famciclovir: 250 mg BID Valacyclovir: 500 mg or 1 g/d	Acyclovir: 500 mg TID or 800 mg BID for 5 d Famciclovir: 125 mg BID for 5 d or 1000 mg BID for 1 d Valacyclovir: 500 mg BID for 3 d or 1000 mg QD for 5 d

BID, twice a day; PO, oral; QD, every day; TID, three times a day.

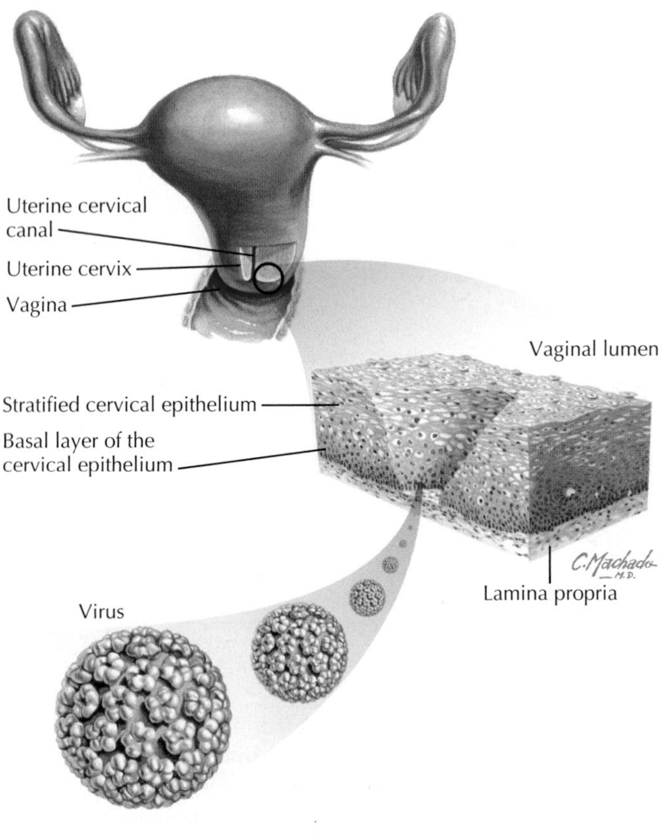

Uterine cervical canal

Uterine cervix

Vagina

Vaginal lumen

Stratified cervical epithelium

Basal layer of the cervical epithelium

Lamina propria

Virus

Figure 89-4 *Human papillomavirus.*

Cervical dysplasia is either low- or high-grade squamous intraepithelial dysplasia (LSIL and HSIL) or cervical intraepithelial neoplasia (CIN). Annually, 2 million women in the United States and 3% to 14% of adolescent females younger than the age of 19 years develop dysplasia. Although most are LSIL that spontaneously regress, some young women develop HSIL or CIN, which are considered precancerous, requiring more aggressive intervention. Although the cervix is the most affected anogenital region, HPV can also cause vulvar or vaginal intraepithelial neoplasia and cancer.

Diagnosis and Management

The diagnosis of genital warts is generally made by visual inspection. If external genital lesions are found in women, an internal examination of the genital tract is warranted. Anoscopy and urethroscopy may be indicated. Cervical dysplasia is diagnosed by Pap smear testing. Currently, Pap smears are recommended within 3 years of sexual initiation or by age 18 years. Testing should be performed yearly until a patient has three consecutive normal tests. Screening can then be performed every 3 years unless the patient is engaging in any high-risk sexual behavior or has had other STIs.

Treatment of genital warts includes multiple patient- and clinician-directed methods (Table 89-8). Treatment of an abnormal Pap smear depends on the degree of cervical dysplasia. For the most recent updates regarding cervical cancer screening, refer to www.asccp.org.

In addition to current cervical cancer screening, a quadrivalent HPV vaccine was approved in 2006 for the prevention of genital lesions and cervical cancers caused by HPV types 6, 11, 16 and 18. The vaccine is recommended for routine administration to 11- and 12-year-old girls and for catch-up vaccination to 13- to 26-year-old girls and women. It has been shown to be highly effective in girls and young women who have not yet been exposed to any of the HPV vaccine types.

CONCLUSION

STIs are an important part of adolescent health care. In a population that may have limited access to STI services, it is important to promote prevention and education and to provide screening during health care encounters. Although this chapter focuses on adolescents, STIs also occur in prepubertal children, and screening for sexual abuse should ensue (see Chapter 12).

Table 89-8 Management of Human Papillomavirus Infections

External genital warts For treatment of vaginal, cervical, or urethral warts, see www.cdc.gov/std/treatment	Patient administered: Podofilox 0.5% solution or gel Imiquod 5% cream Provider administered: Cryotherapy with liquid nitrogen or cryopulse every 1-2 wk until lesions resolve Podophyllin resin 10%-25% TCA or BCA 80%-90%
ASCUS	Repeat Pap smear in 4-6 months. If results remain abnormal, refer for colposcopy. If results are normal, repeat again in 6 months. If the patient has two consecutive normal smear results, can continue routine screening. *or* HPV DNA typing: if high-risk HPV type isolated, refer for colposcopy.
LSIL	If good, follow-up can repeat Pap every 4-6 months. If the patient develops HSIL or if LSIL persists, refer to colposcopy. If follow-up unreliable, refer directly for colposcopy.
HSIL	Refer for colposcopy.

ASCUS, atypical squamous cells of undetermined significance; BCA, bichloracetic acid; CIN, cervical intraepithelial neoplasia; HPV, human papillomavirus; HSIL, high-grade squamous intraepithelial dysplasia; LSIL, low-grade squamous intraepithelial dysplasia; TCA, trichloroacetic acid.

Clinical presentation of genital warts

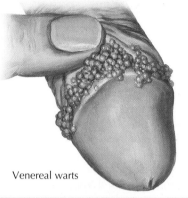

Venereal warts

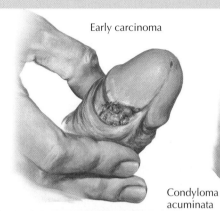

Early carcinoma

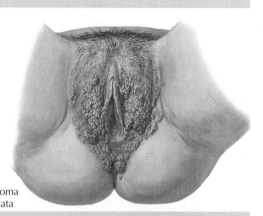

Condyloma
acuminata

Colposcopic views of abnormal cervical changes

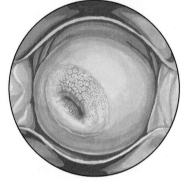

Coarse mosaicism and punctation
in transformation zone

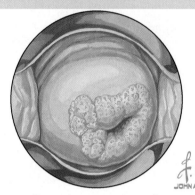

Papilloma of cervix. Some papillomas
may predispose to cervical malignancy

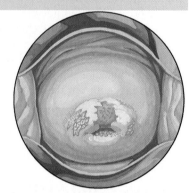

Changes suggestive of carcinoma in situ.
Abnormal vasculature with leukoplakia,
mosaicism, and punctation

Figure 89-5 *Genital warts.*

SUGGESTED READINGS

American Social Health Association: Available at http://www.ashastd.org.

Centers for Disease Control and Prevention: Sexually Transmitted Diseases 2006 Treatment Guidelines, Available at http://www.cdc.gov/std/treatment/2006/toc.htm.

National Institute of Allergy and Infectious Diseases: Sexually Transmitted Infections, Available at http://www3.niaid.nih.gov/topics/sti/default.htm.

Neinstein LS, Gordon CM, Katzman DK, Rosen DS, Woods ER, editors: *Adolescent Health Care: A Practical Guide*, Philadelphia, Lippincott, 2008, Williams & Wilkins.

Pickering LK, Baker CJ, Kimberlin DW, Long SS, editors: *Red Book: 2009 Report of the Committee on Infectious Diseases*, ed 28, Elk Grove Village, IL, 2009, American Academy of Pediatrics.

Skin and Soft Tissue Infections

90

Eric D. Shelov

Skin and soft tissue infections are common problems in the inpatient and outpatient populations. This chapter includes a discussion of localized skin infections, including cellulitis, impetigo, erysipelas, folliculitis, carbuncles, furuncles, and necrotizing fasciitis. The severity of these infections may vary greatly, from simple outpatient care to management in the intensive care setting. There is also the potential for rapid progression in cases where diagnosis and appropriate treatment are not initiated promptly. Children have their own predispositions to skin breakdown and infection, whether through the routine cuts and minor injuries of childhood or difficulty restraining from scratching of insect bites or dry skin. In the vast majority of cases, early recognition and treatment lead to a complete resolution, but infections of the soft tissues have the potential to result in significant morbidity, including arthritis, nephritis, carditis and septicemia.

For clinicians, it is essential to quickly recognize these infections, assess and evaluate their depth and rate of spread, and begin appropriate antimicrobial treatment (Table 90-1).

ETIOLOGY AND PATHOGENESIS

In the majority of cases, infection occurs after there has been breakdown of the skin, allowing bacteria that are normal colonizing flora of the host to invade into the subcutaneous tissues and beyond. Sources of the breakdown include direct trauma to the area, excoriation of an insect bite, or underlying conditions such as atopic dermatitis, which disrupt the integrity of the skin and can be intensely pruritic. The seeding point for the infection may be caused by micro trauma and not clear to the naked eye. After bacteria are beyond the skin barrier, they can invade to varying depths, determining the severity of the infection. Hair follicles and their surrounding glands are other sources of cutaneous infections, as seen in folliculitis, carbuncles, and furuncles. In addition to the level of introduction of the bacteria, host factors play a role in the severity and progression of illness. Children with underlying illness, particularly atopic dermatitis, diabetes mellitus, and renal failure requiring hemodialysis or those who are immunocompromised, are at a higher risk for colonization with pathogenic bacteria and for invasive disease.

Organisms

The vast majority of skin infections are caused by gram-positive organisms that are resident flora on the skin of human beings. Gram-negative organisms may infect the soft tissues but usually in unique circumstances such as bite wounds, patients with extended hospital stays (and thus increased exposure to gram negative bacteria), and immunocompromised hosts. Staphylococci and streptococci make up the majority of gram-positive infections. Whereas staphylococci are more predominant as causes of furuncles and carbuncles and impetigo, streptococci are more common in cellulitis and erysipelas. The predominant

staphylococci species in skin and soft tissue infections is *Staphylococcus aureus*, with methicillin-resistant *S. aureus* (MRSA) of particular concern because it is increasingly being detected in the nonhospitalized population. In addition, children with atopic dermatitis are more commonly colonized with *S. aureus*. The predominant streptococcus group for skin infections is group A (*Streptococcus pyogenes*). Although *S. pyogenes*' primary site of colonization is the oropharynx, it frequently makes transient appearances on the skin via droplets or the fingers of the host. Other organisms that are less frequently the cause of infection include other *Streptococcus* spp., gram-negative organisms such as *Escherichia coli* and *Pseudomonas* spp., and anaerobic bacteria.

CLINICAL PRESENTATION

Nearly all skin and soft tissue infections are characterized by a varying degree of erythema, pain or tenderness, and warmth. For clinicians, after it has been established that there is a likely bacterial infection, the next steps are to determine the depth and degree of the infection and its rate of spread (Figure 90-1).

Folliculitis

Folliculitis is a superficial pustule or local area of inflammation surrounding a hair follicle (Figure 90-2). It can be solitary, but it can also occur in clusters. The most commonly affected areas include those of high moisture and friction, such as the axillae and inguinal creases, but the scalp, extremities, and perioral and paranasal areas are also commonly affected. Poor hygiene and a humid environment are risk factors, as are active drainage from more severe nearby wounds. *S. aureus* is the predominant organism, with the exception of folliculitis that occurs shortly after immersion in a poorly maintained pool or hot tub, in which case *Pseudomonas aeruginosa* is the likely organism. Folliculitis is not usually painful, but if progression to more significant infections takes place, pain can become significant.

Furuncles and Carbuncles

Furuncles (boils) and carbuncles are uncommon in childhood, with the notable exception of children with atopic dermatitis (Figure 90-3). This population, perhaps because of its higher rates of *S. aureus* (the primary causative organism) colonization, is at risk for these infections. Both of these infections can be sequelae of poorly managed folliculitis. A furuncle is an acute infection of the hair follicle, often accompanied by necrosis, that begins as a nodule and then progresses to a pustule. Common locations are the neck, face, axillae, groin, and buttocks, and risk factors are similar to those of folliculitis, with the addition of hyperhidrosis, anemia, and obesity. A carbuncle is a collection of confluent furuncles, often with multiple drainage points. They can be single or multiple, frequently appearing in crops

Table 90-1 Characteristics and Treatment of Common Pediatric Skin and Soft Tissue Infections

Infection	Organism(s)	Key Features	Treatment
Folliculitis	*Staphylococcus aureus* *Pseudomonas aeruginosa* (rare)	Follicular distribution Poor hygiene Moist, friction-prone areas Erythema, painless	Improved hygiene with antibacterial soap Topical or oral antimicrobials for severe or refractory cases
Furuncles and carbuncles	*S. aureus*	Nodular or pustular Prone areas similar to folliculitis Erythema, painful	Similar to folliculitis More severe may require drainage, antimicrobials, and hospital admission if systemic signs are present (rare)
Impetigo	*Streptococcus pyogenes* *S. aureus*	Bullous and nonbullous Epidermal Vesicles, pustules with yellow or brown crust Minimal pain or erythema	Topical or oral antimicrobials Close follow-up Admission and parenteral medication if systemic signs (rare)
Erysipelas	*S. pyogenes* Other *Streptococcus* spp. (rare)	Confined to dermis and superficial lymphatics Prodrome Sharply demarcated borders Warmth, tenderness, induration May progress to vesicles or regional lymphatics	Obtain specimen if vesicles or pustules are present Antimicrobials Consider fluid resuscitation, hospital admission, and parenteral medication if systemic signs are present
Cellulitis or abscess	*S. pyogenes* *S. aureus*, attention to MRSA Gram-negative organisms (certain circumstances)	Warmth, tenderness, induration No prodrome Poorly demarcated borders May progress to systemic illness or deeper tissue involvement	Drain collection (may require imaging to define) Antimicrobials Resuscitation, hospital admission, and parenteral medication if systemic signs are present
Necrotizing fasciitis	*S. pyogenes* Other gram-positive organisms, gram-negative organisms, anaerobes	Recent surgery or trauma Pain out of proportion to superficial exam Necrosis, gas formation (crepitus) May appear well or toxic	ABCs Admission with broad antimicrobial coverage Surgery consult Consider intensive care management

ABCs, airway, breathing, circulation; MRSA, methicillin-resistant *S. aureus*.

in areas similar to furuncles. Both lesions are erythematous and can be painful, and occasionally, carbuncles can progress to the point where the patient develops constitutional symptoms and laboratory evidence of more severe infection.

Impetigo

Impetigo is a superficial bacterial infection that is confined to the outermost layer of skin, the epidermis, and can present in a bullous form, with lesions >1 cm or the more common nonbullous forms. *S. aureus* is the sole agent for bullous impetigo, but it can also cause nonbullous infection. Many species of group A streptococci can lead to nonbullous impetigo. Typically affected are young children, who present with vesicles or pustules, which rupture and form a yellowish-brown crust. The bullous form presents with larger, flaccid lesions that are easily ruptured. Surrounding erythema is minimal and is usually painless or occasionally pruritic, and only in the most severe of cases does the patient have any signs of systemic illness such as fever. In cases in which infection is predisposed by underlying atopic dermatitis, early infection can be difficult to differentiate from the baseline lichenification and excoriation related trauma.

Erysipelas

Erysipelas and cellulitis are skin infections that are both characterized by erythema, warmth, and pain (Figure 90-4).

Erysipelas is the more superficial of the two infections, with invasion confined to the dermis and frequently the superficial lymphatics. *S. pyogenes* is the most common pathogen, but other *Streptococcus* spp. have been isolated. The bacteria are usually established as colonizers in the host's nasopharynx and autoinoculated into a break in the patient's skin. The skin lesions are often preceded by prodromal symptoms of fever, malaise, and chills up to 48 hours before the onset of lesions. Skin lesions begin as brightly erythematous, raised areas with *sharply demarcated*, potentially rapidly advancing borders. Warmth, local edema, and tenderness are nearly universally present, and less frequently, there are signs of lymphatic spread such as streaking and regional lymph node inflammation. Severe infection can lead to the formation of vesicles and skin necrosis.

Cellulitis

Cellulitis is another frequently encountered skin infection, but unlike erysipelas, it extends deeper into the soft tissues below the dermis. It is also frequently seeded by relatively minor wounds or skin breakdown, such as insect bites, atopic dermatitis, tattoos, or blisters. It presents with erythema, tenderness, warmth, and induration of the affected tissues. Unlike erysipelas, the erythema is less clearly demarcated, although the two can frequently coexist, making differentiation more difficult. Lymphatic spread and systemic signs of illness do occur with

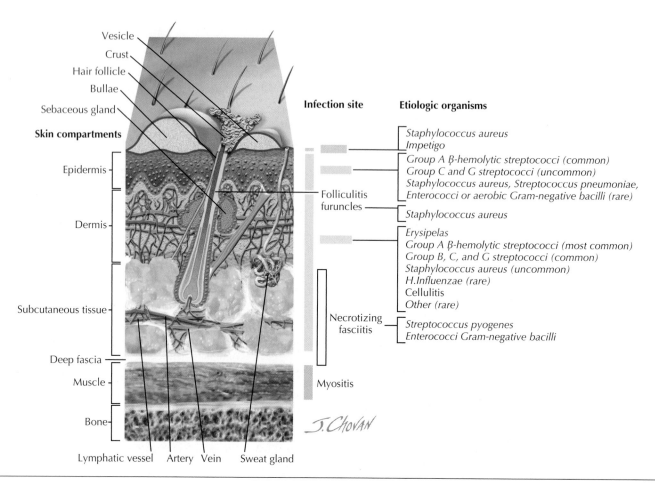

Skin compartments

Vesicle
Crust
Hair follicle
Bullae
Sebaceous gland

Epidermis

Dermis

Subcutaneous tissue

Deep fascia

Muscle

Bone

Lymphatic vessel   Artery   Vein   Sweat gland

Infection site

Etiologic organisms

Staphylococcus aureus
Impetigo

Group A β-hemolytic streptococci (common)
Group C and G streptococci (uncommon)
Staphylococcus aureus, Streptococcus pneumoniae,
Enterococci or aerobic Gram-negative bacilli (rare)

Folliculitis
furuncles

Staphylococcus aureus

Erysipelas
Group A β-hemolytic streptococci (most common)
Group B, C, and G streptococci (common)
Staphylococcus aureus (uncommon)
H.Influenzae (rare)
Cellulitis
Other (rare)

Necrotizing
fasciitis

Streptococcus pyogenes
Enterococci Gram-negative bacilli

Myositis

J. Chovan

Figure 90-1 *Cross-section of the skin showing layers and types of infections.*

Small pustule due
to bacterial invasion
of irritated follicular
opening.

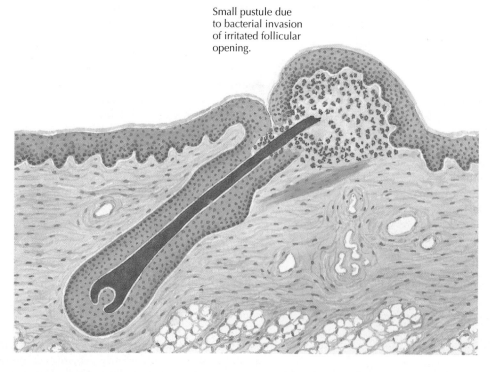

Figure 90-2 *Follicular infection.*

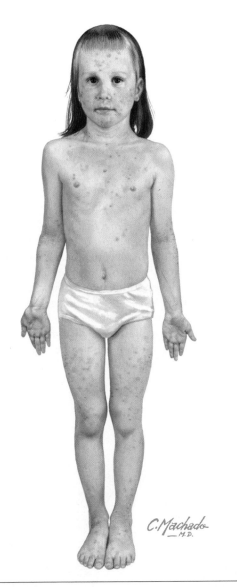

Figure 90-3 *Child with atopic dermatitis, frontal view.*

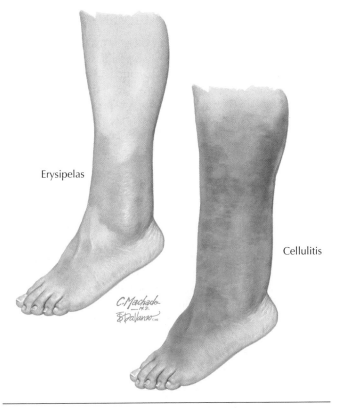

Erysipelas

Cellulitis

Figure 90-4 *Appearance of erysipelas and cellulitis.*

Necrotizing Fasciitis

Necrotizing fasciitis, a severe soft tissue infection that can rapidly progress to severe morbidity or death, is fortunately very rare in the pediatric population. Infection usually begins in the superficial tissues and rapidly spreads along fascial planes into the deeper tissues. Pathogen-produced toxins lead to rapid local necrosis, vascular compromise, peripheral nervous system damage, and potentially profound systemic illness. Cases are most commonly associated with recent trauma, retained foreign bodies, or recent surgical procedures, although spontaneous infections have been reported. The patient initially presents with significant pain, often near the site of recent trauma or surgery. As the infection progresses to involve the peripheral nerves, the pain may progress to anesthesia. Infection can begin with an area of erythema, but other classic signs of local superficial infection such as induration and warmth may be absent. As the infection rapidly spreads to the deeper tissues, there may be evidence of cell necrosis, gas production (crepitus), bullae formation, and discharge, although none of these findings may be apparent in the superficial tissues. Patients may initially seem well-appearing, but because of tremendous toxin production and inflammation, they more frequently show signs of severe illness such as toxic appearance, fever, and cardiovascular instability. Infections can be either mono- or polymicrobial, involving gram-positive, gram-negative, or anaerobic bacteria. Whereas cases with invasive trauma are more likely to involve anaerobes and mixed flora, those caused by minimally apparent trauma are more likely secondary to monomicrobial group A β-hemolytic strep infections.

cellulitis but are less ubiquitous than in erysipelas. Findings that warrant concern for a clinician are evidence of rapid progression, lymphatic streaking or abscess formation, pain out of proportion to the remainder of examination, and signs of systemic illness. Risk factors for infection include recent trauma or local infections such as folliculitis or carbuncles or furuncles and underlying skin conditions such as atopic dermatitis. Risk factors for more severe or recurrent infections include chronic liver or kidney disease, immune compromise, and poorly controlled diabetes mellitus.

As with erysipelas, *S. pyogenes* is a common pathogen, but other gram-positive organisms such as *S. aureus* and other groups of streptococci play a more prominent role. *S. aureus* may be of particular concern when significant purulence is identified on examination. Gram-negative and polymicrobial cellulitis can also occur, but these infections are usually preceded by a more invasive injury such as bite wounds or other forms of penetrating trauma.

EVALUATION AND MANAGEMENT

After it has been determined that there is a skin or soft tissue infection, management consists of several basic principles that vary based on the severity of the infection and include (1) resuscitation of the patient (if indicated), (2) drainage of purulent material (if indicated) and acquisition of specimens for culture, and (3) appropriate antimicrobial coverage. With the exception of antimicrobial choice, which will be discussed separately, evaluation and management are best separated by severity of infection.

Mild Infections

Mild infections are those for which minimal treatment is required and include folliculitis and solitary furuncles. Obtaining a bacterial sample in this cases is of minimal yield because bacterial load in the lesions themselves is minimal and would not be worth the invasiveness of procedures required to obtain a sample. Skin swabs would most likely yield the host's colonizing flora, not the pathogen at the source of infection. Decreasing moisture, the use of antibacterial soap, and improved hand hygiene may be all that is needed, with topical or oral antibiotics reserved for refractory cases.

Moderate Infections

Moderate infections include furunculosis, carbuncles, impetigo, erysipelas, and all but the most severe cases of cellulitis. Although more important in severe infections, initial evaluation and management should focus on the need for any resuscitation. Although there may not be direct toxin-mediated cardiovascular compromise, associated fever (either prodromal or subsequent) and malaise may contribute to a varying degree of dehydration from poor intake and insensible fluid losses, possibly requiring parenteral fluid administration.

Obtaining a specimen, when possible, is very important because it has implications for both management and treatment. Not only will a culture of the material be useful for appropriate antimicrobial selection, but removal of fluid within a collection or abscess is an essential therapeutic step because the likelihood that such lesions would improve with antimicrobials alone is minimal. For many lesions (impetigo, carbuncles), drainage may be spontaneous or may be achieved with soaks and compresses. In other cases, incision and drainage may be required (Figure 90-5). If an abscess or collection is identified on examination, the procedure is straightforward. If a collection is not apparent but the clinician has a high index of suspicion based on history (abscesses in past, duration, fevers) or examination (location,

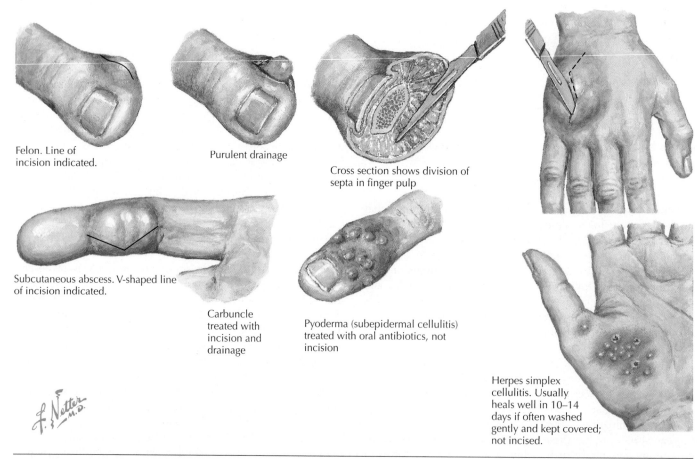

Felon. Line of incision indicated.

Purulent drainage

Cross section shows division of septa in finger pulp

Subcutaneous abscess. V-shaped line of incision indicated.

Carbuncle treated with incision and drainage

Pyoderma (subepidermal cellulitis) treated with oral antibiotics, not incision

Herpes simplex cellulitis. Usually heals well in 10–14 days if often washed gently and kept covered; not incised.

Figure 90-5 *Cellulitis and epidermal abscess.*

size), imaging may be indicated. Optimal modalities vary largely with the location of the lesions: ultrasonography is most useful when the infection is confined to the superficial tissues of an extremity, computed tomography is frequently used when evaluating the head or neck, and magnetic resonance imaging is used when there is the question of bony involvement. When the infection is causing systemic signs and symptoms that require fluid resuscitation and more extensive incision and drainage, the clinician should consider the need for further evaluation, including laboratory testing (blood culture and complete blood count), intravenous antimicrobials, and hospital admission. Inflammatory markers such as C-reactive protein may be used to monitor response to therapy in more severe infections. Blood cultures clearly do not have as high a yield as wound or lesion cultures, but their yield increases when signs of systemic illness are present.

Severe Infections

Severe infections of the skin and soft tissues include any of the moderate infections that have significant cardiovascular instability and necrotizing fasciitis. Evaluation and management of severe infections are similar to those of moderate infections, with more attention to resuscitation as needed. Along with the blood tests mentioned for moderate infections, clinicians should also obtain a complete metabolic panel and coagulation parameters to evaluate for possible end-organ damage and disseminated intravascular coagulation. In suspected cases of necrotizing fasciitis, prompt surgical evaluation with possible exploration and subsequent debridement are essential to minimize morbidity and mortality. If cardiovascular compromise is significant, vasopressors and admission to an intensive care unit may be indicated.

Antimicrobials

For the vast majority of cases, therapy is directed at gram-positive organisms, namely *S. pyogenes* and *S. aureus*, with consideration given to MRSA. For mild infections such as folliculitis, solitary furuncles and mild cases of nonbullous impetigo, topical treatment may be sufficient. Mupirocin is the topical agent of choice, and the infection should be followed closely by the outpatient provider for signs of progression and the need for more aggressive treatment. If the infection requires systemic antimicrobials, there are several factors for the provider to consider, including the severity of infection and presence of systemic illness, appearance of the infection on examination, medical history, risk factors for MRSA (prior MRSA infections, hemodialysis, recent antibiotic usage or hospitalization), and the epidemiology of local bacterial flora. If it is the patient's first infection, there are no MRSA risk factors, and the patient is without any systemic signs of illness, the clinician may choose to provide coverage for β-hemolytic streptococci and methicillin-susceptible *S. aureus* (MSSA) with oral cephalexin or dicloxacillin. If the patient has any risk factors but the severity of the infection is such that outpatient management is preferred, choices for empiric coverage include clindamycin, trimethoprim-sulfamethoxazole, or linezolid. The choice between these agents depends largely on the local patterns of resistance for *S. aureus*, with some areas possible requiring a combination of the two. For parenteral coverage, choices are the same, although the parenteral form of trimethoprim–sulfamethoxazole is caustic and should be avoided. In addition, for those with severe illness or for whom there is concern for hospital-acquired strains of MRSA, vancomycin should be considered as well.

SUGGESTED READINGS

American Academy of Pediatrics, Committee on Infectious Diseases: severe invasive group A streptococcal infections: a subject review, *Pediatrics* 101(1 Pt 1):136-140, 1998.

Fleisher GR, Ludwig S, Henretig FM, eds. *Textbook of Pediatric Emergency Medicine*, 5th ed, Philadelphia, 2005, Lippincott Williams & Wilkins.

Hedrick J: Acute bacterial skin infections in pediatric medicine: current issues in presentation and treatment, *Paediatr Drug* 5(Suppl 1):35-46, 2003.

Oumeish I, Oumeish OY, Bataineh O: Acute bacterial skin infections in children, *Clin Dermatol* 18(6):667-678, 2000.

Zaoutis B, Chiang W: *Comprehensive Pediatric Hospital Medicine*, Philadelphia, 2007, Saunders.

This chapter discusses pneumonia and lower respiratory infections such as bacterial tracheitis. These lower respiratory infections are encountered frequently in children; although up to half of lower respiratory infections in children are viral, bacterial pneumonia is the most common serious bacterial infection in children. The number of diagnostic methods available for identification of the causative pathogen has increased dramatically over the past decade, yet amoxicillin and ampicillin remain the most appropriate first-line therapy for uncomplicated community-acquired pneumonia (CAP).

ETIOLOGY AND PATHOGENESIS

Epidemiology

Definitions of pneumonia vary: the World Health Organization (WHO) uses the clinical symptoms of cough and fast or difficult breathing to define pneumonia, characterizing a respiratory rate greater than 50 breaths/min for children 2 to 12 months old and greater than 40 breaths/min for children 1 to 5 years old as abnormally fast. In the developed world, pneumonia is commonly defined as the presence of fever (temperature >38.0°C) and signs of lower respiratory tract infection (e.g., cough, tachypnea, hypoxia) with or without abnormalities on chest radiograph.

The annual incidence of pneumonia is greatest among children younger than 1 year old and decreases as children age. CAP causes almost 20% of deaths in children younger than 5 years old in the developing world, but fewer than 1% of children hospitalized with pneumonia in the United States die. CAP nonetheless remains a frequent cause of outpatient pediatric visits and hospitalization. Bacterial pneumonia may be complicated by parapneumonic effusion; the term *empyema* is used to describe purulent effusions. Empyema occurs in approximately 10% of children hospitalized with CAP.

Microbiology

The common causes of CAP in healthy children in the developed world vary by age group, although an extensive number of pathogens can cause CAP (Table 91-1). Respiratory viruses such as respiratory syncytial virus (RSV); influenza A and B; parainfluenza 1, 2, and 3; adenovirus; and human metapneumovirus (hMPV) can be identified in up to half of patients admitted to the hospital for CAP. These viral pathogens may be identified alone or as part of a co-infection with bacteria. First described in 2001, hMPV, similar to RSV infection in young children, causes a spectrum of respiratory disease ranging from mild bronchiolitis to severe pneumonia.

Streptococcus pneumoniae is the most common bacterial cause of childhood CAP (Figure 91-1). Randomized trials of the heptavalent pneumococcal conjugate vaccine (PCV7) demonstrated that the incidence of radiographically confirmed pneumonia was reduced by 20% in vaccine recipients compared with placebo recipients, suggesting that *S. pneumoniae* causes at least 20% of CAP cases. Postlicensure epidemiologic studies have shown a 39% decrease in all-cause pneumonia hospitalizations in children younger than 2 years of age but nonsignificant decreases in older children. Thus, the significant role of pneumococcus as a cause of childhood CAP drives the choice of empiric antibiotic therapy for younger children.

Staphylococcus aureus, particularly community-associated methicillin-resistant *S. aureus* (CA-MRSA), has been recognized with increasing frequency as a cause of severe CAP even in previously healthy children without exposure to health care settings. *Mycoplasma pneumoniae*, although previously described as a pathogen limited to adolescents and young adults, is also a common pathogen in school-age children and toddlers. *M. pneumoniae* has been associated with wheezing, identified in one study in half of patients with a first episode of wheezing and 20% of patients admitted for an exacerbation of their known prior asthma.

Less common causes of CAP include *Streptococcus pyogenes*, nontypable *Haemophilus influenzae*, enteric gram-negative pathogens (in cases of aspiration or neurologic compromise), *Mycobacterium tuberculosis*, herpes simplex virus (in newborns), varicella-zoster virus, *Legionella pneumophila*, and endemic mycoses such as *Histoplasma capsulatum*, *Coccidioides immitis*, and *Blastomyces dermatitidis*. Before the introduction of the conjugate *H. influenzae* type b (Hib) vaccine, Hib was a common cause of CAP. In countries and areas where Hib vaccine uptake is low, Hib should still be considered as a common cause of CAP.

Bacterial tracheitis is a serious respiratory infection encountered only rarely, and it is most frequently caused by *S. aureus*, although other organisms such as nontypable *H. influenzae*, *Moraxella catarrhalis*, and anaerobes have been implicated in its pathogenesis. As with bacterial pneumonias, tracheitis often follows an antecedent viral upper respiratory infection.

Pathogenesis

Viral illness alone, such as influenza, can cause severe and necrotizing pneumonia (Figure 91-2). Preceding viral illness may play a part in the pathogenesis of bacterial pneumonia. One study demonstrated that rates of invasive pneumococcal disease each winter season rose in close association with respiratory viral illness diagnoses (RSV, influenza, and hMPV), suggesting that the respiratory damage caused by viral respiratory illness may allow for subsequent bacterial pneumonia. Such data do not prove the direct causation of invasive bacterial pneumonia as a consequence of viral respiratory infection, however. Likewise, a randomized trial of children receiving a pneumococcal vaccine found fewer admissions for both pneumococcal pneumonia and hMPV pneumonia among vaccine recipients compared with

Table 91-1 Common Bacterial and Viral Causes of Community-Acquired Pneumonia by Age in Healthy Children in the Developed World

≤3 Months Old	3 Months to 5 Years Old	≥5 Years Old
Bacteria	**Bacteria**	**Bacteria**
Group B streptococcus Enteric gram-negative bacilli *Streptococcus pneumoniae* *Bordetella pertussis* *Chlamydia trachomatis* *Staphylococcus aureus*	*Streptococcus pneumoniae* *Mycoplasma pneumoniae* *Chlamydophila pneumoniae** *Staphylococcus aureus* *Haemophilus influenzae* (nontypable)	*Streptococcus pneumoniae* *Mycoplasma pneumoniae* *Chlamydophila pneumoniae** *Staphylococcus aureus*
Lower Respiratory Viruses	**Lower Respiratory Viruses**	**Lower Respiratory Viruses**
Respiratory syncytial virus Influenza A and B Parainfluenza viruses 1, 2, 3 Human metapneumovirus Rhinovirus Adenovirus Bocavirus Coronaviruses	Respiratory syncytial virus Influenza A and B Parainfluenza viruses 1, 2, 3 Human metapneumovirus Rhinovirus Adenovirus Bocavirus Coronaviruses	Influenza A and B

*Formerly *Chlamydia pneumoniae.*

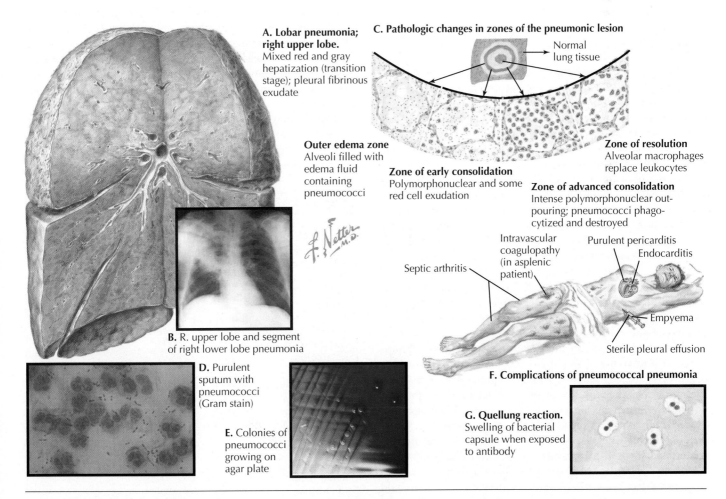

A. Lobar pneumonia; right upper lobe. Mixed red and gray hepatization (transition stage); pleural fibrinous exudate

B. R. upper lobe and segment of right lower lobe pneumonia

C. Pathologic changes in zones of the pneumonic lesion

Normal lung tissue

Outer edema zone Alveoli filled with edema fluid containing pneumococci

Zone of early consolidation Polymorphonuclear and some red cell exudation

Zone of resolution Alveolar macrophages replace leukocytes

Zone of advanced consolidation Intense polymorphonuclear outpouring; pneumococci phagocytized and destroyed

D. Purulent sputum with pneumococci (Gram stain)

E. Colonies of pneumococci growing on agar plate

Intravascular coagulopathy (in asplenic patient)

Septic arthritis

Purulent pericarditis

Endocarditis

Empyema

Sterile pleural effusion

F. Complications of pneumococcal pneumonia

G. Quellung reaction. Swelling of bacterial capsule when exposed to antibody

Figure 91-1 *Pneumococcal pneumonia.*

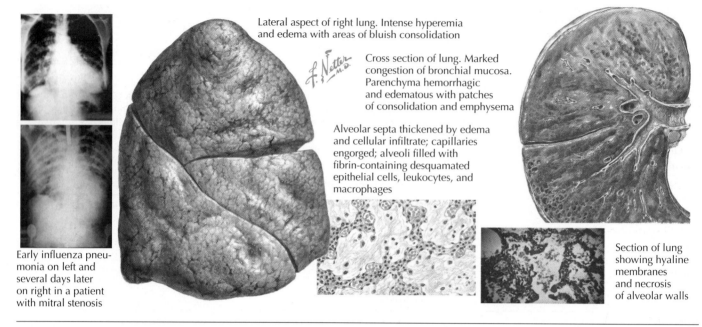

Lateral aspect of right lung. Intense hyperemia and edema with areas of bluish consolidation

Cross section of lung. Marked congestion of bronchial mucosa. Parenchyma hemorrhagic and edematous with patches of consolidation and emphysema

Alveolar septa thickened by edema and cellular infiltrate; capillaries engorged; alveoli filled with fibrin-containing desquamated epithelial cells, leukocytes, and macrophages

Early influenza pneumonia on left and several days later on right in a patient with mitral stenosis

Section of lung showing hyaline membranes and necrosis of alveolar walls

Figure 91-2 *Influenzal pneumonia.*

placebo recipients, suggesting that hospitalizations for hMPV may involve co-infection with pneumococcus.

CLINICAL PRESENTATION AND DIFFERENTIAL DIAGNOSIS

Children with lower respiratory illness classically present with fever, cough, and tachypnea. The spectrum of illness among children with CAP is broad and ranges from mild, well-appearing children to those who require intubation and intensive care. The clinical manifestations of CAP are equally diverse, and few physical examination findings allow for distinction among viral, bacterial, and atypical causes.

The sensitivity of tachypnea alone is up to 74% in identifying children with radiographically confirmed pneumonia. Tachypnea alone has a low specificity for pneumonia, however, because many noninfectious causes of tachypnea exist, so most patients with tachypnea do not have pneumonia. Combinations of multiple physical examination findings, such as tachypnea, rales, and increased respiratory effort, raise the specificity for a clinical diagnosis of pneumonia dramatically but substantially lower the sensitivity, thereby potentially missing many patients with pneumonia. Likewise, the absence of rales on examination does not preclude a pneumonia diagnosis.

Many children with pneumonia also have abdominal symptoms, such as vomiting and abdominal pain. Vomiting may be posttussive, after episodes of severe coughing. Abdominal pain can at times be the most prominent complaint and occurs most commonly in patients with basilar pneumonia. Wheezing and exacerbation of underlying asthma are symptoms more typically encountered in patients with CAP caused by viruses and atypical bacteria such as *M. pneumoniae* and *Chlamydophila pneumoniae* (formerly *Chlamydia pneumoniae*). Children with lower respiratory tract infections caused by atypical bacteria often have mild and nonspecific symptoms such as headache, low-grade fever,

pharyngitis, and cough for 5 to 7 days before their presentation with pneumonia.

Children with bacterial tracheitis are often younger than 5 years of age and most commonly present with barking cough, high fever, and significant respiratory distress, often lending these patients a "toxic" appearance. These patients will not have the drooling or inability to lie flat found in patients with epiglottitis, but they can develop life-threatening respiratory distress nonetheless.

The differential diagnosis of lower respiratory infection includes pulmonary anatomic abnormalities, foreign bodies and chemical irritants, autoimmune diseases, and malignancies, among others (Box 91-1).

Box 91-1 Differential Diagnosis of Pneumonia

Anatomic lesions
• Congenital cystic adenomatoid malformation
• Bronchogenic cyst
• Congenital lobar emphysema
• Pulmonary sequestration
• Congenital diaphragmatic hernia
Aspiration
• Aspirated foreign body
• Inhaled chemical irritants (e.g., hydrocarbons)
Autoimmune diseases
• Sarcoidosis
• Wegener's granulomatosis
• Systemic lupus erythematosus
Malignancies
• Lymphoma
• Primary lung tumor
• Metastatic tumor
Atelectasis
Heart failure
Renal failure
Chylothorax

EVALUATION AND MANAGEMENT

Diagnostic Methods

An etiologic diagnosis is seldom made in cases of childhood CAP because invasive diagnostic procedures such as bronchoalveolar lavage and needle thoracentesis are infrequently performed in young children and because young children cannot provide adequate sputum specimens. However, children 8 years and older with a productive cough are often able to provide adequate sputum specimens for culture after nebulized hypertonic saline treatments (so-called induced sputum cultures).

Bacterial tracheitis is typically diagnosed based on clinical presentation and through culture of sputum or the purulent exudate found in the trachea on bronchoscopy or intubation. Sputum cultures must be nevertheless interpreted cautiously because they can also capture colonizing oropharyngeal flora. A high-quality sputum specimen should have few squamous epithelial cells (≤10 per high power field [hpf]) and many white blood cells (≥25 per hpf) and should arrive within 2 hours to a microbiology laboratory for culture.

Nasopharyngeal aspirates can provide good samples on which to perform polymerase chain reaction (PCR) to identify both viral and bacterial CAP etiologies. PCR on nasopharyngeal aspirates detects respiratory viruses such as RSV and influenza A and B with a sensitivity in the high 90% range, and immunofluorescence on similar specimens has a sensitivity ranging from approximately 50% to 90%, depending on the specific kit. Likewise, PCR from a nasopharyngeal aspirate is the diagnostic method of choice for *Bordetella pertussis* during the first 4 weeks

of illness, but the diagnosis can be confirmed with acute and convalescent serologies in patients with negative PCR results and a high suspicion for the clinical disease. After that time, *B. pertussis* serology can be used to make the diagnosis because the organism is cleared from the nasopharynx over time. Although *B. pertussis* can be cultured during the first 3 weeks of illness, results may not be available for 5 to 7 days.

Chlamydia trachomatis (in neonates) and *C. pneumoniae* can also be detected via PCR, although prolonged shedding can occur, causing PCR test results to remain positive after the initial period of active disease. In neonates and young infants, direct fluorescent antibody testing can also be used on conjunctival and respiratory specimens for the diagnosis of *C. trachomatis*. Both *C. trachomatis* and *C. pneumoniae* can also be diagnosed through use of acute and convalescent serologies. Likewise, *M. pneumoniae* is most reliably detected by serologic testing of paired specimens obtained 2 to 3 weeks apart; a fourfold or greater increase in the antibody titer indicates a recent or current infection. Unfortunately, paired serology testing does not provide a diagnosis quickly enough to influence clinical practice. PCR testing for *M. pneumoniae* has a sensitivity of approximately 80% for pharyngeal specimens and 90% for nasopharyngeal specimens, and specificity is greater than 95% when compared with acute and convalescent serologies.

Tuberculin skin testing should be considered for all patients with appropriate tuberculosis risk factors (i.e., travel to an endemic area, contact with a person with active tuberculosis, or contact with people who work or reside in prison or health care settings) and chest radiography findings (Figure 91-3). Newer

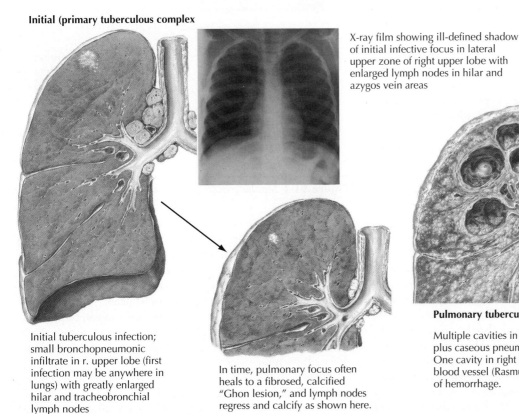

Initial (primary tuberculous complex

X-ray film showing ill-defined shadow of initial infective focus in lateral upper zone of right upper lobe with enlarged lymph nodes in hilar and azygos vein areas

Initial tuberculous infection; small bronchopneumonic infiltrate in r. upper lobe (first infection may be anywhere in lungs) with greatly enlarged hilar and tracheobronchial lymph nodes

In time, pulmonary focus often heals to a fibrosed, calcified "Ghon lesion," and lymph nodes regress and calcify as shown here.

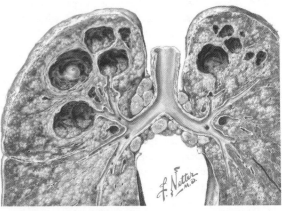

Pulmonary tuberculosis with extensive cavitary disease

Multiple cavities in both lungs with erosion into bronchi plus caseous pneumonitis and fibrosis throughout. One cavity in right lung contains an eroded aneurysmal blood vessel (Rasmussen), which is a common cause of hemorrhage.

Figure 91-3 *Pulmonary tuberculosis.*

diagnostic methods that measure serum interferon-γ released by T-cells stimulated by *M. tuberculosis* antigens are becoming available but are not validated in children, and they cannot distinguish latent from active disease. Of note, children younger than 2 years of age are more likely to have nonspecific chest radiography findings and disseminated or miliary tuberculosis at presentation.

A urine antigen test for *L. pneumophila* exists and can be considered for CAP in immunocompromised children and older adolescents. In patients with an appropriate travel history and chest radiography results, *Histoplasma* serology or urine antigen can be considered. Paired acute and convalescent serologies are useful in diagnosing pneumonia caused by *C. immitis* and *B. dermatitidis*.

Blood culture results are seldom positive (≈2% of cases) in outpatients with CAP and are therefore of little utility in well-appearing patients without hypoxia. Up to 10% of patients requiring admission may have positive blood culture results, and the rate of positive blood cultures may be even higher in those with pneumonia complicated by empyema. Blood cultures in these patient populations may therefore provide useful microbiologic data, including antibiotic sensitivities. Gram stain and bacterial culture of pleural fluid should always be performed in patients with pneumonia with associated pleural effusion that has been drained. Urine antigen testing for *S. pneumoniae* should not, however, be performed routinely because false-positive results may occur as a result of pneumococcal nasopharyngeal colonization in up to 18% of children, and the results are difficult to interpret reliably in the absence of a true gold standard.

Serum white blood cell count and inflammatory markers cannot be used to differentiate between viral and bacterial pneumonia reliably. Although very high circulating neutrophil and C-reactive protein (CRP) levels may be found more commonly in patients with bacterial pneumonia, normal neutrophil and CRP levels do not exclude its possibility. Serum inflammatory markers should therefore be used only to provide supplementary objective measures of disease resolution when tracking the course of a severe pneumonia.

Chest radiography should be considered in highly febrile patients without another identifiable source, especially those with tachypnea or a peripheral blood leukocytosis. Specific chest radiography findings in patients with lower respiratory infection can suggest the etiology. Lobar pneumonia is most common with bacterial pneumonia, although atypical bacterial pathogens occasionally cause lobar infiltrates. Patchy bronchopneumonia with or without effusion or empyema can be seen with *S. aureus* infection (Figure 91-4). Interstitial infiltrates on chest radiography are most frequently seen with viral and atypical bacterial pathogens such as *M. pneumoniae* or *L. pneumophila*. Simple parapneumonic effusions can be seen with almost any pathogen, and severe bacterial pneumonias can also be complicated by complex pleural effusions or empyemas. Hilar lymphadenopathy and nodular disease suggest unusual etiologies such as *M. tuberculosis*; *P. jiroveci*; and endemic mycoses such as *Histoplasma*, *Coccidioides*, or *Blastomyces* spp. Pneumatoceles are air-filled cavities caused by alveolar rupture that can be visualized on chest radiography and can be seen in *S. aureus* pneumonia (and occasionally in pneumonia caused by enteric gram-negative bacilli).

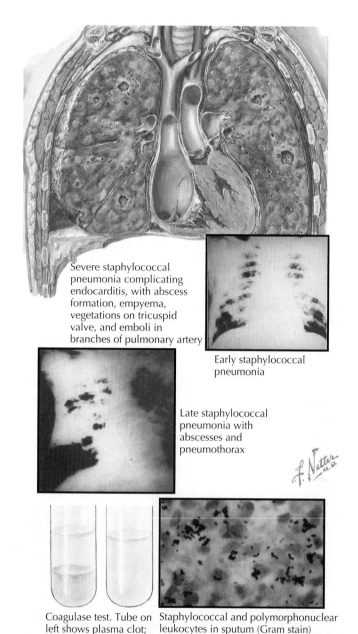

Severe staphylococcal pneumonia complicating endocarditis, with abscess formation, empyema, vegetations on tricuspid valve, and emboli in branches of pulmonary artery

Early staphylococcal pneumonia

Late staphylococcal pneumonia with abscesses and pneumothorax

Coagulase test. Tube on left shows plasma clot; tube on right is control

Staphylococcal and polymorphonuclear leukocytes in sputum (Gram stain)

Figure 91-4 *Staphylococcal pneumonia.*

More detailed imaging with chest computed tomography (CT) should be sought if an underlying pulmonary malformation (e.g., a congenital cystic adenomatoid malformation) is being considered. Bilateral decubitus chest radiographs are also useful in diagnosing aspiration of radiolucent foreign bodies: the foreign body will act as a ball-valve mechanism, trapping air in the affected lung and allowing it to remain paradoxically inflated when it is in the dependent (and therefore typically deflated) position.

Because follow-up chest radiograph results can remain abnormal long after complete clinical recovery, such studies are typically unwarranted in patients with uncomplicated recoveries and seldom change the management of these patients. Chest radiography should be considered for patients who have not

Table 91-2 Treatment Recommendations for Community-Acquired Pneumonia According to Age and Clinical Status in Healthy Children in the Developed World

Age	Outpatient Treatment	Inpatient Treatment	Inpatient Treatment for Complicated Pneumonia*
3 mo and younger	Not recommended	Consider ampicillin and gentamicin IV[†]	Consider ampicillin and cefotaxime IV
3 mo-5 y	*Preferred*: oral amoxicillin (80-100 mg/kg/d in three divided doses)	*Preferred*: IV ampicillin (200 mg/kg/d in four divided doses)	*Preferred*: IV clindamycin and cefotaxime
	Second line: oral clindamycin or third-generation cephalosporin[‡]	*Second line*: IV clindamycin or cefotaxime[‡]	*Second line*: IV vancomycin and cefotaxime (for the most unstable patients)
5 y and older	*Preferred*: oral amoxicillin[‡] (80-100 mg/kg/d in three divided doses)	*Preferred*: IV ampicillin[‡] (200 mg/kg/d in four divided doses)	*Preferred*: IV clindamycin and cefotaxime
	Second line: oral clindamycin, third-generation cephalosporin, or levofloxacin[§]	*Second line*: IV clindamycin, cefotaxime, or levofloxacin[§]	*Second line*: IV vancomycin and cefotaxime (for the most unstable patients)

*Complicated pneumonia is defined as disease in septic-appearing or unstable patients and those with large pleural effusions or necrotizing pneumonia.

[†]Consider adding erythromycin or azithromycin if *Chlamydia trachomatis* or *Bordetella pertussis* is suspected or confirmed.

[‡]Consider azithromycin to cover for atypical pathogens if a diffuse wheeze is present.

[§]Levofloxacin is not approved by the Food and Drug Administration for use in patients younger than 18 years old, but clinical data support its use in these patients.

improved on empiric treatment and who have not yet had any chest imaging. Patients with increasing effusions and worsening symptoms should be referred for diagnostic and therapeutic drainage of the effusion. The findings of hilar lymphadenopathy, cystic or nodular disease, or pulmonary anatomic abnormalities should prompt further diagnostic procedures to identify possible tuberculosis, endemic mycoses, and atypical pathogens; to diagnose certain autoimmune or neoplastic conditions; and to consider underlying immune deficiencies (e.g., chronic granulomatous disease).

Treatment

Distinguishing between viral and bacterial pneumonia clinically can be extremely difficult. It is therefore reasonable to provide empiric antimicrobial therapy to outpatients with a clinical diagnosis of pneumonia. Amoxicillin remains the drug of choice for outpatient pediatric pneumonia (Table 91-2); there are no data to support the choice of empiric standard-dose amoxicillin versus high-dose amoxicillin. If chosen, high-dose amoxicillin or ampicillin should have continued efficacy against resistant *S. pneumoniae*, whose resistance is mediated by alterations in penicillin-binding proteins and can be overcome at higher drug concentrations.

A randomized trial in Pakistan demonstrated fewer failures with amoxicillin treatment compared with trimethoprim–sulfamethoxazole (TMP-SMX) treatment for CAP. Amoxicillin was also specifically more effective in patients under one year of age and those with severe pneumonia, as defined by cough or difficulty breathing with lower chest retractions. Most notably, no patients with pneumococcal bacteremia failed amoxicillin treatment, but almost 30% of such patients treated with TMP-SMX failed treatment. Despite increasing reports of in vitro β-lactam (i.e., amoxicillin or ampicillin) resistance among *S. pneumoniae* isolates, no significant increase in clinical failures

for patients treated with amoxicillin or ampicillin has occurred, underscoring the notion that amoxicillin or ampicillin should be the initial therapy of choice for pediatric CAP. Additionally, since the introduction of PCV7 in 2000, the proportion of pneumococcal isolates resistant to penicillins has decreased.

The incidence of community-acquired MRSA has increased in recent years, and community-acquired MRSA has been recognized as a cause of severe, necrotizing pneumonia. MRSA should be considered as a possible causative pathogen in severely ill hospitalized patients. Although local patterns can vary, community-acquired MRSA is typically susceptible to clindamycin; clindamycin should be considered for use in severe or necrotizing pneumonia in hospitalized patients unless local clindamycin resistance is high among MRSA isolates (>15% of isolates is a common threshold). In such cases, vancomycin should be used. TMP-SMX can also be considered as an alternate treatment for CAP in which MRSA is isolated or suspected, given the high proportion of community-acquired MRSA isolates that are susceptible.

The duration of CAP treatment is unclear but is typically 10 days (or 5 days if azithromycin is used). A randomized, controlled trial of 3 versus 5 days of oral amoxicillin for 2- to 59-month-old patients in Pakistan with nonsevere CAP showed no difference in failure rates or relapse between the two groups, even when the results were limited to those with radiographically confirmed pneumonia. This study's results may be less applicable in the developed world, where there may be greater access to laboratory testing for viral pathogens: this study used the WHO definition of pneumonia and therefore likely included patients with viral illnesses (e.g., 20% of patients in one of these studies had laboratory-confirmed RSV).

Clindamycin is an appropriate alternative treatment choice in patients with penicillin allergies given its excellent pneumococcal coverage. Oral third-generation cephalosporins or macrolides such as azithromycin can also be considered in these patients. These antibiotics are not as effective antipneumococcal agents as the penicillins, however, and there is increasing macrolide resistance among pneumococcal strains. Levofloxacin is a fluoroquinolone effective against most resistant pneumococcal strains and with a broad range of activity in general (including atypical pathogens such as *Legionella* spp. or *M. pneumoniae*). Fluoroquinolones are not recommended in children younger than 18 years of age based on safety concerns for tendon rupture and other musculoskeletal injuries, but data support its safety in these patients, and levofloxacin may be useful in patients with drug allergies or known resistant isolates.

Hospital admission should be considered for any patients younger than 3 months of age, with oxygen saturations less than 92% on room air, severe respiratory distress or grunting, or dehydration or inability to take in oral fluids and oral antibiotics or when providers are unable to monitor patients closely for clinical decompensation.

Patients with persistent symptoms or failure to improve after 48 hours on appropriate empiric therapy should have chest radiography performed or repeated, partly to detect a new or evolving pleural effusion or empyema. Although some patients can have simple parapneumonic effusions requiring no intervention, others require drainage of a significant pleural bacterial infection to speed recovery. Viral diagnostics such as rapid respiratory viral PCR panels should also be considered because positive viral test results often enable providers to discontinue antibiotics. Patients who fail treatment with oral amoxicillin and who have no effusion may receive inpatient treatment with ampicillin, with or without a macrolide. Those admitted to the hospital with an empyema or necrotizing pneumonia should receive broad-spectrum antibiotics that provide coverage against highly resistant *S. pneumoniae* and MRSA isolates (e.g., a combination of clindamycin and cefotaxime).

FUTURE DIRECTIONS

Pneumococcal serotypes not included in the PCV7 vaccine have emerged as more frequent causes of disease in the years after its introduction. Many nonvaccine serotypes have intermediate or high levels of penicillin resistance. There are other pneumococcal vaccines in late clinical trials (e.g., a 13-valent pneumococcal vaccine), and the epidemiology of invasive pneumococcal disease will remain a dynamic process as these vaccines are introduced. Prospective study is needed to identify the most effective empiric antimicrobial treatment for outpatients with CAP. The role and timing of empyema drainage for patients with severe complicated pneumonia need to be fully elucidated. Newer molecular methods of bacterial diagnosis, including PCR using conserved bacterial ribosomal subunits, may increase our diagnostic capabilities in CAP. Little is known about the long-term pulmonary sequelae and residual lung function of those who have recovered from severe pneumonia.

SUGGESTED READINGS

Ampofo K, Bender J, Sheng X, et al: Seasonal invasive pneumococcal disease in children: role of preceding respiratory viral infection, *Pediatrics* 122:229-237, 2008.

Black SB, Shinefield HR, Ling S, et al: Effectiveness of heptavalent pneumococcal conjugate vaccine in children younger than five years of age for prevention of pneumonia, *Pediatr Infect Dis J* 21:810-815, 2002.

Cardoso MR, Nascimento-Carvalho CM, Ferrero F, et al: Penicillin-resistant pneumococcus and risk of treatment failure in pneumonia, *Arch Dis Child* 93:221-225, 2008.

Grant GB, Campbell H, Dowell SF, et al: Recommendations for treatment of childhood non-severe pneumonia, *Lancet Infect Dis* 9:185-196, 2009.

Grijalva CG, Nuorti JP, Arbogast PG, et al: Decline in pneumonia admissions after routine childhood immunisation with pneumococcal conjugate vaccine in the USA: a time-series analysis, *Lancet* 369:1179-1186, 2007.

Haider BA, Saeed MA, Bhutta ZA: Short-course versus long-course antibiotic therapy for non-severe community-acquired pneumonia in children aged 2 months to 59 months. Cochrane Database Syst Rev 2:CD005976, 2008.

Kabra SK, Lodha R, Pandey RM: Antibiotics for community acquired pneumonia in children. Cochrane Database Syst Rev 3:CD004874, 2006.

Kyaw MH, Lynfield R, Schaffner W, et al: Effect of introduction of the pneumococcal conjugate vaccine on drug-resistant *Streptococcus pneumoniae*, *N Engl J Med* 354:1455-1463, 2006.

Madhi SA, Ludewick H, Kuwanda L, et al: Pneumococcal coinfection with human metapneumovirus, *J Infect Dis* 193:1236-1243, 2006.

McIntosh K: Community-acquired pneumonia in children, *N Engl J Med* 346:429-437, 2002.

Michelow IC, Olsen K, Lozano J, et al: Epidemiology and clinical characteristics of community-acquired pneumonia in hospitalized children, *Pediatrics* 113:701-707, 2004.

92

Infections of the Central Nervous System

Sanjeev K. Swami

This chapter discusses infections of the central nervous system (CNS), including meningitis, meningoencephalitis, epidural abscesses, and brain abscesses. Some specific CNS infections are discussed elsewhere and are only briefly mentioned in this chapter.

MENINGITIS AND MENINGOENCEPHALITIS

Meningitis is defined as inflammation of the leptomeninges, and meningoencephalitis is inflammation of the meninges and cerebral cortex.

ETIOLOGY, EPIDEMIOLOGY, AND PATHOGENESIS

Meningitis is usually an acute process that is generally caused by either bacteria or viruses. Meningoencephalitis is predominantly caused by viruses, mostly enteroviruses.

Because enteroviruses are the most common cause of viral meningitis and meningoencephalitis, the incidence of these infections peaks in the summer and fall and wanes in the winter. Herpes family viruses such as herpes simplex virus (HSV) and varicella zoster (VZV) also cause meningoencephalitis, as can a number of other pathogens (Box 92-1).

Historically, the most common causes of bacterial meningitis beyond the neonatal period were *Streptococcus pneumoniae*, *Neisseria meningitidis*, and *Haemophilus influenzae* type b (Hib). Fortunately, there has been a dramatic reduction in the incidence of Hib infections after the introduction of the conjugate Hib vaccine in 1987. Additionally, there has been a reduction in the incidence of meningitis caused by *S. pneumoniae* since the introduction of the heptavalent pneumococcal conjugate vaccine (PCV7); unfortunately, there are serotypes that are not contained in that vaccine that have the ability to cause disease in humans, so the effect of the PCV7has not been as dramatic as the Hib vaccine. The currently licensed vaccine for *N. meningitidis* covers serogroups A, C, W135, and Y. It does not elicit a protective response against serogroup B, which continues to cause both sporadic disease and outbreaks, mostly on college campuses and military bases.

All three of these bacteria colonize the upper respiratory tract (nasopharynx and oropharynx). From there, they are able to invade through the mucosal epithelium, usually when that surface is inflamed because of a viral infection, and enter the bloodstream. The bacteria circulate in the bloodstream and gain access to the CNS via the choroid plexus. The bacteria readily replicate in the subarachnoid space within the cerebrospinal fluid (CSF) because this area is normally sequestered from the immune system. In response to bacterial replication, white blood cells (WBCs) migrate to the CSF, and the ensuing inflammatory response leads to some of the signs and symptoms of meningitis.

In addition to hematogenous seeding of the CSF, bacteria can also gain access to the CNS via direct extension. Congenital malformations, such as dermoid sinuses, or traumatic injuries, including basilar skull fractures and penetrating trauma, can allow bacteria to enter the CSF. Infections of the sinuses, mastoid air cells, or middle ear can also act as portals of entry (Figure 92-1).

Other causes of acute meningitis include *Borrelia burgdorferi*, the etiologic agent of Lyme disease; gram-negative bacilli such as *Citrobacter*, *Salmonella*, and *Pseudomonas* spp.; and fungal pathogens.

CLINICAL PRESENTATION

Neonates and infants with meningitis often present with nonspecific signs and symptoms. The most common parental complaint is fever, and the infants frequently have a history of irritability and poor feeding. They may also develop vomiting and a bulging fontanelle. In more severe cases, infants may present with lethargy or after having a seizure and may have focal neurologic deficits on examination. Although children with meningitis can present in many ways, toddlers and school-aged children are more likely to present with the "classic" signs and symptoms. These include high fever, photophobia, headache, neck stiffness, and vomiting. Of these, fever and headache are the most common. On physical examination, these patients may have nuchal rigidity as well as Kernig's or Brudzinski's signs (Figure 92-2). Children with disseminated *N. meningitidis* infections can have a petechial or purpuric rash. Infants with enteroviral meningitis often have an erythematous, macular rash. Cranial nerve palsies, especially of cranial nerve 7, and papilledema are frequently found in patients with Lyme meningitis but are unusual in other forms of meningitis.

DIFFERENTIAL DIAGNOSIS

The differential diagnosis of meningitis and meningoencephalitis depends on which signs and symptoms are prominent because the presentation of these infections is so varied.

The combination of fever and irritability in an infant or toddler has a very broad differential diagnosis, which includes many infectious and noninfectious etiologies. This is a situation in which a detailed medical history and thorough physical examination are critical in narrowing the differential diagnosis. There will almost always be additional information that helps to focus the differential. A history of vomiting or diarrhea points toward gastroenteritis. Tachypnea or focal findings on lung auscultation

Box 92-1 Causes of Meningitis

Common
- *Neisseria meningitidis*
- *Streptococcus pneumoniae*
- *Borrelia burgdorferi*
- Enteroviruses

Uncommon
- West Nile virus
- Herpes simplex virus

Rare and Special Circumstances
- *Listeria monocytogenes*: neonates, immunocompromised patients
- *Haemophilus influenzae* type b: unimmunized children
- *Staphylococcus aureus*: postoperative wound infection, ventriculoperitoneal shunt
- *Escherichia coli*: neonates
- *Citrobacter* spp.: neonates
- Group b streptococcus: neonates
- Candida spp.: immunocompromised patients
- Cryptococcus: HIV-positive patients
- Mumps
- Eastern equine virus
- Western equine virus
- Poliovirus
- Measles
- Lymphocytic choriomeningitis virus
- HIV
- Varicella zoster virus
- Cytomegalovirus
- Human herpes virus-6
- Epstein-Barr virus

are a sign of pneumonia, either viral or bacterial. Torticollis or other unusual positioning of the head and neck or a history of drooling are concerning for a focal infection in the neck or upper thorax such as a retropharyngeal or peritonsillar abscess. Another consideration in this situation, especially for toddlers with low-grade fevers rather than high fevers, is a foreign body in the upper airway, esophagus, or trachea. Cardiac and metabolic abnormalities are also important considerations in neonates and infants who present with fever, irritability, poor feeding, and vomiting.

Neck stiffness or pain on neck flexion may also be caused by a number of processes. These include peritonsillar or retropharyngeal abscesses, cervical lymphadenitis, muscle strain or spasms, cervical epidural infections, and upper lobe pneumonia.

Seizures as an isolated symptom have many possible causes. These include epilepsy, brain tumors, CNS infections, or metabolic abnormalities (especially hypoglycemia). They may also occur secondarily to trauma.

As patient age increases and they are better able to verbalize their symptoms, the differential diagnosis becomes more focused. However, adolescents who present with fever and altered mental status may not be able to communicate with the medical team to describe their symptoms. The differential diagnosis of fever and altered mental status in an older child includes CNS infections, ingestions or drug use, and metabolic abnormalities including diabetic ketoacidosis.

DIAGNOSTIC APPROACH

The most important diagnostic procedure in the evaluation of a child with suspected bacterial meningitis is a lumbar puncture (LP; see Figure 92-1). An opening pressure should be measured at the time of the LP, and fluid should be sent for at least cell count with differential, gram stain and culture, protein, and glucose. If viral meningitis or meningoencephalitis is suspected, polymerase chain reaction tests for enteroviruses and HSV are useful. Viral culture is an additional way to make the diagnosis of viral meningitis, although many laboratories no longer perform this test. Various CNS infections have typical CSF parameters that can aid the clinician while the results of the CSF culture are pending (Table 92-1). If there is concern for elevated intracranial pressure (ICP) before performing the LP based on clinical signs such as papilledema or focal neurologic findings, it is reasonable to perform either a computed tomography (CT) scan or magnetic resonance imaging (MRI) study. These studies allow the clinician to determine whether there is a space-occupying lesion, such as a brain abscess or brain tumor, or dilatation of the ventricles. These findings indicate that there is a risk of brain herniation if a lumbar puncture were performed.

Blood tests can yield additional information in children with meningitis. Although blood cultures are rarely positive, it is

Table 92-1 Typical Cerebrospinal Fluid Parameters

	Bacterial	Viral	Tuberculosis	Lyme Disease	Epidural Abscess
Opening pressure	Elevated	Normal	Elevated	Normal or mildly elevated	Normal
Gram stain	Occasionally positive	Negative	Negative	Negative	Rarely positive
WBC count	Elevated	Mild elevation	Very elevated	Mild elevation	Normal to mild elevation
WBC differential	Neutrophil predominance	Early: neutrophil predominance Late: lymphocyte and monocyte predominance	Lymphocyte predominance	Lymphocyte and monocyte predominance	Neutrophil predominance
Glucose	Low	Low or normal	Very low	Low or normal	Normal
Protein	High	Normal or mild elevation	Very high	Normal or mild elevation	Normal

WBC, white blood cell.

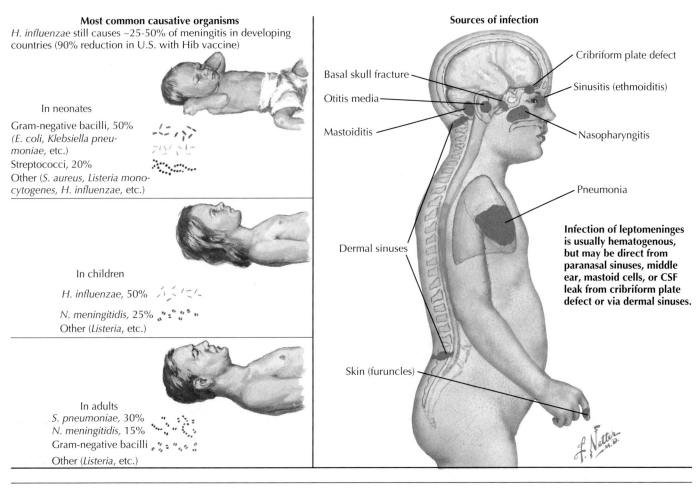

Most common causative organisms
H. influenzae still causes ~25-50% of meningitis in developing countries (90% reduction in U.S. with Hib vaccine)

In neonates
Gram-negative bacilli, 50%
(*E. coli, Klebsiella pneumoniae*, etc.)
Streptococci, 20%
Other (*S. aureus, Listeria monocytogenes, H. influenzae*, etc.)

In children
H. influenzae, 50%
N. meningitidis, 25%
Other (*Listeria*, etc.)

In adults
S. pneumoniae, 30%
N. meningitidis, 15%
Gram-negative bacilli
Other (*Listeria*, etc.)

Sources of infection
Cribriform plate defect
Basal skull fracture
Sinusitis (ethmoiditis)
Otitis media
Mastoiditis
Nasopharyngitis
Pneumonia
Dermal sinuses
Skin (furuncles)

Infection of leptomeninges is usually hematogenous, but may be direct from paranasal sinuses, middle ear, mastoid cells, or CSF leak from cribriform plate defect or via dermal sinuses.

Figure 92-1 *Bacterial meningitis.*

useful to draw a blood culture prior to the administration of antibiotics, especially if there may be a delay in performing the LP. A complete blood count (CBC) occasionally has an elevated WBC count. This is a nonspecific finding, and the remainder of the CBC is usually normal. The results of a basic metabolic panel is rarely abnormal, although some patients develop the syndrome of inappropriate antidiuretic hormone secretion and subsequently have hyponatremia. Inflammatory markers such as an erythrocyte sedimentation rate and C-reactive protein are

rarely helpful and do not reliably differentiate between bacterial meningitis and other causes of meningitis. If Lyme meningitis is suspected, tests for serologic evidence of Lyme exposure are useful as long as there is a confirmatory test included in the laboratory analysis.

MANAGEMENT AND THERAPY

Patients with bacterial meningitis can be critically ill and may require admission to an intensive care unit for management of their airway and circulation. In addition to respiratory and cardiovascular support, antibiotics are the most important intervention in the treatment of patients with bacterial meningitis. In patients in whom the risk of bacterial meningitis is high, antibiotics should not be withheld pending the results of diagnostic procedures or radiographic scans. Empiric antibiotic selection should be made based on local resistance patterns, and the final treatment decision should be made based on the CSF culture and sensitivity reports. In general, the combination of an intravenous (IV) third-generation cephalosporin such as ceftriaxone or cefotaxime plus vancomycin offers excellent activity against the most common pathogens. If gram-negative bacilli are seen on the CSF Gram stain, some experts recommend broader gram-negative coverage with meropenem and consideration of adding an aminoglycoside while awaiting the results

Kernig's sign. Patient supine, with hip flexed 90°. Knee cannot be fully extended.

Neck rigidity (Brudzinski's neck sign). Passive flexion of neck causes flexion of both legs and thighs.

Figure 92-2 *Kernig's sign and Brudzinski's neck sign.*

of the CSF culture. The recommended duration of therapy varies according to the causative pathogen. In general, *N. meningitidis* meningitis is treated for 7 days, Hib meningitis for 7 to 10 days, and pneumococcal meningitis for 14 days.

The treatment of enteroviral meningitis consists of supportive care of the patient. If HSV disease is suspected, IV acyclovir is the drug of choice and is administered in three doses of 20 mg/kg/m^2 per day for 3 weeks. For Lyme meningitis, the current recommendation is 14 to 28 days of ceftriaxone.

The role of dexamethasone in the treatment of children with bacterial meningitis continues to be controversial. Studies of patients with Hib meningitis found that children treated with dexamethasone had decreased morbidity and mortality. This finding has not been reproduced for other causes of bacterial meningitis. Randomized trials have found a suggestion that dexamethasone therapy 1 hour before antibiotic therapy is associated with less hearing loss in children with *S. pneumoniae* meningitis, but this finding did not reach statistical significance.

The most common sequela of bacterial meningitis is sensorineural hearing loss, and all children with meningitis are recommended to have a hearing test after completion of therapy. Most patients with enteroviral meningitis recover with no long-term sequelae. Neonates with HSV meningitis have high rate of morbidity and mortality, and older children with HSV meningitis often have long-term neurologic deficits.

FOCAL SUPPURATIVE INFECTIONS: BRAIN ABSCESS

Brain abscesses are focal infections of the cerebrum or cerebellum.

ETIOLOGY, EPIDEMIOLOGY, AND PATHOGENESIS

Many microbes can form a focal suppurative infection of the CNS, including fungi, parasites, and bacteria, with bacteria being most common. Bacterial brain abscesses are often polymicrobial, and the causative organisms vary by age and pathogenesis. Overall, streptococci are most common, followed by staphylococci and then gram-negative organisms.

Organisms gain access to the brain parenchyma via a number of different mechanisms. These include hematogenous seeding, direct extension from infections of the middle ear or sinuses, or by inoculation after a surgical procedure or penetrating trauma.

Neonates with no predisposing factors can develop brain abscesses after an episode of bacteremia. These infections are usually caused by Enterobacteriaceae such as *Escherichia coli* or *Citrobacter* spp. Infants with cyanotic congenital heart disease are at especially high risk of developing brain abscesses because part of their venous blood flow bypasses the lungs. Infected emboli in the venous system have direct entry into the arterial blood flow and from there can travel to the brain. One large case series of children with brain abscesses found that 25% of the patients had congenital heart disease as a risk factor. Another study estimated that up to 6% of people with cyanotic congenital heart disease develop a brain abscess over the course of their lives.

Box 92-2 Risk Factors and Organisms Associated with Brain Abscesses

Common Organisms
- *Streptococcus milleri*
- *Streptococcus pyogenes*
- *Staphylococcus aureus*
- Anaerobic streptococci
- Peptostreptococcus
- *Citrobacter* spp.
- *Escherichia coli*
- *Enterobacter* spp.
- *Aspergillus* spp.
- *Candida* spp.

Rare Organisms
- *Streptococcus agalactiae*
- Coagulase-negative staphylococci
- *Pseudomonas* spp.
- *Klebsiella* spp.
- *Haemophilus influenzae*
- *Nocardia* spp.

Common Risk Factors
- Cyanotic congenital heart disease
- Sinus or otic infection
- Immunosuppression (solid organ transplant, malignancy)

Rare Risk Factors
- Ventriculoperitoneal shunt
- Trauma
- Dental procedure
- Neurosurgical procedure

Older children are at risk for brain abscesses from direct extension of other infections, specifically sinusitis or otitis media with mastoiditis. Brain abscesses that arise secondary to these infections are often polymicrobial and may include both aerobic and anaerobic organisms. The most commonly isolated organism from these infections is *Streptococcus intermedius*, which is part of the *Streptococcus milleri* group. Other commonly isolated organisms include *Streptococcus viridans* and *Staphylococcus aureus*. Many additional pathogens have been reported as causative agents of brain abscesses (Box 92-2).

Recently, fungal brain infections have become more common in pediatric patients. Almost all patients have some type of immune dysfunction. Many of the patients are on immunosuppressive medications to prevent rejection of a solid organ transplant or are undergoing treatment of a malignancy and had long periods of neutropenia before development of the fungal infection. Primary immunodeficiencies or infection with HIV have not been reported as common risk factors for fungal brain abscesses in children.

CLINICAL PRESENTATION

Children with brain abscesses can have clinical presentation that is similar to patients with meningitis. They often present with fever and headache and may complain of nausea or vomiting. Sometimes they present to medical attention after a seizure or with focal neurologic abnormalities. If the abscess is in a location that affects CSF flow, leading to obstructive

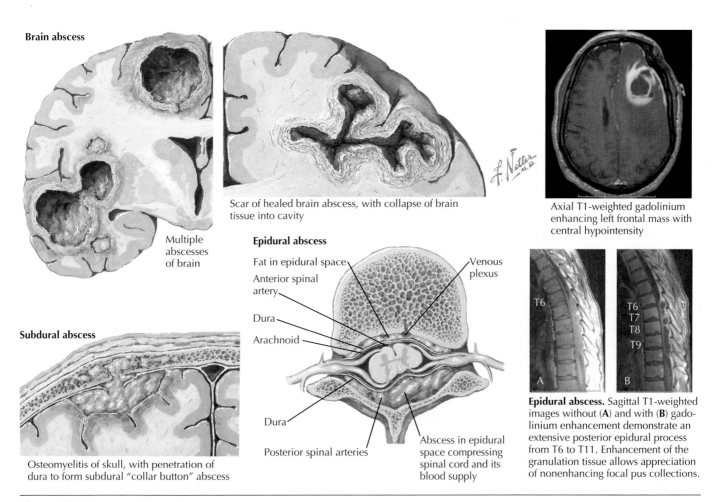

Brain abscess

Multiple abscesses of brain

Scar of healed brain abscess, with collapse of brain tissue into cavity

Axial T1-weighted gadolinium enhancing left frontal mass with central hypointensity

Subdural abscess

Osteomyelitis of skull, with penetration of dura to form subdural "collar button" abscess

Epidural abscess

Fat in epidural space
Anterior spinal artery
Dura
Arachnoid
Dura
Posterior spinal arteries
Venous plexus
Abscess in epidural space compressing spinal cord and its blood supply

Epidural abscess. Sagittal T1-weighted images without (**A**) and with (**B**) gadolinium enhancement demonstrate an extensive posterior epidural process from T6 to T11. Enhancement of the granulation tissue allows appreciation of nonenhancing focal pus collections.

Figure 92-3 *Parameningeal infections.*

hydrocephalus, patients can present with signs of increased ICP, including vital sign abnormalities (bradycardia, hypertension, and abnormal respirations, or Cushing's triad) or papilledema. The clinical presentation of patients with brain abscess differs from the presentation of patients with meningitis because it often lacks nuchal rigidity and Kernig's and Brudzinski's signs.

DIAGNOSTIC APPROACH

The most important diagnostic procedure is brain imaging with contrast, either a CT or MRI (Figure 92-3). The advantages of CT scans are that they are quicker than MRIs and usually do not require sedation for the patient. On CT scans, abscesses appear as rim-enhancing, space-occupying lesions, often with surrounding cerebral edema. After an abscess is found, the patient should be evaluated by a neurosurgeon for drainage of the abscess. Samples should be sent from the operating room to a microbiology laboratory for Gram stain and aerobic and anaerobic culture.

MANAGEMENT AND THERAPY

Surgery and antibiotics are the mainstays of therapy for brain abscesses. If a neurosurgeon is not immediately available,

antibiotics should not be held awaiting surgery for clinical specimens to be sent for culture. Empiric antibiotic therapy should be broad and include activity against anaerobes, streptococci, *S. aureus*, and gram-negative organisms. One possible regimen is vancomycin, a third-generation cephalosporin such as cefotaxime, and metronidazole. β-Lactam and β-lactamase inhibitor combinations or clindamycin should not be used because the β-lactamase inhibitors and clindamycin do not achieve adequate concentrations in the CNS. For a broader spectrum of gram-negative activity, carbapenems such as imipenem or meropenem can be used to replace the third-generation cephalosporin and metronidazole. If the patient shows signs of increased ICP, therapy to reduce this pressure may be necessary before drainage of the abscess.

Most of the time, cultures sent from the abscess reveal the causative organisms, but antibiotics given before the drainage can affect culture results. These infections usually require a prolonged course of IV antibiotics. The decision to stop antibiotics is guided by the patient's clinical response as well as the results of follow-up imaging. Long-term sequelae are difficult to predict and depend on a number of factors including patient comorbidities, location of the abscess, and clinical factors such as increased ICP, seizures, and number of neurosurgical procedures.

SUBDURAL EMPYEMA

Subdural empyema is an infection of the potential space between the dura mater and arachnoid membrane that can spread over the surface of the cerebral cortex.

ETIOLOGY, EPIDEMIOLOGY, AND PATHOGENESIS

Subdural empyema is most commonly associated with infection of the paranasal sinuses and mostly affects children in their second decade of life. It is the most common suppurative complication of sinusitis and affects boys more often than girls (the reported male:female ratio ranges from 1.3:1 to 4.5:1). It can occur via two mechanisms: either direct extension of the infection, usually from the frontal sinus, which passes through the dura into the subdural space, or via thrombophlebitis of the valveless diploic veins. Subdural empyema can also occur after penetrating trauma, after neurosurgery, or as a superinfection of subdural effusions after meningitis in infants.

The microbiology of subdural empyema is determined by the mechanism of the infection. Subdural empyemas which are a complication of paranasal sinusitis are most likely to grow *S. intermedius*. Often, these infections are polymicrobial and include anaerobes such as *Fusobacterium* or *Prevotella* spp. Some data suggest that these anaerobes increase the virulence of *S. intermedius*, which may explain the frequent polymicrobial nature of these infections. Other flora, which commonly cause bacterial sinusitis, including *S. pneumoniae*, *Moraxella catarrhalis*, and nontypable *H. influenzae*, are not common causes of subdural empyema. *S. aureus* is a common cause of subdural empyema after penetrating trauma or neurosurgery. Historically, Hib was a common cause of subdural empyema infecting subdural effusions complicating Hib meningitis, but since the introduction of the Hib vaccine, this entity is now rarely seen.

CLINICAL PRESENTATION

Patients with subdural empyema can present with a spectrum of symptoms. Patients may be asymptomatic; a subdural empyema can be an incidental finding in patients with bacterial sinusitis. The most frequent symptoms associated with subdural empyema are fever, headache, and vomiting. Because vomiting is an uncommon presenting feature of sinusitis, the combination of sinusitis, fever, and vomiting should raise concern for intracranial spread of the infection. Other presenting signs include focal neurologic deficits, seizures, and decreased sensorium. The severity of presentation is usually associated with the extent of the infection and the degree of elevated ICP.

DIAGNOSTIC APPROACH

The most important diagnostic procedure when subdural empyema is suspected is neuroimaging, preferably with an MRI with gadolinium. A CT with contrast may not identify a small subdural collection or may underestimate the extent of involvement of a subdural empyema. An MRI with contrast offers excellent visualization of the subdural space and allows the clinician to differentiate between blood and purulent fluid. It often

contains enough information about localization and the presence of loculations to allow neurosurgeons to decide whether a burr hole is adequate or whether a craniotomy is needed to drain the fluid.

Routine blood work, including CBCs and inflammatory markers, does not give any significant information to aid in the diagnosis of subdural empyema but may be important for overall management of the patient. If antibiotics have not been administered, it is useful to obtain a blood culture. Although bacteremia is uncommon in patients with subdural empyema, it occurs in some of the other processes that are part of the differential diagnosis.

If neuroimaging reveals subdural empyema or signs of elevated ICP or if there is concern about elevated ICP based on the clinical examination findings, an LP should not be performed until the elevated ICP is addressed. An LP is usually not diagnostic of subdural empyema because the infection is sequestered within part of the subdural space. Unlike meningitis, the pathogen does not freely circulate throughout the CSF. If an LP is performed, the CSF often has a mild pleocytosis, but the CSF culture rarely grows an organism.

MANAGEMENT AND THERAPY

After subdural empyema is diagnosed, the most important step in management is neurosurgical consultation. Most patients with this infection require either a burr hole or craniotomy, although there are reports of some patients with small subdural empyemas being managed with medical therapy alone. The fluid drained by the neurosurgeon should be sent for Gram stain, routine culture, and anaerobic culture.

Empiric antibiotic regimens for subdural empyema are the same as the regimens for brain abscesses and should include broad coverage of aerobic and anaerobic streptococci, other oropharyngeal anaerobes, and gram-negative organisms. Antibiotics should be given immediately and should not be delayed awaiting surgical intervention. Patients with subdural empyema require intensive care management even if they do not require surgery. Before surgery, they can have vital sign instability if there is significant elevation of ICP, and they can develop rapid changes in their neurologic function. Postoperatively, they require close monitoring of their cardiorespiratory and neurologic status. The duration of antibiotics depends on their clinical course but usually lasts at least 4 to 6 weeks. Many patients experience some long-term sequelae from these infections, but death is rare.

EPIDURAL ABSCESS

Epidural abscesses are collections of infected fluid that are located between the outermost layer of the meninges (the dura) and the bony structures protecting the CNS (the skull or vertebrae).

ETIOLOGY, EPIDEMIOLOGY, AND PATHOGENESIS

Epidural abscesses can occur either within the cranium or within the spinal canal (see Figure 92-3). The pathogenesis and infectious organisms associated with these infections vary according to the site of infection.

Overall, epidural abscesses are quite rare, and most clinical information about pediatric epidural abscesses consists of case reports and case series. Most intracranial epidural abscesses occur as a complication of sinusitis. The published case series have found an increased incidence during adolescence, which is thought to be attributable to the rapid growth of the sinuses during that time and the increased vascularity of the diploic veins during adolescence. These case series have also described a male predominance, although the etiology is unclear. The frontal sinuses are usually the primary site of infection. It has been hypothesized that epidural abscesses are seen more often in conjunction with frontal sinusitis because of a larger potential space between the frontal sinuses and the cranial vault compared with other locations, where the dura is more adherent to the cranium. Less commonly, epidural abscesses can occur as a complication of otitis media and mastoiditis.

The microbiology of epidural abscesses that are caused by sinusitis is similar to the microbiology of subdural empyema because they have the same primary source of infection. Organisms of the *S. milleri* group, including *S. intermedius*, are the most commonly identified pathogens. These infections can be polymicrobial and include anaerobic bacteria.

Spinal epidural abscesses are less common than intracranial epidural abscesses with an estimated incidence of 0.6 per 10,000 admissions in one large case series. In pediatric patients, the pathophysiology is usually hematogenous seeding of the epidural space with subsequent response by the immune system, leading to abscess formation. These abscesses can occur anywhere from the cervical spine down to the sacrum. Whereas most pediatric patients with spinal epidural abscesses do not have any comorbidities, the majority of adults who develop these infections have an underlying condition that puts them at risk. These conditions include particular disease states (diabetes mellitus, HIV infection), spinal abnormalities (spinal surgery, trauma, degenerative joint disease), or a source of infection (urinary tract infection, epidural anesthesia, IV drug use).

S. aureus is the most common pathogen associated with pediatric spinal epidural abscesses. Many times there is also evidence of osteomyelitis, discitis, or paraspinal pyomyositis. These infections are very rarely polymicrobial, and anaerobes have not been described as part of this syndrome. Other pathogens that have been reported to cause spinal epidural abscesses include *Pseudomonas aeruginosa*, *S. pneumoniae*, *Salmonella* spp. (in children with sickle cell disease), *E. coli*, *Fusobacterium* spp., and *S. viridans*. Children receiving chemotherapy for malignancies or with primary immunodeficiencies have been reported to have infections caused by unusual pathogens, including *Aspergillus flavus*, *Mycobacterium bovis*, and *Candida tropicalis*.

CLINICAL PRESENTATION

The clinical presentation of patients with epidural abscesses depends on the anatomic location of the infection. Patients with epidural abscesses arising from the frontal sinuses typically present with intermittent headaches, which can last for a few days to a few weeks. They may also have fevers, nausea, and vomiting. Occasionally, patients with these infections develop cerebritis and may develop personality changes or other neurologic symptoms. Epidural abscesses can also result from a complication of mastoiditis. In these situations, patients may present with headaches, nausea, and vomiting in addition to the signs and symptoms of mastoiditis. Finally, patients may have epidural abscesses along the spinal cord. The symptoms of this infection are attributable to inflammation of or mass effect on the spinal nerve roots arising in the affected area. Patients with cervical epidural abscesses may present with neck stiffness or focal arm pain or weakness. Patients with epidural abscesses in the lumbosacral region may present with back pain, gait abnormalities, changes in bowel or bladder function, or other symptoms relating to the lower extremities.

DIAGNOSTIC APPROACH

If an epidural abscess is suspected, the first diagnostic step is an MRI with gadolinium or a CT with contrast of the suspected area. Noncontrast studies are less useful because contrast improves the sensitivity of the imaging study and displays a better outline of the abscess. For spinal lesions, MRI is the preferred modality because of its superiority in identifying bone and soft tissue inflammation compared with CT. After an abscess has been identified, a neurosurgeon should be consulted to discuss drainage of the lesion. If sinusitis is also identified on the imaging study, an otolaryngologist should be consulted to discuss whether drainage of the sinuses would also be helpful. Some spinal epidural abscesses may be drained by an interventional radiologist under ultrasound or CT guidance. Occasionally, small abscesses do not require drainage and can be treated with antibiotics alone. If an abscess is drained, samples should be sent for Gram stain and aerobic and anaerobic culture.

MANAGEMENT AND THERAPY

For small epidural abscesses or those that are difficult to approach surgically, medical therapy with antibiotics is the initial step in management. The location of the infection guides empiric antibiotic therapy. The microbiology of epidural abscesses arising from sinusitis or mastoiditis is similar to the microbiology of subdural empyemas and brain abscesses. The combination of a third-generation cephalosporin, vancomycin, and metronidazole offers broad activity with good CNS penetration in the event that there is a subdural component to the infection. Antibiotic therapy can be narrowed based on the results of cultures obtained from the epidural collection. These infections are usually treated for a minimum of 3 weeks, but the total duration depends on the size of the abscess, whether it was drained, and the patient's clinical response. In most cases, there are no long-term sequelae associated with these infections, but the risk of morbidity is increased if there is associated subdural empyema or if the patient presented with focal neurologic signs.

Empiric antibiotic selection for patients with spinal epidural abscesses without any underlying conditions (sickle cell disease, immunodeficiency, or malignancy) should focus on *S. aureus*. Recently, community-acquired methicillin-resistant *S. aureus* (CA-MRSA) has become a common pediatric pathogen, so this must be taken into account when deciding on empiric antibiotics. Clindamycin has good activity against most CA-MRSA isolates and is a good empiric choice. In patients with predisposing conditions, empiric coverage may need to be broader and include gram-negative organisms. The only data about duration of therapy are cases series, and most authors recommend at least 6 weeks of therapy. Factors to take into consideration include the size of the abscess, whether it was drained, whether the patient has a predisposing medication condition, and the patient's response to therapy. Most patients recover fully unless they had focal neurologic findings at the time of presentation.

OTHER INFECTIONS—TUBERCULOSIS MENINGITIS

Meningitis caused by *Mycobacterium tuberculosis* is very uncommon in the developed world but has become more common in areas with a high prevalence of HIV infection (Figure 92-4). It usually occurs in children younger than 2 years of age with tuberculosis (TB) because they are at higher risk of developing extrapulmonary disease (lymphadenitis, osteomyelitis, meningitis). In most cases, the child has a household contact or is in close contact with a caregiver who has active pulmonary TB, which is often undiagnosed.

Unlike bacterial meningitis, TB meningitis (TBM) is often indolent in nature, and most children present with advanced disease. TBM is classified in three stages. Symptoms in stage 1 include irritability, anorexia, fever, personality changes, and listlessness. Stage 2 is characterized by signs of increased ICP and cerebral damage. This can progress to stage 3 disease, which includes coma, irregular pulse and respirations, and rising fever.

Children with suspected TBM should be tested for HIV if their HIV status is unknown. In addition, they should have a tuberculin skin test placed and a chest radiograph. The interpretation of the skin test will depend on the HIV status, age, and nutritional status of the patient. In general, 50% of patients who are HIV positive and have TBM will have a positive skin test result. Chest radiographs are helpful if the results are abnormal, but a normal result does not exclude extrapulmonary TB disease.

If the patient is clinically stable, an LP should be performed. CSF should be sent for the usual tests (gram stain, cell count, protein, glucose, and culture). In addition, CSF should be sent for an acid-fast bacillus (AFB) smear and culture. The sensitivity of the AFB smear can be increased by sending a large volume of CSF (5-10 mL) and centrifuging the sample before examination. The CSF of most patients with TBM will have a lymphocytic pleocytosis with elevated protein and low glucose level. The AFB smear result is often negative, and the culture can take weeks to grow.

TB with involvement of basal cistern with vasculitis and ischemia

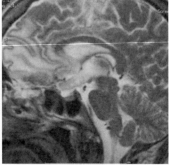

Midsagittal T2-weighted image shows increased T2 signal within ischemic frontal lobe.

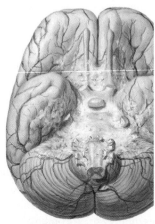

Tuberculous basilar meningitis

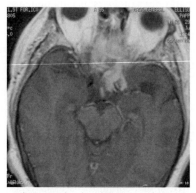

Axial T1-weighted gadolinium-enhanced image with enhancing mass at left basal cisterns and subfrontal region.

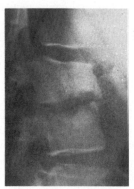

X-ray film: destruction of disk space and adjacent end plates of vertebrae

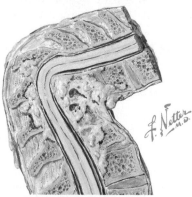

Tuberculosis of spine (Pott's disease) with marked kyphosis

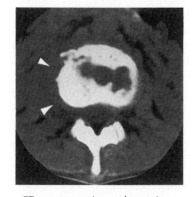

CT scan: paraspinous abscess in addition to bony destruction

Figure 92-4 *Tuberculosis of the brain and spine.*

Management of patients with TBM is outside of the scope of this chapter. Important considerations include the HIV status of the patient and the CD4 count, any other comorbid conditions and medication necessary to treat those conditions, and the sensitivity of the infecting organism. Initial TBM treatment includes four or five drugs, and treatment requires months of medication. TBM is frequently associated with vasculitis, which can lead to strokes. Because of this, many children have permanent disabilities as a consequence of this infection. In addition to meningitis, TB can also cause tuberculomas (tumorlike mass caused by enlargement of a caseous tubercle) and spinal osteomyelitis (Pott's disease).

SUGGESTED READINGS

Adame N, Hedlund G, Byington CL: Sinogenic intracranial empyema in children, *Pediatrics* 116(3):e461-e467, 2005.

Auletta JJ, John CC: Spinal epidural abscesses in children: a 15-year experience and review of the literature, *Clin Infect Dis* 32(1):9-16, 2001.

Bair-Merritt MH, Chung C, Collier A: Spinal epidural abscess in a young child, *Pediatrics* 106(3):E39, 2000.

Bair-Merritt MH, Shah SS, Zaoutis TE, et al: Suppurative intracranial complications of sinusitis in previously healthy children, *Pediatr Infect Dis J* 24(4):384-386, 2005.

Bockova J, Rigamonti, D: Intracranial empyema, *Pediatr Infect Dis J* 19(8):735-737, 2000.

Chavez-Bueno S, McCracken GH Jr: Bacterial meningitis in children, *Pediatr Clin North Am* 52(3):795-810, vii, 2005.

Darouiche RO: Spinal epidural abscess, *N Engl J Med* 355(19):2012-2020, 2006.

de Gans J, van de Beek D: Dexamethasone in adults with bacterial meningitis, *N Engl J Med* 347(20):1549-1556, 2002.

Nguyen TH, Tran TH, Thwaites G, et al: Dexamethasone in Vietnamese adolescents and adults with bacterial meningitis, *N Engl J Med* 357(24):2431-2440, 2007.

Osborn MK, Steinberg JP: Subdural empyema and other suppurative complications of paranasal sinusitis, *Lancet Infect Dis* 7(1):62-67, 2007.

Thwaites GE, Tran TH: Tuberculous meningitis: many questions, too few answers, *Lancet Neurol* 4(3):160-170, 2005.

Tunkel AR, Hartman BJ, Kaplan SL, et al: Practice guidelines for the management of bacterial meningitis, *Clin Infect Dis* 39(9):1267-1284, 2004.

Infections of the Urinary Tract

Eric D. Shelov

93

For patients from infancy to adolescence, infections of the urinary tract are an important topic for pediatric clinicians. As a group, they are the most frequent serious bacterial infections in childhood, with an incidence as high as 20% in certain age groups presenting with a fever. Infection types include those of the lower tract and bladder and those that ascend to the upper tract involving the renal parenchyma (pyelonephritis). Acutely, management of these infections ranges from routine outpatient care to intensive care and hemodialysis, and the long-term sequelae of upper urinary tract infections (UTIs) can involve renal scarring and chronic hypertension. This chapter discusses the etiology, pathogenesis, and risk factors for these infections, the clinical approach to their diagnosis and management, and current recommendations and recent controversies in the management and prevention of recurrent infections.

ETIOLOGY AND PATHOGENESIS

Although some of the mechanisms are unclear, certain populations of children are at higher risk for UTIs. In the neonatal period, uncircumcised boys are at the highest risk of infection followed by girls and circumcised boys. Uncircumcised neonates presenting with fever have an incidence of approximately 20% versus 2% for circumcised boys. Two theories that potentially explain this discrepancy are the unkeratinized skin of the uncircumcised foreskin being more prone to bacterial invasion and relative tightness of the infant foreskin causing possible partial obstruction of the urethral meatus. It should be noted, however, that despite the elevated risk, UTIs are still a rare event in uncircumcised boys. Outside the neonatal period, girls are at higher risk for infection than boys, and the incidence decreases in both sexes with age. Other important host risk factors include familial predisposition, race, sexual activity, underlying anatomy, urinary function, and manipulation of the urinary tract (most commonly in the form of bladder catheterization). Two problems warranting further discussion are dysfunctional elimination syndrome (DES) and vesicoureteral reflux (VUR), the retrograde passage of urine from the bladder into the upper urinary tract.

DES is a very common and often underdiagnosed problem affecting the otherwise healthy pediatric population. It is characterized by abnormal voiding or stooling patterns, incontinence, and observed withholding maneuvers. In school-aged children, evidence suggests that DES plays a significant role in UTIs and the persistence of VUR. VUR is the most common urologic abnormality in children, found in 1% of the population and up to 40% of children with febrile UTIs. VUR is graded 1 to 5 with 95% grade 3 or better, and the majority of mild cases self-resolving by age 1 year. Children with VUR are at increased risk for recurrent UTIs. Furthermore, VUR may also increase the risk of pyelonephritis renal scarring, although evidence has not shown a clear correlation.

Infections of the urinary tract begin with ascension of flora that transiently colonize the lower urinary tract. The most common organism responsible for infection is the enteric gram-negative organism *Escherichia coli*. Other gram-negative organisms include *Klebsiella*, *Proteus*, *Citrobacter*, and *Enterobacter* spp. Gram-positive infections by enterococcus, *Staphylococcus saprophyticus*, and rarely *Staphylococcus aureus* are also known to occur. For infection to take place, the organisms must not only be present in the urinary tract but also needs to attach, adhere to, and invade the mucosa and epithelium. The bacteria are then able to ascend via the epithelial cells to the bladder and kidney (Figure 93-1). It is thought that genetically determined variation in the host's defense against this process may explain the familial association of UTIs among first-degree relatives.

CLINICAL PRESENTATION

UTIs can present in a variety of ways with varying differentials depending on the age of the patient. In general, the older the patient, the more specific the presentation will be. In infants and small children (younger than 2 years of age), UTIs may only present with fever. Certainly, fever without a clear source should prompt the clinician to consider a UTI, but even in infants with another potential source, evaluation of the urine may still be prudent. Other symptoms may include irritability, poor feeding, or failure to thrive. Of note, parental report of "foul-smelling urine" has not been shown to correlate with UTIs. The differential diagnosis, as with all infants with fever and an unknown source, is extensive, but the clinician should primarily be concerned about occult bacteremia, sepsis, and viral infections. Other aspects of the history that may be helpful are the degree and duration of the fever and any history of UTIs in the patient or family.

In older children, presentation is more similar to that of the adult. Symptoms may include fever, abdominal pain, urinary symptoms (dysuria, urgency, incontinence, hematuria, frequency), back pain, or vomiting. The differential diagnosis can vary greatly depending on the presentation. For the urinary symptoms, the differential diagnosis includes urinary calculi, urethritis (chemical, sexually transmitted infection), vaginal foreign body, and DES. The differential for fever and abdominal pain in older children includes group A streptococcus infections, Kawasaki's disease, appendicitis, and gastroenteritis, the first three of which may also present with pyuria. In the patient's history, it is also important to note any history of: UTIs in the patient or family, VUR or DES, constipation, or poor growth.

On physical examination of an infant or child with suspected UTI, it is important to note the degree of fever (if present) and any signs of cardiovascular instability that would reflect severe illness. Other findings on examination, more common in older patients, may include suprapubic or costovertebral tenderness. A complete abdominal examination should be performed to assess for any abdominal masses or abnormal distension of the bladder. A genital examination should look for any signs of

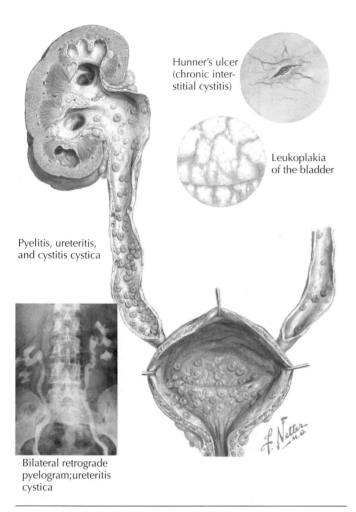

Hunner's ulcer (chronic interstitial cystitis)

Leukoplakia of the bladder

Pyelitis, ureteritis, and cystitis cystica

Bilateral retrograde pyelogram;ureteritis cystica

Figure 93-1 *Cystitis.*

urethritis or vulvovaginitis and for any anatomic abnormalities. If the patient is febrile, attention should also be paid to other potential sources of fever (Figure 93-2).

EVALUATION AND MANAGEMENT
(TABLE 93-1)

Laboratory Evaluation

The appropriate management of a patient with UTI can vary significantly depending on the severity of illness. Those with mild to moderate illness can be effectively managed as outpatients, but those with severe illness may require inpatient or even intensive care and dialysis. Because of the often nonspecific nature of presentation, laboratory analysis of the urine is essential to confirm the diagnosis in all settings. Two important steps for the clinician as they evaluate the patient are (1) whether to obtain a urine sample and (2) how best to do so.

The decision to obtain a urine sample can be very simple, as with the febrile neonate, or in the cases of older children, it can be more complex. Important factors to consider for the clinician evaluating 3- to 24-month-old children are:

- History of a UTI
- Fever: greater than 39°C for longer than 24 hours or without a clear source
- Concerning findings on examination (suprapubic tenderness)
- Ill appearance
- Nonblack race

If one of these risk factors is present for girls and uncircumcised boys or two are present for circumcised boys, it is recommended to obtain a urine sample for urinalysis and culture. One should also obtain samples for girls and uncircumcised boys older than

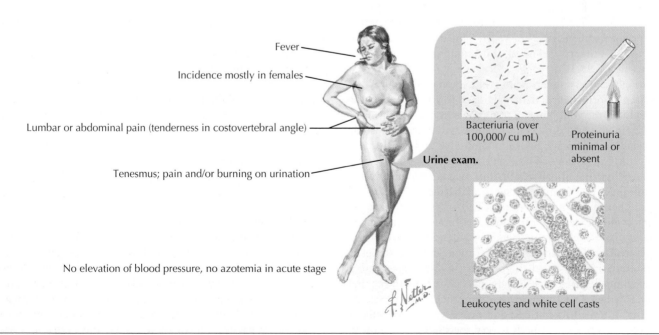

Fever

Incidence mostly in females

Lumbar or abdominal pain (tenderness in costovertebral angle)

Tenesmus; pain and/or burning on urination

No elevation of blood pressure, no azotemia in acute stage

Urine exam.

Bacteriuria (over 100,000/ cu mL)

Proteinuria minimal or absent

Leukocytes and white cell casts

Figure 93-2 *Common clinical and laboratory features of acute pyelonephritis.*

Table 93-1 Summary of Treatment and Workup of Patients at Risk for Urinary Tract Infection

At Risk for UTI?	Obtain Urine? (3-24 months)	Indications for Admission	Routine Workup	Prophylaxis
Uncircumcised male infant DES Prior urine infections VUR or abnormal anatomy Family history, race, sexual activity	History of UTI Fever: >39°C, >24 h or without a clear source Concerning findings on examination (suprapubic tenderness) Ill appearance Nonblack race Circumcised boys: ≥2 (or 1+ suprapubic tenderness) Girls and uncircumcised boys: ≥1 present	Age younger than 2 mo Underlying medical problems Vomiting or unable to tolerate oral medications and maintain hydration Inadequate outpatient follow-up Failed outpatient therapy	UA, culture: all UTI Renal ultrasonography* and VCUG: girls younger than 3 y with first UTI Boys with a first UTI All children with febrile UTI Children with recurrent UTI First UTI with any family history of renal disease	Post-UTI treatment while VCUG results are pending Grades 1-4 reflux demonstrated on VCUG

*Unless documented as normal on prenatal ultrasound done after 30 weeks of gestation.
 DES, dysfunctional elimination syndrome; UA, urinalysis; UTI, urinary tract infection; VCUG, voiding cystourethrography; VUR, vesicoureteral reflux.

2 years of age with any concerning symptom (abdominal pain, back pain, dysuria, frequency, high fever) and circumcised boys older than 2 years with multiple symptoms.

After it has been decided to obtain urine, the clinician must then determine how best to obtain it. For an infant, urine can be obtained by bag specimen, urethral catheterization, and suprapubic aspiration. The bag specimen is the most convenient but is of limited utility and generally not recommended because of the high probability of contamination from skin flora. It cannot be used for culture, and urinalysis is only useful if results are negative. Care must be taken, however, to analyze the sample promptly after voiding because the false results increase as the urine stagnates. Catheterized specimen is the primary means of obtaining urine in the infant for urine culture or enhanced urinalysis. Suprapubic aspiration can also be performed if catheterization is repeatedly unsuccessful or contraindicated, which despite its invasive nature is very well tolerated when performed correctly. For toilet-trained children, a clean catch is the primary means of collection for urinalysis and culture (Figure 93-3).

A urinalysis is a relatively rapid test that can give the provider important information and help initiate treatment while the urine culture, the gold standard test, is performed. The urinalysis exists in several forms. The simplest is the urine dipstick, which has the advantage of being affordable and can be performed in virtually any clinical setting, but it may miss some cases of infection. A urinalysis with microscopic examination can more accurately detect the presence of bacteria, white blood cells, and hematuria. An enhanced urinalysis, available in larger hospitals and academic institutions, examines uncentrifuged specimens and adds Gram staining and a hemocytometer. A positive urine dipstick result can show the presence of leukocyte esterase (higher sensitivity) or nitrites (higher specificity), the centrifuged specimen can show pyuria or bacteriuria, and the uncentrifuged specimen gives a more quantitative analysis of pyuria. Although bacteriuria and pyuria can occur without infection, the presence of both is very specific for infection in the urine.

The gold standard for diagnosis is the urine culture, which not only makes the diagnosis but also helps to guide antimicrobial management. Growth criteria for definite infection are different depending on the means of collection, with any growth significant for a suprapubic aspirate and >50,000 or >100,000 colonies for a catheterization and clean catch, respectively. Although the current American Academy of Pediatrics guidelines recognize 10,000 colonies from a catheterization specimen as significant, recent evidence suggests the 10,000 to 50,000 range be classified as indeterminate and a repeat specimen be obtained. When empiric coverage has already been initiated, however, this may not be practical, and the decision to treat will likely incorporate other factors (clinical presentation, positive or negative urinalysis). In the majority of cases, any growth of nonpathogens or mixed flora indicates contamination and the need for a new specimen (Figure 93-4).

Blood tests are usually not indicated in routine infections of the urinary tract. A blood culture is of little utility because the urine is the source of the infection, and the presence of bacteremia does not alter the course of treatment. Markers of inflammation, such as a C-reactive protein, will certainly be elevated during a UTI, but their utility in differentiating between upper tract (pyelonephritis) and lower tract infection is yet to be supported by evidence. Electrolytes are not routinely drawn if the patient does not have any clinical signs of renal failure (anuria, edema, hypertension).

Hospital Admission

The clinician must also decide if admission to the hospital is necessary. Previously, all young children with pyelonephritis or febrile UTIs were hospitalized. Recent evidence, however, suggests the equal efficacy of oral third-generation cephalosporins compared with their parenteral counterparts. With good outpatient follow-up and hydration, therefore, outpatient management upper UTIs is reasonable. Along with severe illness (urosepsis, renal failure), there are other indications for inpatient care, including:

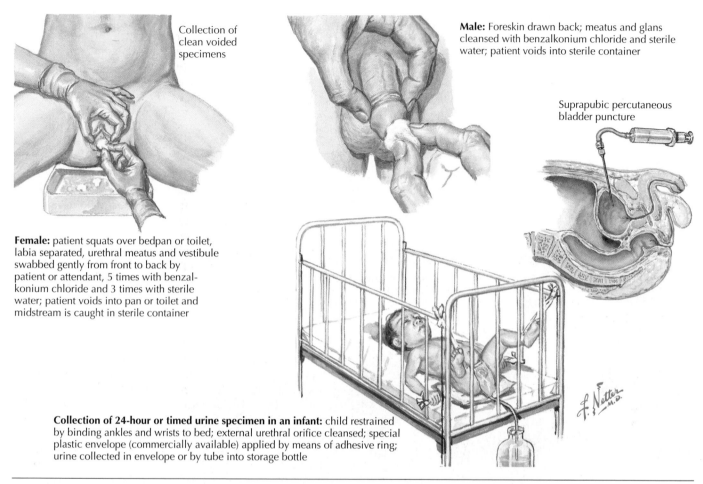

Collection of clean voided specimens

Male: Foreskin drawn back; meatus and glans cleansed with benzalkonium chloride and sterile water; patient voids into sterile container

Suprapubic percutaneous bladder puncture

Female: patient squats over bedpan or toilet, labia separated, urethral meatus and vestibule swabbed gently from front to back by patient or attendant, 5 times with benzalkonium chloride and 3 times with sterile water; patient voids into pan or toilet and midstream is caught in sterile container

Collection of 24-hour or timed urine specimen in an infant: child restrained by binding ankles and wrists to bed; external urethral orifice cleansed; special plastic envelope (commercially available) applied by means of adhesive ring; urine collected in envelope or by tube into storage bottle

Figure 93-3 *Collection of urine specimens.*

- Age younger than 2 months
- Patients with underlying medical problems that may complicate management
- Patients with vomiting or who are unable to tolerate oral medications and maintain hydration
- Patients with inadequate outpatient follow-up
- Patients who have failed outpatient therapy

Antimicrobials

It is important to begin therapy promptly in UTIs because delays in treatment can lead to complications both in the acute illness (pyelonephritis, renal abscess) and chronic sequelae (renal scarring, hypertension). When choosing empiric therapy, the clinician should consider the severity of illness, any history of prior UTIs, and the local patterns of resistance. For empiric coverage while awaiting culture results, the primary organism to consider is *E. coli*, although in certain circumstances (e.g., history of catheterization or manipulation), enterococcus should be covered as well. For routine outpatient care, amoxicillin is no longer adequate for coverage of *E. coli*, and rates of resistance to amoxicillin–clavulanate, first-generation cephalosporins, and trimethoprim–sulfamethoxazole (TMP-SMX) are increasing such that a clinician may not feel comfortable with these agents as well. Resistance patterns will dictate the empiric choice of

antibiotics. Empiric therapy may be initiated with a third-generation cephalosporin such as cefixime, 8 mg/kg given once daily as a reasonable alternative. Note that this does not provide adequate coverage for enterococcus, so if this organism is of concern, amoxicillin should be added.

Inpatient management can be initiated with a third-generation cephalosporin such as cefotaxime, although the clinician also has the option of gentamicin, which is acceptable coverage for *E coli*. Again, neither provides adequate coverage for enterococcus, so ampicillin should be added in those cases, which many providers choose to do for all cases when hospital admission is indicated. The duration of treatment is 10 days for children younger than 2 years of age or older children with febrile UTI; for older afebrile children, a shorter course of 5 to 7 days is acceptable. If imaging studies are to be performed, it is also recommended that children begin prophylactic antibiotics until the results are available.

Imaging

Three modalities of imaging are available to the clinician in the evaluation of UTIs: voiding cystourethrography (VCUG), renal ultrasound, and renal scintigraphy (DMSA [dimercaptosuccinic acid] scan). Intravenous pyelography (IVP) is rarely used in the pediatric population and is not discussed here. Overall, the goals

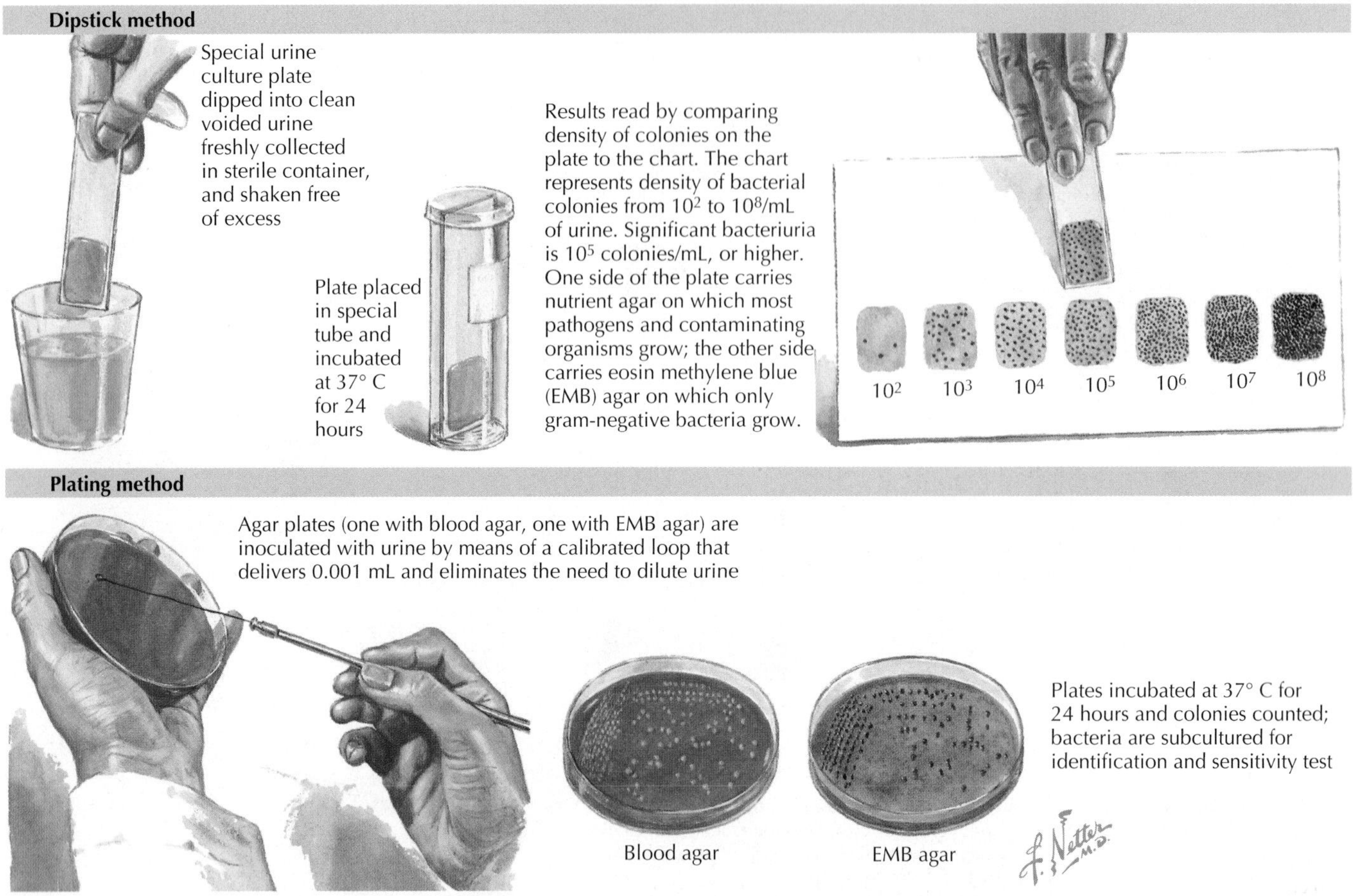

Dipstick method

Special urine culture plate dipped into clean voided urine freshly collected in sterile container, and shaken free of excess

Plate placed in special tube and incubated at 37° C for 24 hours

Results read by comparing density of colonies on the plate to the chart. The chart represents density of bacterial colonies from 10^2 to 10^8/mL of urine. Significant bacteriuria is 10^5 colonies/mL, or higher. One side of the plate carries nutrient agar on which most pathogens and contaminating organisms grow; the other side carries eosin methylene blue (EMB) agar on which only gram-negative bacteria grow.

10^2 10^3 10^4 10^5 10^6 10^7 10^8

Plating method

Agar plates (one with blood agar, one with EMB agar) are inoculated with urine by means of a calibrated loop that delivers 0.001 mL and eliminates the need to dilute urine

Plates incubated at 37° C for 24 hours and colonies counted; bacteria are subcultured for identification and sensitivity test

Blood agar   EMB agar

Figure 93-4 *Bacteriologic examination of urine.*

of these studies are to identify any anatomic abnormalities that may predispose the patient to recurrent infections, evaluate for complications such as renal abscess or lobar nephronia (Figure 93-5), and look for evidence of renal scarring. VCUG, which involves catheterization and subsequent imaging of instilled dye during voiding, is an excellent test to evaluate for the presence and degree of VUR. Renal ultrasound can identify certain anatomic anomalies (e.g., ureteral dilatation, duplication), is noninvasive, and has the benefit of no radiation exposure. It is not able to identify renal scarring or VUR. Current recommendations are for these two studies to be performed in:

- Girls younger than 3 years of age with a first UTI
- Boys of any age with a first UTI
- Children of any age with a febrile UTI
- Children with recurrent UTI
- First UTI in a child of any age with any family history of renal disease

If the patient has required hospitalization, it is usually routine to complete these studies before discharge. Of note, if the patient had normal prenatal ultrasound results after 30 weeks of gestation, it does not need to be repeated, but particularly in the inpatient setting, these results may not be available, and repetition may be necessary.

DMSA scanning is used to detect acute pyelonephritis and renal scarring. It is not routinely recommended for UTIs because children with febrile UTIs are often presumed to have pyelonephritis, and treatment would not change with a positive study result. Times when it may be useful are when evaluating children with recurrent UTIs and possible renal damage or in cases where urine studies have been equivocal.

FUTURE DIRECTIONS

Patients with VUR have been treated both medically and surgically, with the goal of preventing progressive renal damage. Grades 1 to 3 usually resolve spontaneously, but grades 4 to 5 are more likely to need definitive correction, such as surgical ureteral reimplantation. Current recommendations for young children with mild to moderate reflux demonstrated on VCUG are to begin prophylactic antimicrobials, usually TMP-SMX or nitrofurantoin at half dose given daily until the VUR resolves. This approach has been called into question in recent years because of the significant rates of febrile UTIs and renal scarring in patients on prophylaxis. Although there has been no large experimental trial comparing the long-term efficacy of this approach, several multicenter studies are underway and will hopefully provide more guidance for future clinicians.

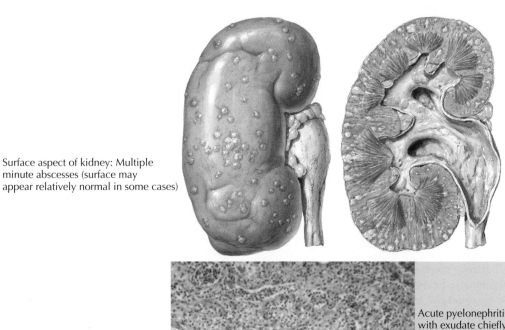

Surface aspect of kidney: Multiple
minute abscesses (surface may
appear relatively normal in some cases)

Cut section: Radiating yellowish gray
streaks in pyramids and abscesses in
cortex; moderate hydronephrosis
with infection; blunting of calyces
(ascending infection)

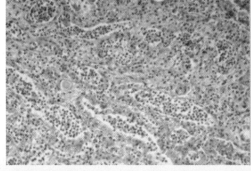

Acute pyelonephritis
with exudate chiefly
of polymorpho-
nuclear leukocytes
in interstitium and
collecting tubules

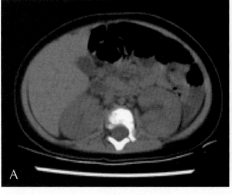
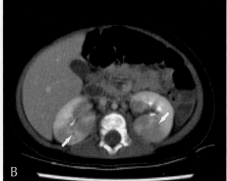

Characteristic precontrast (A)
and contrast-enhanced (B) CT
scans for an 8-month-old patient
who had acute lobar nephronia
and presented with severe
bilateral nephromegaly but
without a focal mass sono-
graphically. No attenuation
area is seen in the kidney
before enhancement. (*From
Cheng CH, Tsau YK, Lin
TY: Effective duration of antimicrobial therapy for the treatment of acute lobar nephronia.
Pediatrics 2006: 117:e84-e89.*)

Figure 93-5 *Acute pyelonephritis and sequelae: pathology.*

SUGGESTED READINGS

Fleisher GR, Ludwig S, Henretig FM, eds. *Textbook of Pediatric Emergency Medicine*, 5th ed, Philadelphia, 2005, Lippincott Williams & Wilkins.

Hodson EM, Willis NS, Craig JC: Antibiotics for acute pyelonephritis in children, *Cochrane Database Syst Rev* 4:CD003772, 2007.

Keren R, Chan E: A meta-analysis of randomized, controlled trials comparing short- and long-course antibiotic therapy for urinary tract infections in children, *Pediatrics* 109(5):E70-0, 2002.

Montini G, Zucchetta P, Tomasi L, et al: Value of imaging studies after a first febrile urinary tract infection in young children: data from Italian Renal Infection Study 1, *Pediatrics* 123(2):e239-e246, 2009.

Pennesi M, Travan L, Peratoner L, et al: Is antibiotic prophylaxis in children with vesicoureteral reflux effective in preventing pyelonephritis and renal scars? A randomized, controlled trial, *Pediatrics* 121(6):e1489-e1494, 2008.

Shaikh N, Morone NE, Lopez J, et al: Does this child have a urinary tract infection? *JAMA* 298(24):2895-2904, 2007.

Zaoutis B, Chiang W: *Comprehensive Pediatric Hospital Medicine*, Philadelphia, 2007, Saunders.

Infections of the Cardiovascular System

94

Deborah Whitney

INFECTIVE ENDOCARDITIS

Infective endocarditis (IE) is an infection of the endocardium, most commonly producing vegetations on heart valves, but also involving perivalvular structures and mural endocardium. Incidence studies, mainly in adults, report 1.4 to 6.2 cases per 100,000 patient years. It is more rare in children, primarily affecting children with predisposing congenital heart lesions and indwelling catheters. Previously, IE mainly affected individuals with abnormal heart valves from rheumatic heart disease, but since the advent of antibiotics for treatment of streptococcal infections, this demographic is extremely rare in industrialized countries. The overall incidence of IE has not changed over the past several decades, but the demographics have. It is increasingly a disease of elderly individuals with degenerative valve sclerosis, intravenous (IV) drug users, patients with intravascular devices, patients on hemodialysis, and patients undergoing invasive procedures at risk for bacteremia.

PATHOGENESIS

Underlying endothelial injury combined with bacteremia leads to the development of vegetations. Heart lesions with high-velocity jets predispose to endothelial injury. The resulting platelet–fibrin coagulum creates a rich environment for the deposition of bacteria and the growth of a vegetation. The bacteria often become fully enveloped by fibrin, allowing the pathogens to evade the host defenses (Figure 94-1). Congenital heart lesions most at risk include unrepaired cyanotic heart disease (including palliative shunts and conduits), any repaired congenital heart defect with prosthetic material or device in the first 6 months after the procedure, and repaired heart defects with residual defects at the site or adjacent to the site of the prosthesis.

Procedures at highest risk for bacteremia involve manipulation of gingival tissue or perforation of oral mucosa. Frequent exposures to random bacteremia from daily activities such as brushing teeth and chewing are more likely to cause endocarditis than are medical procedures. Intravascular catheters also predispose patients to bacteremia. Bacterial colonization of the catheter may prolong periods of bacteremia and creates a risk factor for IE. Nosocomial infections are on the rise. This is troubling because nosocomial infections frequently affect patients without underlying heart conditions, the organisms tend to be more resistant, and there is a high case fatality rate.

The bacteria implicated in IE tend to be those with greatest ability to adhere to damaged tissue. *Staphylococcus* and *Streptococcus* spp. have certain surface adhesins, which facilitate attachment to the endocardium. *Staphylococcus aureus* is the most common pathogen in IE, accounting for more than 50% of cases, especially in those with indwelling catheters, prosthetic

valves, and IV drug use. *Staphylococcus epidermidis*, oral streptococci, and enterococci are also common. In cases of culture-negative endocarditis, the HACEK organisms (a group of fastidious, oral gram-negative bacilli including *Haemophilus* spp., *Actinobacillus actinomycetemcomitans*, *Cardiobacterium hominis*, *Eikenella corrodens*, and *Kingella kingae*) along with *Brucella* spp. and fungus must be considered.

CLINICAL PRESENTATION

Symptoms of IE range from being asymptomatic, to congestive heart failure, to end-organ involvement with septic emboli. History taking should focus on fever, predisposing heart conditions, recent procedures at risk for bacteremia, the existence of indwelling catheters, and symptoms from end-organ involvement. The organs most commonly involved with septic emboli from left-sided IE include the central nervous system, eyes, kidneys, spleen, and skin. Septic pulmonary emboli are seen in cases of right-sided IE. Neurologic complications, which can occur in up to 33% of cases, include stroke, hemorrhage, seizure, abscess, and meningoencephalitis. The physical examination should include a thorough cardiac examination and a search for splenomegaly and for emboli of the fundus, conjunctiva, skin, and digits. Cardiac findings that are most likely to be present include new regurgitant murmurs and signs of congestive heart failure. Physical examination findings that support the diagnosis of IE but are not diagnostic include splinter hemorrhages, Janeway's lesions, Osler's nodes, and Roth's spots (Figure 94-2). These peripheral stigmata of IE are less common in acute IE because patients often present at an earlier stage of disease than those with subacute IE. IE remains a disease with high morbidity and mortality. Cardiac complications occur in up to 30% to 50% of cases. Heart failure is the most common complication and the leading cause of death.

EVALUATION AND MANAGEMENT

The Duke classification remains the most reliable way to diagnose IE (Box 94-1). A definitive diagnosis of IE requires direct histologic evidence of IE, culture of specimens from surgery or autopsy, two major criteria, one major criteria and three minor criteria, or five minor criteria. Blood culture results may be negative in up to 15% of cases. The most common reason for a negative culture result is pretreatment with antibiotics, but one must also consider organisms that are difficult to isolate such as nutritionally variant streptococci, HACEK organisms, fungi, and intracellular bacteria (*Coxiella burnetii*, *Bartonella* spp., *Chlamydia* spp., and *Tropheryma whippelii*). If blood culture results are negative but clinical suspicion remains high, specific culture media or adsorbent resins may be used to isolate these organisms. Cultures should be maintained for up to 2 weeks to

Early lesions

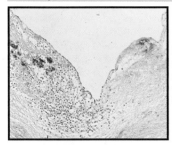

Deposit of platelets and organisms (stained dark), edema, and leukocytic infiltration in very early bacterial endocarditis of aortic valve

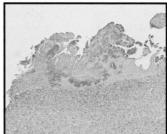

Development of vegetations containing clumps of bacteria on tricuspid valve

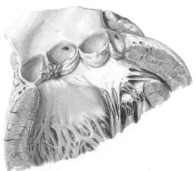

Early vegetations of bacterial endocarditis on bicuspid aortic valve

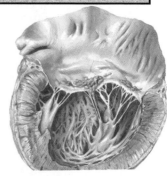

Early vegetations of bacterial endocarditis at contact line of mitral valve

Advanced lesions

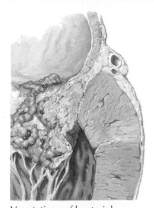

Vegetations of bacterial endocarditis on under-aspect as well as on atrial surface of mitral valve

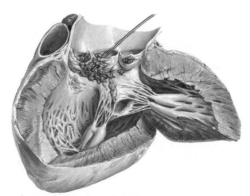

Advanced bacterial endocarditis of aortic valve: perforation of cusp; extension to anterior cusp of mitral valve and chordae tendineae: "jet lesion" on septal wall

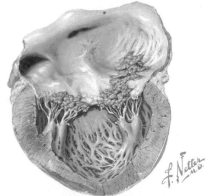

Advanced lesion of mitral valve: vegetations extending onto chordae tendineae with rupture of two chordae; also extension to atrial wall and contact lesion on opposite cusp

Figure 94-1 *Bacterial endocarditis.*

allow slower growing organisms to replicate. Serologic testing may be useful for detecting *C. burnetii* and *Bartonella* spp. and should be performed if cultures are negative. Polymerase chain reaction (PCR) testing from the blood or infected tissue may also prove useful in cases of culture negative IE. Transesophageal echocardiography (TEE) remains more sensitive than transthoracic echocardiography (TTE) and should be used in high-risk groups. For routine screening in low-risk patients, TTE is acceptable, but if clinical suspicion remains high despite a normal finding, TEE may be required.

Antimicrobial therapy for IE should be directed against the isolated organism, with special attention paid to susceptibility testing. In recent years, the development of resistant organisms poses a particular challenge. A full discussion of antibiotic treatments is beyond the scope of this chapter but can be found in the Suggested Readings. Bactericidal IV treatments should be used, usually for a minimum of 4 weeks. An adequate response to therapy can be ascertained by the absence of fever, normalization of inflammatory markers, negative blood culture results, and echocardiography. Surgical intervention is required in up to 20% to 40% of cases of IE. The indications for surgery include refractory cardiac failure from valvular insufficiency, persistent sepsis, abscess, and persistent life-threatening embolization.

The recommendations for antibiotic prophylaxis for procedures have recently changed. Current recommendations for prophylaxis focus on conditions at the highest risk for an adverse outcome, not an overall increased lifetime risk of IE (Box 94-2). Prophylaxis is only recommended for certain dental procedures and is no longer recommended for respiratory, gastrointestinal,

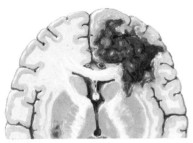

Infarct of brain with secondary hemorrhage from embolism to right anterior cerebral artery; also small infarct in left basal ganglia

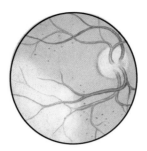

Embolus in vessel of ocular fundus with retinal infarction; petechiae

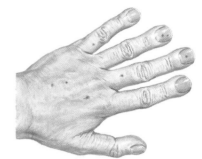

Multiple petechiae of skin and clubbing of fingers

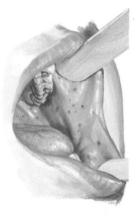

Petechiae of mucous membranes

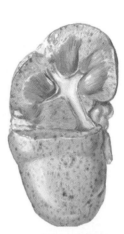

Petechiae and gross infarcts of kidney

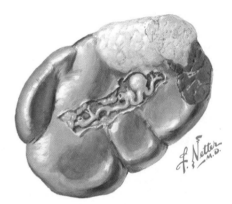

Mycotic aneurysms of splenic arteries and infarct of spleen; splenomegaly

Figure 94-2 *Bacterial endocarditis: remote embolic effects.*

or genitourinary procedures unless contact with infected tissue is expected.

FUTURE DIRECTIONS

Research is underway to evaluate potential vaccines and therapies against bacterial adhesins, which may prevent bacterial adhesion to damaged endocardium. Because IE is increasingly becoming a nosocomial disease in patients with indwelling catheters, modified biomaterials with antiadherence properties are under development. Despite advances and the development of newer antimicrobial therapies, antibiotic resistance will continue to pose a problem in the treatment of IE.

INFECTIOUS MYOCARDITIS

Myocarditis is defined as inflammation of the myocardium. The differential diagnosis in children is broad, including drug hypersensitivity reactions and infectious, rheumatologic, genetic, and metabolic causes. There is much debate over the classification, diagnosis, and treatment of myocarditis. For this reason, the true incidence of myocarditis is unknown. Myocarditis is the

leading cause of dilated cardiomyopathy in children (51.6%). This section focuses on infectious myocarditis (IM).

PATHOGENESIS

IM is mainly caused by viruses, although bacteria, fungi, protozoa, and parasites have been implicated as well (Box 94-3). The most common causes include enteroviruses, adenovirus, human herpes virus-6 (HHV-6), Epstein-Barr virus (EBV), cytomegalovirus (CMV), parvovirus B19, and HIV. Coxsackievirus B was initially the most commonly discovered virus associated with myocarditis, but this shifted to include other enteroviruses and adenovirus in the late 1990s and more recently to HHV-6 and parvovirus B19. *Borrelia burgdorferi* (Lyme disease) should be considered in patients with a history of tick bite, especially if conduction abnormalities are present. Myocarditis is commonly seen in HIV infection—by some reports, up to 50% at autopsy. It is unknown if this is solely because of the viral infection or the effects of long-term antiretroviral therapy.

It is believed that viral pathogens enter cardiac myocytes via specific receptors, and the ensuing immunologic response and inflammation is responsible for much of the damage. However, direct killing from viruses likely takes place because viral genomes have been found in cases of dilated cardiomyopathy in the absence of inflammation or myocarditis. Whether IM is purely an infectious process or also involves an autoimmune component is still under debate.

CLINICAL PRESENTATION

IM can present with a wide range of symptoms, from none at all to sudden death. Patients often have a history of a viral prodrome such as fever, malaise, myalgias, and rash. These symptoms usually precede the cardiac symptoms by several weeks and are often resolved at the time of diagnosis. Typically, cardiac symptoms have only been present for a few weeks before diagnosis. Patients may present with chest pain, dyspnea, exercise intolerance, symptoms of congestive heart failure, arrhythmias, or an acute myocardial infarction–like syndrome. The physical examination should focus on a detailed cardiac examination and stigmata of other diseases known to be associated with myocarditis. Skeletal muscle weakness, dysmorphic facies, hepatosplenomegaly, or multiple organ anomalies may indicate underlying genetic or metabolic causes. History or physical examination findings for particular viral etiologies may help guide the diagnosis. Risk factors for HIV should always be assessed. A history of pharyngitis may point toward EBV or adenovirus, hand or feet lesions may indicate coxsackievirus B, and a history of a "slapped cheek" appearance may implicate parvovirus B19.

EVALUATION AND MANAGEMENT

There is much debate on how to accurately diagnose myocarditis. Historically, diagnosis has relied on endomyocardial biopsy and the Dallas criteria, which state that an inflammatory cell infiltrate with associated myocyte necrosis be present (Figure 94-3). The sensitivity of the Dallas criteria is reported to be as low as 10% to 22%, and to increase sensitivity to 80%, an estimated 17 ventricular biopsy specimens are needed. The low sensitivity can be explained by a number of reasons. The inflammation in myocarditis is often patchy, leading to endomyocardial biopsy sampling error. There is also much variability in the interpretation of histopathologic samples, with differences in opinion among pathologists in interpreting the same specimen. Often, biopsy is not performed because it is thought to be too invasive, and the diagnosis of myocarditis is made on clinical grounds after other cardiac processes are ruled out.

Echocardiographic findings of myocarditis are often nonspecific and are most useful in ruling out other causes of heart failure. Echocardiography may show segmental wall motion abnormalities, thrombus, right ventricular involvement, pericardial effusion, or transient increases in left ventricular thickness as a measure of edema. More recently, cardiac magnetic resonance (CMR) imaging has proven a useful tool in the diagnosis of acute myocarditis, with high sensitivity and

Box 94-3 Causes of Infectious Myocarditis

Viral
- Human herpes virus-6 (HHV6)
- Parvovirus B19
- Enteroviruses (especially coxsackievirus B)
- Adenovirus
- HIV
- Epstein-Barr virus
- Cytomegalovirus
- Hepatitis C virus

Bacterial
- Mycobacterial
- Streptococcal species
- *Mycoplasma pneumoniae*
- *Treponema pallidum*

Fungal
- *Aspergillus* spp.
- *Candida* spp.
- *Coccidioides* spp.
- *Histoplasma* spp.

Protozoal
- *Trypanosoma cruzi*

Parasitic
- Schistosomiasis
- Larva migrans

Adapted from Magnani J, Dec GW: Myocarditis: current trends in diagnosis and treatment. Circulation 113:876-890, 2006.

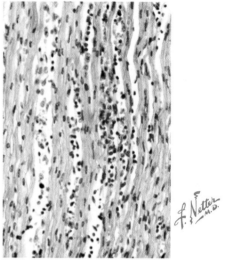

Coxsackie group B virus infection. Diffuse and patchy interstitial edema; cellular infiltration with only moderate muscle fiber destruction (×100)

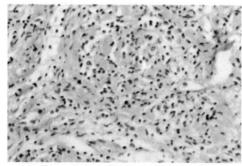

Diffuse cellular infiltration of bundle of His and right and left bundle branches (×100)

Figure 94-3 *Viral myocarditis.*

specificity. It has been used to select endomyocardial biopsy sites, with proven success. Cardiac biomarkers, including creatine kinase and troponins, may or may not be elevated in acute myocarditis. Electrocardiography (ECG) may show nonspecific ST-segment and T-wave abnormalities. If the pericardium is involved, the ECG would show changes consistent with pericarditis.

The search for a viral cause of IM includes testing for specific virus serology as well as viral genomes. Any biopsy specimen should be tested by PCR for coxsackievirus B, echoviruses, parvovirus B19, adenovirus, CMV, EBV, and HHV-6. If an endomyocardial biopsy is not performed, these tests can be sent from the blood. Serologies may also be useful in identifying acute infection. If the history is suggestive of HIV infection, the patient should undergo HIV testing.

Treatment of IM is mainly supportive. Because most patients with viral myocarditis improve over time, therapy is focused on medical management of heart failure until the inflammation improves. This usually includes angiotensin-converting enzyme inhibitors, β-blockers, and diuretics. There may be a need for mechanical circulatory support such as left ventricular assist devices or extracorporeal membrane oxygenation in cases of fulminant myocarditis with profound left ventricular dysfunction. Studies on immunosuppressive therapies for treatment of acute myocarditis have not shown any benefit. Treatment with IV immunoglobulin (IVIG) has proven equally disappointing. A Cochrane review concluded that there was no benefit from the use of IVIG for the management of presumed viral myocarditis in children and adults. Interferon-α and -β have shown some promise in small, single-center studies, but the results need to be confirmed in larger randomized studies. Because the diagnosis of IM often happens weeks after the onset of acute viral infection, it is unlikely that specific viral treatments would significantly alter the course of the disease. Although there is a high rate of spontaneous improvement in IM, the late sequela of chronic dilated cardiomyopathy has significant morbidity, with some patients progressing to a need for cardiac transplantation.

FUTURE DIRECTIONS

CMR is becoming increasingly useful in the diagnosis and management of patients with myocarditis. It is likely to become integral in the diagnosis and follow-up of all patients with myocarditis, perhaps even making biopsies unnecessary. Better understanding of viral pathogenesis and the immune response should help guide therapies in the future, whether it is to halt viral replication or alter the body's immune destruction to minimize damage.

SUGGESTED READINGS

Infective Endocarditis

Baddour LM, Wilson WR, Bayer AS, et al: Infective endocarditis: diagnosis, antimicrobial therapy, and management of complications: a statement for healthcare professionals from the Committee on Rheumatic Fever, Endocarditis, and Kawasaki Disease, Council on Cardiovascular Disease in the Young, and the Councils on Clinical Cardiology, Stroke, and Cardiovascular Surgery and Anesthesia, American Heart Association-Executive Summary: endorsed by the Infectious Disease Society of America, *Circulation* 111:3167-3184, 2005.

Moreillon P, Que Y: Infective endocarditis, *Lancet* 363:139-149, 2004.

Nishimura RA, Carabello BA, Faxon DP, et al: ACC/AHA 2008 guideline update on valvular heart disease: focused update on infective endocarditis, *J Am Coll Cardiol* 52:676-685, 2008.

Paterick TE, Paterick TJ, Nishimura RA, Steckelberg JM: Complexity and subtlety of infective endocarditis, *Mayo Clin Proc* 82(5):615-621, 2007.

Tleyjeh IM, Abdel-Latif A, Rahbi H, et al: A systematic review of population-based studies of infective endocarditis, *Chest* 132(3):1025-1035, 2007.

Infectious Myocarditis

Hartling RJ, Vandermeer B, Klassen TP: Intravenous immunoglobulin for presumed viral myocarditis in children and adults (review). The Cochrane Collaboration, 2009, Issue 2.

Cooper LT Jr: Myocarditis, *N Engl J Med* 360:1526-1538, 2009.

Cox GF, Sleeper LA, Lowe AM, et al: Factors associated with establishing a causal diagnosis for children with cardiomyopathy, *Pediatrics* 118(4):1519-1531, 2006.

Hauck AJ, Kearney DL, Edwards WD: Evaluation of postmortem endomyocardial biopsy specimens from 38 patients with lymphocytic myocarditis: implications for role of sampling error, *Mayo Clin Proc* 64(10):1235-1245, 1989.

Magnani J, Dec GW: Myocarditis: current trends in diagnosis and treatment, *Circulation* 113:876-890, 2006.

Mahrholdt H, Wagner A, Deluigi CC, et al: Presentation, patterns of myocardial damage, and clinical course of viral myocarditis, *Circulation* 114(15):1581-1590, 2006.

Human Immunodeficiency Virus

95

Elizabeth Lowenthal

Worldwide, more than half a million children younger than 15 years of age are infected with HIV. Untreated HIV infection leads to a complex immunosuppressive state that increases the risk of serious morbidities and mortality. A few decades ago, the diagnosis of HIV was thought to be a death sentence. In contrast, children born with HIV today can have essentially normal childhoods. Keeping HIV-infected children healthy requires the long-term administration of highly active antiretroviral therapy (HAART). Effective antiretroviral therapy must be combined with a holistic approach that considers the functioning and quality of life of the child and family.

PATHOGENESIS

HIV is a lentivirus that infects humans chronically, progressively damaging the hosts' immune systems. Two viral types have been characterized in humans: HIV type 1 (HIV-1) and HIV type 2 (HIV-2). Based on viral genetic sequences, HIV-1 isolates have been classified into three groups (M, N, and O). The majority of HIV-1 strains identified worldwide belong to group M. Group M ("main group") is classified into a number of subtypes (also termed *clades*). The subtypes are designated by letters (A, B, C, D, F, G, H, J, and K).

HIV begins its life cycle after entry into the human body when it binds to CD4 receptors and one of two co-receptors (CCR5 or CXCR4) on CD4+ T-lymphocytes and other receptor-containing cells. Binding to appropriate receptors allows the virus to fuse with the host cell, releasing viral RNA and enzymes into the host cell. The genetic material of HIV is single-stranded RNA. The virus also contains three enzymes that are essential to its replication: reverse transcriptase, integrase, and protease. Reverse transcriptase converts the single-stranded RNA into double-stranded DNA. Reverse transcriptase is a "low-fidelity" enzyme, meaning it is prone to making errors. On average, it inserts the wrong base into the growing cDNA chain at least every 4000 bases, producing mutated viral quasi-species. Over time, each infected individual accumulates a number of quasispecies that become "archived" within the host genome. The existence of drug-resistant quasispecies also creates a therapeutic challenge.

After reverse transcription, the double-stranded DNA enters the host cell's nucleus, where viral integrase facilitates its integration into the host DNA. The integrated HIV DNA is referred to as a *provirus*. The provirus can remain inactive for years. Activation of the cell induces transcription of proviral DNA into mRNA. The mRNA migrates into the cytoplasm, where viral proteins are produced by the host cell. The viral protease cleaves the large viral proteins into smaller pieces to create the infectious virus. Two viral RNA strands and the replication enzymes are then surrounded by a capsid of core proteins. The viral capsid acquires a glycopeptide-studded envelope during budding from the host cell. These HIV glycoproteins are necessary for the virus to bind to CD4 and co-receptors. The process of viral replication leads to death of the host cell.

As many as 10 billion HIV virions are produced daily in a single human host. Untreated people typically have 10^3 to 10^6 virions per milliliter of plasma. The concentration of virus in lymph nodes is usually two to three orders of magnitude higher than in plasma. The amount of virus in the plasma is measured using quantitative HIV RNA polymerase chain reaction (PCR) tests, also called "viral loads." Antiretroviral treatment aims to halt HIV replication and get the viral load down to undetectable levels.

DIAGNOSIS

Within 6 to 12 weeks of infection with HIV, people produce HIV-specific antibodies, detectable by commercially available assays. Adults and children older than 18 months of age are typically tested for HIV with antibody-based assays such as rapid HIV immunoassays ("rapid test" or enzyme immunoassay [EIA]) and enzyme-linked immunosorbent assay (ELISA). A positive rapid test or ELISA result is usually confirmed with a Western blot test. These antibody tests are positive in virtually all HIV-infected individuals after the first 3 months of infection. The period during which the person is HIV infected but does not have detectable antibodies is referred to as the *window period*. With the currently available antibody assays, antibodies to HIV are usually detectable by 4 to 6 weeks after infection.

Babies born to mothers with HIV are considered to be HIV exposed and need to undergo testing for HIV. HIV-exposed babies will have positive HIV antibody test results, even if the infants are not HIV infected. Maternal anti-HIV immunoglobulin G (IgG) antibodies cross the placenta and can be detected in babies born to mothers who carry the HIV antibodies. On average, maternal antibodies to HIV persist in the infants for the first 9 to 18 months of life. Therefore, virologic tests are used to confirm the presence of HIV infection in babies who are younger than 18 months of age. Most commonly, HIV DNA PCR or HIV RNA PCR is used for diagnosis during this time. Negative (DNA or RNA) PCR test results done at 1 month and 4 months of age can rule out HIV infection in perinatally HIV-exposed babies who are not breastfeeding. HIV viral culture and p24 antigen assays may also be done for diagnosis but are considered less sensitive and specific than RNA and DNA PCR tests. Early negative HIV virologic test results can be confirmed by obtaining a negative antibody-based test result around 18 months of age.

Table 95-1 summarizes the expected results of HIV diagnostic tests for HIV-exposed and -infected infants and adolescents. Children older than the age of 18 months would have the same test results as adolescents in the same infection or exposure category.

Table 95-1 Expected Diagnostic Test Results for Children by Age

Diagnostic Test	HIV-Infected Infant	HIV-Exposed Uninfected Infant	Infected Adolescent During Window Period	Infected Adolescent After Window Period	HIV-Exposed Uninfected Adolescent
ELISA or Western blot	Positive	Positive	Negative	Positive	Negative
DNA PCR	Positive	Negative	Positive	Positive	Negative
RNA PCR (viral load)	Positive (high viral load)	Negative	Positive (high viral load)	Positive	Negative

ELISA, enzyme-linked immunosorbent assay; PCR, polymerase chain reaction.

CLINICAL MANIFESTATIONS OF HIV INFECTION

The process of HIV replication leads to depletion of CD4+ T lymphocytes. The degree of immunologic suppression is classified based on the number and percent of CD4+ T lymphocytes present in the bloodstream. In young children, the normal number of CD4+ T lymphocytes is much higher than in adults. Therefore, age-specific absolute CD4+ T lymphocyte count ranges should be used to determine the degree of immune suppression in children. CD4+ T lymphocyte percents change less with age and can be used instead of absolute counts to classify the degree of immune suppression in HIV-infected children (Table 95-2).

Along with depletion of CD4+ T lymphocytes, HIV infection leads to functional defects in existing CD4+ T-lymphocytes and defects in B-cell function. These combined immunosuppressive processes lead to a number of clinical manifestations. The most severe and common of these manifestations are outlined in Table 95-3. Opportunistic infections, cancers, hematologic aberrations, and other noninfectious manifestations are among the most severe AIDS-defining conditions.

TREATMENT

Before antiretroviral drugs were available, care for children with HIV focused on prevention and management of HIV-related complications and palliative care. When the first antiretroviral drugs became available in the early 1990s, significant clinical and immunologic benefits were seen. Initially, monotherapy was used. Later, two-drug combinations were introduced. Unfortunately, these had limited durability because viral mutations rapidly led to formation of resistance to the therapies. Currently, combinations of at least three drugs from two different drug classes are recommended for HIV treatment. These combinations are referred to as HAART. Excellent adherence to

appropriate HAART regimens is associated with viral suppression, immunologic recovery, reduction in opportunistic infections and other disease manifestations, and improved survival.

Currently available antiretroviral therapies target various points in the HIV life cycle. The three oldest classes of antiretroviral drugs are nucleoside reverse transcriptase inhibitors (NRTIs), non-nucleoside reverse transcriptase inhibitors (NNRTIs), and protease inhibitors (PIs). The first available antiretroviral therapies were in the NRTI drug class. NRTI's are drugs whose chemical structure is a modified version of a natural nucleoside. NRTI's interfere with the action of reverse transcription by causing premature termination of the proviral DNA chain. NNRTIs act as noncompetitive inhibitors of the HIV-1 reverse transcriptase by binding to the reverse transcriptase catalytic site. PIs block protease from cleaving HIV protein precursors, preventing formation of new infectious virions. HAART consisting of an NNRTI or a PI plus two NRTIs is recommended for treatment of antiretroviral-naïve children. In the United States and other high-resource settings, therapy choices are usually guided by viral resistance testing. When resistance to drugs in the NRTI, NNRTI, and PI classes occurs in children, newer drug classes are sometimes used.

Two newer commercially available drug classes exert activity against viral entry into the host cell by inhibiting viral fusion with the cell membrane or binding to the CCR5 co-receptor. A third drug class inhibits integration of proviral DNA into the human genome. None of these drugs is yet recommended for initial therapy of HIV-infected children because there are not yet sufficient data on pediatric dosing and safety. To allow for long-term effectiveness, three drugs to which the patient's virus has not developed resistance should be given. Therefore, the newer drug classes are sometimes used in highly treatment-experienced children who otherwise have limited treatment options.

Figure 95-1 shows the life cycle as well as the targets of antiretroviral medications.

Table 95-2 Immunologic Categorization Based on Age-Specific CD4+ T-Lymphocyte Counts and Percent of Total Lymphocytes

Immunologic Category	Age <12 Months	Age 1-5 Years	Age 6-12 Years
1: No evidence of suppression	≥1500 cells/μL ≥25%	≥1000 cells/μL ≥25%	≥500 cells/μL ≥25%
2: Moderate suppression	750-1499 cells/μL 15%-24%	500-999 cells/μL 15%-24%	200-499 cells/μL 15%-24%
3: Severe suppression	<750 cells/μL <15%	<500 cells/μL <15%	<200 cells/μL <15%

Table 95-3 Selected Clinical Manifestations of HIV Infection

Severe Manifestations	Description
Pneumocystis jiroveci pneumonia	Definitive diagnosis via microscopy of induced sputum or BAL
Multiple or recurrent serious bacterial infections	Septicemia, pneumonia, meningitis, bone or joint infection, internal organ infections
Kaposi's sarcoma	Characterized by pink or purple lesions on the skin and soft tissues; diagnosis is confirmed with biopsy
Lymphoma	Cerebral or B-cell non-Hodgkin's lymphoma
Mycobacterial infections	Extrapulmonary mycobacterium tuberculosis infection and nontuberculous mycobacterial infections
HIV encephalopathy	Failure to attain or loss of developmental milestones or loss of intellectual ability, impaired brain growth, or acquired symmetric motor deficits lasting for >2 mo without a cause other than HIV
HIV wasting syndrome	Unexplained severe wasting, stunting, or severe malnutrition not adequately responding to standard therapy
Severe herpes simplex infections	Bronchitis, pneumonitis, esophagitis (or mucocutaneous ulcer persisting >1 mo)
Severe candidiasis	Esophageal or pulmonary (including bronchi and trachea)
Moderately Severe Manifestations	
Single episode of serious bacterial infection	Septicemia, pneumonia, meningitis, bone or joint infection, internal organ infections
Lymphoid interstitial pneumonitis	Definitive diagnosis via biopsy but characterized by chronic bilateral reticulonodular interstitial pulmonary infiltrates and hypoxemia
Recurrent or chronic diarrhea	Persistent ≥14 days
Anemia, neutropenia, or thrombocytopenia persisting ≥30 days	Anemia: hemoglobin <8 g/dL Neutropenia: ANC <1000 cells/mm^3 Thrombocytopenia: platelets <100,000 cells/mm^3
Herpes zoster	At least two distinct episodes or more than one dermatome
Herpes simplex virus	Recurrent stomatitis (>two episodes in 1 year)
Complicated varicella	Disseminated or severe chicken pox
Candidiasis	Oropharyngeal lasting for >2 mo
Mild Manifestations	
Lymphadenopathy	≥0.5 cm at more than two sites
Recurrent or persistent upper respiratory tract infections	Including sinusitis or otitis media
Hepatosplenomegaly	Unexplained, persistent
Mucocutaneous lesions	Extensive wart virus infection, extensive molluscum contagiosum, popular pruritic eruptions, recurrent oral ulcers

ANC, absolute neutrophil count; BAL, bronchoalveolar lavage.

Table 95-4 describes key features of the antiretroviral medications most commonly used for treatment of children with HIV. To maintain long-term effectiveness, these drugs must be given in appropriate combinations and adherence to therapy must be excellent. Adherence is sometimes complicated by drug side effects. The PIs often cause gastrointestinal distress, particularly early in therapy, that make medication tolerance challenging. Many of the drugs have significant long-term effects, including hyperlipidemia, body habitus changes, and peripheral neuropathy. Careful monitoring by doctors who are experienced in the treatment of HIV allows for early detection of problems and appropriate adjustment of regimens to help ensure long-term therapeutic success.

For children with severe HIV-related immunosuppression, prophylactic medications should also be given to help prevent opportunistic infections. Common infections in children without HIV are also seen in children with HIV but frequently are more severe. Therefore, routine vaccination of HIV-infected children is essential. Table 95-5 outlines recommended strategies for primary prevention of infectious complications in children with HIV. After treatment of an opportunistic infection, long-term secondary prophylaxis is often given to prevent recurrence of disease, regardless of immunologic recovery.

Comprehensive care of HIV-infected children must include psychosocial support to facilitate excellent lifelong adherence to therapy and overall health. Avoiding resistance to antiretroviral therapies requires excellent adherence to appropriate regimens. Age-appropriate counseling regarding the child's HIV status and strategies to maintain health are essential. Counseling and support must be extended to the child's entire family to ensure that the child's environment will support excellent medication adherence and help the child achieve his or her life goals.

PREVENTION

One of the greatest successes in HIV medicine has been the development of therapies to prevent the mother-to-child

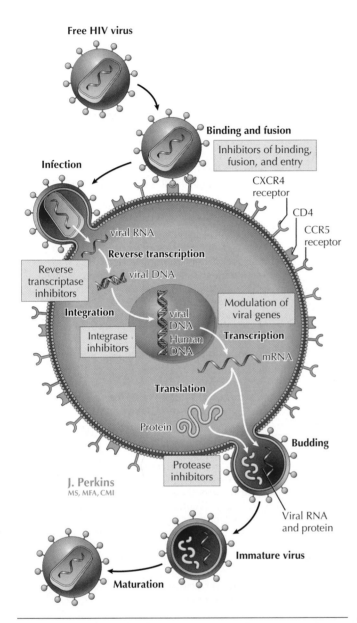

Figure 95-1 *Life cycle of HIV and targets of antiretroviral medications.*

transmission (MTCT) of HIV. Without any intervention, approximately 40% of babies born to breastfeeding HIV-infected mothers will be infected with HIV. When comprehensive preventive methods are adopted, the MTCT risk can be reduced to less than 2%.

Prevention of HIV infection in neonates begins with early identification of HIV infection in pregnant women. HIV testing during the first prenatal visit should be a part of routine prenatal care. This allows for early initiation (<28 weeks of gestation) of HAART to help prevent MTCT of HIV. Repeat HIV testing during the third trimester is recommended for women thought to be at "high risk" of HIV infection because the mother's acquisition of HIV during pregnancy puts the child at especially high risk of infection around the time of delivery. After delivery, the perinatally HIV-exposed baby is often given AZT (Zidovudine) to further reduce the transmission risk.

Additional antiretroviral drugs are sometimes given to the infant when the risk of perinatal infection is thought to be high (e.g., when the mother received no preventive therapy before delivery).

For women in resource-limited settings where HAART cannot be given for all HIV-infected pregnant women, a number of short-course antiretroviral options are considered. In settings where resources are most limited, a single dose of nevirapine is often given to the mother while she is in labor and to the infant right after birth. This single low-cost intervention can decrease the risk of HIV transmission by around 50%.

For women who are HIV infected, a number of nonpharmacologic interventions have proven to be valuable for the prevention of MTCT. Avoiding instrumentation (e.g., forceps and fetal scalp monitors) during deliveries also decreases MTCT risk. Cesarean section deliveries are recommended when the maternal HIV viral load is >1000 copies/mL at the time of delivery and resources are available for safe cesarean sections. Treating other sexually transmitted diseases (e.g., active herpes lesions) also decreases HIV transmission risk. Breastfeeding is another important mode of HIV transmission in some settings. Babies born to HIV-infected mothers therefore are usually recommended to formula feed when such feeding can be made affordable, feasible, accessible, safe, and sustainable.

Prevention of new HIV infections among adolescents is also a challenge in pediatrics. Although abstinence is a sure way to avoid sexual transmission of HIV, abstinence-only education has unfortunately proven to be an unsuccessful preventive approach. The consistent use of condoms is important for avoiding the spread of HIV and other sexually transmitted diseases among sexually active individuals. Male circumcision has also proven to be successful at decreasing the risk of HIV transmission.

SUMMARY

HIV is a major worldwide cause of pediatric morbidity and mortality. Available therapies allow children who are born with HIV to maintain their health into adulthood. Unfortunately, only a minority of HIV-infected children worldwide currently have access to HIV treatment. Effective strategies for the prevention of MTCT of HIV are also available but are currently reaching only a minority of HIV-infected women worldwide.

FUTURE DIRECTIONS

A great deal of work needs to be done to expand prevention and treatment options in low-resource settings where the HIV prevalence is highest. New antiretroviral drugs and pediatric formulations of existing drugs are being developed to facilitate long-term effective treatment. Vaccine development is also a key area of research. The rapid mutation of HIV and its skill at evading antibodies and other immune responses makes it a particularly difficult target for preventive vaccines. Many researchers are also trying to create therapeutic vaccines that would improve the body's ability to fight HIV, augmenting currently available antiretroviral therapies for individuals already infected with the virus.

Table 95-4 Antiretroviral Medications Available for Children

	Pediatric Indication	Main Side Effects	Special Considerations
Nucleoside Reverse Transcriptase Inhibitors			
Abacavir (ABC)	Yes	Potentially fatal hypersensitivity reaction in ≈5% of people	Genetic testing (HLA B*5701) for susceptibility to hypersensitivity is available.
Didanosine (ddI)	Yes	Lipoatrophy, peripheral neuropathy, lactic acidosis	Delayed-release formulation allows for once-daily dosing in older children. Other formulation must be given on an empty stomach.
Emtricitabine (FTC)	Yes	Relatively well tolerated	Also active against hepatitis B. Should not be given with 3TC.
Lamivudine (3TC)	Yes	Relatively well tolerated	Also active against hepatitis B. Should not be given with FTC.
Stavudine (d4T)	Yes	Lipoatrophy, peripheral neuropathy, hyperlipidemia, lactic acidosis	Should not be given with AZT because of antagonism. Should not be given with ddI because of overlapping side effects.
Tenofovir (TDF)	No	Reduced bone mineral density, nephrotoxicity	Sometimes used in very treatment-experienced children. Also active against hepatitis B (nucleotide analog; NtRTI).
Zidovudine (AZT)	Yes	Bone marrow suppression	Given to infants to help prevent MTCT of HIV.
Non-nucleoside Reverse Transcriptase Inhibitors			
Efavirenz (EFV)	≥3 y	Neuropsychiatric; may cause neural tube defects if taken during early pregnancy	Women with childbearing potential should use with caution.
Nevirapine (NVP)	Yes	Hepatoxicity; potentially severe rashes or Stevens-Johnson syndrome early in therapy	Single dose used in low-resource settings for basic prevention of MTCT regimen.
Protease Inhibitors			
Atazanavir	≥6 y	Indirect hyperbilirubinemia; prolonged PR interval on ECG	Must be administered with another protease inhibitor, ritonavir, to obtain therapeutic levels.
Darunavir	Not currently approved	May cause less GI distress than other PIs	Sometimes used in children with highly resistant virus. May maintain activity when resistance to other PIs has occurred.
Fosamprenavir	≥6 y	GI distress; nausea or vomiting; rashes	Must be administered with ritonavir.
Lopinavir/ritonavir (LPV/r)	Yes	GI distress; nausea or vomiting	Lopinavir and ritonavir are co-formulated as a single tablet.
Nelfinavir	≥2 y	Diarrhea	TID dosing for younger children makes this a less desirable option.
Fusion Inhibitor			
Enfuvirtide (T-20, fusion)	Yes	Local injection site reactions	BID SC injections.
CCR5 Receptor Blocker			
Maraviroc	No	Allergic reactions and hepatotoxicity	Limited data on pediatric dosing and safety. For use in CCR5-trophic virus only.
Integrase Inhibitor			
Raltegravir	No	Diarrhea, nausea, headache	Limited data on pediatric dosing and safety.

BID, twice a day; ECG, electrocardiography; GI, gastrointestinal; HLA, human leukocyte antigen; MCTC, mother-to-child transmission; NtRTI, nucleotide analog reverse transcriptase inhibitor; PI, protease inhibitor; SC, subcutaneous; TID, three times a day.

Table 95-5 Primary Prophylaxis of Opportunistic Infection in HIV

Infection	Indications for Prophylaxis	Prevention Strategy
Pneumocystis jiroveci pneumonia	• <1 y: HIV infection or HIV exposure with uncertain HIV infection status • 2-5 y: CD4 <500 cells/mcL or <15% • 6+ y: CD4 <200 cells/mcL or <15%	TMP-SMX twice a day, 3 d/wk
Tuberculosis	Positive TB skin test result (≥5 mm) and no evidence of active TB disease	Isoniazid daily for 9 mo
Mycobacterium avium complex	• <1 y: CD4 <750 cells/mcL • 1-2 y: CD4 <500 cells/mcL • 2-5 y: CD4 <75 cells/mcL • ≥6 y: CD4 <50 cells/mcL	Azithromycin given weekly
Vaccine-preventable illnesses	All children with HIV	All routine recommended childhood immunizations; defer varicella and MMR if CD4 <15%

MMR, mumps, measles, and rubella; TB, tuberculosis; TMP-SMX, trimethoprim–sulfamethoxazole.

SUGGESTED READINGS

Centers for Disease Control and Prevention: Revised guidelines for HIV counseling, testing, and referral and revised recommendations for HIV screening of pregnant women, *MMWR Morbid Mortal Wkly Rep* 50(RR-19):1-110, 2001. Available at http://www.cdc.gov/mmwr/PDF/rr/rr5019.pdf.

Mofenson LM, Brady MT, Danner SP, et al: *Guidelines for Prevention and Treatment of Opportunistic Infections among HIV-Exposed and HIV-Infected Children.* Available at http://aidsinfo.nih.gov/contentfiles/Pediatric_OI.pdf.

HIV Paediatric Prognostic Markers Collaborative Study and the CASCADE Collaboration, Dunn D, Woodburn P, et al: Current CD4 cell count and the short-term risk of AIDS and death before the availability of effective antiretroviral therapy in HIV-infected children and adults, *J Infect Dis* 197(3):398-404, 2008.

Working Group on Antiretroviral Therapy and Medical Management of HIV-Infected Children: *Guidelines for the Use of Antiretroviral Agents in Pediatric HIV Infection.* February 23, 2009, pp 1-139. Available at http://aidsinfo.nih.gov/ContentFiles/PediatricGuidelines.pdf.

World Health Organization: *Antiretroviral Therapy of HIV Infection in Infants and Children in Resource-Limited Settings: Toward Universal Access,* 2006. Available at http://www.who.int/hiv/en.

World Health Organization: *Towards Universal Access: Scaling up Priority HIV/AIDS Interventions in the Health Sector. 2008 Progress Report.* Available at http://www.unicef.org/aids/files/towards_universal_access_report_2008.pdf.

Gastrointestinal Infections

Jennifer J. Wilkes

96

Gastrointestinal (GI) infections, particularly acute gastroenteritis, cause significant pediatric morbidity and mortality worldwide. Gastroenteritis is an infection of the GI tract characterized by vomiting, diarrhea, or both with three or more loose or watery stools a day. The worldwide mortality of diarrheal illness in children has been estimated at 1.8 million. In the United States, it is estimated that gastroenteritis primarily affects children younger than 5 years of age with 21 to 37 million episodes annually, approximately 200,000 hospitalizations, and 300 to 400 deaths per year. More readily accessible treatment has been made through the uptake of aggressive oral rehydration therapy (ORT). The causes of acute diarrhea in children differ by location, time of year, and immunologic status (Figure 96-1). This chapter discusses diarrheal illness caused by bacteria and viruses; parasites are discussed in Chapter 99. Additional infections of the GI tract are briefly addressed, including appendicitis, peritonitis, and intraabdominal abscesses.

ACUTE INFECTIOUS DIARRHEA

ETIOLOGY AND PATHOPHYSIOLOGY

Common viral etiologies of acute infectious diarrhea in immunocompetent children include rotavirus, enteric adenoviruses, noroviruses, and astroviruses. Common bacterial pathogens include *Salmonella* spp., *Escherichia coli*, *Shigella* spp., and *Campylobacter jejuni* (Figure 96-2). *Clostridium difficile* is the most common cause of antibiotic-associated diarrhea, although its role in infants younger than 1 year of age is unclear. Additional causes are discussed in Table 96-1 with further discussion of treatment. These pathogens cause diarrhea by a variety of pathogenic means: (1) osmotic or malabsorptive, (3) inflammatory, and (3) toxigenic. In immunocompromised hosts, cytomegalovirus and herpes simplex virus should also be considered as causes of infectious diarrhea.

CLINICAL PRESENTATION

Patients with gastroenteritis often present with symptoms that include emesis, diarrhea, and abdominal pain, which may be associated with fever. Clinical examination findings are usually nonspecific and do not point toward the etiologic organism.

Electrolyte losses and dehydration account for the high morbidity of acute gastroenteritis. In a systematic meta-analysis conducted by Steiner et al., useful individual clinical signs to predict 5% dehydration in children are an abnormal capillary refill time, abnormal skin turgor, and abnormal respiratory pattern for clinical signs of dehydration. Other studies have found that a combination of clinical signs and symptoms is more reliable in the demonstration of at least 5% dehydration: capillary refill time longer than 2 seconds, absent tears, dry mucous membranes, and ill general appearance.

Certain infectious agents are associated with extraintestinal manifestations. *Shigella* spp. organisms produce a toxin that has been associated with seizure. *Yersinia enterocolitica* infection has been associated with reactive arthritis. Additional extraintestinal manifestations can be seen in Table 96-1.

DIFFERENTIAL DIAGNOSIS

A broad differential diagnosis must be entertained with acute gastroenteritis. Diarrhea can be the presenting symptom of other infections, anatomic, or malabsorptive issues such as bowel obstruction or inflammatory bowel disease. In addition, vomiting may indicate other infections such as meningitis, lower lobe pneumonia, sepsis, or urinary tract infection, as well as metabolic disorders, toxin ingestion, heart failure, and trauma.

EVALUATION AND MANAGEMENT

The laboratory evaluation of children with gastroenteritis is often guided by history and clinical presentation, particularly the degree of dehydration. Assessment and treatment of dehydration is at the forefront of management of gastroenteritis in children. Serum electrolyte testing helps in the management of patients who appear severely dehydrated and in the detection of hyponatremic or hypernatremic dehydration. Hemoccult testing of stool can aid in identifying pathogens that cause bloody diarrhea. Stool culture should be performed in patients in whom a bacterial etiology is suspected, especially in cases lasting longer than 3 days and with bloody diarrhea. Identifying diarrhea-associated *E. coli* can be difficult because most clinical laboratories cannot differentiate diarrhea-associated *E. coli* strains from normal intestinal flora. Bacterial toxin testing is used to identify A and B toxins from *C. difficile*, as well as *Shiga*-type toxins. Viral antigen detection or molecular polymerase chain reaction–based tests can be used to identify rotavirus, adenovirus, and caliciviruses (norovirus).

Treatment of patients with gastroenteritis includes supportive care and fluid management. In some cases of bacterial gastroenteritis, antimicrobial therapy may be helpful, although it is not routinely recommended.

A brief discussion of rehydration is provided here, but more detailed discussions can be found in the Suggested Readings section at the end of the chapter. Current recommendations from the American Academy of Pediatrics encourage use of ORT in managing acute gastroenteritis in children. Oral rehydration occurs in two phases of treatment: a rehydration phase in which water and electrolytes are given in the form of an oral rehydration solution (ORS) for existing losses and a maintenance phase. ORS introduces glucose as well as sodium at the same time to allow for coupled transport. The World Health Organization's components for rehydration solution consist of at least a complex carbohydrate or 2% glucose and 50 to

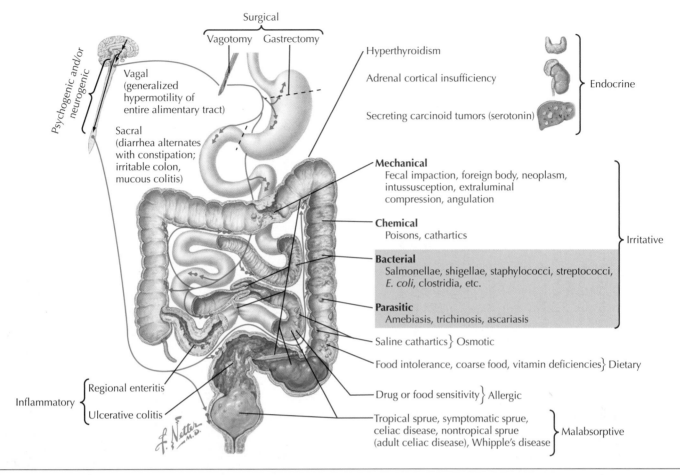

Figure 96-1 *Diarrhea.*

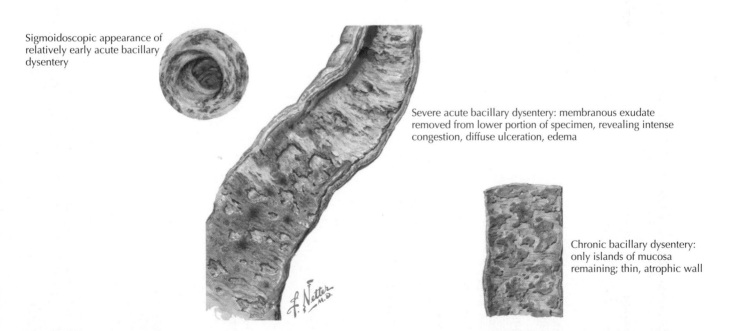

Sigmoidoscopic appearance of relatively early acute bacillary dysentery

Severe acute bacillary dysentery: membranous exudate removed from lower portion of specimen, revealing intense congestion, diffuse ulceration, edema

Chronic bacillary dysentery: only islands of mucosa remaining; thin, atrophic wall

Figure 96-2 *Bacillary dysentery.*

Table 96-1   Common Infectious Causes of Gastroenteritis

Pathogen	Toxin	Course	Presence of Blood?	Extraintestinal Manifestations	Historical Pearls	Treatment in Immunocompetent Patients
Rotavirus	None	Usually fever and vomiting and then followed by watery diarrhea	No	Unusual	Common season is late fall to early spring; virus can persist in stool ≤21 d	Supportive therapy, including rehydration
Enteric adenovirus	None		No	Nonenteric often upper respiratory infections, pharyngoconjunctivitis		Supportive therapy, including rehydration
Astrovirus	None	Diarrhea, self-limited infection	No		Late winter to spring	Supportive therapy, including rehydration
Human calicivirus (norovirus)	None	Mild to moderate diarrhea	No	Myalgia, headache	Isolated vomiting, closed populations (daycare), outbreaks, fecal-oral spread	Supportive therapy, including rehydration
Escherichia coli	Toxins with enterotoxigenic and enterohemorrhagic strains (see text)	Diverse	Possibly	With enterohemorrhagic strains: HUS, TTP, screen for diabetes mellitus	Recent travel, undercooked meats	For traveler's diarrhea in resource-limited setting: azithromycin, fluoroquinolone
Salmonella typhi	None	Diarrhea in children but can present as constipation	Yes	Rose spots: rash on neck or torso, leukopenia, anemia, bacteremia, hepatosplenomegaly, change in mental status	Contaminated food and water, pet amphibians	Infants younger than 3 mo, HIV, hemoglobinopathies, immunocompromised: **ampicillin/amoxicillin, Bactrim** (if strain not resistant); if resistant: **ceftriaxone**
Shigella spp.		Diverse	Yes	Seizures or encephalopathy	Bandemia, child care settings	Oral rehydration, severe disease, dysentery, or immunosuppressed: ceftriaxone, fluoroquinolone, azithromycin (and susceptibility testing)
Campylobacter spp.			Yes	Immunoreactive postinfectious acute idiopathic polyneuritis or Reiter's syndrome; abdominal pain can mimic appendicitis or intussusception	Young pet, erythema nodosum	Rehydration, severe disease: azithromycin, erythromycin, fluoroquinolones
Clostridium difficile	Toxin		No		Recent antibiotic use	Metronidazole, oral vancomycin
Yersinia enterocolitica			Bloody	Pseudoappendicitis syndrome	Erythema nodosum	Sepsis, immunodeficiency: cefotaxime, Bactrim, fluoroquinolones, aminoglycosides

HUS, hemolytic uremic syndrome; TTP, thrombotic thrombocytopenic purpura.
Adapted from Steiner MJ, DeWalt DA, Byerley JS: Is this child dehydrated? JAMA 291(22):2746-2754, 2004.

90 m Eq/L of sodium. Early refeeding is now encouraged after previous losses are corrected. Antimicrobial therapies for certain bacterial etiologies are discussed in Table 96-1.

FUTURE DIRECTIONS

New research into prevention and treatment continues. The use of vaccination for rotavirus may reduce the morbidity and mortality of gastroenteritis in young children. Use of probiotics is an ongoing controversial issue with future research still necessary to see if it aids recovery from gastroenteritis.

APPENDICITIS

Acute abdominal pain in children is a common clinical complaint with a wide differential diagnosis. The most common surgical cause is appendicitis, occurring in about four in 1000 children younger than 16 years of age. In 2002, 77,000 pediatric hospital discharges were for appendicitis and appendiceal disorders. Appendicitis is characterized by inflammation of the appendix caused by obstruction of the lumen of the appendix. In preverbal toddlers, diagnosis by clinical examination is particularly difficult, with appendiceal perforation occurring in many cases. Appendicitis, however, is more common in the second decade of life.

ETIOLOGY AND PATHOGENESIS

The pathogenesis of appendicitis begins with obstruction of the appendiceal lumen, often by lymphoid hyperplasia of the Peyer's patches on the walls of the appendix. These lymphoid tissues increase in size likely because of exposure to infection. With the hyperplasia of the lymphoid tissue, foreign material such as fecal material, food, or parasites are more likely to get caught in the appendix, creating an obstruction. The obstruction leads to thickening of the appendiceal wall, bacterial overgrowth, invasion, inflammation, and ischemia of the appendix. Polymicrobial infection with fecal flora is often reported, with *E. coli*, *Peptostreptococcus* spp., *Bacteroides fragilis*, and *Pseudomonas aeruginosa*.

Perforation with peritonitis is a common complication in children. The appendix is longer and thinner, which makes obstruction and perforation more likely with an omentum that is thinner and less likely to sequester inflammation. Therefore, peritonitis is more likely to be a complication of appendicitis in children than in adults.

CLINICAL PRESENTATION

Appendicitis is often difficult to diagnose clinically in children because the typical signs and symptoms are often absent. The classical presentation of acute appendicitis is abdominal pain that migrates from the periumbilical area to the right lower quadrant of the abdomen (McBurney's point), fever, anorexia, nausea, vomiting, and diarrhea. However, obtaining this history, especially in a preverbal child, is difficult. A recent systematic review tried to identify which historical and clinical examination findings are useful in determining which children warrant

further diagnostic and surgical evaluation. Dysuria can also be a presenting symptom.

Clinical evaluation should include a full head-to-toe examination, including a pelvic examination for sexually active young women. Signs that have been associated with appendicitis in adults (with few pediatric studies) are Rovsing's sign, the psoas sign, and the obturator sign. Rovsing's sign involves palpation of the left lower quadrant, which leads to pain in the right lower quadrant. The psoas sign involves flexing the right hip against resistance. The obturator sign is raising the patient's right leg with knee flexed and then internally rotating. Rectal examination is especially important in infants for whom a rectal mass can be palpated about 30% of the time in the setting of appendicitis.

DIFFERENTIAL DIAGNOSIS

The differential diagnosis for appendicitis is quite broad. Gastroenteritis with abdominal pain can often mimic appendicitis, with *Yersinia* infection known as the great imitator of appendicitis. Other abdominal processes such as mesenteric adenitis, intussusception, and Meckel's diverticulitis are included as well. Urinary tract infection can also cause abdominal pain and vomiting, and urine should be evaluated. In girls, ovarian and pelvic processes, including tubo-ovarian abscess with torsion and pelvic inflammatory disease, can also mimic appendicitis. Nonabdominal processes, particularly right lower lobe pneumonia, can also cause right-sided abdominal pain.

EVALUATION AND MANAGEMENT

In the discussion above about history and physical evaluation, abdominal pain and concerning abdominal examination findings appear to be the most common history and physical findings. Rebound and guarding are concerning for appendiceal rupture or perforation.

Although appendicitis can often be identified by history and physical examination alone, reliance solely on clinical presentation may miss atypical presentations and then can result in delays in treatment and unnecessary hospital admissions. Adjunctive laboratory and radiologic testing can be helpful in the diagnosis of appendicitis.

Although no laboratory test is sensitive and specific for appendicitis, evaluation for signs of inflammation can give adjunctive data to the diagnosis. A complete blood cell count with white blood cell (WBC) count with increased bands or leukocytosis and C-reactive protein (CRP) can help evaluate for inflammation. Urinalysis should be performed because an inflamed appendix overlying the bladder wall may cause pyuria.

Controversy remains as to which radiologic study should serve as an adjunct in the diagnosis of appendicitis. One-view abdominal radiography has limited utility; it can show a calcified fecalith, localized ileus, or free air if perforation is suspected. Ultrasound is often used as the first imaging modality because it can be diagnostic and does not expose the child to X-rays. Findings seen on abdominal ultrasound concerning for appendicitis are dilatation of the appendix, a thickened wall, or free fluid. Abdominal computed tomography (CT) has significantly higher sensitivity for diagnosing appendicitis than ultrasound, with sensitivity of about 94% and specificity of 95%. Recent studies have also shown that intravenous (IV) contrast is equivalent to IV and rectal contrast in the evaluation for acute appendicitis.

The definitive treatment of patients with appendicitis is surgical intervention. In preparation for surgical intervention, broad-spectrum antimicrobials to cover fecal flora can be used and are part of the mainstay of therapy particularly in ruptured appendicitis. A review of pediatric hospital practice of the use of aminoglycoside-based triple therapy versus monotherapy for ruptured appendicitis yielded findings that single-agent antibiotic therapy may be used and may result in decreased lengths of stay and hospital charges.

PERITONITIS AND INTRAABDOMINAL ABSCESSES

Peritonitis is the inflammation of the peritoneum, either from infectious or noninfectious etiologies. Additional causes of abdominal pain in children caused by infection include peritonitis and intraabdominal abscesses, which can present after acute appendicitis or gastroenteritis (Figure 96-3).

ETIOLOGY AND PATHOGENESIS

Primary peritonitis also known as spontaneous bacterial peritonitis (SBP) denotes pathogenic bacteria in the peritoneal fluid

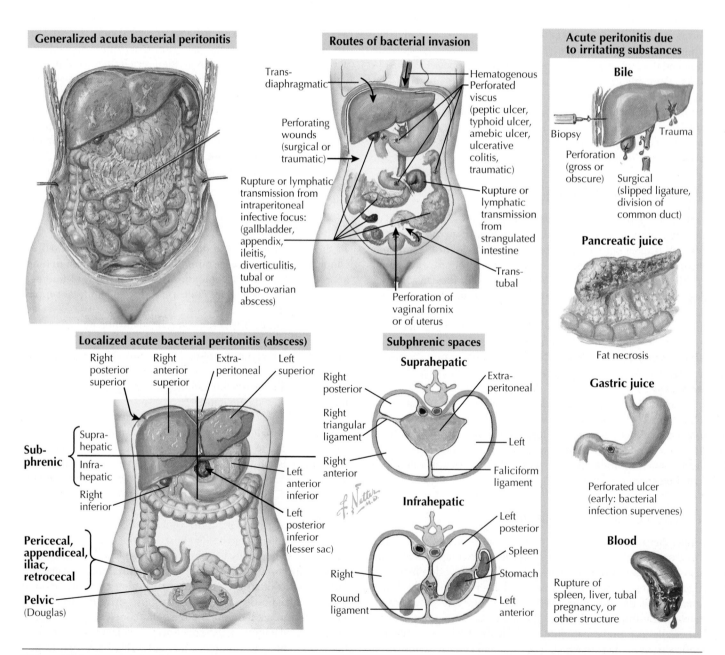

Figure 96-3 *Acute peritonitis.*

Table 96-2 Common Bacterial Causes of Peritonitis

Microbe	Risk Factor	Primary or Secondary	% of Primary
Streptococcus pneumoniae	Previously healthy children	Primary	30-50
Escherichia coli	Appendiceal rupture	Both	25-40
Staphylococcus aureus	Peritoneal dialysis, VP shunts	Both	2-4
Gram-negative enteric bacilli	Cirrhosis	Secondary	
Coagulase-negative Staphylococci	Peritoneal dialysis, VP Shunts	Secondary	
Bacteroides fragilis	Appendiceal rupture	Secondary	

VP, ventriculoperitoneal.

without a clear intraabdominal source. Hematogenous or lymphoid seeding of bacteria into ascites is often how SBP is initiated.

Secondary peritonitis, which is more common, is inflammation from a source such as a perforated viscus or interrupted abdominal wall (as with foreign material catheters). Appendiceal rupture or perforation from appendicitis can occur after gangrene of appendiceal wall and can lead to peritonitis. Foreign materials in the abdomen, particularly chronic peritoneal dialysis catheters and ventriculoperitoneal (VP) shunts, are associated with secondary peritonitis. Peritoneal dialysis catheters provide a track for microorganisms to enter from the environment into the peritoneum. VP shunts can transmit descending intraventricular infections to the abdomen. Risk factors include appendicitis, chronic renal failure, liver failure, peritoneal dialysis, and VP shunts.

Peritonitis may lead to formation of a phlegmon and may then proceed to abscess formation. Additional abscesses in the abdomen may occur within organ structures, especially the liver and spleen, through bacteremia. Amebic abscesses in the liver are discussed in Chapter 99. The microbes involved in peritonitis and abscesses are listed in Table 96-2. The most common targets of therapy are *E. coli* and *Bacteroides* spp.

CLINICAL PRESENTATION

The clinical presentation is nonspecific. As many as 10% of patients with peritonitis and abscesses do not have any symptoms at presentation. Fever, abdominal pain, distension, and lethargy are symptoms commonly associated with peritonitis. The presentation in children with medical devices is often even more elusive. In particular, children who are on immunosuppressive regimens for renal disease may have blunted signs of inflammation and pain. With all patients, complete physical examination is warranted, with particular attention to examination for shifting dullness or fluid in abdominal examination.

Patients with abscesses often present with fever and localization to the viscus that is infected. For example, patients with hepatic pyogenic abscesses present with fever, jaundice, and right upper quadrant pain.

DIFFERENTIAL DIAGNOSIS

As with other GI infections, a broad differential diagnosis must be entertained when concerned for peritonitis. This includes sepsis, gastroenteritis, appendicitis, pyelonephritis, and lower lobe pneumonia.

EVALUATION AND MANAGEMENT

Laboratory and radiologic evaluation are helpful adjuncts in the diagnosis of peritonitis and abdominal abscesses. General evaluation for inflammation through WBC count and CRP may be helpful, but negative test results do not rule out the diagnoses. Blood culture can be positive in about 75% of primary spontaneous peritonitis. Paracentesis can aid in supporting the diagnosis: WBC greater than 250/mm^3, total protein greater than 1 g/L, lactate greater than 25 mg/dL, and glucose less than 50 mg/dL. Fluid should be sent for bacterial, mycobacterial, and fungal cultures, especially in patients undergoing peritoneal dialysis. Radiologic studies are recommended to localize infection and to guide future surgical management. Plain films can reveal free peritoneal air from ruptured viscus. Ultrasound can aid in visualizing free fluid and can be used to guide paracentesis, but it is limited in visualizing all aspects of the abdomen. CT scans with oral and IV contrast provide the most detailed information about the abdominal cavity.

Management of patients with peritonitis targets the microbes believed to be involved. In primary peritonitis, therapy should be directed against *Streptococcus pneumoniae*; usually a third-generation cephalosporin; and in more life-threatening or VP shunt–associated infections, vancomycin can be added to cover *S. aureus* and penicillin-resistant *S. pneumoniae*. The duration of therapy is often 14 days. Aminoglycoside therapy should be added for secondary peritonitis in order to cover *P. aeruginosa*. Alternate regimens include ampicillin–sulbactam, ticarcillin–clavulanate, piperacillin–tazobactam, or carbapenems, which can be used especially if there is concern for drug-resistant nosocomial flora.

Surgical intervention in drainage of abscess formation is recommended to aid in narrowing antimicrobial coverage and more rapid resolution of abscesses.

SUGGESTED READINGS

Bundy DG, Byerley JS, Liles EA, et al: Does this child have appendicitis? *JAMA* 298(4):438-451, 2007.

Goldin AB, Sawin RS, Garrison MM, et al: Aminoglycoside-based triple-antibiotic therapy versus monotherapy for children with ruptured appendicitis, *Pediatrics* 119(5):905-911, 2007.

Gorelick MH, Shaw KN, Murphy KO: Validity and reliability of clinical signs in the diagnosis of dehydration in children, *Pediatrics* 99:E6, 1997.

Hartling L, Bellemare S, Wiebe N, et al: Oral versus intravenous rehydration for treating dehydration due to gastroenteritis in children. Cochrane Database Syst Rev 3:CD004390, 2006.

Kharbanda AB, Taylor GA, Bachur RG: Suspected appendicitis in children: rectal and intravenous contrast-enhanced versus intravenous contrast-enhanced CT, *Radiology* 243:520-526, 2007.

Kim JY: Peritonitis and intra-abdominal abscess. In *Pediatric Infectious Diseases: The Requisites in Pediatrics*, Philadelphia, 2008, Mosby Elsevier.

King CK, Glass R, Bresee JS, Duggan C; Centers for Disease Control and Prevention: Managing acute gastroenteritis among children: oral rehydration, maintenance, and nutritional therapy, *MMWR Morbid Mortal Wkly Rep* 21:52, 2003.

Pickering LK: *Red Book: 2006 Report of the Committee of Infectious Disease*, ed 27, Elk Grove Village, IL, 2006, American Academy of Pediatrics.

Steiner MJ, DeWalt DA, Byerley JS: Is this child dehydrated? *JAMA* 291(22):2746-2754, 2004.

Sundel ER: Abdominal pain and acute abdomen. In *Comprehensive Pediatric Hospital Medicine*, Philadelphia, 2007, Mosby Elsevier.

EPSTEIN-BARR VIRUS

Epstein-Barr virus (EBV) is a common virus: most people become infected sometime in their lives. The clinical syndrome frequently associated with EBV is infectious mononucleosis, or "mono." In socioeconomically disadvantaged areas, infants and children are most commonly affected, but adolescents are more commonly affected in affluent areas.

ETIOLOGY AND PATHOGENESIS

EBV is transmitted by oral secretions and sexual intercourse, thus requiring close contact for transmission. After infection, the virus is excreted for many months and then intermittently for life. The incubation period is usually 30 to 50 days. The virus most likely spreads from the epithelial cells of the buccal mucosa to B-lymphocytes and then disseminates to the entire lymphoreticular system, including the liver and spleen. Similar to other herpesviruses, EBV stays latent in the body for life. EBV has been associated with a spectrum of proliferative disorders such as hemophagocytic syndrome, nasopharyngeal carcinoma, Burkitt lymphoma, and lymphoproliferative disorders.

CLINICAL PRESENTATION

EBV infection causes a wide spectrum of clinical diseases. In many infants and young children, the symptoms are mild or unrecognized. The symptoms of infectious mononucleosis are malaise, fatigue, prolonged fever, sore throat, headache, nausea, and abdominal pain. Patients often have pharyngitis with exudates, lymphadenopathy, hepatomegaly, or splenomegaly. The incidence of dermatitis may be as high as 15% and is even more pronounced in children who were treated with ampicillin or amoxicillin; it is often called "ampicillin rash" (Figure 97-1). Rare complications of mononucleosis include airway obstruction, central nervous system (CNS) disorders, splenic rupture, thrombocytopenia, and hemolytic anemia.

EBV is also associated with Gianotti-Crosti syndrome in which a symmetric rash is seen on the cheeks, extensor surfaces, or buttocks with multiple erythematous papules, which may coalesce into plaques. This may persist for 15 to 50 days and may sometimes look like atopic dermatitis (see Figure 97-1).

DIFFERENTIAL DIAGNOSIS

Several other pathogens may cause a mononucleosis-like illness, including cytomegalovirus (CMV), adenovirus, hepatitis viruses, HIV, rubella, and *Toxoplasma gondii*. Another infection that causes a similar clinical picture is streptococcal pharyngitis; however, it usually is not associated with hepatosplenomegaly.

EVALUATION AND MANAGEMENT

In 90% of cases, there is leukocytosis of 10,000 to 20,000 cells/mm^3 with a predominance of lymphocytes with 20% to 40% atypical lymphocytes. There may be a mild thrombocytopenia but usually no purpura, and mild elevations of transaminases can occur. A nonspecific test for heterophile antibodies (also called Monospot) can be done. These are immunoglobulin M (IgM) antibodies that agglutinate sheep or horse red blood cells (RBCs) and usually appear during the first 2 weeks of illness and gradually disappear over a 6-month period. This test result is often negative in children younger than 4 years old. EBV can also be detected by serologic antibody testing. In the acute phase, there is a rapid immunoglobulin M (IgM) and IgG response to viral capsid antigen (VCA) and IgG to early antigen(EA). Positive Epstein-Barr virus nuclear antigen (EBNA) (nuclear antigen) antibody indicates past infection because this is not usually present until several weeks to months after infection (Table 97-1).

There is no specific treatment for infectious mononucleosis. Patients should not participate in contact sports until they have recovered or until the spleen normalizes. In severe cases with complications, a short course of corticosteroids may be helpful; however, there are no controlled data showing efficacy.

FUTURE DIRECTIONS

Further studies need to be done regarding the safety and efficacy of corticosteroids for treating complicated EBV infections. Research regarding treatment of EBV infections in immunocompromised patients is also needed. Investigations into associations between EBV, malignancies, and lymphoproliferative disorders will help elucidate these disease processes.

MEASLES

In the United States, the current rate of measles infection is less than one case per million people; however, historically, more than 90% of children were infected before the age of 15 years. This change is entirely attributable to the measles vaccine that was introduced in 1963. An outbreak that occurred between 1989 and 1991 resulted in 55,000 cases and prompted implementation of the two-dose vaccine. The majority of cases of measles are imported into the United States from abroad or are import related.

ETIOLOGY AND PATHOGENESIS

Measles is transmitted by direct contact with large droplets or small droplet aerosols that enter through the respiratory tract or conjunctivae. Patients are contagious 3 days before the rash

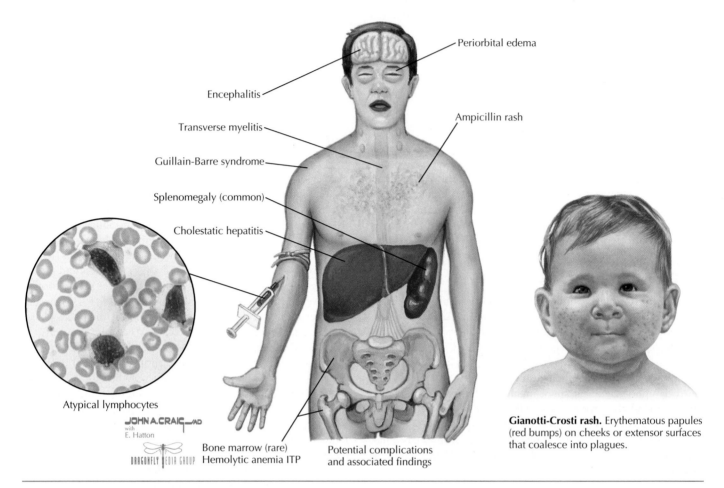

Figure 97-1 *Clinical presentation of Epstein-Barr virus.*

Labels on figure:
- Periorbital edema
- Encephalitis
- Transverse myelitis
- Guillain-Barre syndrome
- Ampicillin rash
- Splenomegaly (common)
- Cholestatic hepatitis
- Atypical lymphocytes
- Bone marrow (rare) Hemolytic anemia ITP
- Potential complications and associated findings
- **Gianotti-Crosti rash.** Erythematous papules (red bumps) on cheeks or extensor surfaces that coalesce into plagues.

JOHN A. CRAIG—AD
with
E. Hatton
DRAGONFLY MEDIA GROUP

and up to 4 to 6 days afterward. The incubation period is 8 to 12 days. It is very contagious and affects 90% of exposed individuals. The virus causes necrosis of epithelium and a small vessel vasculitis of skin and oral mucosa. Infected cells fuse and cause multinucleated giant cells called Warthin-Finkeldey giant cells that are pathognomonic for measles.

CLINICAL PRESENTATION

There are four phases to the infection: incubation period, prodrome, exanthem, and recovery. The prodrome period begins with a mild fever that increases to 103° to 105°F, conjunctivitis, coryza, and cough. Koplik spots appear 1 to 4 days

before the rash. They appear as red lesions with a bluish white spot in the center and are usually on the inner aspects of the cheek. Rash usually appears after 2 to 4 days and begins on the face as discrete erythematous patches and spreads downward often becoming confluent (Figure 97-2). Lesions are also seen on the palms and soles. Rash fades in about 7 days and may leave desquamation of the skin. Cough can last up to 10 days.

Complications include otitis media, pneumonia, laryngotracheobronchitis, seizures, and diarrhea. In rare cases, measles may cause acute encephalitis and subacute sclerosing panencephalitis (SSPE), a degeneration of the CNS usually occurring an average of 7 years later.

Table 97-1 EBV Antibodies in EBV Infection

Infection	Viral Capsid Antigen Immunoglobulin G	Viral Capsid Antigen Immunoglobulin M	Early Antigen	Epstein-Barr Virus Nuclear Antigen
No previous infection	−	−	−	−
Acute infection	+	+	+/−	−
Recent infection	+	+/−	+/−	+/−
Past infection	+	−	+/−	+

From Pickering LK: Red Book: 2006 Report of the Committee of Infectious Disease, ed 27. Elk Grove Village, IL, American Academy of Pediatrics.

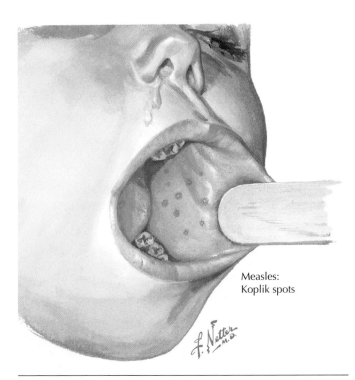

Measles:
Koplik spots

Figure 97-2 *Koplik spots.*

DIFFERENTIAL DIAGNOSIS

Measles may sometimes be confused with other viruses that cause exanthems such as rubella, adenovirus, enterovirus, EBV, human herpesvirus-6 (HHV-6), and parvovirus. *Mycoplasma pneumoniae* and group A streptococci (GAS) can also produce similar rashes. Several clinical findings are similar in Kawasaki's disease, but there is a more prominent cough and no thrombocytosis in measles. Drug reactions should also be in the differential diagnosis.

EVALUATION AND MANAGEMENT

The diagnosis of measles is usually clinical; however, laboratory findings can include decreased white blood cell count, and a normal erythrocyte sedimentation rate and C-reactive protein. IgM antibody can be detected 1 to 2 days after the onset of rash and remains for 1 month and is therefore indicative of acute infection. A fourfold increase in IgG antibodies after 2 to 4 weeks can also be diagnostic. There is no specific treatment for measles; however, low vitamin A levels are associated with increased morbidity and mortality. Therefore, vitamin A supplementation is recommended. No antibiotic prophylaxis is recommended.

PREVENTION

Vaccination is the best form of prevention. The first dose is recommended between 12 and 15 months followed by a second dose at 4 to 6 years of age. Because the vaccine is a live-attenuated vaccine, it should not be given to pregnant women or severely immunocompromised children. The MMR (mumps, measles, and rubella) vaccine can cause fever (6-12 days after), rash (7-12

days after) and rarely a transient thrombocytopenia. Fortunately, several large and well-designed scientific studies have convincingly shown that there is no evidence that the measles vaccine causes autism.

Postexposure prophylaxis can be administered via vaccine if it is less than 72 hours after exposure or immune globulin up to 6 days after exposure.

FUTURE DIRECTIONS

Continued educational efforts need to be undertaken to assure parents about the necessity and the safety of the measles vaccine. Preventing measles from becoming endemic again in the United States will require maintenance of a high level of immunity through vaccination. Eliminating measles from developing countries through vaccines remains a continuing effort.

HERPES SIMPLEX VIRUS

There are 2 types of herpes simplex virus (HSV), type 1 and type 2, that can cause a variety of illnesses depending on the host and the site of infection. A primary herpes infection occurs in those who have never been infected with either HSV-1 or HSV-2. A nonprimary first infection occurs when an individual who was previously infected with one type of HSV then becomes infected with another type. A recurrent infection is a reactivation of the virus from the latent state. HSV can also cause severe neonatal infection (see Chapter 105).

ETIOLOGY AND PATHOGENESIS

HSV is ubiquitous and is transmitted through direct contact with infected mucocutaneous surfaces. Even if a person is asymptomatic, the virus can be intermittently shed; however, the greatest concentration of virus is shed during symptomatic primary infections. Although HSV-1 is thought to infect oral mucosa and HSV-2 is thought to cause genital infections, either type can cause initial infections in any mucosa surface. However, HSV-1 is more likely to cause recurrent oral infections, and HSV-2 is more likely to cause recurrent genital infections.

The virus enters through mucosal surfaces and then spreads via nerve endings to sensory ganglia. Some viruses then establish latency in these sensory neurons (Figure 97-3). The incubation period is usually 2 days to 2 weeks.

CLINICAL PRESENTATION

The most common clinical manifestation of primary infection in children is gingivostomatitis and is usually caused by HSV-1. It causes sudden onset of pain in the mouth often manifested as refusal to eat, drooling, and high fevers. The gums become very swollen, and vesicles that are usually grouped on an erythematous base are seen throughout the oral cavity, including the gums, lips, tongue, palate, tonsils, and pharynx. The vesicles can progress to ulcers, and lymphadenopathy is often seen (see Figure 97-3). The illness usually resolves in 7 to 14 days.

Herpes labialis (common names include cold sores or fever blisters) is a common manifestation of recurrent HSV-1

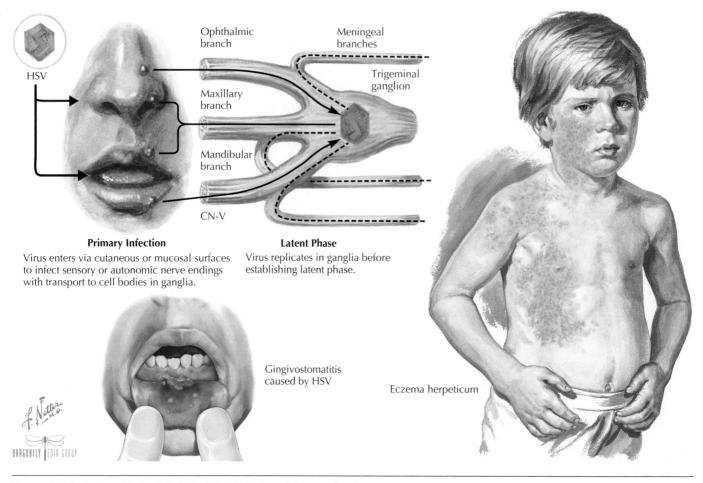

Figure 97-3 *Pathogenesis and clinical presentation of herpes simplex viruses.*

infections. Usually, a burning, tingling, itching sensation is felt several hours or days before the development of a herpetic lesion. It usually begins as a small grouping of erythematous papules that progress to small, thin-walled vesicles. The vesicles then form ulcers or become pustular. The most common site of infection is the vermillion border of the lip. Symptoms usually last 6 to 10 days.

HSV infections can occur on any skin surface that may have breakdown or trauma. *Herpetic whitlow* is a term used for HSV infections of the fingers or toes. Lesions and pain usually last for 10 days, and complete recovery usually occurs in 18 to 20 days. Eczema herpeticum is described in patients with a history of eczema who are superinfected with HSV (see Figure 97-3). In addition to severe rash, patients can present with high fevers, malaise, and lymphadenopathy. Other areas of the body that may be affected by HSV include the conjunctiva, cornea, and retina as well as the CNS, causing encephalitis and aseptic meningitis. Thus, any vesicles around the eyes should prompt an ophthalmologic examination. HSV has also been implicated in erythema multiforme and Bell's palsy.

DIFFERENTIAL DIAGNOSIS

When vesicular lesions are seen, the differential diagnosis should always include infections caused by varicella zoster (VZV). Gingivostomatitis can be confused with hand, foot, and mouth disease caused by coxsackievirus or other causes of pharyngitis such as GAS and infectious mononucleosis. Widespread eczema herpeticum can be confused with Stevens-Johnson syndrome.

EVALUATION AND MANAGEMENT

The diagnosis of HSV infection can be made by detection of viral antigen or viral DNA by polymerase chain reaction (PCR) as well as by viral culture obtained by vigorous rubbing of vesicular base. In HSV encephalitis, there is usually a pleocytosis with predominance of lymphocytes. Electroencephalography and magnetic resonance imaging may show temporal lobe abnormalities as well.

The treatment of HSV includes three antiviral medications, acyclovir, valacyclovir, and famciclovir. For gingivostomatitis, acyclovir started within 72 hours of onset reduces the severity and duration of illness. For herpes labialis, oral treatment can shorten duration of the episode and can also be used to prevent recurrences. Acyclovir has also been shown to be effective in the treatment of eczema herpeticum.

FUTURE DIRECTIONS

Further studies need to be conducted regarding the efficacy of acyclovir for prevention of recurrent HSV infections and treatment of various HSV infection. Currently, valacyclovir and famciclovir have not been approved by the Food and Drug Administration for use in children. If they are approved, alternatives to acyclovir will be available and may be more effective in the treatment of HSV infections in children.

VARICELLA ZOSTER VIRUS

VZV is a very contagious virus that causes chicken pox, and similar to other members of the family Herpesviridae, then remains latent in the body. It can be reactivated to cause herpes zoster or shingles. Before the vaccine was introduced in 1995, most children were infected by age 15 years. In healthy children, chicken pox is usually a mild disease, but there is a higher morbidity and mortality in adolescents, adults, infants, and immunocompromised individuals.

ETIOLOGY AND PATHOGENESIS

The virus is spread through direct contact with respiratory secretions or fluid of skin lesions as well as by airborne spread of respiratory secretions. The incubation period is 10 to 21 days after exposure. Patients are contagious 1 to 2 days before the onset of rash until all of the vesicles have crusted over. The virus then establishes a latent infection in the dorsal root ganglia.

CLINICAL PRESENTATION

Chicken pox is characterized by fever, malaise, anorexia, headache, and a classic rash that starts centrally and then spreads outward. The rash begins as erythematous macules that then become very pruritic and vesicular. It is often described as a "dew drop on a rose petal" (Figure 97-4). Crusting of the lesions then occurs as new ones arise, resulting in different stages of rash. A child who has been previously vaccinated but infected with VZV may have "breakthrough varicella" in which the rash is more atypical. The rash may be maculopapular and less vesicular with fewer lesions. Severe neonatal chicken pox can develop if a mother develops the disease 5 days before delivery or 2 days after.

Complications of varicella include bacterial superinfections of the skin, thrombocytopenia, arthritis, hepatitis, cerebellar ataxia, encephalitis, meningitis, and glomerulonephritis. These complications are more common in adolescents, adults, infants, and immunocompromised patients. The reactivation of latent VZV causes zoster or shingles and manifests as grouped vesicles within one or two dermatomes (see Figure 97-4). Although the lesions can cause intense pain in adults, children commonly have a mild rash with minimal symptoms that usually resolve in 1 to 2 weeks.

DIFFERENTIAL DIAGNOSIS

The differential diagnosis of varicella includes HSV and enterovirus caused by the vesicular lesions. It can often be confused with drug reactions, contact dermatitis, and insect bites.

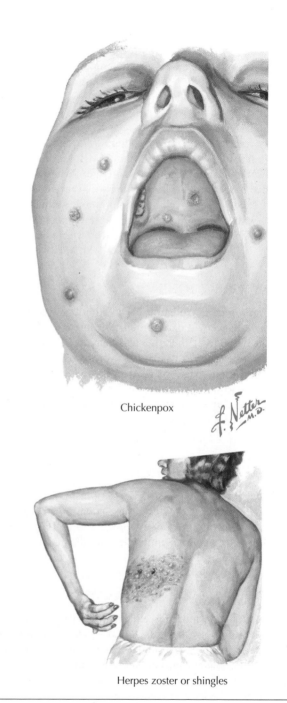

Chickenpox

Herpes zoster or shingles

Figure 97-4 *Clinical presentations of varicella zoster virus.*

EVALUATION AND MANAGEMENT

The diagnosis of VZV can be confirmed using direct fluorescence antigen or PCR. Viral cultures can also be done from tissue sample in 3 to 4 days. A fourfold increase in VZV IgG titer can also be confirmatory. There is usually an initial leukopenia and then a lymphocytosis. In most cases, the liver enzymes are slightly elevated.

Acyclovir can be used to treat varicella infections but is not currently recommended in healthy children. It can be given to adolescents, children older than 12 months old with skin or pulmonary disorders and children receiving chronic salicylates or corticosteroids. Treatment should be started within 72 hours of onset of rash and as soon as possible. Intravenous (IV) acyclovir should be used in any complicated or disseminated cases.

PREVENTION

A varicella vaccine was introduced in 1995 and is currently recommended to be given with the MMR vaccine at 12 to 18 months and again at 4 to 6 years of age. Postexposure prophylaxis can be given to healthy children via vaccine within 3 to 5 days of exposure. Varicella zoster immune globulin can be given as postexposure prophylaxis to immunocompromised children, pregnant women, and newborns within 96 hours of exposure.

FUTURE DIRECTIONS

With the new recommendation for an additional vaccine dose, further surveillance will determine if this increases the efficacy of the vaccine and whether this will increase the incidence of herpes zoster. Because of the atypical presentation of varicella after immunization, diagnosis will rely more heavily on laboratory tests. As with HSV, approval for use of famciclovir and valacyclovir in children may provide alternatives for the treatment of varicella infections.

HUMAN HERPESVIRUS 6

Primary infection with HHV-6 causes nonspecific febrile illnesses as well as roseola (or exanthem subitum, sixth disease). There is a low rate of infection before 6 months of age because of the presence of maternal antibodies, but the majority of children are infected by 2 years of age.

ETIOLOGY AND PATHOGENESIS

HHV-6 is likely transmitted to children via asymptomatic shedding in the secretions (such as saliva) of close contacts. The incubation period is 9 to 10 days. After primary infection, HHV-6 becomes latent in peripheral blood mononuclear cells and persists in salivary glands as well as possibly other tissues such as kidneys, lungs, and CNS.

CLINICAL PRESENTATION

Roseola is characterized by high fever (usually >103°F) that may persist for 3 to 7 days. During this time some infants may be irritable and anorexic, usually without upper respiratory tract infections. Febrile seizure can occur in 10% to 15% of patients. A rose-colored maculopapular rash usually develops on the trunk during defervescence, spreads to the extremities and face, and then fades after 1 to 3 days (Figure 97-5). HHV-6 can also cause nonspecific febrile illnesses without rash accompanied by cervical or post-occipital lymphadenopathy, respiratory or gastrointestinal (GI) symptoms and inflamed tympanic membranes. It is also thought that HHV-6 reactivation may contribute to disease in the immunocompromised host.

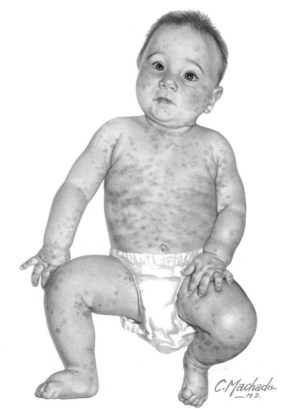

Rose-colored maculopapular rash seen in roseola.

Figure 97-5 *Roseola.*

DIFFERENTIAL DIAGNOSIS

Other illnesses causing fever and rash should be considered, including rubella, measles, scarlet fever, and drug hypersensitivity. If children are very irritable, meningitis and encephalitis need to be ruled out.

EVALUATION AND MANAGEMENT

The diagnosis is usually made clinically but can be confirmed by PCR or serology from the serum. IgM antibodies usually develop on day 5 to 7 of illness and resolves in 2 months, but it can persist in 5% of healthy adults. A fourfold increase in IgG antibody titer can also be used. Plasma PCR has a sensitivity and specificity of 90% and 100%, respectively, for the diagnosis of primary HHV-6 infection in immunocompetent children. There is no recommended antiviral treatment for healthy children except for supportive needs.

FUTURE DIRECTIONS

HHV-6 has been associated with multiple sclerosis, encephalitis in AIDS, glove and sock syndrome (a benign dermatosis), Gianotti-Crosti syndrome, and pityriasis rosea, but more work is required in these areas. Because of the persistence of the virus, current diagnostic tests cannot differentiate between primary versus reactivation versus latent infection; thus, more research is needed in this area. Currently, ganciclovir and cidofovir are used in the treatment of immunocompromised patients with severe disease. Additional research is needed to determine the most effective antiviral therapy in this population.

PARVOVIRUS B19

Parvovirus B19 is the cause of erythema infectiosum or fifth disease, which is most notable for its characteristic "slapped cheek" appearance. Most clinically significant infections occur between the ages of 5 to 15 years of age. By young adulthood, approximately 50% of people are infected.

ETIOLOGY AND PATHOGENESIS

Parvovirus B19 is transmitted by contact with respiratory tract secretions via large droplets from nasopharyngeal viral shedding. Its primary target is the erythroid cell line, leading to progressive depletion of erythroid precursors and a brief decline in erythropoiesis. The incubation period is 4 to 28 days. Children with rash or arthralgia are not considered to be infectious because this usually occurs after viremia. However, individuals with aplastic crisis are considered to be infectious. Populations that are at risk for developing complications secondary to parvovirus infection include those with hematologic disease, immunosuppressed patients, and pregnant women.

CLINICAL PRESENTATION

Erythema infectiosum usually causes fever, malaise, and rhinorrhea during viral shedding, which precedes the distinctive "slapped cheek" facial rash by 7 to 10 days. A maculopapular lacy or reticular rash, often pruritic, can also appear on the trunk and move peripherally. Arthralgia and arthritis occur much less commonly in children than in adults (10% vs. 60%, respectively). Parvovirus can also cause mild respiratory illnesses with no rash or other types of rashes. Patients with hemoglobinopathies or other anemias that depend on reticulocytosis may develop transient aplastic crisis because of cessation of RBC production. They may present with symptoms of severe anemia, including pallor, tachycardia, and lethargy. Parvovirus B19 has also been found to be a cause of nonimmune hydrops fetalis.

DIFFERENTIAL DIAGNOSIS

The differential diagnosis includes rubella, measles, enterovirus infections, and drug reactions. In children with arthritis or arthralgia juvenile rheumatoid arthritis, systemic lupus erythematosus (SLE), serum sickness may be considered.

EVALUATION AND MANAGEMENT

The diagnosis of parvovirus can be confirmed using serologic testing. In an immunocompetent host, diagnosis using IgM antibody is preferred because it can usually be detected by the third day of illness and persists for 6 to 8 weeks. PCR can detect parvovirus in serum for 9 months and thus may not indicate acute infection. However, PCR testing is recommended for detection in immunocompromised patients who may have chronic infections.

The treatment for parvovirus is often supportive, although patients with aplastic crisis may require RBC transfusions. Immunocompromised patients who are at risk for complications can be treated with IV immunoglobulin.

FUTURE DIRECTIONS

There are ongoing studies linking parvovirus B19 to rheumatologic disorders such as SLE and juvenile idiopathic arthritis. Screening for B19 in blood products may help to prevent complications in immunocompromised children, but currently there is insufficient evidence to recommend universal testing.

ENTEROVIRUS (NONPOLIOVIRUS)

Nonpolio enterovirus infections are caused by several viral agents, including coxsackieviruses, echoviruses, and several types of enteroviruses. They cause a broad range of illnesses, including herpangina, hand, foot, and mouth disease , conjunctivitis, and myocarditis. They are more common during the summer and early fall and thus are often called "summer viruses."

ETIOLOGY AND PATHOGENESIS

Enteroviruses are spread by fecal-oral and respiratory routes. They may survive on surfaces for periods of time and thus may be transmitted via fomites. The incubation period is 3-10 days. Virus can be shed in the respiratory tract for 1 to 3 weeks but fecal viral shedding can occur for 7 to 11 weeks. There may be 2 stages of viremia and thus a biphasic pattern can be seen.

CLINICAL PRESENTATION

Enterovirus can cause nonspecific febrile illnesses, which may present as fevers (101°-104°F), malaise, irritability, diarrhea, vomiting, rash, sore throat, or respiratory symptoms. Illness usually lasts for 3 days but can last longer than 1 week. A biphasic pattern may be seen with initial fever for 1 day followed by 2 to 3 days of normal temperatures and recurrence of fever. Rashes vary from maculopapular to urticarial, vesicular, or petechial.

A common manifestation in children is hand, foot, and mouth disease in which children usually have fever, oropharyngeal inflammation, and vesicles with an erythematous ring in the oral cavity usually on the tongue, buccal mucosa, and posterior soft palate. The vesicles can ulcerate and cause anorexia. Often there is also a maculopapular, vesicular, or pustular lesion on the palms, soles, hands, feet, and occasionally buttock and groin (Figure 97-6).

Herpangina is another common condition caused by enteroviruses. It is characterized by high fevers (to 106°F), sore throat, dysphagia, and lesions in the oral cavity that are usually discrete, 1- to 2-mm vesicles and ulcers with an erythematous ring. These are typically seen on the anterior tonsillar pillars, soft palate, and posterior pharynx.

The leading cause of aseptic meningitis is nonpolio enterovirus. Less commonly, enterovirus can also cause a number of other illnesses in the respiratory, cardiac, neurologic, and GI systems as well as severe neonatal multisystemic disease.

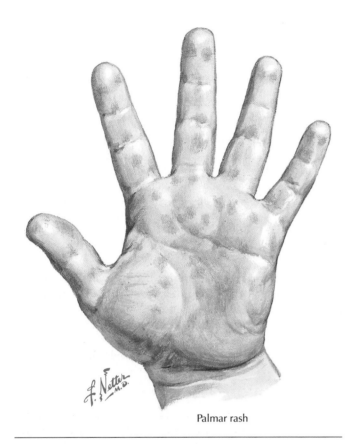

Palmar rash

Figure 97-6 *Hand, foot, and mouth disease.*

DIFFERENTIAL DIAGNOSIS

The differential diagnosis depends on the clinical presentation, but when exanthems are seen, other infectious agents to consider are GAS, *Staphylococcus aureus*, HSV, adenovirus, VZV, EBV, measles, rubella, and HHV-6 or -7.

EVALUATION AND MANAGEMENT

Viral culture or PCR can be done from throat, stool, rectal swab, urine, blood, and cerebrospinal fluid. However, because of long-term shedding of the virus in stool, detection in stool may not indicate acute infection. There is no specific treatment for enterovirus infections, although immune globulin may be used in neonates or immunodeficient patients with severe disease. An antiviral agent called Pleconaril is under evaluation.

FUTURE DIRECTIONS

More studies need to be done to determine the efficacy of immunoglobulin and other antiviral therapies such as Pleconaril for the treatment of nonpolio enterovirus infections.

SUGGESTED READING

Epstein-Barr Virus

Candy B, Hotopf M: Steroids for symptom control in infectious mononucleosis. Cochrane Database Syst Rev 3:CD004402, 2006.

Junker A: Epstein-Barr virus, *Pediatr Rev* 26:79-85, 2005.

Measles

Caldararo S: Measles, *Pediatr Rev* 28:352-354, 2007.

Gerber JS, Offit PA: Vaccines and autism: a tale of shifting hypotheses, *Clin Infect Dis* 48:456-461, 2009.

Papania MJ, Seward JF, Redd SB, et al: Epidemiology of measles in the United States, 1997-2001, *J Infect Dis* 189(Suppl):S61-S68, 2004.

Perry RT, Halsey NA: The clinical significance of measles: a review, *J Infect Dis* 189(Suppl 1):S4-S16, 2004.

Herpes Simplex Virus

Chayavichitsilp P, Buckwalter JV, Krakowski AC, Friedlander SF: Herpes simplex, *Pediatr Rev* 30:110-130, 2009.

Elbers JM, Bitnun A, Richardson SE, et al: A 12 year prospective study of childhood herpes simplex encephalitis: is there a broader spectrum of disease? *Pediatrics* 119:e399-e407, 2007.

Nasser M, Fedorowicz Z, Khoshnevisan MH, et al: Acyclovir for treating primary herpetic gingivostomatitis. Cochrane Database Syst Rev 4: CD006700, 2008.

Varicella Zoster Virus

Gershon AA: Varicella zoster virus infections, *Pediatr Rev* 29:5-11, 2008.

Macartney D, McIntyre P: Vaccines for post-exposure prophylaxis against varicella in children and adults. Cochrane Database System Rev 3:CD001833, 2008.

Nguyen HQ, Jumaan AO, Seward JF: Decline in mortality due to varicella after implementation of varicella vaccination in the United States. *N Engl J Med* 352:450-458, CD001833.

Human Herpes Virus 6

Araujo TD, Berman B: Human herpesviruses 6 and 7, *Dermatol Clin* 20:301-306, 2000.

Caserta MT, Mock DJ, Dewhurst S: Human herpesvirus 6, *Clin Infect Dis* 33:829-833, 2001.

Campadelli-Fiume G, Mirandola P: Human herpesvirus 6: an emerging pathogen, *Emerg Infect Dis* 5:353-366, 1999.

Koch WC: Fifth (human parvovirus) and sixth (herpesvirus 6) diseases, *Curr Opin Infect Dis* 14:343-356, 2001.

Parvovirus B19

Katta R: Parvovirus B19: a review, *Dermatol Clin* 20:333-342, 2002.

Koch WC: Fifth (human parvovirus) and sixth (herpesvirus 6) diseases, *Curr Opin Infect Dis* 14:343-356, 2001.

Smith-Whitley K, Zhao H, Hodinka RL, et al: Epidemiology of human parvovirus B19 in children with sickle cell disease, *Blood* 103:422-427, 2004.

Nonpolio Enterovirus

Stalkup JR, Chiluduri S: Enterovirus infections: a review of clinical presentation, diagnosis, and treatment, *Dermatol Clin* 20:217-223, 2002.

Zaoutis T, Klein JD: Enterovirus Infection, *Pediatr Rev* 19:183-191, 1998.

All Viruses

Pickering LK: *Red Book: 2006 Report of the Committee on Infectious Disease*, ed 27, Elk Grove Village, IL, 2006, American Academy of Pediatrics.

Fungal Infections

98

Melissa Mondello and Jason Y. Kim

Fungi are one of the four major groups of infectious organisms, along with viruses, bacteria, and parasites. They are divided into two morphologic forms, yeasts and molds. Yeasts are unicellular organisms, usually round or oval in shape, that reproduce by budding. In contrast, molds are multicellular organisms composed of hyphae, or tubular structures that grow by extension or branching. Fungi that grow as yeast and mold forms are termed *dimorphic fungi*. Molds also grow by spore formation. In addition to morphologic characteristics, biochemical and molecular assays of fungi are used in laboratory diagnosis to help identify genus and species.

The extent of disease caused by fungal exposure is related to a number of factors, including fungal virulence, inoculum size, and most importantly, the host immune system. The majority of clinically significant fungal infections occur in patients whose defense against infection is either compromised or immature. Dermatophytic infections are an exception and occur in healthy children. Examples of host defense compromise include breaches to the normal skin defenses, such as burns or central catheters, children with decreased neutrophil number (chemotherapy) or function (chronic granulomatous disease), and defects in T-cell functioning (severe combined immunodeficiency or HIV/AIDS). Premature infants comprise another group with increased risk of fungal infections, especially those weighing less than 1000 g because of immature immune function and the complexity of their care, often requiring medical devices.

This chapter discusses the three most clinically significant fungi in childhood—*Candida albicans*, *Aspergillus fumigatus*, and *Cryptococcus neoformans*. Each section contains a brief description of the pathogen, clinical manifestations in the immune competent and immune compromised host, diagnosis, and treatment. Finally, there is a discussion of common dermatophytic infections.

CANDIDA ALBICANS

Candida spp. are yeasts that are ubiquitous in the environment. *C. albicans*, the most common species causing disease in children, is a dimorphic fungus that can be grown in both yeast and hyphal forms, which aids its ability to survive in varied environments, including host tissues. Other species isolated from children include *Candida tropicalis*, *Candida parapsilosis*, *Candida glabrata*, *Candida krusei*, and *Candida guilliermondii*. Nearly 60% of individuals can be colonized with *C. albicans* without symptoms, most commonly in the vaginal and gastrointestinal (GI) tracts. Pregnancy, a state of relative immune compromise, increases the vaginal colonization rate from less than 20% to greater than 30%. Approximately 10% of full-term infants become colonized in the GI and respiratory tracts in the first 5 days of life. The incidence of colonization of infants weighing less than 1500 g can be as high as 30%. Newborn infants can acquire the organism during passage through the birth canal or postnatally. Some forms of locally invasive candidiasis can be found in immune competent children, including vulvovaginitis, laryngeal candidiasis, and chronic draining otitis externa, but usually in the presence of systemic antibiotics. Systemic candidiasis is limited to immune compromised children, including those who are premature.

CLINICAL MANIFESTATIONS AND MANAGEMENT

Oral candidiasis, also known as oral thrush, is a candidal infection of the oral-pharyngeal mucosa (Figure 98-1). It can affect up to 2% to 5% of otherwise healthy newborn infants and present as early as 7 to 10 days of life. In immunocompetent children, it is most common in infants and presents as adherent white plaques on the buccal or gingival mucosa. Removal of these plaques can result in localized bleeding. It can present with no symptoms or with increased fussiness and decreased feeding. Oral thrush is uncommon in children older than 12 months except after antibiotic use. Without recent antibiotic use, one may consider a primary immunodeficiency, diabetes mellitus, or HIV infection. Pseudomembranous candidiasis can be diagnosed clinically or by the identification of yeast cells and pseudohyphae by Gram stain or potassium hydroxide prep. Thrush can be treated with nystatin applied directly to the oral mucosa for 7 to 10 days. Thrush caused by antibiotic use generally resolves as the offending agent is discontinued. Bottle nipples and pacifiers should be sterilized as well to prevent reinfection.

Candidal diaper dermatitis is characterized as beefy red plaques with satellite papules and pustules. It can affect the entire diaper area with a predilection for skin folds unlike other forms of diaper dermatitis. The treatment is with topical nystatin, clotrimazole, or miconazole.

Vulvovaginitis is a locally invasive candidal infection seen most often in postpubertal women and can affect up to 75% of women at some point during their lifetime. Risk factors for presentation at a younger age include systemic antibiotic use, diaper use, diabetes, and immune deficiency. Vulvovaginitis presents as a non-odorous white discharge, classically described as "cottage cheese," from the vagina with associated dysuria, vulvar burning, and pruritus. First-line therapy is generally topical therapy as in diaper dermatitis or systemic fluconazole for recurrent or refractory cases.

Candidal infections in the immunocompromised host can vary from superficial mucocutaneous infections to life-threatening systemic infections. The most serious fungal infection is disseminated candidiasis, in which the organism spreads hematogenously to tissues throughout the body, including the eyes, kidney, bones, meninges, lungs, spleen, or heart valves. Mortality can be as high as 47%. Risk factors include exposure to broad-spectrum antibiotics, central venous catheters, parenteral nutrition, renal replacement therapy in the intensive care

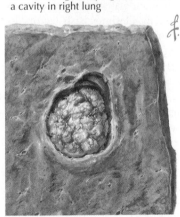

Reprinted with permission from Mandel G (ed): *Essential Atlas of Infectious Diseases*, 2nd Edition., Philadelphia, LWW, 2002, p27.

Figure 98-1 *Pseudomembranous candidiasis of the palate.*

unit, neutropenia, immunosuppression, and prosthetic devices. *Candida* spp. are the fourth leading cause of nosocomial bloodstream infections. Diagnosis requires culturing *Candida* spp. from blood or other sterile body fluids. Recommended treatment of systemic candidiasis includes lipid formulation amphotericin B, caspofungin, or fluconazole with the duration of therapy

determined by the extent of disease and response to therapy. Fluconazole may be added for better penetration into the central nervous system. Prophylactic antifungal medication is recommended in two groups of patients—bone marrow transplant recipients and solid organ transplant recipients because of their prolonged neutropenia and immunosuppression.

ASPERGILLUS FUMIGATUS

Aspergillus is a mycelial fungus, ubiquitous in the environment found in the soil and on decaying plants. *A. fumigatus* is the most common species isolated clinically, followed by *Aspergillus flavus*. Exposure occurs commonly by inhalation of conidia (spores); however inhalation of contaminated aerosols and direct inoculation of skin also occur. Some estimate that most people inhale hundreds of *A. fumigatus* conidia per day. Once inhaled *Aspergillus* can colonize the upper and lower respiratory tract. In an immune competent host, macrophages and neutrophils prevent the development of invasive disease. Immunocompromised children are at risk for invasive respiratory disease and for hematogenous dissemination. Invasive aspergillosis in an otherwise healthy child with no known risk factors should prompt an evaluation for chronic granulomatous disease. *Aspergillus*-related diseases may be hypersensitivity (IgE) mediated, saprophytic (noninvasive), or invasive (Figure 98-2).

Film showing an aspergilloma within a cavity in right lung

Film of same patient as shown at *left*, in left lateral decubitus position, demonstrating shift of fungus ball to dependent portion of cavity

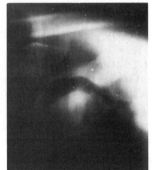

Tomogram of an aspergilloma within a cavity in left upper lobe, demonstrating characteristic radiolucent crescent above fungus ball

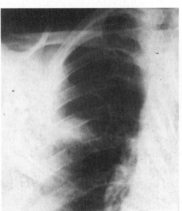

Gross appearance of an aspergilloma in a chronic lung cavity

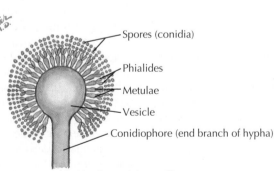

Spores (conidia)

Phialides

Metulae

Vesicle

Conidiophore (end branch of hypha)

Structure of fruiting form of *Aspergillus niger*. Other species of *Aspergillus* vary in configuration, but their general structure is similar

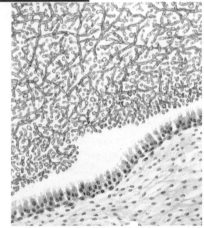

Microscopic structure of an aspergilloma composed of a tangled mass of hyphae within a dilated bronchus. No evidence of tissue invasion

Figure 98-2 *Aspergillosis.*

CLINICAL PRESENTATION AND MANAGEMENT

IgE-Mediated Aspergillus Disease

Allergic bronchopulmonary Aspergillosis (ABPA) is a hypersensitivity reaction to *Aspergillus*. It occurs most commonly in chronic asthmatics (1% to 2%) or cystic fibrosis patients (1% to 15%). Chronic mucosal colonization produces an exaggerated IgE and IgG response, which results in recurrent bronchospasm and transient pulmonary infiltrates. Diagnosis requires reversible episodic bronchial obstruction; immediate scratch test reactivity to *A. fumigatus* antigens, elevated total serum IgE, peripheral blood eosinophilia, precipitating IgG serum antibodies to *A. fumigatus*, and central bronchiectasis. Treatment includes systemic anti-inflammatory medication and bronchodilators.

Saprophytic Aspergillus infection

Cutaneous Aspergillus: Can be classified as primary—inoculated at sites of injury, or secondary—extension or hematologic seeding. It is most commonly found in immune compromised hosts. Proposed mechanisms for primary infection include sites of catheter insertion, burns, wounds, occlusive dressings (tape), or surgery. Neonates are also at increased risk. Cutaneous Aspergillus can present as a tender erythematous plaque and progress to necrotic eschars or ecthyma gangrenosum. Treatment involves systemic anti-fungal therapy and depending on the extent and depth of the lesion, surgical debridement.

Aspergilloma

Aspergillomas, or "fungal balls," may develop in pre-existing cavities or bronchogenic cysts without extension into the surrounding tissue. Aspergillomas complicate up to 2% of the cases of pulmonary tuberculosis with residual cavities greater than 2.5 cm. Other predisposing conditions include congenital heart disease, bronchiectasis, and congenital pulmonary cysts. Children are often asymptomatic. Definitive treatment is surgical resection of the affected lobe.

Invasive Aspergillosis

Risk factors include prolonged neutropenia, graft versus host disease, and impaired phagocytic function (chronic granulomatous disease, immunosuppressive therapy, corticosteroids). Invasive pulmonary aspergillosis is the most common form in immune compromised hosts. Other sites of infection include sinuses, brain, and skin. Less commonly affected are the heart, bones, meninges, eye, or esophagus. Aspergillus causes damage by hyphal infiltration of vascular structures with resultant thrombosis with infarction and necrosis of tissues and dissemination to distant sites. Occasionally vascular destruction results in massive hemorrhage. Pulmonary aspergillosis can present with acute onset fever, cough, dyspnea, and abnormal chest imaging. Diagnosis by bronchial culture is complicated by the presence of airborne spores. Chest radiography or CT scan may show a halo sign or air crescent sign. First-line treatment for invasive aspergillosis is amphotericin B or voriconazole. Voriconazole is preferred for treatment of pulmonary and extrapulmonary invasive aspergillosis. Treatment is continued for at least 12 weeks or until resolution of disease.

CRYPTOCOCCUS NEOFORMANS

Cryptococcus is an encapsulated yeast. *C. neoformans* is the most common form worldwide. It is found in temperate climates in soil contaminated by certain bird droppings. It may also be found on some fruits and vegetables and carried on cockroaches. It grows best at 37 degrees Celsius. Humans come in contact by inhalation of fungal spores.

CLINICAL PRESENTATION AND MANAGEMENT

Pneumonia is the most common form of cryptococcosus and may be asymptomatic in up to one third of immune competent hosts. Symptoms may include fever, pleuritic chest pain, and constitutional symptoms. Chest radiograph may show diffuse interstitial infiltrates and hilar lymphadenopathy (Figure 98-3). Dissemination following pulmonary disease is uncommon except where there is a deficiency in cell mediated immunity—HIV, leukemia, SLE, congenital immunodeficiency, chronic cutaneous candidiasis. HIV infection is the most common immune compromised state for Cryptococcal infection. In addition, Cryptococcus is an AIDS defining infection in HIV patients.

Subacute or chronic meningitis is the most common manifestation of disseminated Cryptococcus and may present only as behavioral change or may present with fever and headache (see Figure 98-3). Signs of increased intracranial pressure are also common and may be life threatening. Focal neurologic signs are present in less than 10%. Classically diagnosis was made by staining CSH with India Ink where encapsulated yeast may be visualized. More recently diagnosis is enhanced by latex agglutination testing for cryptococcal antigen. Treatment of Cryptococcus depends on the status of the host and on the site of infection. Asymptomatic, immune competent hosts may be watched closely or treated with fluconazole daily for 3-12 months. Those with symptomatic or disseminated disease are treated initially with amphotericin B and fluconazole for 2-10 weeks depending on clinical response, then with single therapy with fluconazole for 6-12 months. Children with HIV who complete initial therapy for Cryptococcus should remain on lifelong suppressive therapy with fluconazole.

COMMON TINEA INFECTIONS

Tinea is a superficial infection of the hair, skin, or nails caused by dermatophytic fungi. They invade the stratum corneum layer of the skin and feed on keratin within the skin. There are three genera of dermatophytes that cause infection—Trichophyton, Epidermophyton, and Microsporum—and about 28 species within those genera. Specific organisms tend to cause disease in different body sites. The specific condition is often named by the body site involved.

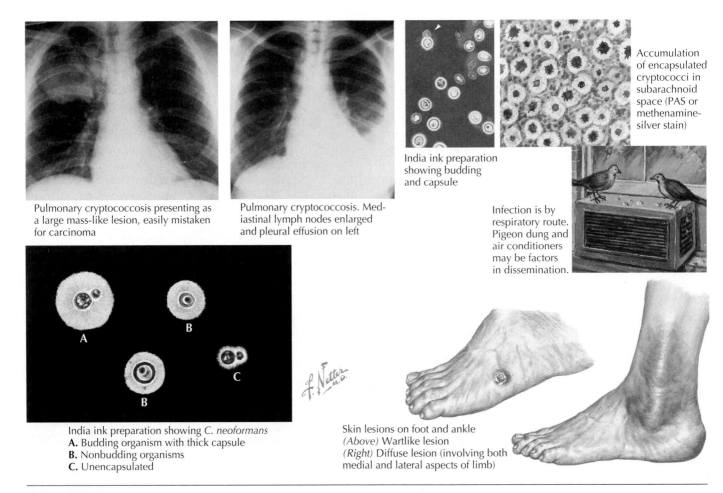

Pulmonary cryptococcosis presenting as a large mass-like lesion, easily mistaken for carcinoma

Pulmonary cryptococcosis. Mediastinal lymph nodes enlarged and pleural effusion on left

India ink preparation showing budding and capsule

Accumulation of encapsulated cryptococci in subarachnoid space (PAS or methenamine-silver stain)

Infection is by respiratory route. Pigeon dung and air conditioners may be factors in dissemination.

India ink preparation showing *C. neoformans*
A. Budding organism with thick capsule
B. Nonbudding organisms
C. Unencapsulated

Skin lesions on foot and ankle
(*Above*) Wartlike lesion
(*Right*) Diffuse lesion (involving both medial and lateral aspects of limb)

Figure 98-3 *Cryptococcus.*

TINEA CAPITIS

Tinea capitis is a dermatophyte infection of the scalp and hair shafts. It is most common in kids younger than 10 with peak occurrence at 3-7 years. The predominant organism causing disease is *Trichophyton tonsurans* in the United States. Infection is spread by infective spores. In addition to direct person-to-person contact, infective spores have been cultured from hairbrushes, clothing, and other inanimate objects. Asymptomatic carries are common and can also perpetuate disease.

Tinea capitis may present in many ways including diffuse scaling, diffuse pustule formation, patchy hair loss, black dot (well-demarcated areas of hair loss with short broken hairs), or with kerion formation (an inflammatory lesion with edematous, boggy swelling). Posterior cervical and suboccipital lymphadenopathy is also common. Topical treatment is not effective as topical medicines do not effectively penetrate the hair shaft. First-line systemic therapy includes griseofulvin for at least 8 weeks. Absorption is improved if taken with fatty foods.

TINEA CORPORIS (RINGWORM)

Tinea corporis is a dermatophyte infection of the glabrous (smooth and hairless) skin. The lesion is typically well demarcated, circular, and slightly erythematous, with a scaly, pustular, or vesicular border and is often pruritic (Figure 98-4). The main causative agents include *Trichophyton rubrum*, *Trichophyton mentagrophytes*, *Trichophyton tonsurans*, *Microsporum canis*, and *Epidermophyton floccosum*. Treatment of tinea corporis is topical with medication applied to the skin at least 2 cm beyond the border of the lesion once or twice daily (depending on the antifungal) for 2 weeks. Persistence of the lesion after 4 weeks of therapy indicates treatment failure and may require systemic therapy. Common topical antifungal therapy for tinea corporis includes miconazole, clotrimazole, terbinafine, ketoconazole, and econazole.

OTHER, LESS COMMON TINEA INFECTIONS

Tinea pedis: Tinea pedis is a superficial infection of the feet, often known as athlete's foot. It often presents with pruritic vesiculopustular or vesicular lesions with associated fissuring and scaling between the toes (Figure 98-5). Tinea pedis may also present in a moccasin distribution with hyperkeratotic scales involving the soles and lateral feet. Treatment is topical. Toenails may be affected (tinea unguium) and require systemic therapy.

Tinea cruris: Tinea infection of the groin and upper thighs, often known as jock itch. Affected skin is erythematous and scaly

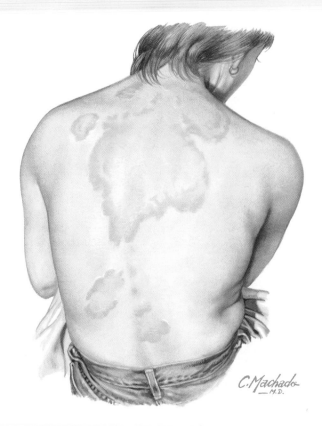

Figure 98-4 *Tinea corporis.*

The two most common forms of tinea pedis are interdigital and moccasin.

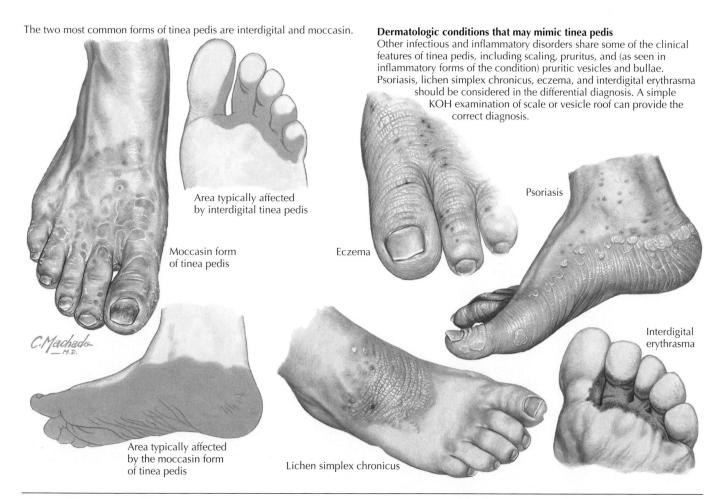

Area typically affected
by interdigital tinea pedis

Moccasin form
of tinea pedis

Area typically affected
by the moccasin form
of tinea pedis

Dermatologic conditions that may mimic tinea pedis
Other infectious and inflammatory disorders share some of the clinical features of tinea pedis, including scaling, pruritus, and (as seen in inflammatory forms of the condition) pruritic vesicles and bullae. Psoriasis, lichen simplex chronicus, eczema, and interdigital erythrasma should be considered in the differential diagnosis. A simple KOH examination of scale or vesicle roof can provide the correct diagnosis.

Psoriasis

Eczema

Interdigital
erythrasma

Lichen simplex chronicus

Figure 98-5 *Tinea pedis.*

with usual bilateral distribution. Tinea cruris is occasionally associated with central clearing and papulovesicular border and is often pruritic. Treatment is twice daily topical antifungal application for 4-6 weeks.

SUGGESTED READINGS

Burgos A, Zaoutis TE, Dvorak CC, et al: Pediatric invasive Aspergillosis: a multicenter retrospective analysis of 139 contemporary cases, *Pediatrics* 121(5):e1286-e1293, 2008.

Committee on Infectious Diseases American Academy of Pediatrics: *Red Book*, ed 27, 2006, American Academy of Pediatrics.

Gershon A, Hotez P, Katz S: *Krugman's Infectious Diseases of Children*, ed 11, St. Louis, 2003, Mosby.

Jeong YJ, Kim KI, Seo IJ, et al: Eosinophilic lung diseases: a clinical, radiologic, and pathologic overview, *RadioGraphics* 27:617-630, 2007.

Kliegman RM, Behrman RE, Jenson HB, Stanton B: *Nelson Textbook of Pediatrics*, ed 18, Philadelphia, 2007, Saunders.

Kokotos F, Henry A: Vulvovaginitis, *Pediatr Rev* 27:116-117, 2006.

Krol D, Keels MA: Oral conditions, *Pediatr Rev* 28(1):15-21, 2005.

Long S, Pickering L, Prober C: *Principles and Practices of Infectious Disease*, ed 3, St. Louis, 2008, Elsevier.

Pappas PG, Kauffman CA, Andes D, et al: Infectious Diseases Society of America: Clinical practice guidelines for the treatment of candidiasis: 2009 update by the Infectious Diseases Society of America, *Clin Infect Dis* 48:503-535, 2009.

Shy R: Tinea corporis and tinea capitis, *Pediatr Rev* 28(5):164-173, 2007.

Parasitic Infections

99

Jennifer J. Wilkes and Jason Y. Kim

*P*arasitic disease causes extensive morbidity and mortality worldwide in children, particularly *Plasmodium falciparum*, which causes 1 to 2.7 million deaths annually. The morbidity of parasitic disease disproportionately affects the developing world with an estimated 39 million disability-adjusted life years attributable to infections with parasitic worms. Children in the United States are still at risk for parasitic infection. More common infections include giardiasis, pinworm infections, and head lice. Contaminated water and pets can serve as exposures to particular parasites including *Giardia lamblia*, *Cryptosporidium parvum*, *Toxoplasma gondii*, and *Toxocara canis*. Although covered in Chapter 89, it should be kept in mind that infection with *Trichomonas* spp. is the most common parasitic infection in the United States with 7.4 million infections each year. A comprehensive review of all parasitic infections in children would exceed the scope of the chapter, so an overview discussion of the most common intestinal parasites, systemic parasites, and specific coverage of malaria is presented.

INTESTINAL PARASITES

ETIOLOGY AND PATHOGENESIS

Intestinal parasites infect millions worldwide, particularly in developing countries with poor access to potable water and in patients with comorbidities. Intestinal parasites that are the most common in children in the United States include: *G. lamblia*, *Entamoeba histolytica*, and *C. parvum*. Table 99-1 reviews additional causes of intestinal parasitic infections (Figures 99-1 and 99-2).

G. lamblia is a flagellated protozoon and the most common cause of parasitic enteritis in the United States. Outbreaks can occur from contaminated water supplies, including pools, because it is resistant to chlorination as well as person to person in daycare centers. The mode of transmission is often fecal–oral or direct person-to-person contact (Figure 99-3).

E. histolytica is a large intestinal amoeba occurring in 1% to 5% of people around the world and causes amebiasis. Cysts are ingested from contaminated water from which they enter and inhabit the colon lumen and may form shallow ulcers. Amebomas can form on the intestinal wall and present with obstruction. With penetration into intestinal wall, invasion of the bloodstream occasionally occurs, leading to *amebic dysentery*. By this mechanism, the parasite can pass to the biliary system in the liver and form amebic abscesses and can be transmitted to other tissues as well. Interestingly, when *E. histolytica* is disseminated to the liver or other tissues, peripheral eosinophilia is not seen on complete blood count.

Cryptosporidium spp. are a worldwide intracellular protozoon seen mostly in immunocompromised patients. The clinical presentation is commonly with diarrhea. Outbreaks occur in healthy individuals as well, especially because *Cryptosporidium* spp. are chlorine resistant and may be spread through infected water and swimming pools. Fecal–oral contamination can transmit the parasite to epithelial cells in the stomach and intestine.

Enterobius vermicularis (pinworm) is the most common helminth of industrialized nations, and causes pruritus ani. Cysts are often ingested by the host via hand contamination. The eggs hatch in the duodenum, and then adult females lay eggs on the perineum.

CLINICAL PRESENTATION

Intestinal infection with parasites is often initially asymptomatic in a carrier state. Children with intestinal parasites can present with failure to thrive, diarrhea, abdominal pain, a protuberant abdomen, anemia, blood in the stool, and delayed development. A careful history with particular attention to travel and food and water intake is valuable. Additional details about sources and geography can be found in Table 99-1

Giardia spp. are often symptomatic in infants and young children with presentations including diarrhea to abdominal cramps with malabsorptive stool. Continued stool output can lead to protein loss and fat soluble vitamin deficiencies. Incubation in older children can occur 3 to 40 days after cyst ingestion until diarrhea. The symptoms and presentation of *Entamoeba* infection can also involve asymptomatic carriage. The symptoms include abdominal cramping, discomfort, anorexia, weight loss, and diarrhea with blood and mucus. Extraintestinal manifestations particularly hepatic abscesses can be seen. *Cryptosporidium* spp. have a variety of presentations depending on the host's immune system. Whereas immunocompetent hosts usually present with watery, self-limited diarrhea, immunocompromised hosts can present with intractable diarrhea, fever, anorexia, and vomiting. *Enterobius vermicularis* infections classically present with perianal pruritus.

DIFFERENTIAL DIAGNOSIS

The differential diagnosis for intestinal parasite infections is broad and includes noninfectious malabsorption and infectious diarrhea caused by viruses or bacteria. Anemia and failure to thrive seen in chronic infection with some parasites can also be misdiagnosed as other etiologies of iron-deficiency anemia and other systemic reasons for failure to thrive. Therefore, chronic infection should be considered in the differential of failure to thrive.

EVALUATION AND MANAGEMENT

Laboratory evaluation for parasitic infection can start with sending stool for ova and parasites (O+P). Several parasites are not found on standard testing such as *Cryptosporidium*, *Cyclospora*, and *Microspora* spp.; if these pathogens are suspected, the microbiology laboratory should be notified. Rapid immunoassays for

Table 99-1 Antiparasitic Recommendations for Intestinal Parasites

Parasite	Geography	Treatment	Alternatives	Clinical Pearls	Associated Foods	Complications
Anisakis	Japan, northern Europe, Pacific coast of South America	Surgical or endoscopic larval removal				
Giardia spp.	Worldwide; more prevalent in developing world	Metronidazole	Nitazoxanide, tinidazole		Uncooked foods, water, ill food handler	
Blastocytosis	Worldwide	If symptomatic, metronidazole	Iodoquinol	Still unclear if pathogenic	Unclear	
Entamoeba		Diloxanide furoate, paromomycin, metronidazole	Nitroimidazoles, ornidazole, tinidazole	Obstruction from ameboma	Uncooked foods, water, ill food handler	Amebic hepatic abscesses
Cryptosporidium	Worldwide	Nitazoxanide in immunocompromised	In HIV, HAART therapy	More severe disease in immunocompromised hosts	Fecal–oral, contaminated water	
Cyclospora	Worldwide, more prevalent in Peru, Nepal, Haiti	TMP-SMX in immunocompromised hosts	Pyrimethamine and folinic acid	Associated with prolonged diarrhea in HIV/AIDS and other immunocompromised states	Fresh produce, water	
Isospora	Southeast Asia, Africa, South America	TMP-SMX	Pyrimethamine and folinic acid			
Enterobius vermicularis (pinworm)	Most common helminth of the industrialized nations	Albendazole once and then again 2 weeks later	Tap water enemas, empiric treatment of contacts	Pruritus ani		
Ascaris lumbricoides	Worldwide, more prevalent in developing world	Albendazole, mebendazole, ivermectin, pyrantel pamoate	Occasionally surgery	Eosinophilia	Contaminated food, soil, raw fruits and vegetables	Has lung phase with cough, hemoptysis
Necator americanus	North and South America, Africa, India	Albendazole	Mebendazole, pamoate, iron therapy	Pica, hypoproteinemia, anemia, and eosinophilia	Soil contamination, infection through skin	

HAART, highly active antiretroviral therapy; TMP-SMX, trimethoprim–sulfamethoxazole.

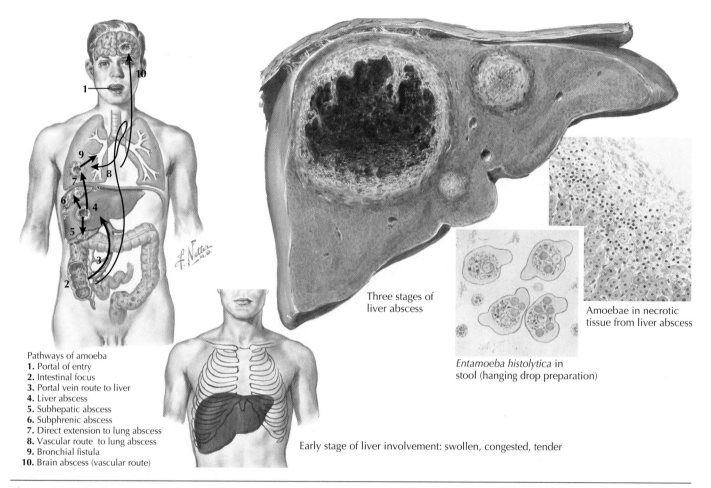

Three stages of
liver abscess

Amoebae in necrotic
tissue from liver abscess

Entamoeba histolytica in
stool (hanging drop preparation)

Pathways of amoeba
1. Portal of entry
2. Intestinal focus
3. Portal vein route to liver
4. Liver abscess
5. Subhepatic abscess
6. Subphrenic abscess
7. Direct extension to lung abscess
8. Vascular route to lung abscess
9. Bronchial fistula
10. Brain abscess (vascular route)

Early stage of liver involvement: swollen, congested, tender

Figure 99-1 *Amebiasis.*

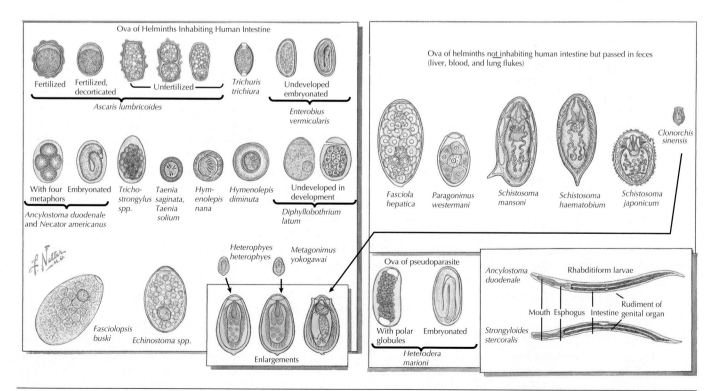

Ova of Helminths Inhabiting Human Intestine

Fertilized   Fertilized,   Unfertilized   *Trichuris*   Undeveloped
              decorticated   *trichiura*   embryonated

Ascaris lumbricoides

*Enterobius
vermicularis*

With four   Embryonated   Tricho-   Taenia   Hym-   Hymenolepis   Undeveloped in
metaphors   strongylus saginata, enolepis diminuta   development
                            spp.   Taenia   nana
                                       solium

*Ancylostoma duodenale
and Necator americanus*

*Diphyllobothrium
latum*

*Heterophyes
heterophyes*   *Metagonimus
                yokogawai*

*Fasciolopsis
buski*

Echinostoma spp.

Enlargements

Ova of helminths not inhabiting human intestine but passed in feces
(liver, blood, and lung flukes)

*Clonorchis
sinensis*

*Fasciola
hepatica*   *Paragonimus
             westermani*   *Schistosoma
                            mansoni*   *Schistosoma
                                        haematobium*   *Schistosoma
                                                        japonicum*

Ova of pseudoparasite

With polar   Embryonated
globules

*Heterodera
marioni*

*Ancylostoma
duodenale*   Rhabditiform larvae

Mouth Esphogus   Intestine   Rudiment of
                              genital organ

*Strongyloides
stercoralis*

Figure 99-2 *Helminths and protozoa infesting the human intestine.*

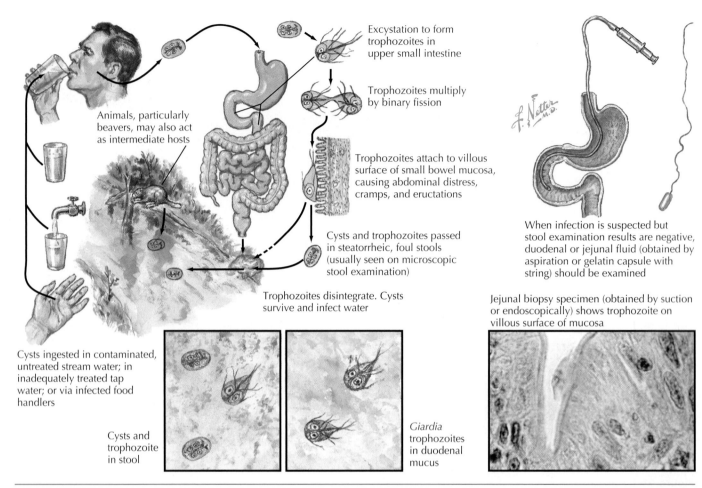

Excystation to form trophozoites in upper small intestine

Trophozoites multiply by binary fission

Trophozoites attach to villous surface of small bowel mucosa, causing abdominal distress, cramps, and eructations

Animals, particularly beavers, may also act as intermediate hosts

Cysts and trophozoites passed in steatorrheic, foul stools (usually seen on microscopic stool examination)

Trophozoites disintegrate. Cysts survive and infect water

When infection is suspected but stool examination results are negative, duodenal or jejunal fluid (obtained by aspiration or gelatin capsule with string) should be examined

Jejunal biopsy specimen (obtained by suction or endoscopically) shows trophozoite on villous surface of mucosa

Cysts ingested in contaminated, untreated stream water; in inadequately treated tap water; or via infected food handlers

Cysts and trophozoite in stool

Giardia trophozoites in duodenal mucus

Figure 99-3 *Giardiasis.*

Giardia spp., *Cryptosporidium* spp., and amebiasis can be sent and are more sensitive than O+P. Pinworms can be diagnosed by tape test to the anus. Mucosal biopsy can aid in diagnosis of *Giardia* spp. and *Entamoeba histolyticum*. Serology can be used for helminthic infections.

In addition to rehydration and supportive care, antimicrobial recommendations for each intestinal parasite covered in this chapter can be found in Table 99-1.

EXTRAINTESTINAL PARASITES

Extraintestinal parasites include bloodborne parasites and parasites that affect other sites of the body. Asymptomatic infection with these agents may underestimate their prevalence in the United States; for example, infection with *Toxoplasma* spp. may be as high as 22% of the United States population. The following sections discuss particular pathogens.

ETIOLOGY AND PATHOGENESIS

The pathogenesis of individual parasites differs by the type of parasite and the mode of transmission. Protozoa are free-living, single-celled eukaryotic organisms. Systemic protozoan infections in humans include *T. gondii*, *Plasmodium* spp., *Babesia* spp.,

Naegleria fowleri, and *Acanthamoeba* spp. A systemic parasite particularly important in pediatrics because of congenital infection is *T. gondii*. *T. gondii* is the third leading cause of death from foodborne illness in the United States. It is estimated that about 22% of the U.S. population has been infected with *Toxoplasma* spp. from undercooked meat or contaminated food or utensils in contact with the parasite, zoonotic transmission often from *Toxoplasma* oocytes shed in cat litter or soil, or newly infected mothers transmitting the organisms to unborn children. *Toxocara* is also a roundworm infection transferred to humans from domestic animals, with estimates of almost 14% of the United States population estimated to be infected.

Leishmania and *Trypanosoma* are bloodborne flagellates that are transmitted by the bite of blood-sucking insects. *Leishmania* spp. are spread by the sandfly. African trypanosomes, the cause of African sleeping sickness, are spread by the tsetse fly, and American trypanosomes, the cause Chagas' disease, are spread by reduviid bugs.

Systemic helminth infections, including *Strongyloides stercoralis*, *Trichinella spiralis*, *Ascaris lumbricoides*, *Toxocara canis*, and *Trichuris trichiura*, are spread via fecal contamination with worms penetrating into the toes of barefoot humans or through ingestion of cysts (Figure 99-4). Discussion of individual parasites is included in Table 99-2.

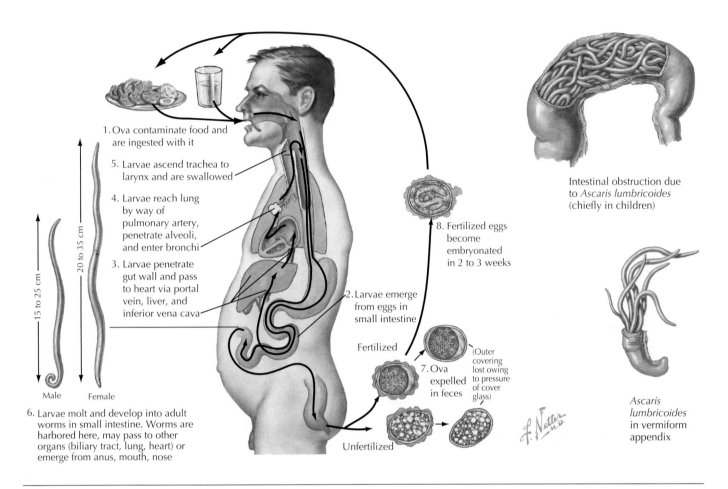

1. Ova contaminate food and are ingested with it

5. Larvae ascend trachea to larynx and are swallowed

4. Larvae reach lung by way of pulmonary artery, penetrate alveoli, and enter bronchi

3. Larvae penetrate gut wall and pass to heart via portal vein, liver, and inferior vena cava

Male   Female

15 to 25 cm

20 to 35 cm

6. Larvae molt and develop into adult worms in small intestine. Worms are harbored here, may pass to other organs (biliary tract, lung, heart) or emerge from anus, mouth, nose

2. Larvae emerge from eggs in small intestine

8. Fertilized eggs become embryonated in 2 to 3 weeks

Fertilized

7. Ova expelled in feces

(Outer covering lost owing to pressure of cover glass)

Unfertilized

Intestinal obstruction due to *Ascaris lumbricoides* (chiefly in children)

Ascaris lumbricoides in vermiform appendix

Figure 99-4 *Parasitic diseases: ascariasis.*

An additional common human ectoparasite includes *Pediculus humanus capitis* or head lice, which can be spread by close contact. Adult lice can live up to 30 days on a person's scalp by feeding on blood.

CLINICAL PRESENTATION

The clinical presentations of many extraintestinal parasites are in Table 99-2. Particular parasites are known for infection within the United States both from zoonotic spread and from international travel. The clinical presentation and burden of disease of *Toxoplasma* and *Toxocara* spp. are discussed. The use of clinical testing can aid in the differential diagnosis of parasitic infection. Malaria is covered in a subsequent section in this chapter.

Toxoplasma spp. are estimated to cause 1.5 million new infections each year, with 400 to 4000 cases of congenital toxoplasmosis yearly in the United States. Primary infection during pregnancy can pass *Toxoplasma* spp. directly to the fetus transplacentally. Potential complications include miscarriage, stillborn birth, or congenital infection. An infant with congenital toxoplasmosis may be asymptomatic at birth but then develop with age vision loss, seizure activity, and developmental delay with intracranial calcifications on imaging. Treatment can be undertaken in the mother as discussed below and in Table 99-2. In addition, more than 1 million people have eye involvement

with toxoplasmosis either from congenital or postnatal infection. An inflammatory lesion of the retina caused by direct infection of *Toxoplasma* spp. can lead to retinal scarring. This infection clinically can present with photophobia, blurred vision, and pain and may over time cause loss of vision, leading to blindness. *Toxoplasma* spp. are known for more severe infection in immunocompromised hosts either through reactivation of latent infection or new primary infection. In particular, *Toxoplasma* spp. Have a tropism for cardiac tissue and the brain, so they are of particular concern in heart transplant recipients. Clinical symptoms from toxoplasmosis usually occur 2 to 24 weeks after transplantation often from reactivation of cysts within a graft. Prophylaxis may be achieved with pyrimethamine or trimethoprim–sulfamethoxazole.

Toxocara infections are most common in those younger than age 20 years, with most infections being asymptomatic. The two major clinical presentations of toxocariasis are visceral larva migrans (VLM) and ocular larva migrans (OLM). VLM involves larval invasion into liver, heart, lungs, brain, or muscle and may cause fever, wheezing, weight loss, and hepatosplenomegaly associated with eosinophilia. Pneumonitis with eosinophilia (Loeffler's syndrome) may occur with VLM. Ocular involvement has very different presentations but often does not have peripheral eosinophilia.

Although the clinical range of parasitic infections is quite broad and overlaps with other infectious diseases, certain clinical

Table 99-2 Clinical Presentations of Extraintestinal Parasites

Parasite	Clinical Presentation	Mode or Endemic Area	Treatment	Clinical Pearls	Complications
Acanthamoeba	Blurry vision, IC: seizures, focal neurologic signs	Fresh water	Pentamidine, 0.1% propamidine isethionate plus neomycin ophthalmic solution	Keratitis in contact lens wearers	Blindness, IC: brain infection
Babesia spp.	Variable: viral-like illness to severe disease in IC, hemolytic anemia	Tickborne, southern New England, New York, Midwest	Clindamycin plus quinine or atovaquone plus azithromycin	Obligate parasite of RBCs	Hemolytic anemia
Leishmania donovani (visceral)	Fever, adenopathy, hepatosplenomegaly	Caribbean	Sodium stibogluconate, amphotericin B	Pancytopenia, hypergammaglobulinemia	
Naegleria fowleri	Acute meningoencephalitis	Fresh water	Intrathecal amphotericin	CSF profile like bacterial infection	Sudden deadly infection
Plasmodium	See text				
Schistosoma	Asymptomatic, fever, cough, abdominal pain, hepatomegaly, hematuria	Skin penetration, Caribbean, Africa, Middle East, Southeast Asia	Praziquantel		
Strongyloides stercoralis	Vomiting, bloating, diarrhea, pruritic rash, wheezing	Worldwide	Ivermectin, thiabendazole	Eosinophilia	
Taenia solium (cysticercosis and neurocysticercosis)	Seizure	Worldwide	Live cysts with seizures: albendazole and steroids and antiseizure medication	Initiate with antiseizure treatment	Potential for neurologic involvement
Toxocara canis, Toxocara cati	Hepatosplenomegaly, wheezing, fever, ocular involvement	Worldwide	Albendazole, mebendazole, steroids with visceral larva migrans	Eosinophilia, puppy, cat exposure or soil ingestion	
Toxoplasma gondii	Cervical lymphadenopathy, flulike illness	Worldwide	Pyrimethamine and sulfadiazine	Severe infection in IC, litter boxes, severe congenital infection	IC: CNS disease, myocarditis, pneumonitis
Trichinella spp.	Nausea, fatigue, abdominal pain, then muscle soreness, weakness	Worldwide	Steroids plus mebendazole	Ingestion of pork	
Trypanosoma cruzi	Fever, malaise, lymph nodes, heart CNS	Southern United States, South America	Nifurtimox, benznidazole	Chagas' disease; Romana's sign: erythema and swelling of periorbital area at bite site	Chronic: heart arrhythmias, megadisease of colon and esophagus
Trypanosoma brucei gambiense, Trypanosoma brucei rhodesiense	Fever, malaise, encephalitis, African sleeping sickness	Sub-Saharan Africa	Pentamidine for gambiense, suramin for rhodesiense	African sleeping sickness; Winterbottom's sign: bilateral occipital lymphadenopathy	Often fatal at encephalitic phase

CNS, central nervous system; CSF, cerebrospinal fluid; IC, immunocompromised child; RBC, red blood cell.

and laboratory presentations are associated with particular parasitic infections. Some of these distinctive features are captured in Table 99-2. With the clinical presentation of pneumonia and peripheral eosinophilia, *Ascaris* spp., hookworms, *Strongyloides* spp., and *Toxocara* spp. should be considered. Isolated eosinophilia can be seen in *Strongyloides*, hookworm, *Schistosomia*, and *Toxocara* infections. *Toxocara* infections are often associated with hepatosplenomegaly.

DIFFERENTIAL DIAGNOSIS

The differential diagnosis for systemic parasites is quite broad. Parasitic infection needs to be considered in returning travelers and those with fever without localizing symptoms. With fever with eosinophilia in returned travelers, schistosomiasis, toxocariasis, hookworm, filariasis, and trichinosis should be entertained. Malaria and leptospirosis needs to be considered in the differential of undifferentiated fever and fever with hemorrhage that also includes meningococcemia and viral hemorrhagic fevers. Fever and splenomegaly include evaluation for malaria, schistosomiasis, toxoplasmosis, trypanosomiasis, leishmaniasis, babesiosis as well as nonparasitic causes, including typhoid, tularemia, rickettsial disease, cytomegalovirus, Epstein-Barr virus, and HIV.

EVALUATION AND MANAGEMENT

The history and physical examination are keys to the evaluation of patients with bloodborne or other systemic parasitic infection. As discussed above in the differential diagnosis section, fever and the presence of localizing symptoms as well as travel history aid in evaluating for parasitic disease. Exposure to animals, water sources, food history, and direct travel should be elucidated.

The diagnosis of extraintestinal parasites is often made through evaluation for peripheral eosinophilia, direct microscopy of the parasite, and serology testing for antibodies against the parasite of concern. Diagnosis of *Toxoplasma* spp. is made by serologic testing for immunoglobulin against *Toxoplasma* spp. or by direct microscopic identification of the parasite. The diagnosis of *Toxocara* infection is presumptive based on clinical presentation, history, and antibodies to *Toxocara* spp.

Treatment of extraintestinal parasitic infections is further described in Table 99-2. Head lice are often treated with pyrethrins or permethrin lotions that are over the counter.

MALARIA

As discussed in the introduction to this chapter, *P. falciparum* is responsible for between 1 and 2.7 million deaths annually in children. In the United States, malaria is often seen in returning international travelers as the most common cause of fever without localizing symptoms.

ETIOLOGY AND PATHOGENESIS

Malaria is caused by protozoa of the genus *Plasmodium* with four species using humans as the intermediary host. These species include *P. falciparum*, *Plasmodium malariae*, *Plasmodium ovale*, and *Plasmodium vivax*. The infectious cycle of *Plasmodium* species can be seen in the attached image. In short, *Plasmodium* spp. is transmitted by arthropod vector, the *Anopheles* mosquito, which is active during nighttime hours. The female *Anopheles* mosquito spreads sporozoites into the human host which then go on to infect liver cells and continue to mature. They then undergo multiplication in the erythrocyte cells, with blood stage parasites causing clinical manifestations of malaria. *P. vivax* and *P. ovale* may stay as liver stage parasites for months and then reactivate (Figure 99-5).

Distribution of *Plasmodium* spp. depends on the correct environment that allows for parasite multiplication in the mosquito. *P. falciparum* is the predominant organism in sub-Saharan Africa, Hispaniola, and New Guinea (50% of cases in United States). *P. vivax* is the next most common and is seen in South Asia, Eastern Europe, Northern Asia, and South America, accounting for 25% of cases in the United States. *P. ovale* is often seen in Western Africa. *P. malariae* is distributed worldwide. Typical incubation periods are 9 to 18 days for *P. falciparum*, *P. vivax*, and *P. ovale* with longer incubation for *P. malariae*.

P. falciparum causes the most severe disease and is associated with the greatest risk of death. The pathogenesis of severe malaria caused by *P. falciparum* is associated with its ability to cause budding on the surface of the erythrocytes. The erythrocyte malformation reduces malleability causing stasis and thrombosis in the visceral capillary beds (i.e., the kidney, liver and brain).

CLINICAL PRESENTATION

Uncomplicated malaria often presents with nonspecific symptoms, particularly fever, chills, headache, weakness, vomiting, diarrhea, and myalgias. The clinical examination may often reveal splenomegaly. Severe malaria, often caused by *P. falciparum*, may involve the following symptoms as described by Griffith et al.: coma, respiratory distress, acidosis, seizures, pulmonary edema, circulatory shock, acute respiratory distress syndrome, jaundice, bleeding, anemia, acute renal failure, hemoglobinuria, parasitemia greater than 5%, and disseminated intravascular coagulation. Cerebral malaria may lead to signs of increased intracranial pressure, and vascular collapse and shock may occur with hypothermia and adrenal insufficiency. *P. vivax* and *P ovale* are known to cause splenomegaly with some reported causes of splenic rupture. *P. malariae* has been associated with nephrotic syndrome caused by immune complex deposition in the kidney.

DIFFERENTIAL DIAGNOSIS

As with other extraintestinal parasites, the differential diagnosis for malaria is broad, including viral and bacterial causes of undifferentiated fever. However, malaria must be considered in all febrile returned travelers from endemic areas.

EVALUATION AND TREATMENT

The evaluation for malaria should be undertaken with any suspicion for infection. A comprehensive discussion and flow chart

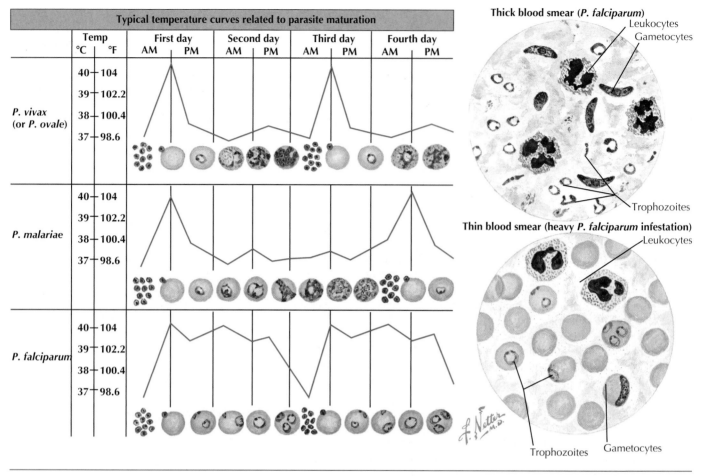

Figure 99-5 *Malaria clinical course and diagnosis.*

for evaluation were undertaken by Griffith et al. In summary, Giemsa-stained thin and thick blood smears should be reviewed microscopically for evaluation of presence of *Plasmodium* spp. within 12 hours of presentation of a patient with suspected malaria. Parasite density in erythrocytes on thin smear will need to be calculated as an indicator of severity of disease. Molecular diagnosis can help identify different species, which may aid in tailoring treatment. If malaria is still clinically suspected despite initially negative thin or thick smears, these should be repeated every 12 to 24 hours for a 72-hour period. The complete blood cell count can also be helpful in looking for thrombocytopenia and hemolysis. If the presentation includes clinical shock or severe infection, the prothrombin time, partial thromboplastin time, and fibrinogen can be helpful.

After infection is identified, treatment should begin immediately. Therapy should be guided by the species of *Plasmodium*, the clinical status of patient, and drug susceptibility of the region where the infection occurred. The clinical status of the patient is important as uncomplicated malaria can be treated with oral antimalarials, but complicated infection has to be more tailored to parenteral therapy. Exchange transfusion may be considered with parasitemia of 10% or evidence of complications, including cerebral malaria. Treatment in areas of chloroquine resistance includes atovaquone and proguanil. Treatment of *P. falciparum*

infection in nonchloroquine-resistant areas includes quinine sulfate plus doxycycline, tetracycline, or clindamycin. *P. vivax* (chloroquine resistant) treatment includes quinine sulfate plus doxycycline. Infection with all other *Plasmodium* spp. may be treated with chloroquine, with parenteral treatment with quinidine. For up-to-date recommendations and dosing, please refer to the Centers for Disease Control and Prevention's website (www.cdc.gov).

Malaria is a reportable disease, and local health departments should be notified with any infections.

TRAVELER PROPHYLAXIS

Travelers to endemic areas are at high risk for acquiring malaria and should take chemoprophylaxis beginning 1 week before travel to endemic region for mefloquine and 1 to 2 days for doxycycline and atovaquone-proguanil. Prevention of chloroquine-resistant malaria includes treatment with atovaquone/proguanil, doxycycline, or mefloquine. Atovaquone/proguanil is not approved for children who weigh less than 11 kg. Mefloquine can be considered for children, despite FDA approval only for children who weigh more than 5 kg and older than 6 months of age, and needs to be taken for 4 weeks after travel is over.

FUTURE DIRECTIONS

Understanding of transmission of parasitic disease and public and physician awareness in a world with increased international travel are important for further prevention and treatment. Prevention of malaria including prophylaxis and netting to prevent inoculation with *Plasmodium* spp. are current efforts to decrease infections. There are many efforts at preventive malaria vaccines underway.

SUGGESTED READINGS

American Academy of Pediatrics' Committee of Infectious Diseases: *Red Book: 2006 Report of the Committee of Infectious Diseases*, ed 27, Elk Grove Village, IL, 2006, American Academy of Pediatrics.

Bergelson JM, Shah SS, Zaoutis TE: *Pediatric Infectious Diseases: The Requisites in Pediatrics*, Philadelphia, 2008, Mosby.

Centers for Disease Control and Prevention: Parasites. Available at http://www.cdc.gov/ncidod/dpd.

Freedman DO: Clinical practice: malaria prevention in short-term travelers, *N Engl J Med* 359(6):603, 2008.

Freedman DO, Weld LH, Kozarsky PE, et al: Spectrum of disease and the relation to place of exposure among returning travelers, *N Engl J Med* 354(2):119, 2006.

Griffith KS, Lewis LS, Mali S, Parise ME: Treatment of malaria in the United States: a systematic review, *JAMA* 297(20):2264, 2007.

Long SS, Pickering LK, Prober CG: *Principles and Practice of Pediatric Infectious Diseases*, ed 3, Philadelphia, 2009, Saunders.

Won K, Kruszon-Moran D, Schantz P, Jones J: National seroprevalence and risk factors for zoonotic *Toxocara* spp. infection. In *Abstracts of the 56th American Society of Tropical Medicine and Hygiene*. Philadelphia, 2007.

David A. Munson

SECTION
XVI

Neonatal Medicine

Kristin N. Ray

Although most infants experience a transient increase in their bilirubin levels during the first week of life, a subset of infants experiences a more severe and potentially pathologic degree of hyperbilirubinemia. Early identification and treatment of these infants is required to reduce the potential for *kernicterus*, which is permanent neurologic harm from excessive unconjugated bilirubin. Most cases of severe hyperbilirubinemia and kernicterus are preventable through universal assessment of risk for severe hyperbilirubinemia, arrangement of close follow-up, and timely intervention when necessary. Although unconjugated hyperbilirubinemia is more common in infancy, some infants experience conjugated hyperbilirubinemia, which requires a separate process of evaluation and management from that of unconjugated hyperbilirubinemia.

ETIOLOGY AND PATHOGENESIS

Bilirubin is produced from the breakdown of heme. Heme is released from hemoglobin in the red blood cells (RBCs), metabolized to an intermediate product called biliverdin, and then metabolized further into *unconjugated bilirubin*, which circulates in the bloodstream primarily bound to albumin. Unconjugated bilirubin is then taken up by the liver, where it is bound to glucuronic acid by the enzyme uridine diphosphate glucuronyltransferase (UDPGT), creating water-soluble *conjugated bilirubin*, which can then be excreted into the gastrointestinal (GI) tract through the bile ducts. When stool has a delayed transit time, conjugated bilirubin can be broken down in the GI tract and reabsorbed into the bloodstream, a process known as *enterohepatic circulation*.

Most infants have at least a transient increase in their bilirubin levels in the first week of life, referred to as *physiologic jaundice*. This is attributable to relatively low activity of UDPGT at birth, large RBC mass, and the relatively short duration of survival of a newborn's RBCs. Physiologic jaundice generally peaks during the first week of life, with levels rarely requiring treatment.

Because of multiple different etiologies, some infants develop more severe hyperbilirubinemia. Increased bilirubin production can occur in infants with increased RBC breakdown (G6PD [glucose-6-phosphate dehydrogenase] deficiency, ABO incompatibility, cephalohematoma) or elevated total body RBC stores (polycythemia, infants of diabetic mothers). Decreased bilirubin conjugation also contributes to hyperbilirubinemia in some infants because of decreased activity of UDPGT in Crigler-Najjar and Gilbert's syndromes. Additionally, *breastfeeding jaundice* can occur early in the neonatal period in the setting of poor breast milk supply and associated dehydration and decreased stool output in an exclusively breastfed infant. In contrast, *breast milk jaundice* usually peaks during the second week of life and may take several more weeks to resolve completely. The mechanism of this process is not entirely understood but may involve components of breast milk inhibiting hepatic conjugating enzymes or increasing enterohepatic circulation. All of the aforementioned processes, because of their position in the bilirubin pathway, cause *unconjugated hyperbilirubinemia* (Box 100-1 and Figure 100-1).

Conjugated hyperbilirubinemia occurs when the defective step exists after the conjugation of bilirubin, specifically involving defects in bile flow resulting in neonatal cholestasis (see Figure 100-1). The differential diagnosis of neonatal cholestasis is vast, including structural anomalies such as biliary atresia, choledochal cysts, and Alagille syndrome, metabolic disorders, including α-1 antitrypsin deficiency, galactosemia, and tyrosinemia, and endocrinopathies such as hypothyroidism (Figure 100-2). Additionally, infectious causes include viral (cytomegalovirus, HIV, herpes simplex virus), and bacterial (sepsis, urinary tract infections), and parasitic infections have been associated with conjugated hyperbilirubinemia. Other causes of conjugated hyperbilirubinemia include inherited deficiencies in excretion (Dubin-Johnson and Rotor's syndromes), chromosomal disorders, parenteral nutrition, vascular and neoplastic processes, and idiopathic neonatal hepatitis (see Box 100-1).

The primary toxicity of bilirubin results from unconjugated bilirubin crossing the blood–brain barrier. Neurotoxicity appears to be most closely related to the amount of free or unbound bilirubin in the bloodstream. Patients with low albumin levels or who have elevated levels of other substances competing for albumin binding sites (including medications such as ceftriaxone) may have increased levels of free unconjugated bilirubin, increasing their risk of toxicity.

CLINICAL PRESENTATION

Unconjugated Hyperbilirubinemia

Jaundice often is first evident in the face, particularly in the sclera and the frenulum, and can be noted more caudally at increased levels of hyperbilirubinemia. Estimations of the degree of hyperbilirubinemia have been made based on the level of jaundice observed but are unreliable and require more objective measurement. Many patients with neonatal hyperbilirubinemia are identified through recommended routine screening in the newborn nursery, where the patient's bilirubin level should be systematically compared with nomograms to determine whether the current level requires intervention. In addition to obtaining routine screening levels, bilirubin levels should be obtained for all infants with jaundice evident in the first 24 hours of life, jaundice that is extensive, or jaundice that appears to be rapidly worsening.

Important historical information in a newborn with jaundice includes feeding and stooling patterns. Dehydration caused by poor feeding or poor maternal milk supply can exacerbate hyperbilirubinemia caused by hemoconcentration and increased enterohepatic circulation. For prevention of hyperbilirubinemia, the American Academy of Pediatrics (AAP) recommends

Box 100-1 Selected Differential Diagnosis of Unconjugated and Conjugated Hyperbilirubinemia

Unconjugated Hyperbilirubinemia

Physiologic Increased Bilirubin Production
- Hemolytic anemia
  - ABO incompatibility
  - Rh disease
  - G6PD deficiency
- Polycythemia
  - IDM
- Blood extravasation
  - Cephalohematoma
  - Caput succedaneum

Decreased Bilirubin Clearance
- Defects of conjugation
  - Crigler-Najjar, Gilbert's syndromes
- Increased enterohepatic circulation
  - Breastfeeding jaundice
  - Breast milk jaundice

Decreased Albumin Binding Capacity
- Medications
- Comorbid conditions

Conjugated Hyperbilirubinemia

Structural
- Biliary atresia
- Choledochal cyst
- Alagille syndrome
- Neonatal sclerosing cholangitis

Toxins
- Parenteral nutrition

Endocrinopathy
- Hypothyroidism

Genetic Disorders
- Trisomy 21
- Cystic fibrosis
- Dubin-Johnson, Rotor's syndrome
- α-1 antitrypsin deficiency

Metabolic Diseases
- Galactosemia
- Tyrosinemia

Vascular Disorders
- Neonatal asphyxia
- Budd-Chiari syndrome

Infection
- TORCH infections
- Sepsis
- UTI

Neoplastic Disease

G6PD, glucose-6-phosphate dehydrogenase; IDM, infant of a diabetic mother; TORCH, toxoplasmosis or Toxoplasma gondii, other infections, rubella, cytomegalovirus, and herpes simplex virus; UTI, urinary tract infection.

that breastfeeding mothers should nurse their infants at least 8 to 12 times daily for the first several days of life. In addition to detailed feeding and stooling histories, other important parts of the history include level of arousal, presence of fever, and frequency and appearance of urination.

The prenatal and perinatal histories are likewise important. Infants born earlier than 38 weeks of gestational age, of East Asian descent, exclusively breastfed, or with a sibling with a history of neonatal hyperbilirubinemia are at increased risk of hyperbilirubinemia. The mother's prenatal laboratory study results, including blood type, are also useful if they can be obtained. Jaundice noted before discharge from the newborn nursery, especially if noted within the first 24 hours of life, further elevates the patient's risk of severe hyperbilirubinemia. Additionally, G6PD deficiency increases the risk of hyperbilirubinemia caused by increased hemolysis after birth and might be noted in the family history. Physical examination findings consistent with hemolytic processes, such as pallor or tachycardia, might increase clinical concern for unconjugated hyperbilirubinemia. Birth trauma resulting in cephalohematomas or significant bruising can lead to increased RBC breakdown, further increasing the infant's risk. Elevated or low temperature and other signs of infection should also be noted because sepsis is a cause of hyperbilirubinemia.

At severe levels of hyperbilirubinemia, infants may have signs of *acute bilirubin encephalopathy*, with early signs that include lethargy, hypotonia, decreased activity, and poor suck. Untreated, this can progress over the course of days as infants become irritable, stuporous, and eventually comatose, with decreased or no feeding, hypertonia, retrocollis, opisthotonus, fever, apnea, and a shrill cry. Prolonged severe hyperbilirubinemia results in *kernicterus*, which is permanent neurologic damage caused by unconjugated hyperbilirubinemia, most notably in the basal ganglia and cranial nerve nuclei. Kernicterus is characterized by athetoid cerebral palsy, auditory disturbances, impaired upward gaze, and dysplasia of the primary teeth (Figure 100-3). Cognitive damage may also occur. Although the risk of kernicterus increases with increased levels of bilirubin, other clinical features appear to modify the risk, including prematurity, albumin binding capacity, duration of hyperbilirubinemia, and the presence of comorbid conditions. Although kernicterus decreased in frequency over the course of the 20th century, new cases continue to be reported, with shortened hospital stays and a resurgence of breastfeeding now requiring a high level of vigilance and the implementation of universal systematic monitoring protocols to avoid further cases of this devastating but preventable disease.

Conjugated Hyperbilirubinemia

Conjugated bilirubin does not cross the blood–brain barrier, so the primary clinical concern in conjugated hyperbilirubinemia is not the risk of kernicterus but rather the risks associated with a significant underlying disease. Patients with neonatal cholestasis may present with prolonged jaundice, pale stools, and dark urine. Jaundice in these infants may appear greener in tone than infants with unconjugated hyperbilirubinemia. Pertinent findings on physical examination may include jaundice, hepatomegaly, abnormal neurologic examination results caused by infectious or metabolic etiologies, or dysmorphisms suggestive of an underlying syndrome or intrauterine infection. The patient may also exhibit evidence of coagulopathy because of underlying liver disease.

EVALUATION AND MANAGEMENT

Unconjugated Hyperbilirubinemia

Transcutaneous or serum bilirubin levels should be measured in all jaundiced infants. A high level on transcutaneous testing should be confirmed with total, unconjugated (indirect), and conjugated (direct) bilirubin levels. Additionally, infant blood type, direct Coombs testing, a complete blood count with smear, and reticulocyte count should be performed in patients requiring phototherapy and in those whose bilirubin levels are increasing rapidly to evaluate for the possibility of a hemolytic process. If hemolysis is suspected in a male infant, G6PD testing should also be considered. A basic metabolic panel can be helpful in a child with associated clinical concern for dehydration. A type and screen as well as an albumin level should be obtained if there is a possibility that the infant needs exchange transfusion.

For unconjugated hyperbilirubinemia, the infant's total bilirubin level should be plotted according to hour of life on the

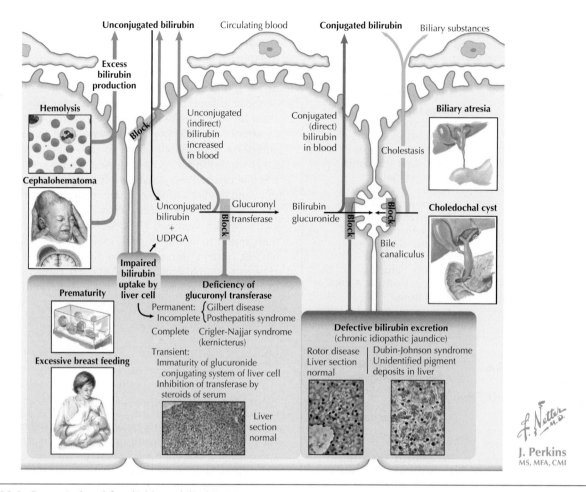

Figure 100-1 *Congenital and familial hyperbilirubinemias.*

nomogram developed by Bhutani et al. in 1999 and available in the AAP 2004 guidelines (Figure 100-4). This nomogram determines the age-specific bilirubin level at which phototherapy or exchange transfusion should be initiated in infants who are 35 weeks gestational age or greater. The treatment threshold is based on hour of life, total serum bilirubin level, and presence of additional risk factors, including gestational age, isoimmune hemolytic disease, G6PD deficiency, asphyxia, significant lethargy, unstable temperatures, acidosis, sepsis, or hypoalbuminemia. The conjugated bilirubin level should not be subtracted from the total bilirubin level when using the nomogram. However, providers should be aware of the risk of *bronze baby syndrome*, a usually benign discoloration of the skin that occurs in infants with cholestasis receiving phototherapy, and if conjugated bilirubin exceeds 50% of the total bilirubin in an infant requiring phototherapy, expert consultation is advised.

Based on this nomogram, phototherapy should be initiated at moderate levels of hyperbilirubinemia to aid in clearance by photoisomerizing unconjugated bilirubin into a water-soluble form that can be excreted in the bile and urine without further conjugation. Phototherapy is most effective with appropriate wavelengths of light (ideally 460–490 nm), appropriate distance and irradiance, and maximal skin exposure. Phototherapy can be toxic to the immature retina, requiring protective eye shields during treatment (Figure 100-5).

Exchange transfusion is initiated at severe levels of hyperbilirubinemia also based on the infant's hour of life (see Figure 100-4) and in any infant exhibiting signs of acute bilirubin encephalopathy. Severe hyperbilirubinemia requiring exchange transfusion should be treated as a medical emergency and requires immediate admission to a neonatal intensive care unit for further care (see Figure 100-5). Intravenous γ-globulin may be considered in infants with isoimmune hemolytic disease who are approaching the exchange transfusion threshold.

In addition to these specific treatments for hyperbilirubinemia, it is important to respond appropriately to any concomitant issues, such as dehydration, anemia, or sepsis. Additionally, if hyperbilirubinemia is determined not to require treatment at the time of evaluation, it is important to determine when the total serum bilirubin level should next be obtained, provide the patient's parents with education about jaundice, and ensure appropriate follow-up for reevaluation.

Conjugated Hyperbilirubinemia

Conjugated hyperbilirubinemia is defined as conjugated bilirubin greater than 1 mg/dL or greater than 20% of the total bilirubin level if total bilirubin is greater than 5 mg/dL. Initial evaluation requires obtaining a thorough history and physical examination as described above, as well as fractionated bilirubin

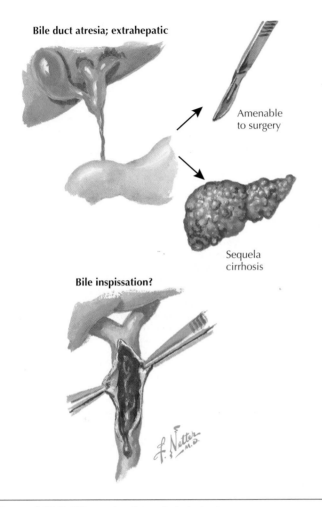

Bile duct atresia; extrahepatic

Amenable
to surgery

Sequela
cirrhosis

Bile inspissation?

Figure 100-2 *Biliary atresia and cholestasis.*

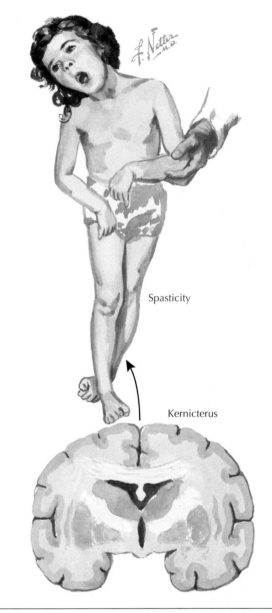

Spasticity

Kernicterus

Figure 100-3 *Kernicterus.*

levels and liver function tests, including alanine aminotransferase, aspartate aminotransferase, alkaline phosphatase, γ-glutamyl transferase, albumin, and prothrombin time. Evaluation should then occur in a stepwise fashion, focusing first on disease processes requiring urgent treatment, such as sepsis, urinary tract and TORCH (toxoplasmosis or *Toxoplasma gondii*, other infections, rubella, cytomegalovirus, and herpes simplex virus) infections, hypothyroidism, and metabolic disorders. Next, imaging studies should be considered to localize whether the anatomic site of dysfunction is either intrahepatic or extrahepatic. Ultrasound can provide useful information about the gallbladder; hepatobiliary scintigraphy, however, has better sensitivity for biliary atresia. If no etiology has been found, additional evaluation for other specific etiologies, such as cystic fibrosis and α-1 antitrypsin deficiency, may be helpful.

Therapy for neonatal cholestasis varies depending on the underlying cause. Sepsis requires antibiotic therapy (see Chapter 105), and inborn errors of metabolism require dietary modification or enzyme supplementation. Biliary atresia requires urgent surgical treatment because prognoses are markedly better when the Kasai procedure is performed within the first 60 days of life. In contrast, treatment of patients with many other causes focuses more on supportive care such as nutritional support with caloric and fat-soluble vitamin supplementation along with use of

ursodeoxycholic acid, which aims to enhance bilirubin excretion and may reduce associated pruritus. Further management should be conducted in consultation with the appropriate specialist and is beyond the scope of this chapter.

FUTURE DIRECTIONS

Although clear guidelines for term and near-term infants presenting with unconjugated hyperbilirubinemia are available based on the best current evidence and expert opinion, less consensus exists currently in treatment recommendations for premature and low-birth-weight infants, making further study necessary to optimize treatment for these at-risk populations. Additionally, further work is necessary to improve our understanding of bilirubin neurotoxicity at both a cellular and population-based level, so we can better target screening and treatment to those most at risk. Improving our ability to use

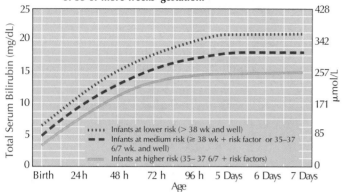

Guidelines for phototherapy in hospitalized infants of 35 or more weeks' gestation.

- Infants at lower risk (> 38 wk and well)
- Infants at medium risk (≥ 38 wk + risk factor or 35–37 6/7 wk. and well)
- Infants at higher risk (35– 37 6/7 + risk factors)

· Use total bilirubin. Do not subtract direct reacting or conjugated bilirubin.
· Risk factors = isoimmune hemolytic disease, G6PD deficiency, asphyxia, significant lethargy, temperature instability, sepsis, acidosis, or albumin < 3.0 g/dL (if measured).
· For well infants 35–37 6/7 wk can adjust TSB levels for intervention around the medium risk line. It is an option to intervene at lower TSB levels for infants closer to 35 wk and at higher TSB levels for those closer to 37 6/7 wk.
· It is an option to provide conventional phototherapy in hospital or at home at TSB levels 2–3 mg/dL (35–50 mmol/L) below those shown, but home phototherapy should not be used in any infant with risk factors.

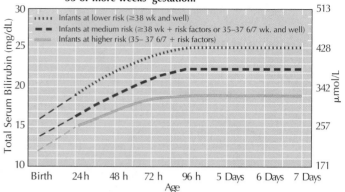

Guidelines for exchange transfusion in infants of 35 or more weeks' gestation.

- Infants at lower risk (≥38 wk and well)
- Infants at medium risk (≥38 wk + risk factors or 35–37 6/7 wk. and well)
- Infants at higher risk (35– 37 6/7 + risk factors)

· The dashed lines for the first 24 hours indicate uncertainty due to a wide range of clinical circumstances and a range of responses to phototherapy.
· Immediate exchange transfusion is recommended if infant shows signs of acute bilirubin encephalopathy (hypertonia, arching, retrocollis, opisthotonos, fever, high-pitched cry) or if TSB is ≥5 mg/dL (85 μmol/L) above these lines.
· Risk factors - isoimmune hemolytic disease, G6PD deficiency, asphyxia, significant lethargy, temperature instability, sepsis, acidosis.
· Measure serum albumin and calculate B/A ratio.
· Use total bilirubin. Do not subtract direct reacting or conjugated bilirubin.
· If infant is well and 35–37 6/7 wk (median risk) can individualize TSB levels for exchange based on actual gestational age.

Reprinted with permission from Subcommittee on Hypebilirubinemia. Management of Hyperbilirubinemia in the Newborn Infant 35 or More Weeks of Gestation. Pediatrics 2004;114:297-316.

Figure 100-4 *American Academy of Pediatrics guidelines for phototherapy and exchange transfusion.*

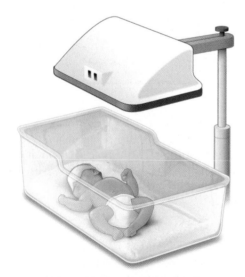

Jaundiced infant under phototherapy (with eye proctection)

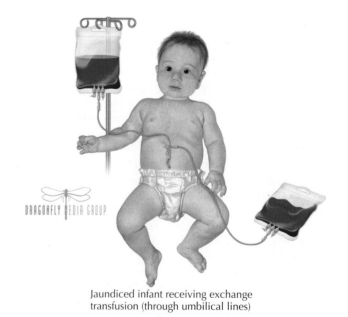

Jaundiced infant receiving exchange transfusion (through umbilical lines)

Figure 100-5 *Phototherapy and exchange transfusion.*

noninvasive testing such as transcutaneous bilirubin measurements and brainstem auditory evoked responses to monitor for hyperbilirubinemia and for bilirubin-induced neurotoxicity will further enhance our targeting of therapy, as would the ability to measure free bilirubin, a test that is not currently available. Furthermore, pharmacologic treatment for hyperbilirubinemia, although not currently available, would greatly enhance our therapeutic options and might increase the opportunity for effective treatment in resource-poor countries as well. Finally, in addition to refining current guidelines for treatment as more evidence becomes available, it is important to ensure that these guidelines are translated into universal clinical practice to maximize prevention of the permanent consequences of severe hyperbilirubinemia.

SUGGESTED READINGS

Bhutani VK, Johnson LH, Shapiro SM: Kernicterus in sick and preterm infants (1999–2002): a need for an effective preventive approach, *Semin Perinatol* 28(5):319-325, 2004.

Bhutani VK, Johnson L, Sivieri EM: Predictive ability of a predischarge hour-specific serum bilirubin for subsequent significant hyperbilirubinemia in healthy term and near-term newborns, *Pediatrics* 103(1):6-14, 1999.

Bhutani VK, Maisels MJ, Stark AR, Buonocore G; Expert Committee for Severe Neonatal Hyperbilirubinemia; European Society for Pediatric Research; American Academy of Pediatrics: Management of jaundice and prevention of severe neonatal hyperbilirubinemia in infants >or=35 weeks gestation, *Neonatology* 94(1):63-67, 2008.

Ip S, Chung M, Kulig J, et al: An evidence based review of important issues concerning neonatal hyperbilirubinemia, *Pediatrics* 114(1):e130-e153, 2004.

Maisels MJ, McDonagh AF: Phototherapy for neonatal jaundice, *N Engl J Med* 358(9):920-928, 2008.

Subcommittee on Hyperbilirubinemia: Management of hyperbilirubinemia in the newborn infant 35 or more weeks of gestation, *Pediatrics* 114(1):297-316, 2004.

Venigalla S, Gourley GR: Neonatal cholestasis, *Semin Perinatol* 28(5):348-355, 2004.

Disorders of the Nervous System

101

Ryan J. Felling and David A. Munson

The neonatal period is an important time for development of the nervous system. Interruption of normal development through disease or injury often leads to permanent neurologic sequelae. As our ability to care for critically ill neonates improves, neurologic disorders continue to be a significant cause of morbidity and mortality. It is crucial to identify neonates at risk for neurologic disorders through careful history taking and physical examination so that problems can be prevented or treated early.

ETIOLOGY AND PATHOGENESIS

Hypoxic-Ischemic Encephalopathy

With dramatic advances in neonatal critical care, hypoxic-ischemic encephalopathy (HIE) has emerged as the primary cause of neurologic morbidity in the newborn period. This injury can occur both in premature neonates and term neonates. HIE is a consequence of poor delivery of oxygen to the brain, with hypoperfusion and ischemia likely being the most important mechanism. Much of the injury actually occurs during reperfusion of the ischemic brain. HIE can result from any mechanism that results in poor blood flow to the fetal brain in utero including chorioamnionitis, placental abruption, nuchal cord, and chronic maternal hypertension. It can also occur in the setting of severe postnatal cardiorespiratory compromise, including respiratory or cardiac arrest. In premature neonates, it is often associated with intraventricular hemorrhage (IVH).

Intraventricular Hemorrhage

Although the premature cerebrovasculature has reasonable capacity for autoregulation within the normal range of blood pressure, this mechanism quickly becomes inadequate as blood pressures fluctuate outside the norm, predisposing the brain to ischemic injury during times of hypotension and hemorrhagic injury during times of hypertension. The periventricular germinal matrix of the premature brain is at high risk for hemorrhagic injury because of the presence of a rich but relatively immature capillary network. This region is particularly critical because it harbors the neural stem and progenitor cell population that provides precursors necessary for future myelination and development of the brain. Figure 101-1 demonstrates patterns of hemorrhagic injury that can occur in both premature and term infants.

Neonatal Seizures

Neonatal seizures are often a manifestation of underlying neurologic disease or injury (Table 101-1). In each case, the metabolic or structural abnormalities cause disorganized electrical activity that can lead to epileptogenic foci.

Neonatal Hypotonia

Hypotonia is a common sign of neurologic disease in newborns that can be caused by dysfunction anywhere along the neuromuscular axis. These may arise from genetic defects causing protein dysfunction in either nerve or muscle cells, loss of cerebral regulation of tone secondary to global central nervous system (CNS) dysfunction as in many chromosomal disorders or injuries, or disturbed signal transmission at the neuromuscular junction. The more common causes of hypotonia can be organized by the location of the primary defect (Figure 101-2).

CLINICAL PRESENTATION

Hypoxic-Ischemic Encephalopathy

In his classic text, Volpe describes a "neurologic syndrome" that summarizes an infant who has sustained a hypoxic-ischemic insult to the brain. In severe cases, the infant progresses through several clinical phases. During the first 6 to 12 hours, the baby will have depressed consciousness and may even be comatose. This time is often characterized by apnea or periodic breathing and minimal movement, but the patient usually has intact pupillary and oculomotor reflexes. Seizures commonly occur during this initial period. The next 12 to 24 hours are often characterized by apparent clinical improvement. The newborn may appear more alert. Jitteriness is common and may be misinterpreted as seizures, although a considerable number of patients also develop true seizures during this time window. The apparent improvement is likely a consequence of excitatory neurotransmitter cascades that are characteristic of this phase of reperfusion injury. The next 24 to 72 hours often see a return of stupor or coma; respiratory failure; and more significant loss of central reflexes, including oculomotor disturbances.

Intraventricular Hemorrhage

In a premature baby in the first few days of life, acute IVH may be characterized by subtle signs such as new-onset apnea or decreased activity. However, a catastrophic bleed may make itself evident by a dramatic change in mental status along with cardiovascular collapse. If enough blood is lost into the brain, the baby may become anemic and develop severe hypotension and respiratory failure. Metabolic acidosis may become refractory to therapy if systemic perfusion is inadequate because of anemia and hypotension. Hydrocephalus is a common consequence of IVH as the blood obstructs the flow of cerebrospinal fluid (CSF). This manifests clinically as increasing head circumference, which may develop acutely or slowly depending on the size of the hemorrhage.

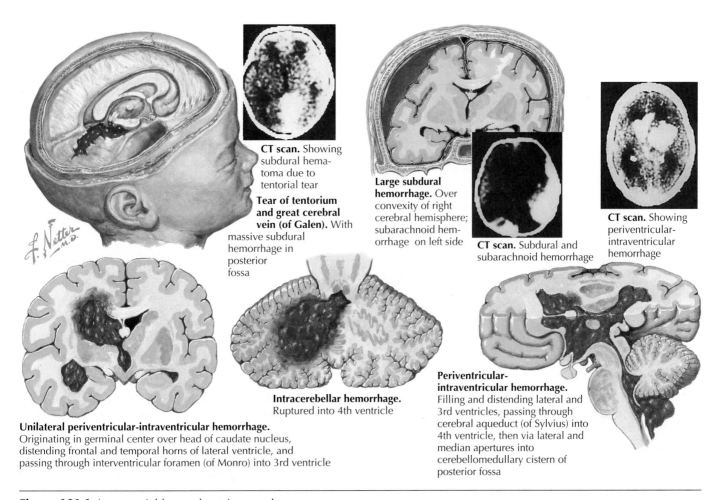

CT scan. Showing subdural hematoma due to tentorial tear

Tear of tentorium and great cerebral vein (of Galen). With massive subdural hemorrhage in posterior fossa

Large subdural hemorrhage. Over convexity of right cerebral hemisphere; subarachnoid hemorrhage on left side

CT scan. Subdural and subarachnoid hemorrhage

CT scan. Showing periventricular-intraventricular hemorrhage

Intracerebellar hemorrhage. Ruptured into 4th ventricle

Periventricular-intraventricular hemorrhage. Filling and distending lateral and 3rd ventricles, passing through cerebral aqueduct (of Sylvius) into 4th ventricle, then via lateral and median apertures into cerebellomedullary cistern of posterior fossa

Unilateral periventricular-intraventricular hemorrhage. Originating in germinal center over head of caudate nucleus, distending frontal and temporal horns of lateral ventricle, and passing through interventricular foramen (of Monro) into 3rd ventricle

Figure 101-1 *Intracranial hemorrhage in a newborn.*

Neonatal Seizures

The newborn brain remains immature, particularly with regard to myelination. This immature anatomic organization makes neonatal seizures difficult to recognize and classify and often presents problems in selecting therapy and gauging efficacy. The fact that normal newborn infants often exhibit unusual movements confounds the diagnosis of neonatal seizures. With these difficulties, neonatal seizures often experience a paradoxical combination of overdiagnosis and underdiagnosis.

Neonatal seizures have a variety of manifestations and a variety of normal mimics (Box 101-1). Clonic seizures can occur either focally or multifocally and are repetitive high-amplitude, low-frequency jerking movements. Tonic seizures are constant stiffening of a portion of the body and may be focal or generalized. Myoclonic seizures include sudden extension or flexion of

Table 101-1 Common Causes of Neonatal Seizures

Vascular Injuries	Structural Malformations	Infection	Metabolic Disorders	Genetic Epilepsy Syndromes
Hypoxic-ischemic encephalopathy	Neuronal migration defects	Meningitis	Transient	Benign familial neonatal convulsions
Intraventricular hemorrhage	Neurocutaneous syndromes	Encephalitis	• Hyponatremia	Idiopathic benign neonatal seizures
Perinatal arterial stroke	Tumors		• Hypoglycemia	Early myoclonic encephalopathy
Sinus venous thrombosis	Vein of Galen malformations		• Hypocalcemia	Ohtahara's syndrome
Subdural hemorrhage			• Hypomagnesemia	
Subarachnoid hemorrhage			Persistent	
			• Inborn errors of metabolism	
			• GLUT-1 deficiency	
			• Pyridoxine-dependent epilepsy	

GLUT-1, glucose transporter protein type 1.

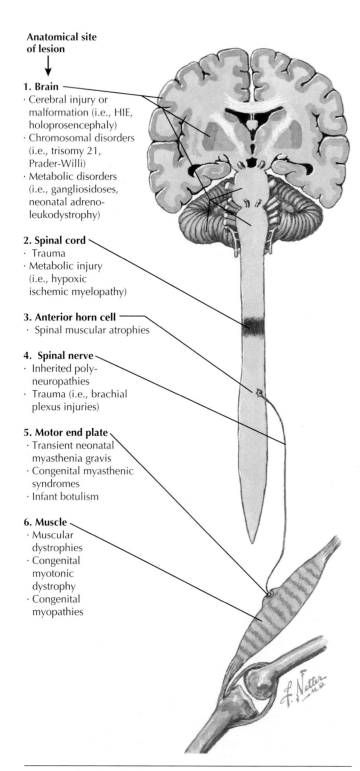

Anatomical site of lesion

1. Brain
· Cerebral injury or malformation (i.e., HIE, holoprosencephaly)
· Chromosomal disorders (i.e., trisomy 21, Prader-Willi)
· Metabolic disorders (i.e., gangliosidoses, neonatal adreno-leukodystrophy)

2. Spinal cord
· Trauma
· Metabolic injury (i.e., hypoxic ischemic myelopathy)

3. Anterior horn cell
· Spinal muscular atrophies

4. Spinal nerve
· Inherited poly-neuropathies
· Trauma (i.e., brachial plexus injuries)

5. Motor end plate
· Transient neonatal myasthenia gravis
· Congenital myasthenic syndromes
· Infant botulism

6. Muscle
· Muscular dystrophies
· Congenital myotonic dystrophy
· Congenital myopathies

Figure 101-2 *Primary sites of motor disorders.*

part of the body. Subtle seizures encompass other small abnormal movements that do not fit into the previously listed seizure types, including eye deviation, lip smacking, and tongue thrusting, among others. Subtle seizures and generalized tonic seizures often do not have electroencephalographic (EEG) correlates and are thought to emanate from deeper subcortical brain regions, a theory supported by animal studies.

Box 101-1	Appearance of Neonatal Seizures

Neonatal Seizure Classification
• Clonic
  • Focal
  • Multifocal
• Tonic
  • Focal
• Generalized
  • Myoclonic
  • Subtle

Neonatal Seizure Mimics
• Jitteriness
• Benign myoclonus
• Opisthotonus
• Apnea

Several other unusual movements frequently seen in newborns must be considered in the differential diagnosis of seizures. These may occur in normal infants or may suggest other underlying disease. Jitteriness is a hypersensitivity to stimulus and may be suggestive of underlying abnormalities such as drug withdrawal; hypoxic-ischemic injury; or metabolic disease, particularly hypoglycemia. Benign myoclonus is a sudden, brief, jerking movement of the extremities that occurs during sleep in many normal infants. Opisthotonus is a tonic stiffening of the body, often resulting in arching of the back and neck. This is a common finding associated with gastroesophageal reflux (Sandifer's syndrome). Neonatal apnea may or may not be associated with seizures, but it is frequently an independent clinical event in premature infants.

Neonatal Hypotonia

Hypotonia is a cardinal sign associated with many neurologic abnormalities that is characterized by decreased resistance of muscle to passive stretch. Hypotonia presenting in the newborn period has a similar clinical appearance regardless of where along the neuromuscular axis the disease originates. Figure 101-3 shows the characteristic appearance of hypotonic infants. These infants often appear in a frog leg posture with hips abducted and knees flexed when lying supine. Spontaneous movements are decreased compared with their healthy counterparts. Useful physical examination maneuvers to test for hypotonia are traction and prone suspension (Figure 101-4). With traction, a healthy full-term infant should demonstrate flexion at the shoulders and elbows and should be able to slightly flex the neck to keep the head in line with the body as it is brought up. Hypotonic infants show no flexion of the upper extremities, and their head fall to full extension as they are lifted. Similarly, in prone suspension, a healthy infant should show flexion of the extremities and some neck extension in an effort to maintain a horizontal position. Hypotonic infants lie draped over the examiner's hand.

Depending on the severity and duration of hypotonia in utero, neonates may have significant compromise at birth. Chest wall abnormalities caused by a lack of muscle tone necessary to keep the thoracic cavity expanded are frequently accompanied by respiratory distress. Infants with neuromuscular disease can

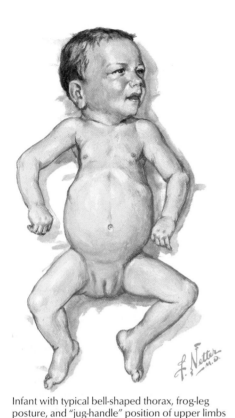

Infant with typical bell-shaped thorax, frog-leg posture, and "jug-handle" position of upper limbs

Figure 101-3 *Clinical presentation of neonatal hypotonia.*

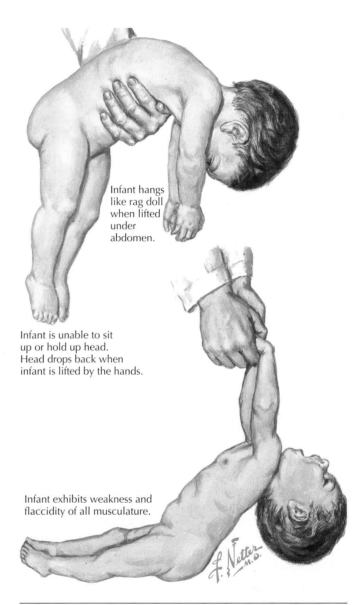

Infant hangs like rag doll when lifted under abdomen.

Infant is unable to sit up or hold up head. Head drops back when infant is lifted by the hands.

Infant exhibits weakness and flaccidity of all musculature.

Figure 101-4 *Floppy infant.*

also exhibit difficulty feeding because of a combination of easy fatigue and poorly coordinated suck and swallow function. This can also impede the body's natural airway protection, leading to an inability to clear secretions and potentially aspiration. As hypotonia progresses and becomes more prolonged, musculo-skeletal contractures may occur.

EVALUATION AND MANAGEMENT

Neurologic Assessment

HISTORY AND PHYSICAL EXAMINATION

Many neurologic disorders share a common set of symptoms in the neonatal period; therefore, the tools for evaluating these infants are discussed here collectively. A thorough history and physical examination should always be the initial investigation into an infant with neurologic disease. The history should encompass the pregnancy, including gestational age and the results of any prenatal testing. Details of any previous pregnancies are also helpful. Frequent pregnancy losses could suggest the presence of an underlying genetic abnormality or a hyper-coagulable disorder that may cause placental insufficiency. The neurologic examination of a neonate is an art that requires practice; however, numerous studies have demonstrated its value for both localization of pathology and prognosis. The clinician should always measure the head circumference and examine the fontanelles, sutures, and general shape of the head. Molding of the skull, overlapping sutures, and extracranial hemorrhages

including caput succedaneum and cephalohematomas are common abnormalities but do not portend underlying brain anomalies. A tense fontanelle and widely patent sutures are sug-gestive of hydrocephalus or infection. Testing of cranial nerves should focus on pupillary responses, extraocular movements, sucking, and swallowing. The motor examination includes assessment of overall tone and spontaneous movements as well as primitive reflexes, including the Moro, grasp, and asymmetric tonic neck reflex. All three reflexes should be present by 28 weeks of gestation but become stronger as the infant nears term. The sensory examination should describe the type of stimulus and characterize the response. For example, whereas flexion of an extremity to a painful stimulus may be a reflex response, crying and specific withdrawal to such stimulus indicate intact cortical processing of pain.

Details obtained from the history and physical examination can help prioritize the use of adjunctive studies to determine the underlying cause of the disease. For example, whereas a history of fetal depression in utero might indicate HIE as the source of symptoms, a normal pregnancy with a particularly difficult delivery could suggest the possibility of an intracranial hemorrhage. Dysmorphic features often raise concern for a genetic syndrome that may involve structural brain anomalies.

ELECTROENCEPHALOGRAPHY

As discussed in the Clinical Presentation section, neonatal seizures are difficult to identify and thus present a diagnostic dilemma for clinicians. A critical tool in the evaluation of suspected seizures is EEG. EEGs measure electrical activity between electrodes placed in an array over the scalp. These can be combined with video monitoring to correlate the brain's electrical activity with the clinical presentation of the patient. This is an indispensable tool for distinguishing seizure activity from other nonepileptic movements and for quantifying seizure activity. EEG can also identify particular brain regions that are prone to epileptic activity. Certain types of epilepsy exhibit characteristic patterns on EEG. Examples of this include burst-suppression in Ohtahara's syndrome and hypsarrhythmia in infantile spasms.

LUMBAR PUNCTURE

Analysis of the CSF is an important test for several reasons. Sepsis must always be near the top of the differential diagnosis list for ill neonates. Meningitis is indicated by a pleocytosis in the CSF, and culture of the CSF can help to identify a pathogen and direct antimicrobial therapy. Furthermore, blood in the CSF that does not clear can demonstrate the presence of a subarachnoid hemorrhage. Other CSF measurements can also be helpful. A significantly low glucose relative to serum glucose level may be indicative of GLUT-1 (glucose transporter protein type 1) transporter deficiency, and an elevated lactate level could suggest metabolic disease or indicate the presence of hypoxic-ischemic injury to the brain.

NEUROIMAGING

Neuroimaging offers many modalities that are of use in assessing the neonatal brain. Ultrasound is a readily available tool that can identify the presence of hemorrhage in the neonatal brain; however, it provides relatively poor anatomic definition. Magnetic resonance imaging (MRI) has become more common in the neonatal neurologic assessment. This modality provides excellent anatomic resolution and more precisely defines the location of pathologic lesions. Furthermore, it can provide metabolic information through the use of MR spectroscopy and vascular anatomy with MR angiography or venography. The ability to use MRI can be limited by availability and the clinical stability of the patient; however, ultrasound can be easily performed at the bedside. Computed tomography is rarely used in neonates because of the increasing availability of MRI, the ease of ultrasound, and the risks associated with radiation exposure to the newborn brain.

ADDITIONAL TESTING

Many additional studies are helpful in the diagnosis of neurologic disorders but are less commonly used. These are particularly relevant to infants with seizures or hypotonia of uncertain etiology. Genetic and metabolic studies can help identify inherited disorders. The proliferation of gene array studies has been helpful in this regard, although if specific disorders are suspected, targeted gene studies are more helpful. Typical metabolic screening tests include plasma amino acids, lactate, pyruvate, and urine organic acids. CSF can also be analyzed with these studies. Nerve conduction studies and electromyography can be performed to help localize the source of hypotonia. Finally, nerve and muscle biopsies can be helpful to identify particular myopathies and metabolic disorders.

Management

HYPOXIC-ISCHEMIC ENCEPHALOPATHY

Early identification of neonates at risk for HIE is important to optimize management. One of the more recent advances that has shown promise in term infants with HIE is hypothermia. Hypothermia reduces the cerebral metabolic demand and may interrupt the excitatory cascade contributing to brain injury in the 72 hours that follow the inciting event. Several trials have demonstrated beneficial outcomes of this therapy, and large centers throughout the world are continuing to evaluate its efficacy. Other management issues focus on addressing the comorbidities associated with HIE. Seizure management may provide protection against further injury by reducing metabolic demand (excitotoxic injury) and preserving oxygenation of the brain.

INTRAVENTRICULAR HEMORRHAGE

Little can be done to help a baby after significant IVH has occurred, so prevention is the mainstay. Limiting fluid boluses and carefully adjusting medications to maintain normal blood pressure may help in this regard. The use of prophylactic indomethacin for closure of patent ductus arteriosus in the smallest babies (those <1000 g) has been shown to decrease the rate of severe IVH. Its use remains controversial, however, because this decrease has not yet correlated to improved long-term outcome.

If a baby does develop IVH, acute management is focused on supporting the baby through the cardiovascular collapse. If the patient survives, he must be monitored closely for the development of hydrocephalus over the ensuing weeks. This is routinely done through serial head circumference measurements and intermittent cranial ultrasound. In severe cases of hydrocephalus, neurosurgical intervention may be required through placement of a ventricular shunt to divert the flow of CSF. Babies who have had severe IVH are at significant risk for neurodevelopmental impairment, so long-term follow-up is necessary. Supportive services such as physical therapy, occupational therapy, and speech therapy are invaluable in terms of maximizing the patient's future functionality.

NEONATAL SEIZURES

Although the field of epilepsy overall has robustly expanded its armament of therapeutics, the treatment of neonatal seizures has been comparatively slow to evolve. The difficulty of accurately identifying neonatal seizures and the risk associated with

Table 101-2 Intravenous Dosages of Common Antiepileptics in Neonates

	Loading Dose	Maintenance Dose
Phenobarbital	20 mg/kg	3–4 mg/kg/day divided BID
Fosphenytoin	20 mg/kg	3–4 mg/kg/day divided BID
Lorazepam	0.05 mg/kg	repeated loading as needed

BID, twice a day.

many antiepileptic medications fueled controversy in the past regarding how aggressive clinicians should be in treating neonatal seizures. Accumulating evidence suggests, however, that repeated seizures in the neonatal period are independently associated with poor neurologic outcomes. These data and the tremendous improvements in neonatal care warrant early therapy.

Treatment of neonatal seizures should always focus on correction of the underlying etiology if possible. Transient metabolic disturbances should be addressed specifically. In the absence of such abnormalities, phenobarbital continues to be the mainstay of treatment for neonatal seizures by both neonatologists and neurologists. Second-line agents include phenytoin (or its preferred precursor fosphenytoin) and benzodiazepines, with lorazepam being the most common medication chosen from the latter class. Typical doses are listed in Table 101-2. The most significant risks associated with these drugs are sedation, respiratory depression, and hypotension, and neonates should be monitored closely during initiation these therapies. Clearance of these drugs from the neonatal system is notoriously variable, and infants must be closely monitored for signs of toxicity with clinical observation and drug levels.

The use of traditional antiepileptics provides moderate control of seizures at best, and given concerns regarding the effect of these medications on the developing brain, it is essential to develop more effective treatments. Newer antiepileptics are available, but data on their safety and effectiveness in neonates are scarce. In animal models, several of these, including topiramate and levetiracetam, appear to have fewer detrimental effects on the CNS than the traditional antiepileptics, but further investigation is necessary. It is also important to consider some of the rarer causes of refractory seizures in neonates, particularly if there are no identifiable risk factors. Some of these children may respond to alternative therapies such as pyridoxine or the ketogenic diet, although in-depth discussion of these topics is beyond the scope of this text.

Neonatal Hypotonia

The treatment of neonatal hypotonia generally involves managing the comorbidities associated with the underlying disease. Ventilatory support is sometimes required and generally infers a poor prognosis. Nutritional support through tube feeding while continuing to encourage oral feeding is a necessity. Physical therapy is also an essential component of management to improve strength and feeding ability and to prevent contractures. Although clinicians can offer only supportive care for the vast majority of neuromuscular disorders of infancy, several diseases have specific treatment and therefore warrant mention here. The first is transient neonatal myasthenia gravis, which can be treated with neostigmine (0.05–0.1 mg/kg intramuscularly before feeding). Patients with congenital myasthenic syndromes can benefit from different therapies depending on the underlying defect (acetylcholinesterase inhibitors, 3,4-diaminopyridine, and acetylcholine receptor blockers). Finally, patients with disorders with evidence of neuropathy may benefit from steroid treatment (prednisone 2 mg/kg/d divided twice daily).

FUTURE DIRECTIONS

Basic science has provided extraordinary information regarding the nervous system in recent decades, and clinicians have seen tremendous benefit in terms of diagnostic potential. Much of this information, however, has yet to be translated into therapeutic interventions. Clearly, clinical studies of newer antiepileptics in newborns are necessary to improve the management of patients with seizures. Neuroprotection is another active area of research, and further understanding will help identify strategies to reduce morbidity and mortality associated with neurologic injury. Regenerative medicine is a rapidly developing area as well, and research on neural stem cell physiology will hopefully yield therapies targeted to improve development after neurologic injury. Genetic medicine also holds promise for inherited disorders such as spinal muscular atrophy in which the underlying genetic defects have been identified.

SUGGESTED READINGS

Aranda JV, Thomas R: Systematic review: intravenous Ibuprofen in preterm newborns, *Semin Perinatol* 30(3):114-120, 2006.

Booth D, Evans DJ: Anticonvulsants for neonates with seizures. *Cochrane Database Syst Rev* (4):CD004218. 2004.

Fenichel GM: *Clinical Pediatric Neurology—A Signs and Symptoms Approach*, ed 5, Philadelphia, 2005, Elsevier.

Glass HC, Glidden D, Jeremy RJ, et al: Clinical neonatal seizures are independently associated with outcome in infants at risk for hypoxic-ischemic brain injury, *J Pediatr* 155(3):318-323, 2009.

Jacobs S, Hunt R, Tarnow-Mordi W, et al: Cooling for newborns with hypoxic ischaemic encephalopathy. *Cochrane Database Syst Rev* (4):CD003311, 2007.

Painter MJ, Scher MS, Stein AD, et al: Phenobarbital compared with phenytoin for the treatment of neonatal seizures, *N Engl J Med* 341(7):485-489, 1999.

Schmidt B, Davis P, Moddemann D, et al: Long-term effects of indomethacin prophylaxis in extremely-low-birth-weight infants, *N Engl J Med* 344(26):1966-1972, 2001.

Volpe JJL: *Neurology of the Newborn*, ed 5, Philadelphia, 2008, Elsevier Saunders.

Disorders of the Respiratory System

Lori A. Christ and David A. Munson

102

A dvancements in the treatment of respiratory distress in newborns have significantly reduced infant mortality in the United States over the span of 40 years. Neonatal morbidity persists despite major progress and includes maternal–infant separation caused by prolonged hospitalizations and need for specialized hospital care, multiple diagnostic studies, advanced respiratory support, and an increased likelihood of developing chronic lung disease. In addition, respiratory distress in newborns remains a significant cause of neonatal morbidity and mortality in the developing world.

ETIOLOGY AND PATHOGENESIS

Several well-defined events are necessary for the transition to extrauterine life, including establishment of spontaneous respirations, clearance of amniotic fluid from the airway, surfactant release and function, and a decrease in pulmonary vascular resistance to aid in pulmonary blood flow. Impediments to one or more of these events generally manifest as respiratory distress in the newborn. The differential diagnosis of respiratory distress in neonates is broad, and nonrespiratory etiologies are varied (Table 102-1).

Respiratory Distress Syndrome

Respiratory distress syndrome (RDS), also known as hyaline membrane disease, is the end result of a relative surfactant deficiency that, when combined with the compliant chest wall of the neonate, promotes alveolar atelectasis and prevents newborns from developing a normal functional residual capacity (Figure 102-1). The most significant risk factor for RDS is prematurity because surfactant production begins between 24 and 28 weeks of gestation and does not become fully functional until at least 35 weeks. Other risk factors for the development of RDS include maternal diabetes; early-onset sepsis; and less commonly, congenital surfactant deficiency. Fifty percent of infants with birth weights between 500 and 1500 g develop some degree of respiratory distress; however, survival is greater than 90% with the use of exogenous surfactant and antenatal steroids.

Transient Tachypnea of the Newborn

Transient tachypnea of the newborn (TTN) is one of the most common respiratory disorders of newborns with an incidence of 5.7 per 1000 deliveries. TTN occurs as a result of delayed reabsorption and clearance of fetal alveolar fluid from the airways. Throughout gestation, epithelial cells in the lung secrete alveolar fluid. In the late gestational period, epithelial ion channels shift from active secretion of sodium and chloride to active reabsorption caused by high circulating levels of maternal epinephrine. At birth, inspired oxygen increases gene expression of the sodium transporter, which further facilitates fluid shifts from the airways to the interstitium and intravascular space. Passive fluid reabsorption is also postulated to play a role. However, the accumulation of fluid in the interstitium can decrease lung compliance and prevent the establishment of functional residual capacity.

Factors that increase the likelihood of TTN include nonreassuring fetal status, instrumentation at delivery, Apgar score less than 7 at 1 minute, male sex, in vitro fertilization, multiple gestation, and macrosomia. Relevant maternal characteristics include history of maternal asthma, maternal diabetes, and nulliparity. Cesarean section poses a theoretical risk because of the absence of a "squeeze" effect created by passage through the vagina, which may increase the passive absorption of alveolar fluid. The risk of TTN in the setting of cesarean section increases with absence of labor before delivery and with delivery before 39 weeks.

Meconium Aspiration Syndrome

Meconium aspiration syndrome (MAS) is defined as respiratory distress in a newborn in the setting of meconium-stained amniotic fluid, whose distress cannot be otherwise explained. Meconium is a combination of amniotic fluid, bile, water, intestinal epithelial cells, lanugo, and mucous, all of which are swallowed by the fetus. A fetus in distress is likely to pass meconium because the stress response results in a relaxation of the anal sphincter and subsequent release of meconium. Fetal distress, when prolonged, can provoke fetal gasping and increase the likelihood of aspiration. When aspirated into the airway, meconium contributes to respiratory distress by obstructing the airway, inactivating surfactant, and producing an inflammatory response that damages the respiratory epithelial barrier and predisposes the neonate to serious bacterial infection. The inflammatory response leads to vasoconstriction and persistent pulmonary hypertension in 20% of infants, with an increased risk in infants who experience chronic intrauterine hypoxemia. Meconium staining occurs in 10% to 20% of all deliveries and accounts for 2% of all perinatal mortality.

Bronchopulmonary Dysplasia

Bronchopulmonary dysplasia (BPD) is defined as oxygen dependency in a premature infant continuing past 36 weeks corrected gestational age. An exaggerated inflammatory response occurs soon after birth in the incompletely developed lung, which is exacerbated by positive-pressure ventilation and prolonged mechanical ventilation, which can result in barotrauma and further lung damage over time. There are currently two descriptions of BPD in the literature. The first is seen in premature infants resuscitated as the field of neonatology initially expanded,

Table 102-1 Differential Diagnosis of Neonatal Respiratory Distress

System	Category	Diagnoses
Respiratory	Airway obstruction	Pierre Robin sequence
	Parenchymal disease	Choanal atresia
	Congenital lung malformations	Nasal stenosis
	Air leak syndromes	Vascular ring or sling
		Hemangioma
		Tracheomalacia
		Transient tachypnea of the newborn
		Respiratory distress syndrome
		Pneumonia
		Congenital surfactant deficiency
		Meconium aspiration syndrome
		Congenital cystic adenomatoid malformation
		Congenital diaphragmatic hernia
		Neoplastic processes
		Bronchopulmonary sequestration
		Arteriovenous malformation
		Congenital lobar emphysema
		Pneumothorax
		Pulmonary interstitial emphysema
		Pneumomediastinum
Cardiac	Acyanotic lesions	Patent ductus arteriosus
	Cyanotic lesions	Interrupted aortic arch
		Critical aortic stenosis
		Coarctation of the aorta
		Transposition of the great arteries
		Tetralogy of Fallot
		Truncus arteriosus
		Total anomalous pulmonary venous return
		Tricuspid atresia
		Ebstein's anomaly
		Pulmonary atresia
Neurologic		Birth trauma
		Meningitis
		Venous sinus thrombosis
		Hypoxic ischemic encephalopathy
		Seizure disorder
		Apnea
		Neuromuscular weakness
		Intraventricular hemorrhage
Metabolic		Inborn error of metabolism
		Hypoglycemia
		Maternal medication effect

with the majority of lung damage attributable to mechanical ventilation and its effects (barotrauma, endotracheal bacterial colonization, high inspired oxygen concentration). As mechanical ventilation of neonates has become more refined over time, histologic examination has revealed a changing pattern of lung damage, including fewer and larger alveoli with abnormal septation and an otherwise normal airway. This pattern is best conceptualized as an arrest in development with simplified architecture. As resuscitation techniques have permitted neonates of earlier gestational ages to survive, these changes are attributable not only to mechanical ventilation but also to the effects of sepsis and extreme prematurity. The role of a persistent patent ductus arteriosus continues to be the subject of considerable debate and research. The risk of a premature infant with RDS progressing to BPD decreases linearly with increasing gestational age. Antenatal steroid administration also decreases the risk of BPD.

Pneumothorax

Air leak syndromes, as the name implies, result from rupture of the alveolar sac with subsequent flow of air into the interstitial spaces of the lung, and they occur in the setting of a rapid change in intrathoracic pressure. In term infants, pneumothorax is the most common result of an air leak and occurs in 1% of all deliveries (Figure 102-2). Risk factors include positive-pressure ventilation with high peak inspiratory pressures (>20–25 mm Hg) and surfactant administration. Pneumothorax may occur spontaneously at birth even without application of positive-pressure ventilation.

A. Risk factors for development of respiratory distress syndrome (RDS) of newborn

Prematurity
Birth wt. >2.5 kg; RDS not likely
Birth wt. <2.5 kg; likelihood of
RDS increases in relation to lower
wt. (if viable)

Perinatal asphyxia
(2nd born
of twins
∴ more
susceptible)

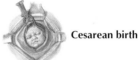
Cesarean birth

Diabetes mellitus (maternal)

B. Surfactant effects during lung inflation in the neonate

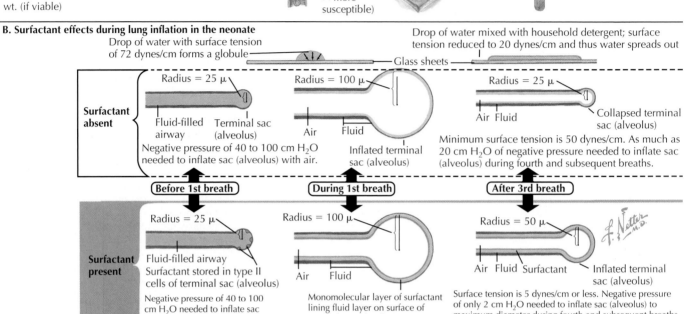

Drop of water with surface tension of 72 dynes/cm forms a globule

Drop of water mixed with household detergent; surface tension reduced to 20 dynes/cm and thus water spreads out

Glass sheets

Surfactant absent

Radius = 25 μ — Fluid-filled airway Terminal sac (alveolus)
Negative pressure of 40 to 100 cm H_2O needed to inflate sac (alveolus) with air.

Radius = 100 μ — Air Fluid Inflated terminal sac (alveolus)

Radius = 25 μ — Air Fluid Collapsed terminal sac (alveolus)
Minimum surface tension is 50 dynes/cm. As much as 20 cm H_2O of negative pressure needed to inflate sac (alveolus) during fourth and subsequent breaths.

Before 1st breath — **During 1st breath** — **After 3rd breath**

Surfactant present

Radius = 25 μ — Fluid-filled airway Surfactant stored in type II cells of terminal sac (alveolus)
Negative pressure of 40 to 100 cm H_2O needed to inflate sac (alveolus) with air.

Radius = 100 μ — Air Fluid
Monomolecular layer of surfactant lining fluid layer on surface of terminal sac (alveolus)

Radius = 50 μ — Air Fluid Surfactant Inflated terminal sac (alveolus)
Surface tension is 5 dynes/cm or less. Negative pressure of only 2 cm H_2O needed to inflate sac (alveolus) to maximum diameter during fourth and subsequent breaths.

The initial inflation of the collapsed lungs of a neonate requires high negative pressure (40 to 100 cm H_2O), but surface tension is reduced in subsequent breaths as surfactant lines the alveoli and small airways, reducing the work required to inflate the lungs. Premature birth is often associated with surfactant deficiency and respiratory distress.

Figure 102-1 *Respiratory distress syndrome of the newborn.*

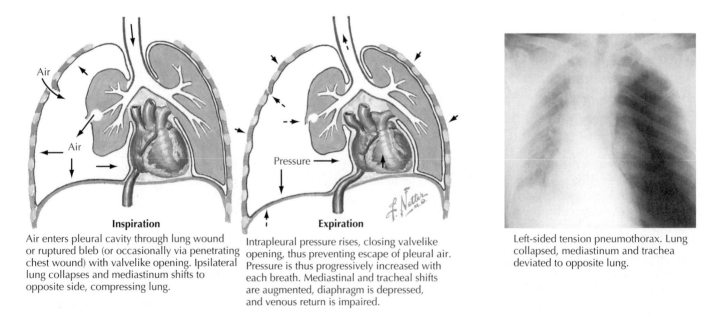

Inspiration
Air enters pleural cavity through lung wound or ruptured bleb (or occasionally via penetrating chest wound) with valvelike opening. Ipsilateral lung collapses and mediastinum shifts to opposite side, compressing lung.

Expiration
Intrapleural pressure rises, closing valvelike opening, thus preventing escape of pleural air. Pressure is thus progressively increased with each breath. Mediastinal and tracheal shifts are augmented, diaphragm is depressed, and venous return is impaired.

Left-sided tension pneumothorax. Lung collapsed, mediastinum and trachea deviated to opposite lung.

Figure 102-2 *Pneumothorax.*

Anatomic Abnormalities

Congenital anomalies of the pulmonary system may or may not be prenatally diagnosed and include the following disorders: choanal atresia, a congenital blockage of the posterior nares; trachea-esophageal fistula; congenital diaphragmatic hernia (CDH), a patent pleuroperitoneal canal that allows the intestines to occupy the pleural space and results in pulmonary hypoplasia (Figure 102-3); congenital cystic adenomatous malformation (CCAM); bronchopulmonary sequestration, in which a segment of lung parenchyma is not supplied by the pulmonary blood supply and does not communicate with the bronchial tree (see Figure 102-3); bronchogenic cysts; congenital lobar emphysema, which results in air trapping in one lung segment; vascular rings and slings; and Pierre Robin sequence and other maxillofacial malformations. A full exploration of these

disorders is beyond the scope of this chapter, but it is important to keep them in mind when faced with an infant with respiratory distress without risk factors for the more common disorders described above.

CLINICAL PRESENTATION

Pertinent aspects of the maternal history include antenatal complications such as infection, hypertension, diabetes, medication and substance use, abnormal prenatal sonography, oligo- or polyhydramnios, history of preterm labor and steroid administration, and parity. A birth history significant for prolonged rupture of membranes, birth trauma, nonreassuring fetal heart tracings, and meconium-stained amniotic fluid may also provide clues to a diagnosis. Infants in respiratory distress present with

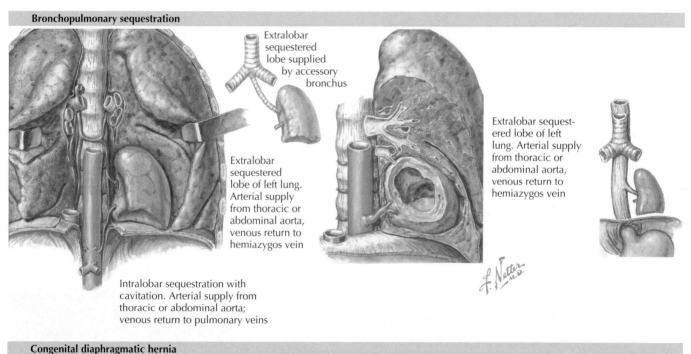

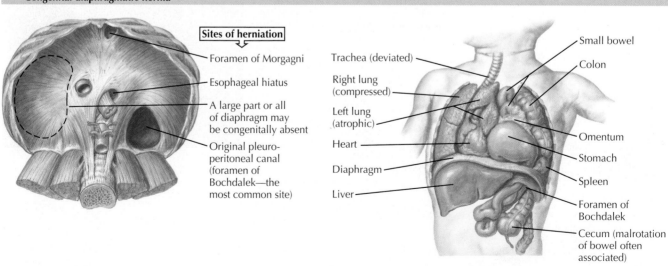

Figure 102-3 *Anatomic abnormalities.*

some degree of the following: tachypnea (respiratory rate > 60 breaths/min), intercostal and subcostal retractions, grunting, cyanosis, and nasal flaring.

MAS presents soon after birth, with tachypnea and hypoxemia worsening over several hours. There is always a history of meconium-stained amniotic fluid, and meconium may be visualized in the oropharynx or below the vocal cords if endotracheal suctioning is attempted per the Neonatal Resuscitation Program guidelines (see below). Signs of respiratory distress are the presenting features, and a barrel-shaped chest with palpable liver and spleen caused by hyperinflation may be noted.

TTN presents within 6 hours after birth. Cyanosis is uncommon but responds readily to inspired oxygen when present. TTN is self-limited and resolves on average within 72 hours.

RDS is most common in premature infants as a result of surfactant deficiency and lung immaturity. Symptoms progress over the first 48 to 96 hours after birth.

Asymmetric chest wall movement and asymmetric breath sounds characterize pneumothorax on examination. Transillumination of the chest wall may reveal hyperlucency of the affected side. In term infants, the presentation can vary based on the size of the air leak from mild tachypnea or oxygen requirement to marked respiratory distress and even cardiovascular collapse if a tension pneumothorax develops.

Other physical findings pertinent to the differential diagnosis include a full cardiac examination with specific attention to murmurs, the precordium, and perfusion. Maxillofacial abnormalities are generally readily noticeable, and an inability to pass a suction catheter through the nose into the nasopharynx raises concern for choanal atresia. CDH must be considered in the infant with a scaphoid abdomen. Signs of impending respiratory failure may include cyanosis, stridor, gasping, marked retractions, poor perfusion, and apnea.

EVALUATION AND MANAGEMENT

Initial Evaluation

Chest radiography is the best test to differentiate between RDS and TTN, the most common causes of respiratory distress in newborns. Whereas fluid in the interlobar fissure, with perihilar streaking, indicates TTN, a uniform reticulogranular pattern ("ground-glass appearance") and peripheral air bronchograms suggest RDS (Figure 102-4). Chest radiography is also useful to evaluate for pneumonia, congenital heart disease, pneumothorax, and CDH. Radiographic findings of pneumothorax are air in the pleural cavity resulting in hyperlucency with absence of pulmonary markings in the affected area. A more subtle chest radiography finding suggestive of pneumothorax is a downward displacement of the diaphragm, which can be verified with a cross-table lateral chest radiograph as an anterior mediastinal collection of air.

Arterial blood gas analysis is useful to guide therapy in a variety of causes of respiratory failure. Elevated carbon dioxide levels indicate a need for increased respiratory support. Extremely low partial pressure of oxygen in the face of high inspired oxygen is a marker of severe pulmonary disease or intracardiac shunting of blood in the setting of congenital heart disease. Alkalosis in the setting of tachypnea may indicate a neurologic cause. A metabolic acidosis most commonly indicates significant systemic illness with inadequate delivery of oxygen and nutrients to end organs but can also suggest an inborn error of metabolism.

Other evaluation and management of respiratory distress should be pursued as the clinical history and examination indicate. Pulse oximetry, screening and treatment for sepsis, and blood sugar measurement are all appropriate first-line interventions. Neonates with an elevated respiratory rate should not

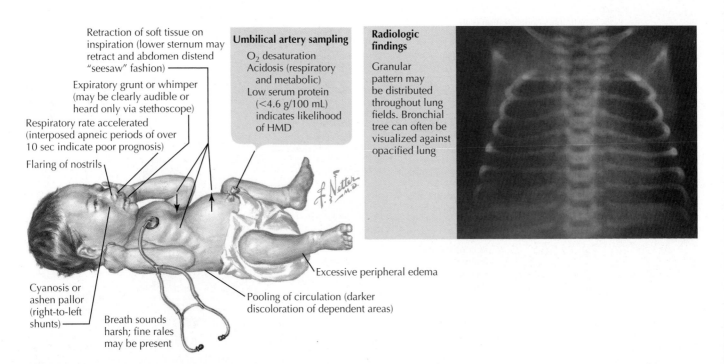

Figure 102-4 *Manifestations of hyaline membrane disease in the newborn.*

feed by mouth because of increased risk of aspiration and may require intravenous fluids or nasogastric feeding. Echocardiography is warranted if the cardiac examination, persistent cyanosis, and vital signs suggest congenital heart disease.

Disease-Specific Management

Respiratory distress syndrome is a result of surfactant deficiency, and if distress or hypoxemia is severe, surfactant administration can significantly reduce distress and the need for invasive ventilation. The use of surfactant has also been noted to decrease the incidence of intraventricular hemorrhage in preterm infants.

The management of an infant with meconium-stained amniotic fluid occurs per the Neonatal Resuscitation Program guidelines. If vigorous, infants with meconium-stained amniotic fluid may be observed for signs of respiratory distress; suctioning in vigorous infants has not prevented MAS in large, prospective, randomized trials. If amniotic fluid is meconium stained and the newborn is not vigorous at delivery, immediate nasopharyngeal suctioning at the perineum is not indicated. Instead, endotracheal intubation for the purpose of suctioning meconium from the trachea before the onset of respiration is recommended to remove all gross particulate meconium from the airway. This prevents meconium from being further aspirated into the lungs and may prevent progression to MAS. Patients with MAS and persistent pulmonary hypertension may require a high level of respiratory support, including high-frequency oscillatory ventilation, inhaled nitric oxide, and endotracheal administration of surfactant. Extracorporeal membrane oxygenation (ECMO) may be indicated, and infants should be referred to an ECMO center for evaluation. Overall, despite an intensive hospital course, survival from MAS is approximately 90%.

Transient tachypnea of the newborn is made retrospectively as a diagnosis of exclusion. Care is supportive; prospective randomized, controlled trials have shown no benefit to using furosemide or inhaled racemic epinephrine treatments. TTN generally resolves within 72 hours; prolonged tachypnea (>60 rpm) or deteriorating clinical status should prompt further evaluation.

The degree of respiratory distress dictates the management of pneumothorax. Infants with mild distress may require little more than oxygen supplementation and close monitoring. Moderate to severe distress warrants emergent decompression and chest tube placement until the infant is clinically stable. Hemodynamic instability indicates a tension pneumothorax that should be immediately decompressed.

FUTURE DIRECTIONS

The early ventilatory management of preterm neonates with respiratory distress syndrome is a topic of ongoing research; optimal timing of surfactant administration and the role of noninvasive ventilation are two areas of intense debate. Furthermore, new strategies for the prevention and management of meconium aspiration and the role of ECMO continue to be refined.

SUGGESTED READINGS

Dargaville PA, Copnell P; Australian and New Zealand Neonatal Network: The epidemiology of meconium aspiration syndrome: incidence, risk factors, therapies, and outcome, *Pediatrics* 117(5):1712-1721, 2006.

Engle WA; American Academy of Pediatrics Committee on Fetus and Newborn: Surfactant-replacement therapy for respiratory distress in the preterm and term neonate, *Pediatrics* 121(2):419-432, 2008.

Niermeyer S, Kattwinkel J, Van Reempts P, et al: International Guidelines for Neonatal Resuscitation: an excerpt from the Guidelines 2000 for Cardiopulmonary Resuscitation and Emergency Cardiovascular Care: International Consensus on Science. Contributors and Reviewers for the Neonatal Resuscitation Guidelines, *Pediatrics* 106(3):e29, 2000.

Roberts D, Dalziel S: Antenatal corticosteroids for accelerating fetal lung maturation for women at risk of preterm birth. Cochrane Database Syst Rev 3:CD004454, 2006.

Stevens TP, Harrington EW, Blennow M, Soll RF: Early surfactant administration with brief ventilation vs. selective surfactant and continued mechanical ventilation for preterm infants with or at risk for respiratory distress syndrome. Cochrane Database Syst Rev (4):CD003063, 2007.

Takaya A, Igarashi M, Nakajima M, et al: Risk factors for transient tachypnea of the newborn in infants delivered vaginally at 37 weeks or later, *J Nippon Med Sch* 75(5):269-273, 2008.

Wiswell, TE, Gannon CM, Jacob J, et al: Delivery room management of the apparently vigorous meconium-stained neonate: results of the multicenter, international collaborative trial, *Pediatrics* 105(1 Pt 1):1-7, 2000.

103

Disorders of the Gastrointestinal System

John J. Flibotte

Gastrointestinal (GI) disorders are common causes of serious illness in the neonatal population. Necrotizing enterocolitis (NEC) affects 1% to 8% of all infants in neonatal intensive care units (NICUs), and population-based reports not limited to the NICU indicate that anywhere from one in 700 to one in 10,000 infants will experience GI obstruction. Neonatal GI disorders share many common and nonspecific presenting signs. However, careful history regarding the timing of symptom onset, relation to initiation of feeds, and maternal and perinatal factors can direct an efficient diagnostic evaluation and initial management.

NECROTIZING ENTEROCOLITIS

ETIOLOGY AND PATHOGENESIS

Necrotizing enterocolitis (NEC) is one of the most common GI conditions affecting premature neonates. Despite advances made in the diagnosis and treatment of other conditions associated with prematurity, rates of NEC have increased in the past several decades because of the increased survival of infants at younger gestational ages. Mortality associated with NEC remains significant, ranging from 10% to 50%.

Although the pathogenesis of NEC is not clear, the concurrence of multiple conditions seems to result in NEC. Prematurity is the most consistently identified risk factor. The association of NEC with initiation of feeds, osmolarity of feeds, and rate of feed increases suggests that immature gut mucosa is injured in a way that allows intestinal bacterial translocation. This results in an immune response that may progress to a systemic inflammatory response and shock. Clusters of NEC cases in NICUs and the isolation of bacteria from infants affected by NEC suggests that microbial infection may play a role in either initiating or propagating the above cascade of events. Bacteria isolated from infants affected by NEC include *Klebsiella pneumoniae*, *Pseudomonas aeruginosa*, *Escherichia coli*, and *Enterobacter* spp.

CLINICAL PRESENTATION

Early signs of NEC are nonspecific, and a high index of suspicion is required for early identification. Feeding intolerance, abdominal distension, lethargy, and temperature instability are early harbingers of evolving NEC. Later findings include bloody stools; worsening abdominal distension; abdominal skin redness and necrosis and; in severe cases, findings associated with viscus perforation and fulminant sepsis.

EVALUATION AND MANAGEMENT

Radiographic findings associated with NEC are variable. Early NEC can present with isolated bowel loop distension. The most classic sign of NEC seen on abdominal radiographs is pneumatosis intestinalis (i.e., intramural air). In the most severe cases, abdominal free air becomes evident. In cases in which microperforation results in release of air into the venous system, the only radiographic finding that may be detected is portal venous gas.

The most common laboratory finding is a low white blood cell count. However, thrombocytopenia, acidosis, and hypoglycemia are also seen. In cases that evolve to septic shock, laboratory study results may be consistent with disseminated intravascular coagulation.

The majority of infants affected by NEC are managed medically, the principles of which include supportive care followed by a period of bowel rest and slow reintroduction of feeds. Patients should be followed closely for progression of disease, which is evident from enlarging abdominal circumference, declining clinical status, and evolution of radiographic findings. Because physical findings may be subtle, repeated abdominal imaging is often performed in the early stages of NEC to identify evolving disease.

Intubation and ventilatory support may be required. Acidosis is a marker of progressive disease and inadequate perfusion of end organs. When needed, pressors should be initiated to maintain hemodynamic stability. After blood cultures are drawn, empiric antibiotic treatment for intestinal flora should be started. Although ampicillin, gentamicin, and Flagyl have been the first-line choice of treatment, local antibiotic susceptibilities should guide therapy. Infants should receive no enteral nutrition for a period of time, typically 7 to 14 days, after which feeds should be gradually introduced.

Approximately one-third to one-half of patients with NEC require surgical management. Indications for surgical management include intestinal perforation or bowel necrosis. The preferred approach in infants weighing more than 1500 g is resection of necrotic bowel and temporary diversion to a mucocutaneous fistula, with reanastomosis after approximately 6 weeks. In patients weighing less than 1500 g, primary peritoneal drainage is used because of significant morbidity and mortality associated with resection and diversion.

Several complications are associated with NEC. The most common is intestinal stricture, which presents with feeding intolerance about 1 to 2 weeks after the resolution of NEC. This should be distinguished from recurrence of NEC, which is seen in about 6% of NEC survivors. Other long-term

Table 103-1 Localizing Features of Intestinal Obstruction

Sign or Finding	Proximal or Distal	Specific Site (When Applicable)
Nonbilious vomiting	Proximal	Proximal to the ampulla of Vater
Bilious vomiting	Proximal or distal	Distal to the ampulla of Vater
Scaphoid abdomen	Proximal	Often preduodenal
Distended abdomen	Distal	
Maternal polyhydramnios	Proximal	

complications include neurodevelopmental delay as well as total parenteral nutrition–associated cholestasis in infants who are on prolonged parenteral nutrition during treatment for NEC. Importantly, if a lengthy section of intestine required resection, infants can experience short gut syndrome.

INTESTINAL OBSTRUCTION

ETIOLOGY AND PATHOGENESIS

Intestinal obstruction is possible at any point along the GI tract. Causes of obstruction are subdivided into mechanical and functional causes. Mechanical causes result from a failure of development of the GI tract. Examples include intestinal and anal atresias, which are caused by a failure of recanalization of the alimentary tract; malrotation, which is caused by a failure of complete rotation of the GI tract during development; and pyloric stenosis, which is caused by overgrowth of the pyloric muscle after birth. Functional causes of obstruction include meconium plug syndrome, Hirschsprung's disease, and small left colon syndrome, all of which result from impairment of the normal peristaltic movements.

CLINICAL PRESENTATION

Intestinal obstruction in a neonate, regardless of the underlying cause, presents with the following common signs:

- Vomiting or feeding intolerance
- Abdominal distension
- Failure to pass meconium

Subtle differences in presentation can suggest the location of the obstruction along the alimentary tract (Table 103-1). These unique features are highlighted below as each disorder is discussed.

Esophageal Atresia

The esophagus can be obstructed in the form of esophageal atresia (EA), which is caused by a failure of separation of the esophagus from the trachea during normal development. Pure EA is rare and often coexists with tracheoesophageal fistula (TEF). A standard classification scheme describes the relationship between the atresia and the coexistent TEF (Figure 103-1). The most common combination is EA with distal TEF (type

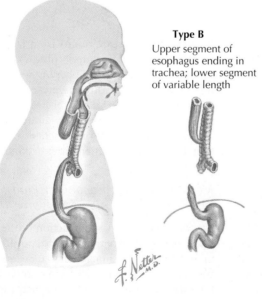

Type C

Most common form (90% to 95%) of tracheo-esophageal fistula. Upper segment of esophagus ending in blind pouch; lower segment originating from trachea just above bifurcation. The two segments may be connected by a solid cord

Type B

Upper segment of esophagus ending in trachea; lower segment of variable length

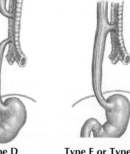

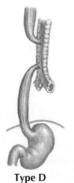

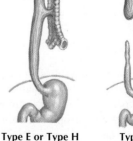

Type D
Double fistula

Type E or Type H
Fistula without esophageal atresia

Type A
Esophageal atresia without fistula

Figure 103-1 *Tracheoesophageal fistula.*

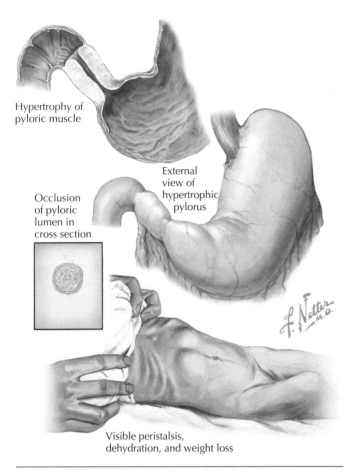

Hypertrophy of pyloric muscle

External view of hypertrophic pylorus

Occlusion of pyloric lumen in cross section

Visible peristalsis, dehydration, and weight loss

Figure 103-2 *Hypertrophic pyloric stenosis.*

C). The most difficult to recognize and diagnose is "H-type," which refers to isolated TEF without EA.

EA presents early in the newborn period with intolerance of feeds. Infants with EA have copious oral secretions that are difficult to control. They display nonbilious vomiting after the first feed and do not tolerate any additional feeds. Whether or not the abdomen is distended depends on the presence of TEF. If there is no connection between the trachea and distal portion of the esophagus, the abdomen will be gasless; if there is a distal connection, the stomach and abdomen will be distended. Infants with H-type EA or TEF tolerate feeds without difficulty and instead present with more subtle signs of tachypnea or recurrent pneumonia from pulmonary aspiration of feeds.

Pyloric Stenosis

Obstruction at the level of the pylorus from congenital abnormalities, such as webs or membranes, is rare in the immediate neonatal period. However, approximately one in 500 infants will develop hypertrophic pyloric stenosis (HPS) during the first month of life (Figure 103-2). The classic presentation of HPS is a 3- to 4-week-old infant with persistent nonbilious projectile vomiting after each feed. Although found in male and female infants of all ethnicities, first-born male white infants seem to be disproportionately affected. Use of the antibiotic

erythromycin in the neonatal period is a known risk factor as well. Infants with HPS appear irritable and hungry, and in some cases, a mass in the shape of an olive can be palpated in the right upper quadrant, representing the hypertrophic pyloric sphincter. Immediately after feeding, a reverse peristaltic wave may be seen just before vomiting. The abdomen may appear scaphoid before air and feeds are not able to pass beyond the level of the pylorus.

Intestinal Atresias and Stenosis

Intestinal atresias are possible at any point along the GI tract. Jejunoileal atresia is the most common atresia followed by duodenal atresia and finally colonic atresia. Presenting signs and symptoms are nonspecific and similar to those of other obstruction syndromes. Duodenal and jejunal atresias generally present with bilious emesis. More distal obstruction often still have emesis but may present with more subtle signs of feeding intolerance, including abdominal distension. In addition, the time to onset of symptoms and the presence of maternal polyhydramnios can suggest the location of stenosis. More distal obstructions take longer to present, and it is less likely that the mother will have had polyhydramnios because amniotic fluid is absorbed in the proximal small bowel.

Malrotation and Volvulus

Malrotation refers to a disruption of the normal rotational process of the midgut, resulting in abnormal fixation of the duodenum. This creates a stalk around which the gut can twist intermittently, creating bowel obstruction and ischemia. The peak time of presentation is within the first month of life, and there is a 2 : 1 male predominance. Symptoms at the time of presentation are as highlighted above for obstruction syndromes, but bilious emesis in a neonate should prompt immediate concern for volvulus. Malrotation without volvulus can manifest simply as reflux or feeding intolerance.

Hirschsprung's Disease

Hirschsprung's disease results from failure of the ganglion cells to develop in the myenteric plexus of the colon, resulting in dysfunctional peristalsis. There is a wide range of severity, and infants with severe cases may present with the signs of obstruction outlined above. Mildly affected infants often have a delayed presentation characterized by failure to pass meconium within the first 24 hours of life or intractable constipation. On examination, the abdomen is often distended but is generally not tender.

Meconium Ileus, Meconium Plug Syndrome, and Small Left Colon Syndrome

Meconium ileus refers to impaction of the distal ileum by inspissated meconium from birth. The specific terminology of meconium ileus refers to impaction that occurs in a patient with cystic fibrosis (CF). This results from high viscosity of meconium in CF patients because of a lack of pancreatic enzyme activity along with abnormal mucous secretion. Meconium plug syndrome and small left colon syndrome both appear to be related to poor gut motility rather than intrinsic obstruction, and both are seen most often in the setting of infants of diabetic mothers. Presenting signs and symptoms in all cases include abdominal distension shortly after birth. This may be followed by emesis and intolerance of feeds.

Imperforate Anus

Imperforate anus results from a failure of the normal development of the hindgut. The presence of imperforate anus should be apparent on physical examination and may be associated with other congenital anomalies (i.e., VACTERL [vertebral anomalies, anal atresia, cardiovascular anomalies, tracheoesophageal fistula, esophageal atresia, renal or radial anomalies, and limb defects] association; see Chapter 120).

EVALUATION AND MANAGEMENT

In all cases of suspected intestinal obstruction, evaluation should proceed quickly. After stabilizing the patient, confirmation of the presence of obstruction with abdominal radiography or other imagining modality and consultation with pediatric surgeons should ensue. Initial stabilization should include eliminating oral feeds, correcting any electrolyte or metabolic abnormalities, administering intravenous (IV) fluid boluses for unstable patients and starting maintenance fluids, and placement of a nasogastric (NG) or orogastric (OG) tube to decompress the abdomen. Blood cultures should also be sent and empiric antibiotic coverage for intestinal flora initiated. There are specific diagnostic options and management steps to consider based on the suspected obstruction syndrome, as discussed below. Finally, specific causes of intestinal obstruction may be components of genetic syndromes and should prompt complete evaluation to rule out associated conditions (Table 103-2).

Esophageal Atresia

In cases of suspected EA, initial abdominal radiographs may reveal a gasless abdomen. Placement of a NG or OG tube may be met with resistance. Injection of air through the NG tube can be used as contrast before chest radiographs are performed, thereby highlighting a blind-ended esophageal pouch. In cases of suspected H-type TEF, a dedicated upper GI radiography

Table 103-2 Site of Obstruction and Associated Genetic Syndromes

Type of Obstruction	Genetic Association
Esophageal atresia	VACTERL
Duodenal atresia	Down syndrome
Colonic atresia	Eye, heart, and abdominal wall anomalies
Meconium ileus	Cystic fibrosis
Small left colon syndrome	Diabetic mother

VACTERL, vertebral anomalies, anal atresia, cardiovascular anomalies, tracheoesophageal fistula, esophageal atresia, renal or radial anomalies, and limb defects.

series may be required to confirm diagnosis. After diagnosis is confirmed, surgical repair via thoracotomy and reanastomosis of the esophagus is required. In the presence of a TEF, the fistula should be repaired early in the hospital course to prevent ongoing soiling of the lungs. In cases with other associated anomalies, surgical repair may be delayed or performed in several stages to allow for adequate growth.

Pyloric Stenosis

Initial stabilization of infants suspected of having HPS should include hydration with IV fluids, determination of electrolytes, and imaging. Hypochloremic hypokalemic metabolic alkalosis is the electrolyte abnormality associated with HPS. Abdominal ultrasound is the definitive diagnostic test for HPS, and criteria for the diagnosis of HPS are a pyloric canal longer than 1.4 cm in length or a thickness of 0.3 cm or greater. Definitive management requires surgical pyloromyotomy.

Intestinal Atresias

The initial workup for intestinal atresia should proceed as highlighted above. In addition to abdominal plain radiography, contrast studies including upper GI studies with follow-through may be needed to identify the level of intestinal obstruction before surgical repair.

Malrotation and Volvulus

When an infant presents with bilious emesis, an upper GI series must be performed emergently because the time from presentation to operation will determine the amount of viable intestine saved when there is a volvulus. Malrotation is diagnosed when the upper GI series demonstrates an abnormal point of attachment of the ligament of Treitz. Surgical management with a Ladd's procedure is required to release the mesentery. This topic is covered in greater detail in Chapter 109.

Hirschsprung's Disease

Abdominal plain radiographs may reveal dilated bowel loops or the presence of stool in the colon, and a barium enema may show a transition point in affected patients (Figure 103-3). Definitive diagnosis is made with a suction rectal biopsy to evaluate for the presence of ganglion cells. Surgical repair is required to remove the aganglionic section of bowel and restore normal peristalsis.

Meconium Ileus, Meconium Plug Syndrome, and Small Left Colon Syndrome

These entities have similar diagnostic workup that includes abdominal radiography. Key findings include intestinal distension proximal to the site of obstruction and possibly calcifications within the meconium. Barium enema may be used to better identify the point of obstruction, and it may also be therapeutic in the setting of meconium plug syndrome. In meconium ileus, contrast enema will demonstrate a small, unused colon and meconium pellets in the distal ileum. Because

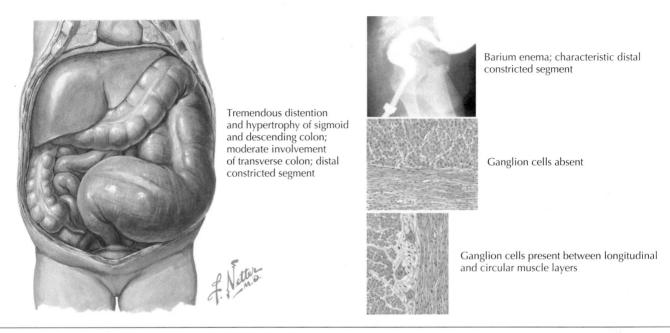

Tremendous distention
and hypertrophy of sigmoid
and descending colon;
moderate involvement
of transverse colon; distal
constricted segment

Barium enema; characteristic distal
constricted segment

Ganglion cells absent

Ganglion cells present between longitudinal
and circular muscle layers

Figure 103-3 *Hirschsprung's disease.*

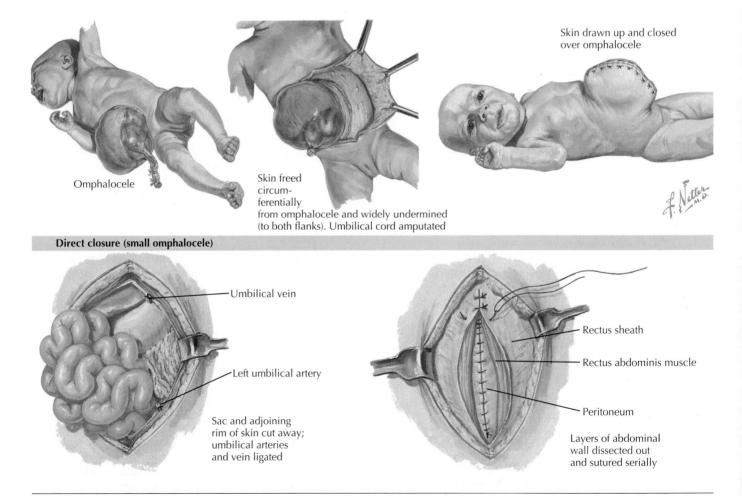

Skin drawn up and closed
over omphalocele

Omphalocele

Skin freed
circum-
ferentially
from omphalocele and widely undermined
(to both flanks). Umbilical cord amputated

Direct closure (small omphalocele)

Umbilical vein

Left umbilical artery

Sac and adjoining
rim of skin cut away;
umbilical arteries
and vein ligated

Rectus sheath

Rectus abdominis muscle

Peritoneum

Layers of abdominal
wall dissected out
and sutured serially

Figure 103-4 *Omphalocele.*

of the specificity of this disease for CF, genetic testing should be undertaken (see Chapter 41). If water-soluble enema fails to relieve the obstruction or if the obstruction is complicated by proximal volvulus, surgical intervention is indicated.

Imperforate Anus

Surgical reconstruction is necessary for patients with imperforate anus. Often a perianal fistula will allow for a contrast enema that may clarify the severity of the imperforate anus. The distance from the end of the large intestine to the perineum will dictate the complexity of surgical repair. A diverting colostomy may be required to allow the patient to grow before definitive repair.

ABDOMINAL WALL DEFECTS

ETIOLOGY AND PATHOGENESIS

The two most common abdominal wall defects in neonates are gastroschisis and omphalocele. Both result from a failure of closure of the abdominal wall after extraabdominal development and rotation of the GI tract.

CLINICAL PRESENTATION

The presence of gastroschisis or omphalocele is readily apparent on physical examination, and both are often diagnosed prenatally on ultrasound (Figure 103-4). Omphalocele is characterized by an overlying membrane and a central location. Gastroschisis is displaced to the right of the umbilicus and does not have an overlying membrane.

EVALUATION AND MANAGEMENT

Gastroschisis and omphalocele require surgical correction (see Figure 103-4). Before surgical intervention, the defects should be covered and kept moist. Infants may require additional fluids given their higher-than-normal insensible losses. Preterm infants may need to be supported during a period of growth until they are large enough to undergo closure. Omphalocele has a high association with genetic syndromes; therefore, a careful physical examination and genetic evaluation are indicated.

FUTURE DIRECTIONS

Ongoing research is being performed to further elucidate strategies for preventing NEC. Areas of interest include evaluating the timing and source of feeds for premature infants. Early initiation of breast milk has been identified as one protective factor. In addition, the belief that NEC partly results from an imbalance in the intestinal flora of neonates has led to some promising studies evaluating the role of probiotics in preventing NEC.

SUGGESTED READINGS

Claud EC, Walker WA: Bacterial colonization, probiotics, and necrotizing enterocolitis. *J Clin Gastroenterol* 42(suppl 2):S46-S52, 2008.

Dimmitt RA, Moss RL: Clinical management of necrotizing enterocolitis. *NeoReviews* 2:e110-e116, 2001.

Hajivassiliou CA: Intestinal obstruction in neonatal/pediatric surgery. *Semin Pediatr Surg* 12(4):241-253, 2003.

Jesse N, Neu J: Necrotizing enterocolitis: relationship to innate immunity, clinical features, and strategies for prevention. *NeoReviews* 7:e143-e149, 2006.

Many hematologic disorders, both hereditary and acquired, manifest during the first week of life. Early recognition of disease processes, an understanding of their pathogenesis, and prompt institution of necessary (and often lifesaving) therapies are vital.

RBC DISORDERS

Hemolytic Anemias

ETIOLOGY AND PATHOGENESIS

ABO incompatibility primarily occurs in blood group O mothers with fetuses who have blood group A or B. All group O individuals have anti-A and anti-B antibodies that are produced as a result of immune stimulation by the A or B antigens contained in food and bacteria. Interactions between these maternal isoantibodies and fetal red blood cells (RBCs) result in hemolysis. Fifteen percent of pregnancies are ABO incompatible, yet evidence of ABO incompatibility disease is found in only 3% of pregnancies and necessitates exchange transfusion (ET) in fewer than 1% of pregnancies. This is because ABO hemolytic disease tends to occur in newborns whose mothers have high levels of immunoglobulin G (IgG) antibody. Although anti-A and anti-B antibodies are found in the plasma as IgA, IgM, and IgG, only the latter can cross the placenta and interact with fetal RBCs.

Rh incompatibility affects one of every 15 pregnancies and causes a wide variety of symptoms in the fetus, ranging from mild to severe hemolytic anemia and hydrops fetalis. Sensitization to the Rh (D) antigen is the result of exposure of an Rh-negative mother to Rh-positive blood. Possible exposures include prior pregnancy with an Rh-positive fetus, fetomaternal hemorrhage, and obstetric procedures (e.g., amniocentesis, chorionic villus sampling, abortion). Unlike A or B antigens, which are expressed on a number of different tissues, Rh antigens are expressed only on RBCs. Thus, maternal anti-Rh (anti-D) IgG antibodies (Rh-negative mother) cross the placenta and interact with a greater number of fetal RBCs (Rh-positive infant), resulting in significant fetal hemolysis.

CLINICAL PRESENTATION AND DIFFERENTIAL DIAGNOSIS

Both ABO incompatibility and Rh disease are associated with jaundice within the first 24 hours of life. In cases of severe hemolytic disease (i.e., erythroblastosis fetalis), infants also present with signs of hydrops fetalis (ascites, pleural or pericardial effusions, edema), pallor (secondary to anemia), petechiae or purpura (caused by thrombocytopenia), and hepatosplenomegaly (result of extramedullary hematopoiesis and splenic sequestration) (Figure 104-1). Each manifestation has a long list of possible causes, but the combination of jaundice and anemia with any of the above findings should focus clinical attention on diseases associated with hemolysis.

The differential diagnosis of neonatal anemia includes chronic or acute blood loss, congenital disorders of erythrocyte production (e.g., Fanconi's anemia, Diamond-Blackfan), erythrocyte membrane defects (e.g., hereditary spherocytosis, hereditary elliptocytosis), congenital enzyme deficiencies (e.g., G6PD [glucose-6-phosphate dehydrogenase], pyruvate kinase), infection, and hemoglobin disorders (Figure 104-2). Of the hemoglobinopathies, α-thalassemias are the most common and severe. The switch from fetal ($\alpha_2\gamma_2$) to adult ($\alpha_2\beta_2$) hemoglobin occurs during the first year of life. As a result, defects in α-globin synthesis manifest in utero, whereas defects in β-globin synthesis become apparent in late infancy. Deletion of three (hemoglobin H disease) or four (hemoglobin Barts) α-globin genes can cause significant hemolytic anemia and present as hydrops fetalis. Newborn screening enables early detection and treatment of infants with major hemoglobinopathies and therefore reduces the mortality and morbidity associated with these conditions.

DIAGNOSTIC APPROACH

Hemolytic disease of newborns is associated with rapidly progressive or prolonged indirect hyperbilirubinemia, signs of hemolysis on peripheral blood smear (e.g., schistocytes and spherocytes), an elevated reticulocyte count, and anemia. Blood group testing reveals evidence of ABO or Rh incompatibility between the mother and newborn. Direct and indirect Coombs' testing is positive in Rh disease but only weakly positive in ABO incompatibility. Infants with Rh disease should be monitored for thrombocytopenia (caused by liver dysfunction or disseminated intravascular coagulation [DIC]), hypoglycemia (secondary to islet cell hyperplasia of the pancreas), and direct hyperbilirubinemia (may be the result of hepatocellular damage).

MANAGEMENT AND THERAPY

Phototherapy and ET are the primary modes of treatment for infants with hemolytic disease. In Rh incompatibility, intensive phototherapy should be started immediately after birth. Prompt initiation of phototherapy might prevent the need for ET.

Treatment of neonatal hyperbilirubinemia with ET was introduced in the early 1950s. Although ET is proven to reduce mortality and the risk of kernicterus, it is associated with serious complications, including hemodynamic instability, apnea, coagulopathies, electrolyte imbalance, vascular thromboses, sepsis, arrhythmias, and necrotizing enterocolitis (NEC) (see Chapter 100). Efforts to reduce perinatal mortality and the need for ET have led to the development of several prenatal care strategies, including RhoGAM, use of Doppler ultrasound to detect fetal anemia, and intrauterine blood transfusions.

The use of RhoGAM (anti-D prophylaxis) in Rh-negative women has led to a marked decline in Rh sensitization and hemolytic disease of the newborn. Studies have demonstrated that

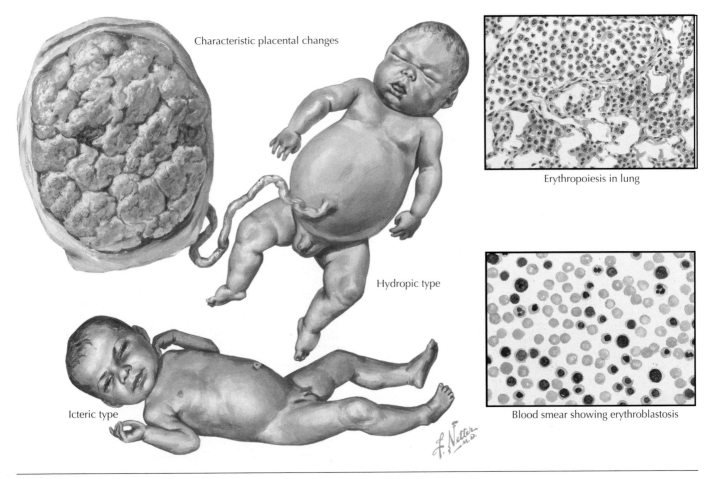

Characteristic placental changes

Erythropoiesis in lung

Hydropic type

Icteric type

Blood smear showing erythroblastosis

Figure 104-1 *Erythroblastosis fetalis.*

of all Rh-sensitized pregnancies with Rh-positive fetuses, 51% require no treatment, 31% require treatment after full-term delivery, 10% are delivered early and need ET, and 9% require intrauterine fetal transfusion. In developed countries, a high proportion of clinically significant hemolytic disease is now caused by antibodies to antigens other than D (i.e., anti-C, anti-E, or anti-Kell) and therefore is not preventable with RhoGAM.

Intravenous immunoglobulin (IVIG) is a supplemental therapy that may be effective in reducing the need for ET in infants with immune-mediated hemolytic disease. In isoimmune hemolysis, RBCs are destroyed by an antibody-dependent cytotoxic process directed by Fc receptor–bearing cells of the reticuloendothelial system. IVIG's mechanism of action is postulated to be attributable to nonspecific blockade of Fc receptors. Potential benefits of IVIG over ET include relative ease of administration, reduced invasiveness, and improved safety profile. Preliminary studies have demonstrated lower maximum bilirubin levels and shorter durations of hospitalization among patients receiving IVIG treatment.

Polycythemia

ETIOLOGY AND PATHOGENESIS

Polycythemia can be subdivided into three categories based on the underlying etiology: (1) increased RBC mass and plasma volume secondary to maternal diabetes or "blood transfusion" (e.g., delayed cord clamping, twin–twin, or maternal–fetal transfusion); (2) increased RBC mass and normal plasma volume related to a congenital syndrome (trisomies 13, 18, and 21); and (3) increased RBC mass and normal or decreased plasma volume caused by intrauterine growth retardation, placental insufficiency, maternal hypertension, or smoking. The incidence of polycythemia is 1% to 5% in all neonates versus 10% to 15% in neonates who are small for gestational age.

CLINICAL PRESENTATION AND DIFFERENTIAL DIAGNOSIS

Polycythemic infants appear ruddy and plethoric with sluggish capillary refill and poor peripheral perfusion. Hyperviscosity of blood results in increased resistance to blood flow and decreased oxygen delivery. Although most neonates with polycythemia are asymptomatic, it can cause abnormalities in central nervous system function (lethargy, apnea, tremors or jitteriness, poor feeding, and hypotonia), decreased renal function (oliguria, proteinuria, and hematuria), cardiorespiratory distress (tachypnea, cyanosis, and cardiomegaly), and coagulation disorders. Rare complications include strokes, seizures, congestive heart failure, renal vein thrombosis, DIC, and NEC. Studies have also noted associations between hyperviscosity and long-term motor and cognitive neurodevelopmental disorders.

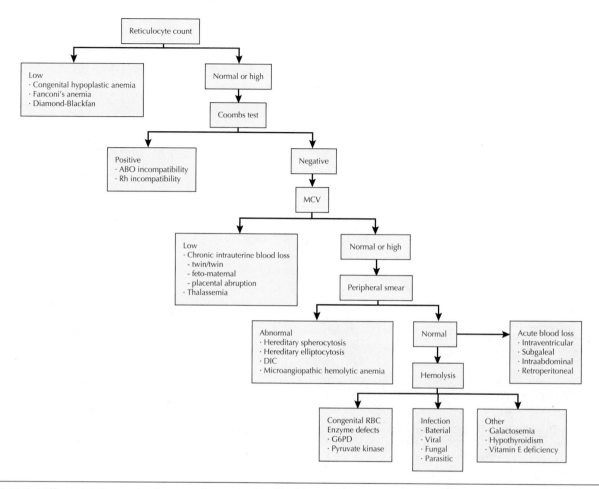

Figure 104-2 *Differential diagnosis of neonatal anemia.* (Modified from Blanchette VS, Zipursky A. Assessment of anemia in newborn infants. *Clin Perinatol* 11(2):489-510, 1984.)

DIAGNOSTIC APPROACH

Polycythemia is defined as a venous hematocrit above 65%. In neonates, hematocrit (Hct) levels peak at 2 hours of life and then progressively decrease, stabilizing by 6 to 24 hours of life. Capillary Hct values are significantly higher than venous values, and arterial and umbilical vessel values are generally lower. Infants should also be monitored for hypoglycemia, hypocalcemia, hyperbilirubinemia, and thrombocytopenia.

MANAGEMENT AND THERAPY

Partial ET (PET) is used as a method to lower Hct and treat hyperviscosity. Studies have shown that PET reduces pulmonary vascular resistance and increases cerebral blood flow velocity. PET should be performed in symptomatic infants with Hct greater than 65% or asymptomatic infants with Hct greater than 70%. Either crystalloid (normal saline) or colloid (albumin) solution may be used. The volume to be exchanged is based on the observed and desired Hct (generally 50%–55%). Exchange volume (mL) = Blood volume × (Observed Hct – Desired Hct)/Observed Hct. Blood volume is estimated to be 80 to 90 mL/kg. During this procedure, blood is removed using a central venous or arterial line and replaced with fluid infused via a peripheral intravenous line. Complications of PET are thought to be similar to a single- or double-volume ET (Figure 104-3).

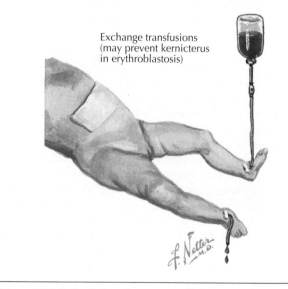

Exchange transfusions (may prevent kernicterus in erythroblastosis)

Figure 104-3 *Partial exchange transfusion.*

Future Directions

Further research into the role of IVIG in the treatment of neonatal hemolytic disease is needed. Trials must focus on the safety and efficacy of IVIG, the need for ET, and long-term neurodevelopmental outcomes.

PLATELET DISORDERS AND COAGULOPATHIES

Thrombocytopenia

ETIOLOGY AND PATHOGENESIS

Thrombocytopenia is diagnosed in 1% to 5% of newborns and 22% to 35% of infants admitted to neonatal intensive care units. The most frequent cause of early-onset thrombocytopenia (<72 hours of life) is reduced megakaryopoiesis secondary to chronic fetal hypoxia from maternal diabetes, pregnancy-induced hypertension (PIH), or intrauterine growth restriction. Late-onset thrombocytopenia (>72 hours of life) is caused by sepsis (e.g., bacterial infection with group B β-hemolytic streptococci, *Escherichia coli*, *Enterococcus* spp.) or NEC in more than 80% of cases. Less common disorders that present with thrombocytopenia at birth include congenital viral infections (e.g., cytomegalovirus [CMV]), perinatal asphyxia, aneuploidy (e.g., trisomies 13, 18, and 21), neonatal alloimmune thrombocytopenia (NAIT), and neonatal autoimmune thrombocytopenia. NAIT results from the transplacental passage of maternal IgG antibodies directed against fetal platelet antigens inherited from the father and absent on maternal platelets. Neonatal autoimmune thrombocytopenia affects one or two per 1000 pregnancies and is associated with the transplacental passage of maternal platelet autoantibodies in mothers with idiopathic thrombocytopenic purpura (ITP) or systemic lupus erythematosus.

CLINICAL PRESENTATION AND DIFFERENTIAL DIAGNOSIS

Affected neonates may be asymptomatic, present with petechiae or purpura, or have symptoms of bleeding. Early-onset thrombocytopenia is generally mild to moderate and self-limiting (usually resolves within 10 days). Late-onset thrombocytopenia develops rapidly over 1 to 2 days, can be severe (platelets <30 × 10^9/L) depending on the cause, and may take several weeks to recover. NAIT often occurs in the first pregnancy (almost 50% of cases), is extremely severe (platelets <20 × 10^9/L), and may result in major bleeding (intracranial, pulmonary, renal). Intracranial hemorrhage (ICH) is seen in 10% to 20% of pregnancies with untreated NAIT versus fewer than 1% of mothers with ITP. Bleeding risk is highest in patients with NAIT followed by sepsis or NEC and chronic fetal hypoxia.

DIAGNOSTIC APPROACH

Thrombocytopenia is defined as a platelet count below 150 × 10^9/L. Neonates with thrombocytopenia secondary to chronic fetal hypoxia have additional hematologic abnormalities including transient neutropenia, increased circulating nucleated RBCs with or without polycythemia, elevated erythropoietin levels, and evidence of hyposplenism (spherocytes, target cells, Howell-Jolly bodies). The diagnosis of NAIT is made by demonstrating platelet antigen incompatibility between the mother and baby serologically or by polymerase chain reaction.

MANAGEMENT AND THERAPY

Platelet transfusion is the only specific therapy for neonatal thrombocytopenia. Clear indications for transfusion include active bleeding in association with thrombocytopenia, neonates in the first week of life with platelets below 50 × 10^9/L, and severe thrombocytopenia (platelets <30 × 10^9/L). Infants of mothers with autoimmune disease should have their platelet counts determined at birth. In those with thrombocytopenia, a platelet count should be repeated after 2 to 3 days (time of platelet nadir). If severe thrombocytopenia develops, treatment with IVIG (1 g/kg) for 2 days is usually effective.

Management of pregnancies with NAIT remains controversial, although most centers now rely on noninvasive strategies. A recent study of women with known human platelet antigen incompatibility treated with IVIG alone at a dose of 1 g/kg weekly (beginning at 16 weeks of gestation if the previous sibling had an ICH and 32 weeks if not) resulted in live births, no ICH, and no neonatal deaths. Because of the high risk of ICH in neonates with NAIT, platelet counts should be maintained above 50 × 10^9/L for the first 2 weeks of life, and all infants with severe thrombocytopenia should undergo a head ultrasound to look for evidence of ICH. Transfusion of PLA1-negative platelets is usually required to achieve an increase in platelet count.

Hemorrhagic Disease of the Newborn

ETIOLOGY AND PATHOGENESIS

Hemorrhagic disease of the newborn (HDN) is caused by low plasma levels of vitamin K–dependent clotting factors (II, VII, IX, X), which are synthesized in the liver. Concentrations of these factors in neonates are 30% to 60% of those in adults. In the absence of prophylactic vitamin K, HDN occurs in 1 in 200 to 400 infants. Although placental transfer of vitamin K does occur, it is not always adequate. As a result, infants with insufficient enteral intake of vitamin K can quickly become deficient. Breast milk contains lower amounts of vitamin K than formula, thus increasing the risk of vitamin K deficiency in breastfed infants.

CLINICAL PRESENTATION AND DIFFERENTIAL DIAGNOSIS

Classic HDN is observed on days 1 to 7 of life and associated with bleeding from the gastrointestinal tract, cutaneous sites (e.g., circumcision), and nasal passages. Late HDN occurs during weeks 2 to 12. Common sites of bleeding include intracranial, cutaneous, and gastrointestinal.

DIAGNOSTIC APPROACH

Vitamin K deficiency results in a prolonged prothrombin time (PT) and an International Normalized Ratio (INR) above 1. PT depends on various clotting factors, several of which are vitamin K dependent. INR compares the blood coagulation status of

Table 104-1 Coagulation Test Norms in Healthy Infants*

	Full-Term			Premature (30-36 Weeks)		
	Day 1	Day 5	Day 30	Day 1	Day 5	Day 30
PT (sec)	13.0 (10.1-15.9)	12.4 (10.0-15.3)	11.8 (10.0-14.3)	13.0 (10.6-16.2)	12.5 (10.0-15.3)	11.8 (10.0-13.6)
INR	1.00 (0.53-1.62)	0.89 (0.53-1.48)	0.79 (0.53-1.26)	1.0 (0.61-1.7)	0.91 (0.53-1.48)	0.79 (0.53-1.11)
aPTT (sec)	42.9 (31.3-54.5)	42.6 (25.4-59.8)	40.4 (32.0-55.2)	53.6 (27.5-79.4)	50.5 (26.9-74.1)	44.7 (26.9-62.5)
Fibrinogen (g/L)	2.83 (1.67-3.99)	3.12 (1.62-4.62)	2.70 (1.62-3.78)	2.43 (1.50-3.73)	2.80 (1.60-4.18)	2.54 (1.50-4.14)

*All measurements are recorded as a mean value followed by the lower and upper boundaries encompassing 95% of the population.

aPTT, activated partial thromboplastin time; INR, International Normalized Ratio; PT, prothrombin time.

Adapted from Andrew M, Paes B, Johnston M: Development of the hemostatic system in the neonate and young infant. Am J Pediatr Hematol Oncol 12:95, 1990.

an individual to that of the normal population. Thus, an INR greater than 1 indicates that coagulation is slower than in the control group (Table 104-1).

MANAGEMENT AND THERAPY

A single dose (1 mg) of intramuscular vitamin K after birth is effective in preventing classic HDN. Oral vitamin K prophylaxis has been shown to improve indices of coagulation status at 1 to 7 days but has not been tested in randomized trials. Because it takes approximately 2 hours for systemically administered vitamin K to increase levels of vitamin K–dependent factors, infants with bleeding secondary to vitamin K deficiency should also be treated with plasma.

FUTURE DIRECTIONS

Randomized, controlled trials are needed to define the safe lower limit for platelet counts in sick newborns and provide evidence that platelet transfusion improves neonatal outcomes. With regard to HDN, a trial comparing multiple oral doses of vitamin K with a single intramuscular dose could potentially provide a cost-effective and less invasive alternative to vitamin K injection at birth.

LEUKOCYTE DISORDERS

Neutropenia

ETIOLOGY AND PATHOGENESIS

When evaluating neonates with neutropenia, it is important to first determine whether the cytopenia results from a defect in cellular production or peripheral destruction or is of mixed etiology (Box 104-1). The most common causes of neonatal neutropenia are maternal PIH, sepsis, and congenital viral infections (e.g., CMV, parvovirus, HIV, hepatitis B, rubella). Infants with severe and prolonged neutropenia should be evaluated for immune-mediated conditions and inherited genetic mutations.

CLINICAL PRESENTATION AND DIFFERENTIAL DIAGNOSIS

The neutropenia of maternal pregnancy-induced hypertension and sepsis is generally transient, rarely persisting for more than 72 hours. In contrast, infants with immune-mediated and inherited disorders show evidence of severe neutropenia for many weeks to months and can have recurrent bacterial infections. Clinical signs of neutropenia in this population include ulcerations of the oral mucosa or gingival inflammation. Otitis media, skin infections (cellulitis, pustules, abscesses), adenitis, pneumonia, and bacterial sepsis can also occur. The most common offending organisms are *Staphylococcus aureus* and gram-negative bacteria derived from the child's skin or bowel flora.

DIAGNOSTIC APPROACH

Normal values for the absolute neutrophil count (ANC) vary by age, particularly during the first weeks after birth. The lower limit of normal is 6000/μL during the first 24 hours after birth, 5000/μL for the first week, 1500/μL during the second week, and 1000/μL between 2 weeks and 1 year of age. Severe neutropenia is defined as an ANC of less than 500/μL.

The initial evaluation of an infant with severe neutropenia should include a thorough history and physical examination. It

Box 104-1 Causes of Neonatal Neutropenia

Decreased Production
Bone marrow failure syndromes
- Kostmann's syndrome
- Cartilage-hair hypoplasia
- Reticular dysgenesis
- Shwachman-Diamond syndrome
Maternal pregnancy-induced hypertension
Viral infections
Copper deficiency
Organic acidemias
Glycogen storage disease type 1b

Increased Destruction
Alloimmune
Maternal autoimmune
Fetal or neonatal autoimmune

Mixed Etiology
Prematurity
Drug-induced neutropenia
Necrotizing enterocolitis
Bacterial or fungal sepsis

is critical to know whether there is a family history of neutropenia or associated congenital anomalies suggestive of an inherited syndrome. If additional evaluation is warranted, antineutrophil antibody titers (elevated in immune-mediated neutropenias) and immunoglobulin quantification (decreased levels in underlying immunodeficiency) may be performed. Neonates with severe and prolonged neutropenia should be referred to a hematologist for bone marrow examination and possible genetic testing.

MANAGEMENT AND THERAPY

Infants with fever and severe neutropenia should be hospitalized and started on parenteral broad-spectrum antibiotics. Specific recommendations for antibiotic coverage depend on the prevalence of organisms in each community or hospital and their susceptibility patterns.

If recovery from neutropenia is not expected, as in inherited syndromes, granulocyte colony-stimulating factor (G-CSF) administration or stem cell transplantation may be necessary. G-CSF has been shown to mobilize preformed neutrophils from the bone marrow, promote neutrophil precursor proliferation, and enhance phagocytic bactericidal function. However, there is currently insufficient evidence to support the use of G-CSF in neutropenic neonates with systemic infection or as prophylaxis to prevent systemic infection in high-risk neonates.

FUTURE DIRECTIONS

Although children with inherited bone marrow failure syndromes often respond to treatment with G-CSF, many physicians remain concerned that it may increase the risk of malignant transformation. Further research is needed to help elucidate the mechanisms by which such transformations occur and to monitor long-term clinical outcomes.

SUGGESTED READINGS

RED BLOOD CELL DISORDERS

Aher S, Malwatkar K, Kadam S: Neonatal anemia. *Semin Fetal Neonatal Med* 13(4):239-247, 2008.

Alcock GS, Liley H: Immunoglobulin infusion for isoimmune haemolytic jaundice in neonates. *Cochrane Database Syst Rev* (3):CD003313, 2002.

Sarkar S, Rosenkrantz TS: Neonatal polycythemia and hyperviscosity. *Semin Fetal Neonatal Med* 13(4):248-255, 2008.

Soll R, Schimmel MS, Ozek E: Partial exchange transfusion to prevent neurodevelopmental disability in infants with polycythemia (protocol). *Cochrane Database Syst Rev* (1):CD005089, 2009.

Steiner LA, Gallagher PG: Erythrocyte disorders in the perinatal period. *Semin Perinatol* 31(4):254-261, 2007.

PLATELET DISORDERS AND COAGULOPATHIES

Puckett RM, Offringa M: Prophylactic vitamin K for vitamin K deficiency bleeding in neonates. *Cochrane Database Syst Rev* (4):CD002776, 2000.

Roberts I, Stanworth S, Murray NA: Thrombocytopenia in the neonate. *Blood Rev* 22(4):173-186, 2008.

van den Akker ES, Oepkes D, Lopriore E, et al: Noninvasive antenatal management of fetal and neonatal alloimmune thrombocytopenia: safe and effective. *BJOG* 114(4):469-473, 2007.

LEUKOCYTE DISORDERS

Carr R, Modi N, Doré C: G-CSF and GM-CSF for treating or preventing neonatal infections. *Cochrane Database Syst Rev* (3):CD003066, 2003.

Rivers A, Slayton WB: Congenital cytopenias and bone marrow failure syndromes. *Semin Perinatol* 33(1):20-28, 2009.

Segel GB, Halterman JS: Neutropenia in pediatric practice. *Pediatr Rev* 29(1):12-23, 2008.

Neonatal Infections

Lori A. Christ

105

Neonates are uniquely susceptible to bacterial and viral infections because of deficiencies in immune function, including neutrophil function and humoral and cellular immunity. Before the introduction of antibiotics, mortality from neonatal sepsis approached 90%; however, even with the advent of antibiotics and identification of common causative organisms, mortality remains 20% to 50%. With continually updated guidelines for maternal screening, the rates of maternally transmitted infections also continue to fall; however, because of significant morbidity, pediatricians must continue to have a high index of suspicion for these infections.

NEONATAL SEPSIS

ETIOLOGY AND PATHOGENESIS

Overall, the incidence of neonatal sepsis is 3 to 4 per 1000 births; it accounts for 25 of 1000 preterm live births. The overall mortality rate is approximately 25%. To aid in identification of likely pathogens, neonatal sepsis is divided into two classifications, early- and late-onset sepsis.

Early-onset sepsis represents infection acquired from the maternal genital tract, whether via ascension into the uterus following rupture of membranes or during passage through the vaginal canal during the birth process. As such, it generally presents within the first five to seven days of life with a sudden onset and fulminant course. Ports of entry include the conjunctivae, respiratory tract, umbilicus, skin, and oropharynx. Implicated organisms include group B β-hemolytic streptococci (GBS), *Escherichia coli*, and less commonly other gram-negative enteric organisms and *Listeria monocytogenes*.

GBS infections account for a large number of cases of early-onset sepsis and have been a focus of Centers for Disease Control and Prevention guidelines because of significant mortality. GBS colonizes the genital tract of 30% of women, and all pregnant women are screened for vaginal and rectal colonization at 35 to 37 weeks of gestation. Colonized women are treated with intrapartum penicillin chemoprophylaxis when delivering vaginally; since the institution of these guidelines, mortality from GBS disease has declined by 80%.

Late-onset sepsis may represent organisms acquired from the maternal genital tract but more often are transmitted horizontally by caregivers. Late-onset disease is more common after the first week of life and is more likely to present with urinary tract infection or meningitis caused by hematogenous seeding of end organs. The most common organisms are gram-positive organisms, such as *Staphylococcus aureus* and GBS, in addition to *E. coli* and other gram negative organisms. In the community, viral infection should also be included in the differential diagnosis. For hospitalized infants, the most common pathogen is *Staphylococcus epidermidis*; other organisms to consider include

Pseudomonas aeruginosa, *Candida* spp., anaerobes, and methicillin-resistant *S. aureus*.

CLINICAL PRESENTATION

Neonatal sepsis may present as a constellation of nonspecific symptoms including one or more of the following: progressive lethargy or irritability, apnea, temperature instability, poor feeding, changes in tone, abdominal distension, vomiting or loose stools, or decreased urine output. Fever in a neonate is defined as a temperature of 38.0°C or greater. Clinicians should have a very high index of suspicion for sepsis in an ill-appearing or febrile infant.

EVALUATION AND MANAGEMENT

A thorough birth history should be obtained including the following: gestational age (prematurity is the most significant risk factor in the evaluation of neonatal sepsis); duration of rupture of membranes; presence of meconium stained amniotic fluid; indicators of chorioamnionitis, including maternal fever in the peripartum period, fundal tenderness, and foul-smelling amniotic fluid; and invasive procedures such as fetal scalp electrodes. For reasons that are unclear, male infants are four times as likely as female infants to develop early-onset sepsis. The antepartum history is equally as important and should include maternal infections or exposures during pregnancy, the duration of prenatal care, and results of prenatal testing if available. The U.S. Preventative Services Task Force recommends routine screening of mothers for the following: syphilis (rapid plasma reagin [RPR]), hepatitis B (hepatitis B surface antigen [HBsAg]), rubella (titers), HIV, gonorrhea, chlamydia, and GBS.

A thorough physical examination should be performed with special attention to the following findings: growth parameters including head circumference, overall appearance of the infant, presence of a bulging fontanel, eye discharge and ophthalmologic examination, nasal discharge, hydration status, respiratory symptoms, perfusion and cardiac examination, abdominal distension, organomegaly, erythema or drainage from the umbilicus, skin lesions including petechiae and vesicles, jaundice, and the overall neurologic examination, including tone.

Newborns with historical factors putting them at significant risk for early-onset sepsis should receive serial screening complete blood counts (CBCs) and C-reactive protein levels in the newborn nursery, regardless of their clinical appearance. For infants who are septic appearing in the first days of life, a complete evaluation, including blood culture and lumbar puncture with cerebrospinal fluid (CSF) culture, should be obtained and the infant initiated on appropriate antibiotic coverage until culture results are negative for at least 48 hours. GBS and *Listeria* coverage with a β-lactam and gram-negative coverage with an aminoglycoside (usually ampicillin and gentamicin) is recommended. Antibiotic therapy may be tailored to cover organisms common to a particular nursery, as indicated.

Infants who present after 5 to 7 days of life with any of the symptoms detailed above should be evaluated for late-onset sepsis. Blood, urine, and CSF studies, including cultures before the initiation of antibiotics, should be obtained. Exact laboratory criteria for the diagnosis of late-onset sepsis is somewhat controversial; however, an elevated white blood cell count on an enhanced urinalysis specimen, CSF specimen, or peripheral blood sample is concerning for serious bacterial infection. As in early-onset sepsis, infants should be started on appropriate antibiotics until all culture results are negative. Because meningitis features more prominently in late-onset sepsis, a third-generation cephalosporin (usually cefotaxime) may be substituted for gentamicin if concern for meningitis is high based on clinical examination or lumbar puncture results.

TORCH INFECTIONS

ETIOLOGY AND PATHOGENESIS

The TORCH (toxoplasmosis or *Toxoplasma gondii*, other infections, rubella, cytomegalovirus [CMV], and herpes simplex virus [HSV]) infections are congenital infections that are transmitted transplacentally from mother to fetus. As a rule, the likelihood of transmission to a fetus is greatest when primary maternal infection occurs. Gestational age at the time of exposure determines the severity of the disease. Neonates who appear most severely infected at birth have most likely been infected during the first trimester; exposure during the first few weeks of gestation may also result in intrauterine demise. TORCH is an acronym that represents the most common pathogens responsible for transplacentally transmitted infections. Historically, these include toxoplasmosis or *T. gondii*, other infections, rubella, CMV, and HSV.

Toxoplasma gondii

This is an obligate intracellular protozoan of which cats are the primary host. Maternal infection occurs by ingestion of oocytes via contaminated food or water, and infection persists in the tissues of the human host. Thirty percent of fetuses acquire infection at the time of primary maternal acquisition, resulting in 3500 newly infected infants per year.

Other: Syphilis, Hepatitis B, and HIV

Neonatal HIV infection occurs transplacentally (≤40% of cases), during delivery, and via breastfeeding postnatally. The risk of transmission increases with high maternal viral load. In the United States, 150 to 300 infants with HIV are born yearly, representing a significant decrease over the past 10 years because of the availability of antiretroviral therapy for pregnant women.

Hepatitis B is a DNA-containing hepadnavirus that is transmitted vertically during delivery in almost all cases, and risk is highest with high circulating viral titers.

The spirochete *Treponema pallidum* is the causative agent of syphilis. Rates of primary and secondary syphilis infection continue to decrease within the United States. Maternal factors associated with infection include lack of prenatal care and cocaine use.

Rubella

Rubella is an RNA virus in the Togaviridae family. The incidence of neonatal rubella has declined 99% since the immunization program began in the 1960s and includes 400 new cases per year.

Cytomegalovirus

A member of the herpesvirus group, CMV is the most common TORCH infection in the developing world, with an incidence of 30,000 new cases per year.

Herpes Simplex Virus

A total of 2% to 3% of women acquire HSV during pregnancy, with primary maternal infection again posing the highest risk to neonates.

CLINICAL PRESENTATION

TORCH infections are often part of a large differential diagnosis and share many overlapping features. These infections may result in dysmorphic facies, developmental delay, or symmetric intrauterine growth retardation. Other signs and symptoms common to vertically transmitted infections are hepatosplenomegaly, micro- or macrocephaly, and abnormal tone.

Toxoplasmosis generally presents within the second or third decade of life with visual and learning difficulties. Eighty-five percent of affected infants appear normal at birth. The most severe form is noted in the first month of life with intrauterine growth restriction, hepatosplenomegaly, micro- or macrocephaly, abnormal tone, or seizures. The classic triad of chorioretinitis, intracranial calcifications, and hydrocephalus presents in fewer than 10% of infants.

Congenital syphilis is similar to the acquired form of syphilis in that it presents with early and late manifestations. Most cases are detected by routine maternal screening. Early syphilis presents within the first 2 years of life, with one-third of patients symptomatic at birth. Symptoms can affect almost any organ system and include the following: hepatosplenomegaly, jaundice, Coombs'-negative hemolytic anemia, thrombocytopenia, rhinitis (snuffles), condylomatous skin or mucous membrane lesions, diffuse mucocutaneous rash involving the palms and soles, osteochondritis presenting as pain and refusal to move the affected limb (pseudoparalysis of Parrot), periosteitis, chorioretinitis, failure to thrive, or renal disease (Figure 105-1). Late manifestations are not detailed here but result from chronic tissue inflammation, most commonly involving the central nervous system (CNS), bones, and teeth, and present within the first 2 decades of life.

With an incubation of 2 to 6 months, hepatitis B is an unlikely cause of neonatal cholestasis and can remain asymptomatic for years. After 2 months of age, hepatitis B presents with self-limited hepatitis, fulminant hepatitis, or insidious onset of cirrhosis and progression to liver failure.

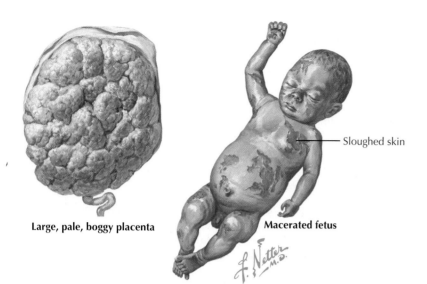

Large, pale, boggy placenta   Macerated fetus — Sloughed skin

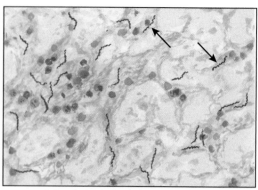

Spirochetes in fetal tissue (Levaditi stain)

Figure 105-1 *Manifestations of congenital syphilis.*

HIV screening is recommended for all pregnant women because of advances in antiretroviral prophylaxis. The median age of onset in infants who acquire the virus perinatally is 12 to 18 months if left untreated, and it carries a 20% mortality rate in the first 4 years of life. Briefly, the clinical presentation can vary from mild systemic symptoms with recurrent fever or failure to thrive, recurrent mild infections, to serious bacterial infections and AIDS-defining illnesses.

Congenital rubella presents with many of the common symptoms of TORCH infections. Unique features include patent ductus arteriosus and extramedullary hematopoiesis, resulting in the characteristic rash known as "blueberry muffin baby."

Cytomegalic inclusion disease is apparent at birth and is the most severe form of CMV disease, representing 10% of all cases. Other features of TORCH infections are also present, including intrauterine growth restriction, hepatosplenomegaly, thrombocytopenia, and dermal erythropoiesis. CNS manifestations include ventriculomegaly, microcephaly, chorioretinitis, and sensorineural hearing loss.

Infection with HSV acquired in the perinatal period presents within the first 4 weeks of life with one of three presentations. Approximately 45% of patients present with skin, eye, and mouth disease; other presentations include CNS involvement only (seizures, hypotonia) and disseminated disease (CNS, liver, adrenal, and pulmonary disease). Congenital HSV represents intrauterine infection and presents at birth with microcephaly, vesicular lesions, and micro-ophthalmia.

EVALUATION AND MANAGEMENT

Toxoplasmosis

If in utero infection is suspected based on prenatal ultrasonographic findings, amniotic fluid can be sent for *Toxoplasmosis* polymerase chain reaction (PCR). Postnatally, the recommended workup includes ophthalmologic, neurologic, and audiologic evaluations, as well as CSF PCR testing for Toxoplasma and head computed tomography (CT). For infected newborns, treatment with pyrimethamine, sulfadiazine, and leucovorin is the most widely accepted regimen and results in improved ocular outcomes. All pregnant women should be counseled to avoid changing cats' litter boxes and to wear gloves when in contact with soil (Figure 105-2).

Hepatitis B

Prevention is the most important aspect of disease management because 95% of vertically transmitted cases can be prevented. Management includes both active and passive immunoprophylaxis. Infants born to mothers with positive or unknown HBsAg status should receive the hepatitis B vaccine within 12 hours of life. Hepatitis B vaccination should then proceed as recommended by the current immunization schedule. If the mother is positive, hepatitis B immunoglobulin (HBIG) should be administered with vaccine. If maternal status is unknown and the infant is born at term, HBIG should be administered within the first 7 days of life pending results of maternal testing. If the infant weighs less than 2 kg, HBIG should be administered within the first 12 hours of life even if maternal testing is still pending, and these infants should receive 4 total doses of hepatitis B vaccine.

Syphilis

All pregnant women should be screened with a serum RPR; positive test results should be confirmed with antitreponemal testing with either the fluorescent antitreponemal antibody absorption test (FTA-ABS) or microhemagglutination assay for antibodies to *T. pallidum* (MHA-TP). RPR titers can be used to follow disease activity. Serum RPR or Venereal Disease Research Laboratory test (VDRL) should be done on all infants of mothers with a positive screen, and full evaluation should be

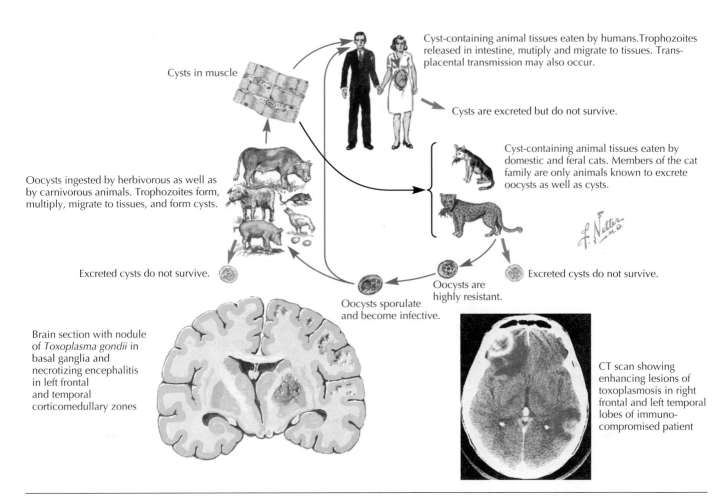

Cyst-containing animal tissues eaten by humans. Trophozoites released in intestine, mutiply and migrate to tissues. Transplacental transmission may also occur.

Cysts in muscle

Cysts are excreted but do not survive.

Cyst-containing animal tissues eaten by domestic and feral cats. Members of the cat family are only animals known to excrete oocysts as well as cysts.

Oocysts ingested by herbivorous as well as by carnivorous animals. Trophozoites form, multiply, migrate to tissues, and form cysts.

Excreted cysts do not survive.

Excreted cysts do not survive.

Oocysts are highly resistant.

Oocysts sporulate and become infective.

Brain section with nodule of *Toxoplasma gondii* in basal ganglia and necrotizing encephalitis in left frontal and temporal corticomedullary zones

CT scan showing enhancing lesions of toxoplasmosis in right frontal and left temporal lobes of immunocompromised patient

Figure 105-2 *Life cycle of* Toxoplasma gondii.

performed on infants with abnormal examination results, whose RPR titers are fourfold greater than maternal titers, or if maternal treatment is unknown, with an antibiotic other than penicillin or given within 1 month of delivery or if maternal titers have not fallen before delivery. Full evaluation includes a CBC, CSF for cell count, protein and VDRL, and long bone radiographs. Standard treatment is with penicillin for 10 days.

HIV

To decrease the rate of vertical transmission of HIV, delivery via caesarian section before rupture of membranes is recommended, with complete avoidance of breastfeeding. Maternal therapy with zidovudine (AZT) should begin during the first trimester, with intravenous (IV) therapy during delivery and administration of AZT to the newborn as soon as possible (within hours) after birth and continuing until at least 6 weeks of age. In neonates with suspected HIV infection, HIV PCR testing is recommended because of transplacental transmission of anti-HIV antibodies to the infant, which may result in false-positive test results. Thirty percent of infants tested using detection of nucleic acid will have a positive test result within the first 48 hours of life, and almost all have detectable viral load by 1 month of age. If both test results are negative, the absence of

HIV infection can be confirmed between 12 and 18 months of age by HIV antibody testing.

Rubella

No specific treatment for rubella is available; however, infection is ongoing, and infants should be considered infectious until 1 year of age. Current guidelines recommend serum immunoglobulin M (IgM) in neonates and serial measurements of rubella-specific IgG at 3, 6, and 12 months. Increasing titers are indicative of ongoing infection.

CMV

The diagnosis of CMV requires isolation of virus (PCR testing) from urine, respiratory secretions, stool, or CSF obtained within 3 weeks of birth. Head imaging with head ultrasound or CT scan should be performed in suspected cases, and periventricular calcifications are predictive of later neurologic outcomes. Hearing screening may not identify associated sensorineural hearing loss until several months after birth. Ganciclovir may be used in infants with demonstrated CNS involvement and has been shown to decrease sensorineural hearing loss in this specific population.

Herpes Simplex Virus

If present, vesicles should be unroofed and fluid sent for HSV PCR and culture. Suspicion for disseminated HSV should be high in all ill-appearing neonates younger than 1 month of age, and serum and CSF HSV PCR testing should be considered. IV acyclovir is the treatment of choice and should be continued for 14 to 21 days depending on the extent of infection.

OTHER INFECTIONS

ETIOLOGY AND PATHOGENESIS

Neisseria gonorrhoeae is a gram-negative diplococcus that resides intracellularly. The gonococcus is transmitted when the neonate passes through the vaginal canal. *Chlamydia trachomatis* is an obligate intracellular bacteria with 18 serologic variants. Neonatal acquisition from the vaginal canal is approximately 50%, and the nasopharynx is the most commonly primarily infected site.

CLINICAL PRESENTATION

Gonococcal infection generally presents as purulent unilateral or bilateral eye discharge and conjunctival erythema, termed *ophthalmia neonatorum* (Figure 105-3). Scalp abscess after fetal monitoring has also been noted. Less commonly, meningitis or disseminated disease can present and should be included in the differential diagnosis of a septic-appearing infant. Similarly, chlamydial disease presents as purulent eye discharge and may form a membrane on the conjunctivae. Neonatal pneumonia is another classic presentation of neonatal chlamydial infection, presenting with staccato cough, tachypnea, and occasionally nasal congestion within the first 2 to 3 months of life.

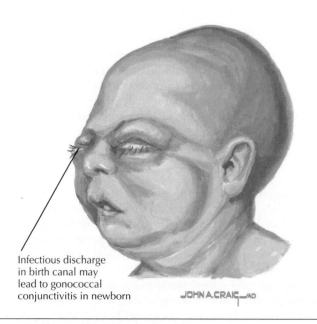

Infectious discharge in birth canal may lead to gonococcal conjunctivitis in newborn

JOHN A.CRAIG—AD

Figure 105-3 *Gonococcal ophthalmia.*

ETIOLOGY AND MANAGEMENT

Neisseria gonorrhoeae

Gram-negative diplococci may be visualized on Gram stain from samples taken from eye drainage, blood, or CSF. Nuclear acid amplification is the most sensitive mode of testing and can be used on a variety of body fluid samples. Prophylaxis with erythromycin or tetracycline eye ointment within 1 hour of delivery is effective at preventing neonatal ophthalmia. Treatment with an extended-spectrum cephalosporin (ceftriaxone or cefotaxime) in addition to frequent eye irrigation is recommended.

Chlamydia trachomatis

Birth prophylaxis with eye ointment as above is not as effective in preventing Chlamydia ophthalmia. Nuclear acid amplification is also a sensitive method of testing for chlamydial infection from body fluids. including eye discharge. If an infant is positively diagnosed with chlamydial infection of the eye, the infant should receive a 14-day course of oral erythromycin for presumed chlamydial pneumonia, which may present days later.

FUTURE DIRECTIONS

The laboratory criteria for diagnosis, hospital admission, and antibiotic administration in the setting of suspected neonatal sepsis continue to undergo rigorous evaluation, as are new laboratory markers for sepsis. Clinicians should maintain a high suspicion in all infants presenting with parental concerns as above because neonatal sepsis can have devastating consequences.

SUGGESTED READINGS

Baker MD, Bell LM, Avner JR: Outpatient management without antibiotics of fever in selected infants. *N Engl J Med* 329(20):1437-1441, 1993.

Gordon A, Jeffery HE. Antibiotic regimens for suspected late onset sepsis in newborn infants. *Cochrane Database Syst Rev* (3):CD004501, 2005.

Hammerschlag MR, Cummings C, Roblin PM, et al: Efficacy of neonatal ocular prophylaxis for the prevention of chlamydial and gonococcal conjunctivitis. *N Engl J Med* 320(12):769-772, 1989.

Kimberlin DW, Lin CY, Jacobs RF, et al: Natural history of neonatal herpes simplex virus infections in the acyclovir era. *Pediatrics* 108(2):223-229, 2001.

Lee C, Gong Y, Brok J, Boxall EH, Gluud C: Effect of hepatitis B immunisation in newborn infants of mothers positive for hepatitis B surface antigen: systematic review and meta-analysis. *BMJ* 332(7537):328-336, 2006.

Lopez A, Dietz V, Wilson M, Narvin T, Jones JL: Preventing congenital toxoplasmosis. MMWR *Morbid Mortal Wkly Rep* 49(RR02):57-75, 2000.

Mofenson LM: U.S. Public Health Service Task Force recommendations for use of antiretroviral drugs in pregnant HIV-1 infected women for maternal health and for interventions to reduce perinatal HIV-1 transmission in the United States. *MMWR Morbid Mortal Wkly Rep* 51(RR18):1-38, 2002.

Pickering LK, editor: *Red Book: 2009 Report of the Committee on Infectious Diseases*, ed 27, Elk Grove Village, IL, 2009, American Academy of Pediatrics.

Schrag SJ, Gorwitz R, Fultz-Butts K, Schuchat A: Prevention of perinatal group B streptococcal disease. Revised guidelines from CDC. MMWR *Morbid Mortal Wkly Rep* 51(RR-11):1-22, 2002.

Schrag SJ, Zell ER, Lynfield R, et al: A population-based comparison of strategies to prevent early-onset group B streptococcal disease in neonates. *N Engl J Med* 347(4):233-239, 2002.

Neonatal Resuscitation

Shazia Bhat

106

R esuscitation of newborns has been documented as far in the past as the 16th century BC, at which time descriptions were recorded of newborns that were likely to survive versus those who were not. The development of assisted ventilation, endotracheal intubation, and oxygen delivery can be traced through the writings of physicians and midwives dating back to the 1600s. In current times, approximately 10% of neonates require some assistance with initiating respiration at birth, and 1% of neonates have need of more aggressive interventions. Neonatal resuscitation has been standardized by the Neonatal Resuscitation Program (NRP), but recognizing the reasoning behind this algorithm requires an understanding of the transition between fetal and neonatal circulation.

ETIOLOGY AND PATHOGENESIS

Fetal Circulation

In fetuses, the placenta performs the primary gas exchange function rather than the lungs, and several circulatory adaptations exist to facilitate flow of oxygenated blood through the body and placenta. Deoxygenated blood from the body of the fetus flows to the placenta via the umbilical artery and becomes oxygenated through gas exchange with maternal blood. The oxygenated blood then flows back to the fetus via the umbilical vein (Figure 106-1). The umbilical vein deposits the blood to the inferior vena cava via the ductus venosus, which subsequently delivers it to the right atrium of the heart. In the right atrium, the blood partially mixes with blood from the superior vena cava, and the majority of it streams across the foramen ovale to the left atrium because of the high pulmonary vascular resistance. From the left atrium, blood flows through the left ventricle to the aorta, thereby delivering the most oxygenated blood to the brain via the carotid arteries. The remaining blood in the right atrium, largely from the superior vena cava, flows into the right ventricle and then into the pulmonary artery. A small amount of blood perfuses the lungs and then travels to the left atrium via the pulmonary veins. Most of the blood, however, is diverted across the ductus arteriosus to the descending aorta, where it joins the blood from the left ventricle. From the aorta, the blood is distributed via branches off the aorta and ultimately reaches the umbilical artery and the low pressure placenta again (Figure 106-2).

Transition to Neonatal Circulation

This system changes dramatically when the infant is born. Because of the stress of labor and delivery, the baby experiences a catecholamine surge at birth. Catecholamines regulate fluid resorption in the lungs, surfactant release into the alveoli, temperature, glucose mobilization, and blood flow to the brain and vital organs. When the umbilical cord is clamped, the placenta is removed from the circulation, causing a large increase in systemic vascular resistance. When the infant takes his or her first breath, the pulmonary vascular resistance decreases precipitously, causing blood to travel through the right atrium to the right ventricle and then the lungs rather than through the foramen ovale to the left atrium. The lower pulmonary pressures also result in less blood flow across the ductus arteriosus and more flow from the pulmonary artery to the lungs. The ductus venosus, ductus arteriosus, and umbilical vessels eventually constrict, leaving the infant with a fully intact neonatal circulatory system (see Figure 106-2). The initial breaths taken by the infant also must inflate the lungs and effect a change in vascular pressures so lung water is absorbed into the pulmonary arterial system and cleared from the lung.

Asphyxia

Fetuses are relatively hypoxemic compared with neonates; fetal partial pressures of arterial oxygen are between 20 and 25 mm Hg. Therefore, fetuses are particularly vulnerable to asphyxia. However, several adaptations exist to protect fetuses. Fetal hemoglobin has a higher affinity for oxygen than adult hemoglobin, and fetal tissues are more efficient at extracting oxygen than adult tissues. In addition, the "diving reflex" allows for blood flow to be distributed preferentially to the brain, adrenal glands, and heart and away from the lungs, gut, liver, spleen, kidney, and extremities to decrease oxygen consumption in the event of asphyxia.

In some cases, the fetal reserve is not enough to protect the infant from difficulties with transition. Neonatal asphyxia can result from multiple factors, both maternal and fetal (Table 106-1), and may begin in utero. The initial response to asphyxia is a brief period of rapid breathing followed by "primary apnea." During primary apnea, stimulation such as drying or slapping the feet will restart breathing. If the apnea is prolonged, the infant loses muscle tone and becomes cyanotic and then bradycardic. After a few gasping respirations, the neonate enters "secondary apnea." At this point, ventilatory support must be provided for the newborn to survive. In this situation, an infant requires resuscitative efforts to aid in the transition to extrauterine life.

EVALUATION AND MANAGEMENT

Neonatal Resuscitation Guidelines

The NRP was introduced in 1987; its goal is to ensure that a health care professional trained in providing care to newborns just after delivery is present at every birth in the United States. To accomplish this goal, the NRP has compiled an algorithm standardizing neonatal resuscitation techniques, which was last revised in 2005 (Figure 106-3).

The first step in neonatal resuscitation is the initial evaluation of the infant, beginning with assessment of four parameters: the

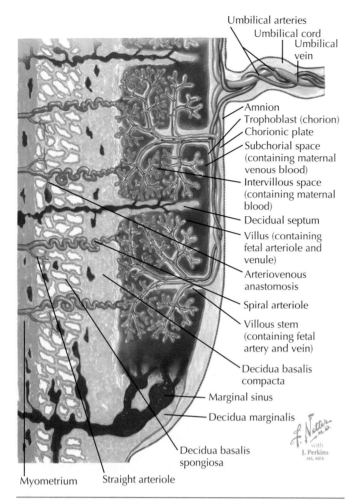

Umbilical arteries
Umbilical cord
Umbilical vein

Amnion
Trophoblast (chorion)
Chorionic plate
Subchorial space (containing maternal venous blood)
Intervillous space (containing maternal blood)
Decidual septum
Villus (containing fetal arteriole and venule)
Arteriovenous anastomosis
Spiral arteriole
Villous stem (containing fetal artery and vein)
Decidua basalis compacta
Marginal sinus
Decidua marginalis
Decidua basalis spongiosa
Myometrium   Straight arteriole

Figure 106-1 *Circulation in placenta.*

Table 106-1 Conditions Predisposing to Neonatal Asphyxia

Maternal	
Uterus	Uterine malformations, hypertonus, rupture
Infection	Chorioamnionitis
Blood	Anemia, hemoglobinopathy
Vascular	Diabetes, hypertension, preeclampsia, hypotension
Medications	Narcotics, magnesium
Placenta	Uteroplacental insufficiency, placental abruption, placenta previa, postmature placenta
Fetal	
Umbilical cord	Compression, prolapse, knot, nuchal cord, thrombosis
Blood	Anemia
Other	Infection, fetal hydrops, malformations, multiple gestations, inborn error of metabolism

infant's gestational age, the presence or absence of breathing, respiratory effort or crying, and muscle tone. See below for a discussion of meconium and the resuscitation of premature infants.

If an infant is not breathing or has poor muscle tone, the first steps in resuscitation are to provide warmth, clear the airway, position the infant so that the airway is open, and dry and stimulate the baby.

After 30 seconds, the baby's respiratory rate, heart rate, and color should be reevaluated. If the baby is apneic or the heart rate is less than 100 beats/min, positive-pressure ventilation should be initiated at a rate of 40 to 60 breaths/min. If the baby is breathing and has a heart rate greater than 100 beats/min but is cyanotic, supplemental oxygen should be provided. If the baby remains cyanotic despite this intervention, positive-pressure ventilation must commence. Positive-pressure ventilation should be administered via a bag and mask; endotracheal intubation can also be considered at this point to facilitate ventilation. Effective ventilation is the most important step in neonatal resuscitation; the baby will not be able to generate adequate cardiac output if the lungs are not adequately inflated. High inflating pressures (25-40 cm H_2O) may be necessary initially because the lungs remain filled with fluid, but with expansion, pressures must be decreased to only that which adequately moves the chest wall.

Thirty seconds later, if the heart rate remains less than 60 beats/min with effective positive-pressure ventilation, chest compressions should be initiated with the two-thumb technique. The chest should be compressed to one-third to one-half the anteroposterior diameter of the chest at a ratio of three compressions to one breath given (Figure 106-4). Chest compressions continue until the heart rate rises above 60 beats/min. If, after 30 seconds, the heart rate does not rise, then epinephrine should be administered. Epinephrine can be administered through the endotracheal tube or intravenously (often via the umbilical vein); the intravenous route is preferred because the endotracheal route yields lower serum concentrations. The dose is 0.01 to 0.03 mg/kg of epinephrine diluted to a 1:10,000 concentration. Thirty seconds later, the heart rate should be assessed again; if the heart rate remains less then 60 beats/min, epinephrine can be repeated every 3 to 5 minutes until the heart rate increases.

The Apgar scores are also assessed during this time; the infant is given a score at 1 and 5 minutes of life but should continue to be scored every 5 minutes until a score of 7 is achieved (Table 106-2).

Volume expansion is indicated if the baby still does not respond to resuscitative efforts and appears pale with delayed capillary refill or weak pulses. Hypovolemic shock can result from an acute hemorrhage from a placental abruption or placenta previa or blood loss from the umbilical cord (Figure 106-5). Isotonic, crystalloid solutions, including normal saline and lactated Ringer's solution, are best for acutely treating hypovolemia. O-negative, Rh-negative packed red blood cells can also be given if there is evidence of fetal anemia or severe fetal blood loss. Volume expansion should be accomplished with small volumes, 10 mL/kg at a time, to decrease the risk of intraventricular hemorrhage.

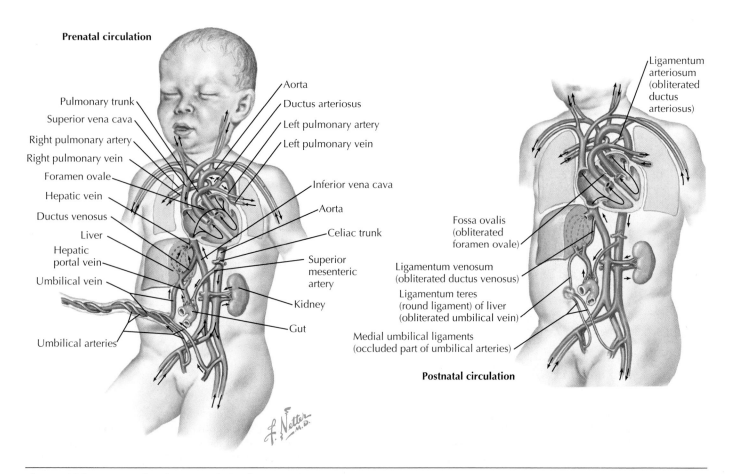

Prenatal circulation

Aorta
Pulmonary trunk
Superior vena cava
Right pulmonary artery
Right pulmonary vein
Foramen ovale
Hepatic vein
Ductus venosus
Liver
Hepatic portal vein
Umbilical vein
Umbilical arteries

Ductus arteriosus
Left pulmonary artery
Left pulmonary vein
Inferior vena cava
Aorta
Celiac trunk
Superior mesenteric artery
Kidney
Gut

Ligamentum arteriosum (obliterated ductus arteriosus)
Fossa ovalis (obliterated foramen ovale)
Ligamentum venosum (obliterated ductus venosus)
Ligamentum teres (round ligament) of liver (obliterated umbilical vein)
Medial umbilical ligaments (occluded part of umbilical arteries)

Postnatal circulation

Figure 106-2 *Prenatal and postnatal circulation.*

Consideration of anatomic or structural abnormalities affecting the airway is necessary if the baby remains depressed after these interventions. The presence of pneumothorax, congenital diaphragmatic hernia (CDH), congenital heart disease, and airway malformations would require adjusted therapies to resuscitate the infant.

Table 106-2 Apgar Scores			
	Score		
Sign	**0**	**1**	**2**
Heart rate	None	<100 beats/min	>100 beats/min
Respiration	None	Irregular, slow, gasping	Vigorous, crying
Muscle tone	Limp	Some flexion	Active motion
Reflex irritability	None	Grimace	Cough, sneeze, pulls away
Color	Blue or pale	Pink body, pale or blue extremities	Completely pink

Resuscitation of Premature Infants

Premature infants, particularly extremely premature infants (weight <1000 g) require special attention during resuscitation. The same algorithm is followed, with some additions to account for their specific needs. Premature infants are more likely to develop respiratory distress than term infants. As a result, assisted ventilation must be provided effectively but gently. Endotracheal intubation is usually necessary for surfactant administration. Premature infants are much more fragile than term infants; therefore, they must be gently handled to avoid inducing injury or intraventricular hemorrhage. Because premature infants have a much larger relative surface area and less well-developed skin, careful attention must be paid to drying the infant immediately and keeping the infant warm, usually via a radiant warmer bed.

Ventilation of preterm infants also warrants particular consideration. Prevention of lung overinflation is crucial; hyperexpansion of the lungs can lead to interstitial emphysema and pneumothorax. In addition, rapid fluctuations in blood carbon dioxide levels can predispose infants to developing intraventricular hemorrhage and periventricular leukomalacia. Hyperoxia should also be avoided; oxygen toxicity can increase the risk of retinopathy of prematurity, necrotizing enterocolitis, and bronchopulmonary dysplasia. Moreover, preterm infants are likely to have respiratory distress syndrome; surfactant therapy can help mitigate that risk.

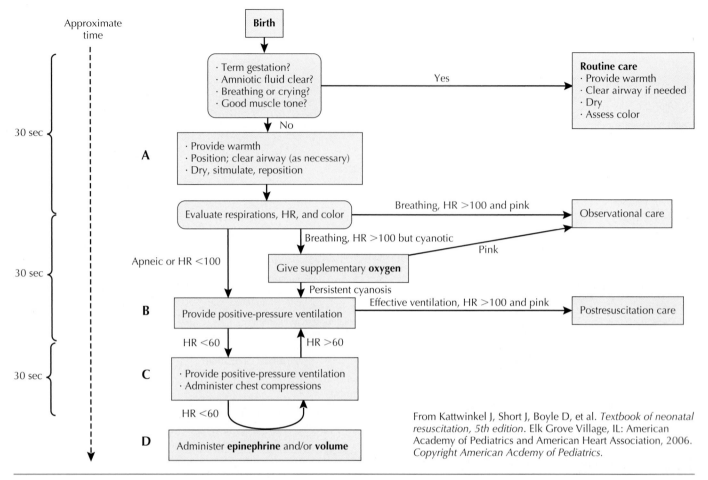

Approximate time

30 sec

30 sec

30 sec

Birth

· Term gestation?
· Amniotic fluid clear?
· Breathing or crying?
· Good muscle tone?

Yes → **Routine care**
· Provide warmth
· Clear airway if needed
· Dry
· Assess color

No

A
· Provide warmth
· Position; clear airway (as necessary)
· Dry, sitmulate, reposition

Evaluate respirations, HR, and color

Breathing, HR >100 and pink → Observational care

Breathing, HR >100 but cyanotic

Apneic or HR <100

Give supplementary **oxygen** — Pink → Observational care

Persistent cyanosis

B
Provide positive-pressure ventilation

Effective ventilation, HR >100 and pink → Postresuscitation care

HR <60   HR >60

C
· Provide positive-pressure ventilation
· Administer chest compressions

HR <60

D
Administer **epinephrine** and/or **volume**

From Kattwinkel J, Short J, Boyle D, et al. *Textbook of neonatal resuscitation, 5th edition.* Elk Grove Village, IL: American Academy of Pediatrics and American Heart Association, 2006. *Copyright American Acdemy of Pediatrics.*

Figure 106-3 *Overview of neonatal resuscitation.*

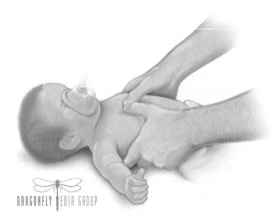

External cardiac compressions in an infant using the two-handed thumb technique. The compressor's hands encircle the patient's chest to provide countertraction, while the two thumbs are placed over the lower half of the patient's sternum to compress the chest.

Figure 106-4 *Bag and mask ventilation and chest compressions.*

Umbilical vessel catheterization is often beneficial during the resuscitation of premature infants. Arterial access allows for monitoring of blood gas values and central blood pressures. Central venous access via the umbilical vein allows for administration of fluids, drugs, and blood as needed during the resuscitation.

Special Circumstances

Meconium passage occurs during approximately 11% of deliveries; 2% of infants have aspiration syndrome as a result. Meconium obstructs the large airways and induces inflammation of the small airways, and the sequelae of meconium aspiration syndrome can range from mild initial tachypnea to development of pulmonary hypertension. To thwart this outcome, direct suctioning of the trachea is recommended if meconium is present at a delivery and the infant has decreased respiratory effort, heart rate, and tone. Tracheal suctioning is not recommended for vigorous infants born through meconium.

Infants born with CDH have small, underdeveloped lungs caused by compression by the herniated intestines and abdominal organs. As a result, CDHs typically present with immediate marked respiratory distress, a scaphoid abdomen, and the presence of bowel sounds in the chest. After a CDH is recognized,

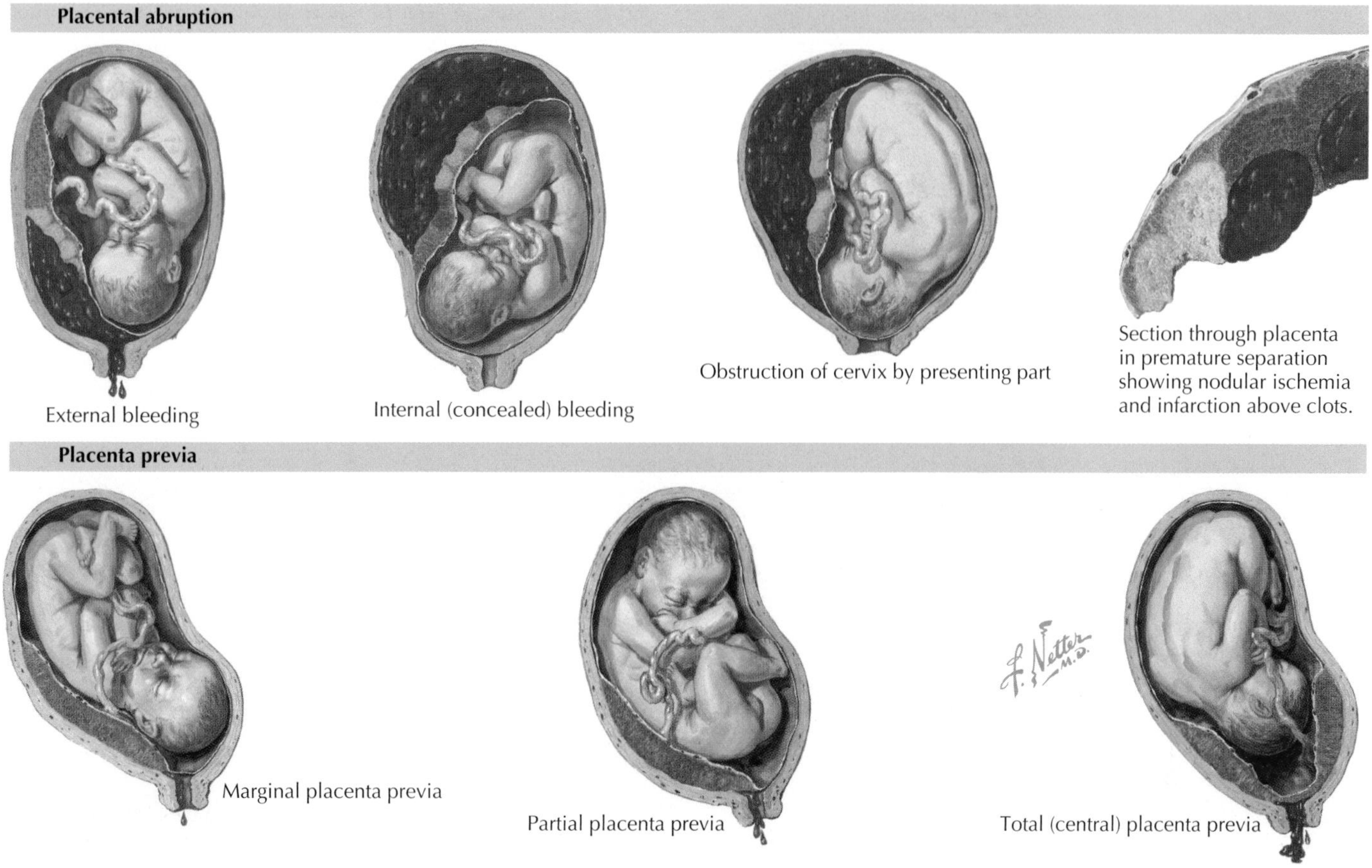

Placental abruption

External bleeding

Internal (concealed) bleeding

Obstruction of cervix by presenting part

Section through placenta in premature separation showing nodular ischemia and infarction above clots.

Placenta previa

Marginal placenta previa

Partial placenta previa

Total (central) placenta previa

Figure 106-5 *Placental abruption and previa.*

the duration of positive-pressure ventilation via bag and mask should be limited to avoid gaseous distension of the stomach and intestines and further constriction of the lungs. To this end, endotracheal intubation should occur rapidly, and an orogastric tube should be placed to decompress the gastrointestinal tract.

Several other malformations require different additional techniques for delivery room resuscitation. Infants with Pierre Robin sequence should be placed prone if possible so that the tongue can fall forward and clear the airway; a jaw thrust can also be performed until a more stable airway can be established, usually via the nasopharynx. Neonates with myelomeningocele should be placed in the decubitus position, and the defect must be covered with sterile plastic to prevent infection, desiccation, and trauma. Omphalocele or gastroschisis is initially treated in a similar way; infants born with either of these malformations should be placed in a sterile plastic bag up to the chest to cover the abdominal defect and prevent trauma and insensible water loss.

Postresuscitation Care

Infants who are stressed enough to require resuscitation at birth also require close monitoring after birth for signs and symptoms of further complications. These infants are at higher risk of developing pulmonary hypertension, systemic infections, hypotension, seizures, hypoglycemia, acute tubular necrosis of the kidney, necrotizing enterocolitis, electrolyte abnormalities, and difficulties with feeding because of ischemia and depression at birth. As a result, after an infant is resuscitated, the focus of care shifts to include several other parameters, including temperature regulation to achieve normothermia, assessments of blood glucose and electrolytes, and close monitoring of vital signs in anticipation of further complications that may occur.

FUTURE DIRECTIONS

The neonatal resuscitation algorithm continues to include the use of 100% oxygen; however, available and emerging evidence does support the option to provide positive-pressure ventilation with room air because of the risks of oxygen toxicity, especially in preterm infants. In addition, the role of hypothermia for cerebral protection in asphyxiated infants continues to be studied.

SUGGESTED READINGS

American Heart Association and American Academy of Pediatrics: 2005 American Heart Association (AHA) guidelines for cardiopulmonary resuscitation (CPR) and emergency cardiovascular care (ECC) of pediatric and neonatal patients: neonatal resuscitation guidelines, *Pediatrics* 117(5):e1029-e1038, 2006.

International Liaison Committee on Resuscitation: 2005 International Consensus on cardiopulmonary resuscitation and emergency cardiovascular care science with treatment recommendations. part 7: neonatal resuscitation, *Resuscitation* 67(2-3):293-303, 2005.

Kattwinkel J, Perlman JM, Aziz K, et al: Neonatal resuscitation: 2010 American Heart Association Guidelines for Cardiopulmonary Resuscitation and Emergency Cardiovascular Care, *Circulation* 122:876-908, 2010.

Kattwinkel J, Short J, Boyle D, et al: *Textbook of Neonatal Resuscitation*, ed 5, Elk Grove Village, IL, 2006, American Academy of Pediatrics and American Heart Association.

Obladen M: History of neonatal resuscitation. part 1: artificial ventilation, *Neonatology* 94(3):144-149, 2008.

Rajani AK, Chitkara R, Halamek LP: Delivery room management of the newborn, *Pediatr Clin North Am* 56(3):515-535, 2009.

Stevens TP, Sinkin RA: Surfactant replacement therapy, *Chest* 131(5):1577-1582, 2007.

Taeusch HW, Ballard R, Gleason C: *Avery's Diseases of the Newborn*, ed 8, Philadelphia, 2005, Elsevier, pp 349-363.

Rose C. Graham and Joshua R. Friedman

SECTION
XVII

Disorders of the Digestive System

The esophagus is a muscular tube connecting the pharynx and the stomach. Its role is to move material from the mouth to the stomach. It does not produce any digestive enzymes and has no active role in digestion. Disorders of the esophagus can present with chest or abdominal pain, difficulty swallowing, abnormal movement of gastric contents, or gastrointestinal (GI) bleeding. Disorders involving the esophagus include developmental anomalies, motility disorders, gastroesophageal reflux (GER), esophagitis, and traumatic injury.

DEVELOPMENTAL ANOMALIES

Congenital disorders of the esophagus occur in approximately 1 in 3000 to 5000 births. These disorders commonly occur during embryogenesis as the trachea separates from the esophagus, and include atresia with or without tracheoesophageal fistula (TEF), esophageal stenosis, esophageal duplication, esophageal webs and rings, esophageal diverticulum, and esophageal or bronchogenic cysts.

ETIOLOGY AND PATHOGENESIS

The esophagus forms from a small ventral diverticulum of the embryonic foregut. This diverticulum separates into the esophagus and trachea around the fourth gestational week of fetal development. Anomalies can occur with abnormalities in any step in esophageal formation and development. One of the most common anomalies is TEF with or without atresia. This occurs when there is a disruption in the elongation and separation of the trachea from the esophagus. There are five types of TEF. The most common is type C in which there is atresia of the proximal esophagus with a fistula from the trachea to the distal esophagus (Figure 107-1). Other categories of TEF, in descending frequency, include isolated esophageal atresia without TEF, isolated TEF, esophageal atresia with proximal TEF, and esophageal atresia with proximal and distal TEF.

Congenital disorders of the esophagus are often associated with polyhydramnios as a result of the infant's inability to swallow and absorb amniotic fluid and with prematurity. As many as 70% of children with esophageal abnormalities may have other congenital anomalies, including imperforate anus, vertebral anomalies, duodenal atresia, and annular pancreas. The VACTERL association is a combination of defects that are commonly found together: vertebral anomalies, anorectal atresia, cardiac anomalies, tracheoesophageal fistula, esophageal atresia, renal anomalies, and limb anomalies.

CLINICAL PRESENTATION

A neonate with an esophageal congenital anomaly may present with episodes of respiratory distress worsened by feeding, regurgitation, a history of multiple episodes of pneumonia, or failure to thrive. Older children may present with dysphagia, regurgitation, halitosis, or respiratory symptoms. The severity of symptoms depends on the degree of esophageal compression or obstruction.

EVALUATION AND MANAGEMENT

Esophageal atresia or complete esophageal obstruction can be diagnosed by an inability to pass an orogastric or nasogastric tube into the stomach. TEF may be suggested on abdominal or chest radiograph; however, an isolated TEF (H-type) is best detected by esophagography with contrast. Barium swallow or endoscopy can be useful in diagnosing stenosis or incomplete obstruction from a web, ring, cyst, or diverticulum. Surgical correction is required to treat most congenital anomalies.

MOTILITY DISORDERS OF THE ESOPHAGUS

The esophagus relies on a coordinated motility effort to drive food forward into the stomach and to clear acidic and bilious secretions that may leak upward from the stomach. If a motility disorder disturbs this muscular endeavor, proper delivery of food and clearance of gastroesophageal fluids cannot occur.

ETIOLOGY AND PATHOGENESIS

Striated muscle makes up the upper esophageal sphincter along with the proximal one-third of the esophagus. Smooth muscle composes the remaining two-thirds. The lower esophageal sphincter (LES) is a physiologic sphincter. There is a rich nerve supply to the esophagus. Motility problems can arise from muscular disorders (polymyositis, dermatomyositis, muscular dystrophy, myasthenia gravis), neurologic disorders (stroke, multiple sclerosis, lead poisoning), systemic illness (lupus, scleroderma, sarcoidosis, thyroid disease, diabetes), or infection (tetanus, botulism, *Trypanosoma cruzi* infection).

Achalasia

Achalasia is a progressive motor disorder of the esophagus resulting in increased lower esophageal pressure, impaired relaxation of the LES during swallowing, and impaired esophageal peristalsis. This produces a functional obstruction at the esophagogastric junction. It is an uncommon disorder in the pediatric population. In the United States, childhood-onset achalasia is most often idiopathic, but systemic disease should be considered in determining the etiology. Histologic changes seen with achalasia include loss of ganglion cells, a decrease in the number of myenteric plexus nerve fibers, and degeneration of the vagus nerve.

1. **Tracheoesophageal fistula**

Most common form (90% to 95%) of tracheo-esophageal fistula. Upper segment of esophagus ending in blind pouch; lower segment originating from trachea just above bifurcation. The two segments may be connected by a solid cord

2. **Variations of tracheoesophageal fistula and rare anomalies of trachea**

Upper segment of esophagus ending in trachea; lower segment of variable length

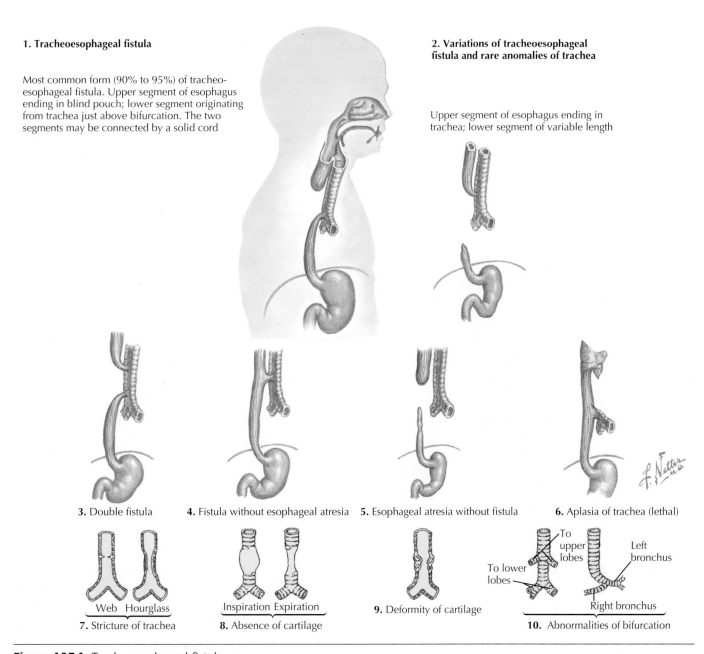

3. Double fistula   4. Fistula without esophageal atresia   5. Esophageal atresia without fistula   6. Aplasia of trachea (lethal)

Web   Hourglass
7. Stricture of trachea

Inspiration   Expiration
8. Absence of cartilage

9. Deformity of cartilage

To upper lobes   Left bronchus
To lower lobes   Right bronchus
10. Abnormalities of bifurcation

Figure 107-1 *Tracheoesophageal fistula.*

Spastic Motility Disorders

Spastic esophageal disorders occur from diffuse esophageal spasm (contraction of more than one esophageal site at the same time), nutcracker esophagus (esophageal contractions of amplitude >180 mm Hg and duration >6 sec), or a hypertensive LES (lower esophageal pressure >44 mm Hg).

CLINICAL PRESENTATION

Achalasia

Symptoms of achalasia include food and liquid dysphagia, regurgitation, vomiting, choking and coughing episodes, a sense of "food getting stuck," a gurgling noise coming from the chest, postprandial and nocturnal chest pain, recurrent episodes of

pneumonia, and loss of weight. Leiomyoma of the distal esophagus, anorexia nervosa, rumination syndromes, Chagas' disease, and candidal esophagitis are other diseases with similar symptoms that need to be considered in the differential diagnosis. Allgrove's syndrome is an autosomal recessive disorder that includes achalasia, alacrima, and adrenocorticotropic hormone insensitivity.

Spastic Motility Disorders

Spastic motility disorders present with dysphagia and substernal chest pain. Unlike cardiac chest pain, pain associated with esophageal dysfunction is nonexertional, occurs at night, is affected by ingestion of food, and responds to antacids. Loss of weight is not usually seen with these disorders.

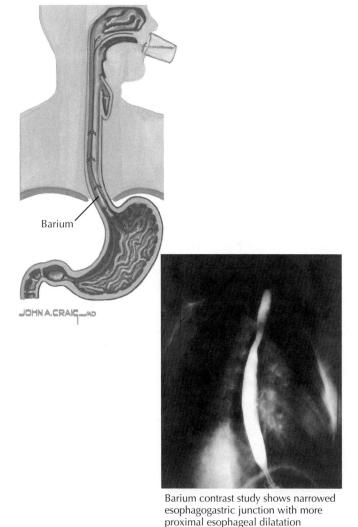

Barium

JOHN A.CRAIG—AD

Barium contrast study shows narrowed esophagogastric junction with more proximal esophageal dilatation

Figure 107-2 *Barium swallow findings seen with achalasia.*

EVALUATION

Achalasia

Chest radiograph may show widening of the mediastinum, loss of the gastric air bubble, or an esophageal air-fluid level. Barium swallow will show impaired contrast movement, abnormal peristalsis, and tapering of the distal esophagus known as the "bird's beak" sign (Figure 107-2). Endoscopy should always be performed and often shows esophageal dilatation, erythema, and ulceration from stasis. Esophageal manometry assesses LES pressures and function in addition to esophageal contraction and motor pattern. In achalasia, manometry shows increased lower esophageal pressure, abnormal peristalsis, and elevated intraesophageal pressures.

Spastic Motility Disorders

Barium swallow may reveal nonperistaltic contractions intermixed with normal peristaltic contractions. Manometry reveals similar pathologic findings observed in achalasia.

MANAGEMENT

Achalasia

Treatment of patients with achalasia includes pneumatic dilatation, surgical myotomy, botulinum toxin injection to inhibit acetylcholine release at the neuromuscular junction, and drug therapy (smooth muscle relaxants such as nitrates and calcium channel blockers). A long-term complication of achalasia may be the development of squamous cell carcinoma.

Spastic Motility Disorders

Spastic motility disorders are not progressive or threatening. Treatment should be aimed at reducing symptoms. Acid suppression and behavioral antistress modifications may be helpful.

GASTROESOPHAGEAL REFLUX

Gastroesophageal reflux (GER) is the intermittent movement of gastric contents into the esophagus. Infrequent GER is a normal process in all age groups. However, GER becomes pathologic when it causes clinical symptoms and is then labeled gastroesophageal reflux disease (GERD). GERD is the most common esophageal disorder in children of all ages. Emesis from GER occurs in 67% of all 4-month-old infants, and heartburn and epigastric pain from GERD occur in 1% to 8% of children. The incidence of GERD is increased in the population of children born prematurely and in those children with neurologic, pulmonary, and developmental disorders.

ETIOLOGY AND PATHOGENESIS

Reflux of stomach contents into the esophagus is prevented by normal LES function and pressure in addition to normal transit of stomach contents into the intestine. GER occurs when the LES is not maintained at a pressure greater than 4 mm of Hg as a result of functional or mechanical defects or when peristalsis of the esophagus is inhibited.

CLINICAL PRESENTATION

GER and GERD manifest differently in infants and children. In infants, the most common symptoms of GER are regurgitation and emesis. When associated with additional symptoms of irritability, arching, respiratory distress, refusal of food, or failure to thrive, this may be considered GERD. Infantile GER and GERD usually begin to improve after 6 months of age and typically disappear by 2 years of age. In children, GERD most commonly manifests as abdominal pain or substernal heartburn after meals. Children with GERD may also experience cough, dysphagia, odynophagia, or nocturnal worsening of their asthma. GERD may be associated with sore throat, otalgia, oral cavity disease, wheezing, and hoarseness in some children. In infants with chronic vomiting, one must consider food allergies, anatomic abnormality (pyloric stenosis, malrotation, volvulus, rings, webs, and stenosis), infection, metabolic disorder, rumination, toxic ingestion, or increased intracranial pressure in the differential diagnosis.

Box 107-1 Concerning Symptoms in Vomiting Infants and Children

- Bilious emesis
- Bulging fontanelle, lethargy, morning emesis
- Hematemesis or hematochezia
- Failure to thrive
- Respiratory distress or history of multiple episodes of pneumonia
- Fever or systemic symptoms
- Skin lesions
- Hepatosplenomegaly

EVALUATION

The diagnosis of GERD can most often be made clinically with a thorough medical and dietary history and a physical examination. Diagnostic studies should be reserved for those with atypical or concerning symptoms (Box 107-1), symptoms unresponsive to therapy, or symptoms suggestive of anatomic abnormality or tissue damage (hematemesis, bloody stool, anemia). An upper GI study with barium swallow is used to demonstrate anatomic anomalies. Scintigraphy (also known as milk scan or gastric emptying study) can show delayed gastric emptying. Upper endoscopy assesses for mucosal injury, inflammation, or dysplasia and may distinguish GERD from eosinophilic esophagitis. Esophageal pH monitoring is helpful to evaluate the frequency of acid reflux events, and multichannel intraluminal impedance studies can demonstrate non–acid reflux events. These measurements are also correlated with symptoms to help establish or refute the relationship between clinical symptoms and GERD.

MANAGEMENT

The goals of treatment of GERD are to reduce symptoms; heal esophageal mucosal injury; and prevent complications, including esophagitis, Barrett's esophagus (metaplasia of the lower esophagus), and stricture formation (Figure 107-3). In infants with GER who are not bothered by emesis and who are growing appropriately, no therapy is necessary. Initial therapy for symptomatic infants with GERD is lifestyle modification, including thickening of feeds, giving smaller volume frequent feeds, frequent burping, and maintaining upright position for longer duration after feeds. Pharmacologic therapy for GERD includes antacids to buffer existing acid and H2 receptor antagonists

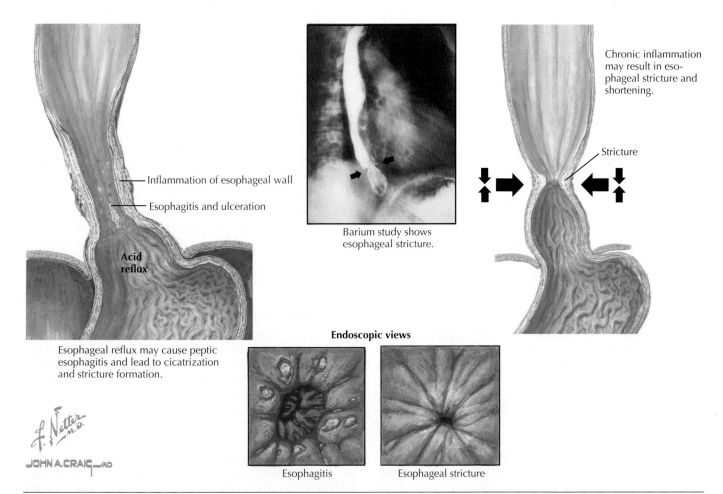

Inflammation of esophageal wall

Esophagitis and ulceration

Acid reflux

Esophageal reflux may cause peptic esophagitis and lead to cicatrization and stricture formation.

Barium study shows esophageal stricture.

Chronic inflammation may result in esophageal stricture and shortening.

Stricture

Endoscopic views

Esophagitis

Esophageal stricture

Figure 107-3 *Complications of gastroesophageal reflux disease.*

(e.g., ranitidine) or proton pump inhibitors (PPIs; e.g., omeprazole) to decrease secretion of acid from parietal cells. PPIs have been shown to be the most effective pharmacologic therapy for GERD. However, they are not always necessary and may be associated with adverse effects such as an increased risk of community-acquired pneumonia and acute gastroenteritis. Prokinetic use (e.g., metoclopramide) has declined because of unfavorable side effect profiles. Surgical fundoplication, a procedure in which the fundus is wrapped around the distal esophagus, is an option for children who are unresponsive to pharmacologic treatment and for those who develop respiratory compromise or stricture. Side effects of fundoplication are not inconsequential and include bloating, dysphagia, dumping syndrome, hernia, small bowel obstruction, and recurrence requiring a second fundoplication.

ESOPHAGITIS

Esophagitis (inflammation of the squamous epithelium of the esophagus) has a variety of causes in the pediatric population. Esophagitis may occur from chemical irritation, infection, immunologic response, trauma, or systemic disease or may be idiopathic in nature.

ETIOLOGY AND PATHOGENESIS

Chemical Esophagitis

Chemical esophagitis may occur from acid that is refluxed from the stomach into the esophagus (GER) or from ingestion (accidental or intentional) of caustic substances. GERD is the most common cause of esophagitis in children. Common causes of caustic esophagitis include household alkaline substances, non-steroidal antiinflammatory drugs (NSAIDs), and anti-acne medications (doxycycline, tetracycline, clindamycin).

Infectious Esophagitis

Infectious esophagitis most frequently occurs in immunocompromised children. Infections that commonly cause esophagitis include herpes simplex virus (HSV); cytomegalovirus, Candida; and less frequently, varicella zoster virus, *Helicobacter pylori*, and human immunodeficiency virus (HIV). HSV is the most common cause of esophagitis in immunocompetent patients.

Immunologic Esophagitis

Although multiple food antigens can induce esophagitis, cow's milk protein is the most common cause of allergic esophagitis in children.

Traumatic Esophagitis

Traumatic injury to the esophagus may be accidental, iatrogenic, or intentional. Esophagitis may occur after procedures such as nasogastric tube placement or gastric suctioning. Radiation esophagitis usually occurs within 1 to 2 weeks; however, radiation-induced esophageal strictures may occur years later.

Systemic Disease

Esophagitis may be seen in any systemic disease that causes GER. Esophagitis may also be seen separately from GER in Crohn's disease, glycogen storage disease, chronic granulomatous disease, scleroderma, Behçet's disease, graft-versus-host disease, and vasculitic disorders.

Idiopathic Eosinophilic Esophagitis

Idiopathic eosinophilic esophagitis (EoE) is a dense esophageal eosinophilic infiltrate in the absence of any recognized cause of eosinophilic inflammation. EoE can occur at any age.

CLINICAL PRESENTATION

Esophagitis can present with irritability, dysphagia, odynophagia, food regurgitation, epigastric pain, chest pain, and food impaction. Children with infectious esophagitis may have a concurrent fever, skin lesions, oral ulcers, or thrush.

EVALUATION

Endoscopy with biopsy is the main diagnostic modality for esophagitis. Macroscopic visualization of the esophagus may reveal erythema, erosions, or ulcerations; however, a normal macroscopic appearance of the esophagus does not exclude histologic esophagitis. Histology, electron microscopy, and immunohistochemistry can help distinguish the different causes of esophagitis (Table 107-1).

MANAGEMENT

Management of esophagitis depends on the etiology. The treatment of GERD has been discussed previously and involves behavioral modification, antacids, H2 blockers, and PPIs. Infectious esophagitis requires the appropriate antiviral, antifungal, or antibiotic therapy for the specific infection, especially in immunosuppressed hosts. However, eradication of *Helicobacter pylori* gastritis does not improve esophagitis. Treatment of EoE centers around removal of all offending dietary antigens. Often, it is difficult to identify the exact offending agents, so an elemental diet may need to be initiated until the esophagus heals with subsequent sequential reintroduction of foods.

TRAUMATIC INJURIES TO THE ESOPHAGUS

Traumatic injury to the esophagus during childhood may occur as a result of ingestion of caustic substances or foreign bodies, blunt or penetrating injury, medical procedures, or child abuse.

Esophageal Foreign Body

Foreign bodies are most frequently ingested by children younger than the age of 3 years and by children with neurologic disease or developmental delay. Whereas young children most frequently ingest coins, toy parts, and jewelry, older children and

Table 107-1 Characteristic Histological Findings for Various Causes of Esophagitis

Finding	Etiology
Eosinophils	
<20/hpf	Primary GER
>20/hpf	Idiopathic EoE
Macroscopic shallow ulcers	Herpes simplex esophagitis
Mononuclear infiltrate	
Multinucleate giant cells	
Basophilic nuclear inclusions	Cytomegalovirus esophagitis
Macroscopic white plaques	Candidal esophagitis
Pseudohyphae and budding yeast	
Polymorphonuclear infiltrate, vessel thrombosis, granulation tissue	Corrosive esophagitis

EoE, eosinophilic esophagitis; GER, gastroesophageal reflux; hpf, high-power field.

adolescents more frequently choke on food particles. These items may become lodged in the esophagus at the thoracic inlet, the level of the aortic arch, or the gastroesophageal junction. Food impaction should raise suspicion for anatomic abnormality, including stricture or vascular ring. With impaction, children may be asymptomatic or may experience dysphagia, odynophagia, drooling, wheezing, or hoarseness. A high index of suspicion is necessary. Chest radiograph may identify radiopaque, but not radiolucent, objects that may be seen using computed tomography. Esophagoscopy is often the primary diagnostic tool when suspicion is high but imaging is inconclusive. Endoscopic removal is often necessary and can also evaluate the esophagus after removal of the foreign body. Timing of endoscopic removal is based on the presence or absence of symptoms, the type and location of the suspected object, and the duration since ingestion. In general, patients who have ingested button batteries or sharp objects, as well as symptomatic patients with any object type, should undergo emergent removal. Asymptomatic patients with ingestion of noncaustic, blunt objects can be observed for 12 to 24 hours to allow for spontaneous passage. Most objects retained after 24 hours should be removed endoscopically. In general, after the object passes into the stomach, endoscopic removal is not necessary unless symptoms develop, the object is large (longer than 5 cm or wider than 2 cm), or multiple magnets were ingested. After they are in the stomach, most objects will pass uneventfully through the entire GI tract within 2 to 3 weeks. Monitoring the stool and, if necessary, follow-up imaging, can document complete passage of the object.

Caustic Injury

The ingestion of caustic substances can cause immediate and long-lasting damage to the esophagus, including perforation, stricture formation, stenosis, and squamous cell carcinoma.

ALKALINE SUBSTANCES

Household alkaline substances are responsible for 70% of corrosive ingestions and include ammonia, bleach, dishwashing detergent, drain cleaners, and disc batteries. Alkaline substances cause liquefaction necrosis with fat and protein digestion.

ACIDIC SUBSTANCES

Acidic household substances include toilet bowl cleaners, drain cleaners, stain removers, and swimming pool additives. Acids are less commonly ingested and cause a more superficial mucosal coagulation necrosis. The stomach is more affected by acidic ingestions than the esophagus.

Symptoms of caustic ingestion include burning of the oropharynx, dysphagia, odynophagia, drooling, or respiratory distress. Symptoms do not always correlate with the severity of the burn. Initially, the child should get chest and abdominal radiographs, and oral intake should be prohibited. Vomiting should *not* be induced. Endoscopy should be performed to assess the extent of damage.

Pill Esophagitis

Medications, including NSAIDs, potassium, iron, and antibiotics, can cause esophageal damage, particularly in patients with delayed esophageal motility. Symptoms of odynophagia can occur immediately after ingestion or can be delayed. Endoscopy will reveal inflammation and provides the opportunity to remove the pill if still retained.

Mallory-Weiss Syndrome

Mallory-Weiss syndrome is a spontaneous longitudinal tear in the esophageal mucosa that occurs after forceful or prolonged vomiting. Most commonly, the tear is located near the gastroesophageal junction. Patients present with a history of vomiting or retching followed by an episode of hematemesis. The vast majority of the time, the bleeding of a Mallory-Weiss tear is self-limited. However, an upper endoscopy may be useful to confirm this diagnosis and rule out other diagnoses if the bleeding does not stop spontaneously.

Esophageal Rupture

Esophageal rupture is a life-threatening event and can result from severe vomiting (Boerhaave's syndrome), thoracic or abdominal trauma, instrumentation, or ulcer perforation. Patients with esophageal rupture present with chest, neck, or abdominal pain; dysphagia; hematemesis; subcutaneous emphysema; or signs of shock. Chest and abdominal radiographs may reveal air in the subcutaneous tissue, mediastinum, thorax, or abdomen. Treatment is often surgical.

SUGGESTED READINGS

Hassall E: Step-up and step-down approaches to treatment of gastroesophageal reflux disease in children, *Curr Gastroenterol Rep* 10:324-331, 2008.

Nelson SP, Chen EH, Syniar GM, Christoffel KK: Prevalence of symptoms of gastroesophageal reflux during childhood: a pediatric practice-based survey. Pediatric Practice Research Group, *Arch Pediatr Adolesc Med* 154:150-154, 2000.

Pediatric Gastroesophageal Reflux Clinical Practice Guidelines: Joint Recommendations of the North American Society for Pediatric Gastroenterology, Hepatology, and Nutrition (NASPGHAN) and the European Society for Pediatric Gastroenterology, Hepatology, and Nutrition (ESPGHAN). *J Pediatr Gastroenterol Nutr* 49:498-547, 2009.

Spergel JM, Brown-Whitehorn TF, Beausoleil JL, et al: 14 years of eosinophilic esophagitis: clinical features and prognosis, *J Pediatr Gastroenterol Nutr* 48(1):30-36, 2009.

Wilsey MJ Jr, Scheimann AO, Gilger MA: The role of upper gastrointestinal endoscopy in the diagnosis and treatment of caustic ingestion, esophageal strictures, and achalasia in children, *Gastrointestinal Endoscopy Clin North Am* 11(4):767-787, 2001.

Gastritis and Gastrointestinal Bleeding

108

Andrew Chu

Numerous potential etiologies, combined with the gastrointestinal (GI) tract's extensive surface area, can make the assessment and management of GI bleeding exceptionally challenging. Observations of several key clinical features assist clinicians in formulating rational differential diagnoses. Gastritis is an important cause of GI bleeding and abdominal pain that deserves particular attention. Although the inability to arrive at a definitive diagnosis (i.e., obscure GI bleeding) remains a significant problem, the growing arsenal of diagnostic modalities is making it increasingly possible to isolate the source of bleeding and construct a successful treatment strategy.

ETIOLOGY AND PATHOGENESIS

The causes of GI bleeding are diverse (Figure 108-1). Although the sheer number of causes may seem intimidating, grouping them into pathophysiologic categories aids in constructing a differential diagnosis. Note that underlying disorders of coagulation (e.g., hemophilias, vitamin K deficiency in neonates) and hepatic dysfunction (caused by the liver's role in producing coagulation factors) can exacerbate any of these causes.

Direct Mechanical Injury

Blunt and penetrating trauma can initiate bleeding from any part of the GI tract. Ingestion of certain foreign bodies (e.g., coin batteries) may result in mucosal injury and even bowel perforation. Repeated vomiting or retching may create esophageal mucosal defects called Mallory-Weiss tears that can bleed. Surgical interventions, such as dental procedures and tonsillectomy, may result in blood loss that is swallowed and subsequently vomited.

Mucosal Erosion

The GI tract has a robust and sophisticated mucosal defense mechanism designed to prevent erosion. These protective elements include (1) the superficial "unmixed" layer of mucus, bicarbonate, and other factors that form a neutralizing barrier against acid, enzymatic, and abrasive injury; (2) the epithelial cells that generate this superficial layer; (3) continuous cell renewal coupled with (4) uninterrupted nutrient blood flow to the mucosa and (5) sensory innervation that optimizes this blood flow; and (6) endothelial production of prostaglandins and nitric oxide, which synergize to promote all of the aforementioned mechanisms. Disruption of any of these factors may predispose a given region of mucosa to erosion, local loss of vascular integrity, and resultant bleeding.

DRUG-INDUCED

A number of drugs can precipitate mucosal erosions, the most notorious being those from the nonsteroidal antiinflammatory drug (NSAID) class, which inhibit cyclooxygenase-mediated prostaglandin synthesis. Other culprits include corticosteroids, alcohol, caffeine, and nicotine. Chemotherapeutic agents, such as vincristine, methotrexate, and 5-fluorouracil, may cause GI bleeding via inflammation and mucosal erosion (termed *mucositis*) anywhere along the GI tract by inhibiting epithelial cell turnover, recruiting inflammatory cells, and making the mucosa more susceptible to infectious insults.

INFLAMMATION

Disruption of mucosal integrity may occur in disorders that promote the recruitment of inflammatory cells, such as lymphocytes and neutrophils, which injure the epithelium by direct cell-to-cell contact or via secreted immunologic factors, such as cytokines. Examples include autoimmune enteropathy and eosinophilic gastroenteritis. Another important example is inflammatory bowel disease, a complex autoimmune disease that encompasses Crohn's disease, which can cause full-thickness inflammation anywhere along the GI tract, and ulcerative colitis, which causes mucosal ulcerations in the colon (see Chapter 110). Children who have undergone bone marrow transplant may experience a form of rejection called graft-versus-host disease (GVHD). When it affects the GI tract, GVHD causes diarrhea, vomiting, fever, abdominal pain, and GI bleeding. Certain immunodeficiencies, such as common variable immunodeficiency, precipitate inflammation because of dysregulated immunity that leads to autoimmune responses (see Chapter 21).

INFECTION

Infections disrupt mucosal integrity by direct cytotoxicity and/or by promoting inflammation. For example, herpes simplex virus is known to cause florid esophagitis, particularly in immunocompromised individuals, with nearly one-third of these patients experiencing an acute upper GI bleed. Additionally, infections may elicit specific peculiar responses. For example, cytomegalovirus is occasionally associated with massive gastric epithelial proliferation leading to a hypertrophic gastropathy called Menetrier's disease. This causes protein wasting (including coagulation factors) from the leaky mucosa, as well as a higher risk of mucosal erosion and bleeding. *Helicobacter pylori* is perhaps the most infamous of the infectious

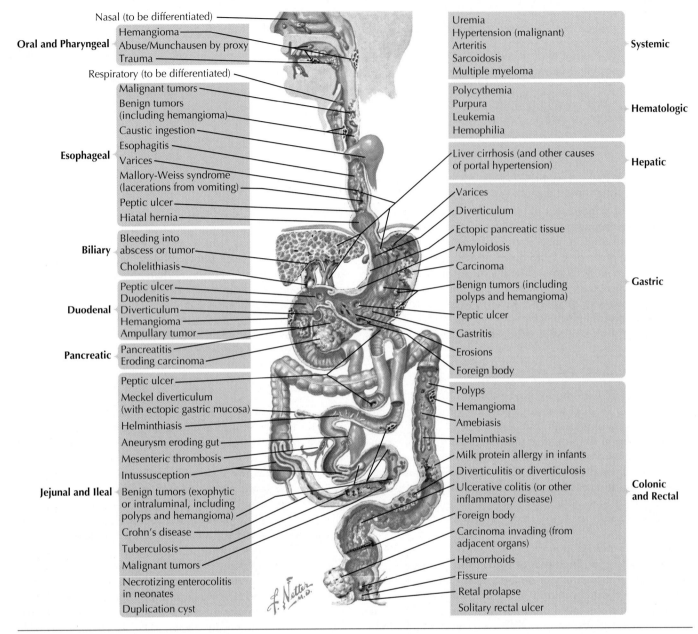

Figure 108-1 *Gastrointestinal hemorrhage.*

causes of gastritis and duodenitis because of its chronicity, high prevalence (especially in certain populations of children, such as immigrants, the poor, and those attending daycare centers), its associations with peptic ulcers and adenocarcinoma of the stomach and duodenum, and its resistance to eradication (Figure 108-2).

CAUSTIC INGESTIONS

Ingestion of acid substances causes a coagulation necrosis that results in ulcers and mucosal bleeding. Alkali ingestions can create significantly worse complications through liquefaction necrosis and mucosal sloughing, which can lead to severe ulceration, perforation, and eventual luminal stenosis.

ISCHEMIA

Loss of blood flow to the bowel can lead to ischemic injury and necrosis. Examples of conditions in which this may occur are mesenteric arterial thrombosis; vascular malformations that create regions of suboptimal blood flow; and drug-induced bowel injury, as can occur with the use of certain chemotherapeutic agents such as vincristine and cisplatin. Depending on the severity of the occlusion, microscopic or frank bleeding may occur, typically accompanied by severe postprandial abdominal pain. Stress-related mucosal disease is a form of gastritis encountered in critically ill patients. The systemic hypotension frequently experienced in this population leads to local mucosal ischemia, causing erosions and subepithelial hemorrhage.

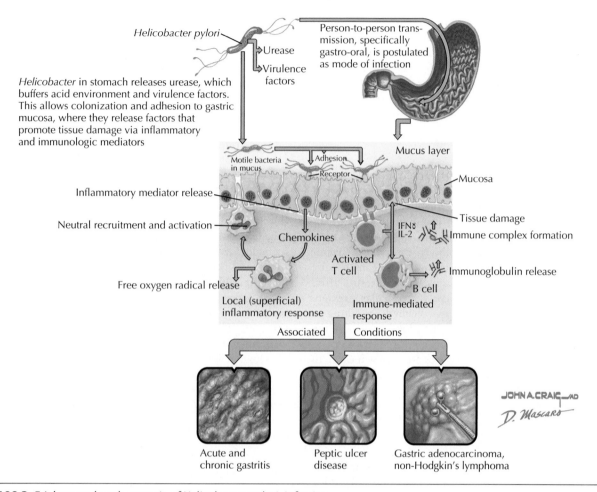

Helicobacter pylori

Urease
Virulence factors

Helicobacter in stomach releases urease, which buffers acid environment and virulence factors. This allows colonization and adhesion to gastric mucosa, where they release factors that promote tissue damage via inflammatory and immunologic mediators

Person-to-person transmission, specifically gastro-oral, is postulated as mode of infection

Motile bacteria in mucus
Adhesion
Receptor
Mucus layer
Mucosa

Inflammatory mediator release

Neutral recruitment and activation

Chemokines

IFNδ
IL-2
Tissue damage
Immune complex formation

Free oxygen radical release

Activated T cell

Immunoglobulin release

B cell

Local (superficial) inflammatory response

Immune-mediated response

Associated   Conditions

JOHN A.CRAIG—AD
D. Mascaro

Acute and chronic gastritis

Peptic ulcer disease

Gastric adenocarcinoma, non-Hodgkin's lymphoma

Figure 108-2 *Etiology and pathogenesis of* Helicobacter pylori *infection.*

INFILTRATION

Although rare in children, tumors involving the GI tract, such as lymphoma, may promote bleeding by direct invasion and by inflammatory cells that may also damage the mucosa.

HYPERSECRETION

Several rare disorders may result in excessive or ectopic acid secretion. For example, gastrinomas are uncommon tumors arising in the stomach or pancreas that are a major cause of Zollinger-Ellison syndrome, in which pathologically elevated gastrin production promotes excess gastric acid secretion and the formation of peptic ulcers in almost all affected patients. Duplication cysts are developmental disorders in which ectopic gastric tissue within the cyst may cause inappropriate acid secretion in a relatively unprotected portion of the GI tract (potentially anywhere, most commonly the ileum), resulting in erosion and bleeding. They can also cause GI bleeding through other mechanisms, such as by acting as lead points for intussusception, with resultant ischemia, or through the rare development of a malignancy at the cyst site. Meckel's diverticulum is another developmental disorder resulting from incomplete involution of the vitelline duct that can harbor ectopic gastric mucosa (features summarized by the rule of twos: 2% of the population, 2 feet

from ileocecal valve, 2 inches long, most commonly presents around age 2 years, and boys are two times as likely to be affected).

Polyps

Polyps are mucosal projections into the intestinal lumen caused by disordered epithelial growth. Various spontaneous and familial polyposis entities exist. Regardless of the specific underlying process, they are a source of bleeding (generally painless) secondary to mechanical irritation or wholesale shearing by passing fecal material. In contrast to adults, the vast majority of polyps in children are juvenile polyps. These non-neoplastic polyps are typically composed of many cystic, dilated glands; copious inflammation; and surface erosions, the last of which is the cause of bleeding. Juvenile polyps have a peak incidence from 2 to 6 years of age, represent more than 90% of all pediatric polyp diagnoses, and are found in about 1% of school-age children.

Vascular Abnormalities

Congenital vascular defects may result in fragile vascular arrangements vulnerable to erosive and mechanical insults. Whereas hemangiomas represent proliferative vessel abnormalities that may regress, true malformations (including disorders such as arteriovenous malformations, blue rubber bleb nevus syndrome, and Osler-Rendu-Weber syndrome) are non-proliferative and do not regress. Processes that compromise the full thickness of bowel, such as Crohn's disease and bowel surgery, may result in vessel-to-bowel fistulas associated with significant bleeding. Vasculitides, such as Henoch-Schönlein purpura, may result in occlusion of mesenteric vessels and intestinal ischemia (see Chapter 28).

Portal Hypertension

The final common pathway for many chronic liver diseases is cirrhosis, in which the underlying disease causes excessive production of extracellular matrix; destruction of normal liver architecture; and, ultimately, severe organ dysfunction. Cirrhosis is the most common cause of portal hypertension. Other potential causes include portal venous thrombosis, veno-occlusive disease in patients receiving chemotherapy, and hepatic vein thrombosis (Budd-Chiari syndrome). Backpressure from the high-resistance liver increases the intravascular pressure experienced by the portal vein and its collaterals, resulting in esophageal varices (abnormally dilated venous system in the distal esophagus) and portal gastropathy (increased venous pressure throughout the gastric wall). Varices are a known cause of catastrophic GI bleeds. The bleeding from these engorged vessels is only exacerbated by inadequate hepatic synthesis of coagulation factors.

Blood from Extrinsic Sources

In neonates, swallowed maternal blood from delivery or breast-feeding is a potential cause of bloody emesis or stool. Blood swallowed from the airway in patients with frequent, severe coughing (e.g., pneumonia, cystic fibrosis, tuberculosis) may be mistaken for hematemesis. Rarely, hepatic injury from trauma or an abscess may cause hemobilia, with blood draining from the biliary system into the duodenum.

CLINICAL PRESENTATION

The clinician's first priority is to establish the patient's stability; the initial impression can provide valuable clues. Pallor, lethargy, and diaphoresis are all immediately concerning signs of significant blood loss. However, the absence of these signs in a seemingly well-appearing individual with a history of hematemesis, melena, or hematochezia should not automatically comfort the clinician. Indeed, tachycardia combined with normal blood pressure for age could indicate compensated shock (see Chapter 2). The most definitive physical examination indicator of significant blood loss is orthostatic hypotension, defined as a decrease in systolic blood pressure of at least 20 mm Hg or diastolic blood pressure of at least 10 mm Hg within 3 minutes of standing.

The clinician should then focus on addressing several key questions:

What Are the Route and Appearance of the Bleeding?

Visible GI bleeding presents in different forms depending on the location of origin. Traditionally, authors have grouped causes of GI bleeding into upper and lower sources divided by the ligament of Treitz. In 2007, the American Gastroenterological Association promoted the refinement of this classification into upper, middle, and lower GI tract bleeding, with the dividing point between the upper and middle tract being the ampulla of Vater (pancreatic outlet into the duodenum) and the dividing point between the middle and lower tract being the ileocecal valve.

Hematemesis, which is vomiting of either fresh blood or coagulated, denatured blood ("coffee grounds"), indicates upper GI bleeding. Coffee-ground hematemesis generally represents old blood or bleeding that is occurring at a slow rate, as opposed to red blood, which raises concern for active bleeding. *Melena* (black, tarry, foul-smelling stool containing oxidized blood) usually comes from the upper GI tract, but it can emanate from a middle GI source if the transit rate is not rapid. *Hematochezia* (red blood per rectum) generally suggests middle or lower GI bleeding, although it may also represent a massive upper GI bleed. Indeed, hematemesis combined with melena or hematochezia is an ominous combination that must be investigated promptly. Therefore, in any patient with bloody stool, the clinician must be convinced that there is no evidence of upper GI bleeding. It is important to remember that many cases of GI bleeding are *occult* (i.e., microscopic), which are not visible to the eye and can occur anywhere along the GI tract. It is also essential to determine whether the blood could be emanating from a non-GI source, epistaxis and menstruation being two common examples.

What Is the Age of the Patient?

Most causes can present in a variety of ages. However, some disorders tend to present more commonly in specific age groups. For example, juvenile polyps have a peak incidence in young school-age children. Inflammatory bowel disease, although it can present at almost any age, is generally rare in very young children, and when it does occur in that group, its presence prompts concerns of a possible immunodeficiency.

Several disorders appear almost exclusively in neonates and infants. In newborns, particularly premature infants, necrotizing enterocolitis is a life-threatening emergency in which segments of bowel become inflamed and necrotic, leading to hematochezia, melena, or both; abdominal distension; and fever. Neonates at delivery or breastfeeding infants may also swallow blood (the latter from cracked maternal nipples), which can then appear in reflux or emesis. The Apt test can help distinguish maternal blood from that of the patient. Milk protein allergy most often presents in the first few months of life as fussiness and mild hematochezia in an otherwise well-appearing infant who has been exposed to cow's milk proteins, either through formula or indirect transmission via the mother's breast milk.

Is the Bleeding Acute or Chronic?

A history of repeated bleeding episodes over a period of time suggests causes that have the potential for chronicity. For example, inflammatory bowel disease does not typically present with sudden, catastrophic bleeds but tends to have a more insidious course marked initially with other symptoms such as weight loss or diarrhea. Peptic ulcers are another example in which bleeding may begin as occult but worsen over time if left untreated or exacerbated by other factors such as NSAID use. In such cases, a patient may exhibit pallor and fatigue but can remain functional, at least for a time, because of the body's adaptation to the progressive anemia. On the other hand, rapid onset of significant bleeds should sway the clinician toward other causes. For example, two significant causes of sudden melena or hematochezia are Meckel's diverticulum and vascular malformations. In patients with known liver disease, esophageal varices are a critical consideration.

Is the Bleeding Associated with Pain?

Abdominal pain associated with GI bleeding may suggest structural compromise. Bleeding coincident with pain in the epigastric region may be caused by peptic disease or necrotizing pancreatitis. If the pain is associated with distension or vomiting, the clinician should be concerned for causes of intestinal obstruction potentially associated with bleeding, such as intussusception, although upper GI blood itself can stimulate vomiting. If significant bleeding of rapid onset occurs with generalized abdominal pain disproportionate to the rest of the physical examination, ischemia may be the contributing cause. Bowel inflammation, as occurs with ulcerative colitis, can cause cramping pain. An ill-appearing patient with peritoneal signs (involuntary guarding, rebound tenderness, exquisite pain with movement) may be experiencing bowel perforation and requires urgent medical and surgical evaluation.

What Is the Relationship Between the Blood and Stool?

The answer to this question can help guide the physician toward a region of pathology as long as one keeps in mind the limitations of these generalizations. Melena indicates bleeding from an upper or middle GI source. If the patient is having frequent, watery stool containing melena, this suggests small bowel pathology, as in Crohn's disease. Pure melena without watery diarrhea suggests other causes, such as peptic ulcers or esophageal varices. If the patient has profuse diarrhea with cramping and hematochezia (dysentery), this is more suggestive of colitis, as can occur with ulcerative colitis and many infectious causes, such as *Clostridium difficile*, *Yersinia* spp., *Shigella* spp., and *Campylobacter* spp. If the patient has pure hematochezia, infectious and inflammatory causes are still possible, but one also needs to consider other causes such as Meckel's diverticulum, polyps, or vascular malformations, particularly if the bleeding is painless. If the patient has formed stool coated with blood (rather than permeating it), this suggests a distal cause such as solitary rectal ulcer (caused by mucosal erosion in the rectum from hard stool) or an anal fissure.

Does the Patient Have Other Prominent Abnormalities by History or Examination?

Any associated findings may provide clues to the etiology. Cutaneous hemangiomas raise the possibility of internal hemangiomas affecting the GI tract. A history of failure to thrive or weight loss raises concern for small bowel dysfunction, such as occurs with Crohn's disease, or, less commonly, malignancy. Inflammatory bowel disease can also be associated with a host of other extraintestinal findings, such as erythema nodosum and episcleritis. Polyps may often be a part of syndromes with other findings, a classic example being Peutz-Jeghers syndrome, in which hamartomatous polyps occur with mucocutaneous macules. Stigmata of liver disease, including jaundice, icterus, spider angiomas, and hepatosplenomegaly, may raise concerns for esophageal varices.

EVALUATION AND MANAGEMENT

The clinician's first priority is to triage the patient based on the acuity and severity of a patient's bleeding and ensure hemodynamic stability. Each case needs to be assessed individually, but if the amount of blood reported or witnessed is significant (more than just a streak), there is repeated bleeding, or there is any concern for hemodynamic instability, the patient should be sent to the emergency department for further evaluation. Extra caution should be paid to infants unless an obvious cause combined with very small amounts of bleeding can be identified (e.g., stool covered with streaks of blood in a patient with anal fissure). When the patient has presented for medical attention, management should contain the elements discussed in the following paragraphs.

Determine Hemodynamic Status

Rapid comprehensive assessment of the patient, starting with the ABCs (airway, breathing, circulation) and including general appearance, vital signs, signs of injury, and mental status, should be performed first to determine the patient's stability and the next step in management.

ESTABLISH THE PRESENCE OF BLOOD

Many ingested products can mimic the appearance of blood: red-colored foods, drinks, candies, and beets can appear as hematemesis, and licorice, spinach, blueberries, bismuth, and iron supplements can mimic melena. It is therefore important at the outset to confirm that the substance is truly blood using an appropriate guaiac test: Hemoccult for stool and Gastroccult for gastric contents. These cards are quick and generally reliable, but occasionally, the presence of significant amounts of vitamin C, hemoglobin, or myoglobin (from meat) in the test sample can produce a false-positive result. The Apt test, which capitalizes on biochemical differences between fetal and adult hemoglobin, can delineate whether the source is from the mother or baby when it is unclear if bleeding is caused by swallowed maternal blood.

Determine High-Risk Historical Factors

The clinician must determine whether there are exogenous factors that have contributed to the patient's clinical picture, including a history of trauma, ingestion, drug use, and other illnesses.

Table 108-1 Diagnostic Modalities for Gastrointestinal Bleeding*

	Modality	GI Region Assessed	Question Addressed	Notes
Clinical	Nasogastric lavage	Upper GI tract	Is active upper GI bleeding occurring?	Concern for esophageal varices not a contraindication; use of ice-cold fluid not shown to inhibit bleeding
	Apt test	Upper GI tract	Is the origin of hematemesis the mother or the baby?	Pink = fetal Hgb; yellow-brown = adult Hgb
Radiologic	Radiography ("plain film")	All	Is there a foreign body or evidence of perforation?	Use limited to rapid screening early in assessment
	CT with contrast	Abdomen or pelvis	Are there structural lesions that may be responsible? And when performed as CT angiography, is a vascular defect the source?	High level of structural detail; CT angiography provides vascular data; study of choice in trauma and severely ill patients; may be useful in patients with persistent obscure GI bleeding; significant radiation burden
	Bleeding scan (Tc-99m tagged RBC scan)	All	Where is the source of GI bleeding?	Nuclear studies may have limited availability; lower limit of bleeding rate detection = 0.1 mL/min; poor sensitivity and specificity; only helpful in setting of brisk bleeding
	Meckel scan (Tc-99m pertechnetate scan)	All	Is ectopic gastric mucosa present in the ileum?	Nuclear studies may have limited availability; positive scan results justify bypassing endoscopy and proceeding to surgery
	Angiography	Targeted assessment of bowel vasculature	Is a vascular defect the source of bleeding?	Lower limit of bleeding rate detection = 0.5 mL/min; invasive and associated with risk of internal hemorrhage; may be used for therapeutic intervention
	Ultrasound	Liver or pancreas	Is there structural evidence of liver or pancreatic disease?	Helpful if concerned for hepatic disease, hemobilia, or pancreatitis
	Barium enema	Colon	Is a mucosal defect of the colon responsible?	Rarely used in this context given the overall superiority of colonoscopy; exception is evaluation of intussusception, in which it can also be therapeutic
	Upper GI series with small bowel follow-through*	Proximal GI tract to terminal ileum	Is a mucosal defect or anatomic defect of the bowel from the esophagus to the terminal ileum responsible?	Defects can only be inferred by abnormalities in lumen contour but allows noninvasive evaluation of the small bowel; also detects malrotation
	Enteroclysis (fluoroscopic or CT) MRI*	Small bowel Abdomen or pelvis	Are there structural lesions that may be responsible? And when performed as MR angiography, is a vascular defect the source?	High level of structural detail; SBFT may be superior for evaluation of mucosal defects; no radiation burden; not appropriate for acute evaluation; young patients may need sedation
			Is an intestinal mucosal defect responsible?	Permits more complete examination than SBFT; requires introduction of catheter into small intestine; associated radiation burden; most useful for investigation of occult bleeding
Endoscopic	Upper endoscopy (esophagogastroduodenoscopy)	Proximal GI tract to duodenum	Is a mucosal defect of the upper GI tract responsible?	Gold standard evaluation; direct visualization of lesions capable of obtaining biopsies for tissue diagnosis; capable of therapeutic interventions
	Lower endoscopy (colonoscopy)	Colon, terminal ileum	Is a mucosal defect of the colon or terminal ileum responsible?	Gold standard evaluation; direct visualization of lesions capable of obtaining biopsies for tissue diagnosis; capable of therapeutic interventions
	Capsule endoscopy*	Duodenum through terminal ileum	Is a mucosal defect of the small bowel responsible?	Allows direct visualization of the mucosa; no ability to guide the capsule or biopsy tissue
	Balloon enteroscopy*	Proximal GI tract to terminal ileum	Is a mucosal defect of jejunum or proximal ileum responsible?	Limited availability; technically difficult
Surgical	Exploratory laparotomy	Clinician-defined	Where is the source of this major bleed?	Reserved for catastrophic bleeds with goal of surgical intervention
	Push enteroscopy	Jejunum, ileum	Is there a mucosal defect of the jejunum or proximal ileum?	Reserved for evaluation of persistent obscure GI bleeding after endoscopy and radiologic assessments have been repeatedly negative

*Studies not suitable for the acute-care setting.
CT, computed tomography; GI, gastrointestinal; Hgb, hemoglobin; MRI, magnetic resonance imaging. RBC, red blood cell; SBFT, small bowel follow-through; Tc-99m, technetium-99m.

INITIAL MANAGEMENT IN THE EMERGENCY DEPARTMENT

Any patient with evidence of significant bleeding should receive supplemental oxygen, be placed on constant hemodynamic monitoring, and have at least two large-bore intravenous catheters placed. If rapid hemodynamic resuscitation is indicated, isotonic fluids may be required, but blood is the preferred product if there is clear evidence of significant blood loss (see Chapter 2).

Although it is associated with patient discomfort, nasogastric lavage is a valuable tool in assessing patients with GI bleeding. When bleeding is self-limited in a well-appearing patient who is hemodynamically stable and when bleeding is clearly from a discernible source such as epistaxis, lavage may not be necessary. However, if the patient has had hematemesis, lavage assesses whether bleeding is ongoing, which would increase the urgency for endoscopic evaluation. In melena and hematochezia, lavage can help determine whether there is upper GI bleeding, although a clear aspirate does not definitively exclude this. When performed, a sump-type catheter (not feeding tube) should be used, the patient's head should be at 30 degrees to reduce the risk of aspiration, and the liquid should be room temperature normal saline. The clinician should infuse 1 to 2 oz for infants, 4 to 6 oz for school-age children, or 1 L for adult-sized children per infusion and allow the liquid to stand for 2 to 3 minutes before aspirating and repeating until the aspirate is clear. If the lavage does not clear after three attempts, there is limited utility to continuing, and the tube can be left to gravity or low intermittent suction.

Consultation with a gastroenterologist will assist with guiding the evaluation. Intensive care physicians and surgeons should be consulted in cases of significant blood loss or hemodynamic instability.

Laboratory Evaluations

Initial laboratory studies assess the patient's hematologic status, screen for underlying contributory factors, and prepare for potential procedures. They should include a complete blood count (including platelet count), reticulocyte count, prothrombin and partial thromboplastin times, liver function tests (including aspartate aminotransferase, alanine aminotransferase, total and unconjugated bilirubin, and serum albumin), serum chemistries, and type and screen. The blood urea nitrogen may be elevated relative to the serum creatinine because of the absorption of amino acids produced by the enzymatic degradation of hemoglobin. As discussed earlier, the presence of blood should be confirmed by Hemoccult (stool) or Gastroccult (gastric aspirate), and the Apt test may be indicated in the neonatal setting if there is suspicion of swallowed maternal blood.

Additional Evaluations

Radiologic, endoscopic, and surgical evaluations are summarized in Table 108-1. The approach depends on the bleeding acuity and the setting in which the patient is seen. In general, when the source of bleeding is unclear, the goal is to get the patient to endoscopy, in which a fiberoptic camera is inserted into the mouth (upper endoscopy) or anus (lower endoscopy) to directly visualize the intestinal lumen. Endoscopy is the gold standard given its relative safety and its ability to directly visualize the mucosa, obtain tissue for pathologic diagnosis, and potentially administer therapy. However, other diagnostic methods offer particular advantages and may be indispensable to the patient's assessment before endoscopy. Indeed, certain diagnoses, such as Meckel's diverticulum or intussusception, may permit bypassing the need for endoscopy, and when bleeding is heavy, the ability to visualize the lumen is severely hampered.

Therapeutic Interventions

Patients with significant anemia (hemoglobin <8 gm/dL), active bleeding, or symptomatic anemia should receive blood replacement with packed red blood cells at a dose of 10 to 15 mL/kg per transfusion. If coagulation abnormalities are found, they should be corrected with vitamin K, fresh-frozen plasma, or both depending on the clinical context. All patients with GI bleeding should presumptively be started on acid-suppression therapy, preferably with a proton pump inhibitor, until the patient is stable and an upper GI cause has been excluded. Additional interventions depend on the underlying cause. Endoscopy is capable of administering internal therapies, depending on the context (e.g., sclerotherapy or banding of varices, electrocautery or argon plasma coagulation for ulcers, clipping or injection for vessels). In severe bleeding, more drastic interventions such as continuous octreotide infusion or surgery may be required.

FUTURE DIRECTIONS

Capsule endoscopy and balloon enteroscopy have been exciting additions to the diagnostic arsenal, but the availability of these studies and the expertise required are limited, particularly in pediatrics. With time, these should become more widely accessible. Furthermore, radiologic techniques such as computed tomography (CT) angiography and magnetic resonance angiography or venography are becoming more refined, and CT radiation loads are gradually falling compared with the past.

SUGGESTED READINGS

AGA Institute Clinical Practice and Economics Committee: American Gastroenterological Association (AGA) Institute Technical Review on Obscure Gastrointestinal Bleeding, *Gastroenterology* 133:1697-1717, 2007.

Gold BD, Colletti RB, Abbott M, et al, North American Society for Pediatric Gastroenterology and Nutrition: *Helicobacter pylori* infection in children: recommendations for diagnosis and treatment, *J Pediatr Gastroenterol Nutr* 31(5):490-497, 2000.

Laine L, Takeuchi K, Tarnawski A: Gastric mucosal defense and cytoprotection: bench to bedside, *Gastroenterology* 135:41-60, 2008.

Intestinal Obstruction and Malrotation

Andrew Chu

109

In its most simplistic conceptualization, the gastrointestinal (GI) tract is a long, flexible tube designed for active, unidirectional flow, with its only openings to the outside world being the mouth for input and the anus for output. Any impediment to the forward progress of ingested contents results in luminal distension proximal to the obstruction and eventual vomiting or perforation. A variety of congenital and acquired defects may cause throughput failure, with clinical presentations ranging from subtle findings that go undiagnosed for years to acute clinical deterioration. The clinician's first responsibilities are to triage the severity of the obstruction and provide relief of the obstruction to prevent further complications, most notably intestinal perforation, peritonitis, sepsis, and death.

ETIOLOGY AND PATHOGENESIS

The many etiologies that cause intestinal obstruction ultimately result in a final common pathophysiologic pathway (Figure 109-1). Anything that prevents forward progress of intestinal contents sets into motion this sequence of events, leading to worsening distension, vomiting, and systemic dysfunction. Not only do the resulting dehydration and electrolyte imbalances create significant complications, bacterial proliferation within the static intestinal contents and compromised mucosal integrity set the stage for bacterial translocation across the intestinal wall, with consequent bacteremia and sepsis.

Although many disorders may cause obstruction (Figure 109-2), they can be summarized by several pathophysiologic categories that aid in constructing a rational differential diagnosis.

Extrinsic Compression

Because the bowel is a flexible organ, anything that compresses it externally can decrease the intraluminal diameter and precipitate obstruction. For example, adhesions are fibrous bands of tissue that spontaneously arise within the peritoneum in reaction to insults, such as peritonitis or abdominal surgery, and can encircle and constrict loops of bowel. They are relatively common after surgery, with up to a 25% 5-year readmission rate caused by adhesions, depending on the type of operation.

Intraabdominal masses, such as Wilms' tumor, can compress and obstruct bowel by their sheer size ("mass effect"). Annular pancreas is an anatomic variant in which a ring of pancreatic tissue encircles and can cause duodenal obstruction. Superior mesenteric artery (SMA) syndrome results from compression of the third duodenal segment by the artery against the aorta. It is sometimes seen in patients who have had precipitous weight loss with resultant loss of the mesenteric fat pad that protects the duodenum from compression; external body cast application; or after intestinal or orthopedic surgery that results in traction upon the SMA, pulling it down upon the duodenum. Another example

is closed loop obstruction (internal hernia), in which a loop of bowel passes through a mesenteric defect or similar orifice (e.g., inguinal hernia) and becomes lodged within it, resulting in occlusion of both the proximal and distal ends of the loop.

Intrinsic Decrease in Lumen Caliber

CONGENITAL DEFECTS

Children can be born with an abnormally reduced lumen caliber that leads to obstruction. For example, atresias and webs represent a spectrum of disorders potentially affecting any region of the GI tract from the esophagus to the colon. In some cases, mucosal membranes within the lumen precipitate obstruction (web). In other instances, there is total or near-total discontinuity of a segment of bowel (atresia). Hirschsprung's disease is a disorder of the rectum and colon in which absence of enteric neurons caused by defective migration during development leads to smooth muscle dysfunction in the affected regions and severe constipation.

ACQUIRED DEFECTS

Chronic bowel inflammation can, over time, lead to narrowing of the lumen. An important example is Crohn's disease, in which there is discontinuous full-thickness bowel inflammation anywhere from the mouth to the anus (see Chapter 110). Over time, inflamed areas may stricture and obstruct. Another example of this is eosinophilic esophagitis, an entity that lies within the spectrum of food allergies and atopic disease. Because of persistent eosinophilic inflammation in the presence of the offending antigen, the esophagus can eventually stricture over time, leading to dysphagia and the need for esophageal dilatation to relieve the obstruction. Malignancy, although relatively uncommon in children compared with adults, is another important cause of decreased lumen caliber. For example, the GI tract is the most common extranodal site affected in non-Hodgkin's lymphoma. Infiltration of the bowel wall by tumor leads to decreased effective luminal diameter and a higher risk of obstruction. Achalasia causes functional esophageal obstruction caused by aperistalsis and inadequate lower esophageal sphincter relaxation. An example of gastric outlet obstruction caused by decreased diameter is hypertrophic pyloric stenosis, a disease primarily affecting infants in the first few months of life in which smooth muscle hypertrophy leads to occlusion of the pylorus (Figure 109-3).

Internal Blockage

A wide variety of etiologies may be associated with internal blockage of the GI tract. Areas that are inherently narrow relative to

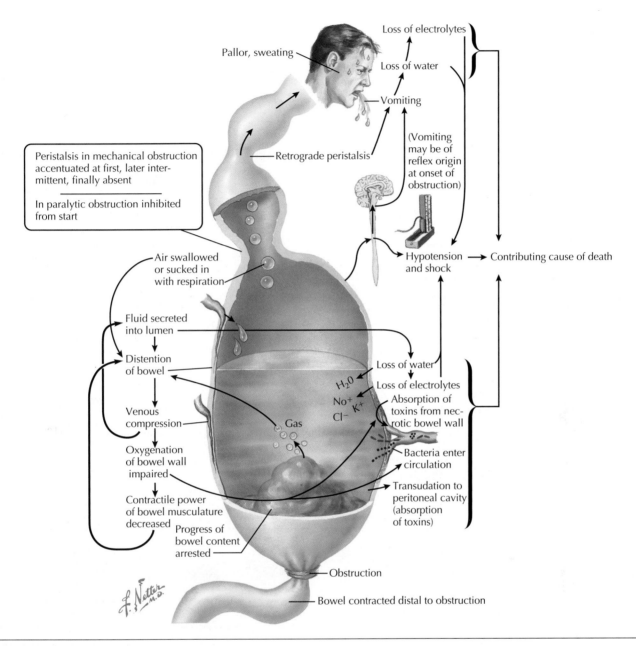

Figure 109-1 *Intestinal obstruction, adynamic ileus.*

the rest of the GI tract (upper esophageal sphincter, esophagus adjacent to the carina, lower esophageal sphincter, pylorus, ileocecal valve) are at more risk of becoming obstructed by large foreign bodies. In a special example of this, bezoars are accumulations of indigestible material (e.g., hair, fiber from vegetables) that become trapped in the GI tract (typically the stomach) and can cause obstruction when they grow large enough. Injury to the wall of the small intestine from blunt abdominal trauma, as can occur when bicycle handlebars injure a child's duodenum, may instigate a hematoma, which can obstruct the small intestine because of its small caliber.

In neonates, meconium ileus is a cause of distal GI obstruction shortly after birth. Meconium is a conglomeration of sloughed intestinal mucosa, bile salts, and other debris that

accumulates during fetal development. It is normally passed within the first day of life, but when it is exceedingly inspissated, as occurs in cystic fibrosis, patients may be unable to expel it, leading to obstructive symptoms. In young children, intussusception is an example in which the bowel obstructs itself because of telescoping of one portion of bowel into the adjacent region of bowel.

Defects in Bowel Arrangement

Malrotation is an important entity that clinicians must be aware of when evaluating intestinal obstruction of unknown etiology. Malrotation is a congenital defect typically involving both the small and large intestines that occurs when the bowel assumes

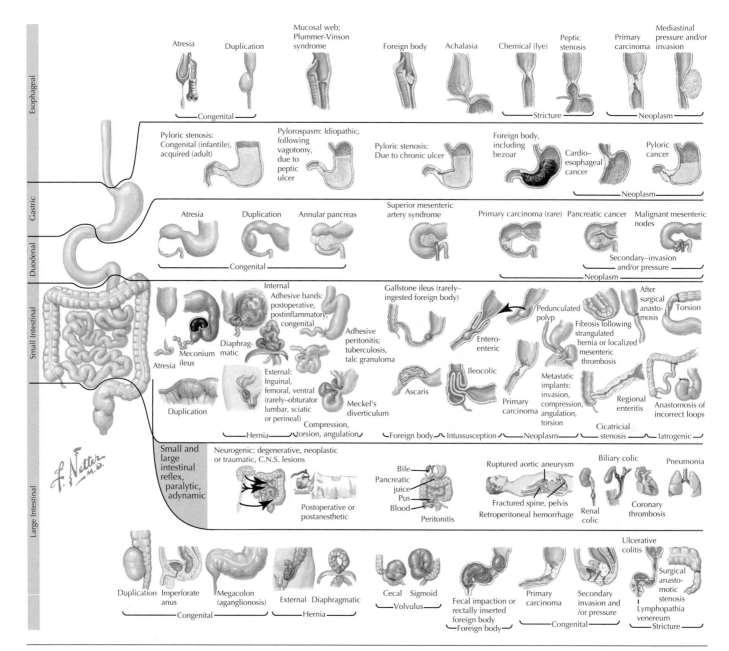

Figure 109-2 *Alimentary tract obstruction.*

an abnormal spatial arrangement within the abdomen. Intestinal development is a complex, continuous process spanning the fourth fetal week to birth that takes the primitive gut, which begins as a short, straight tube, and transforms it into a long, highly specialized organ. As part of this process, the intestinal tract, after rotating 270 degrees, becomes fixed in a specific arrangement such that the duodenum ends at the ligament of Treitz in the left upper quadrant and the cecum is found in the right lower quadrant. When this final arrangement fails to take place properly, the bowel is malrotated. Although this may not result in any clinical symptoms in mild cases, the most feared complication is volvulus, a surgical emergency in which the bowel, as a result of its inappropriate positioning and lack of usual support, twists upon its mesenteric stalk, causing not only

intestinal obstruction but also ischemia (Figure 109-4). Ladd's bands, intraperitoneal fibrous bands that can encircle and obstruct the duodenum, are also associated with malrotation.

Motility Failure

Even when there is not an occlusive obstruction of the intestine, failure of appropriate peristalsis can nonetheless create obstructive symptoms. A common example is postinfectious ileus, which is an interruption in normal intestinal motility and forward propulsion of contents without physical occlusion that most often occurs after viral gastroenteritis. It is usually mild and self-limited, but in rare instances, it can result in severe and prolonged gastroparesis, feeding intolerance, and the need for

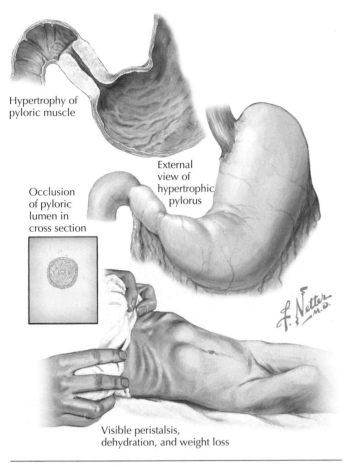

Hypertrophy of pyloric muscle

External view of hypertrophic pylorus

Occlusion of pyloric lumen in cross section

Visible peristalsis, dehydration, and weight loss

Figure 109-3 *Hypertrophic, pyloric stenosis.*

postpyloric nasogastric enteral feeding until it resolves. Intestinal surgery can cause postoperative ileus, a temporary disruption of normal motility, particularly when combined with narcotics, which have intrinsic antimotility effects.

Another important consideration is intestinal pseudoobstruction, which is a spectrum of congenital and acquired disorders involving the small or large bowel (or both) that ultimately results from failure of either the enteric nervous system or the intestinal smooth muscle to coordinate appropriate peristalsis. Examples of factors that can trigger pseudoobstruction are trauma, electrolyte abnormalities, sepsis, orthopedic and cardiovascular surgery, and pregnancy.

CLINICAL PRESENTATION

Patients with obstruction may experience a wide range of symptoms depending on the nature and severity of the etiology. The physician's primary responsibility at first contact with any patient is to triage the severity of illness and prevent the further progress of medical complications. Patients with obstruction may exhibit severe pain, abdominal distension (unless involvement is in the proximal GI tract), diaphoresis, stigmata of dehydration, and vomiting with inability to tolerate oral input. The patient may be tachycardic (both from pain and hypovolemia). The blood pressure can be difficult to interpret, with high values being most likely a response to pain; a normal blood pressure should not be taken as a necessarily reassuring sign without a measure of skepticism. Indeed, a normal value in the context of an ill-appearing, tachycardic patient may be indicative of compensated shock (see Chapter 2). Fever raises concerns for intestinal ischemia, perforation, and peritonitis.

There are many potential causes of GI obstruction (see Figure 109-2). However, because the clinical presentation of the patient is governed by the specific characteristics of the

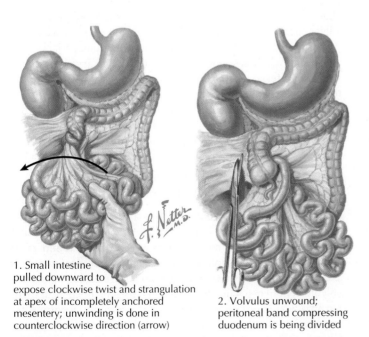

1. Small intestine pulled downward to expose clockwise twist and strangulation at apex of incompletely anchored mesentery; unwinding is done in counterclockwise direction (arrow)

2. Volvulus unwound; peritoneal band compressing duodenum is being divided

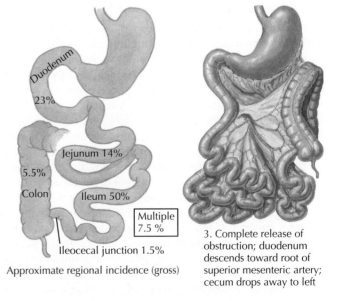

Duodenum 23%

Jejunum 14%

5.5% Colon

Ileum 50%

Multiple 7.5 %

Ileocecal junction 1.5%

Approximate regional incidence (gross)

3. Complete release of obstruction; duodenum descends toward root of superior mesenteric artery; cecum drops away to left

Figure 109-4 *Malrotation and volvulus.*

obstructive etiology, attention to the patient's particular symptom complex can yield clues helpful to constructing a rational differential diagnosis. Several key questions help to organize the approach to the patient.

What Is the Age of the Patient?

Although many etiologies cross age lines, the age of a patient can raise the level of suspicion for particular problems. The neonatal period is when many congenital disorders, such as atresias and webs, become evident. Although malrotation can present at any point in life, most are diagnosed within the first year in patients with recurrent or bilious vomiting. Meconium ileus becomes evident within the first few days of life and prompts concern for cystic fibrosis. Hypertrophic pyloric stenosis presents within the first few months of life as nonbilious "projectile" vomiting. Intussusception most often presents within the first few years of life as recurrent bouts of vomiting associated with intense pain that both completely resolve between episodes.

Is the Patient Ill Appearing?

One of the first priorities of the physician is to determine the severity of the patient's illness. Although any patient who has comorbid conditions or who has had prolonged obstruction may be ill appearing (e.g., pallor, lethargy, diaphoresis, restlessness), the ill appearance itself should prompt concern that the patient has a complication of the obstruction. In this regard, an important way of classifying an obstruction is whether it is simple or strangulated. Whereas *simple obstruction* implies preserved blood flow to the bowel in the setting of obstruction, a *strangulated obstruction* denotes an obstructive process complicated by bowel ischemia. Certain etiologies, such as volvulus and internal hernia, have a high risk of strangulation. Strangulated obstruction is an emergency that requires prompt attention and surgical evaluation.

What Is the Character of the Vomitus?

Obstruction can occur anywhere from the esophagus to the anus, with the location being an important influence on the symptom pattern that the patient experiences. If the obstruction is in the esophagus, the patient may experience dysphagia (difficulty swallowing) or outright inability to intake orally. Low-grade esophageal obstruction can hinder the swallowing of solids, and high-grade obstruction can also interfere with the ingestion of liquids, which results in drooling and frequent spitting. Gastric outlet obstruction, as in pyloric stenosis, causes nonbilious vomiting because bile is secreted by the liver into the duodenum at the ampulla of Vater beyond the point of obstruction.

Small bowel obstruction leads to abdominal distension, cramping discomfort in the middle or upper abdomen, and repeated episodes of bilious vomiting. Symptoms often have a rapid onset after the obstructive process has begun. If there is total obstruction, patients eventually become obstipated (i.e., cease to pass stool). Fluid and electrolyte disturbances are relatively common. Abdominal pain raises concerns for bowel ischemia. Large bowel obstruction, on the other hand, tends to have symptoms that are milder and slower in onset compared with small bowel obstruction. Vomiting does not invariably occur,

although the bowel does become distended. Patients may have lower abdominal cramping. On rectal examination, if the obstruction is high in the colon, the rectum will be devoid of stool, but hard stool in the rectum may be present if the patient has fecal impaction. Explosive stooling may be precipitated by rectal examination in a patient with Hirschsprung's disease. Fluid and electrolyte disturbances do not tend to develop as precipitously as in small bowel obstruction.

Are the Symptoms Constant or Intermittent?

Partial obstruction occurs when the effective intraluminal diameter through which intestinal contents may pass is narrowed to the point of reducing, but not eliminating, flow. In these cases, patients may experience waxing and waning symptoms, and older patients who have repeated episodes of partial small bowel obstruction, such as those with a Crohn's disease–associated stricture, may even adapt themselves by limiting oral intake at the moment they detect characteristic symptoms. *Complete obstruction* results from a total inability of the bowel to propel its load forward past the blockage point. When such a process has begun, symptoms typically continue until the patient has been mechanically decompressed and the obstruction has been relieved.

Has the Patient Had a Chronic History of Severe Reflux or Abdominal Pain?

If a patient has had a long-standing history of severe reflux or abdominal pain, it raises suspicion for malrotation, as well as mild forms of other congenital anomalies such as webs.

Has the Patient Had Previous Abdominal Surgery (or other Peritoneal Insults)?

In any patient with obstructive symptoms who has had previous abdominal surgery, the clinician should suspect the presence of adhesions. Such concern should also arise in patients who have had other forms of peritoneal injury. For example, patients with advanced liver disease and associated ascites are at risk for spontaneous bacterial peritonitis. Repeated episodes may lead to the formation of adhesions. In patients who have had peritoneal dialysis for renal failure, there have been rare cases of a disorder called sclerosing encapsulating peritonitis in which the entire bowel becomes progressively encased in fibrotic tissue.

Does the Child Have Other Historical or Physical Examination Abnormalities?

The presence of other abnormalities may raise suspicion for particular etiologies. Trisomy 21 is one of many congenital disorders that can be associated with intestinal atresia and other anomalies such as malrotation (see Chapter 117). Heterotaxy is associated with malrotation, which can lead to Ladd's bands and volvulus. Patients who have recently had Henoch-Schönlein purpura, an acquired form of vasculitis, are at risk for intussusception, as are those with polyps and duplication cysts (see Chapter 28). Crohn's disease is a common cause of intestinal stenosis (see Chapter 110).

EVALUATION AND MANAGEMENT

Initial Care in the Emergency Department

Patients reporting symptoms concerning for obstruction should be directed to emergency care. The goal of the initial evaluation in the emergency department is to determine the acuity and severity of the child's illness. The clinician should rapidly obtain a general sense of the patient's predicament through the general appearance, ascertaining clinical signs such as lethargy, diaphoresis, pallor, and restlessness. The first pass on physical examination should quickly acquire information regarding the patient's critical features, beginning with the ABCs (airway, breathing, and circulation). Vital signs should be evaluated for fever (in the setting of obstruction, concerning for ischemia), tachycardia, hypotension (worrisome for decompensated shock), and low-normal blood pressure with widened pulse pressure (concerning for compensated shock). On the second pass, the clinician should perform a thorough but expedient head-to-toe examination that includes assessments of mental status, level of dehydration, signs of trauma, and stigmata of disease. The abdominal examination must assess for distension (and whether it is caused by gas or fluid), bowel sounds (early obstruction results in hyperactive sounds, but ischemic bowel will be silent), the presence of masses, and the presence and location of pain. If peritoneal signs are present (involuntary guarding, rebound tenderness to palpation, exquisite sensitivity to movement), there should be immediate concern for perforation. In addition, the assessment should include a rectal examination to check stool for the presence of blood via stool guaiac testing and to screen for low-lying pathologies such as distal intussusception, Hirschsprung's disease, fecal impaction, and pelvic masses.

After the patient's status has been determined, initial interventions should be initiated without delay while the workup continues. Patients with vomiting should receive nothing by mouth (NPO) and should have an intravenous (IV) line started for maintenance fluids. If there are signs of dehydration, isotonic fluid boluses are appropriate until the patient is hemodynamically stable. Patients with repeated emesis should also receive a nasogastric tube using a sump-type catheter (which is more rigid, larger in caliber, and less likely to collapse than a feeding tube), which can then be placed on low intermittent suction. If the sump aspirates large volumes, it is important to replace those losses via IV fluid administration. Indeed, without decompression, even when a patient is NPO, vomiting may continue because of the significant volume of fluid that the GI tract produces in the form of secretions. If the patient is ill appearing or has fever in the context of suspected obstruction, the physician should strongly consider initiating IV antibiotic therapy with adequate coverage for common gut flora (gram-negative and anaerobic organisms) after obtaining a blood culture. Early in this process, the team should contact a surgeon to evaluate the need for operative intervention. If patients are determined in the course of their workup to have partial small bowel obstruction, they may be admitted for observation and continued decompression before further evaluation and management. Those with complete obstruction or other complications, such as ischemia and perforation, require surgical management.

It is essential to keep in mind that many illnesses can initially present with a constellation of signs and symptoms resembling obstruction. This can make the assessment of the vomiting child challenging. On the more benign end of the spectrum, viral gastroenteritis is an example of a disorder that can cause repeated vomiting. What distinguishes this from obstruction is that there is typically a history of ill contact, the vomiting is nonbilious (or perhaps "highlighter" green after repeated vomiting episodes, as opposed to the "spinach green" color of truly bilious emesis in obstructed patients), diarrhea is present, and the patient's abdomen is not distended. *On the other end of the spectrum are several pitfalls that are important for the physician not to miss*:

- *Intracranial lesions*: Although malignancy is generally rare in children, it is critical not to miss brain tumors, which can present with recurrent emesis (see Chapter 57). Distinguishing characteristics may include a concurrent history of neurologic symptoms (e.g., headaches, vision changes, or loss of motor coordination) or changes in other psychological parameters (e.g., loss of milestones or changes in speech). The vomiting typically occurs without abdominal pain or even nausea, and other signs of obstruction such as distension should also be absent. The physical examination should include a funduscopic examination and neurologic assessment. If there is clinical concern, the team should obtain intracranial imaging (typically computed tomography [CT] in the emergency setting because of its short scan time, although magnetic resonance imaging may eventually be required because of its higher resolution and superiority in detecting posterior fossa lesions).
- *Other medical illness*: A variety of medical conditions, including hypoglycemia, diabetic ketoacidosis, hypokalemia, and certain drug ingestions, can cause ill appearance and repeated vomiting. A number of metabolic diseases, such as fatty acid oxidation disorders and urea cycle defects, can create multiple disturbances that lead to this clinical picture as well. Obstruction of the urinary tract by renal stones can create abdominal pain and recurrent vomiting that mimics intestinal obstruction. Pancreatitis causes epigastric pain and vomiting, particularly with food intake.
- *Pregnancy*: Postmenarchal women who are pregnant may have a palpable uterus, along with vomiting that is caused by morning sickness or hyperemesis gravidarum.
- *Abuse*: In children, the physical examination must always screen for signs of abuse. Intracranial hemorrhage from a strike to the head can produce symptoms mimicking obstruction, as discussed above. Blunt abdominal trauma may result in a duodenal hematoma, leading to obstruction. In Munchausen's syndrome by proxy, a caretaker may secretly be making his or her young child ill via ingestions or other methods.

Using the clinical questions presented in the previous section, the clinician can begin to localize and characterize the nature of the symptoms to construct a differential diagnosis based on data that addresses those questions.

Laboratory Tests

Although clinical suspicion should ultimately determine the full set of laboratory tests ordered, initial laboratory studies should generally include a complete chemistry panel (with blood urea nitrogen and creatinine), glucose, hepatic function panel (to screen for metabolic abnormalities), amylase and lipase (to screen for pancreatic involvement, although an isolated amylase elevation could be attributable to bowel injury from ischemia), complete blood count (to ensure tachycardia is not attributable to anemia and to assess for leukocytosis), and urinalysis (to check for evidence of urinary tract infection or hematuria as evidence of stones). If there is concern for drug ingestion, appropriate drug testing should be considered. In postmenarchal women, pregnancy testing should be included. If the patient is ill appearing and has a fever, a blood culture should be done before administration of antibiotics. In a deteriorating patient, blood gas measurement may also be helpful in determining whether there is a metabolic acidosis, which would heighten concern for bowel ischemia.

Radiologic Tests

All patients with signs consistent with obstruction should have initial flat and upright abdominal radiographs to assess the bowel gas pattern and to screen for other pathologies, such as intraabdominal free air, foreign bodies, volvulus, and masses. Air-fluid levels denote stasis of intraluminal contents, either from obstruction or ileus. Obstruction is generally associated with significant proximal intestinal distension, either with fluid or air, and the portions of bowel that are distended may help locate the obstruction. For example, an image that shows gas in the stomach but not in any distal regions suggests gastric outlet obstruction or, less likely, gastric volvulus. The "double-bubble" sign, in which air is seen both in the stomach and in the proximal duodenum but not distally, is suggestive of duodenal atresia.

Real-time fluoroscopic contrast studies greatly enhance the radiologic ability to discern anatomic features of the bowel and thus are of considerable value in determining the region of obstruction in stable patients. Furthermore, fluoroscopy provides dynamic information about the function of the bowel. Historically, the contrast agent has been barium, but in the setting of evaluating obstruction, it is more appropriate to use a water-soluble contrast agent. This is because barium that extravasates into the peritoneum through a perforation can create severe peritonitis, and stagnant barium that becomes trapped at the obstruction will solidify over time, potentially creating further complications. When a patient is medically unstable, fluoroscopic contrast studies are inadvisable given that they involve introduction of a foreign substance into the GI tract, and they do not provide enough information about extraintestinal pathology that may be contributing to the clinical picture.

If the individual has primarily esophageal symptoms, an esophagram can delineate the site and nature of defect, as well as evaluate esophageal function (see Chapter 107). In a stable patient with small bowel obstructive symptoms, the study of choice is the upper GI series, in which the contrast is followed to the ligament of Treitz. This study assesses for malrotation or volvulus in addition to a host of other anatomic defects. It is essential that any child younger than 1 year of age with bilious vomiting must be assessed for malrotation and volvulus. A variant on the upper GI series is the upper GI with small bowel follow-through, in which the radiologist assesses the bowel to the terminal ileum. This study is inappropriate for the acute setting given the length of time required to perform the study and the need to use barium, which is required because endogenous secretions dilute water-soluble contrast as it passes through the GI tract, making it ineffective for delineating the distal small bowel. However, this is a valuable tool when the suspicion is that a defect beyond the ligament of Treitz may be causing partial small bowel obstruction.

In limited settings, contrast enemas help to delineate causes of colonic obstruction. For example, the unprepped barium enema is an essential tool in the workup of Hirschsprung's disease. In the rare case of colonic tumors (a far more common problem in adults), it is also helpful. It is unnecessary in the evaluation of fecal impaction, which can be diagnosed by clinical assessment. A special case is the air-contrast enema study, which is used in the setting of suspected intussusception. In this situation, air is the contrast agent used to diagnose the area involved. After the radiologist identifies the intussusception, this modality becomes useful as a therapeutic tool because the air then serves as a means to reduce the intussusception.

In patients who are medically unstable, who have a history of trauma, or who have a suspected perforation, the study of choice is the CT scan because of its rapid throughput and ability to provide the clinical team with large amounts of information about the intestinal anatomy as well as extraintestinal pathologies. The drawback to CT is its radiation burden, which is equal to many plain radiographs and is at least twice that of an upper GI series with small bowel follow-through. However, this consideration is outweighed by its benefits in the acute setting, and newer pediatric protocols have reduced the radiation load significantly.

In limited situations, ultrasound is a useful tool when specific etiologies are suspected. For example, it is widely used in the assessment of pyloric stenosis and intussusception. Because it does not create a radiation burden, it is also finding use at some centers in the form of small bowel evaluation of strictures that may cause partial small bowel obstruction, as can occur in Crohn's disease.

Additional Evaluation

Although it is not indicated in the acute setting, GI endoscopy is a useful tool for diagnosing mucosal disorders that may not be obvious on radiologic imaging, and it offers the advantage of allowing therapeutic intervention in some cases. Endoscopy involves a gastroenterologist inserting an endoscope into either the mouth or anus, depending on the region of interest. The instrument allows direct visualization of the mucosa and provides the ability to sample the tissue for histologic diagnosis. For example, an older patient who has had a long-standing history of intermittent abdominal pain and poor weight gain and is found to have small bowel strictures causing partial small bowel obstruction could have Crohn's disease, which requires mucosal biopsies for definitive diagnosis. In progressive esophageal strictures, eosinophilic esophagitis is an important consideration; this also requires histologic diagnosis from biopsies.

Surgical evaluation is critical at all stages of the assessment of children with obstruction. After enough clinical information is available to determine whether the child should go to the operating room, the surgical team will proceed with exploratory laparotomy or, at some centers, laparoscopy. Although the most invasive of all diagnostic modalities, it provides definitive diagnosis of the obstruction, and it is lifesaving and absolutely indicated in patients with complete obstruction and who have evidence of bowel ischemia or perforation.

FUTURE DIRECTIONS

Refinements in CT protocols show promise in further reducing the radiation loads. In addition, with the proliferation of surgeons who are trained in laparoscopic techniques, some centers are finding laparoscopy to be a reasonable initial intervention in

obstructed patients that offers good outcomes in most situations with reduced lengths of stay and morbidity compared with open laparotomy.

SUGGESTED READINGS

Applegate KE, Anderson JM, Klatte EC: Intestinal malrotation in children: a problem-solving approach to the upper gastrointestinal series, *Radiographics* 26:1485-1500, 2006.

Grant HW, Parker MC, Wilson MS, et al: Adhesions after abdominal surgery in children, *J Pediatr Surg* 43:152-157, 2008.

Zerey M, Sechrist CW, Kercher KW, et al: The laparoscopic management of small-bowel obstruction, *Am J Surg* 194:882-888, 2007.

Inflammatory Bowel Disease

Jessica Wen and Rose C. Graham

110

*I*nflammatory bowel disease (IBD) is an idiopathic, likely immune-mediated, inflammatory disease involving the gastrointestinal (GI) tract. There are two subtypes, ulcerative colitis (UC) and Crohn's disease. In the pediatric population, Crohn's disease is more common than UC, with the majority of children diagnosed in adolescence, although some are much younger. Worldwide, the incidence of IBD is higher in developed countries than developing countries. Persons living in urban areas have increased rates of IBD compared with persons living in rural areas. Currently, there is no cure for IBD, and the goal of therapy in the pediatric population is maintenance of long-term remission and normal growth and nutritional status.

ETIOLOGY AND PATHOGENESIS

The etiology of IBD remains elusive and is thought to be multifactorial with probable contributions from genetics and the environment. There is a high incidence of disease among first-degree relatives. Genetic linkage analysis reveals multiple susceptibility loci. The *IBD1* locus contains the *NOD2/CARD15* gene, which is normally involved in NF-κB activation in response to bacterial polysaccharides. The effects of mutations in this pathway suggest that IBD may result from defective immune tolerance to luminal bacteria, a process mediated by proinflammatory cytokines including tumor necrosis factor-α (TNF-α), interleukin-1 (IL-1), IL-6, interferon-γ, and IL-23.

The role of infectious agents in IBD pathogenesis is unclear. Atypical mycobacteria, *Escherichia coli*, *Listeria* spp., *Streptococcus* spp., and measles have all been suspected as antigenic stimuli, although none is proven. Clinically, IBD patients with intercurrent enteric bacterial or viral infection often experience an exacerbation of their disease.

CLINICAL PRESENTATION

The differential diagnosis for IBD is extensive and largely depends on the presenting symptoms (Table 110-1).

Ulcerative Colitis

Ulcerative colitis (UC) is characterized by diffuse colonic mucosal inflammation that begins at the anal verge and extends proximally to a variable extent. The disease is limited to the colon, although distal ileal involvement ("backwash ileitis") may occur. The most common symptoms are rectal bleeding, diarrhea, abdominal pain, urgency to defecate, and tenesmus. The majority of children with UC present with mild to moderate disease and a lack of systemic symptoms of fever, weight loss, or growth failure, although these may occur. Some patients may present with severe hemorrhage, toxic megacolon, or perforation. In addition, some patients may present with extraintestinal

manifestations, such as arthropathy, skin findings, or liver disease.

On physical examination, children with mild to moderate UC often have mild lower abdominal tenderness. Stools may have streaks of blood or be occult blood positive. About 10% to 15% of children with UC present with fulminant colitis, which may include severe cramping, abdominal pain, fever, frequent diarrhea, rectal bleeding, abdominal distension, orthostatic hypotension, and tachycardia. Toxic megacolon is a true emergency and may require surgical intervention.

Crohn's Disease

Crohn's disease is characterized by transmural inflammation that may involve any segment of the intestinal tract from the mouth to the anus. Disease presentation is primarily determined by the location and extent of involvement. In children, the most common presenting distribution is ileocolonic disease (Figure 110-1) followed by small bowel disease alone and then colonic disease alone. Gastroduodenal disease is found in 30% of children with Crohn's disease. Patients with ileocecal disease often present with right lower quadrant abdominal pain and diarrhea. In such patients, loops of bowel or fullness may be palpable in the right lower quadrant. Bloody stool is more common in colonic disease. Epigastric pain may occur with gastroduodenal disease. Dysphagia can be seen with esophageal involvement. Many children with Crohn's disease have diarrhea, nocturnal defecation, low-grade intermittent fever, oral ulcers, weight loss, and decelerated growth velocity.

Crohn's disease is categorized into three subtypes: inflammatory, stricturing, and fistulizing. Inflammatory disease is that described above. Stricturing disease involves luminal narrowing, which may be accompanied by prestenotic dilatation or signs of intestinal obstruction. This most commonly occurs in the small bowel but may involve the colon. Perianal or perirectal fistulae and abscesses or intraabdominal fistulae, phlegmon, or abscesses characterize fistulizing disease (Figure 110-2).

Extraintestinal Manifestations

About a third of patients with IBD also have extraintestinal manifestations involving rheumatologic, cutaneous, ocular, vascular, hepatobiliary, renal, and skeletal systems (Figure 110-3). Arthralgia and arthritis are the most common extraintestinal symptoms and may involve both axial and peripheral joints. Joint manifestations may precede GI tract disease, so IBD should be in the differential diagnosis of isolated arthralgia or arthritis. Juvenile rheumatoid arthritis and ankylosing spondylitis are associated with IBD.

Skin manifestations of IBD are common in the pediatric population and include erythema nodosum and pyoderma

Table 110-1 Differential Diagnosis of Inflammatory Bowel Disease

Abdominal Pain	Diarrhea	Hematochezia	Abdominal Obstruction	Growth Failure or Weight Loss
Functional abdominal pain	Infection-bacterial, parasitic, protozoan, *Clostridium difficile*	Polyp	Lymphoma	Endocrinopathy
Constipation	Carbohydrate intolerance	Meckel's diverticulum	Intussusception	Anorexia
Irritable bowel syndrome	Celiac disease	Intestinal AV malformation	Volvulus	Constitutional growth delay
GERD	Laxative abuse	Anal fissure	Postsurgical adhesions	Parasitic infection
Appendicitis	Allergic colitis	Hemorrhoids		Neoplasms
Ischemic colitis	Immune deficiency-CGD, CVID	Infections		
Ovarian cyst		Solitary rectal ulcer		
Mesenteric lymphadenitis				
Pelvic inflammatory disorder				
Vasculitis				

AV, arteriovenous; CGD, chronic granulomatous disease; CVID, common variable immune deficiency; GERD, gastroesophageal reflux disease.

gangrenosum. Red, raised, tender nodules located along the anterior shins characterize erythema nodosum. Its course correlates with the severity of GI tract inflammation. Deep necrotic ulcers (often on the legs) characterize pyoderma gangrenosum, with a course that is not related to intestinal disease.

The most common hepatobiliary diseases associated with IBD are primary sclerosing cholangitis and autoimmune

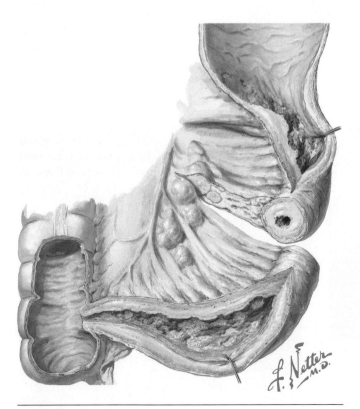

Figure 110-1 *Ileocolonic Crohn's disease.*

hepatitis. Primary sclerosing cholangitis is more commonly associated with UC but can also be found in patients with Crohn's disease. Its activity is not associated with intestinal disease activity, and its onset may occur years before or after IBD diagnosis. Other associated hepatobiliary disorders include hepatic abscess, hepatic granuloma, cholelithiasis, and cholecystitis. Cholelithiasis in IBD is caused by terminal ileal inflammation or resection, which leads to interrupted enterohepatic circulation of bile acids, causing lithogenic bile. Patients with ileal disease also have increased risk of kidney stones because of malabsorption of fat, which binds calcium and leaves oxalate to be absorbed and excreted in the urine.

Ocular findings associated with IBD include episcleritis, uveitis, and iritis. They are more common in Crohn's disease patients compared with those with UC. Uveitis may be asymptomatic, so patients should have routine ophthalmologic examinations.

There is an increased incidence of thromboembolic disease in both Crohn's disease and UC patients compared with the general population. This hypercoagulable state is likely attributable to chronic inflammation and may result in deep venous thrombosis, pulmonary embolism, and cerebrovascular disease.

IBD-associated osteopenia is multifactorial with contributions from malabsorption, malnutrition, inadequate calcium and vitamin D intake, chronic steroid use, inactivity, and chronic inflammation.

EVALUATION AND MANAGEMENT

A thorough history, including family history, is very important in the evaluation process. Review of potential extraintestinal symptoms should be carefully conducted. Review of the growth chart may reveal subtle growth failure. A careful physical examination may reveal fullness in the right lower quadrant, skin findings, clubbing, or stomatitis. Inspection of the perianal area and perineum for skin tags and fistulae and a digital rectal examination with stool guaiac are necessary.

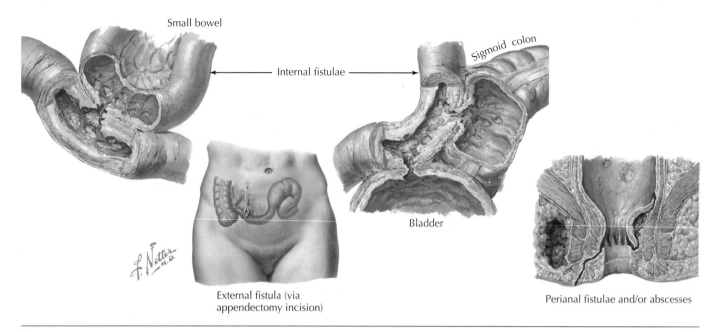

Small bowel

Internal fistulae

Sigmoid colon

Bladder

External fistula (via appendectomy incision)

Perianal fistulae and/or abscesses

Figure 110-2 *Types of fistulae in Crohn's disease.*

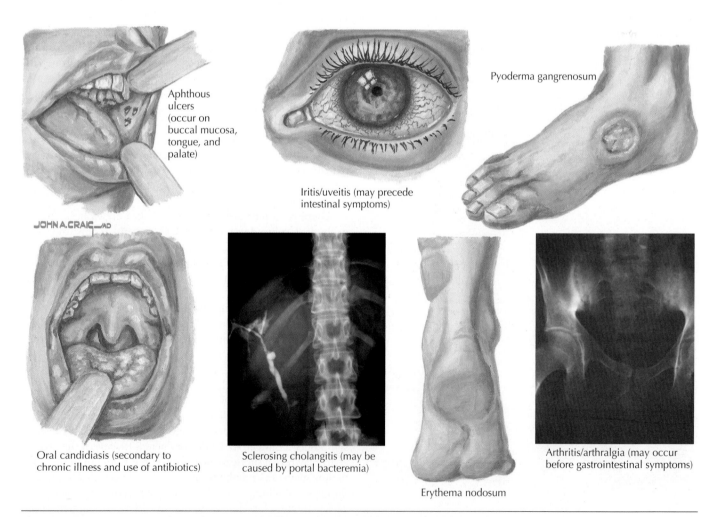

Aphthous ulcers (occur on buccal mucosa, tongue, and palate)

Iritis/uveitis (may precede intestinal symptoms)

Pyoderma gangrenosum

Oral candidiasis (secondary to chronic illness and use of antibiotics)

Sclerosing cholangitis (may be caused by portal bacteremia)

Erythema nodosum

Arthritis/arthralgia (may occur before gastrointestinal symptoms)

Figure 110-3 *Extraintestinal manifestations of inflammatory bowel disease.*

Stool studies for bacterial pathogens, parasites, *Clostridium difficile*, *Cryptosporidium* spp., and *Giardia* spp. are indicated to differentiate infectious diarrhea from IBD. In addition, patients with IBD have an increased incidence of *C. difficile* infection. On routine laboratory studies, patients may have anemia, elevated erythrocyte sedimentation rate, elevated C-reactive protein, hypoalbuminemia, and thrombocytosis. If toxic megacolon is present, studies may demonstrate leukocytosis with bandemia. Anti-neutrophil cytoplasmic antibody (pANCA) and anti–*Saccharomyces cerevisiae* antibody (ASCA) have low positive and negative predictive values and thus are of limited use in diagnosing IBD.

The most important diagnostic tests for IBD are upper endoscopy and colonoscopy. Findings of erythema, aphthous ulcers, cobblestone appearance, pseudopolyps, and mucosal friability are all consistent with IBD (Figure 110-4). In UC, there will be signs of inflammation starting in the rectum, extending proximally in a continuous fashion. In Crohn's disease, rectal sparing and skip lesions are often noted. Microscopically, inflammatory infiltrates with crypt distortion and crypt abscesses consistent with chronic active inflammation are diagnostic for IBD. Occasionally, granulomas, which are consistent with Crohn's disease and not with UC, may be noted.

In addition to upper endoscopy and colonoscopy, an upper GI series with small bowel follow-through is routinely used to evaluate for small bowel disease. In Crohn's disease, there may be nodularity and thickened bowel loops in the terminal ileum. Occasionally, fistulous tracts and luminal narrowing can be seen. Computed tomography is often used in the emergency department to evaluate patients presenting with severe abdominal pain for a surgical abdomen, such as acute appendicitis (see Chapter 5). This may reveal thickened bowel loops, fistulous tracts, and intraabdominal abscesses in patients with IBD. Abdominal ultrasound may reveal thickening or vascular congestion within the bowel wall or intraabdominal abscess, raising suspicion for

IBD. Magnetic resonance imaging is especially valuable in the context of perirectal disease and may help delineate the extent of perirectal fistulae and abscesses.

Recently, wireless capsule endoscopy, in which a pill capsule containing a camera is swallowed by the patient, has become widely available and may be useful to visually assess for small bowel ulcers in patients suspected of Crohn's disease when conventional studies have been unrevealing. It is crucial that the small intestine is already known to be patent (most often by using small bowel follow-through imaging) before the patient undergoes a capsule study. This large capsule is typically swallowed but can be placed endoscopically into the stomach or duodenum in a patient who cannot swallow it. The capsule study does not allow for tissue pathology because biopsies are not possible.

Treatment

Medical management of Crohn's disease and UC are very similar with subtle differences. The aminosalicylates, including sulfasalazine and mesalamine, are frequently used in mild to moderate IBD and act locally in the GI tract with limited systemic absorption. They function by inhibiting the cyclooxygenase and lipoxygenase pathways of arachidonic acid metabolism, which alters mucosal prostaglandin production. The various preparations differ in their locations of action based on their release mechanism. In addition to the oral form, a rectal suppository and retention enema can be useful in distal colonic disease. The main side effects are headache, nausea, vomiting, diarrhea, abdominal pain, and rash. Less common side effects include hepatotoxicity, pancreatitis, nephritis, and pericarditis.

Systemic corticosteroids are typically effective in symptom control in all distributions of IBD and remain the mainstay of therapy for acute exacerbations. Oral prednisone is usually initiated at 1 to 2 mg/kg/d, with a maximum dose of 60 mg/d. Corticosteroid dependence, defined as recurrent symptoms

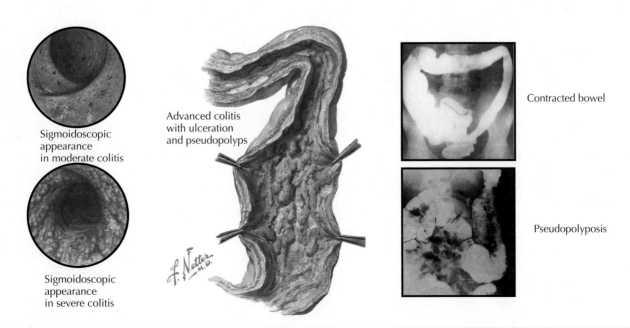

Sigmoidoscopic appearance in moderate colitis

Sigmoidoscopic appearance in severe colitis

Advanced colitis with ulceration and pseudopolyps

Contracted bowel

Pseudopolyposis

Figure 110-4 *Findings typical of ulcerative colitis on colonoscopy and fluoroscopy study.*

when the dose is gradually tapered, is a common occurrence and may require an increased dose or additional therapy with immunomodulators (see below). Corticosteroid resistance may occur over time and together with the many side effects of corticosteroids make them inappropriate for long-term therapy.

Budesonide is a synthetic steroid that has extensive first-pass hepatic metabolism, resulting in fewer side effects and less adrenal suppression than prednisone. Entocort EC, budesonide formulated to release in the terminal ileum, is sometimes used in patients with terminal ileal or cecal disease for short-term therapy, typically less than 3 months.

Antibiotic therapy is sometimes used to treat complications of Crohn's disease, such as *C. difficile* infection and perianal fistulae. It may also be used as part of a maintenance regimen. The most common antibiotics in IBD are metronidazole and ciprofloxacin, used separately or in combination. Side effects with long-term use include peripheral neuropathy associated with metronidazole and potential cartilage damage with ciprofloxacin.

There are several different classes of immunomodulators used to treat moderate to severe IBD. Six-mercaptopurine (6-MP) and its prodrug, azathioprine, are some of the most commonly used drugs in IBD. In active disease, these are often used in conjunction with corticosteroids to induce remission. They may be used as monotherapy for maintenance after the disease is in remission. The side effects of these medications include leucopenia, thrombocytopenia, hepatitis, infection, pancreatitis, and allergic reaction. There have also been cases of malignancy reported in patients taking these medications. 6-MP is metabolized by the enzyme thiopurine methyltransferase (TPMT), and the TPMT phenotype is commonly tested before initiating therapy. After therapy is initiated, patients should be monitored closely for

toxicity. Furthermore, the therapeutic effect and its potential for toxicity can be measured with 6-MP metabolite levels.

Methotrexate is another class of immunomodulator that may be used long term to maintain remission. Limited data are available on the use of methotrexate in the pediatric IBD population. It can be given by the oral or subcutaneous route, although the oral form may have less bioavailability when there is small bowel inflammation and poor absorption. Common side effects include nausea, vomiting, diarrhea, alopecia, headache, hepatotoxicity, bone marrow suppression, and allergic reactions. Folic acid supplementation should be given concurrently to minimize side effects.

Infliximab is a humanized, chimeric, monoclonal anti–TNF-α antibody used to treat severe and fistulizing IBD. It is given as an infusion of 5 mg/kg at 0, 2, and 6 weeks for induction therapy and subsequently given approximately every 8 weeks. The dose can be increased to 10 mg/kg if needed. In the past, this medication was reserved for patients who failed immunomodulators in combination with corticosteroids. However, more recently, it has been used as first-line therapy in conjunction with corticosteroids for patients presenting with moderate to severe disease. Studies are underway to assess these different approaches in the use of biologic therapy. Adalimumab is a closely related, fully humanized, monoclonal anti–TNF-α antibody that is given as a subcutaneous injection every 2 weeks. It is often used in patients who have had an allergic reaction to infliximab. Both of these medications have side effects that include opportunistic infections, serum sickness, and rare cases of malignancy. Furthermore, infusion reaction may occur with infliximab, necessitating premedication with corticosteroids and diphenhydramine.

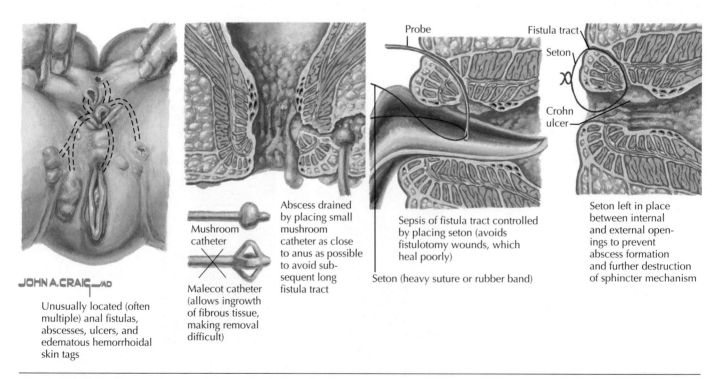

JOHN A. CRAIG—AD

Unusually located (often multiple) anal fistulas, abscesses, ulcers, and edematous hemorrhoidal skin tags

Mushroom catheter

Malecot catheter (allows ingrowth of fibrous tissue, making removal difficult)

Abscess drained by placing small mushroom catheter as close to anus as possible to avoid subsequent long fistula tract

Sepsis of fistula tract controlled by placing seton (avoids fistulotomy wounds, which heal poorly)

Seton (heavy suture or rubber band)

Probe

Fistula tract

Seton

Crohn ulcer

Seton left in place between internal and external openings to prevent abscess formation and further destruction of sphincter mechanism

Figure 110-5 *Treatment of perianal disease in Crohn's disease.*

Nutritional therapy is an important part of medical management in patients with IBD with malnutrition. In children with growth failure and predominant small bowel Crohn's disease, exclusive enteral nutrition therapy with special formulas can help patients achieve remission and decrease corticosteroid use. Formulas are best tolerated by nasogastric tube because most formulas are not very palatable. Bowel rest with total parenteral nutrition (TPN) may sometimes be required in patients with severe, steroid-refractory disease. However, it carries significant risks such as central venous line infection and TPN-associated liver disease.

Surgical therapy in IBD may be indicated when medical therapy fails. Surgical therapies are targeted toward the symptoms and may include small bowel resection, colectomy, abscess drainage, and seton placement in the case of perianal abscess (Figure 110-5). Indications for surgery include bowel stricture or obstruction, uncontrollable GI bleeding, intraabdominal abscess, perianal abscess, and fistula(e). Although surgical colectomy for UC is curative and eliminates the risk for future malignancy, surgery for Crohn's disease often results in temporary relief of symptoms, and disease frequently recurs. Therefore, bowel resections should be considered carefully in Crohn's disease patients. In addition, patients with indeterminate colitis or young patients with presumed UC require thorough repeat evaluations, including esophagogastroduodenoscopy, colonoscopy, and small bowel imaging before colectomy.

FUTURE DIRECTIONS

There is currently much research effort put into expanding the therapeutic repertoire for medical management of IBD. Effectiveness of other types of immunomodulators, such as granulocyte-macrophage colony-stimulating factor (GM-CSF) and other biologic therapies, are undergoing clinical trials. Furthermore, alternative therapies such as probiotics and omega-3 fatty acids are being studied. There is also great interest in the genetic factors of IBD and how they may affect aggressiveness of disease as well as response to certain therapies. The future of IBD therapy may become much more individualized as genetic factors and their implications are better understood.

SUGGESTED READINGS

Bousvaros A, Sylvester F, Kugathasan S, et al, Challenges in Pediatric IBD Study Groups: Challenges in pediatric inflammatory bowel disease, *Inflamm Bowel Dis* 12(9):885-913, 2006.

Escher JC, Taminiau JA, Nieuwenhuis EE, et al: Treatment of inflammatory bowel disease in childhood: best available evidence, *Inflamm Bowel Dis* 9:34-58, 2003.

Kleinman RE, Baldassano RN, Caplan A, et al; North American Society for Pediatric Gastroenterology, Hepatology and Nutrition: Nutrition support for pediatric patients with inflammatory bowel disease: a clinical report of the North American Society for Pediatric Gastroenterology, Hepatology and Nutrition, *J Pediatr Gastroenterol Nutr* 39(1):15-27, 2004.

Diarrhea

111

Anna Hunter and Rose C. Graham

*A*cute diarrhea accounts for more than 1.5 million outpatient visits, 200,000 hospitalizations, and approximately 300 deaths annually among children in the United States. It is estimated that diarrhea admissions in the United States cost $1 billion per year. In developing countries, diarrhea is a common cause of mortality among children younger than 5 years of age, with approximately 2 million deaths annually.

PATHOPHYSIOLOGY

A total of 8 to 9 L of fluid enters the healthy intestines on a daily basis. Only 1 to 2 L are derived from food and liquid intake; the rest is from salivary, gastric, pancreatic, biliary, and intestinal secretions. Each day, about 90% of this fluid is absorbed in the small intestine, 1 L enters the colon, and about 100 mL is excreted in stool. Normal stool output is approximately 100 to 200 g/d. Diarrhea is defined as stool output greater than 200 g/d in children older than 2 years of age and greater than 10 mL/kg/d in children younger than 2 years of age. It is also described more practically as an increase in liquidity and frequency of bowel movements. Diarrhea can be categorized by duration, as either *acute* (≤2 weeks) or *chronic* (>2 weeks), or by mechanism, as *osmotic* or *secretory*. It can also be categorized by the presence or absence of malabsorption (Figure 111-1).

Both secretory and osmotic diarrhea are caused by defective or impaired mucosal absorption. In osmotic diarrhea, excess amounts of nonabsorbed substances, such as lactose, lactulose, fructose, or sorbitol, remain in the intestinal lumen, causing luminal water retention. After these luminal substances enter the colon, they are processed by colonic flora, producing large amounts of organic acids, increased flatulence, and faster transit. The fecal osmolar gap [290 mOsm/L − {2 × (measured stool sodium + measured stool potassium)}] is usually greater than 50 mOsm/L in the setting of osmotic diarrhea. When an abnormal gap is found, reducing substances, stool pH, and fecal fat should be measured. Osmotic diarrhea improves with fasting. Examples of osmotic diarrhea include lactase deficiency, celiac disease, and short bowel syndrome. Secretory diarrhea is the result of abnormal ion transport in epithelial cells, leading to decreased absorption of electrolytes and increased secretion of fluid. The fecal osmolar gap is less than 50 mOsm/L, and the diarrhea persists despite fasting. Examples include congenital chloride and sodium diarrhea, cholera, and neuroendocrine tumors.

Another important underlying mechanism of diarrhea is dysmotility. For example, pseudo-obstruction may result in bacterial stasis, overgrowth and resultant diarrhea, while hyperthyroidism may be associated with diarrhea because of rapid intestinal transit.

The character of the stool can help to determine the origin of diarrhea. Watery, voluminous, nonbloody stool with few or no white blood cells (WBCs) and low pH (<5.5) is likely to emanate from disease of the small intestine. Low-volume, mucusy, often bloody diarrhea with a large number of WBCs and higher pH often originates from the colon. The most common electrolyte abnormalities related to diarrhea include hypokalemic metabolic acidosis caused by bicarbonate and potassium losses in stool.

Bloody diarrhea is a concerning symptom. The most common cause is infection, especially in a setting of fever and acute onset. If bloody diarrhea is progressive and persistent, chronic inflammatory causes should be considered. The age of the patient is also important. In infants, milk protein–induced enterocolitis is a common cause of bloody stools.

ACUTE DIARRHEA

ETIOLOGY AND PATHOGENESIS

The most common cause of acute diarrhea is infection (see Chapter 96). In young children, this is most often viral, with the most common agents being rotavirus, adenovirus, astrovirus, and norovirus. Norovirus causes 60% to 90% of nonbacterial gastroenteritis in the United States, affecting 23 million Americans each year. Rotavirus is a leading cause of death in children younger than 5 years of age worldwide. In immunocompromised hosts, viruses, including cytomegalovirus, Epstein-Barr virus, and BK virus, should be considered. It is estimated that 70% of infectious diarrhea is foodborne, and thus a detailed history of exposures is very important (Table 111-1). Exposure to untreated water may cause giardiasis. Use of public swimming pools poses a risk of *Shigella, Giardia, Cryptosporidium,* and *Entamoeba* infection, with the last three being chlorine resistant. Home pets can transmit infections. For example, turtles carry *Salmonella* spp. History of foreign travel may narrow exposures based on the specific destination. The most common etiology of traveler's diarrhea remains enterotoxigenic *Escherichia coli. Cryptosporidium* and *Giardia* spp. are responsible for most parasitic infections in developed countries. Cyclospora outbreaks have occurred in the United States. *Clostridium difficile* infection, previously thought to affect only hospitalized patients or those taking antibiotics, is now responsible for 40% of community-acquired diarrhea. A recent increase in *C. difficile* infections has been observed, some attributable to the resistant strain, BI/NAP1. An overgrowth of toxin-producing *Clostridium* organisms causes pseudomembranous colitis, which may be a potentially life-threatening condition. *Vibrio cholerae* remains a cause of illness and death in war zones and developing countries. The mechanism of infectious diarrhea is primarily secretory. It can quickly lead to electrolyte abnormalities and acidosis. Infection may result in villous atrophy, which can add an osmotic component. Mucosal healing after infection may lead to transient postinfectious diarrhea.

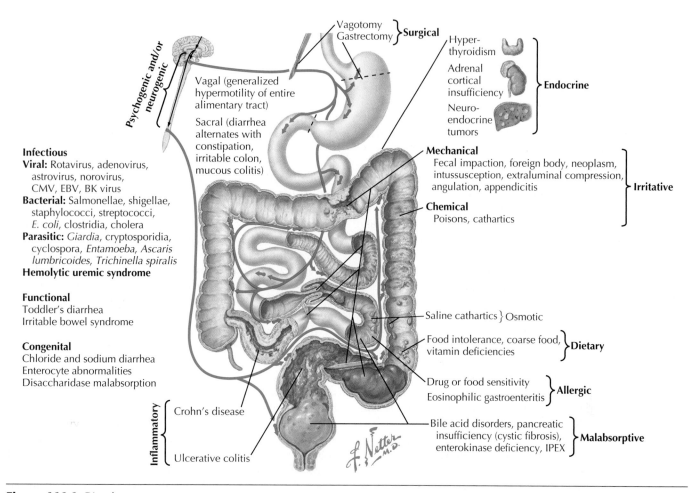

Figure 111-1 *Diarrhea.*

Several other causes of acute diarrhea, particularly in afebrile children, may be particularly concerning. Intussusception, a telescoping of two segments of bowel that occurs mostly in children between 6 months and 2 years of age, may present with bloody diarrhea (see Chapter 109). The typical presentation is colicky abdominal pain, vomiting, and an abdominal mass. "Currant jelly" stools do not occur in all patients with intussusception but are pathognomonic for the condition. Hemolytic-uremic syndrome (HUS) is an uncommon but potentially fatal illness that may present with acute bloody diarrhea. HUS begins as a mild gastroenteritis that evolves into hematochezia, microangiopathic hemolytic anemia, thrombocytopenia, and acute renal failure (see Chapter 64). Less commonly, appendicitis may present with abdominal pain and diarrhea as a result of colonic irritation from the inflamed appendix (see Chapter 5).

Other acute causes of diarrhea include inflammatory bowel disease (IBD; see Chapter 110), overfeeding (caused by increased osmotic loads), antibiotic-associated diarrhea (likely caused by changes in bowel flora), extraintestinal infections (otitis media, urinary tract infection, pneumonia), and toxic ingestions.

CLINICAL PRESENTATION

In any patient presenting with acute diarrhea, a thorough history and physical examination should guide the immediate and subsequent evaluation and therapy. It is important to quantify the duration and frequency of stooling in addition to emesis, liquid intake, and urine output to assess for hydration status. A travel history should be obtained. Recent antibiotic use may suggest pseudomembranous colitis with *C. difficile*. The presence of abdominal pain may occur in infectious enteritis; however, it may also be indicative of intussusception (colicky, episodic) or appendicitis (periumbilical, right lower quadrant). Bloody diarrhea is usually typical in bacterial enteritis but may be seen in viral illness, HUS, or colitis. Associated vomiting suggests viral

Table 111-1 Foodborne Infectious Agents

Food	Associated Infectious Agent
Eggs	Salmonella
Dairy	*Campylobacter jejunii*
Vegetables	*Clostridium perfringens*
Pork	*Clostridium perfringens*
	Yersinia enterocolitica
Seafood	*Aeromonas* spp.
	Vibrio spp.
	Plesiomonas spp.
Rice	*Bacillus cereus*
Beef	Enterohemorrhagic *Escherichia coli*

gastroenteritis. In infectious diarrhea, there is usually a 1- to 8-day incubation period with a sudden onset of symptoms. There may be associated fever, vomiting, crampy abdominal pain, bloody stools, tenesmus, loss of appetite, and dehydration. The immune state of the child should be determined because an immunocompromised child may present with more unusual organisms.

The physical examination begins with the general appearance of the child—does the child look malnourished or has he or she lost weight? Vital signs then help to guide evaluation and management. Fever usually indicates infection. Pulse and blood pressure changes may indicate dehydration, shock, or sepsis. A careful abdominal examination should look for bowel sounds (to evaluate for obstruction) and masses (to evaluate for intussusception). A stool sample should be guaiac tested for microscopic blood.

EVALUATION AND MANAGEMENT

Patients should be assessed for hydration status and electrolyte abnormalities, with correction as indicated. Acute viral gastroenteritis often requires aggressive rehydration with intravenous fluids or oral rehydration solutions. Stool should be sent for viral polymerase chain reaction, culture, and *C. difficile* toxin assay. Most gastrointestinal (GI) infections, except for *C. difficile*, do not require treatment. Antibiotics tend to prolong diarrhea and result in a carrier state. There are special circumstances, such as *Salmonella* enteritis in young infants and immunocompromised patients, for which antibiotic therapy is indicated. Most infections resolve in 14 days in healthy children. Antidiarrheal agents are typically not effective and should be avoided in children. Serious complications, such as sepsis, HUS, pancreatitis, urinary tract infection, and perforation, are uncommon.

CHRONIC DIARRHEA (Figure 111-2)

ETIOLOGY AND PATHOGENESIS

Chronic diarrhea manifesting as two to eight large, loose bowel movements per day, occurring during the daytime, in an otherwise healthy and normally growing child is usually attributable to functional diarrhea. Chronic nonspecific diarrhea of childhood (toddler's diarrhea) most commonly affects young children 6 months to 5 years of age and is typically due to excessive fluid or carbohydrate intake, low fat intake, or rapid transit. Irritable bowel syndrome (IBS) is another cause of functional diarrhea in older children with a prevalence of 11% and is two times more common in girls than boys. Functional diarrhea is mainly caused by osmotic effects of carbohydrates such as sorbitol and fructose or dysmotility with rapid transit.

Congenital diarrheas are rare causes of voluminous, watery stools that present at birth. These disorders include chloride and sodium diarrhea, structural enterocyte abnormalities (e.g., microvillus inclusion disease and intestinal epithelial dysplasia or tufting enteropathy), and disaccharidase malabsorption (e.g., congenital sucrase-isomaltase deficiency and glucose–galactose transporter deficiency). Sodium and chloride diarrhea are autosomal recessive disorders that present at birth with secretory

diarrhea in the presence of normal mucosa. In chloride diarrhea, the Cl/HCO_3 exchanger in the brush border membrane is defective, leading to excessive chloride loss in the stool. Sodium diarrhea, which is exceedingly rare, is likely the result of an impaired Na/H exchanger leading to excessive loss of sodium in stool. Microvillous inclusion disease likely involves an intracellular trafficking defect. Congenital disaccharidase deficiencies derive from gene mutations of the involved proteins.

Lactose intolerance (hypolactasia) is an inherited disorder caused by reduced genetic expression of the enzyme lactasephlorizin hydrolase, which results in carbohydrate malabsorption. It is most common among American Indians and Asians and is least prevalent among Northern Europeans. Congenital hypolactasia is exceedingly rare. Lactase deficiency (a form of disaccharidase deficiency) in enterocytes results in the rapid passage of ingested lactose to the colon, where it is processed by bacterial flora and converted to short-chain fatty acids and hydrogen gas. Lactose malabsorption can also be a secondary process caused by mucosal injury, bacterial overgrowth, or inflammation.

Malabsorption of fat may also result in chronic diarrhea (Figure 111-3). Digestion of protein and fat begins in the oral cavity by salivary amylase and lipase and continues in the duodenum by pancreatic enzymes. Pancreatic enzymes are initially secreted as inactive proenzymes, which are activated by enterokinase, a brush border membrane protease. Enterokinase activates trypsinogen to its active form trypsin, which in turn activates the rest of the digestive enzymes. Lack of enterokinase, colipase, or lipase results in maldigestion of fats, failure to thrive, and steatorrhea. In cystic fibrosis, the secretion of pancreatic enzymes is diminished by hyperviscosity and mucous plugging of ducts. Bile acids participate in fat digestion and absorption by emulsifying long chain fatty acids, allowing them to form chylomicrons, which are then transported to the liver through lymphatics.

Fat malabsorption can be secondary to bile acid disorders or pancreatic insufficiency. Bile acid disorders include chronic cholestasis, terminal ileum resection, bacterial overgrowth, and primary bile acid malabsorption. Pancreatic insufficiency can result in both fat and protein malabsorption. It can result from cystic fibrosis, recurrent severe inflammation, and syndromes such as Shwachman-Diamond syndrome (short stature, pancreatic insufficiency, neutropenia, skeletal abnormalities). Enterokinase deficiency in the brush border may result in malabsorption caused by impaired activation of pancreatic proenzymes. Abetalipoproteinemia presents shortly after birth with steatorrhea and failure to thrive and if untreated may result in neurologic damage. Diarrhea with protein loss can be caused by a wide spectrum of disorders, including IBD, celiac disease, IPEX (immune dysregulation, polyendocrinopathy, enteropathy, X-linked) syndrome, and lymphangiectasia.

Several conditions causing chronic diarrhea are the result of an abnormal immune response to antigens in food or in the GI tract itself. Celiac disease is caused by gluten sensitivity, causing inflammation of the small intestine (see Figure 111-3). In celiac disease, exposure to gluten and its active component gliadin results in an abnormal immune activation. This dietary glutentriggered immune process leads to villous blunting or flattening, crypt elongation, and lymphocytic infiltration of the lamina

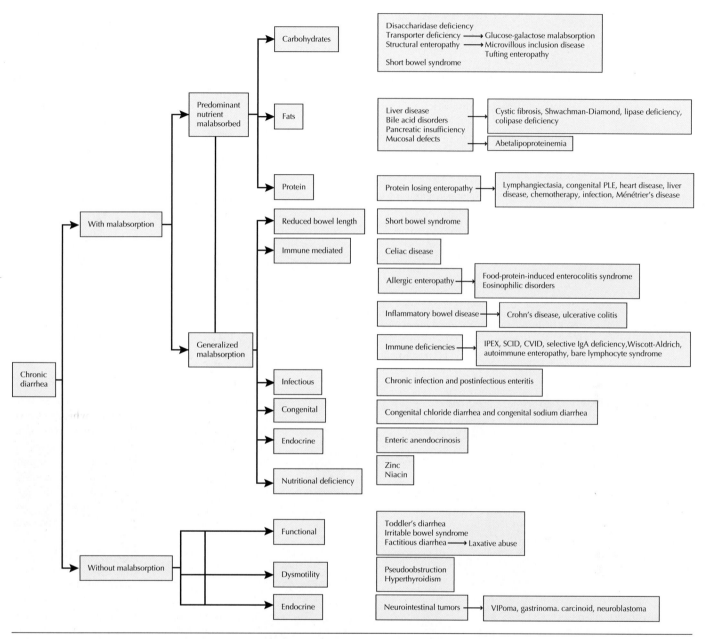

Figure 111-2 *Differential diagnosis of chronic diarrhea.*

propria. This disease affects about 1% of the population and can present any time between infancy and adulthood. It is associated with higher prevalence of HLA DQ2/DQ8; therefore, family history is important. It is also more common in the setting of Down's syndrome, type 1 diabetes, IgA deficiency, Turner's syndrome, William's syndrome, and autoimmune thyroiditis. Chronic IBD, including Crohn's disease and ulcerative colitis, usually presents with slow-onset, sometimes bloody, diarrhea (see Chapter 110). *Allergic colitis*, which is often the result of milk or soy allergy, may present as bloody or nonbloody diarrhea in infants. Food allergies resulting in malabsorption may be caused by eosinophilic gastroenteritis (Figure 111-4). This disorder is often associated with multiple food proteins and other atopic conditions, such as asthma, eczema, and allergic rhinitis. Mechanisms of eosinophilic disorders that are associated with

eosinophilic infiltration of various parts of the GI tract are poorly understood. They seem to involve an interaction among genetic predisposition, environmental exposures to foods and allergens, immunoglobulin E (IgE)–mediated activation of the immune system, and possible interaction with GI microbiota. Rare immune deficiencies that cause diarrhea include IPEX syndrome, severe combined immune deficiency, and autoimmune enteropathy. IPEX syndrome is caused by a mutation in the *FoxP3* gene in T-regulatory cells, resulting in a lack of immune homeostasis. Autoimmune enteropathy, which is associated with antienterocyte antibodies, may occur as part of IPEX but can also be isolated.

Neuroendocrine tumors, such as gastrinoma (Zollinger-Ellison syndrome), carcinoid, and VIPoma (pancreatic cholera), are rare in children and cause secretory diarrhea as a result of

Physical findings

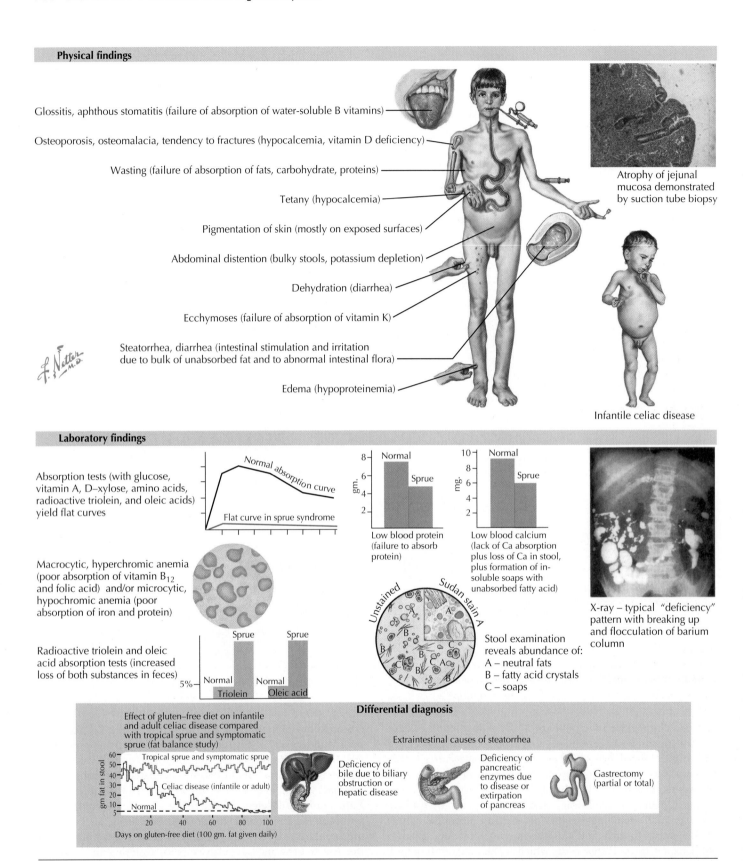

Glossitis, aphthous stomatitis (failure of absorption of water-soluble B vitamins)

Osteoporosis, osteomalacia, tendency to fractures (hypocalcemia, vitamin D deficiency)

Wasting (failure of absorption of fats, carbohydrate, proteins)

Tetany (hypocalcemia)

Pigmentation of skin (mostly on exposed surfaces)

Abdominal distention (bulky stools, potassium depletion)

Dehydration (diarrhea)

Ecchymoses (failure of absorption of vitamin K)

Steatorrhea, diarrhea (intestinal stimulation and irritation due to bulk of unabsorbed fat and to abnormal intestinal flora)

Edema (hypoproteinemia)

Atrophy of jejunal mucosa demonstrated by suction tube biopsy

Infantile celiac disease

Laboratory findings

Absorption tests (with glucose, vitamin A, D–xylose, amino acids, radioactive triolein, and oleic acids) yield flat curves

Normal absorption curve

Flat curve in sprue syndrome

Macrocytic, hyperchromic anemia (poor absorption of vitamin B$_{12}$ and folic acid) and/or microcytic, hypochromic anemia (poor absorption of iron and protein)

Radioactive triolein and oleic acid absorption tests (increased loss of both substances in feces)

Sprue / Normal Triolein   Sprue / Normal Oleic acid   5%

Normal / Sprue — Low blood protein (failure to absorb protein)

Normal / Sprue — Low blood calcium (lack of Ca absorption plus loss of Ca in stool, plus formation of insoluble soaps with unabsorbed fatty acid)

Unstained / Sudan stain

Stool examination reveals abundance of:
A – neutral fats
B – fatty acid crystals
C – soaps

X-ray – typical "deficiency" pattern with breaking up and flocculation of barium column

Differential diagnosis

Effect of gluten–free diet on infantile and adult celiac disease compared with tropical sprue and symptomatic sprue (fat balance study)

Tropical sprue and symptomatic sprue

Celiac disease (infantile or adult)

Normal

Days on gluten-free diet (100 gm. fat given daily)

Extraintestinal causes of steatorrhea

Deficiency of bile due to biliary obstruction or hepatic disease

Deficiency of pancreatic enzymes due to disease or extirpation of pancreas

Gastrectomy (partial or total)

Figure 111-3 *Malabsorption and celiac disease.*

Symptoms • Dyspepsia
• Malnutrition and malabsorption
• Diarrhea
• Weight loss
• Allergy symptoms (asthma)

Biopsy appearance

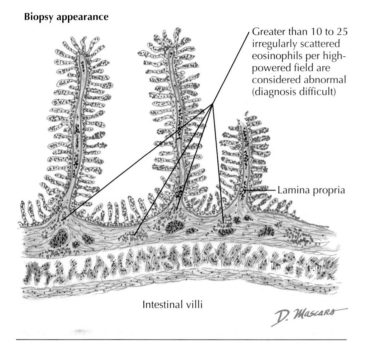

Greater than 10 to 25 irregularly scattered eosinophils per high-powered field are considered abnormal (diagnosis difficult)

Lamina propria

Intestinal villi

D. Mascaro

Figure 111-4 *Eosinophilic gastroenteritis.*

overproduction of intestinal hormones. Intestinal anendocrinosis is a rare autosomal recessive disorder that causes severe diarrhea and is associated with type 1 diabetes. In this condition, mutation of neurogenin 3 results in deficient enteroendocrine cells perturbing the balance of fluid secretion and absorption, which in turn results in malabsorptive diarrhea.

Motility disorders are both diagnostically and therapeutically complex. They can be primary or secondary processes. Intestinal motility is controlled by the enteric nervous system which interacts with multiple hormones, neurotransmitters, and extraintestinal stimuli. Hyperthyroidism is a common cause of alterations in intestinal dysmotility leading to mild to moderate diarrhea. Rapid transit time may be the result of increased neuronal stimulation. Lack of proper peristalsis may lead to bacterial overgrowth with associated diarrhea. Hyperthyroidism is associated with rapid transit, hypersecretion, increased adrenergic stimulation, and possibly a small degree of fat malabsorption secondary to rapid transit.

CLINICAL PRESENTATION AND EVALUATION

Functional Diarrhea

Functional diarrhea in young children does not result in malabsorption or weight loss. IBS with diarrhea predominance presents with a wide range of symptoms, including abdominal pain and diarrhea characterized by frequent loose stools during

waking hours, mostly in the morning and postprandially. The Rome III criteria are currently used for the diagnosis of IBS and are based on symptoms of abdominal pain associated with altered bowel pattern and improvement with defecation in the absence of inflammatory, anatomic, metabolic, or neoplastic processes that would otherwise explain the symptoms.

Congenital Diarrhea

Congenital chloride and sodium diarrhea present with voluminous stool output, high in chloride or sodium, respectively, which does not improve with fasting. Polyhydramnios may be noted prenatally. Diarrhea quickly leads to dehydration and acidosis. Structural abnormalities, such as tufting enteropathy and microvillous inclusion disease, present at birth with intractable secretory diarrhea and require endoscopic biopsies for diagnosis. Congenital disaccharidase deficiency usually presents with osmotic diarrhea when foods are introduced to the infant's diet and should be suspected if the stool contains reducing substances and the pH is low (<5.5). It is also associated with severe diaper rash. The diagnosis is made by disaccharidase analysis of duodenal tissue.

Carbohydrate Malabsorption

Symptoms after the ingestion of lactose include abdominal pain; bloating; flatulence; diarrhea; and, particularly in adolescents, vomiting. The stools tend to be bulky, frothy, and watery. In older children, the hydrogen produced by intestinal bacteria can be measured by a breath hydrogen test. Enzyme activity can also be determined by small bowel biopsy. Stool-reducing substances are present, and stool pH is low (<5.5).

Fat Malabsorption

Patients with fat malabsorption usually present with steatorrhea and failure to thrive. Fat-soluble vitamins (A, D, E, K) may be deficient. Protein loss may result in hypoalbuminemia, which may present clinically as edema or anasarca.

Celiac Disease and Immune-Mediated Diarrhea

Celiac disease may present with a wide range of symptoms, including diarrhea, steatorrhea, constipation, abdominal distension, failure to thrive, iron-deficiency anemia, dermatitis herpetiformis, arthritis, and ataxia, or may be asymptomatic. Celiac disease is diagnosed by a combination of serologic testing and histopathologic findings. Serology should include antitissue transglutaminase antibodies (anti-tTG) and endomysial antibodies. For children younger than 2 years of age, antigliadin antibodies should also be measured. Most serologic testing is IgA based, but about 10% of patients with celiac disease are IgA deficient, so testing should include a total IgA level to aid in interpretation. In the event of IgA deficiency, the antibodies can be tested using IgG-based assays. Upper endoscopy with duodenal biopsy remains the gold standard for the diagnosis of celiac disease. Eosinophilic GI disease may present with diarrhea, poor growth, and bloody stools. Peripheral eosinophilia may not be present. The diagnosis is based on histopathologic evaluation of endoscopic biopsies. IPEX syndrome presents with chronic diarrhea, failure to thrive, food allergies, endocrinopathies such as type 1 diabetes and thyroiditis, hematologic disorders, and dermatitis. Suspected immune deficiencies require specialized evaluation with immunoglobulin levels, lymphocyte activities, WBC function tests, and genetic testing.

Endocrine-Mediated Diarrhea

VIPomas present with watery diarrhea, hypokalemia, and hypochlorhydria. Stool volumes are high and may lead to dehydration. Episodic symptoms in VIPoma and carcinoid may be related to sudden intermittent release of large quantities of hormones. Other associated symptoms include skin flushing caused by the vasodilator effects of VIP (vasoactive intestinal peptide) and secretin (commonly produced by carcinoid). The diagnosis is made by clinical symptoms and the presence of high hormone levels in the blood or metabolites in the urine. Gastrinoma (Zollinger-Ellison syndrome) causes large gastric secretion volumes that cannot be reabsorbed by the small intestine, thus leading to diarrhea.

Dysmotility

Diarrhea caused by dysmotility requires a thorough evaluation including motility evaluation, endoscopy and investigation into extraintestinal causes.

MANAGEMENT

Functional Diarrhea

Eliminating fruit juices and dietary sorbitol, reducing fluid intake if excessive, and liberalizing fat intake are the initial therapies for functional diarrhea in toddlers and young children. IBS treatment starts with dietary modifications to eliminate sorbitol and increase fiber intake. Other therapies may include antidepressants to increase the pain threshold and slow transit, antispasmodic agents to relax intestinal smooth muscle, and behavioral health techniques to manage anxiety and stress.

Congenital Diarrhea

Nutritional support, including parenteral and enteral nutrition, is necessary. Congenital chloride and sodium diarrhea require chronic electrolyte supplementation. Congenital disaccharidase deficiency is managed by eliminating the offending sugar from the diet or in the case of sucrase-isomaltase deficiency, sucrosidase replacement may be used.

Carbohydrate Malabsorption: Disaccharidase Deficiency

Treatment involves an elimination diet, lactase enzyme supplementation, or both. If the disaccharidase deficiency is secondary, treatment of the underlying condition may help to restore enzyme activity.

Fat Malabsorption

Fat malabsorption is detected by a 72-hour quantitative fecal fat. Fat-soluble vitamins should be measured in serum. Pancreatic insufficiency can be screened for using a fecal elastase level. Pancreatic enzyme collection and activity measurement can also be performed endoscopically by collection of pancreatic secretions after secretin administration. If enzyme activity is low, pancreatic enzyme supplementation is indicated. If abetalipoproteinemia is suspected, serum very low-density lipoprotein and β-lipoprotein levels should be measured. In a patient with diarrhea and peripheral edema, protein loss should be evaluated by concurrent measurement of stool and serum α-1 antitrypsin (AAT). Because AAT is not digested while passing through the GI tract, its amount in stool is a good indicator of protein losses.

Celiac Disease and Immune-Mediated Diarrhea

Treatment of celiac disease is currently limited to a strict gluten-free diet. Dietary adherence is measured by periodic anti-tTG level measurement. Management of eosinophilic disorders involves allergy testing for specific food sensitivities with use of elimination or elemental diets (or both). Sequential endoscopies may be useful to assess treatment success. Antiinflammatory and antiallergy agents have been tried with variable success. Treatment of immune deficiency is determined by the specific disorder and may require a bone marrow or stem cell transplant. Supportive nutritional therapy is indicated.

Endocrine-Mediated Diarrhea

Surgical removal of the offending endocrinologic tumor is optimal. Supportive therapy with somatostatin analogs may be required. Postcancer surveillance is required after treatment.

Dysmotility

Motility disorders remain a therapeutic challenge. If bacterial overgrowth is a cause of diarrhea, it should be treated with antibiotics. Antiadrenergics such as propranolol have been successfully used in hyperthyroidism to slow down transit and improve absorption.

SUGGESTED READINGS

Holtz LR, Neill MA, Tarr PI: Acute bloody diarrhea: a medical emergency for patients of all ages, *Gastroenterol* 136(6):1887-1898, 2009.

Pawlowski SW, Warren CA, Guerrannt R: Diagnosis and treatment of acute or persistent diarrhea, *Gastroenterol* 136(6):1874-1886, 2009.

Setty M, Hormaza L, Guandalini S: Celiac disease: risk assessment, diagnosis, and monitoring, *Mol Diagn Ther* 12(5):289-298, 2008.

Szajewska H, Setty M, Mrukowicz J, Guandalini S: Probiotics in gastrointestinal diseases in children: hard and not-so-hard evidence of efficacy, *J Pediatr Gastroenterol Nutr* 42(5):454-475, 2006.

Constipation

Melissa Kennedy

112

Constipation is an extremely common complaint in children, accounting for 3% to 5% of all visits to general pediatric clinics and as many as 30% of visits to pediatric gastroenterologists. The North American Society of Gastroenterology and Nutrition defines constipation as "a delay or difficulty in defecation, present for 2 weeks or more, and sufficient to cause significant distress to the patient." The majority of children meeting this definition do not have an underlying medical condition and are thus labeled as having functional constipation, which is the focus of this chapter.

ETIOLOGY AND PATHOGENESIS

Functional constipation is usually caused by painful bowel movements, which then results in voluntary withholding of stool. This withholding then leads to prolonged fecal stasis in the colon, reabsorption of fluids, and increased size and hardened consistency of the stools. The fear of passing large, hard stools that may stretch the anus and cause pain leads to further withholding and avoidance of all defecation. Over time, the rectum gradually accommodates the enlarging fecal mass, the urge to defecate decreases, and this retentive behavior becomes automatic. Fecal soiling, or encopresis, can occur as the rectal wall stretches and causes loss of rectal sensitivity and the urge to defecate.

CLINICAL PRESENTATION

The aforementioned North American Society of Gastroenterology and Nutrition definition is one of several definitions proposed for constipation. The Paris Consensus on Childhood Constipation Terminology defines it as "a period of 8 weeks with at least 2 of the following symptoms: defecation frequency less than 3 times per week, fecal incontinence frequency greater than once per week, passage of stools so large that they obstruct the toilet, palpable abdominal or rectal fecal mass, stool withholding behavior, or painful defecation." The Rome III criteria include separate definitions for infants and toddlers and for children ages 4 to 18 years. Constipation in infants and toddlers is defined as at least two of the following for at least 1 month: two or fewer defecations per week, at least one episode of incontinence after the acquisition of toileting skills, history of excessive stool retention, history of painful or hard bowel movements, the presence of a large fecal mass in the rectum, or a history of large-diameter stools that may obstruct the toilet. In children ages 4 to 18 years of age, constipation is defined as at least two of the following present for at least 2 months: two or fewer defecations per week, at least one episode of fecal incontinence per week, a history of retentive posturing or excessive volitional stool retention, a history of painful or hard bowel movements, the presence of a large fecal mass in the rectum, or a history of large-diameter stools that may obstruct the toilet.

Children with functional constipation can present with decreased stooling; decreased oral intake; and abdominal pain, distension, or cramping. They may also report painful, hard bowel movements, and the parents may report withholding behaviors. Encopresis may also develop if the constipation is severe. Functional constipation often develops around the time of weaning or dietary transition in infants, toilet training in toddlers, or school entry in older children. The physical examination may reveal palpable stool in the abdomen, as well as an enlarged rectum with palpable stool just beyond the anal verge.

Differential Diagnosis

Although the majority of children with constipation have functional disease, it is important to consider the broad differential diagnosis of constipation in the pediatric population (Box 112-1). Patients with an organic disease usually present with a range of symptoms or physical findings in addition to constipation. Children with *Hirschsprung's disease* (Figure 112-1) often do not pass meconium during the first 36 hours of life and have problems with constipation beginning in infancy (Table 112-1). On examination, the rectum is generally very small and empty of stool. Patients with constipation secondary to *hypothyroidism* generally have other symptoms and findings, including lethargy, hypotonia, a large fontanelle if presenting in infancy, short stature, cold intolerance, dry skin, feeding problems, and a palpable goiter (see Chapter 68). *Celiac disease* can also present with constipation in addition to poor growth and abdominal pain. Children with *lead poisoning* can present with constipation in addition to vomiting and intermittent abdominal pain. Patients with a *tethered spinal cord* may have a sacral dimple and motor deficits of the lower extremities on physical examination. In general, patients with constipation secondary to an organic illness rather than functional constipation have some additional finding or red flag on the history or physical examination to warrant further investigation.

History

A thorough history is important in discriminating between functional constipation and that caused by an organic illness. It is important to determine the timing of the child's first bowel movement (i.e., how soon after birth did the baby first stool?), the onset of the constipation, the frequency and consistency of bowel movements, the presence or absence of blood in the stool, tenesmus (ineffectual straining with defecation), withholding behaviors, and encopresis. The history should probe for red flags such as fever, vomiting, bloody diarrhea, failure to thrive, weight loss, or signs or symptoms that are consistent with the disorders listed in the differential diagnosis above. It is also important to elicit a thorough dietary history because many children with constipation have inadequate fiber and fluid intake.

Box 112-1 Differential Diagnosis of Constipation in Children

- Functional constipation
- Hirschsprung's disease
- Hypothyroidism
- Celiac disease
- Cow's milk intolerance
- Tethered spinal cord
- Cystic fibrosis
- Lead poisoning
- Infantile botulism
- Hypercalcemia
- Hypokalemia
- Neurofibromatosis
- Cerebral palsy
- Anorectal anomalies:
  - Imperforate anus, anal atresia
  - Anal stenosis
- Mitochondrial disorders
- Anal achalasia

Table 112-1 Distinguishing Functional Constipation from Hirschsprung's Disease

	Functional Constipation	Hirschsprung's Disease
Onset	Rare in infancy	Common in infancy
Delayed passage of meconium	Rare	Common
Encopresis	Common	Unusual
Stool size	Very large	Small, ribbonlike
Failure to thrive	Rare	Common
Abdominal distension	Variable	Common
Painful defecation	Common	Rare
Stool in rectal vault	Common	Rare
Anal tone	Open, distended	Tight

Adapted from Graham-Maar RC, Ludwig S, Markowtiz J: Constipation. In Fleisher, Ludwig (eds): Textbook of Pediatric Emergency Medicine, ed 5. Philadelphia, Lippincott, Williams & Wilkins, 2006 and Behrman RE, Kliegman RM: Nelson Essentials of Pediatrics, ed 4. St. Louis, Saunders, 2002.

Physical Examination

The physical examination should include a thorough abdominal examination; external examination of the perianal region, including assessment of the anal wink reflex (contraction of the anus elicited by stroking the perianal area); and a digital rectal examination. Upon digital rectal examination, the size of the anal canal and rectum should be noted in addition to the presence or absence of stool and the consistency of the stool. It is recommended that a test for occult blood be performed in all infants with constipation and in any child who also has abdominal pain, failure to thrive, intermittent diarrhea, or a family history of colon cancer or colonic polyps.

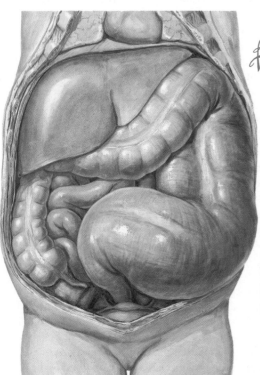

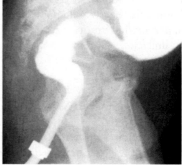
Barium enema; characteristic distal constricted segment

Tremendous distention and hypertrophy of sigmoid and descending colon; moderate involvement of transverse colon; distal constricted segment

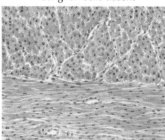
Ganglion cells absent

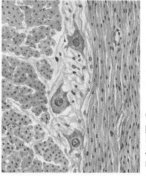
Ganglion cells present between longitudinal and circular muscle layers

Hirschsprung disease, or congenital aganglionic megacolon, is caused by the congenital absence of ganglion cells in the rectosigmoid region and can lead to the onset of constipaton in early infancy and the development of a bowel obstruction and megacolon. Diagnostic evaluation includes an unprepared barium enema that can demonstrate a transition zone (top right, above) and rectal biopsy that demonstrates the absence of ganglion cells (lower middle above). Lower right image depicts the presence of ganglion cells.

Figure 112-1 *Megacolon (Hirschsprung's disease).*

EVALUATION AND MANAGEMENT

Because the majority of children with constipation have functional constipation, an extensive medical workup is often not necessary. If Hirschsprung's disease is a concern, an *unprepared* barium enema to look for a transition zone and a rectal biopsy to detect ganglion cells are indicated. Other tests that might be indicated based on the history and physical examination findings may include thyroid function tests, celiac antibodies, a lead level, a calcium level, a sweat test, and magnetic resonance imaging or ultrasound of the lumbar spine.

If organic disease has been ruled out or deemed unlikely by the history and physical examination findings, no laboratory or radiologic investigation is absolutely necessary at the outset. The clinician might consider an abdominal plain radiograph to further illustrate the degree of fecal impaction or a Sitz marker study (a pill with radiopaque markers is swallowed and their progress through the gastrointestinal [GI] tract is tracked by radiography) after the patient is completely cleaned out to assess the patient's colonic motility.

Treatment of functional constipation generally involves determining whether a fecal impaction is present, treating the impaction, initiating maintenance treatment with oral medication, and educating the patient and the family. Fecal impaction (Figure 112-2) is defined as a hard mass in the lower abdomen on physical examination, a dilated rectum filled with a large amount of hard stool on rectal examination or excessive stool on abdominal radiography. Disimpaction must occur before maintenance therapy can be effective and is best accomplished by the rectal route with phosphate enemas, saline enemas, or mineral oil enemas. An oral approach to disimpaction is slower and less effective than rectal disimpaction, but if necessary, it can be attempted with high doses of polyethylene glycol electrolyte solutions or with high-dose magnesium hydroxide, magnesium citrate, lactulose, sorbitol, senna, mineral oil, or bisacodyl.

After disimpaction is complete, maintenance therapy should focus on prevention of recurrence. Maintenance therapy is generally a combination of behavioral modification, dietary changes, and laxatives. Effective medications include osmotic laxatives such as polyethylene glycol, magnesium hydroxide, lactulose, Kristalose, and sorbitol. Stimulant laxatives such as senna, bisacodyl, or Dulcolax can be used for short intervals; the prolonged use of stimulant laxatives in children is not recommended. Dietary interventions generally consist of increased dietary fiber and increased fluid intake. Behavioral modification is focused on instilling regular toilet habits and includes regularly scheduled toilet sitting and can be combined with a reward system. Successful treatment of functional constipation often takes 3 to 6 months.

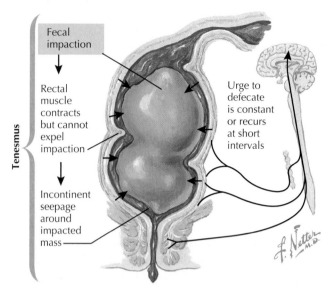

Fecal impaction, or a large amount of hard stool in the distal rectum obstructing the anal outlet. The presence of a fecal impaction can lead to encopresis as more proximal fecal matter seeps around the impacted fecal mass.

Figure 112-2 *Pathophysiology of defecation.*

FUTURE DIRECTIONS

Future advances in the treatment of functional constipation may include improved laxatives for the pediatric age group. In addition, because the field of GI motility is constantly progressing, new advances in motility therapy and investigation are likely to emerge.

SUGGESTED READINGS

Baker SS, Liptak GS, Colletti RB, et al: Constipation in infants and children: evaluation and treatment. A medical position statement of the North American Society for Pediatric Gastroenterology and Nutrition. *J Pediatr Gastroenterol Nutr* 29(5):612-626, 1999.

Benninga M, Candy DC, Catto-Smith AG, et al: The Paris Consensus on Childhood Constipation Terminology (PACCT) Group. *J Pediatr Gastroenterol Nutr* 40(3):273-275, 2005.

Borowitz SM, Cox DJ, Kovatchev B, et al: Treatment of childhood constipation by primary care physicians: efficacy and predictors of outcome. *Pediatrics* (115):873-877, 2005.

Evaluation and treatment of constipation in children: summary of updated recommendations of the North American Society for Pediatric Gastroenterology, Hepatology and Nutrition. North American Society for Pediatric Gastroenterology, Hepatology and Nutrition. *J Pediatr Gastroenterol Nutr* 43(3):405-407, 2006.

Hernias

113

Benjamin A. Sahn and Rose C. Graham

*H*ernias—defined as a protrusion of a structure or part of a structure through tissues normally containing it—are encountered frequently in pediatric clinical practice. In children, external hernias represent the vast majority and are typically in, but not limited to, the inguinal and umbilical regions. Umbilical hernias are very common, most notably in premature infants, infants of African and African American descent, and infants with certain diseases or genetic syndromes. It is estimated that inguinal hernias occur in roughly 1% to 5% of all children, with an increased incidence in specific populations such as those with a family history of inguinal hernia and premature infants, who can have an incidence near 30% in those with birth weights less than 1000 g. Inguinal hernias can cause significant morbidity because of incarceration and strangulation, making it essential that general practitioners and subspecialists alike understand how to approach the condition and recognize when emergent therapy is required.

Congenital diaphragmatic hernia (CDH) and hiatal hernia are the two most common internal hernia types among children. CDH is a neonatal surgical emergency that presents with a scaphoid abdomen, cyanosis, and respiratory distress within minutes of birth as a result of the herniation of abdominal contents into the thoracic cavity (Figure 113-1; see Chapter 102). Hiatal hernias, in which intraabdominal portions of the esophagus, the stomach, or both pass into the thorax, are less common in children than adults but remain an important consideration in certain clinical circumstances. Other internal hernias, including paraduodenal and mesenteric hernias, occur within the abdominal cavity. These are largely the result of congenital abnormalities and in rare circumstances become clinically relevant in childhood.

ETIOLOGY AND PATHOGENESIS

External Hernias

INGUINAL HERNIA

Indirect inguinal hernias are congenital in origin, arising from incomplete embryogenesis. In boys, the testes are initially in a retroperitoneal position. A portion of peritoneum called the processus vaginalis attaches to the testes and precedes the testicular descent through the internal inguinal ring into the scrotal sac. The testes are located at the internal inguinal ring by 28 weeks of gestation and reach their final destination by 36 weeks with the left side completing its descent slightly earlier than the right. The processus vaginalis creates a patent conduit between the abdomen and the scrotum via the inguinal canal and typically obliterates between 36 and 40 weeks of gestation or in the postnatal period. If the processus vaginalis remains patent, abdominal contents may escape through the internal inguinal ring into the inguinal canal and the scrotum (Figure 113-2).

In girls, the ovaries also start in a retroperitoneal position; however, their descent is modified, and they do not leave the abdominal cavity. The processus vaginalis extends through the inguinal canal with the round ligament to the labia majoris and usually obliterates between 32 and 36 weeks of gestation. This embryologic difference is likely why indirect inguinal hernias occur six times more commonly in boys than girls.

Patients with cryptorchidism (failure of one or both testicles to descend into the scrotum), urogenital malformations, and increased intraabdominal pressure are at increased risk for developing indirect inguinal hernias. Direct inguinal hernias are rare in children, entering the inguinal canal through a defect in the posterior wall of the canal medial to the inferior epigastric vessels. Femoral hernias, also rare in children, penetrate an acquired muscular defect in the abdominal wall posterior to the inguinal ligament. Patients with connective tissue disorders and those who have had previous surgery to correct an inguinal hernia have greater risk for femoral or direct inguinal hernias.

UMBILICAL HERNIA

All newborns have a natural defect at the umbilicus, allowing the cord with the umbilical vessels to pass through. In most infants, the umbilical ring closes spontaneously. In some, an anatomic defect persists, increasing the likelihood of herniation. The umbilical vein obliterates and becomes the ligamentum teres, which usually attaches to the umbilical ring inferiorly. A superior attachment may occur, leaving an area of potential weakness. The umbilical ring is also supported by the transversalis fascia and peritoneum. A natural thickening of the transversalis fascia occurs at the umbilicus, which may fail to cover the entire ring, leaving an area of relative weakness. The closure of the ring is most likely multifactorial as suggested by significant racial differences in incidence of hernia and increased frequency in children with Beckwith-Wiedemann syndrome; Hurler's syndrome; trisomies 13, 18, and 21; and congenital hypothyroidism.

ABDOMINAL WALL HERNIAS

Epigastric hernias occur above the umbilicus through a defect in the linea alba and most commonly contain preperitoneal fat. Such a defect develops when there is failure of complete approximation of the midline during the final stages of abdominal wall formation. Incisional hernias, resulting from incomplete healing of a surgical incision, can occur anywhere on the abdomen. Any process that increases intraabdominal pressure, obesity, and postoperative wound infections are major risk factors for incisional hernias. Spigelian hernias, reported rarely in children, occur in an area of natural weakness at the lateral edge of the rectus abdominus muscle and below the arcuate line where only transversalis fascia lies posterior to the rectus abdominus (Figure 113-3).

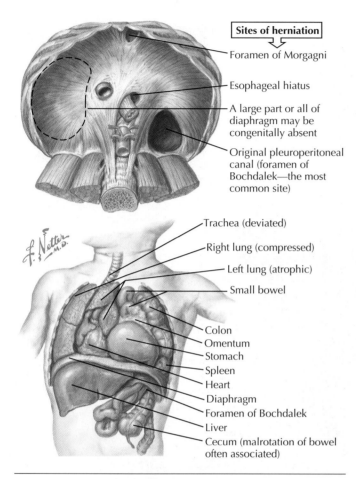

Sites of herniation
Foramen of Morgagni
Esophageal hiatus
A large part or all of diaphragm may be congenitally absent
Original pleuroperitoneal canal (foramen of Bochdalek—the most common site)
Trachea (deviated)
Right lung (compressed)
Left lung (atrophic)
Small bowel
Colon
Omentum
Stomach
Spleen
Heart
Diaphragm
Foramen of Bochdalek
Liver
Cecum (malrotation of bowel often associated)

Figure 113-1 *Congenital diaphragmatic hernia.*

Internal Hernias

HIATAL HERNIA

The intraabdominal esophagus and the stomach are secured in place by numerous fascial and ligamentous elements. At its entry into the abdomen, the esophagus is supported by fibroelastic tissue called the phrenoesophageal membrane. This membrane, as well as many other supporting structures, can be structurally deficient at birth or gradually weaken with time and stress, causing laxity of the support and widening of the muscular hiatus. During inspiration, the transdiaphragmatic pressure differential causes the esophagus and stomach to be pulled upward. Depending on the areas of weakness, the gastroesophageal junction may slide into the posterior mediastinum or a portion of the stomach may pass through the hiatus alongside the esophagus with the lower esophageal sphincter maintained in its correct anatomic position (Figure 113-4).

OTHER INTERNAL HERNIAS

Paraduodenal hernias occur when small bowel protrudes through a fossa created by abnormal mesenteric attachments to the ascending or descending colon. A congenital or acquired defect in the mesentery itself may accept a loop of bowel anywhere along its tract known as a mesenteric hernia.

CLINICAL PRESENTATION

External hernias classically present with the history of an intermittent or persistent swelling without associated pain, which may disappear spontaneously and are most noticeable with crying or straining.

Inguinal hernias can present at birth or any time during childhood. The history may include a description of the bulge extending to the scrotum or labia majora. The differential diagnosis of an inguinal-scrotal or labial swelling also includes incarcerated inguinal hernia, hydrocele, torsion of an undescended testis, and inguinal lymphadenitis. History and a detailed gastrointestinal (GI) and genitourinary examination should differentiate between these entities (Table 113-1). Observing the mass increasing in size during a period of increased intraabdominal pressure and decreasing in size during relaxation or gentle taxis strongly suggests the diagnosis of inguinal hernia. A firm, smooth mass is often palpable at the external inguinal ring. The smooth sensation of the herniated sac rolling over itself when palpated at the pubic tubercle is known as the "silk glove sign" and supports the diagnosis of hernia. Transillumination is not specific for hydroceles and should be used with caution as a tool to differentiate from hernias. Hernias may transilluminate as well, especially in the incarcerated state with excess bowel wall edema. Close inspection of the contralateral inguinal region is important because 10% of patients have bilateral inguinal hernias. Determining if the hernia is indirect or direct is frequently difficult on examination and is often not confirmed until surgery. A femoral hernia is clinically seen as a swelling in the femoral canal inferior to the inguinal ligament but may also be confused for an inguinal hernia.

Umbilical hernias typically present with the history of an external hernia described above. The physical examination reveals a soft mass covered by skin protruding from the umbilicus, increasing in size with increased intraabdominal pressure, and reducing easily and completely in all but the rarest of circumstances. The differential diagnosis for an umbilical mass in a young child also includes umbilical pyogenic granuloma, umbilical polyp, omphalocele, and an omphalomesenteric duct remnant. The umbilical granuloma and polyp are readily differentiated from hernia by the lack of skin covering the mass, reddish color, and serous drainage that may be present. Omphalocele should be detected at birth, if not earlier, with intestine protruding from the umbilicus covered only by a membranous sac. Exceedingly rare umbilical tumors, such as teratomas and sarcomas, have been reported; these are not soft or reducible on examination.

Internal hernias are frequently asymptomatic and may come to the clinician's attention during an unrelated investigation. When symptomatic, the presentation is variable and depends on the site of herniation.

The cardinal symptoms of a sliding hiatal hernia are regurgitation and heartburn, which are manifestations of gastroesophageal reflux (GER; see Chapter 107). When a hiatal hernia is the underlying cause, GER may be associated with complications such as pulmonary infections secondary to aspiration, vomiting, and failure to thrive. Dysphagia may also be described but tends to be a later finding. Paraesophageal hiatal hernias can present in similar fashion to a sliding hernia; however, dysphagia, early satiety, and chest pain tend to be more prominent with paraesophageal hernias. Sliding and paraesophageal hiatal

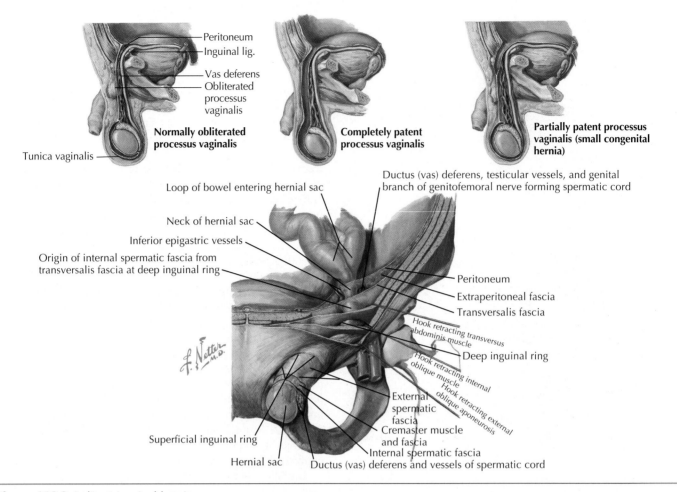

Figure 113-2 *Indirect inguinal hernia.*

hernias should be considered as part of the differential diagnosis for any of these presenting symptoms. The physical examination may provide insight to the presence of GER but is not helpful in making the diagnosis of either type of hiatal hernia.

Paraduodenal, mesenteric and other types of internal hernias contained within the abdominal cavity rarely cause symptoms during childhood. When problematic, these hernias usually present with a constellation of symptoms, including abdominal pain, vomiting, decreased stooling, and irritability as manifestations of acute or recurrent intestinal obstruction.

EVALUATION AND MANAGEMENT

External Hernias

INGUINAL HERNIAS

If the diagnosis remains uncertain, ultrasonography is the imaging test of choice in differentiating a patent processus vaginalis or hydrocele from inguinal hernia. Infrequently, direct visualization with laparoscopy is needed to confirm the diagnosis. After the diagnosis of inguinal hernia has been made, the first step is to determine if the hernia is reducible or incarcerated. Incarceration of the hernia sac has occurred if it cannot be

easily reduced into the abdominal cavity. An incarcerated sac is a surgical emergency and can proceed rapidly to strangulation, in which blood flow to the contents of the sac is compromised, resulting in ischemia. If the spermatic cord and testis or fallopian tube and ovary are affected, sterility of the involved organ may result. A strangulated bowel viscus is at risk for ischemia and perforation.

If the hernia is incarcerated without strangulation and the patient is in stable condition, manual reduction is often successful and should be attempted. The patient must be relaxed to perform this maneuver; analgesics or sedatives are frequently useful. Placing the patient in slight Trendelenburg position is also beneficial. Mild continuous pressure (taxis) is applied to the hernia inferiorly and laterally. After relieved from its fixed position at the external inguinal ring, upward pressure is applied to return the hernia sac into the abdominal cavity. If successful reduction cannot be achieved, intravenous fluids and broad-spectrum antibiotics are administered while awaiting emergent surgical correction before strangulation occurs. If successful, however, definitive surgical repair of the hernia may be delayed for 24 to 48 hours to decrease operative complications as bowel wall edema subsides. During this period, the child is usually observed as an inpatient to ensure feedings are tolerated and symptoms of bowel necrosis do not develop.

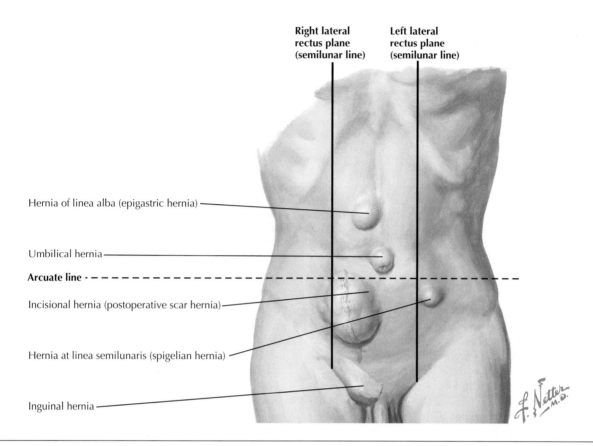

Figure 113-3 *Abdominal wall hernias.*

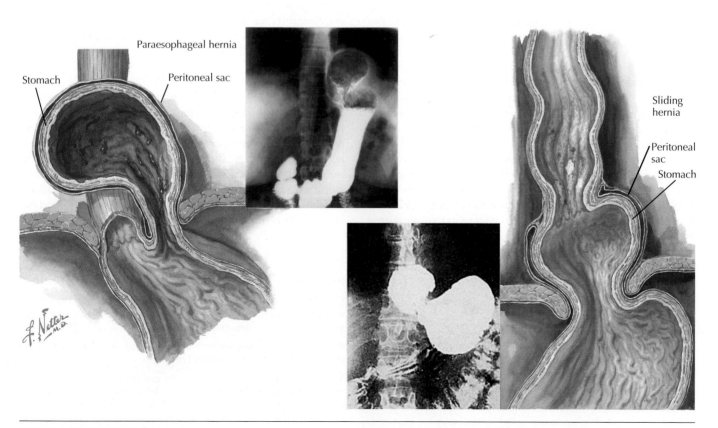

Figure 113-4 *Hiatal hernias.*

Table 113-1 Differential Diagnosis of Inguinal-Scrotal or Labial Swelling

Clinical Condition	Distinguishing Characteristics
Reducible inguinal hernia	Crying or straining enlarges mass
	Relaxation or gentle pressure reduces mass
	Smooth, firm, mobile inguinal mass palpable at external ring
Incarcerated inguinal hernia	Intestinal obstructive symptoms present
	Mass with significant swelling and lack of mobility
Hydrocele	Gradual onset of swelling, often larger in the evening while the child is ambulating
	Intestinal obstructive symptoms absent
	+/− reducible, mobile mass
Torsion of undescended testis	Painful, erythematous groin mass
	Absence of testicle in scrotum on the ipsilateral side
Inguinal lymphadenitis	Infected or crusted skin lesion possible
	Multiple discrete palpable nodes in the inguinal region
	No thickening of spermatic cord or testis

On initial evaluation, if the inguinal hernia is freely reducible, timely operative management is indicated to prevent incarceration from occurring. Inguinal hernias do not resolve without surgery. Children younger than 1 year of age are at highest risk for incarceration, and surgery at the earliest appropriate time is indicated. Premature infants with low birth weight in the neonatal intensive care unit found to have an inguinal hernia should have surgical repair before discharge home unless other medical conditions make the procedure unsafe.

UMBILICAL HERNIAS

As long as the umbilical hernia is asymptomatic and reducible, observation alone will initially suffice. Anticipatory guidance can be given to the parent about the likelihood of the hernia's self-resolving based on the child's age and the size of the defect. Small defects smaller than 1 cm have greater than 80% chance to close spontaneously by age 5 years. Referral to a surgeon is recommended at that time if the defect is still open. If the defect is larger than 1.5 cm in diameter, it will rarely close, making operative closure appropriate by 2 years of age. Defects ranging 1 to 1.5 cm in diameter should be observed for a gradual decrease in size during the first 2 to 3 years of life, and surgical referral should be made at that time if the defect fails to become smaller. The practice of strapping any material over the hernia to maintain it in a reduced position does not assist in facilitating closure. If a patient with umbilical hernia is undergoing an unrelated procedure under general anesthesia, surgical closure may be discussed at that time with risks and benefits examined on a case-by-case basis.

Internal Hernia

HIATAL HERNIA

Children with persistent dysphagia or GER symptoms unresponsive to medical management require evaluation with imaging studies. If an upright chest radiograph has been performed as part of the initial workup, retrocardiac air-fluid levels are highly suggestive of a hiatal hernia. The most important initial test is a contrast upper GI series to define the anatomy. The presence of a portion of the stomach in the thorax confirms the diagnosis. If a sliding hiatal hernia is observed, both medical and surgical management options should be considered. An upper GI endoscopy may be helpful in guiding therapy by assessing for esophagitis or strictures. If optimal medical management—acid blockade pharmacotherapy and appropriate dietary changes—does not control symptoms or significant esophageal disease is found on endoscopy, the next step is a surgical evaluation for a fundoplication. The presence of paraesophageal hiatal hernia on contrast radiography is an indication for surgical repair. The gastric fundus herniating through the diaphragm is at high risk for incarceration, volvulus, or perforation—feared complications that carry significant potential for morbidity and mortality.

OTHER INTERNAL HERNIAS

For patients with signs and symptoms of intestinal obstruction, plain radiographs and contrast studies, including computed tomography scans, may give clues to the presence of an internal hernia; however, these often fail to confirm this etiology as the cause for the obstruction. More frequently, an internal hernia is found intraoperatively where the herniated bowel can be reduced and the defect can be repaired. Strangulation and bowel necrosis are possible complications requiring swift treatment.

SUGGESTED READINGS

Brandt ML: Pediatric hernias. *Surg Clin North Am* 88(1):27-43, 2008.

Curci JA, Melman LM, Thompson RW, et al: Elastic fiber depletion in the supporting ligaments of the gastroesophageal junction: a structural basis for the development of hiatal hernia. *J Am Coll Surg* 207(2):191-196, 2008.

Snyder C: Current management of umbilical abnormalities and related anomalies. *Semin Pediatr Surg* 16:41-49, 2007.

Vandenplas Y, Hassall E: Mechanisms of gastroesophageal reflux and gastroesophageal reflux disease. *J Pediatr Gastroenterol Nutr* 35(2):119-136, 2002.

Melissa Kennedy

Disorders of the pancreas (Figure 114-1) are rare in childhood but can be associated with significant morbidity and mortality. Pancreatitis occurs less frequently in children than in adults and can be either acute or chronic in nature. It can be complicated by shock, hypocalcemia, pseudocyst formation, or necrosis, but these complications are rare. Pancreatic insufficiency (PI), defined as insufficient lipase secretion resulting in fat malabsorption, affects about 80% to 90% of patients with cystic fibrosis (CF). Congenital anomalies of the pancreas, such as pancreas divisum and annular pancreas, are found in approximately 10% of the general population and are generally asymptomatic but can be associated with pancreatitis (pancreas divisum) or duodenal obstruction (annular pancreas).

ETIOLOGY AND PATHOGENESIS

Pancreatitis

The frequency of pancreatitis (i.e., inflammation of the pancreas) in children and adolescents has been increasing over the past 10 to 15 years. There are several common causes of pancreatitis, including blunt abdominal trauma; infections such as enterovirus, Epstein-Barr virus, hepatitis A, rubella, Coxsackie virus B, cytomegalovirus, HIV, and influenza; congenital anomalies of the pancreas; choledochal cysts; and choledocholithiasis. Medications, including azathioprine, 6-mercaptopurine, glucocorticoids, valproate, and L-asparaginase, can cause pancreatitis. Pancreatitis can also be the result of systemic diseases and metabolic abnormalities, including CF, diabetic ketoacidosis, hypercalcemia, hyperlipidemia, and hemolytic-uremic syndrome.

Pancreatitis occurs when intracellular trypsinogen and other digestive enzymes are activated, leading to damage of the pancreatic acinar cells. This damage leads to pancreatic edema (Figure 114-2), a local inflammatory response, and the initiation of autodigestion of the pancreas. These pancreatic secretions may form a collection that becomes walled off by granulation tissue to form a pseudocyst.

Chronic pancreatitis occurs with recurrent episodes of acute pancreatitis, leading to chronic inflammation as well as end-stage fibrosis (see Figure 114-2). The most common causes of chronic pancreatitis in children are CF, hereditary pancreatitis including mutations in the *SPINK1*, *CFTR*, and *PRSS1* genes, and idiopathic causes.

Cystic Fibrosis

Pancreatic insufficiency in patients with CF is caused by dysfunction of the *CFTR* gene (Figure 114-3). This leads to impaired transport of sodium and chloride and subsequent obstruction of the pancreatic ducts with viscous exocrine fluid. These patients have diminished secretion of amylase, lipase, colipase, and phospholipases, as well as a decreased concentration of bicarbonate in their pancreatic secretions.

Congenital and Inherited Anomalies

Congenital anomalies of the pancreas arise during fetal development. The pancreas forms from fusion of dorsal and ventral buds, which develop from the embryonic foregut. The ventral process rotates at about the eighth week of gestation and settles posterior and inferior to the dorsal portion of the pancreas. Pancreas divisum is the most common pancreatic anomaly and occurs when the dorsal and ventral portions fail to fuse. Annular pancreas occurs when the ventral bud fails to rotate with the duodenum and instead surrounds it (Figure 114-4).

Pancreatic disease may present as part of an inherited syndrome. This category includes CF and hereditary pancreatitis (see above). In addition, Schwachman-Diamond syndrome is caused by mutations in *SDS* and is characterized by short stature, variable neutropenia, and PI. The latter often improves as patients grow older. Finally, the spectrum of abnormalities seen in Johanson-Blizzard syndrome includes progressive PI.

CLINICAL PRESENTATION

Pancreatitis

Pancreatitis in children most commonly presents with nausea, vomiting, and epigastric abdominal pain that may radiate to the back. Additional symptoms include fever, tachycardia, hypotension, and jaundice. Physical examination findings include abdominal distention, hypoactive bowel sounds, and epigastric tenderness, rebound, or guarding. Patients with a pseudocyst may present with abdominal distention and a palpable and tender epigastric mass. Acute hemorrhagic pancreatitis is a rare entity in children and is life threatening when it occurs. These patients may present in shock and have physical examination findings that include a bluish discoloration of the flanks (Grey Turner's sign) or periumbilical area (Cullen's sign).

Cystic Fibrosis

Pancreatic insufficiency in patients with CF becomes more common with increasing age, with only about 60% of neonates affected as compared with 80% to 90% of older children. These children generally present with symptoms of fat malabsorption and malnutrition and have decreased serum levels of pancreatic digestive enzymes, but elevated levels of salivary and brush border amylase.

Congenital and Inherited Anomalies

Congenital anomalies of the pancreas are often asymptomatic and are typically found incidentally on imaging or at autopsy. Pancreas divisum is the most common pancreatic congenital anomaly. This condition can lead to pancreatitis in a subset of patients and therefore should be on the differential diagnosis for patients with pancreatitis of unknown etiology. Annular

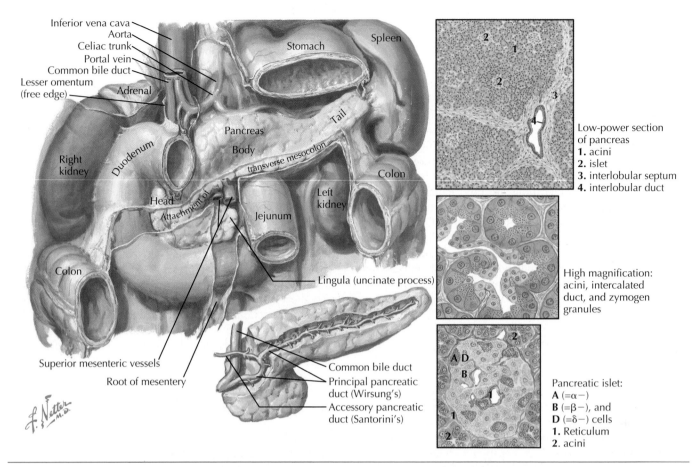

Figure 114-1 *Anatomy and histology of the pancreas.*

pancreas is the second most common congenital anomaly of the pancreas and can cause duodenal obstruction in some patients. This obstruction can present with a range of symptoms depending on the degree of obstruction; the range includes feeding difficulty, vomiting, and abdominal distension in a newborn with severe obstruction to postprandial fullness, nausea, and weight loss in an older child with a lower grade obstruction.

The differential diagnosis of pancreatitis includes disorders of the stomach, intestines, gallbladder, kidneys, lungs, and liver (Box 114-1).

EVALUATION AND MANAGEMENT

Pancreatitis

A thorough history is important to distinguish pancreatitis from other causes of acute abdominal pain. It is important to determine

Box 114-1 Differential Diagnosis of Pancreatitis

- Peptic ulcer disease
- Gastroenteritis
- Acute cholecystitis
- Biliary colic
- Small bowel obstruction
- Renal colic
- Basilar pneumonia
- Early appendicitis

the onset and the character of the pain, as well as any other associated symptoms. A complete list of current medications is important to obtain because many medications may cause pancreatitis, including nonsteroidal antiinflammatory drugs, corticosteroids, antibiotics (sulfonamides, tetracyclines), diuretics (thiazides, furosemide), azathioprine, and mercaptopurine, to name a few. The laboratory evaluation should include amylase and lipase levels, which may be elevated more than three times the upper limit of normal but can be unreliable because they may be elevated for reasons other than pancreatitis (Table 114-1). An ultrasound may reveal an enlarged pancreas with an alteration in echogenicity and can also identify the presence of a pseudocyst. Other findings on ultrasound may include gallstones or biliary sludge in the case of gallstone pancreatitis, pancreatic calcifications, choledochal cysts, dilated pancreatic ducts, or dilated common or hepatic bile ducts. Magnetic resonance cholangio-pancreatography can be helpful in further identifying ductal abnormalities. In patients with recurrent or chronic pancreatitis, genetic testing for *SPINK1*, CF, and cationic trypsinogen (*PRSS1*) can be helpful. Additionally, an elevated triglyceride level may indicate hyperlipidemia as a cause of recurrent pancreatitis.

Treatment of children with pancreatitis is generally supportive and includes pancreatic and bowel rest with nothing per mouth, intravenous (IV) fluids, gastric acid blockade, and pain management. Nevertheless, physicians should remain vigilant for signs of severe complications such as shock, peritonitis, or hypocalcemia. Amylase and lipase values may be followed, although treatment decisions should be based primarily on the

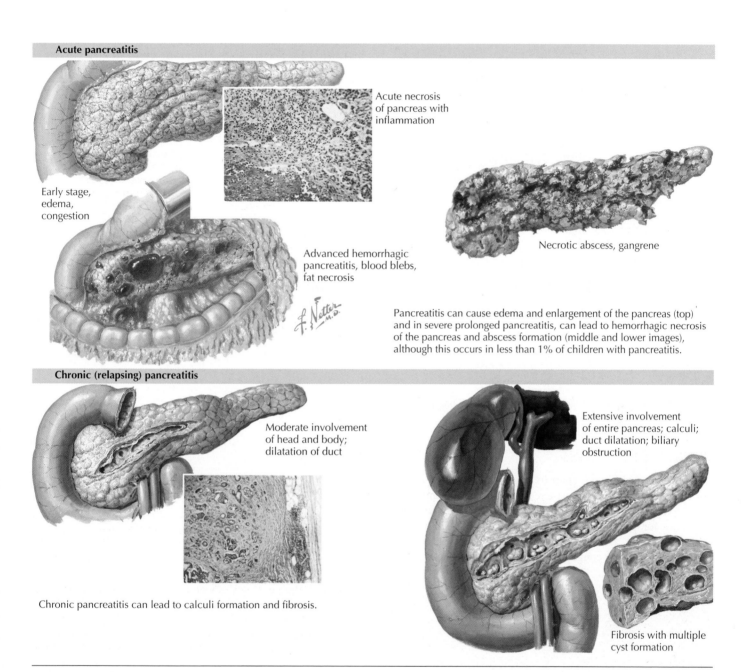

Acute pancreatitis

Early stage, edema, congestion

Acute necrosis of pancreas with inflammation

Advanced hemorrhagic pancreatitis, blood blebs, fat necrosis

Necrotic abscess, gangrene

Pancreatitis can cause edema and enlargement of the pancreas (top) and in severe prolonged pancreatitis, can lead to hemorrhagic necrosis of the pancreas and abscess formation (middle and lower images), although this occurs in less than 1% of children with pancreatitis.

Chronic (relapsing) pancreatitis

Moderate involvement of head and body; dilatation of duct

Extensive involvement of entire pancreas; calculi; duct dilatation; biliary obstruction

Chronic pancreatitis can lead to calculi formation and fibrosis.

Fibrosis with multiple cyst formation

Figure 114-2 *Pancreatitis.*

patient's clinical status and symptoms. In patients who cannot tolerate oral intake for more than 48 hours, nasojejunal feeding can be used to safely provide nutrition as an alternative to IV hyperalimentation. In the approximately 13% of patients who develop a pseudocyst, drainage may be required if it does not resolve spontaneously. Cholecystectomy is indicated in patients with gallstone pancreatitis or biliary sludge. An endoscopic retrograde cholangiopancreatography (ERCP) may be required if there is evidence of acute biliary or pancreatic duct obstruction or in cases of recurrent pancreatitis in which there is concern for a ductal or structural abnormality. Pancreatic necrosis occurs in fewer than 1% of children with pancreatitis and may require surgical intervention for pancreatic debridement or necrosectomy. A number of surgical procedures are also available for patients with chronic pancreatitis.

Cystic Fibrosis

In patients with CF who develop PI, it is helpful to know the pancreatic phenotype because it is a major determinant of prognosis. Homozygotes for ΔF508 most frequently have PI. Patients with PI have a lower median survival age than those with normal pancreatic function. The treatment for PI generally consists of enzyme supplementation.

Congenital Anomalies

Management of patients with congenital anomalies of the pancreas depends on their degree of clinical significance. If an annular pancreas leads to a duodenal obstruction, it can be surgically repaired with a bypass surgery of the annulus. In patients with pancreas divisum who have recurrent episodes

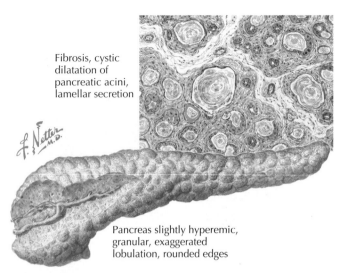

Fibrosis, cystic dilatation of pancreatic acini, lamellar secretion

Pancreas slightly hyperemic, granular, exaggerated lobulation, rounded edges

In cystic fibrosis, sodium and chloride transport is impeded leading to obstruction of the pancreatic ducts with viscous exocrine fluid. This results in cystic dilatation and pancreatic fibrosis.

Figure 114-3 *Pancreatic disease in cystic fibrosis.*

of pancreatitis as well as a narrowing of the minor papilla, surgical or endoscopic intervention may be an option.

FUTURE DIRECTIONS

There are no current therapies to arrest the cascade of pancreatic autodigestion seen in pancreatitis. Further advances and techniques in the field of ERCP may contribute to improved outcomes for patients with pancreatitis. Genetic studies such as genome-wide association studies may reveal causative or modifying alleles for congenital and other pancreatic diseases.

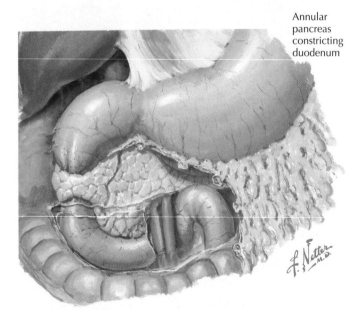

Annular pancreas constricting duodenum

Annular pancreas occurs when the ventral bud fails to rotate with the duodenum and instead surrounds it. This may resutlt in duodenal obstruction.

Figure 114-4 *Annular pancreas.*

Table 114-1 Causes of Elevated Amylase and Lipase Levels

Amylase	Lipase
Pancreatitis and resulting complications	Pancreatitis
Pancreatic ductal obstruction	Pancreatic duct obstruction or calculus
Intestinal disease (perforation, obstruction)	Intestinal disease (perforation, obstruction)
Peritonitis	Duodenal ulcer or perforated peptic ulcer
Celiac disease	Celiac disease
Severe gastroenteritis	Gastroenteritis
Biliary tract disease (choledocholithiasis and cholecystitis)	Acute cholecystitis
	Macrolipasemia
Macroamylasemia	Renal disease
Decreased amylase clearance (renal, liver disease or failure)	Pancreatic trauma (blunt trauma, abdominal surgery, ERCP)
Pancreatic trauma (blunt trauma, abdominal surgery, ERCP)	Pancreatic malignancies
Malignancies	AIDS
AIDS	Drugs
Drugs	Diabetic ketoacidosis
Female reproductive tract disease and pregnancy	
Acidosis	
Parotitis	
Cystic fibrosis	
Pneumonia	
Burns	
Anorexia nervosa and bulimia	
Abdominal aortic aneurysm	

ERCP, endoscopic retrograde cholangiopancreatography.

SUGGESTED READINGS

De Matos V, Mascarenhas M: Cystic fibrosis. In Liacouras C, Piccoli D, editors: *Pediatric Gastroenterology: The Requisites in Pediatrics*, St. Louis, 2008, Mosby Elsevier, pp 315-316.

Gelrud D, Gress F: Approach to the patient with elevated serum amylase or lipase. www.uptodate.com/contents/approach-to-the-patient-with-elevated-serum-amylase-or-lipase.

Lowe ME, Greer JB: Pancreatitis in children and adolescents. *Curr Gastroenterol Rep* 10(2):128-135, 2008.

Nousia-Arvanitakis S: Cystic fibrosis and the pancreas: recent scientific advances. *J Clin Gastroenterol* 29(2):138-142, 1999.

Sreedharan R, Mamula P: Congenital anomalies. In Liacouras C, Piccoli D, editors: *Pediatric Gastroenterology: The Requisites in Pediatrics*, St. Louis, 2008, Mosby Elsevier, pp 307-313.

Verma R, Wong T: Pancreatitis. In Liacouras C, Piccoli D, editors: *Pediatric Gastroenterology: The Requisites in Pediatrics*, St. Louis, 2008, Mosby Elsevier, pp 322-328.

Zyromski NJ, Sandoval JA, Pitt HA et al: Annular pancreas: dramatic differences between children and adults. *J Am Coll Surg* 206(5):1025-1027, 2008.

Hepatobiliary Disease

Melissa Leyva-Vega

115

Hepatobiliary disease in children is relatively uncommon but accounts for significant morbidity. The liver is the most commonly transplanted solid organ in children. The diagnosis of many liver diseases in children can be difficult given their rarity. Data on the incidence of liver disease and the economic burden associated with liver disease are limited in children. In adults, liver disease is the second most costly digestive disease.

NORMAL ANATOMY AND PHYSIOLOGY

The liver arises from endoderm between the third and fourth weeks of gestation. The liver is important in the production of bile, synthesis of coagulation factors, metabolism of proteins and glucose, and biotransformation of drugs and toxins. It consists of four lobes: right, left, caudate, and quadrate. An understanding of the liver's blood supply is useful when considering the consequences of portal hypertension (Figure 115-1). The portal vein and hepatic artery bring blood to the liver. The portal vein, which receives its supply from the splenic vein and mesenteric veins, carries about 75% of the liver's blood supply. The hepatic artery receives its blood supply from the celiac axis. Blood exits the liver through the hepatic vein, which empties into the inferior vena cava. Bile exits the liver by way of the intrahepatic bile ducts that lead to the right and left hepatic ducts, which merge to form the common hepatic duct. The common hepatic duct merges with the cystic duct from the gallbladder to form the common bile duct, which allows drainage of bile into the duodenum.

ETIOLOGY AND PATHOGENESIS

The most common pediatric liver diseases reflect infectious, metabolic, anatomic, autoimmune, and toxic etiologies. Metabolic liver diseases include Crigler-Najjar syndrome, galactosemia, tyrosinemia, hereditary fructose intolerance, urea cycle defects, bile acid synthetic disorders, and α-1-antitrypsin (AAT) deficiency. Anatomic liver diseases may be congenital (e.g., choledochal cysts, Alagille's syndrome) or acquired (e.g., cholelithiasis, Budd-Chiari syndrome). Common infections include hepatitis A, Epstein-Barr virus (EBV), and cytomegalovirus (CMV). Toxins or medications that frequently injure the liver include acetaminophen, ethanol, chemotherapeutic agents, and total parenteral nutrition (TPN). The most common autoimmune diseases of the liver are autoimmune hepatitis and primary sclerosing cholangitis. Systemic processes, such as hypothyroidism or panhypopituitarism and obesity (and nonalcoholic fatty liver disease [NAFLD]) also may affect the liver.

Two common manifestations of hepatobiliary disease are elevations in liver transaminases and jaundice. Elevations of aspartate aminotransferase (AST) and alanine aminotransferase (ALT) arise from hepatocyte injury. Elevations of γ-glutamyl transpeptidase (GGT) and alkaline phosphatase (ALP) result from impaired bile flow. Jaundice results from an elevation in conjugated or unconjugated bilirubin. Unconjugated hyperbilirubinemia occurs in about 60% of full-term infants and is most commonly physiologic jaundice partly caused by the immaturity of the bilirubin conjugation process (see Chapter 100). Unconjugated hyperbilirubinemia may also arise from hemolytic anemia (leading to overproduction of bilirubin) or abnormal bilirubin conjugation. Conjugated hyperbilirubinemia is always considered pathologic (see below).

CLINICAL PRESENTATION

Hepatobiliary diseases can present as acute fulminant liver failure or can be quiescent with an insidious onset. A thorough history can be very helpful in narrowing down the differential diagnosis of liver disease. Knowledge of the time of onset of all symptoms, including jaundice, is helpful. Breast milk jaundice develops after the seventh day of life, in contrast to breastfeeding jaundice, which occurs in the first week of life. Both of these entities present with unconjugated hyperbilirubinemia. Infants who have conjugated hyperbilirubinemia from the first day of life most likely have a pathologic process. The medical provider should ask about medications taken by the child or the mother (in the case of a breastfed infant). Dark urine, abdominal enlargement, easy bruising, epistaxis, and pruritus may be reported in the history of a patient with liver disease. A patient with portal hypertension may present with hematemesis from an esophageal variceal bleed (Figure 115-2). It is important to ask about potential exposures to viral hepatitis and recent travel. Family history is important to address the possibility of hepatitis B or C transmission.

All patients should undergo a thorough physical examination focusing on some key features. Scleral icterus occurs secondary to hyperbilirubinemia (conjugated or unconjugated). Skin jaundice is sometimes difficult to ascertain in dark-skinned children; therefore, careful attention to the sclera is important. Evaluation of the skin may also reveal bruises secondary to coagulopathy in a patient in liver failure or petechiae secondary to thrombocytopenia resulting from portal hypertension and hypersplenism. Heart murmurs can occur secondary to persistent pulmonic stenosis, which occurs in Alagille's disease. The lung examination may reveal signs of pleural effusions in a patient with liver disease who has significant ascites.

Abdominal inspection may reveal distension secondary to ascites or hepatosplenomegaly or prominent superficial abdominal veins in a patient with portal hypertension. Auscultation of the abdomen may reveal bruits in hepatic arteriovenous malformations. Hepatomegaly can be present, but a cirrhotic liver may actually be small in size. In the case of portal hypertension, the liver may be very firm or enlarged, and splenomegaly may be present. To get an accurate assessment of the size of the liver

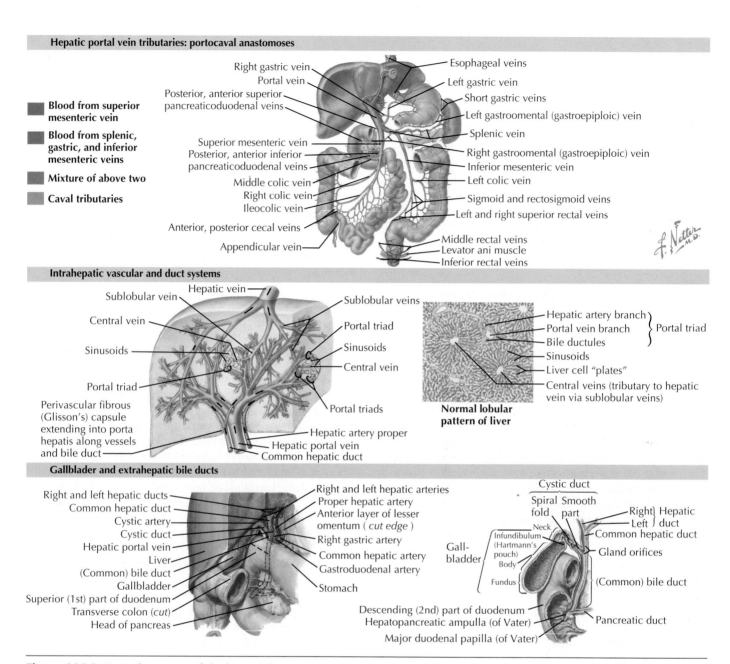

Figure 115-1 *Normal anatomy of the hepatobiliary system.*

and spleen, it is important to palpate the abdomen from the pelvis toward the costal margins because hepatomegaly can be missed if palpation of the liver edge begins too high in the abdomen. Right upper quadrant tenderness may occur in cholecystitis, choledocholithiasis, or acute hepatitis.

Differential Diagnosis

The differential diagnosis is vast and can be divided by age (Table 115-1). The provider should always focus on quickly diagnosing diseases requiring urgent treatment. In the Pediatric Acute Liver Failure Registry, the most common diagnosis is indeterminate (49%); additionally, acetaminophen intoxication accounts for 14%, metabolic disease accounts for 10%,

autoimmune hepatitis and infectious causes each account for 6%, and non-acetaminophen drug-induced liver disease accounts for 5% of cases. Data from the United Network for Organ Sharing show that the most common diagnoses in children who received a liver transplant from 1995 to 1999 were biliary atresia (BA; 35.6%), viral hepatitis (13%), metabolic liver disease (11.4%), intrahepatic cholestasis (7.9%), TPN (5.4%), and idiopathic cirrhosis (4.8%).

NEONATES AND INFANTS

Inborn errors of metabolism generally present in the neonatal period, as do congenital TORCH (toxoplasmosis or *Toxoplasma gondii*, **o**ther infections, **r**ubella, **C**MV, and **h**erpes simplex virus)

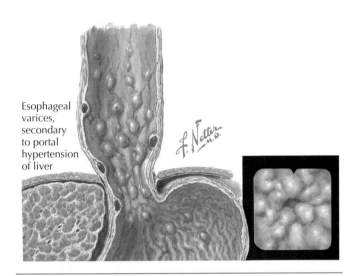

Esophageal varices, secondary to portal hypertension of liver

Figure 115-2 *Esophageal varices as a result of portal hypertension.*

infections. Urinary tract infections (UTIs) can cause cholestasis with conjugated hyperbilirubinemia. Neonatal hemachromatosis usually presents in the first few days of life with liver failure, cirrhosis, and splenomegaly. Patients with cystic fibrosis (CF) may have neonatal jaundice and benefit from early enzyme replacement therapy and nutritional intervention. Hereditary fructose intolerance can present in the infant after introduction of fruit juices, sucrose, or sorbitol.

BA is specific to neonates because it occurs only in the first several weeks of life. Although it is rare, early diagnosis and treatment are imperative to a good outcome. BA is a progressive, idiopathic, necroinflammatory process involving the biliary tree, which leads to obstruction of bile flow (Figure 115-3). At presentation, most infants are thriving and appear quite well despite being jaundiced. BA is treated surgically with hepatoportoenterostomy (see Figure 115-3). Despite this intervention, BA is still the most common reason for liver transplantation in children. To facilitate early detection of BA, it is very important that the evaluation of jaundiced infants beyond the first few days of life includes a fractionated bilirubin level. Any infant with a conjugated bilirubin greater than 2 mg/dL or more than 20% of the total bilirubin level requires a thorough evaluation (Figure 115-4).

OLDER CHILDREN AND ADOLESCENTS

Infectious causes are the most common reason for liver disease in children beyond infancy. Autoimmune hepatitis can present as either acute fulminant hepatitis or chronic hepatitis. Cholecystitis and choledocholithiasis should be considered in any child presenting with acute right upper quadrant pain. Patients with hemolytic syndromes are at increased risk for gallstones. Because of the obesity epidemic, an increasing number of children are diagnosed with NAFLD. These patients typically present with mild elevation in their transaminases. Over time, NAFLD can lead to cirrhosis.

Use of various prescribed (isoniazid, valproate, other antiseizure medications) or recreational (cocaine, "Ecstasy") drugs can

lead to acute liver failure. Intentional or nonintentional overdose of acetaminophen is a common cause for acute liver failure in older children and adolescents. Acetaminophen overdose accounts for 21% of all patients 3 years and older who present with acute liver failure (see Chapter 9).

Wilson's disease should be in the differential diagnosis of acute or chronic hepatitis in children and adolescents. The disease results from impaired biliary copper excretion that leads to progressive accumulation of copper in the liver. Over time, the liver becomes overloaded with copper, and copper begins to accumulate in the nervous system, corneas, and other organs. The presentation is variable; 25% of patients present with acute hepatitis, and a minority of patients present with acute liver failure, requiring liver transplantation. Some patients may first come to medical attention because of neuropsychiatric symptoms, such as fatigue and worsening school performance.

EVALUATION

Although the laboratory evaluation of a child with suspected hepatobiliary disease can be quite extensive, there are studies that should be performed at the beginning of every evaluation (Table 115-2). A complete cell count may reveal a low platelet count or a low white blood cell (WBC) count, which may be seen with cirrhosis and hypersplenism. An elevated WBC count may indicate an infectious process. AST and ALT levels are usually elevated in liver disease, but in liver failure, the transaminases may decrease because of near-total hepatocyte loss. In this case, the synthetic function of liver is compromised, and the prothrombin time is prolonged. High GGT and ALP levels are seen with cholestatic processes, with the rare exception of some types of bile acid synthetic disorder or progressive familiar intrahepatic cholestasis. AAT deficiency can present at any age and can have a variable presentation, including neonatal cholestasis, asymptomatic hepatomegaly, or advanced liver disease. A low AAT level can be suggestive of AAT deficiency, but protease inhibitor (PI) typing is necessary to make the diagnosis of AAT deficiency. Abdominal ultrasonography is a noninvasive way to exclude anatomic abnormalities, such a choledochal cyst, choledocholithiasis, tumors, or vascular anomalies. Ultrasound is also useful in assessing hepatosplenomegaly, especially in patients with ascites in whom the physical examination may be difficult. Lack of visualization of the gallbladder may occur in diseases that involve the biliary system, such as BA and Alagille's syndrome.

Neonates and Infants

As mentioned earlier, the evaluation of neonates with conjugated hyperbilirubinemia should focus on exclusion of disorders requiring immediate treatment, such as BA (see Figure 115-4). The evaluation for BA should take no more than 4 to 5 days. The newborn screen should be reviewed because it may help to exclude thyroid abnormalities, galactosemia, CF, and rare metabolic disorders. A catheterized urine culture should be obtained because UTIs can lead to cholestasis. In addition to a urine culture, a number of other urine tests should be obtained in the evaluation of a neonate with cholestasis, including urine succinylacetone (present in tyrosinemia), urine organic acids

Table 115-1 Differential Diagnosis of Hepatobiliary Disease in Children*

All Ages	Patients (%)
Viral infection: EBV; CMV; hepatitis A, B, and C; herpes simplex virus, echovirus, enterovirus, rubella, parvovirus, adenovirus, toxoplasmosis, syphilis, HIV, varicella	12.0
Bacterial infection: sepsis, UTI, tuberculosis, *Listeria*, treponema pallidum	
Extrahepatic obstruction: choledochal cyst, bile duct stricture or tumor, cholelithiasis)	
Drugs (valproate, isoniazid, acetaminophen)	1.1
Parenteral nutrition	5.4
ECMO	
CF	1.9
Ischemia secondary to congenital heart disease, asphyxia, cardiac surgery	
Metabolic: AAT deficiency, fatty acid oxidation defect, urea cycle disorders	11.4
Intrahepatic cholestasis: PFIC 1, 2, and 3; Alagille's syndrome	7.9
Idiopathic	4.8

Neonates and Infants	
See All Ages	
Biliary atresia	35.6
Endocrine (hypothyroidism, panhypopituitarism)	
Metabolic: galactosemia, glycogen storage disease, hereditary fructose intolerance, tyrosinemia	
Disorders of lipid metabolism: Wolman's disease, Niemann-Pick disease, Gaucher's disease	
Bile acid synthesis defects	
Idiopathic neonatal hepatitis	
Mitochondrial disorders	
Neonatal lupus erythematosus	
Neonatal hemachromatosis	
Congenital hepatic fibrosis and autosomal recessive polycystic kidney disease	2.1
Peroxisomal disorders (Zellweger's syndrome)	

Young Children	
See All Ages	
Autoimmune hepatitis	2.6
Malignancy	3.5

Older Children and Adolescents	
See All Ages and Young Children	
Acetaminophen overdose	
NAFLD	
Primary sclerosing cholangitis (≈68% have IBD)	1.8
Wilson's disease	1.1
Fatty liver disease of pregnancy	

*Percentages of total cases of liver transplant recipients (UNOS 1995–1999) identified as having the listed diagnosis are shown.

AAT, α-1-antitrypsin; CF, cystic fibrosis; CMV, cytomegalovirus; EBV, Epstein-Barr virus; ECMO, extracorporeal membrane oxygenation; IBD, inflammatory bowel disease; NAFLD, Nonalcoholic fatty liver disease; NANB, non-A, non-B; PFIC, progressive familial intrahepatic cholestasis; UTI, urinary tract infection.

(abnormal in organic acidemias, peroxisomal diseases), and urine bile acids (bile acid synthetic defects). An ophthalmologic examination by a pediatric ophthalmologist may reveal posterior embryotoxon, which is seen in Alagille's syndrome. A sweat test should also be obtained if CF is not part of the state's newborn screen.

If BA is suspected, the infant should be promptly referred to a pediatric gastroenterologist. In selecting the referral center, one should remember that research has shown that the success of a hepatoportoenterostomy depends on the expertise of the center. The diagnostic approach varies by institution and may include hepatobiliary scintigraphy, liver biopsy, or both. Because the histologic changes in BA can mimic other diseases (e.g., TPN cholestasis and AAT), it is extremely important that biopsies be read by an experienced pathologist in the context of the patient's history and workup. All patients suspected of having BA should have a cholangiogram, which is the gold standard in the diagnosis of BA. Most commonly, the cholangiogram is done intraoperatively, but an interventional radiologist can also do it percutaneously.

Children and Adolescents

All patients in this age group should be tested for viral hepatitis (EBV, CMV, enterovirus, hepatitis A, B, and C). One should also obtain an autoimmune hepatitis panel, which includes autoantibodies to constituents of the nucleus, liver-kidney-microsome antigens, and smooth muscle. In older children and adolescents, a low ceruloplasmin is suggestive of Wilson's disease and should be followed up with a 24-hour urine collection for

Biliary atresia

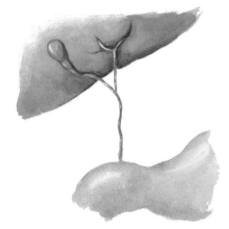

Hepatoportoenterostomy

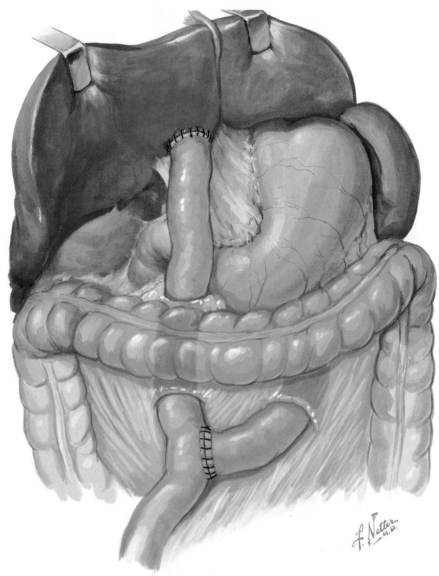

Figure 115-3 *Biliary atresia.*

copper measurement. A sweat test should be considered, especially in a child with failure to thrive or lung disease. Ultrasound is the best initial imaging test for biliary stones. Magnetic resonance cholangiopancreatography can be used to diagnose primary sclerosing cholangitis. Children with persistent cholestasis or hepatitis and otherwise negative workup results should undergo a liver biopsy. Liver biopsy may not only be helpful in making the diagnosis, but it can also assist in staging the disease by showing the presence or absence of fibrosis.

MANAGEMENT

Many liver diseases are managed supportively and ultimately require liver transplantation. However, a number of hepatobiliary diseases may respond to specific therapies (Table 115-3).

Only a few hepatobiliary diseases are treated with endoscopic intervention or surgically. Endoscopic retrograde cholangiopancreatography can be therapeutic in choledocholithiasis; these patients should undergo cholecystectomy. Patients with acute liver failure should be admitted to an intensive care unit for monitoring of fluids, glucose, electrolytes, coagulation abnormalities, and encephalopathy. *N*-acetylcysteine has been shown to improve survival in acetaminophen-induced liver injury.

Some of the complications associated with cirrhosis or portal hypertension are gastrointestinal bleeding, ascites, and hypersplenism. An esophageal variceal bleed can occur secondary to portal hypertension (see Figure 115-2). After they are hemodynamically stable, these patients usually undergo endoscopic intervention, such as sclerotherapy or banding. Diuretics are commonly used in the management of ascites. Abdominal

Table 115-2 Laboratory Evaluation of Hepatobiliary Disease

Test	Significance
AST, ALT, LDH	Elevation results from injury of hepatocytes
GGT, ALP	Elevation results from impaired bile flow
Fractionated bilirubin	Elevation of conjugated bilirubin in cholestasis
Complete metabolic panel	Albumin is low in compromised liver synthetic function
PT and PTT	PT prolongation may reflect abnormal synthetic function or vitamin K deficiency
CBC	Thrombocytopenia and lymphopenia in advanced liver disease with hypersplenism
Ammonia	Elevated in advanced liver disease; important to assess this in liver patients with altered level of consciousness
Sweat test	Many state newborn screens include test for the more common CF mutations only; therefore, sweat test should be obtained if CF is suspected
AAT serum level and PI type	Serum level is low in AAT deficiency; PI type is needed to make the definitive diagnosis

AAT, α-1-antitrypsin; ALP, aspartate aminotransferase; ALT, alanine aminotransferase; AST, aspartate aminotransferase; CBC, complete cell count; CF, cystic fibrosis; GGT, γ-glutamyl transpeptidase; LDH, lactate dehydrogenase; PI, protease inhibitor; PT, prothrombin time; PTT, partial thromboplastin time.

paracentesis may be diagnostic (if spontaneous bacterial peritonitis is suspected) and therapeutic. β-Blockers and portosystemic shunts are sometimes used in pediatric patients with portal hypertension.

In the management of patients with cholestasis, the most commonly used choleretic agent is ursodeoxycholic acid. Some patients develop severe pruritus secondary to the accumulation of biliary salts. These patients may benefit from rifampin, phenobarbital, or surgical biliary diversion. The increased metabolic needs of chronic liver disease and malabsorption of fat secondary to cholestasis may lead to poor nutritional status in

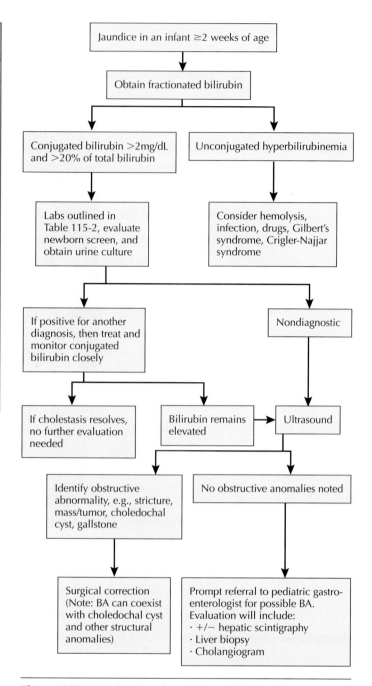

Figure 115-4 Evaluation of a newborn with jaundice.

Table 115-3 Examples of Specific Therapies for Liver Diseases

Disease	Therapy
Chronic hepatitis B	Lamivudine, IFN-α
Chronic hepatitis C	Ribavirin, IFN-α
Galactosemia	Elimination of dietary galactose
Acetaminophen overdose	N-acetylcysteine
Wilson's disease	Chelation
Autoimmune hepatitis	Corticosteroids, azathioprine, 6-MP
Nonalcoholic fatty liver disease	Weight loss and control

IFN, interferon; MP, mercaptopurine.

patients with liver disease. Growth and nutritional status should be monitored carefully. The levels of fat-soluble vitamins should be measured, and vitamins should be supplemented as needed.

Liver transplantation is the ultimate treatment for many hepatobiliary diseases. Children account for about 12% of all liver transplant recipients.

FUTURE DIRECTIONS

Currently, the outcomes of pediatric liver transplantation are quite good, although further improvements in antirejection therapies are needed. There is currently active research in the use of antifibrotic agents that may be useful in extending the time to transplant in patients with chronic liver disease.

N-acetylcysteine is also currently being studied as a treatment in non-acetaminophen acute liver failure.

SUGGESTED READINGS

Arya G, Balistreri WF: Pediatric liver disease in the United States: Epidemiology and impact. *J Gastroenterol Hepatol* 17:521-525, 2002.

Haber BA, Russo P: Biliary atresia. *Gastroenterol Clin North Am* 32:891-911, 2003.

Squires RH, Shneider BL, Bucuvalas J, et al: Acute liver failure in children: the first 348 patients in the Pediatric Acute Liver Failure Study Group. *J Pediatr* 148:652-658, 2005.

Suchy, FJ, Sokol RJ, Balistreri WF: *Liver Disease in Children*, ed 3, New York, 2007, Cambridge University Press.

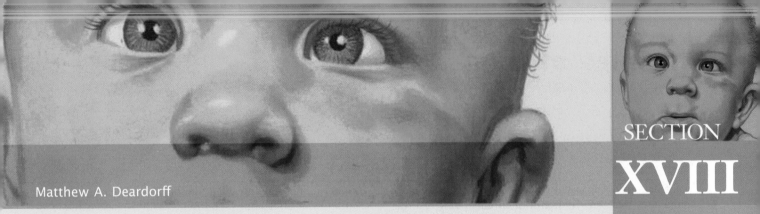

Matthew A. Deardorff

Genetic and Metabolic Disorders

116

Principles of Human Genetics

Kathryn Chatfield

Recent data have suggested that 71% of pediatric hospital admissions were for children with an underlying disorder with a significant genetic component, including 34% with a clear genetic etiology. These genetic disorders comprise chromosomal abnormalities (0.4%-0.6%), diseases caused by a disruption of a single gene (4%-7%), disorders with a genetic association (4%-22%), and malformations of unclear etiology (14%-19%).

Approximately 6500 specific genes have been associated with human disease. As a result of sequencing the human genome, our understanding of human genetics has grown at a rapid pace. Analysis of our genome indicates that there are 20,000 to 25,000 individual genes that determine structure and function of human fetuses, children, and adults, and theoretically, a mutation that disrupts the normal function of any one of these genes could result in human disease. As we learn more about the relationships among genes and human disease, it is clear that an understanding of modes of inheritance and the role of genetic testing will be critical for the care of pediatric patients.

CHROMOSOME STRUCTURE AND NOMENCLATURE

The human genome is composed of deoxyribonucleic acid (DNA), the genetic code for all organisms. Chromosomes are located in the cell nucleus and are composed of DNA packaged with proteins that exist in 23 pairs in every human diploid cell—22 pairs of autosomes (numbered 1-22) and one pair of sex chromosomes (X and Y). Each pair of chromosomes is connected at a region called the *centromere*, creating two arms for each pair of chromosomes (Figure 116-1). In most chromosomes, the centromere is located closer to one end than the other, forming a short *p* arm and a longer *q* arm. Chromosomes can be visualized under a microscope when they are captured during the metaphase stage of the cell cycle. Using a special technique known as Giemsa staining, metaphase chromosomes can be used to determine a *karyotype* for an individual (see Figure 116-1). A karyotype result indicates the total number of chromosomes identified in the cell, typically 46, followed by the sex chromosomes observed, usually XX or XY. Therefore, a normal female karyotype is 46,XX, and a normal male karyotype is 46,XY.

Giemsa staining also allows chromosomal structural differences, and *aneuploidy*, or imbalance in genetic material, to be identified. The most easily identified forms of aneuploidy include *monosomy*, the presence of only one of two normal copies of a pair of chromosomes, and *trisomy*, three copies of a chromosome. Karyotypes are performed on 20 or more cells to determine whether aneuploidy is present in all cells from a patient. To denote aneuploidy, a "+" or "−" is used to indicate an extra or missing chromosome or portion of a chromosome. For example, a female with trisomy 21 would be denoted 47,XX,+21.

Another monosomy involving the short arm of chromosome 4, causing Wolf-Hirschhorn syndrome, would be designated in an affected male as 46,XY,4p-. Smaller chromosomal alterations that result from duplicated or deleted region of a chromosome are designated as *dup* or *del* followed by the chromosome segment that is missing or extra [e.g., 46,XY del(1)(p36)].

METHODS OF DETECTING ANEUPLOIDY

With advances in molecular biology, more specific techniques for evaluating aneuploidy have been developed. In the late 1980s, fluorescent in situ hybridization (FISH) was developed as a method to detect specific chromosomal deletions (Figure 116-2). A fluorescent-labeled DNA sequence that is complementary to a known region of a chromosome is hybridized to a set of chromosomes in a cell. If two copies of the chromosome sequence are present, two fluorescent probes are visualized; if only one probe is seen, it is inferred that one copy of the chromosomal segment is deleted. FISH is used to confirm karyotype findings or to detect deletions too small to be visualized with a standard karyotype. FISH also permits analysis of uncultured cells, permitting diagnoses to be made more rapidly.

Duplicated or deleted regions of the genome must be more than 3 million base pairs in size to be visualized via karyotyping and more than 100 kilobases to be visualized by FISH. Recently, more sophisticated methods of identifying chromosomal alterations of 10 to 100 kilobases to be detected have been introduced. These array-based methods use bacterial artificial chromosome (BAC) probe comparative genomic hybridization (CGH) or synthetic oligonucleotide hybridization probes or single nucleotide polymorphism (SNP) probes. All approaches analyze DNA from a test subject and compare the amount of signal at 5000 with 2 million positions across the genome with that of a normal reference patient's sample. Often, both pathologic and normal variants are noted and collectively are called *copy number variants* (CNVs). Those that are believed to cause disease have been termed *copy number alterations* (CNAs).

MITOSIS, MEIOSIS, AND GAMETE FORMATION

Diploid cells are maintained through the process of *mitosis* in dividing somatic cell types. Typical cells have four stages to their growth and division cycle (Figure 116-3). The first stage, G1 (for growth 1 or gap 1), is largely composed of growth and has no active cell division. During the next stage (S), DNA is replicated or synthesized to form a four-copied, or tetraploid, genome. After another growth phase (G2) during which the replicated genome is surveyed to correct any aberrations, a division phase (D), during which mitosis occurs, results in two new daughter cells. During mitosis, the replicated tetraploid genome is divided so that each daughter cell receives a diploid

Karotypes

Normal male

♂

Normal female

♀

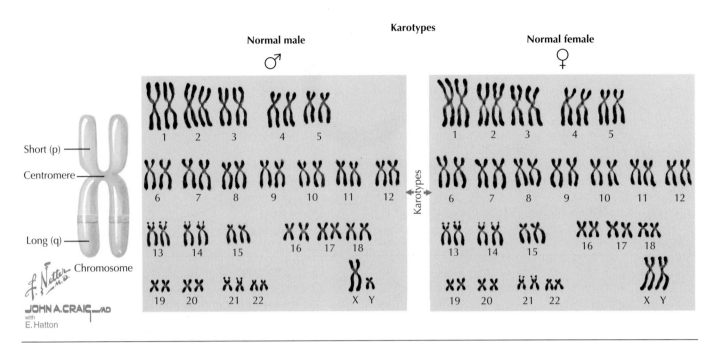

Short (p)

Centromere

Long (q)

Chromosome

JOHN A. CRAIG—AD
with
E. Hatton

Figure 116-1 *Chromosome structure and karyotype.*

complement of chromosomes after cell division. Mitosis is divided into four stages—prophase, metaphase, anaphase, and telophase. At the beginning of prophase, the duplicated chromosomes are elongated and appear as a single chromosome, although two sister chromatids have already been formed by this stage. At the end of prophase, the sister chromatids have become more condensed, and the centrioles are seen at opposite poles

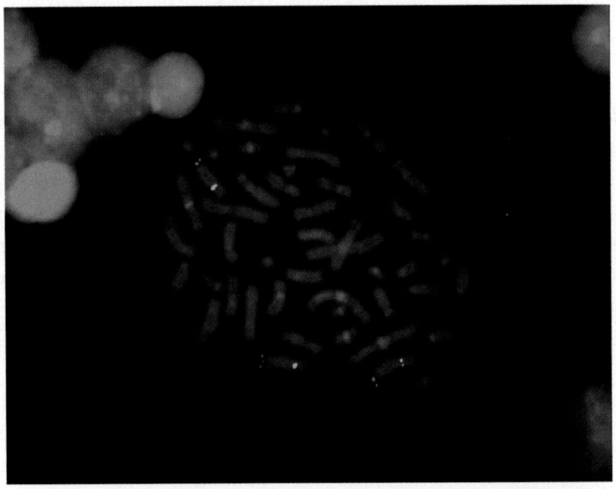

The photograph demonstrates fluorescence in situ hybridization (FISH) carried out on a metaphase spread demonstrating trisomy 8 in this cell. The chromosome 8 centromere is labeled in green, and a chromosome 8q subtelomeric probe is labeled in red. Note the presence of three copies of chromosome 8 in this cell. *(Courtesy Nancy B. Spinner, CytoGenomics Laboratory, The Children's Hospital of Philadelphia).*

Figure 116-2 *Fluorescent in situ hybridization (FISH) detection of aneuploidy.*

of the nucleus. During metaphase, the nuclear membrane disintegrates, and the formation of the mitotic spindle made up of fibers that connect each chromatid of a sister chromatid pair to opposite centrioles, causing them to align in the middle of the nucleus. The centromere of each chromosome also divides in preparation for migration of sister chromatids to opposite centriole spindles. It is during metaphase that chromosomes are typically viewed under the microscope because this is when the chromosomes are most condensed and the mitotic spindle can be arrested with the chemical colchicine. During anaphase, sister chromatics are segregated and migrate toward opposite poles along the spindle. Telophase is marked by the arrival of chromosomes at opposite poles, the disintegration of the spindle, and reformation of a nuclear membrane.

Haploid cells are generated via a special type of germ cell division called *meiosis*, so that each egg or sperm contributes half of the genetic material to an embryo (see Figure 116-3). A haploid complement of chromosomes consists of one of every *autosome* (a non-sex chromosome) and an X *or* Y. In this way, each parent contributes 23 chromosomes to produce a full complement of 46 in an embryo. Meiosis also permits some exchange of genetic material, thus creating genetic variability between gametes. Recombination events, usually at least one per chromosome, result in no two haploid gametes being identical. Recombination events are thought to occur twice as frequently in females as in males. Meiosis is divided into two stages, meiosis I and II. In meiosis I, similar to mitosis, a cell replicates its genome and then divides to create two cells with a full complement of 23 chromosome pairs. In meiosis II, daughter chromatids are divided among daughter cells, such that each contains a single copy of each of the 22 autosomes and an X *or* Y sex chromosome. In males, all four resulting haploid cells differentiate into sperm. In females, only one of these four haploid set of chromosomes ends up as an ova; the other products become *polar bodies*. A common cause of aneuploidy is thought to arise

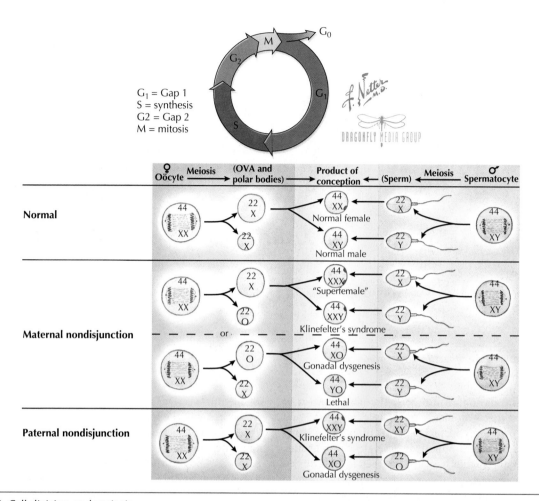

G_1 = Gap 1
S = synthesis
G2 = Gap 2
M = mitosis

Figure 116-3 *Cell division and meiosis.*

from nondisjunction, or failure of the chromosomes to divide equally between daughter cells during meiosis.

GENE STRUCTURE

DNA is a double-stranded macromolecule composed of complementary pairs of the purine bases, adenosine and guanine, and the pyrimidine bases, thymine and cytosine (Figure 116-4). The entire haploid genome is composed of some 3 billion base pairs, with each chromosome composed of 50 to 150 million base pairs. Of the entire genome, only about 2% is *coding* sequence (i.e., encodes genes that are transcribed into proteins). The remainder of the genome is *noncoding* sequence presumably involved in structural integrity of chromosomes or control of gene expression. A typical gene is *transcribed* into RNA (RNA), which in turn is *translated* into a functional protein composed of amino acids. Elements of the genomic DNA surrounding a gene, known as promoters and enhancers, serve to regulate the location, timing. and level of transcription. Before translation, transcribed RNA is processed to form messenger RNA (mRNA) by removing or splicing out intervening sequences known as introns to result in a mature mRNA containing only exons. Mature mRNA moves from the nucleus to the cytoplasm of a cell, where it can be translated into protein in a structure called the ribosome. The ribosome scans the mRNA codons, triplets

of nucleotides that encode a specific amino acid, or a start or stop signal. Using the mRNA as a template, ribosomal RNA (rRNA), ribosomal proteins, and transfer RNA (tRNA), the ribosome delivers the appropriate amino acid into the chain of amino acids in the formation of a translated protein. At any stage in the process of transcription or translation, several types of errors can occur, resulting in alterations of protein structure, function, or both (see Figure 116-4).

MODES OF INHERITANCE

An individual inherits genetic material from the mother and father when an egg and sperm fuse during fertilization. Thus, both a maternal and paternal copy of every gene, or *alleles*, are present in the genome. There are exceptions to this rule, as is evident in males, because the Y chromosome does not carry a matching allele for every gene on the X chromosome. The combination of two specific alleles determines the *genotype*. The nature of the interaction between two alleles of a given gene determines the *mode of inheritance* of a disorder caused by mutations in that gene.

Genetic diseases can also be partially inherited as illustrated by the principles of *penetrance* and *expressivity*. *Penetrance* is the likelihood that an individual who carries a disease-causing gene will manifest signs and symptoms of the disorder. A highly

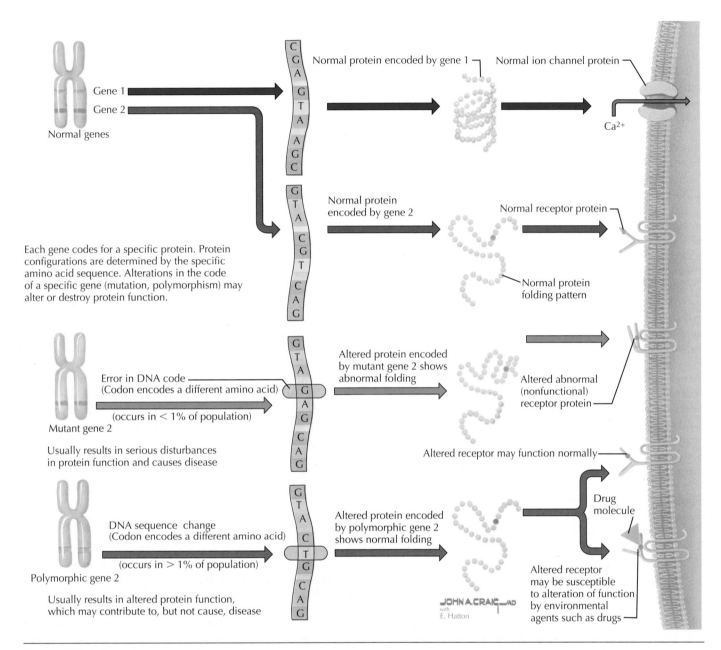

Figure 116-4 *Gene structure and expression.*

penetrant disorder will manifest in nearly all individuals who carry the gene. *Expressivity* describes the variation in the phenotype, or clinical presentation, that results from a gene alteration, or *genotype*. Expressivity can be variable, meaning that individuals with the same genotype may have significantly different manifestations in their phenotype or in the severity of their disease.

Autosomal Dominant Inheritance

In some genetic disorders, a single altered copy of a gene is sufficient to cause disease. This is called *dominant* inheritance and often means that the parent and the progeny who inherited the defective gene are affected. *Autosomal dominant* implies that the gene is on a non-sex chromosome. Although one allele of

the gene may be functional, the allele with the disease-causing mutation is "dominant" over the normal allele. Examples of autosomal dominant disorders include neurofibromatosis type I, achondroplasia, and Huntington's disease. In addition, the affected individual is typically *heterozygous*, meaning the two alleles of the gene are not identical (i.e., one normal and one mutated).

Autosomal Recessive Inheritance

Autosomal recessive disorders result from alterations present in both alleles of a gene. Most autosomal recessive disorders are the result from inheritance of one defective gene from each parent. Individuals with an autosomal recessive disorder, therefore, typically have parents who are heterozygous *carriers* for the disease-causing gene. Carriers are usually unaffected because one functional copy of the gene is often sufficient to mask the effect of the mutant allele. When each allele of the gene has exactly the same mutation, the individual is *homozygous* for the mutation. However, unique disease-causing mutations can be inherited from each parent as well. Such an individual would manifest disease as the result of being a *compound heterozygote* for the recessive disorder. An example of an autosomal recessive disorder is sickle cell disease. In sickle cell disease, one can be homozygous for a disease-causing mutation as in sickle cell SS disease. One can also be a compound heterozygote as in sickle cell SC disease.

Sex-Linked Inheritance

A majority of inherited diseases are the result of disease-causing mutations in autosomal genes. However, a number of diseases are known to occur from a defective gene carried on one of the sex chromosomes, typically the X chromosome. X-linked disorders primarily affect males because the Y chromosome does not carry a matching allele for every gene present on the X chromosome. Therefore, a mutation in a gene present on the X chromosome in a male often behaves like a recessive trait because there is only one allele, termed *X-linked recessive*. X-linked disorders do not typically affect females because their normal allele masks a recessive trait. However, it is common for females to manifest signs and symptoms of an X-linked disorder as a result of *skewed X inactivation*. In every cell that carries two (or more) X chromosomes, one of the X chromosomes is inactivated, such that most of the alleles on that chromosome are not expressed. If in a female carrier of an X-linked disorder, a disproportionate number of normal or non-mutation-carrying X chromosomes are inactivated, she may manifest mild symptoms of the disease. The phenotype of a female carrier of an X-linked disorder with skewed X inactivation is usually mild compared with an affected male.

Mitochondrial Inheritance

The vast majority of human genes reside in the nucleus of the cell. However, 37 genes are found within mitochondria in a double-stranded DNA molecule (mtDNA). Each mitochondrion carries two to 10 copies of mtDNA encoding 13 proteins, 22 transfer RNAs, and two subunits of ribosomal RNA. As in nuclear-encoded DNA, mutations causing disease can be found in mitochondrial DNA. A unique feature of disorders caused by mitochondrial DNA mutations is that they are inherited maternally because the mitochondria in an embryo are almost universally derived from the 100,000 to 1 million copies of mtDNA in the egg. Another unique feature of mitochondrial genetics is called *heteroplasmy*, in which both normal and abnormal mitochondria can be present within the same cell, which can lead to a high degree of variability in disorders caused by defects in the mitochondria.

Uniparental Disomy

Normal embryos are derived from maternal and paternal copies of each chromosome. Occasionally, both chromosomes and allelic regions of chromosome pairs can be derived from either the maternal or paternal contribution. This is called *uniparental disomy* (UPD) and can be either *isodisomy*, in which both chromosomes inherited from one parent are identical, or *heterodisomy*, in which both of the different chromosomes from one parent are inherited. UPD may result in autosomal recessive disease if the isodisomic chromosome carries a recessive allele. UPD can also result in disease when *imprinting*, or the parent-specific expression of the maternal or paternal alleles of a gene is required for normal expression. For example, Prader-Willi syndrome can be caused by maternal UPD of the q arm of chromosome 15, and Angelman's syndrome is caused by paternal UPD of the same region.

Mosaicism

Mosaicism is a condition in which not all cells in an individual are genetically identical. Mosaicism can occur when chromosomal aneuploidy or a gene mutation arises after conception in a single cell of an early-stage embryo. As this single cell divides, it creates a subset of cells in the developing fetus that carry the chromosomal abnormality or mutation, but the rest do not. This results in heterogeneity of genotype *within* the various tissues of the individual. An example of a disorder that is only seen in mosaic form is tetrasomy 12p, or Pallister-Killian syndrome. Mosaicism is diagnosed when aneuploidy is identified in some tissues, such as skin fibroblasts, but is absent from other tissues, such as white blood cells from peripheral blood. Mosaicism can thus be missed on a routine karyotype. Down syndrome can also be found in a mosaic form. At times, the severity of the disorder can be inferred by the percentage of mosaic cells found.

Polygenic-Multifactorial Inheritance

Not all congenital anomalies can be explained by a chromosomal alteration or single gene mutation yet the anomalies are still related to genetic differences found within families. These anomalies are thought to be the result of multiple genes that are important in embryologic development of organs and physical features. In the same way that polygenic traits determine height, facial features, and age of pubertal changes, groups of genes inherited from parents can influence the likelihood of organ malformation and craniofacial abnormalities. Examples of polygenic traits that can have a risk of recurrence in families are congenital heart defects, urogenital tract and renal anomalies, cleft lip and palate, and spina bifida.

EVALUATION AND DIAGNOSIS OF GENETIC SYNDROMES
Categories of Dysmorphic Disorders

A genetic syndrome is often suspected in children who have multiple congenital anomalies or who have *dysmorphic*, or atypically formed, facial or physical features. A pattern of changes that results from a common cause is termed a *syndrome*. Genetic syndromes result from the expression of a gene in more than one tissue of the body, and mutations subsequently affect different organs of different embryologic origins. A pattern of malformations arising from embryologically distinct tissues in nonrandom fashion with no clear cause is known as an *association*. This is different from a *field defect* or complex, which describes a series of malformations that arise from disruption of a single embryologic tissue. Malformation of specific organ systems can also be the result of *dysplasia*, the disorganization of a specific tissue on a cellular level that can be localized or general and can be system specific or organ specific.

When a primary embryologic defect leads to multiple additional and consequent defects, it is called a *sequence*. A well-recognized malformation sequence is Pierre-Robin sequence, which involves a small jaw, a large U-shaped cleft palate, and a large protruding tongue. The jaw malformation is thought to lead to upward displacement of the tongue and failure of the palate to form appropriately. Although Pierre-Robin sequence can be an isolated sequence not related to a genetic syndrome, it can also be found in syndromes with genetic causes.

Congenital malformations and dysmorphology can be genetic in origin, but it is important to recognize that they can also be caused by nongenetic mechanisms. A group of anomalies and dysmorphic features can occur as the result of environmental in utero exposures, or teratogens. Common exposures that result in recognized dysmorphology and malformations include alcohol, valproic acid, and TORCH (toxoplasmosis or *Toxoplasma gondii*, other infections, rubella, cytomegalovirus, and herpes simplex virus) infections.

Malformations can also be caused by an isolated *disruption* or *deformation* during embryogenesis unrelated to a genetic defect or teratogens (Figure 116-5). Disruption is a mechanical factor that can occur in utero, resulting in an isolated or in a series of structural abnormalities. An example of a disruption event that can lead to congenital anomalies is amniotic band syndrome. Limb and craniofacial defects are thought to arise from either a vascular disruption or strangulation of fetal digits or extremities by strands of a partially disrupted amniotic sac. Deformation describes an abnormal shape or form caused by mechanical forces from within the fetus or outside the fetus in the intrauterine environment. Examples of deformation include clubfoot and congenital dislocation of the hip. Deformations can occur as the result of crowding in the uterus, as in twin gestations.

Evaluation of Children with Dysmorphism

Although genetic testing is often used for definitive diagnosis of a genetic syndrome, other information must be collected to effectively generate a differential diagnosis to guide management and testing. First, a careful history should be obtained that includes the prenatal course, birth history, medical history preceding diagnostic evaluation, and assessment of the motor and cognitive development. Second, a complete family pedigree should be obtained to determine possible heredity or familial risk factors pertaining to a diagnosis. Third, a full physical examination, including anthropomorphic measurements and careful attention to dysmorphic features, is necessary (Table 116-1). With all of this information collected, literature review is often needed to assist in generating an appropriate differential diagnosis. Comparison of findings with similar cases is of particular value with the rarer conditions. Finally, cytogenetic,

Malformation

Myelomeningocele

Deformation

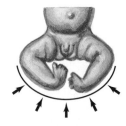

Clubfoot

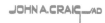

Disruption

Limb reduction deficit

Figure 116-5 *Errors in morphogenesis.*

molecular diagnostic testing, and specific gene testing are used to confirm or exclude a clinical diagnosis.

FUTURE DIRECTIONS

Human genetics is a dynamic and rapidly evolving field in basic science and in clinical medicine. As our knowledge of the organization of the human genome expands and technologies for deciphering the genetic code are refined, we will improve our understanding of how genetic differences cause or influence disease. Rapid, high-throughput methods of genetic analysis have already made it possible to assess children with major and minor malformations both before and after birth and to identify previously unrecognized causes of syndromes and disorders. Emerging technologies such ultra-high-resolution arrays and whole genome sequence analysis are on the cusp of clinical utilization. These breakthroughs will not only further our fundamental understanding of genetic variability in humans but will also be critical for understanding more complex genetic interactions that cause human disease, how they create phenotypic variability, and how environmental factors may modify disease presentation.

Table 116-1 The Dysmorphology Examination

System	Features	Examples
Growth parameters	Weight	Overgrowth, failure to thrive
	Length	Small or large for gestational age
	Head circumference	Microcephaly, macrocephaly
Head	Size	Microcephaly, microcephaly
	Shape	Dolichocephaly, brachycephaly, premature fusion of sutures
	Fontanelles	Size, number, premature or prolonged closure
	Hair	Sparse, hirsuit, unusual hairline, whorls
	Forehead	Bossed, temporal narrowing
	Jaw	Micrognathic, retrognathic
Eyes	Shape	Almond
	Spacing	Hypoteloric (narrow), hyperteloric (wide)
	Structure	Sclera color, cataract, coloboma
	Palpebral fissures	Small, lengthened, upslanted, downslanted, epicanthus
	Setting	Deep set, proptotic
	Eyebrows	Synophrys
Ears	Placement	Low set, posteriorly rotated
	Form	Short, long, square, overfolded or crumpled helix
	Pre- and postauricular surface	Preauricular pits or tags, postauricular pits
Nose	Tip	Small, bulbous
	Alae nasi	Hypoplastic
	Bridge	Depressed, broad
	Choanae	Atretic, stenotic
	Philtrum	Long, short, smooth
Mouth	Size and shape	Small, bow shaped,
	Lips	Thin, thick, downturned, cleft
	Frenulum	Absent, tight
	Teeth	Natal, absent, single central incisor, enamel defects
	Tongue	Macroglossia, protuberant
	Palate	Hard or soft cleft, high, narrow
	Uvula	Wide, bifid
Neck	Length	Short
	Skin	Webbed, excess nuchal
Chest	Cardiac	Murmurs
	Lung	Absent breath sounds, stridor, wheeze, bowel sounds
	Sternum	Pectus deformity
	Shape	Narrow, barrel shaped
	Nipple placement	Wide or narrow, supernumerary
Abdomen	Umbilicus	Hernia, omphalocele, two-vessel cord
	Organs	Hepatomegaly, splenomegaly
Back	Shape	Scoliosis
	Sacrum	Dimple, tuft, myelomeningocele
Genitourinary	Phallus or clitoris	Hypospadias, chordee, clitoromegaly, ambiguous genitalia
	Labia, scrotum, or testes	Bifid scrotum, undescended testes
Extremities	Limb form	Brachymelia (short), rhizomelia (shortening of proximal limbs), mesomelia (shortening of intermediate segments of long bones), acromelia (shortening of distal limbs)
	Digit form	Clinodactyly, camptodactyly
	Digit number	Polydactyly, preaxial, postaxial, oligodactyly
	Digit fusion	Syndactyly
Dermatoglyphics	Digits	Predominance of arches or whorls
	Palm	Single crease, distal triradius
Skin	Pigmentation	Café-au-lait macules, hypopigmented macules, pigmentary variation
	Vasculature	Hemangioma, telangiectasia, port-wine stain
	Sweat glands	Absent
Neurologic	Mental status	Alertness, lethargy, unresponsiveness
	Tone	Hypertonic, hypotonic
	Movements	Seizures, chorea, fasciculations, symmetry
	Vision and hearing	Response to vision and auditory stimuli

SUGGESTED READINGS

Baird PA, Anderson TW, Newcombe HB, et al: Genetic disorders in children and young adults: a population based study. *Am J Med Genet* 42:677-693, 1988.

Hall JG, Powers EK, McIlvaine RT, Ean VH: The frequency and financial burden of genetic disease in a pediatric hospital. *Am J Med Genet* 1(4):417-436, 1978.

Lander ES, Linton, LM, Birren B, et al: Initial sequencing and analysis of the human genome. *Nature* 409:860-921, 2001.

McCandless, SE, Brunger JW, Cassidy SB: The burden of genetic disease on inpatient care in a children's hospital. *Am J Hum Genet* 74:121-127, 2004.

Scriver CR, Neal JL, Saginur R, et al: The frequency of genetic disease and congenital malformation among patients in a pediatric hospital. *Can Med Assoc J* 108:1111-1115, 1973.

Stevenson DA, Carey JC: Contribution of malformations and genetic disorders to mortality in a children's hospital. *Am J Med Genet A* 126A(4):393-397, 2004.

U.S. Department of Energy: Genomic Science Program. Available at http://genomics.energy.gov.

Wang ET, Sandberg R, Luo S, et al: Alternative isoform regulation in human tissue transcriptomes. *Nature* 456(7221):470-476, 2008.

Nilika B. Shah

*D*own syndrome, or trisomy 21, is the most common chromosomal abnormality among live-born infants and is the most frequent microscopically identifiable genetic cause of mental retardation. An extra copy of chromosome 21 results in an overexpression of the genes found on this chromosome to result in the phenotypic differences seen in patients with Down syndrome. This disorder is characterized by a variety of dysmorphic features, congenital malformations, and medical problems (Figures 117-1).

ETIOLOGY AND PATHOGENESIS

Although trisomy 21 is responsible for 1:150 first-trimester spontaneous abortions, the live-born incidence is approximately 1:800-1:1000, and its incidence is highly correlated with advanced maternal age. The additional copy of chromosome 21 usually occurs from meiosis I nondisjunction, when the pair of homologous chromosomes 21 fail to separate. Errors that occur during meiosis are nearly always maternal in origin, and the incidence increases with advancing maternal age. This is likely attributable to the years from oocyte formation during maternal embryogenesis to the time of fertilization that the oocyte spends suspended in meiosis I.

Although trisomy of chromosome 21 (e.g., 47,XY, +21) in which a complete extra copy of chromosome 21 is present, causes approximately 94% of cases, other causes are also seen. Approximately 2% to 3% of cases of trisomy 21 can present with mosaicism (e.g., 47,XY, +21 [50%] or 46,XY[50%]) in which there is a mixture of trisomic cells and normal cells. This can lead to an attenuated phenotype, but it depends on the relative mosaicism of different tissues. Finally, approximately 3% to 4% of cases are caused by a Robertsonian translocation, in which the q arm of chromosome 21 is translocated onto another chromosome. This results in a fetus with 46 chromosomes but three copies of the long arm of chromosome 21, which carries all of the functional genes of this chromosome (e.g., 46,XY,der(15:21)(q10;q10), +21; Figure 117-1). Although most Robertsonian translocations are new mutations and occur regardless of maternal age, it is important to distinguish the cause and rule out a translocation carrier parent, which substantially increases the risk of recurrence.

The risk of recurrence for parents of children with Down syndrome varies according to maternal age at the time of birth of the affected infant. Mothers who were of advanced maternal age maintain their age-related risk, but mothers younger than 30 years old have a sixfold increased risk compared with their age-related peers. The reason for this increased risk is not entirely clear, although it may be related to a lower rate of spontaneous abortion of affected fetuses or an increased risk of nondisjunction that is unrelated to age. Furthermore, some evidence suggests a higher incidence of early pregnancy losses in mothers of children with Down syndrome, although, second- and third-degree relatives of individuals with trisomy 21 are not

at an elevated risk of having children with Down syndrome. Parents of children with de novo translocations are not at increased risk of having another affected child; however, a man carrying balanced Robertsonian translocation has a 3% to 5% risk, but a woman has a 10% to 15% risk for recurrence. Of note, parents carrying a balanced 21;21 translocation have a 100% recurrence risk.

CLINICAL PRESENTATION AND DIFFERENTIAL DIAGNOIS

The diagnosis of trisomy 21 is often made by prenatal screening. When no prenatal diagnosis has been made, Down syndrome is usually recognized from the characteristic phenotype present in the newborn. The diagnosis is confirmed with a karyotype.

Phenotypic Features

The pathogenesis of the characteristic appearance of infants with trisomy 21 and associated malformations of Down syndrome are presumably related to dosage effects of genes on chromosome 21, specifically those in a 5Mb region on 21q22. Certain malformations occur more frequently than others, thus supporting the concept that certain genes rather than a specific embryologic event are involved. The diagnosis of Down syndrome is often straightforward and is based on the overall appearance and characteristics of individuals. Neonates with Down syndrome are typically hypotonic and have poor developmental reflexes. Neonates can also have redundant nuchal skin folds. The skull may be mildly microcephalic with a small occiput and large fontanelles. The eyes are almond shaped with epicanthal folds and upslanting palpebral fissures, and the irises may demonstrate Brushfield spots. The nose is usually short with a low nasal bridge. Usually, the mouth is downturned, and because the oral cavity is small, the tongue often protrudes. The ears may be low set with an overfolded superior helix. The hands are short and commonly have the characteristic single palmar crease.

Developmental Impairment

Nearly all individuals with Down syndrome have some degree of cognitive impairment, although the range is quite wide. Most affected are mildly to moderately mentally retarded, with IQ in the 50 to 70 or 35 to 50 ranges, respectively. Some may be severely impaired with IQ ranges from 20 to 35. Cognitive impairment is evident within the first year of life. Developmental milestones are met typically at twice the age compared with the average population with sitting at around 11 months, creeping at around 17 months, and walking around 26 months. The sequence of the development of language is the same, but the rate is much slower. First words are spoken on average at around

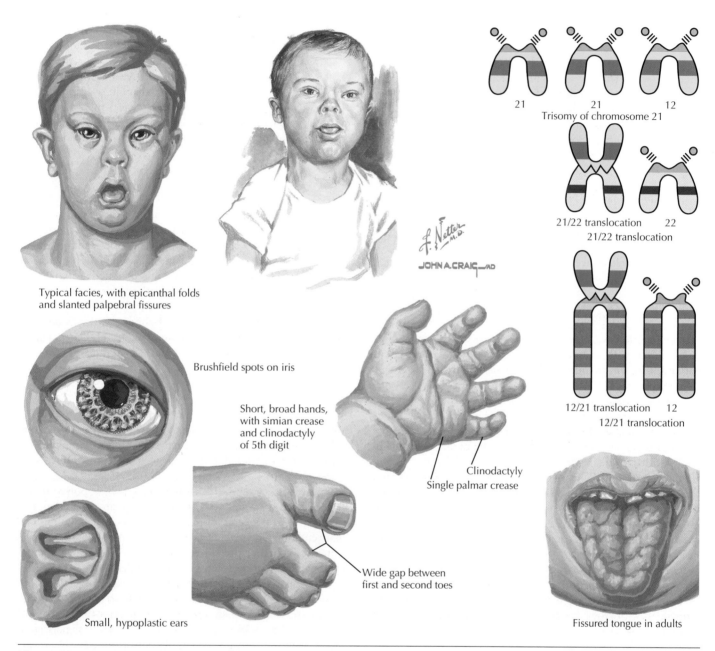

Typical facies, with epicanthal folds
and slanted palpebral fissures

Brushfield spots on iris

Short, broad hands,
with simian crease
and clinodactyly
of 5th digit

Clinodactyly
Single palmar crease

Wide gap between
first and second toes

Small, hypoplastic ears

Fissured tongue in adults

21   21   12
Trisomy of chromosome 21

21/22 translocation   22
21/22 translocation

12/21 translocation   12
12/21 translocation

Figure 117-1 *Trisomy 21 (Down syndrome).*

18 months. Affected children will still gain new skills, but the IQ tends to decline through childhood and plateaus in adolescence.

In more than 60% of children, the profile of cognitive impairment is one in which language comprehension is equal to mental age, and language production is more delayed. However, in about a third of children with Down syndrome, language comprehension, mental age, and language production are equal.

Comorbidities

Several important comorbidities are associated with Down syndrome. Among these, it is important to recognize heart disease, gastrointestinal abnormalities, growth problems, eye problems, hearing loss, hematologic disorders, immune deficiency, endocrine disorders, reproductive disorders, atlanto-axial instability (AAI), sleep apnea, skin disorders, and behavior disorders.

Heart Disease

Approximately 50% of children with Down syndrome have congenital heart disease that includes atrioventricular septal (ASDs), atrioventricular canal or endocardial cushion defects (45%), ventricular septal defects (35%), isolated secundum ASDs, (8%), isolated patent ductus arteriosus (7%), and tetralogy of Fallot (4%). Furthermore, asymptomatic children without congenital structural heart disease may develop valve abnormalities, including mitral valve prolapse, mitral regurgitation, and aortic regurgitation.

Gastrointestinal Disease

Gastrointestinal tract abnormalities occur in about 5% of children with trisomy 21 with the most common being duodenal atresia or stenosis (2.5%), sometimes occurring with an annular pancreas. The characteristic radiographic finding associated with duodenal atresia or stenosis is the "double-bubble" sign. Other anomalies, although less frequently seen, include imperforate anus and esophageal atresia with tracheo-esophageal fistula. Conversely, nearly 30% of patients with duodenal atresia or stenosis and 20% with annular pancreas have Down syndrome. Hirschsprung disease is more common in trisomy 21 compared with the general population, although the risk is less than 1%. Trisomy 21 appears to be strongly associated with celiac disease with an incidence of between 5% and 16%, which is five- to 16-fold greater than the general population.

Growth and Stature

Head circumference, length, and weight are all lower in infants and children with trisomy 21 than unaffected children. Compared with their siblings, at birth, children with trisomy 21 weigh on average 0.2 to 0.4 kg less. The rate of growth of children with trisomy 21 is reduced, especially during infancy and adolescence, and is more severely reduced in children with congenital heart disease. In adolescence, the growth spurt of affected children occurs earlier, further blunting the ultimate height. In adults with Down's syndrome, the average height in men and women is 61.7 and 57 inches (157 and 144 cm), respectively, and the average weight is 157 and 140 lb (71 and 64 kg), respectively.

The cause of trisomy 21–associated growth retardation remains unknown. In some patients, low serum levels of insulin-like growth factor 1 (IGF-1) and lower spontaneous and induced secretion of growth hormone (GH) have been reported. Hypothalamic dysfunction may lead to suboptimal endogenous GH production. Selective deficiency of IGF-1 has been seen in individuals with Down syndrome who are older than the age of 2 years.

Obesity

The prevalence of obesity (body mass index >27.8 kg/m^2 in men and >27.3 kg/m^2 in women) is higher in individuals with trisomy 21 than in the general population. When comparing people with Down syndrome with the general population, obesity rates are 45% versus 33% for males, and 56% versus 36% for females. It is thought that children and adults with trisomy 21 have a reduced resting metabolic rate that results in a majority of children becoming obese by 3 to 4 years of age.

Disturbances of Vision

Ophthalmologic disorders that require monitoring and intervention affect the majority of children with trisomy 21. These include refractive errors (myopia, hyperopia, astigmatism) in 35% to 75%, strabismus, in 25% to 55%, and nystagmus in 18% to 22%.

Cataracts can also occur in up to 5% of newborns. Starting in the second decade of life, many children develop corneal opacities and may also develop glaucoma. The frequency of ocular disorders increases with age, and eye abnormalities have been reported to increase from fewer than 40% of infants 2 to 12 months of age up to 80% of children age 5 to 12 years. The development of ocular anomalies continues to increase into adulthood and is thought to be prevalent in nearly all adults with Down syndrome.

Disturbances of Hearing

Hearing impairment affects 40% to 80% of individuals with trisomy 21. In 50 children with Down syndrome 2 months to 3.5 years of age, auditory brainstem response testing demonstrated unilateral loss in 28%, bilateral loss in 38%, and normal hearing in 34%. The hearing loss was conductive in 19 ears, sensorineural in 16, and mixed in 14 with the extent of loss being mild, moderate, and severe to profound in 33, 13, and three ears, respectively. About 50% to 70% of children with Down syndrome develop otitis media. Because of its high prevalence, monitoring for this condition is crucial to the maintenance of hearing.

Hematologic Disorders

Abnormalities affecting all hematopoietic lineages, red blood cells, white blood cells, and platelets are common in people with trisomy 21. Most notably, the risk of leukemia in Down syndrome is 1% to 1.5%.

Nearly 65% of newborns with trisomy 21 have polycythemia that has been suggested to be attributable to an elevated plasma erythropoietin concentration. This suggests that ongoing fetal hypoxemia may contribute to the increased incidence of polycythemia. Whether the chronic hypoxia is related to placental insufficiency or other factors remains unclear.

Children with trisomy 21 often have macrocytosis. The mean corpuscular volume (MCV) in children with trisomy 21 between ages 2 to 6 years has been reported to be greater than in control subjects (86.9 vs. 80.6 fL), with MCVs above the 95th percentile for age seen in 66% versus 11% of control subjects.

Oncologic Disorders

TRANSIENT LEUKEMIA

Transient leukemia, also known as transient myeloproliferative disorder (TMD), is a form of leukemia that almost exclusively affects newborns with trisomy 21, with an incidence of about 20%. Usually, affected infants are asymptomatic, and the disorder resolves spontaneously by 2 to 3 months of age. Vesicopustular skin eruptions filled with blasts may be associated but also resolve by 3 months of age. In the rare cases that result in death, infants are often antenatally affected with fetal hydrops. The disorder is characterized by the presence of blast cells in the peripheral blood, typically with hemoglobin, platelet, and neutrophil counts being normal, although morphology may be different. Giant platelets and fragments of megakaryocytes may be seen. Bone marrow biopsy of transient leukemia demonstrates a lower percentage of blasts in bone marrow than in peripheral blood, and cytogenetic analysis reveals no clonal abnormalities in the marrow other than trisomy 21.

Life-threatening complications of transient leukemia occasionally occur. A Pediatric Oncology Group study of nearly 50 children with transient leukemia reported seven patients who developed hepatic fibrosis and two who developed cardiopulmonary failure. In retrospective analyses, the clinical features associated with early death of children with transient leukemia included preterm delivery, white blood cell count of 100,000 cells/µL or greater, direct bilirubin of 4.8 mg/dL (83 µmol/L) or greater, ascites, and bleeding disorders. Hepatic fibrosis presents as progressive obstructive jaundice and results in death in approximately 50% of cases. Cardiopulmonary disease presents most commonly as whole-body edema, with pulmonary edema, pericardial effusions, and ascites; the mechanism is unknown.

ACUTE MEGAKARYOBLASTIC LEUKEMIA

Up to 25% of infants with transient leukemia later develop acute megakaryoblastic leukemia (AMKL), also known as the FAB M7 subtype of acute myeloid leukemia (AML-M7). AML-M7 occurs in 0.5% to 2% of children with Down syndrome, and the incidence is nearly 500 times greater in children with trisomy 21. Usually, AML-M7 develops during the first 4 years of life, and 20% to 70% of affected patients present with myelodysplastic syndrome, consisting of progressive thrombocytopenia and anemia. Neutropenia is not commonly seen. Some children develop hepatomegaly and liver failure secondary to fibrosis. Treatment issues are complicated, and children with Down syndrome affected with either acute lymphoblastic leukemia (ALL) or AML are subject to increased rates of treatment-related mortality.

ACUTE LYMPHOBLASTIC LEUKEMIA

The risk of developing ALL is approximately 10 to 20 times higher in those with trisomy 21. The clinical presentation is similar to that of children without trisomy 21, and at presentation, includes similar leukocyte count and leukemic cell mass, slightly older age of trisomy 21 patients (median age, 6 vs. 4.7 years), less frequent mediastinal mass (1.6% vs. 8.9%), and central nervous system leukemia (0% vs. 2.7%), both of which are favorable prognostic signs. Less favorable prognostic signs seen in patients with trisomy 21 include lower rates of T-cell leukemia, higher rates of translocation of (9;22) or t(4;11), and less hyperdiploidy.

Importantly, children with trisomy 21 with ALL often respond to chemotherapy as well as do children without trisomy 21.

Immune Deficiency

Down syndrome is associated with a variety of immunologic deficiencies that likely contribute to susceptibility to infection, autoimmune disorders, and malignancies. These immunologic impairments include chemotactic defects, decreased immunoglobulin G (IgG) levels, specifically IgG4, and abnormalities of T- and B-cell systems. It has yet to be established whether these represent intrinsic or secondary immune deficiencies.

Endocrinologic Disorders

The most common endocrine abnormalities in individuals with trisomy 21 include thyroid dysfunction and diabetes. The prevalence of thyroid disease varies depending on the population examined, and hypothyroidism has ranged from 3% to greater than 50%. Hyperthyroidism is also relatively common in adults with trisomy 21, occurring in 2.5%. Thyroid disease is also seen in children with Down syndrome, and even in patients younger than 25 years of age, 35% have been shown to have hypothyroidism, with 50% developing the disorder before age 8 years.

Recent data have suggested that the risk of type 1 diabetes in trisomy 21 is three times greater than in the general population. Furthermore, the prevalence of type 1 diabetes in affected children up to 9 years of age is thought to be eight times greater than in age-matched control subjects.

Reproductive Concerns

Women with trisomy 21 are fertile and may become pregnant. Offspring may or may not be affected by trisomy 21, depending on the type of mutation. As always, counseling should be provided for managing menstruation and contraception. Alternatively, nearly all men with trisomy 21 are infertile because of impairment of spermatogenesis, although fathers with trisomy 21 producing offspring have been reported.

Atlantoaxial Instability

AAI, which is excessive mobility of the joint between the atlas (C1) and the axis (C2), may lead to cervical spine subluxation. Although 13% of individuals with trisomy 21 are asymptomatic, spinal cord compression caused by AAI affects approximately 2%. Lateral neck radiographs of neutral position, flexion, and extension help to confirm the diagnosis. Spinal cord compression may present as neck pain, torticollis, gait abnormalities, loss of bowel or bladder control, and quadriparesis or quadriplegia. If such symptoms arise, immediate stabilization may be required. Asymptomatic individuals appear to remain so whether or not physical activity is restricted.

Sleep Apnea

About 30% to 75% of children with trisomy 21 have obstructive sleep apnea, independent of obesity. This is likely because of soft tissue and skeletal causes of upper airway obstruction. Chronic intermittent hypoxemia may contribute to pulmonary hypertension, which may further deteriorate mental capacities.

Skin Disorders

Most children with trisomy 21 have benign skin changes, which may include palmoplantar hyperkeratosis, seborrheic dermatitis, cutis marmorata, fissured or geographic tongue, and xerosis. Skin problems often worsen in adolescence, with half developing folliculitis.

Behavior Disturbances

Behavior and psychiatric disorders are more common in trisomy 21 than typical children but not as common than in those with other reasons for mental retardation. Psychiatric disorders have been reported to affect nearly 20% of individuals with trisomy 21 younger than 20 years of age. These include behavioral disorders such as attention-deficit hyperactivity disorder, conduct or oppositional disorder, and aggressive behavior as well as psychiatric disorders (most often major depressive illness or aggressive behavior); these disorders affect 25% of adults with trisomy 21. Autism occurs in as many as 7% of children with trisomy 21, and when compared with children without trisomy 21, the diagnosis is often delayed.

RECENT ADVANCES AND FUTURE DIRECTIONS

Numerous recent advances in genomics have led to an increased understanding of trisomy 21. The number of genes currently known on chromosome 21 is around 400, and this number is expected to increase. One of the major focuses of research into the pathology of trisomy 21 is to identify which of the genes on chromosome 21 lead to the various Down syndrome–associated phenotypes. To facilitate this understanding, mouse models of trisomy 21 have been developed to further understand pathologic mechanisms and dosage-sensitive genes. Ongoing discoveries similar to those outlined below are helping us to understand the pathology of trisomy 21 on the brain, heart, and hematopoietic anomalies.

Learning and Memory

All people with trisomy 21 have some degree of learning disability. A number of genes located on chromosome 21 that are overexpressed, including *DYRK1A*, synaptojanin 1, and *SIM2*, have been shown to contribute to learning and memory deficits in mouse models. In addition, extra copies of neuronal channel proteins such as GIRK2 may also contribute to learning difficulties.

Alzheimer Disease

Individuals affected by trisomy 21 have a notably increased risk of early-onset Alzheimer disease compared with unaffected individuals. It has been shown that amyloid precursor protein is encoded on chromosome 21, and overexpression of this gene likely contributes to the 50% to 70% of people with trisomy 21 who develop dementia by age 60 years.

Cancer

As noted above, trisomy 21–affected people have a much higher risk of developing AMKL and ALL. Recent evidence has suggested that AML-M7 may result from a mutation in the GATA-1 transcription factor that is required for normal differentiation of megakaryocytes. It is thought that these mutations are acquired in utero and that finding such mutations at birth might serve as a biomarker for an increased risk of transient leukemia and subsequent AMKL. Furthermore, mutations in Janus Kinase 3 (JAK3) have been noted in some populations of patients with TMD/AMKL. Because JAK3 has been a target of pharmacologic development, JAK3 inhibitors may be a potential source of therapy for these disorders in patients with trisomy 21, although further work needs to be done to elucidate if JAK3 mutations are loss-of-function or gain-of-function in AKML before therapeutic evaluation.

Cognitive Ability

Most recent therapeutic work for people with trisomy 21 has centered on treatment to enhance cognitive ability. In a trisomy 21 mouse model, picrotoxin and pentylenetetrazole improved learning associated with the hippocampus, even after treatment stopped. These therapeutics decrease γ-aminobutyric acid–mediated inhibition in the hippocampus as their mechanism of improving cognitive ability. Furthermore, in the same mouse model, cognition is improved by treatment with N-methyl-D-aspartic acid receptor (NMDAR) antagonist memantine. The biggest contributor for identifying treatments for people with Down syndrome will be to determine which genes specifically contribute to specific cognitive phenotypes. To accomplish this, standardized multicenter protocols will be necessary to assess sufficient numbers of patients. Large-scale collaboration has been successful in other medical fields in developing treatment algorithms, and the same principles can be used to treat trisomy 21. Mouse studies currently being used to model trisomy 21 in humans will be a first step in the development of new therapeutics.

Despite the past, when Down syndrome was thought to be untreatable because of its genetic complexity, marked advances in the understanding of Down syndrome have occurred and will likely usher in new treatment approaches for improving the cognition, health, and well-being of these patients.

SUGGESTED READINGS

American Academy of Pediatrics: Health supervision for children with Down syndrome. *Pediatrics* 107:442, 2001.

Epstein, CJ: Down syndrome (trisomy 21). In Scriver CR, Beaudet AL, Sly WS, Valle D, editors: *The Metabolic and Molecular Bases of Inherited Disease*, ed 8, New York, 2001, McGraw-Hill, pp 1223.

Kumin L: Speech and language skills in children with Down syndrome. *MRDD Res Rev* 2:109, 1996.

Massey GV, Zipursky A, Chang MN, et al: A prospective study of the natural history of transient leukemia (TL) in neonates with Down syndrome (DS): Children's Oncology Group (COG) study POG-9481. *Blood* 107:4606, 2006.

Myrelid A, Gustafsson J, Ollars B, et al: Growth charts for Down's syndrome from birth to 18 years of age. *Arch Dis Child* 87:97, 2002.

Weijerman, ME, van Furth, AM, Vonk Noordegraaf A, et al: Prevalence, neonatal characteristics, and first-year mortality of Down syndrome: a national study. *J Pediatr* 152:15, 2008.

118

Chromosomal Abnormalities

Bettina Mucha-Le Ny and Reena Jethva

*S*ince the discovery in 1959 that Down syndrome is caused by trisomy of chromosome 21, multiple syndromes have been found to have an identifiable chromosomal abnormality. These range from triplication of a complete chromosome as in Edwards syndrome (trisomy 18) to monosomies such as Turner syndrome (45,X) and to a growing number of smaller duplication and deletion syndromes. Several of the more common or illustrative chromosomal aberrations are discussed in this chapter.

TRISOMY 18 (EDWARDS SYNDROME)

ETIOLOGY AND PATHOGENESIS

Trisomy 18 (Edwards syndrome) is most commonly caused by meiotic nondisjunction, and the risk is related to maternal age. However, Edwards syndrome can also result from an unbalanced translocation. If the parents of an affected infant have a normal karyotype (i.e., neither is a balanced translocation carriers), the recurrence risk for trisomy 18 in a subsequent pregnancy is no greater than the age-related risk.

CLINICAL PRESENTATION

Trisomy 18 is one of the more common malformation syndromes, with an incidence of 0.3 in 100 newborn infants. On prenatal ultrasound, increased nuchal translucency may be seen early in gestation. At birth, reduced birth weight, a small placenta, and fetal distress may be noted along with multiple other clinical features (Table 118-1).

PROGNOSIS

The median survival of infants with trisomy 18 is 2 weeks, with 5% to 10% of patients living through the first year. Surviving children exhibit severe physical and mental retardation with vision and hearing impairment. Poor feeding often makes nasogastric tube feedings necessary. Growth is poor, and specific growth charts are available.

TRISOMY 13 (PATAU SYNDROME)

ETIOLOGY AND PATHOGENESIS

Most cases of Patau syndrome are caused by trisomy 13, which also demonstrates an increased incidence with advancing maternal age. Similarly, chromosomal studies should be performed to rule out an unbalanced translocation because recurrence is higher in a parent with a balanced translocation.

CLINICAL PRESENTATION

Trisomy 13 occurs with an incidence of approximately 1 in 5000 births. Early prenatal detection is possible with a combined screening protocol that includes maternal age, nuchal translucency, and maternal serum markers. The mean birth weight is reduced, and multiple dysmorphic features may be observed (see Table 118-1).

PROGNOSIS

The median survival of a newborn with Patau syndrome is less than 1 week, and only 3% live to 6 months of age. Survivors have profound mental retardation, seizure disorders, behavioral problems, and feeding difficulties.

TURNER'S SYNDROME (45,X)

ETIOLOGY AND PATHOGENESIS

Turner's syndrome is diagnosed in a female by the absence of a second normal sex chromosome caused by the complete or partial deletion of an X or Y chromosome. The loss is not associated with advanced maternal age and may happen during spermatogenesis, oogenesis, or postzygotic nondisjunction. The resulting karyotype is 45,X in approximately half of patients with Turner syndrome, but isochromosomes with duplication of the long arm of the X chromosome, ring and marker chromosomes, and mosaicism are frequently observed.

Turner syndrome occurs in 1 in 2500 to 1 in 3000 female live births and is caused by the absence of a second normal sex chromosome. The incidence of 45,X is actually higher in pregnancy losses.

CLINICAL PRESENTATION

Females with Turner syndrome may present prenatally with features of lymphedema/hydrops and/or a congenital heart defect, in puberty due to short stature or in adulthood with premature ovarian failure (Figure 118-1). Multiple organ systems may be involved, but no single feature is pathognomonic or universally present.

Several physical features are found as a consequence of lymphatic abnormalities that include webbed neck, puffy hands and feet, dysplastic finger- and toenails, protuberant ears, and a broad chest.

Up to 45% of patients have a cardiac anomaly identified by echocardiography, most often a bicuspid aortic valve or aortic coarctation, but other cardiac anomalies such as partial anomalous pulmonary venous connection can also occur. Renal

Table 118-1 Frequent Clinical Features in Trisomies 18 and 13

	Trisomy 18	Trisomy 13
Head and CNS	Microcephaly, prominent occiput	Microcephaly, parieto-occipital scalp defect, holoprosencephaly (≈66%)
Eyes	Short palpebral fissures	Anophthalmia or microphthalmia
Ears	Low set, posteriorly rotated	Abnormal helices
Mouth	Small, micrognathia	Cleft lip or palate
Hands	Index finger overlapping third and fourth digit	Polydactyly
	Nail hypoplasia	Camptodactyly
	Dermatoglyphics: arches (>6/10)	Hyperconvex narrow fingernails
Feet	Rocker-bottom feet	Prominent heels
Hips	Small pelvis	Small pelvis
Cardiac	VSD, PDA, pulmonary hypertension	ASD, VSD, PDA
Renal	Abnormalities in 10%-50%	Large cystic kidneys
Genitalia	Cryptorchidism	Cryptorchidism, bicornuate uterus

ASD, atrial septal defect; CNS, central nervous system; PDA, patent ductus arteriosus; VSD, ventricular septal defect.

anomalies are equally frequent (40%), including renal agenesis and horseshoe kidney. Hypothyroidism may develop in 5% to 10% of girls in mid to late childhood and affects up to one-third of adult women.

Growth delay begins in childhood, but short stature may not be noticed until 5 to 10 years of age or in puberty with a blunted growth spurt. Growth hormone treatment may lead to improvement, but adult height is usually reduced.

Gonadal dysgenesis is a hallmark of Turner syndrome and typically leads to ovarian failure. Puberty occurs spontaneously in 10% of patients, and hormonal replacement therapy is necessary to achieve development of secondary sexual characteristics as well as to avoid osteoporosis and other postmenopausal complications. Nonetheless, spontaneous pregnancy has been observed in about 2% to 4% of women with Turner syndrome.

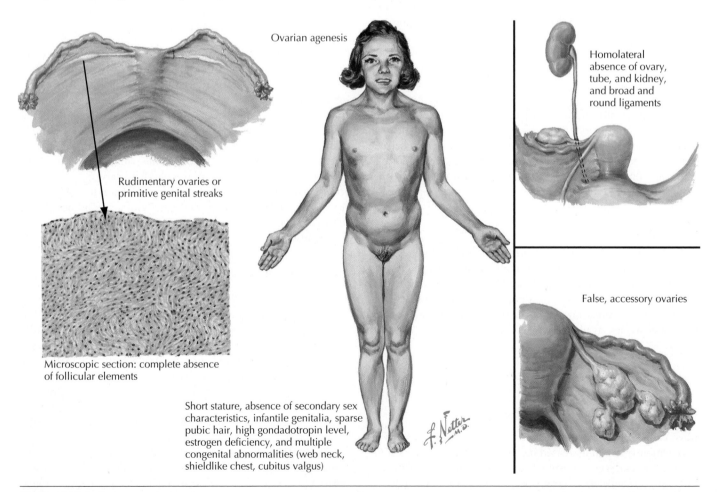

Ovarian agenesis

Rudimentary ovaries or primitive genital streaks

Microscopic section: complete absence of follicular elements

Homolateral absence of ovary, tube, and kidney, and broad and round ligaments

False, accessory ovaries

Short stature, absence of secondary sex characteristics, infantile genitalia, sparse pubic hair, high gonadotropin level, estrogen deficiency, and multiple congenital abnormalities (web neck, shieldlike chest, cubitus valgus)

Figure 118-1 *Turner syndrome.*

Most girls with Turner syndrome have normal developmental milestones and intelligence. About 10% of individuals experience specific learning disabilities, mental retardation, motor deficits, or difficulties with attention, maturity, and social skills. Correlation has been observed between the intellectual phenotype and the karyotype, and girls with a marker or ring chromosome have a higher prevalence of mental retardation.

PROGNOSIS

Cardiovascular disease confers the highest risk for mortality in females with Turner syndrome. Developmental difficulties and immature behavior may lead to an older age for women to attain independence. Pregnancy can be successful using donor egg programs.

KLINEFELTER SYNDROME

ETIOLOGY AND PATHOGENESIS

Klinefelter syndrome is caused by a 47,XXY or 46,XY/47,XXY karyotype with mosaic men exhibiting a milder phenotype. Nondisjunction of the sex chromosomes is equally derived from either parent with only a small association with maternal age.

With an incidence of 1 in 500 to 1 in 1000 male infant births, Klinefelter syndrome is the most common sex chromosome aneuploidy.

CLINICAL PRESENTATION

Newborns with 47,XXY do not have any significant dysmorphic features. In fact, 10% of boys are identified incidentally during chorionic villus sampling or amniocentesis for advanced maternal age. In rare cases, chromosomal studies are initiated in the newborn period for cryptorchidism, hypospadias, or a small phallus. About 25% of affected individuals are diagnosed in childhood, adolescence, and adulthood. A large fraction of 47,XXY men are thought to remain undiagnosed.

In childhood, language delay, learning differences, or behavioral problems may bring a boy to medical attention. Physical symptoms start to develop in adolescence with increased height, narrower than average shoulders, broader than average hips, and scoliosis or kyphosis.

Although the age and onset of puberty is unchanged in boys with Klinefelter syndrome, testicular growth is arrested, leading to oligospermia or azoospermia and low testosterone levels. A small fraction of men present with gynecomastia, eunuchoid habitus, and decreased hair (Figure 118-2). Muscle strength may be decreased. Testosterone replacement therapy aims

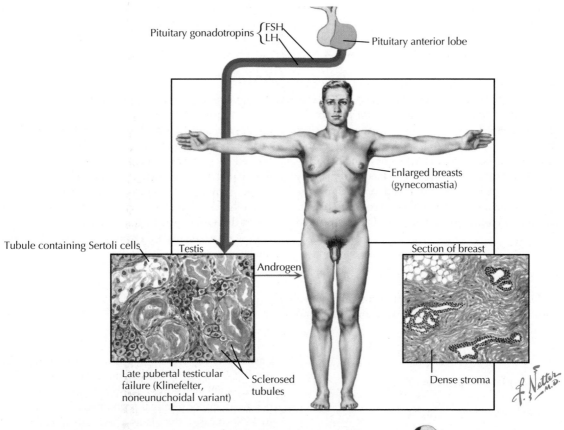

Pituitary gonadotropins { FSH LH }

Pituitary anterior lobe

Enlarged breasts (gynecomastia)

Tubule containing Sertoli cells

Testis

Androgen

Section of breast

Late pubertal testicular failure (Klinefelter, noneunuchoidal variant)

Sclerosed tubules

Dense stroma

Nuclear chromatin often positive (female); usually XXY chromosomal pattern but XXX Y , XXXX Y , XXY Y , and mosaic patterns have been described

 XXY

Figure 118-2 *Klinefelter syndrome.*

at increasing muscle mass, libido, energy, and improving mood through support of androgen-dependent processes. Fertility is rarely preserved except in mosaic men.

Development is normal in most infants, although hypotonia and delayed acquisition of language milestones can occur. The mean IQ in individuals with Klinefelter syndrome falls into the normal range, but wide variability has been observed, and verbal IQ is consistently lower, often benefitting from speech and language therapy. Temperamental differences may manifest as shyness, lower activity, and insecurity.

Prognosis

Men with Klinefelter syndrome have a higher risk for breast cancer and extragonadal germ cell tumors. In addition, increased incidences of deep venous thrombosis, pulmonary embolism, vascular insufficiency, elevated cholesterol levels, and autoimmune disorders have been observed.

1P36 DELETION SYNDROME

ETIOLOGY AND PATHOGENESIS

Monosomy for the distal short arm of chromosome 1 occurs in approximately 1 in 10,000 live births, but the incidence is likely to be higher with improved diagnostic tests. Most deletions are de novo caused by a terminal or interstitial deletion, a complex rearrangement, or a derivative chromosome.

CLINICAL PRESENTATION

Distinctive facial features include microbrachycephaly, frontal bossing, large anterior fontanelle, marked midface hypoplasia, deep-set eyes, straight eyebrows, long philtrum, and abnormally shaped ears. Mental retardation with poor or absent speech, hypotonia, short feet, brachycamptodactyly, and brain abnormalities (dilatation of the large ventricles, atrophy, and hypoplasia) are present in more than 75% of patients. In addition, many have congenital heart defects, seizures, and ophthalmologic abnormalities. Sensorineural deafness, hypothyroidism, behavioral problems, and cardiomyopathy have also been associated with a 1p36 deletion.

PROGNOSIS

Approximately 90% of patients have severe to profound mental retardation, with only 25% being able to walk unassisted and absent language in 75%.

WOLF-HIRSCHHORN SYNDROME (4p-)

ETIOLOGY AND PATHOGENESIS

Wolf-Hirschhorn syndrome (WHS) is caused by partial monosomy for the short arm of chromosome 4 (4p-) and occurs with an estimated incidence of 1 in 50,000 live births. The deletion arises de novo in 75% of patients, with ring chromosome 4 and unbalanced translocations making up much of the remainder. The diagnosis can be made by conventional karyotype for deletions larger than 5 Mb (megabases) or by using a specific FISH (fluorescence in situ hybridization) probe or high-resolution array for smaller deletions.

CLINICAL PRESENTATION

Wolf-Hirschhorn syndrome and Pitt-Rogers-Dank syndrome are clinical manifestations of a phenotypical spectrum caused by monosomy 4p. Individuals with WHS demonstrate typical facial features characterized as a "Greek warrior helmet" appearance. These include microcephaly, frontal bossing with a high frontal hairline and prominent glabella, a broad nasal bridge and beaked nose, hypertelorism, epicanthal folds, highly arched eyebrows, downturned mouth with short upper lip and short philtrum, micrognathia, and low-set, large ears often with pits or tags. Low birth weight with subsequent failure to thrive and growth restriction is common. More than 75% of patients have severe mental retardation, hypotonia, seizures, structural brain abnormalities, and feeding difficulties. Craniofacial asymmetry, ptosis, abnormal dentition, antibody deficiency, and skeletal and skin abnormalities can be found in 50% to 75%. Closure defects of the face, including cleft lip or palate, iris coloboma, cardial septal defects, and genitourinary tract abnormalities (e.g., cryptorchidism, renal agenesis or malformation), are less common, but any organ system can be involved, and a thorough clinical evaluation, including imaging studies, is recommended.

PROGNOSIS

All patients experience global developmental delay, with 65% demonstrating severe cognitive impairment, 25% with a moderate degree, and 10% with a mild degree. Only 45% walk independently or with support. Expressive language is frequently limited to guttural or disyllabic sounds and only occasionally modulated in a communicative way, with 6% able to pronounce simple sentences. About 93% have been reported to develop generalized tonic-clonic seizures within the first 3 years of life. Heart defects are usually not complex, but antibody deficiencies may lead to recurrent respiratory tract infections and otitis media.

CRI DU CHAT SYNDROME (5p-)

ETIOLOGY AND PATHOGENESIS

Partial deletion of the short arm of chromosome 5 results in cri du chat syndrome (CdCS) and is estimated to occur in 1:15,000 to 1:50,000 newborns. Most are paternally derived de novo deletions, either terminal or interstitial, of variable size. In 10% to 15% of cases, the phenotype is attributable to familial or de novo translocations. Genotype–phenotype correlation studies have mapped characteristic symptoms to specific critical regions and genes on 5p.

CLINICAL PRESENTATION

The name of the syndrome refers to the characteristic high-pitched catlike cry of the affected newborn, which is caused by laryngeal abnormalities. Other clinical findings are low birth weight, microcephaly, round face, large nasal bridge, hypertelorism, epicanthal folds, downslanting palpebral fissures, downturned corners of the mouth, low-set ears, and micrognathia. Facial features change with age, and the catlike cry disappears within the first year of life. Other organ systems are rarely involved, but stunted growth, mostly affecting head circumference and weight, is common.

PROGNOSIS

Many infants do not survive early childhood. Patients with CdCS have severe psychomotor retardation, although they can attain milestones such as walking, talking in short sentences, and feeding themselves late in childhood. With intensive early intervention, the resulting social and psychomotor development reaches the level of a 5- to 6-year old unaffected child.

WILLIAMS SYNDROME

ETIOLOGY AND PATHOGENESIS

Williams syndrome (WS) is a sporadic contiguous gene deletion disorder caused by an interstitial deletion of the long arm of chromosome 7 encompassing the Williams-Beuren syndrome critical region (WBSCR). Among the genes in the WBSCR is elastin, which is deleted in 90% of WS patients. Hemizygosity for elastin is associated with cardiovascular disease, also termed *elastin arteriopathy*. Occasionally, autosomal dominant transmission from a parent to a child is observed. Penetrance is 100%, but phenotypic expression is variable. The incidence of WS is estimated to be 1 in 20,000 to 1 in 50,000 newborns.

CLINICAL PRESENTATION

Features include congenital heart disease (supravalvular stenosis and peripheral pulmonary stenosis), failure to thrive secondary to feeding difficulties, and hypotonia. Distinctive facial characteristics consist of a broad brow, bitemporal narrowing, periorbital fullness, a stellate or lacy iris pattern, strabismus, short nose, full nasal tip, malar hypoplasia, long philtrum, full lips, wide mouth, malocclusion, small jaw, and prominent earlobes. The face typically becomes more coarse with age. Connective tissue abnormalities lead, among other symptoms, to a hoarse voice, hyperextensible joints, and hernias. Most individuals have some degree of mental retardation, which can range from severe to mild with notable strengths in verbal short-term memory and language and weakness in visual–motor integration. Patients with WS have a unique personality and are typically over-friendly, empathic, and gregarious, which has also been termed the "cocktail party" personality. Hypercalcemia occurs in about 15% of patients and early puberty in 50%. Linear growth is stunted, and the mean adult height is below the third percentile.

Adults are at risk for severe cardiovascular disease secondary to elastin arteriopathy, sudden death, hypertension, progressive sensorineural hearing loss, hypothyroidism, and diabetes mellitus. Annual surveillance is recommended.

MILLER-DIEKER SYNDROME

ETIOLOGY AND PATHOGENESIS

Miller-Dieker syndrome (MDS) is caused by variable deletions of the distal end of the short arm of chromosome 17 (17p13.3), including the gene *LIS1*, which plays a significant role in neuronal development. Smaller submicroscopic deletions or other sequence variations of *LIS1* cause isolated lissencephaly sequence (ILS). Most cases of MDS occur sporadically, with the remaining 20% caused by a parental balanced translocation that increases the recurrence risk for subsequent pregnancies. The diagnosis can be made using FISH, high-resolution array, sequence analysis, or multiplex ligation-dependent probe amplification (MLPA) analysis of *LIS1*.

CLINICAL PRESENTATION

Lissencephaly is defined as a cortical malformation secondary to deficient neural migration, resulting in a "smooth brain" with absent gyri (agyria) or abnormally wide gyri (pachygyria). On magnetic resonance imaging, the severity can be graded with grade 1 being the most severe (lissencephaly) to the mildest form, grade 6 (subcortical band heterotopia). MDS is distinguished from ILS through characteristic facial features consisting of high and prominent forehead, bitemporal narrowing, short nose with upturned nares, protuberant upper lip with downturned vermillion border, and small jaw. Intrauterine, poor swallowing may lead to polyhydramnios. Postnatally, severe growth restriction and microcephaly develop, and seizures occur in 90% within the first 6 months of life. Some children have an omphalocele or congenital heart defects. Hypotonia and feeding difficulties are common.

The developmental prognosis is poor for all affected children. Even with good seizure control, most children only reach the developmental milestones of a 3- to 5-month-old child. Life span is shortened, with most children with MDS dying within the first 2 years of life. Complications arise from respiratory tract infections caused by poor airway control.

SMITH-MAGENIS SYNDROME

ETIOLOGY AND PATHOGENESIS

Interstitial deletions on the short arm of chromosome 17 involving 17p11.2, including the *RAI1* gene, are causative for Smith-Magenis syndrome (SMS) and arise on both paternal and maternal chromosomes. Most deletions are de novo and cytogenetically visible. Most smaller deletions can be identified by commercially available FISH probes. The birth incidence is estimated to be 1 in 25,000 newborns.

CLINICAL PRESENTATION

The distinctive facial features in individuals with SMS progress with age and include brachycephaly, midface hypoplasia with a broad nasal bridge, prognathism, a tented upper lip, deep-set, close-spaced eyes, and dental anomalies. More than 75% have short, broad hands and laryngeal anomalies, including polyps, nodules, edema, partial vocal cord paralysis, velopharyngeal insufficiency, or structural vocal fold abnormalities. The latter findings lead to a hoarse voice and may contribute to the significant delays in speech development. Facial features in older patients become more coarse with heavy eyebrows and persistent midface hypoplasia.

Infants have mild to moderate hypotonia and feeding difficulties that result in failure to thrive. They are developmentally delayed with speech, and fine and gross motor skills are affected. Older individuals exhibit a wide variability in cognitive and adaptive functioning, usually with mild to moderate mental retardation.

Other common features occurring in 50% to 75% of individuals are ocular abnormalities (iris anomalies, microcornea), sleep disturbances (difficulty falling and staying asleep, REM sleep abnormalities), constipation, and hypertriglyceridemia or hypercholesterolemia.

The neurobehavioral phenotype is distinctive in people with SMS and usually becomes recognizable after 18 months of age. More than two-thirds of individuals with SMS demonstrate self-injurious behavior; nail pulling (onychotillomania) and insertion of foreign objects into body orifices (polyembolokoilamania) are especially distinctive of SMS. Self-injurious behaviors, stereotypic behaviors (self-hugging, hand-licking, and page flipping), and maladaptive behaviors (frequent outbursts or temper tantrums, attention seeking, impulsivity, distractibility, disobedience, aggression, toileting difficulties) become more severe with age or significant life cycle events (e.g., school, onset of puberty).

PROGNOSIS

If no major organ system is involved, life expectancy in patients with SMS is expected to be comparable to other patients with mental retardation, although thorough longitudinal studies have not been performed. Behavioral problems persist but seem to improve slightly in adulthood.

22q11.2 DELETION SYNDROME

ETIOLOGY AND PATHOGENESIS

Multiple different clinical syndromes are caused by a microdeletion on the long arm of chromosome 22, including DiGeorge's syndrome, velocardiofacial syndrome, and conotruncal anomaly syndrome. The deletion involving 22q11.2 arises de novo in about 93% of patients but can be inherited in an autosomal dominant pattern from an affected parent with 100% penetrance. The diagnosis is made by FISH analysis or high-resolution array. The incidence of 22q11.2 deletion syndrome (del22q11.2) ranges from 1 in 4000 to 1 in 6000 live births but

may be underestimated secondary to marked phenotypic variability. Inter- and intrafamilial clinical variability has been observed in patients with the same deletion, and genotype–phenotype correlation is difficult.

CLINICAL PRESENTATION

The suspicion for del22q11.2 in a newborn is often raised by the presence of one or more of a constellation of physical findings that include congenital heart disease, especially conotruncal malformations, hypocalcemia, immune deficiency, and characteristic facial features. Frequently observed dysmorphisms include overfolded or squared-off ear helices, small and protuberant ears with preauricular pits or tags, a prominent nasal root and bulbous nasal tip, hooded eyelids, ocular hypertelorism, cleft lip and palate, asymmetric crying facies, and craniosynostosis (Figure 118-3). Infants often have feeding difficulties secondary to severe dysphagia and palatal abnormalities. In older patients, learning difficulties, growth hormone deficiency, autoimmune disease, and psychiatric illness may become apparent. Other organ systems can be involved, and a renal ultrasound to evaluate for renal abnormalities and chest radiography to assess for vertebral malformations should be performed.

The majority of children with del22q11.2 experience significant developmental delay and attain motor and language milestones later than their peers. The prevalence of autism or disorders of the autistic spectrum is approximately 20%. In older individuals, full-scale IQ scores are lower than the normal population, although they have a significantly higher verbal IQ than performance IQ, evidence of stronger verbal than visual memory skills and stronger reading than math skills.

PROGNOSIS

The mortality of patients with del22q11.2 is largely determined by the severity of the congenital heart defect. The impairment

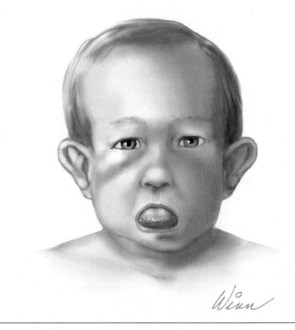

Figure 118-3 *22q11.2 deletion syndrome.*

of T-cell–mediated immune function rarely requires treatment and improves over time. In adults, the incidence of psychiatric disorders, including schizophrenia, bipolar disorder, anxiety, and depression, is increased.

FUTURE DIRECTIONS

The advent of high-resolution genome array analysis has further enhanced our ability to identify microdeletion syndromes in patients with dysmorphic features, multiorgan involvement, and developmental delay. As these continue to be refined, we will surely identify and characterize many additional disorders with much smaller chromosomal deletions or duplications.

SUGGESTED READINGS

Battaglia A, Filippi T, Carey JC: Update on the clinical features and natural history of Wolf-Hirschhorn (4p-) syndrome: experience with 87 patients and recommendations for routine health supervision. *Am J Med Genet C Semin Med Genet* 148C(4):246-251, 2008.

Loscalzo M: Turner syndrome. *Pediatr Rev* 29(7):219-227, 2008.

Mainardi PC: Cri du chat syndrome. *Orphanet J Rare Dis* 1:33, 2006.

National Center for Biotechnology Information: GeneReviews. Available at http://www.ncbi.nlm.nih.gov/sites/GeneTests/review?db=GeneTests.

Disorders of Sexual Development

Chad R. Haldeman-Englert and Jennifer M. Kalish

119

The development of the internal and external male and female reproductive systems from early embryogenesis through puberty involves a highly complex series of genetic and hormonal influences. Differentiation between these systems occurs in early fetal life (first trimester), and the components of sexual differentiation have classically been divided into three main categories: chromosomal sex (XX vs. XY), gonadal sex (ovary vs. testis), and phenotypic sex (female vs. male reproductive organs). Abnormalities of one or more of these important developmental stages may result in a disorder of sexual development with several possible phenotypic outcomes, such as ambiguous genitalia to complete discordance between the chromosomal sex and phenotypic features.

Changes in the classification and nomenclature of these disorders have occurred in more recent years. Terms such as *intersex*, *hermaphrodite*, and *pseudohermaphrodite* can be perceived as derogatory and confusing when used to discuss a newborn's abnormalities. Therefore, this terminology has been replaced with the designation *disorders of sexual development* (DSD), which is a broader descriptor that reflects the fact that a patient has discordance between the internal reproductive organs and external genitalia because of various mechanisms. Current categories are now considered as sex chromosome DSDs, 46,XY DSDs, and 46,XX DSDs. This chapter focuses on our current understanding of the development of internal and external reproductive organs, with a focus on the causes, evaluation, and management of the more common DSDs.

NORMAL SEXUAL DEVELOPMENT

The normal development of the reproductive organs in humans begins with the differentiation of primordial structures and ends with the completion of secondary sexual characteristics that begins during puberty (see Chapter 67 for a discussion on puberty). Around the fifth week of gestation, the genital ridge develops into the appropriate gonads based on the chromosomal sex (XX or XY) established at conception. A complex series of genetic events must occur to establish the appropriate differentiation to an ovary or testis. It was clear that genes on the Y chromosome were involved in this differentiation because the presence of a Y chromosome resulted in male sexual characteristics, such as in XY or XXY individuals. Before these genes were known, they were referred to as "testis-determining factor" (TDF) because their presence led to testis formation. Ovaries and other female-specific reproductive organs were believed to develop by "default" because of the absence of Y chromosome material or TDF. Accordingly, research in mice and humans with X-Y translocations determined that the *SRY* gene (sex-determining region, Y) encoded for a transcription factor that is necessary for male reproductive organ development. Additional genes have also been identified for testis formation (Figure 119-1), and mutations in any of these genes (e.g., *SOX9*,

DMRT1) have been associated with sex-reversal in XY patients. It is also important to note that more recent data have demonstrated an active role of several genes (*FOXL2*, *WNT4*, *RSPO1*) in ovary development in XX individuals, contradicting the older "default" female development notion.

After the development of the gonads, the genital ducts must differentiate into the appropriate internal structures necessary for reproduction (Figure 119-2). In the undifferentiated stage, both mesonephric (Wolffian) and paramesonephric (Müllerian) ducts are present. In males, the newly formed testes secrete anti-Müllerian hormone (AMH), inhibin B, and testosterone between weeks 7 and 11, causing the Müllerian ducts to regress and the Wolffian ducts to persist, eventually becoming the seminal vesicles, vas deferentia, and epididymis. The opposite occurs in females, in whom the absence of testicular secretions causes the mesonephric ducts to regress and the Müllerian ducts to persist, forming the fallopian tubes, uterus, and upper third of the vagina

The undifferentiated genital tubercle, labioscrotal swellings, and urethral folds are present around gestational week 4, and the external genitalia begin to become more distinguishable during weeks 9 to 13. In males, the presence of testosterone and the testosterone derivative dihydrotestosterone (converted by 5-αreductase) causes the genital tubercle to form the glans penis, stimulating the urethral folds to fuse ventrally and form the spongy urethra and resulting in part of the penile shaft and labioscrotal swellings to fuse and form the scrotum (Figure 119-3). The absence of testosterone and dihydrotestosterone in females causes the genital tubercle to form the glans clitoris and the urethral folds and labioscrotal swelling to remain unfused (except posteriorly) to form the labia minora and labia majora, respectively. In males, testicular descent begins during the twelfth week of gestation and finishes during the third trimester.

ETIOLOGY, PATHOGENESIS, AND CLINICAL PRESENTATION

Because of the myriad genes associated with urogenital development, many genetic abnormalities may alter the structure and function of the reproductive organs. As noted above, these DSDs have been recently subtyped into sex chromosome DSDs, 46,XY DSDs, and 46,XX DSDs (Table 119-1). Sex chromosome DSDs are caused by various mechanisms (Figure 119-4) and include Klinefelter syndrome (47,XXY) and variants, Turner syndrome (45,X) and variants, and other types of XX/XY mosaicism, as discussed in Chapter 118, and typically result in largely normal prenatal sexual development but reduced function of the gonads during and after puberty. Most other genetic abnormalities may include point mutations, frameshift mutations, or deletions of specific genes that cause the protein product to be nonfunctional and thereby affect gonad differentiation, leading

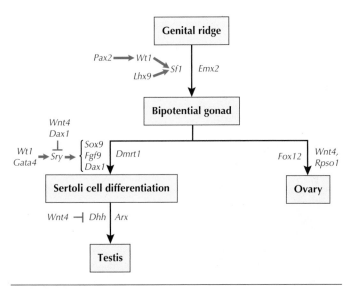

Figure 119-1 *Genes associated with testicular and ovarian differentiation.*

to a disparity between the chromosomal sex (XX or XY) and gonad development (ovary or testis).

46,XY Disorders of Sexual Development

The clearest example of 46,XY DSDs is still *SRY*, which is important for testis development, and when mutated, results in

the undifferentiated gonad to develop into an ovary. Other abnormalities involving *SRY* include balanced chromosomal translocations between the *SRY*-containing portion of the Y chromosome (Yp11.31) and another chromosome in a father that could lead to an imbalance in the child, causing either a 46,XY DSD caused by *SRY* deficiency or a 46,XX DSD if there is ectopic *SRY* expression.

Other genes that may be associated with various 46,XY DSDs are listed in Table 119-1. *SOX9* is a transcription factor that along with *SF1* regulates transcription of AMH. *SOX9* is also involved in chondrocyte differentiation, and mutations of this gene cause a skeletal disorder called camptomelic dysplasia (Figure 119-5), where about 67% of XY patients develop as phenotypic females with abnormalities that include gonadal dysgenesis; the presence of Müllerian structures such as a uterus, fallopian tubes, and vagina; and external female genitalia. *WT1* is another transcription factor involved in testis formation and synergizes with *SF1* to induce AMH. Mutations of *WT1* are seen in patients with Denys-Drash syndrome, in which XY patients have various urogenital anomalies, including ambiguous genitalia. In addition, larger deletions that include *WT1* cause WAGR syndrome (Wilms' tumor, aniridia, genitourinary anomalies, and mental retardation). *DHH* is an important signaling molecule involved in various areas of morphogenesis, including male gonadal development, and mutations in *DHH* are associated with XY gonadal dysgenesis.

Other 46,XY DSDs involve abnormalities with androgen synthesis or action. Smith-Lemli-Opitz syndrome is a multiple congenital anomaly disorder of cholesterol biosynthesis caused

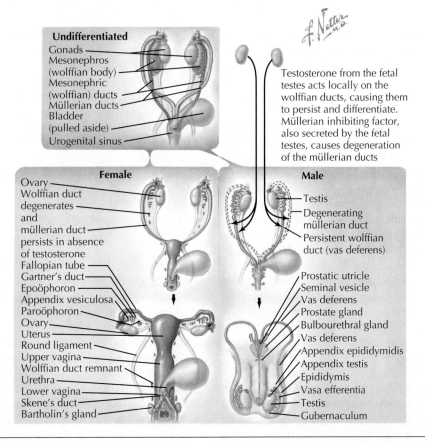

Figure 119-2 *Gonad and genital duct formation.*

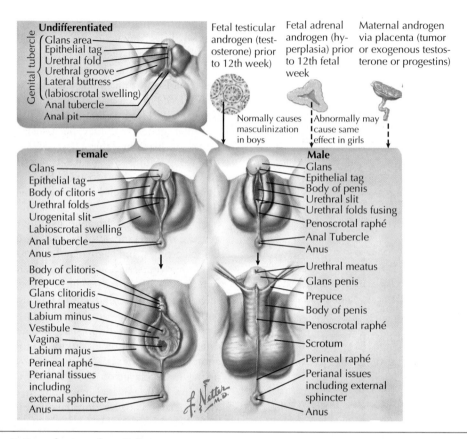

Figure 119-3 *Differentiation of external genitalia.*

by mutations of the sterol δ-7-reductase (*DHCR7*) gene and resulting in decreased androgen production. Abnormalities typically involve ambiguous genitalia but may involve the presence of other female reproductive organs. Other mutations along the cholesterol biosynthesis pathway that cause a DSD in XY individuals include those of 17-αhydroxylase (*CYP17A1*) and cholesterol side-chain cleavage (*CYP11A1*). Defects in these genes present with a spectrum of abnormalities such as ambiguous genitalia, female internal and external genitalia, and adrenal hyperplasia and insufficiency. Patients with 5-α reductase 2 deficiency have normal-appearing female genitalia at birth because testosterone is not converted to dihydrotestosterone, an important effector hormone in male external genital development. However, at puberty, when testosterone levels surge, these patients develop clitoromegaly and virilization. Androgen insensitivity syndrome is caused by a defect in the androgen receptor gene (*AR*) that is unresponsive to testosterone binding. Patients have female external genitalia, breast development, inguinal or abdominal testes, and a blind vaginal pouch but no uterus or fallopian tubes.

46,XX Disorders of Sexual Development

46,XX DSDs may also be attributable to gene defects or, more commonly, androgen excess. As mentioned previously, XX individuals who express *SRY* develop testes during gonadal differentiation. Duplication of *SOX9* can also cause a similar phenotype with testis development and male external genitalia.

The most common 46,XX DSD is caused by androgen excess from congenital adrenal hyperplasia (CAH), a group of disorders where the basic defect is in the conversion of cholesterol to cortisol. 21-Hydroxylase (*CYP21A2*) is the most common cause of CAH, involved in more than 90% of cases. Masculinization occurs when there is an increase in testosterone production, which is mostly seen in patients with 21-hydroxylase and 11-β hydroxylase deficiencies (*CYP11A2*). The external genitalia appear male in females but normal in males. The decrease in cortisol production also causes the adrenal glands to enlarge and salt wasting to occur, which can be life threatening in the neonatal period. Additional causes of masculinization of females can occur with exposure of the fetus to androgens either by maternal tumors that produce androgens (luteomas) or via an exogenous source.

Several genetic syndromes are also associated with 46,XX DSDs. MURCS (Müllerian duct aplasia, renal agenesis or ectopia, and cervical somite dysplasia) is a sporadic condition associated with an absent or hypoplastic uterus as well as the proximal two-thirds of the vagina caused by aplasia of the Müllerian ducts. Female patients with MODY5 (maturity-onset diabetes of the young, type 5), caused by mutations of the *TCF2* gene, have been found to have vagina aplasia and uterine anomalies such as a rudimentary or bicornuate uterus. Finally, vaginal abnormalities such as aplasia, transverse vaginal membrane, hydrometrocolpos, and rectovaginal fistula have been seen in females with *MKKS* mutations that cause McKusick-Kaufman syndrome.

Table 119-1 Classification of Disorders of Sexual Differentiation

Sex Chromosome DSDs	46,XY DSDs	46,XX DSDs

A. 47,XXY
B. 45,X
 	
C. 45,X/46,XY
D. 46,XX/46,XY mosaicism
	A. Disorders of testicular development
	  1. Complete or partial gonadal dysgenesis (e.g., *SRY, SOX9, SF1, WT1, DHH*)
	  2. Ovotesticular DSD
	  3. Testis regression
	B. Disorders of androgen synthesis
	  1. LH receptor mutations
	
	  2. Smith-Lemli-Opitz (cholesterol biosynthesis defect)
	  3. Cholesterol side-chain cleavage (CYP11A1)
	  4. 17-α hydroxylase (CYP17)
	  5. P450 oxidoreductase (POR)
	  6. 5-α reductase 2
	C. Disorders of androgen action
	  1. Androgen insensitivity syndrome
	  2. Drugs and environmental modulators
	
	D. Other
	  1. Syndromic associations of male genital development (cloacal anomalies, Robinow, Aarskog, hand-foot-genital)
	  2. Persistent Müllerian duct syndrome
	  3. Vanishing testis syndrome
	  4. Isolated hypospadias
	  5. Congenital hypogonatropic hypogonadism
	  6. Cryptorchidism (*INSL3, GREAT*)
	  7. Environmental influences
		A. Disorders of ovarian development
		  1. Gonadal dysgenesis
		
		  2. Ovotesticular DSD
		  3. Testicular DSD (SRY+, dup SOX9)
		B. Androgen excess
		  1. Fetal (3-β hydroxysteroid dehydrogenase 2), 21-hydroxylase (CYP21A2), P450 oxidoreductase (POR), 11-β hydroxylase (CYP11B1), glucocorticoid receptor mutations
		  2. Fetoplacental (aromatase [CYP19], oxidoreductase [POR])
		  3. Maternal (virilizing tumors [luteoma], androgenic drugs)
		
		C. Other
		  1. Syndromic associations (cloacal anomalies)
		  2. Müllerian agenesis or hypoplasia (MURCS)
		  3. Uterine abnormalities (MODY5)
		  4. Vaginal atresia (McKusick-Kaufman)
		  5. Labial adhesions

DSD, disorders of sexual development; LH, luteinizing hormone; MURCS, Müllerian duct aplasia, renal agenesis or ectopia, and cervical somite dysplasia; MODY5, maturity-onset diabetes of the young.
Adapted from Hughes IA: Disorders of sex development: a new definition and classification. Best Pract Res Clin Endocrinol Metab 22:119-134, 2008.

EVALUATION AND MANAGEMENT

Although the introduction of routine prenatal ultrasound screening has allowed for the discovery and evaluation of ambiguous genitalia in a fetus, most DSDs present at birth in a newborn with ambiguous genitalia. Unfortunately, as difficult as it might be for the parents and health care team, gender assignment should be postponed until a thorough assessment has been completed. The health care team may consist of several members beyond the nursery or neonatal care unit, including endocrinology, surgery, urology, genetics, psychology, and social work. Input from all involved is critical in providing not only a methodical approach to the diagnosis and treatment of the child but also to offer appropriate family support during this difficult period.

Diagnosis

A comprehensive evaluation begins with a detailed history and physical examination. Historical information should focus on the gestational age at the time of birth (preterm neonates may have some degree of phallic ambiguity); discordance between a known prenatal karyotype and phenotypic features; maternal exposures, medications, or ingestions; and family history of any consanguinity, genital or urologic abnormalities, infant deaths, and amenorrhea or other issues with puberty or fertility. Examination findings that suggest the presence of a DSD include ambiguous genitalia in which neither male or female sex assignment can be made; apparent female genitalia with clitoromegaly; posterior labial fusion; an inguinal or labial mass; or male genitalia with nonpalpable testes, hypospadias, or micropenis. Other physical findings may focus on the presence of dysmorphic features, such as short stature, a broad neck, and wide nipples in Turner's syndrome, syndactyly between the second and third toes in Smith-Lemli-Opitz syndrome, aniridia in *WT1* deletions, or abnormal curvature of the limbs as seen in camptomelic dysplasia.

Laboratory and radiologic studies vary for each patient and are based on the historical and physical findings (Figure 119-6). The genetic investigation focuses on determining the number

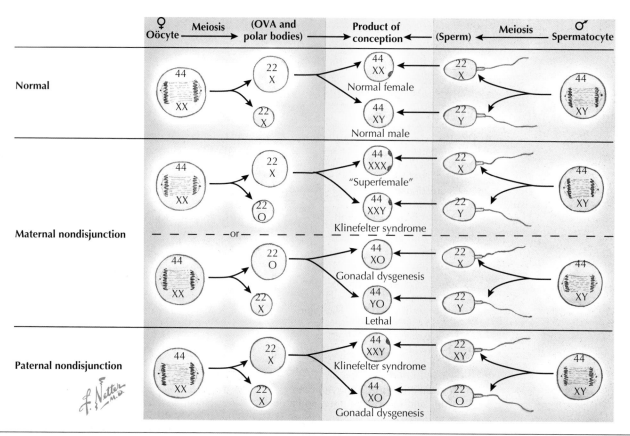

Figure 119-4 *Errors in chromosomal sex.*

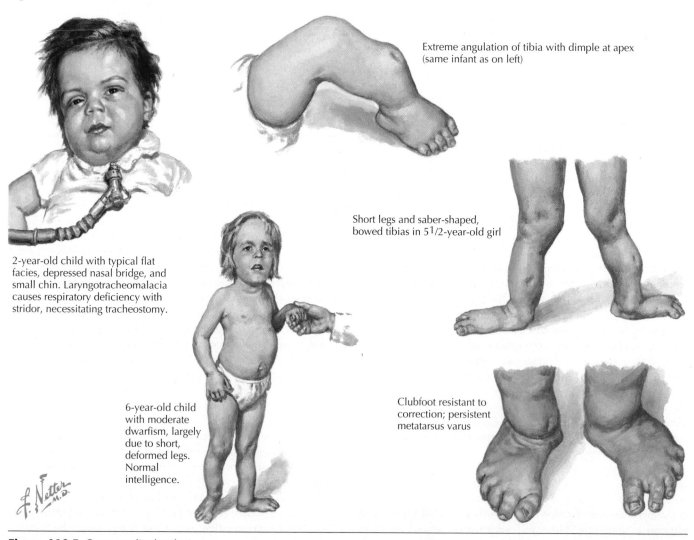

Extreme angulation of tibia with dimple at apex (same infant as on left)

2-year-old child with typical flat facies, depressed nasal bridge, and small chin. Laryngotracheomalacia causes respiratory deficiency with stridor, necessitating tracheostomy.

6-year-old child with moderate dwarfism, largely due to short, deformed legs. Normal intelligence.

Short legs and saber-shaped, bowed tibias in 5$\frac{1}{2}$-year-old girl

Clubfoot resistant to correction; persistent metatarsus varus

Figure 119-5 *Campomelic dysplasia.*

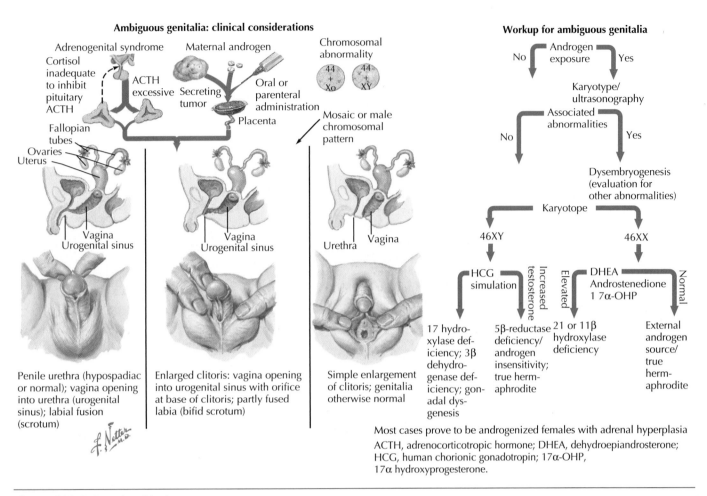

Ambiguous genitalia: clinical considerations

Adrenogenital syndrome

Cortisol inadequate to inhibit pituitary ACTH

ACTH excessive

Maternal androgen

Secreting tumor

Oral or parenteral administration

Placenta

Chromosomal abnormality

44 + Xo   44 + XY

Mosaic or male chromosomal pattern

Fallopian tubes
Ovaries
Uterus

Vagina
Urogenital sinus

Vagina
Urogenital sinus

Urethra   Vagina

Penile urethra (hypospadiac or normal); vagina opening into urethra (urogenital sinus); labial fusion (scrotum)

Enlarged clitoris: vagina opening into urogenital sinus with orifice at base of clitoris; partly fused labia (bifid scrotum)

Simple enlargement of clitoris; genitalia otherwise normal

Workup for ambiguous genitalia

No ← Androgen exposure → Yes

Karyotype/ ultrasonography

No ← Associated abnormalities → Yes

Dysembryogenesis (evaluation for other abnormalities)

Karyotope

46XY   46XX

HCG simulation   Increased testosterone   Elevated   DHEA Androstenedione 1 7α-OHP   Normal

17 hydroxylase deficiency; 3β dehydrogenase deficiency; gonadal dysgenesis

5β-reductase deficiency/ androgen insensitivity; true hermaphrodite

21 or 11β hydroxylase deficiency

External androgen source/ true hermaphrodite

Most cases prove to be androgenized females with adrenal hyperplasia
ACTH, adrenocorticotropic hormone; DHEA, dehydroepiandrosterone; HCG, human chorionic gonadotropin; 17α-OHP, 17α hydroxyprogesterone.

Figure 119-6 *Sexual ambiguity.*

of X and Y chromosomes by karyotype, fluorescence in situ hybridization, or microarray analysis to determine the chromosomal sex (e.g., 46,XY, 46,XX, 45,X, 46,XX/46,XY) and any evidence of mosaicism. Specific genes can also be analyzed for mutations based on other associated findings on the physical examination or serum chemistries. Serum electrolytes are necessary to evaluate sodium concentration in cases of suspected CAH. Other CAH studies include the levels of 17-OH-progesterone (elevated in CAH) and 11-deoxycortisol (high in 11-β hydroxylase deficiency; low in 21-hydroxylase deficiency). If 17-OH-progesterone is normal, testosterone and dihydrotestosterone levels (after human chorionic gonadotropin [hCG] stimulation) may help elucidate the cause of some 46,XY DSDs (e.g., high testosterone to low dihydrotestosterone is seen in 5-α reductase 2 deficiency). hCG stimulation may also determine anorchia if there is no significant change in androgen levels combined with elevated luteinizing hormone and follicle-stimulating hormone levels. An ultrasound should be the first radiologic procedure performed because it may determine the Müllerian anatomy and possibly the presence and location of the gonads. Computed tomography or magnetic resonance imaging may also assist in clarifying these structures further. Finally, infants with intraabdominal or nonpalpable gonads may require exploratory laparoscopy with biopsy to determine if dysgenetic gonads, ovotestes, or streak testes are present.

Management

Management of patients with DSDs depends on the clinical history and physical examination, as well as any relevant laboratory, radiologic, and surgical results. If a specific genetic abnormality is discovered, evaluation of the parents for carrier status is important for assessing their risk for additional affected children. In CAH, electrolyte abnormalities should be corrected and appropriate hormone replacement initiated.

One of the most challenging aspects of treating patients with DSDs is the timing and type of gender assignment surgery. There is no clear consensus, and each case should be evaluated independently based on the patient data and diagnosis, patient input (if old enough), family requests, likelihood of fertility, and feasibility of the corrective surgery. Early female assignment may be most appropriate in patients who have 46,XX CAH with ambiguous genitalia and normal ovaries and uterus, bilateral testicular dysgenesis with the presence of a vagina and uterus, and complete androgen insensitivity syndrome. Patients with partial androgen insensitivity and 5-α reductase 2 deficiency should be considered for male assignment for various reasons, but particularly because if there is presence of significant testosterone exposure during fetal development, these patients show fewer signs of typical female behaviors in adolescence and adulthood. Because it is sometimes difficult to predict the gender and sexual identity that a newborn with a DSD might display later in life, there are instances in which it may be beneficial to delay assignment surgery, if possible, to align the patient's preferences with the anatomic structures while still maintaining fertility. However, in any newborn with a 46,XY DSD who will be raised as a girl, it is important to remove the gonads (testes) to decrease the chance of developing a gonadal tumor.

FUTURE DIRECTIONS

Patients with DSDs often present a difficult and challenging array of historical and clinical findings, diagnostic possibilities, and treatment options. Further research into the various causes of DSDs at the genetic and molecular levels will likely increase not only our understanding of these conditions but also improve the diagnostic yield and therefore risk counseling available to our patients and their families. Last, a focus on maintaining open communication between the patient (if older), family, and health care team needs to continue to provide the best possible outcomes.

SUGGESTED READINGS

Achermann JC, Hughes IA Disorders of sexual development. In Kronenberg HM, Melmed S, Polonsky KS, Larsen PR, editors: *Williams Textbook of Endocrinology*, ed 11. Philadelphia, Saunders Elsevier, 2008, pp 783-848.

Burke LW: Female genital system. In Stevenson RE, Hall JG, editors: *Human Malformations and Related Anomalies*, ed 2, New York, Oxford Press, 2006, pp 1279-1306.

Hughes IA: Disorders of sex development: a new definition and classification. *Best Pract Res Clin Endocrinol Metab* 22:119-134, 2008.

Kolon TF: Disorders of sexual development. *Curr Urol Rep* 9:172-177, 2008.

Martin RA: Male genital system. In Stevenson RE, Hall JG, editors: *Human Malformations and Related Anomalies*, ed 2, New York, Oxford Press, 2006, pp 1251-1278.

Moore KL, Persuad TVN, editors: The urogenital system. In *The Developing Human*, ed 8, Philadelphia, 2008, Saunders Elsevier, pp 243-284.

Genetic Syndromes

120

Jennifer M. Kalish and Chad R. Haldeman-Englert

Diagnosis of genetic syndromes is based on a systematic approach using a thorough medical history, pedigree analysis, detailed physical examination, pattern recognition, and literature and database consultation. This strategy guides testing for disorders for which a genetic cause has been identified. Although correction of the gene defect is currently available for very few disorders, specific diagnosis enables proper management of complications and recurrence counseling.

One of the specific approaches to diagnosis of genetics syndromes is the incorporation of major malformations (e.g., cleft lip or palate, brain or cardiac anomalies) as well as more common minor malformations (e.g., downslanting palpebral fissures, flat nasal bridge, syndactyly, or clinodactyly; see Chapter 116) to lead the diagnostician toward a specific diagnosis. The goal of this chapter is to illustrate a systematic approach using categories of major or unique findings. Only one or two of the more common or classic syndromes are illustrated for each major category.

VERY SMALL OR SHORT STATURE

Cornelia de Lange Syndrome

Cornelia de Lange syndrome (CdLS) has a prevalence of around 1:10,000 and is characterized by prenatal and postnatal growth retardation, hirsutism, and upper limb reduction defects. Craniofacial abnormalities include synophrys, arched eyebrows, long eyelashes, a small, upturned nose, small, widely spaced teeth, and microcephaly (Figure 120-1). Patients have moderate to severe mental retardation (MR), and many show autistic and self-destructive behaviors. Upper limb abnormalities range from severe deficiencies to merely proximally placed thumbs or fifth digit clinodactyly. Patients classically have growth failure as well as feeding difficulties, which include regurgitation, projectile vomiting, and swallowing difficulties. Hearing loss and speech delay are common. CdLS has dominant inheritance usually caused by de novo mutations in NIPBL (50%), SMC1A (5%), and SMC3 (<1%).

Rubenstein-Tabyi Syndrome

Rubenstein-Tabyi syndrome (RTS) has a prevalence of around 1:100,000 and is characterized by postnatal short stature, moderate to severe MR with speech difficulty, downslanted palpebral fissures, hypoplastic maxilla with narrow palate, prominent or beaked nose with columella extending below the nares, highly arched palate, grimacing smile, talon cusps, broad great thumbs and toes with radial angulation, and hirsutism. Patients have normal prenatal growth, and obesity occurs in childhood or adolescence. Developmental milestones are significantly delayed, with reading limited to the first grade level. Many patients have gastroesophageal reflux, constipation, recurrent ear infections, and dental problems secondary to tooth overcrowding in the small jaw. Most cases are caused by dominant sporadic mutations in the CREB binding protein (CBP) gene in 60% of cases and the functionally related EP300 gene in about 3% of cases.

Russell-Silver Syndrome

Russell-Silver syndrome (RSS) has a prevalence of about 1:100,000 and includes intrauterine growth retardation, postnatal growth deficiency, delayed bone age, normal head circumference, limb-length asymmetry, and fifth digit clinodactyly (Figure 120-2). A typical face in RSS is small and triangular with a broad and prominent forehead, downturned corners of the mouth, and micrognathia. Café-au-lait spots are sometimes present, and patients can sweat extensively. Nearly 40% of cases have been shown to have abnormal imprinting of chromosome 11p15.5, and 10% of cases demonstrate uniparental disomy (UPD) for chromosome 7. Growth hormone may benefit patients for whom growth plateaus early.

Noonan Syndrome

Noonan syndrome (NS) has been suggested to occur with a prevalence of around 1:2000 and demonstrates a combination of short statue, congenital heart disease, and variable developmental delay. In the neonate, the typical face has a tall forehead, hypertelorism with downslanting palpebral fissures, epicanthal folds, ptosis, vivid blue or blue-green irises, low-set posteriorly rotated ears with thickened helices, a depressed nasal root, a deeply grooved philtrum, a protruding upper lip, and retrognathia. In adolescence, the facial shape suggests an inverted triangle with a pointed chin, and the neck lengthens to accentuate the webbed appearance. Other features may include a low posterior hairline, a broad chest with superior pectus excavatum and inferior pectus carinatum, and pulmonic stenosis. Postnatal short stature is seen in half of the patients, and skeletal abnormalities, including cubitus valgus and scoliosis, may be seen. Cardiomyopathy or congenital heart disease (CHD) is present in 50% to 80% of patients with the most common anomaly being pulmonary valve stenosis. About one-third of affected individuals have a coagulation or platelet pathway defect. Skin café-au-lait spots and lentigines are prevalent. Mild MR is present in about 30% of patients. Molecular testing has demonstrated dominant mutations in the Ras signaling pathway that include PTPN11 (50%), SOS1 (13%), RAF1 (3%–17%) and KRAS (5%).

PREMATURE AGING

Hutchinson-Gilford Progeria Syndrome

Hutchinson-Gilford Progeria syndrome (HGPS) occurs in between 4 and 8 million births and is a composite of features

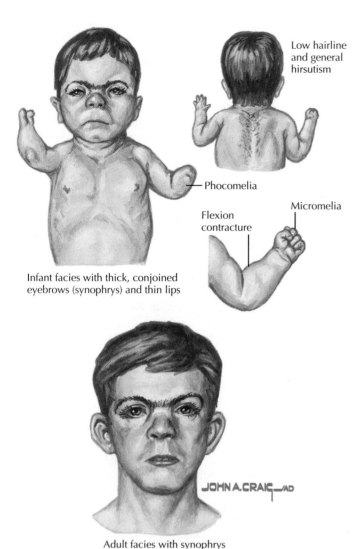

Low hairline and general hirsutism

Phocomelia

Micromelia

Flexion contracture

Infant facies with thick, conjoined eyebrows (synophrys) and thin lips

Adult facies with synophrys and long eyelashes

Figure 120-1 *Profile of the face in a patient with Cornelia de Lange syndrome.*

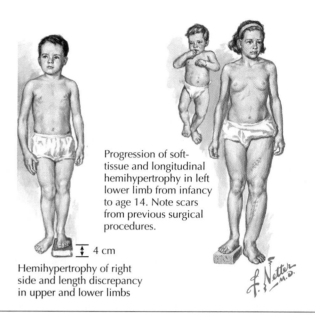

Progression of soft-tissue and longitudinal hemihypertrophy in left lower limb from infancy to age 14. Note scars from previous surgical procedures.

4 cm

Hemihypertrophy of right side and length discrepancy in upper and lower limbs

Figure 120-2 *Hemihypertrophy: limb length discrepancy.*

that develop in childhood that are reminiscent of accelerated aging (Figure 120-3). These include alopecia, diminished subcutaneous fat, stiffness of joints, bone changes, and an abnormal tightness of the skin over the abdomen and upper thighs that emerge during the second to third year of life. Facial features include a pinched nose, thin lips, protruding ears, and a thin, high-pitched voice. Skeletal manifestations include distal phalangeal osteolysis, delayed fontanelle closure, a pear-shaped thorax, micrognathia, short dystrophic clavicles, a "horse-riding" stance, thin limbs, and tightened joint ligaments. Cognitive development is normal. Patients typically develop severe atherosclerosis requiring electrocardiography, echocardiography, and carotid duplex scans every 6 months. Yearly lipid profiles and medical treatment for cardiovascular disease and elevated lipids are recommended. Hip dislocations and contractures are common and should be managed conservatively with physical and occupational therapy. Classical HGPS is caused by de novo dominant splice site mutations in the *LMNA* gene for which genetic testing is available.

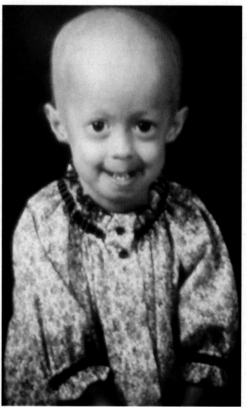

Reprinted with permission from *Hutchinson-Gilford Progeria syndrome: A Pathologic Study.* Jeanne Ackerman; Enid Gilbert-Barness. Fetal and Pediatric Pathology, 1551-3823, Volume 21-1, 1-13, 2002.

Figure 120-3 *Progeria.*

OVERGROWTH SYNDROMES

Fragile X Syndrome

Fragile X syndrome (FXS) is seen in patients with a *FMR1* full mutation and is characterized by moderate MR in males and mild MR in females. Males are macrocephalic, with long faces, prominent foreheads and chins, protruding ears, and large testes after puberty (Figure 120-4). Developmental milestones are delayed, and behavioral features such as tactile defensiveness, poor eye contact, perseverative speech, difficulty with impulse control, and distractibility become more prominent with age. More than 99% of patients with FXS have a loss-of-function mutation in the *FMR1* gene at Xq27.3 that results from more than 200 repeats of a CGG tri-nucleotide (normal 0-40 repeats) and subsequent aberrant methylation of the gene. Individuals with 59 to 200 trinucleotide repeats are considered to have an *FMR1* premutation and can have late-onset, progressive cerebellar ataxia and intention tremor in males and premature ovarian failure in females but with normal appearance and intellect. FXS demonstrates a phenomenon known as anticipation, in which the trinucleotide repeat becomes larger and the phenotype more pronounced with passage from one generation to the next. Molecular epidemiology has suggested 16 to 25 in 100,000 males affected and about half of that prevalence for females.

Beckwith-Wiedemann Syndrome

Beckwith-Wiedemann Syndrome (BWS) is a growth disorder characterized by macrosomia, macroglossia, visceromegaly, omphalocele, neonatal hypoglycemia, ear creases or pits, and a risk for embryonic tumors that includes hepatoblastoma and Wilms' tumors (Figure 120-5). Partial overgrowth, or hemihyperplasia, may occur in tissues, organs, or body segments (see Figure 120-2). Nearly 60% of people with BWS have methylation abnormalities or mutations in the imprinted 11p15 region. Mutations in the *CDKN1C* gene, a growth-regulating gene in this region, are seen in 40% of familial cases and 5% to 10% of nonfamilial cases of BWS. Methylation abnormalities in *KCNQ1OT1* are present in 50% to 60% of the cases and in *H19* in 2% to 7% of the cases. Because of the risk of tumors, abdominal ultrasonography is recommended every 3 months until age 8 years, and serum α-fetoprotein concentration is monitored during the first 3 years.

NEUROLOGIC FINDINGS

Prader-Willi Syndrome and Angelman Syndrome

Prader-Willi syndrome (PWS) is characterized by hypotonia and difficulty feeding early in infancy followed by hyperphagia, beginning from 12 months to 6 years, that leads to central obesity. The face has a narrow bifrontal diameter, almond-shaped eyes, and a downturned mouth (Figure 120-6). Motor and language development is delayed because of cognitive impairment. Hypogonadism with incomplete pubertal development and infertility occurs. Behavioral outbursts (temper tantrums, obsessive-compulsiveness, stubbornness, and manipulation), sleep disturbances, short stature, hypopigmentation,

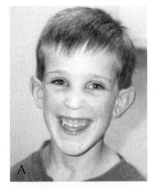

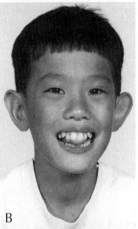

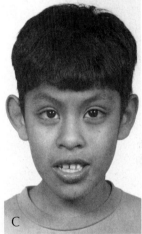

Boys with fragile X syndrome. Note the long faces, prominent jaws, large ears, and similar characteristics of children from different ethnic groups. Caucasian (A), Asian (B), and Hispanic (C). *Reprinted with permission from Jorde LB, Carey JC, Bamshad MJ, White RL. Medical Genetics, 3rd Edition. Mosby, Elsevier. Philadelphia 2003, pg 99, Figure 5-13.*

Figure 120-4 *Fragile X syndrome.*

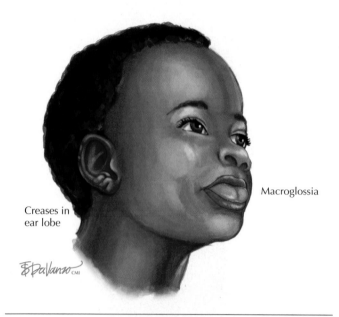

Creases in ear lobe

Macroglossia

Figure 120-5 *Macroglossia in a patient with Beckwith-Wiedemann syndrome.*

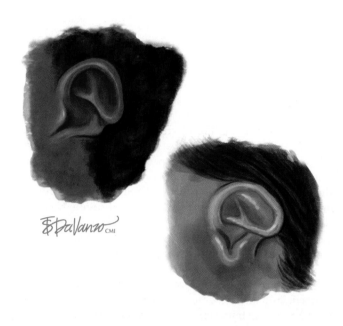

Figure 120-7 *CHARGE (coloboma, heart defects, choanal atresia, retarded growth and development, genital abnormalities, and ear anomalies) syndrome.*

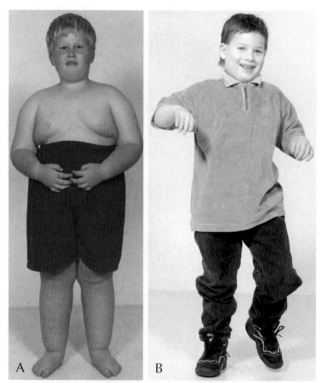

Illustration of the effect of imprinting on chromosome 15 deletions. **A.** Inheritance of the deletion from the father produces Prader-Willi syndrome (note the inverted V-shaped upper lip, small hands, and truncal obesity). **B.** Inheritance of the deletion from the mother produces Angelman syndrome (note the characteristic posture). *(Reprinted with permission from Jorde LB, Carey JC, Bamshad MJ, White RL. Medical Genetics, 3rd Edition. Mosby, Elsevier. Philadelphia 2003, page 78, figure 4.20.)*

Figure 120-6 *Prader-Willi syndrome.*

small hands and feet, skin picking, and articulation difficulties are also seen. Treatment with growth hormone is recommended for those with PWS, and patients may thrive in settings where behavior and food intake are closely monitored.

Diagnosis is made by DNA methylation studies for imprinting on chromosome 15q11. Lack of paternal imprinting leads to PWS, but lack of maternal imprinting leads to a distinctly different disorder called Angelman's syndrome (AS), which demonstrates severe developmental delay, gait ataxia, inappropriately happy demeanor (frequent laughing, smiling, excitability), microcephaly, and seizures.

Deletion of one imprinted parental copy of this region causes 70% of PWS and AS. Mutations in the methylation control region and parental translocations can also cause either syndrome. Risk to siblings is up to 50% for mutations of the imprinting control center but only 1% for UPD. Although PWS is the result of dysregulation of multiple genes, AS can also be caused by mutations in the maternally expressed *UBE3A*.

CHARGE Syndrome

CHARGE syndrome (CHARGE) is an acronym for the combination of coloboma, heart defects, choanal atresia, retarded growth and development, genital abnormalities, and ear anomalies that occurs in 1:8500 to 1:10,000 births. Major diagnostic criteria include colobomas, choanal atresia, and cranial nerve abnormalities. The outer ear is distinctive with its short, wide appearance with a minimal lobe and "snipped off" helix (Figure 120-7). Other ear deformities include ossicle and cochlea malformations, temporal bone abnormalities, and absent semicircular canals. A variety of additional features include hypogonadotropic hypogonadism, developmental delay, cardiovascular malformations, growth deficiency, orofacial clefts, tracheo-esophageal fistulae, and suggestive facies.

Although there are rare dominant familial cases, CHARGE is typically sporadic with mutations in the *CHD7* gene found in 60% to 65% of patients. Management of patients is based on systematic care for each affected organ system.

FACE AND LIMB COMBINATIONS

Townes-Brock Syndrome

Townes-Brock syndrome (TBS) is characterized by imperforate anus, dysplastic ears with overfolded superior helices or preauricular tags, sensorineural or conductive hearing loss, and thumb anomalies consisting of triphalangeal thumbs, duplication, or hypoplasia. Renal impairment with or without structural abnormalities, congenital heart disease, genitourinary malformations, and foot malformations may also occur. Mental retardation occurs in 10% of cases. Nearly half of cases are caused by dominant de novo mutations in *SALL1*. Management of TBS must include cardiac and ophthalmologic evaluations and renal ultrasound. Surgical intervention may be required for an imperforate anus or thumb malformations.

Trichorhinophalangeal Syndrome

Trichorhinophalangeal syndrome (TRPS) is a composite of a bulbous nose, sparse hair, and epiphyseal coning. Growth is usually between the third and tenth percentiles, and the face has a pear-shaped nose with a long, prominent philtrum, a narrow palate, large, prominent ears, small carious teeth with dental malocclusion, and a horizontal groove on the chin. The hair is sparse, thin, and hypopigmented from birth. The nails are thin, and the metacarpals and metatarsals are short and middle phalangeal joints have cone-shaped epiphyses that are broadened, and there are split distal radial epiphyses. The osseous changes are seen in childhood and may progress to degenerative hip disease in young adulthood. The majority of patients with TRPS, type 1 have dominant mutations in *TRPS1* on 8q24.1.

TRPS type II (TRPS II) includes the above features plus multiple bony exostoses. Affected individuals can also present with mild postnatal growth deficiency, microcephaly with mild to severe MR, delayed onset of speech, and sensorineural hearing loss. TRPS II is caused by contiguous gene deletions that span from the *TRPS1* gene to *EXT1*.

Hay-Wells Syndrome of Ectodermal Dysplasia

Hay-Wells syndrome (HWS) is a compilation of ankyloblepharon (bridging of eyelids), ectodermal dysplasia, and cleft lip and palate. Patients have an oval face, maxillary hypoplasia, cleft lip and palate, conical, widely spaced teeth, and hypodontia or partial anodontia. Their skin is notable for palmar and plantar keratoderma, peeling, erythematous eroded skin at birth, partial anhidrosis, hyperpigmentation, and absent or dystrophic nails and hair that ranges from wiry and sparse to alopecia. They often require surgical removal of the eyelid lesions and cleft lip and palate repair. Patients have normal intelligence but often have

heat intolerance because of a reduced number of sweat glands. Inheritance is autosomal dominant with variable expression caused by mutations of the *TP63* gene on chromosome 3q27.

LIMB ANOMALIES

Holt-Oram Syndrome

Holt-Oram syndrome (HOS) comprises upper limb defects, cardiac anomalies, and narrow shoulders. Patients may have absent, hypoplastic, triphalangeal, or bifid thumbs with syndactyly between the thumb and second digit. Phocomelia occurs in 10% of patients. The clavicle, scapula, and sternum can all be affected, resulting in decreased range of motion at the shoulders and sloping or narrow shoulders. Cardiovascular anomalies include ostium secundum, atrial septal defects, and ventricular septal defects. About one-third of patients have other CHD or conduction defects. Autosomal dominant mutations in *TBX5* are seen in 25% of familial cases and 50% of sporadic cases. There is variation within families, although there is a suggestion that the severity may increase with successive generations. Rare mutations in *SALL4* are also seen.

TAR Syndrome

TAR syndrome (TS) is a combination of thrombocytopenia and an absent radius (Figure 120-8). The thrombocytopenia is most severe in infancy and occurs with a constellation of hypoplasia of megakaryocytes, "leukemoid" granulocytosis, eosinophilia, or anemia. Limb defects are usually bilateral and range from complete absence to mildly hypoplastic radii or humeri, with ulnar deficiencies being less common. The thumbs are always present. Leg abnormalities are seen in 50% and may include hip dislocation, patellar abnormalities, dislocation, absent fibulas, small feet, or abnormal toe placement. Congenital heart defects (22%-33%), renal anomalies (23%), and mental retardation (7%) are also seen. Nearly 40% of patients die in infancy because of hemorrhage. The inheritance pattern is complex, and TAR syndrome can be diagnosed by prenatal ultrasound.

SKELETAL DYSPLASIAS

Achondroplasia

Achondroplasia is a combination of short stature caused by abnormal bone growth with disproportionately short arms and legs, a large head, frontal bossing, and midface hypoplasia. It is seen in ~1:20,000 births (Figure 120-9). Hypotonia and delayed motor milestones are seen in infancy, but intelligence and lifespan are normal. There is an increased risk of death in infancy caused by compression on the spinal cord and upper airway obstruction. The diagnosis is made based on rhizomelic limb shortening, trident hands, and thoracolumbar gibbus in infancy, and radiologic findings include narrowing of interpedicular distance of the caudal spine and a notchlike sacroiliac groove. Achondroplasia-specific *FGFR3* gene mutations are seen in 99% of affected patients. Inheritance is autosomal dominant, and most mutations are de novo. Management includes monitoring growth, avoiding obesity, monitoring for spinal cord

Patterns of Multiple Anomalies: Syndrome Versus Sequence

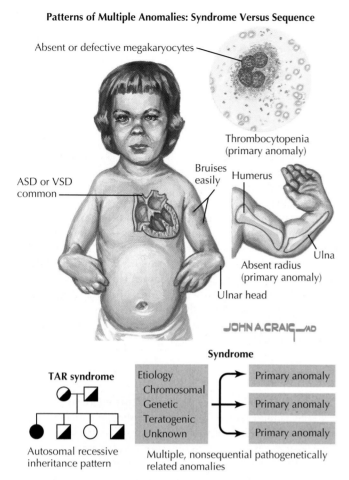

TAR syndrome. Includes two anomalies: thrombocytopenia (T) and absent radius (AR). May be associated with congenital heart anomalies; autosomal recessive transmission

Figure 120-8 *TAR (thrombocytopenia, absent radius) syndrome.*

compression, corrective measures for sleep apnea, and suboccipital decompression for lower limb hyperreflexia, clonus, or central hypopnea.

Leri-Weill Dyschondrosteosis

Leri-Weill Dyschondrosteosis (LWD) represents the severe end of a spectrum of short stature homeobox (*SHX*)-related haploinsufficiency disorders. LWD is characterized by short stature, mesomelia, and Madelung's deformity. Mesomelia is a shortening of the middle limb portion relative to the proximal portion. Madelung's deformity is the abnormal alignment of the radius, ulna, and carpal bones at the wrist developing in childhood and more common in females (Figure 120-10). Three different subphenotypes can all be found within one family: (1) the classic deformity, dorsal subluxation of the distal ulna leading to a "dinner fork" deformity; (2) the reverse deformity, volar subluxation of the distal ulna; and (3) the chevron carpus, which maintains wrist alignment but leads to painful impingement of the lunate bone on the distal radius. Patients with LWD have

normal intelligence and can display muscle hypertrophy, short fourth metacarpals, scoliosis, and exostoses. Deletions or mutations of the *SHOX* genes on the pseudoautosomal regions of X and Y are found in 70% of patients with LWD. Growth hormone treatment and gonadotrophin-releasing hormone agonist improve the final adult height and can help offset an estrogen-blunted growth spurt. Wrist splinting and supports help decrease wrist discomfort but may require physiolysis of the ulnar side of the distal radius and excision of the Vickers ligament in childhood to decrease wrist pain and restore function.

CRANIOSYNOSTOSES

There are eight FGFR-related craniosynostosis disorders (FRCDs). Facial features shared by all of the FRCD except for Muenke's syndrome and FGFR2-related isolated coronal synostosis include hypertelorism, proptosis, midface hypoplasia, and prognathism. High-arched palates, developmental delay, sensorineural hearing loss, and visual problems are common.

Patients with Apert syndrome, which is characterized by a turribrachycephalic skull shape, moderate to severe midface hypoplasia, soft tissue and bony "mitten glove" syndactyly, and medial deviation of the fingers and toes with a variable number of digits, have a 50% chance of developmental delay (Figure 120-11).

Individuals with Muenke syndrome have normal intelligence, uni- or bilateral coronal craniosynostosis, a range of midface hypoplasia, hypertelorism and variable extremity involvement including carpal-tarsal fusion, brachydactyly, carpal bone malsegregation, or coned epiphyses.

Individuals with Crouzon syndrome have normal intellect, proptosis, external strabismus, mandibular prognathism, normal extremities, progressive hydrocephalus, and acanthosis nigricans in 5%.

Individuals with Jackson-Weiss syndrome also have normal intellect, prognathism, broad, medially deviated great toes, normal hands, short first metatarsals, calcaneocuboid fusion, and abnormally formed tarsals.

There are three types of Pfeiffer syndrome (PS). Individuals with type 1 PS, the least severe subtype, have normal intelligence, moderate to severe midface hypoplasia, broad and medially deviated thumbs and great toes, brachydactyly, hearing loss, and hydrocephalus. Those with type 2 PS have developmental delays or MR, a cloverleaf skull, proptosis, broad and medially deviated thumbs and great toes, choanal stenosis or atresia, laryngotracheal abnormalities, seizures, and sacrococcygeal inversion. These patients are at risk for early death. Type 3 PS differs from type 2 PS only in the skull shape's being turribrachycephalic rather than cloverleaf shaped.

Beare-Stevenson cutis gyrata patients all have MR, midface hypoplasia, abnormal ears, natal teeth, furrowed palms and soles, widespread cutis gyrata, acanthosis nigricans, a bifid scrotum, prominent labial raphe, rugated labia majora, pyloric stenosis, and an anteriorly placed anus.

Most of the craniosynostosis disorders are caused by mutations in *FGFR2*, with the exceptions of type 1 PS, which is caused by mutations in *FGFR1*, and Muenke and Crouzon syndrome with acanthosis nigricans, which are caused by

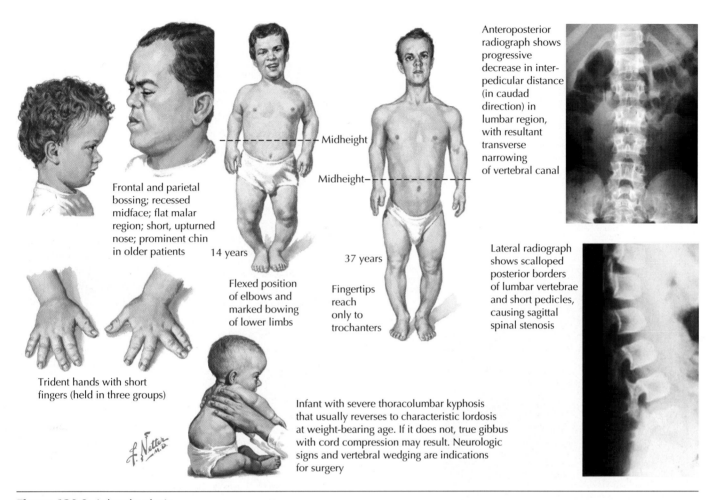

Frontal and parietal bossing; recessed midface; flat malar region; short, upturned nose; prominent chin in older patients

14 years

Midheight

Midheight

37 years

Flexed position of elbows and marked bowing of lower limbs

Fingertips reach only to trochanters

Trident hands with short fingers (held in three groups)

Infant with severe thoracolumbar kyphosis that usually reverses to characteristic lordosis at weight-bearing age. If it does not, true gibbus with cord compression may result. Neurologic signs and vertebral wedging are indications for surgery

Anteroposterior radiograph shows progressive decrease in inter-pedicular distance (in caudad direction) in lumbar region, with resultant transverse narrowing of vertebral canal

Lateral radiograph shows scalloped posterior borders of lumbar vertebrae and short pedicles, causing sagittal spinal stenosis

Figure 120-9 *Achondroplasia.*

mutations in *FGFR3*. The overall incidence of craniosynostosis is ~1:2500 live births. The incidence of coronal synostosis is 1:16,000 in males and 1:8000 in females. The incidence of each of the FGFR-related craniosynostoses is roughly 1:100,000.

CONNECTIVE TISSUE

Osteogenesis Imperfecta

Osteogenesis imperfecta (OI) is a disorder with a growing number of definable subtypes that lead to fractures with minimal trauma. They represent a continuum from perinatal lethality with severe skeletal deformation to mild predisposition to fractures and a normal lifespan. The diagnosis is based on history of fractures; grey-blue sclera; dentinogenesis imperfecta; progressive hearing loss after puberty; and radiographic findings of fractures at different stages of healing, wormian bones, and osteopenia (Figure 120-12). Skin, bone, and chorionic villus biopsies can be used to test the quality and structure of the type I collagen. Molecular testing for *COL1A1* and *COL1A2* mutations can also be used to test for certain dominant types of OI. Types I to V are inherited in an autosomal dominant fashion, and type VII is autosomal recessive. Because of the variable

range of clinical presentations, OI should be considered in suspected cases of child abuse.

Marfan Syndrome

Marfan syndrome is a connective tissue disorder with a range of clinical variability that includes the ocular, skeletal, and cardiovascular systems and has a prevalence of 1:5000 to 1:10,000 (Figure 120-13). The diagnosis is made based on family history and defined diagnostic criteria, which are outlined in Table 120-1.

Management includes blood pressure reduction to reduce the hemodynamic stress of the aortic wall. Yearly echocardiography is recommended, with more frequent monitoring for increased aortic diameters or increased rate of dilatations. Antibiotic prophylaxis before dental work is recommended. Surgical intervention is recommended when the aorta is greater than 5 cm in older children and the rate of enlargement is 1 cm per year or progressive aortic regurgitation is occurring. Morbidity and mortality are closely linked with the cardiovascular manifestations, most commonly a dilated aorta with predisposition for tear and rupture. Marfan syndrome is caused by dominant mutations in *FBN1*, which can also lead to a broad continuum of additional phenotypes.

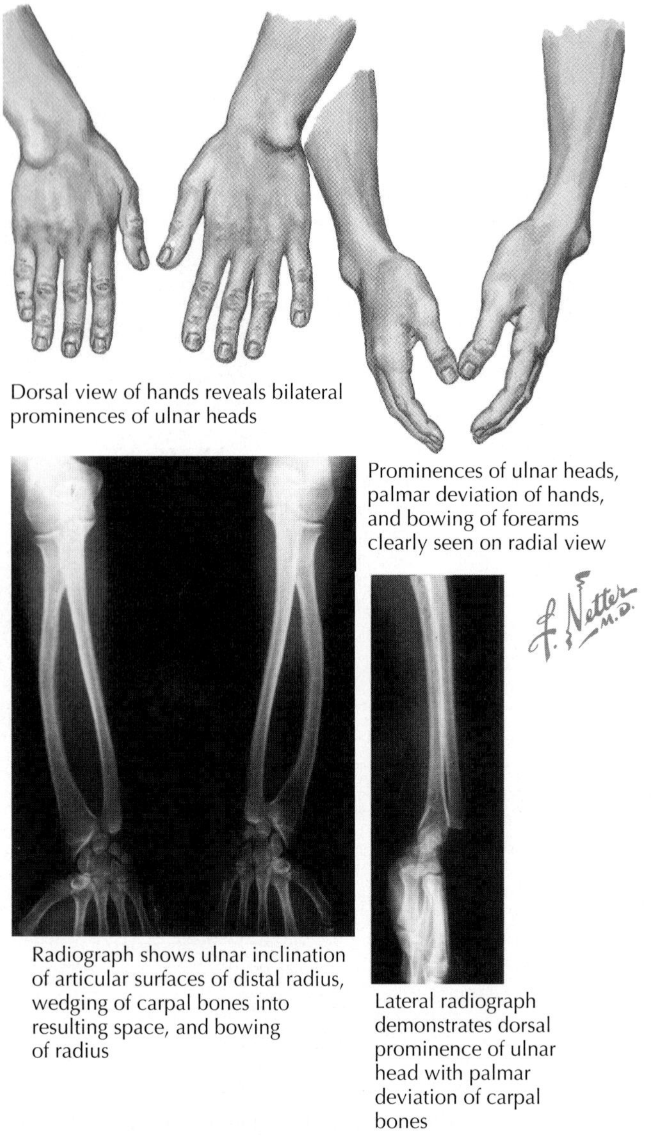
Dorsal view of hands reveals bilateral prominences of ulnar heads
Prominences of ulnar heads, palmar deviation of hands, and bowing of forearms clearly seen on radial view
Radiograph shows ulnar inclination of articular surfaces of distal radius, wedging of carpal bones into resulting space, and bowing of radius
Lateral radiograph demonstrates dorsal prominence of ulnar head with palmar deviation of carpal bones
F. Netter M.D.

Figure 120-10 *Madelung deformity.*

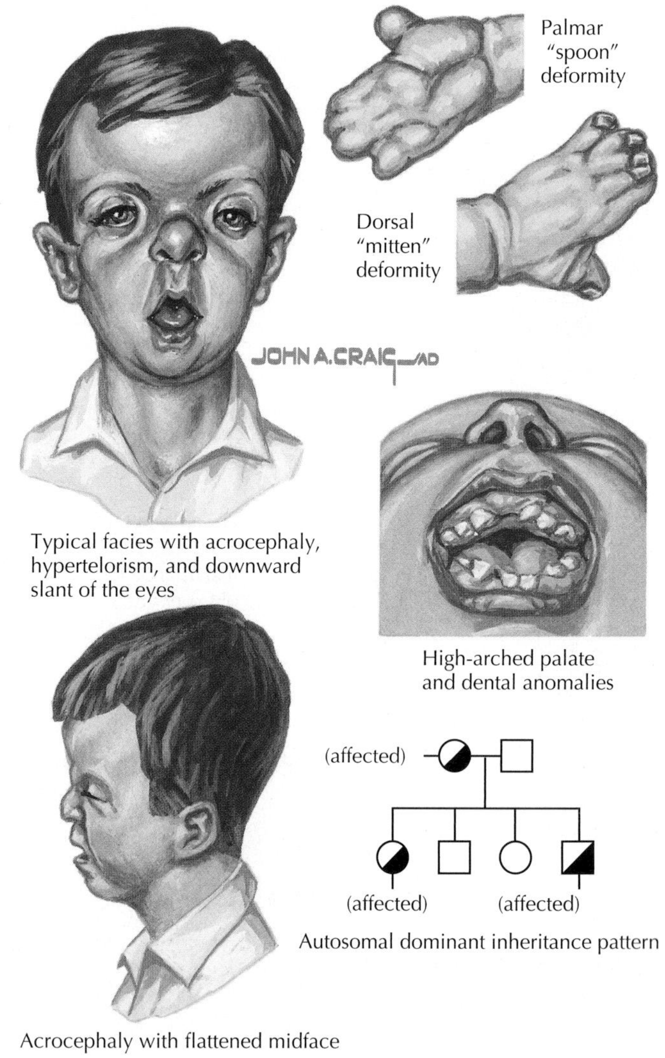
Palmar "spoon" deformity
Dorsal "mitten" deformity
JOHN A.CRAIG—AD
Typical facies with acrocephaly, hypertelorism, and downward slant of the eyes
High-arched palate and dental anomalies
(affected)
(affected)
(affected)
Autosomal dominant inheritance pattern
Acrocephaly with flattened midface

Figure 120-11 *Apert syndrome.*

HAMARTOSES/NEUROCUTANEOUS SYNDROME

Neurofibromatosis

Type 1 neurofibromatosis (NF), or von Recklinghausen disease, is an autosomal dominant disorder characterized by café -au-lait spots and fibromatous tumors of the skin. NF1 is one of the most common dominantly inherited genetic disorders with a prevalence of one in 3000. Diagnostic criteria include at least two of the following: six or more café-au-lait spots, axillary or inguinal freckling, two or more discrete dermal neurofibromas or a plexiform neurofibroma, and two or more of iris Lisch nodules, an optic glioma, a distinctive osseous lesion, or a first-degree relative with NF1 (Figure 120-14).

Children with NF usually develop café-au-lait spots during infancy in 95% of cases and meet the criteria above by 8 years of age. Any child with multiple café-au-lait spots should be given a thorough physical and ophthalmologic examination to look for other features of NF. The parents of that child should also be thoroughly examined for signs of NF. Café-au-lait macules are counted if they are larger than 5 mm in prepubertal individuals and larger than 15 mm in postpubertal individuals.

Diffuse plexiform neurofibromas on the face or neck appear in the first year and on other parts of the body after adolescence. Neurofibromas can occur anywhere and usually appear late in childhood. Half of patients with NF have learning disabilities. Bony complications include vertebral dysplasia, leading to mild scoliosis that may develop between ages 6 and 10 years, pseudarthroses, and overgrowth.

Plexiform neurofibromas, optic and central nervous system gliomas, malignant peripheral nerve sheath tumors, osseous lesions, and vasculopathy are less common. The most common neoplasms seen in NF besides the neurofibromas are optic gliomas in childhood and peripheral nerve sheath tumors that may develop in adolescents or adults. Several brain tumors have been reported, and leukemia (juvenile chronic myelogenous

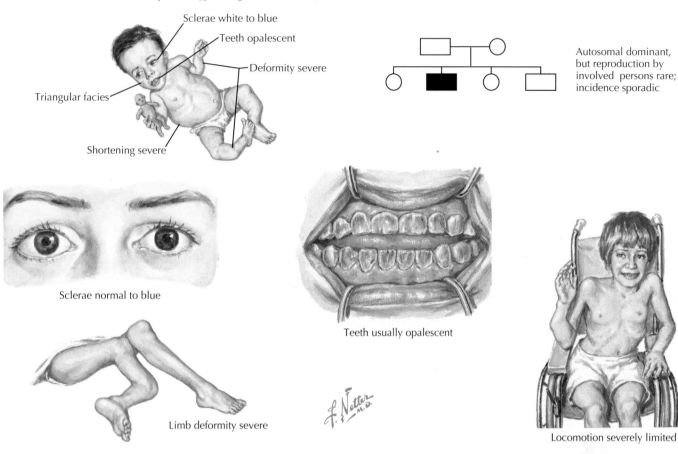

Sclerae white to blue

Teeth opalescent

Deformity severe

Triangular facies

Shortening severe

Autosomal dominant, but reproduction by involved persons rare; incidence sporadic

Sclerae normal to blue

Teeth usually opalescent

Limb deformity severe

Locomotion severely limited

Figure 120-12 *Osteogenesis imperfecta.*

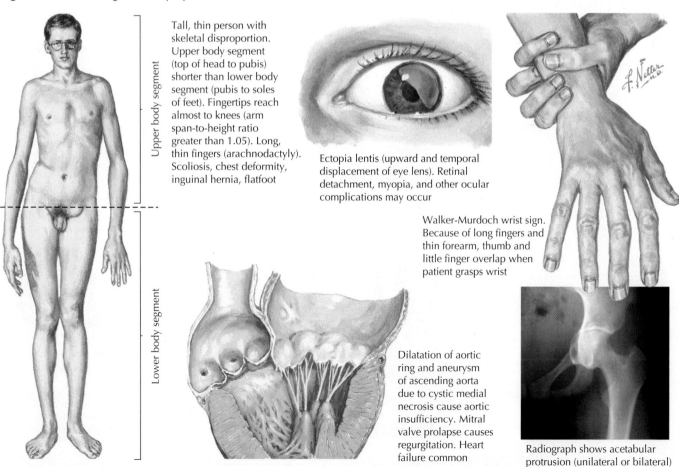

Tall, thin person with skeletal disproportion. Upper body segment (top of head to pubis) shorter than lower body segment (pubis to soles of feet). Fingertips reach almost to knees (arm span-to-height ratio greater than 1.05). Long, thin fingers (arachnodactyly). Scoliosis, chest deformity, inguinal hernia, flatfoot

Upper body segment

Lower body segment

Ectopia lentis (upward and temporal displacement of eye lens). Retinal detachment, myopia, and other ocular complications may occur

Walker-Murdoch wrist sign. Because of long fingers and thin forearm, thumb and little finger overlap when patient grasps wrist

Dilatation of aortic ring and aneurysm of ascending aorta due to cystic medial necrosis cause aortic insufficiency. Mitral valve prolapse causes regurgitation. Heart failure common

Radiograph shows acetabular protrusion (unilateral or bilateral)

Figure 120-13 *Marfan syndrome.*

Table 120-1 Diagnostic Criteria for Marfan Syndrome

Major Criteria	Minor Criteria
Skeletal findings • Major pectus carinatum • Increased limb length • Wrist and thumb signs • Scoliosis • Reduced elbow extension • Protrusion acetabulae	Facial appearance • Dolichocephaly • Malar hypoplasia • Enophthalmos • Retrognathia • Downslanting palpebral fissures • Highly arched palate
Ocular findings • Ectopia lentis	Ocular findings • Abnormally flat cornea • Increased axial length of globe • Hypoplastic iris or ciliary muscle
Dilatation of the ascending aorta	Joint hypermobility
Lumbosacral dural ectasia	Moderate pectus excavatum
Family history	Less specific findings: mitral valve prolapse, dilatation of the main pulmonary artery or descending aorta, spontaneous pneumothorax, apical blebs, striae atrophicae, recurrent hernia

leukemia and myelodysplastic syndromes) is more common in children with NF than in the general population.

The diagnosis of NF is based on clinical findings and detection of dominant heterozygous mutations in the *NF1* gene. The mutation rate for the *NF1* gene is 1:10,000, among the highest known mutation rates for any human gene.

Hereditary Hemorrhagic Telangiectasia

Hereditary hemorrhagic telangiectasia (HHT) is characterized by multiple arteriovenous malformations (AVMs) without intervening capillaries. These AVMs that are close to the surface may bleed with minimal trauma and are included in the diagnostic criteria for HHT, which include three of the following: epistaxis, mucocutaneous telangiectases, AVMs, and a family history of a first-degree relative with HHT. Large AVMs can be symptomatic in the brain, lung, or gastrointestinal tract. HHT is caused by dominant mutations in the *ENG* and *ACVRL1* genes.

Treatment involves managing bleeding and anemia. Pulmonary AVM surveillance should be done every 1 to 2 years in childhood and then every 5 years. Hepatic AVMs are treated with liver transplant. Screening for anemia and neurologic changes should be done annually. Antibiotic anaphylaxis is recommended for dental and other surgery.

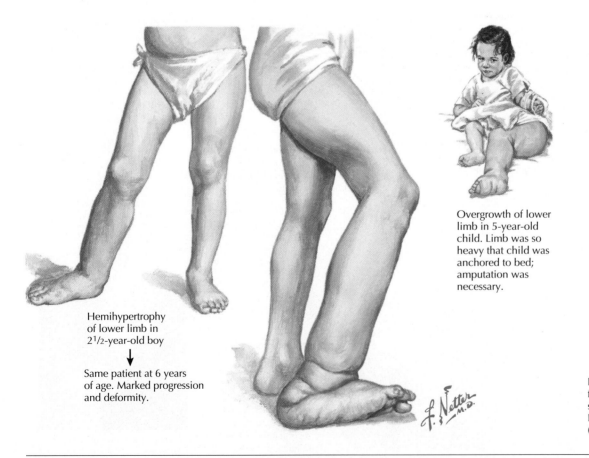

Hemihypertrophy of lower limb in 2½-year-old boy

↓

Same patient at 6 years of age. Marked progression and deformity.

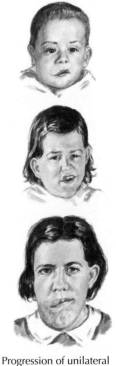

Overgrowth of lower limb in 5-year-old child. Limb was so heavy that child was anchored to bed; amputation was necessary.

Progression of unilateral facial deformity. Note skin pigmentation. Infancy (top); 2½ years (center); 17 years (bottom).

Figure 120-14 *Bone overgrowth and erosion in neurofibromatosis.*

Although these disorders represent but a few of the over more than 2500 described human genetic disorders for which a molecular basis is known, they serve to illustrate a number of the key categories of pediatric disease and the role that accurate diagnosis plays in the proper management of a wide range of pediatric conditions.

SUGGESTED READINGS

Cahill RA, Wenkert D, Perlman SA, et al: Infantile hypophosphatasia: transplantation therapy trial using bone fragments and cultured osteoblasts. *J Clin Endocrinol Metab* 92:2923-2930, 2007.

Davenport SL, Hefner MA, Thelin JW: CHARGE syndrome. Part I. External ear anomalies. *Int J Pediatr Otorhinolaryngol* 12:137-143, 1986.

Firth HV, Hurst JA, Hall JG: *Oxford Desk Reference Clinical Genetics*, New York, 2005, Oxford University Press.

Gunay-Aygun M, Schwartz S, Heeger S, et al: The changing purpose of Prader-Willi syndrome clinical diagnostic criteria and proposed revised criteria. *Pediatrics* 108:E92, 2001.

Jones KL: *Smith's Recognizable Patterns of Human Malformation*, ed 6, Philadelphia, 2006, WB Elsevier Saunders.

University of Washington: *GeneTests: Medical Genetics Information Resource*, 1993-2009. Available at http://www.genetests.org.

Whyte MP, Kurtzberg J, McAlister WH, et al: Marrow cell transplantation for infantile hypophosphatasia. *J Bone Miner Res* 18:624-636, 2003.

Reena Jethva

Inborn errors of metabolism (IEM) are a subgroup of genetic disorders in which biochemical pathways are blocked or have significantly decreased activity, often leading to abnormal accumulation of a substrate or deficiency of a product of an enzyme reaction. In this chapter, a general discussion of IEM is followed by more detailed descriptions of individual categories of disorders.

Individually, IEM are rare, but they collectively make up a significant source of disease, particularly in infants and children. Most diseases are autosomal recessive, but autosomal dominant, X-linked, and mitochondrial inheritance patterns exist (see Chapter 115).

Although metabolic physicians typically manage disorders with abnormal biochemical findings in body fluids that include plasma amino acid and urine organic acid profiles, the true definition of IEM includes a wide array of diseases. Many of these, such as α-1-antitrypsin (AAT) deficiency and congenital adrenal hyperplasia, affect a specific organ system and are often followed by specialists in other specialties. This chapter focuses on pediatric IEM typically managed by metabolic specialists that should be considered in the differential diagnoses of common pediatric presentations.

The advent of newborn screening (NBS) methods has facilitated early detection and management of many of these disorders, with dramatically improved outcomes. The earliest NBS efforts included bacterial inhibition assays for phenylketonuria (PKU), but recent technology such as tandem mass spectrometry, permits highly sensitive rapid detection of metabolites. The challenge of NBS currently lies in deciding which diseases to screen based on available technology, detection rates, cost of follow-up, and the clinical benefits of early management.

The survival rate and quality of life for many patients with IEM is improving, and there is greater recognition of later-onset variants of diseases; thus, physicians who treat both pediatric and adult patients have more contact with affected individuals than in the past. Although management is frequently coordinated by specialists, generalists should be prepared to identify potential new cases, initiate therapy, and assist in general medical management. Even in metabolic disorders for which few therapeutic options exist, making an accurate diagnosis is important for anticipatory guidance, reproductive counseling, and improved decisions about the care of the patient.

CLINICAL PRESENTATION

Although variations in genotype, diet, and lifestyle choices can lead to variable presentations for many IEM, illness or fasting typically exacerbates the disease process because of increased catabolism. Hence, a significant portion of IEM presents in infants, who have both increased metabolic demands associated with growth and a limited capacity to respond to illness. Clinical features can include nonspecific sepsis-like presentations such as poor feeding and growth, vomiting, lethargy, hypothermia,

seizures, and irritability, and before NBS, undiagnosed IEM probably contributed to a significant proportion of unexplained infantile deaths. In older children with metabolic disorders associated with intellectual disabilities or behavioral problems, affected patients may not be able to convey the nature of their symptoms. Therefore, because of potential nonspecific presentations, IEM should be considered in all critically ill newborns or children with developmental delays, seizures, persistent vomiting, severe liver disease, metabolic acidosis, ketosis, hypoglycemia, hyperammonemia, or disease-specific findings common to a particular disorder.

To accomplish this, a thorough history and physical examination will narrow the differential diagnosis before diagnostic testing. A complete dietary history may reveal symptoms instigated by certain food types or fasting. Food preferences or aversions may also be instructive. Other important information includes the frequency of and severity of response to illness, pattern of developmental delays, presence of consanguinity, and distinct body fluid odors. Although there are many physical examination and laboratory findings characteristic of specific disorders (Figure 121-1), several findings help to indicate general categories. For example, Kussmaul's respirations may be found with metabolic acidosis or hyperventilation with hyperammonemia or cerebral edema. Organomegaly may also be evident as the result of a storage defect or organ dysfunction. Several disorders, such as the peroxisomal disorder Zellweger's syndrome, have characteristic patterns of dysmorphia.

EVALUATION AND MANAGEMENT
Diagnostic Testing

When an IEM is suspected, it is often important to initiate treatment measures while an investigative workup is underway because a delay in therapy may affect the clinical outcome. Blood, urine, and cerebrospinal fluid (CSF) can be useful in the laboratory evaluation, and several laboratory studies are particularly helpful when an IEM is suspected in an ill child (Box 121-1). Serum electrolytes and blood gas analysis evaluate the acid-base status and anion gap. Ketone levels in urine, and sometimes blood, should be determined. Serum ammonia, lactate, and pyruvate, which can be tested in most hospitals, can also be informative, particularly in ill newborns. Metabolic laboratory studies such as plasma amino acids, plasma acylcarnitines, and urine organic acids, which provide important diagnostic information, must often be sent to specialized centers. Finally, one should consider other disease-specific testing, such as complete blood counts, to evaluate for bone marrow suppression in some organic acidurias. Molecular DNA testing and enzyme assays may require biopsy of specific tissues.

Key to interpretation of testing, some laboratories require special collection methods. For example, blood for ammonia for lactate levels should be drawn from a free-flowing vessel,

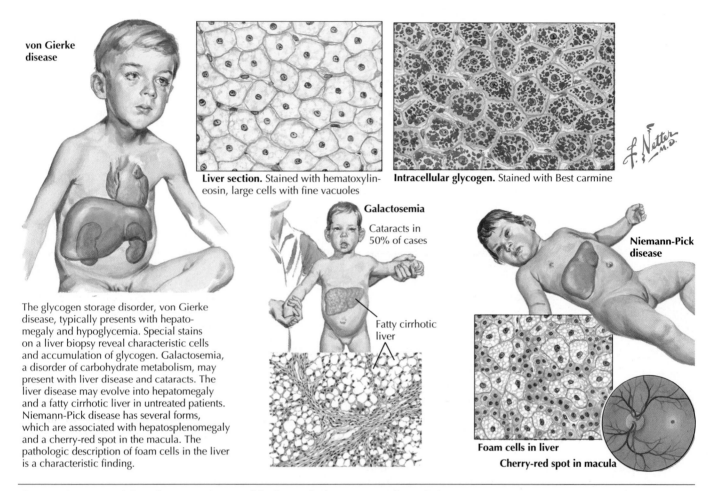

von Gierke disease

Liver section. Stained with hematoxylin-eosin, large cells with fine vacuoles

Intracellular glycogen. Stained with Best carmine

Galactosemia

Cataracts in 50% of cases

Fatty cirrhotic liver

Niemann-Pick disease

The glycogen storage disorder, von Gierke disease, typically presents with hepatomegaly and hypoglycemia. Special stains on a liver biopsy reveal characteristic cells and accumulation of glycogen. Galactosemia, a disorder of carbohydrate metabolism, may present with liver disease and cataracts. The liver disease may evolve into hepatomegaly and a fatty cirrhotic liver in untreated patients. Niemann-Pick disease has several forms, which are associated with hepatosplenomegaly and a cherry-red spot in the macula. The pathologic description of foam cells in the liver is a characteristic finding.

Foam cells in liver

Cherry-red spot in macula

Figure 121-1 *Variability of presentations and findings of inborn errors of metabolism.*

transported to the laboratory on ice, and tested soon after collection or values may be falsely elevated. The metabolic workup is most appropriately performed in a focused, tiered fashion, starting with testing for the most likely and treatable disorders.

Special efforts are necessary to arrive at a diagnosis in patients suspected of having IEM who are dying or recently deceased because clear confirmation of an IEM greatly assists with genetic and reproductive counseling for families. In a dying patient, consider collection and freezing of urine and separated plasma

---

Box 121-1 Initial Evaluation in a Critically Ill Patient with Suspected Inborn Errors of Metabolism

Serum electrolytes
Blood gas analysis
Blood glucose level
Urinalysis (including ketones)
Urine-reducing substances
Plasma amino acids
Urine organic acids
Plasma acylcarnitines
Plasma lactate and pyruvate
Other testing specific for the suspected condition

---

as well as a skin biopsy to be stored in tissue culture medium at room temperature for isolation of skin fibroblasts. One may also consider a liver biopsy (frozen sample for enzyme assays and fresh tissue for electron microscopy).

Common Presentations

Although IEM have a broad range of manifestations, common presentations and laboratory findings can lead one to consider a metabolic disorder. Because IEM are individually rare, a practical, generalized approach to common presentations is valuable.

HYPOGLYCEMIA

In general, hypoglycemia can be induced by lack of adequate glucose intake, poor homeostatic controls, iatrogenic causes, infection, and inborn errors of glucose metabolism. The brain is particularly dependent on glucose for energy but can alternatively use ketone bodies. Symptoms of hypoglycemia include lethargy, sweating, pallor, seizures, and mental status changes. Central to determining a metabolic cause of hypoglycemia is its onset after a carbohydrate load. For example, whereas early postprandial symptoms are more likely to be related to hyperinsulinism and glycogenoses, defects in fatty acid oxidation,

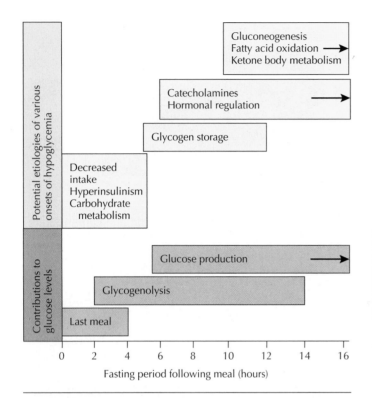

Figure 121-2 *Contributions to and factors influencing fasting glucose levels.*

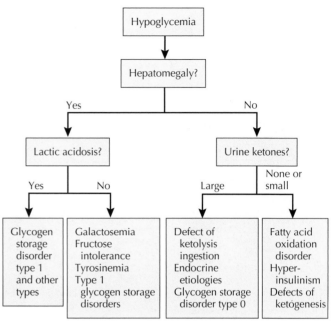

Figure 121-3 *Diagnostic pathway for hypoglycemia.*

ketone body synthesis, gluconeogenesis, and other IEM tend to take longer to present with hypoglycemia (Figure 121-2). Diagnostic pathways to approach the metabolic differential diagnosis for hypoglycemia are useful (Figure 121-3). A focused evaluation for an IEM may include electrolytes, glucose level, urine ketones, urine-reducing substances, ammonia, lactate, urine organic acids, and plasma acylcarnitines. One should also consider evaluation for non-IEM causes of hypoglycemia such as infection, drugs or toxins, and abnormal counterregulatory hormone mechanisms.

METABOLIC ACIDOSIS

Acid-base status is affected by several buffering systems. Whereas fast-acting buffering is accomplished by proteins and the bicarbonate-carbonic acid system, slower acting mechanisms include renal bicarbonate resorption. Metabolic acidosis generally results from bicarbonate losses or an increased presence of acid. These can be distinguished by bicarbonate losses leading to a non-anion gap metabolic acidosis in which chloride levels increase in compensation. Renal tubular acidosis and diarrhea are common causes of non-anion gap metabolic acidosis. A non-anion gap acidosis does not exclude IEM, such as in metabolic disorders with renal tubular acidosis, but many IEM are associated with anion gaps because of buildup of acid metabolites, particularly during periods of illness or stress. Determining which acid is accumulating is important for diagnosis. Lactic acid is commonly elevated in many metabolic diseases. In contrast, acidoses of other organic acids should be suspected in anion gap metabolic acidoses with ketosis, a normal response to

lack of adequate glucose and utilization of fatty acid stores. Ketosis may also contribute to acidosis, as classically seen in diabetes mellitus.

KETOSIS

Ketone production is a common physiologic response to fasting. Infants, however, rarely produce urine ketones even in a fasting state, making the finding highly suggestive of an IEM in this population. In children and adults, ketosis may indicate a biochemical disorder when present with metabolic acidosis or in a nonfasted state, but a lack of sufficient ketones with hypoglycemia suggests a fatty acid oxidation disorder (FAOD) or ketogenesis disorder.

HYPERAMMONEMIA

Ammonia is a product of protein metabolism that, in elevated levels, is toxic to the central nervous system (CNS), resulting in cerebral edema. Normally, ammonia is converted to urea in the liver via the urea cycle and is excreted in the urine. When the nitrogen load exceeds the clearance capacity of the liver, ammonia accumulates. The nitrogen load increases with dietary protein intake and endogenous protein breakdown, both of which can cause hyperammonemia in patients with primary or secondary urea cycle defects. Symptoms of hyperammonemia include vomiting, seizures, lethargy, coma, and hyperventilation associated with respiratory alkalosis. Nonspecific episodes of headache, vomiting, and mental status changes may be the only signs in later-onset cases. For extremely high ammonia levels, such as during neonatal presentations of urea cycle disorders (UCDs), dialysis to rapidly reduce the toxic levels may be necessary in addition to less invasive therapies. Nonmetabolic causes

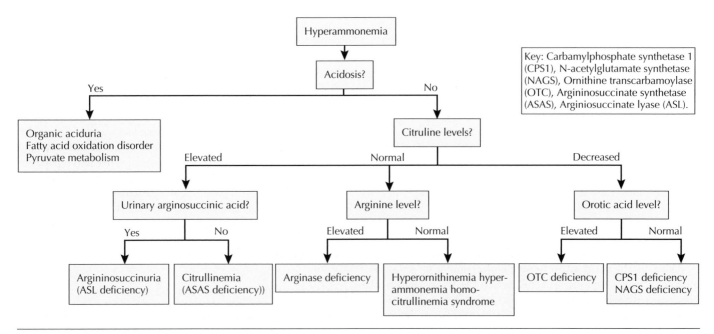

Figure 121-4 *Diagnostic pathway for hyperammonemia.*

of hyperammonemia include sepsis; liver failure; use of medications such as valproate; and transient hyperammonemia of the newborn, a disorder associated with severe neonatal hyperammonemia that resolves perinatally, although residual neurologic sequelae may result. Classic metabolic causes of hyperammonemia include UCDs, organic acidurias, FAODs, hyperornithinemia-hyperammonemia-homocitrullinemia syndrome, pyruvate carboxylase deficiency, and hyperammonemia-hyperinsulinemia syndrome. Several of these disorders, including organic acidurias and FAODs, cause secondary urea cycle inhibition. Whereas hyperammonemia without metabolic acidosis and hypoglycemia is suggestive of UCD, an anion gap metabolic acidosis should arouse suspicion for an organic aciduria. Diagnostic pathways for biochemical causes of hyperammonemia are depicted in Figure 121-4.

Treatment

In most IEM, long-term treatment goals focus on tight intake regulation of the offending substrate within the defective pathway, pharmacologic reduction of metabolite toxicity, and replacement of deficient metabolites. In some disorders, supplementation of cofactors to optimize residual enzyme activity, enzyme replacement, and tissue transplantation are also possible.

In disorders associated with hypoglycemia, hyperammonemia, and acidosis, patients may present critically ill or be at risk for rapid decompensation. Therefore, prompt management must be instituted to prevent long-term systemic sequelae. Oral intake of substrates or metabolites that are harmful in the disease must be restricted (e.g., protein restriction in UCDs). If hypoglycemia is detected, a bolus of intravenous (IV) glucose should be provided (often starting with 2-4 mL/kg of 10% dextrose). Continuous IV hydration with dextrose should be started with a glucose infusion rate of 6 to 9 mg/kg of dextrose per minute

and further titrated to keep the patient euglycemic. This provides calories and an alternative safe energy source to reduce catabolism. An IV fluid rate of 1.5 to 2 times maintenance with 10% dextrose is often used, although alternative rates or concentrations may be required in the presence of fluid-restricted conditions such as heart disease. Furthermore, although dextrose administration is a primary therapy in most acute presentations of IEM, it is important to remember that it may be harmful in a few primary lactic acidosis syndromes (in which glucose is the harmful substrate).

In some situations, with the notable exception of FAODs, IV lipids are also used as an additional energy source to provide calories and decrease catabolism.

In addition to the critical provision of calories, other approaches, based on disease and presentation, are used. Management of metabolic acidosis may also require bicarbonate therapy. In UCDs, nitrogen scavenger therapy is given to reduce demand on the urea cycle. Dialysis may be necessary in some critically ill metabolic patients with very high levels of ammonia. Although other methods of dialysis have been used in the past, hemodialysis is currently the recommended standard. In acutely ill patients undergoing diet restriction, it is usually important to reintroduce the restricted substrate as the patient improves. For example, the essential amino acids required for normal metabolism can become deficient if a patient remains completely protein restricted for longer than 24 to 48 hours, increasing the risk for catabolism with breakdown of endogenous protein stores. After confirmation of a diagnosis, other disease-specific management goals exist, some of which are discussed below.

SPECIFIC INBORN ERRORS OF METABOLISM

This section covers some of the more common and well-described IEM encountered by metabolic physicians. A simplified diagram of some of the major biochemical pathways in the liver cell can be referred to as a visual aid (Figure 121-5).

Disorders of Carbohydrate Metabolism

Inborn errors of carbohydrate metabolism are disorders of intermediary metabolism. Disease results from energy deficiency or toxicity of metabolites. Presentations can vary from acute intermittent onset during infancy to a gradual progression of symptoms and signs. Acute episodes are often precipitated by catabolic states, such as intercurrent illness and fasting.

GALACTOSEMIA

Classic galactosemia is an autosomal recessive disorder caused by defects in the pathway for hepatic conversion of galactose to glucose. Three enzymes, galactokinase (GALK), galactose-1-phosphate uridyltransferase (GALT), and UDP galactose-4-epimerase, are involved and cause variable disease in deficient states. Classic galactosemia (GALT deficiency) is the most common and the most severe. It leads to galactose-1-phosphate buildup in liver, brain, and renal tubules with resulting hepatic

parenchymal disease, intellectual impairment, and renal tubular dysfunction. Upon exposure to lactose in milk, neonates present with vomiting, jaundice, and hepatomegaly within a few weeks of birth and may be predisposed to *Escherichia coli* sepsis. Cataracts may result from galactitol accumulation in the lens. Positive urine-reducing substances, particularly during the prediagnosis period, are a classic finding but may not always be present. Treatment simply involves a lactose-free diet, which dramatically improves and prevents many manifestations. However, even in presymptomatically treated patients, speech delay, learning difficulties, and ovarian failure have been noted. Most U.S. NBS panels detect galactosemia and confirmatory testing is used to verify deficient GALT enzyme activity and elevated galactose-1-phosphate in red blood cells and elevated urine galactitol, with possible proteinuria or aminoaciduria.

HEREDITARY FRUCTOSE INTOLERANCE

Hereditary fructose intolerance (HFI) is caused by a deficiency of fructose-1,6-bisphosphate aldolase. Infants typically present with poor growth, vomiting, loose stools, jaundice, hepatomegaly, and renal tubular acidosis as sucrose or fructose is introduced in the diet. Laboratory findings include hypoglycemia, elevated transaminases, positive urine-reducing substances, proteinuria, and generalized aminoaciduria. Fructose tolerance tests are not advised without appropriate supervision in a hospital setting because enzyme assays and molecular testing are available. Good outcomes are associated with strict exclusion of dietary fructose and sucrose.

GLYCOGEN STORAGE DISORDERS

Glycogen is a branched polymer of glucose monomers used for storage in the liver and muscle. Several enzyme defects in the biosynthesis and breakdown of glycogen make up the collective group of autosomal recessive glycogen storage disorders (GSDs). Type I (von Gierke disease; glucose-6-phosphatase deficiency), type III (debrancher enzyme deficiency), and type VI (hepatic phosphorylase deficiency) are the most well-known hepatic forms. Type I is the most common and presents with varied features, including failure to thrive, hepatomegaly, and fasting hypoglycemia. Type Ib has been associated with neutropenia and inflammatory bowel disease. Treatment involves regular feedings, restricted intake of lactose and sucrose, and ingesting safe amounts of uncooked cornstarch to balance prevention of hypoglycemia with the risk of additional glycogen storage. Type III is often accompanied by significant muscle disease. Type V (muscle phosphorylase deficiency) and VII (phosphofructokinase deficiency) are classic muscle forms associated with later-onset exercise intolerance and myopathy. Type II (Pompe's disease; acid maltase deficiency) is unique as a lysosomal enzyme deficiency that tends to present with cardiomegaly during infancy. Enzyme replacement therapy has had variable effects on patients with type II disease. Laboratory findings of GSDs may include fasting hypoglycemia, ketosis, lactic acidosis, creatine kinase, hyperlipidemia, and hyperuricemia. Glucagon tolerance tests, specific enzyme assays from affected tissues, and molecular testing narrow the diagnosis.

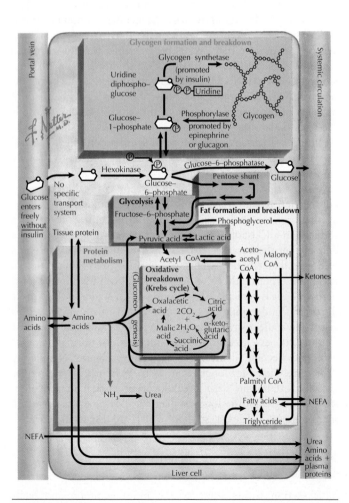

Figure 121-5 *Intermediary metabolism of the liver cell.*

Disorders of Amino Acid Metabolism

These inborn disorders of intermediary metabolism tend to have characteristic abnormalities on plasma amino acid studies. They present with a variety of acute and chronic presentations with acute episodes often precipitated by catabolic states such as intercurrent illness and fasting. PKU is unique because it has a nonacute progressive neurologic course.

UREA CYCLE DISORDERS

The urea cycle converts ammonia, a product of protein breakdown, to water-soluble urea, which is excreted in urine. If deficient, ammonia elevations result in toxicity to the CNS. Several enzymes are involved in the hepatic mitochondrial urea cycle, each of which causes disease if deficient (Figure 121-6). Other than arginase deficiency, which has a chronic progressive neurologic presentation, the UCDs present during infancy with poor feeding, vomiting, and lethargy. Neonates classically manifest symptoms after 12 to 24 hours of life, presumably because of the toxic accumulation of ammonia. In addition, the effect of ammonia on brainstem respiratory control typically results in hyperventilation and respiratory alkalosis. However, patients with more residual enzyme activity may not be diagnosed until childhood or adulthood. All UCDs are autosomal recessive except for ornithine transcarbamoylase (OTC) deficiency, which is X-linked and the most common. Accordingly, a family history of male newborn deaths suggestive of X-linked disease is suggestive of OTC deficiency. The hair condition trichorrhexis nodosa is unique in argininosuccinate lyase deficiency.

Classic patterns of biochemical findings assist with diagnosis. A low citrulline level (see Figure 121-6) is suggestive of enzymatic defects upstream in the urea cycle, of which only OTC deficiency has elevated urinary orotic acid, a product of accumulated carbamylphosphate. In contrast, citrulline levels are high in patients with downstream defects of the urea cycle. Molecular DNA analysis is available for many of the disorders.

Acute management of hyperammonemia includes nitrogen scavengers such as sodium benzoate and sodium phenylacetate that convert ammonia sources into renally cleared metabolites. In severe cases, dialysis is used to rapidly remove ammonia. Long-term management focuses on the prevention of hyperammonemia. This is accomplished by balancing protein restriction with provision of essential amino acids to allow normal growth. Arginine, which becomes an essential amino acid in UCD, is often supplemented. Of note, heterozygous affected female carriers of OTC deficiency often require therapy. Liver transplantation is another therapeutic option. Most patients with UCD have varying degrees of neurologic impairment, but prognoses are generally better with aggressive early treatment.

PHENYLKETONURIA

Classic PKU results from deficient phenylalanine hydroxylase, which converts phenylalanine to tyrosine. Rare cases may be caused by deficiency of the cofactor tetrahydrobiopterin or by defects in biopterin synthesis that require additional treatment with various neurotransmitters. Untreated patients present with progressive brain disease that manifests as acquired microcephaly, developmental delays, seizures, behavioral problems, and intellectual disabilities. A fair complexion, eczema, and a mousy or musty odor (caused by increased levels of phenylacetic acid) have also been noted. Classic PKU is associated with persistently elevated phenylalanine levels above 20 mg/dL with normal or low tyrosine and characteristic urinary derivatives. In variants with persistent hyperphenylalaninemia, phenylalanine levels range from 4 to 10 mg/dL.

Patients with classic PKU and other variants with elevated phenylalanine require phenylalanine-restricted diets to maintain

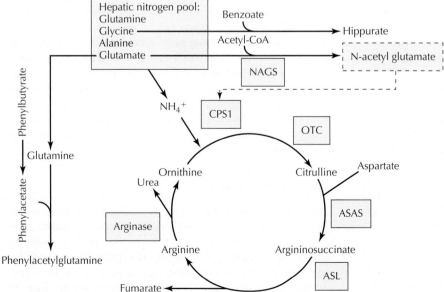

Carbamylphosphate synthetase 1 (CPS1), which requires the activator N-acetylglutamate, catalyzes the first step, the synthesis of carbamylphosphate from ammonia. The enzyme N-acetylglutamate synthetase (NAGS) is necessary for synthesis of the activator from acetyl-CoA and glutamate. Ornithine transcarbamoylase (OTC) catalyzes the condensation of carbamylphosphate (containing a nitrogen atom) and ornithine to make citrulline. Citrulline then reacts with aspartate (which introduces another waste nitrogen atom into the cycle) to make argininosuccinate, a reation catalyzed by argininosuccinate synthetase (ASAS). Argininosuccinate lyase (ASL) catalyzes the formation of arginine and fumarate from argininosuccinate, after which arginase converts arginine to urea and reforms ornithine to replenish the cycle. Urea is cleared by the kidneys. Nitrogen scavenger medications, including sodium benzoate, sodium phenylbutyrate, and sodium phenylacetate, can convert nitrogen sources into renally excretable metabolites (hippurate and phenylacetylglutamine) via the reactions shown in the diagram.

Figure 121-6 *The urea cycle.*

goal levels of 2 to 6 mg/dL. Patients diagnosed via NBS who start restrictions within the first month and achieve appropriate control of levels have normal intellectual and neurologic development. NBS performed before 24 hours of age has a risk of false-negative results and should always be repeated. Of note, women with PKU are fertile, and maternal PKU is a teratogenic condition requiring strict metabolic control before and during pregnancy.

MAPLE SYRUP URINE DISEASE

Maple syrup urine disease is caused by a deficiency of branched-chain 2-keto dehydrogenase complex involved in the early steps of branched-chain amino acid (BCAA; e.g., leucine, isoleucine, and valine) metabolism in mitochondria. Most cases are the classic form in which neonates present with nonspecific symptoms of poor feeding, changes in tone, and lethargy after several days of cumulative milk ingestion. Accumulating ketoacids result in a sweet odor resembling burnt sugar in urine and other body substances. The ketoacid of leucine is neurotoxic and causes seizures, encephalopathy, and coma. Laboratory findings include metabolic acidosis; ketosis; and significantly elevated plasma BCAAs, particularly leucine. Alloisoleucine, an isoleucine pathway metabolite, is a pathognomonic finding. Treatment includes dietary restriction of BCAA to reduce disease toxicity but allow normal growth and BCAA deficiency, which results in rash and anemia. Prompt management of acute episodes is important to prevent neurologic sequelae.

HEREDITARY TYROSINEMIA TYPE 1

Defects of the tyrosine metabolism pathway cause several types of tyrosinemia. Transient tyrosinemia is a commonly diagnosed type in premature and newborn infants and results from delayed hepatic maturation that improves with age. Hereditary tyrosinemia type 1, in contrast, leads to severe liver disease. It is prevalent in French Canadians and presents with hepatomegaly, coagulation defects, failure to thrive, or jaundice during infancy or with gradual hepatic parenchymal disease. It is caused by a deficiency of fumarylacetoacetate hydrolase (FAH), which catalyzes a reaction late in the phenylalanine and tyrosine pathway. Despite the name, tyrosine levels are not always very elevated. Patients often develop hepatocellular carcinoma. In addition to liver disease, patients have renal tubular acidosis that may lead to hypophosphatemic rickets.

Laboratory findings reveal severe liver disease, generalized aminoaciduria, hypermethioninemia, and tyrosine metabolites. Increased urine succinylacetone is pathognomonic. Dietary management includes phenylalanine and tyrosine restriction. Nitisinone therapy has significantly reduced liver and renal morbidity. It inhibits the step before FAH to decrease toxic fumarylacetoacetate and succinylacetone accumulation. Liver transplantation remains the only truly curative therapy.

NONKETOTIC HYPERGLYCINEMIA

Nonketotic hyperglycinemia is an autosomal recessive defect of glycine metabolism. Secondary inhibition results from ketotic hyperglycinemia and valproate. Excessive glycine accumulation in the brain is associated with encephalopathy. The most severe forms present acutely in infants with hypotonia, intractable seizures, and hiccups caused by diaphragmatic spasms. Laboratory findings include CSF glycine elevation out of proportion to the blood level, low serine levels (the product the enzyme), and an increase in the ratio of glycine to serine in body fluids. The disease is not associated with acidosis or ketosis. Efforts to find effective therapy are ongoing.

Disorders of Organic Acid Metabolism

These disorders of intermediary metabolism are associated with accumulation of characteristic urine organic acids. These organic acids differ from amino acids because of a lack of an α-amino group. Similar to disorders of amino acid metabolism, presentations may be acute or chronic, and many of these disorders present with metabolic acidosis and encephalopathy.

THE KETOTIC HYPERGLYCINEMIAS: PROPIONIC AND METHYLMALONIC ACIDEMIA

Propionic acidemia (PA) and methylmalonic acidemia (MMA) were initially termed *ketotic hyperglycinemias* to distinguish them from nonketotic hyperglycinemias. The deficient enzymes act sequentially downstream in threonine, valine, methionine, and isoleucine metabolism. MMA may also result from defects in the synthesis of its cofactor, adenosyl-cobalamin. Although variable phenotypes exist, the classic presentation occurs within the first week of life with poor feeding, vomiting, lethargy, and liver enlargement. Patients with PA are predisposed to cardiomyopathy, and those with MMA are predisposed to renal tubulopathy. Both can develop pancreatitis and brain lesions, particularly in the basal ganglia. Acute laboratory findings for both disorders include anion gap metabolic acidosis, ketosis, hyperammonemia (from secondary urea cycle inhibition), and hyperglycinemia or hyperglycinuria. Thrombocytopenia, leukopenia, or anemia may occur secondary to bone marrow suppression. Urinary propionylglycine and methylcitrate (metabolites of propionate) are seen in patients with PA. Urinary methylmalonic acid is seen in classic MMA. Enzyme assays can be performed for PA, MMA, or cobalamin defects. Long-term management requires dietary restriction of precursor amino acids and adequate calories to optimize growth but prevent toxicity. Some patients with MMA respond well to cobalamin supplementation. Periodic administration of antimicrobials may help reduce gut bacteria, a source of propionate production. Patients need urgent management for acute presentations of disease often precipitated by intercurrent viral illness.

ISOVALERIC ACIDEMIA

Isovaleric acidemia is caused by a deficiency of isovaleryl-CoA dehydrogenase in the leucine oxidative pathway. Infants often present in the first week of life with poor feeding, vomiting, lethargy, and seizures. A pungent odor resembling sweaty feet may result from accumulated isovaleric acid. A later-onset chronic intermittent form consists of periodic metabolic crises induced by protein intake or illness. Similar to ketotic hyperglycinemias, laboratory findings include anion gap metabolic acidosis, ketosis, hyperammonemia (from secondary urea cycle inhibition), and evidence of bone marrow suppression. Biochemical findings include urinary isovalerylglycine and 3-hydroxyisovaleric acid. Long-term management requires dietary restriction with adequate supplies to optimize growth but prevent toxicity. Glycine therapy may promote production of the nontoxic compound isovalerylglycine and reduce levels of isovaleric acid in body fluids. Patients need urgent management for acute presentations of disease.

MULTIPLE CARBOXYLASE DEFICIENCY

Multiple carboxylase deficiency is a disorder of biotin metabolism resulting from one of two possible enzyme deficiencies—holocarboxylase synthetase, which couples biotin to four different carboxylase enzymes, or biotinidase, which recycles biotin after degradation of the enzymes. Whereas holocarboxylase synthetase deficiency may present in neonates with hypotonia, patients with biotinidase deficiency tend to present later during infancy with ataxia, neurologic symptoms, and seborrhea. The diagnosis is made by measurement of the carboxylase enzyme activities. Other laboratory findings include an anion gap metabolic acidosis, with elevated lactate, 3-methyl-crotonylglycine, and propionate metabolites. Treatment involves biotin, often in supratherapeutic doses, to overcome lower affinity enzyme-deficient states.

GLUTARIC ACIDEMIA TYPE 1

Glutaric acidemia type 1, prevalent in some Canadian and Amish populations, is caused by deficiency of glutaryl-CoA dehydrogenase in the lysine, hydroxylysine, and tryptophan metabolism pathways. Although macrocephaly is often present at birth, patients tend to present acutely with encephalopathy during infancy and develop progressive extrapyramidal symptoms, including dystonia and athetosis. Imaging may reveal bilateral brain damage in the basal ganglia, subdural hygromas or hemorrhages, and widening of the sylvian fissures. The course is highly variable. Laboratory findings include urinary glutaric acid and 3-hydroxyglutaric acid and decreased enzyme activity. Treatment involves dietary restriction of precursor amino acids and management of movement disorders. Aggressive management of acute episodes to reduce catabolism may help reduce long-term neurologic morbidity.

Disorders of Energy Metabolism

Collectively, these disorders result from defects in pyruvate metabolism, the Krebs cycle, the mitochondrial respiratory chain, fatty acid oxidation, ketone body metabolism, and cytoplasmic energy defects (e.g., disorders of glycolysis, gluconeogenesis, creatine deficiency, and the pentose phosphate pathway).

PRIMARY LACTIC ACIDOSIS

Lactate is formed from pyruvate during anaerobic glucose metabolism. Lactate and pyruvate exist in equilibrium and are affected by the redox state of cells and the generation of electron donors such as NADH (nicotinamide adenine dinucleotide), which contribute to oxidative phosphorylation. Oxidative phosphorylation occurs along the mitochondrial respiratory or electron transport chain (ETC). It couples the donation of electrons to acceptors (e.g., oxygen) with the transport of protons across a membrane, which then forms a proton gradient whose release is associated with adenosine triphosphate generation (Figure 121-7). Lactate accumulates because of blocks in pathways leading up to the ETC or defects along the ETC itself (which may result from circulatory collapse or hypoxia in addition to IEM). Primary lactic acidemias include defects in the mitochondrial respiratory chain, Krebs cycle, pyruvate metabolism, and several disorders of gluconeogenesis, and secondary lactic acidemias result from organic acidurias, FAODs, and UCDs that affect cellular redox potential or conversion of pyruvate to lactate. Several of these disorders can be inherited via maternal mitochondrial inheritance, as discussed in Chapter 115.

Primary disorders, particularly those involving pyruvate and ETC metabolism, are associated with neurodevelopmental and multiorgan disease, but the extent of systemic involvement, severity, age of onset, and prognosis can vary greatly, even between patients with the same disease. Laboratory testing for the various defects includes lactate and pyruvate levels in various body fluids, muscle biopsy for histopathology and electron microscopy, and molecular DNA analysis or enzyme assays (often using blood, muscle, liver, or skin). Treatment options often have limited effectiveness, but patients may receive various cofactors that promote flux through pathways and symptomatic therapies.

DISORDERS OF FATTY ACID OXIDATION

Disorders of fatty acid oxidation (FAOD) are caused by deficiencies in enzymes that participate in mitochondrial β-oxidation of fatty acids. General signs and symptoms include hypoketotic hypoglycemia, vomiting, lethargy, and liver disease. Medium-chain acyl-CoA dehydrogenase deficiency is the most common FAOD and tends to present during infancy after a precipitating event such as fasting or illness. In the past, fatal cases have been diagnosed as sudden infant death syndrome, but with NBS, the mortality associated with the disease, particularly in the first presentation, has decreased significantly. Long-chain FAODs are associated with cardiomyopathy and rhabdomyolysis.

The finding of low ketones with fasting is an inappropriate response and a classic finding suggestive of FAOD. Characteristic patterns of accumulated plasma acylcarnitines and urinary acylglycines are useful in the diagnosis; however, abnormal laboratory findings may be intermittent or absent during well states. Enzyme assays are available, and common mutations for several of the disorders have been described. Treatment focuses on dietary fat restriction, frequent carbohydrate feedings, avoidance of fasting, and prompt management during catabolic states. Medium-chain fatty acid supplementation may be beneficial for long-chain defects.

DEFECTS IN KETONE METABOLISM

Ketone bodies are products of fatty acid metabolism that are used as an energy source for the heart and brain, particularly during fasting. Defects in ketone metabolism lead to variable

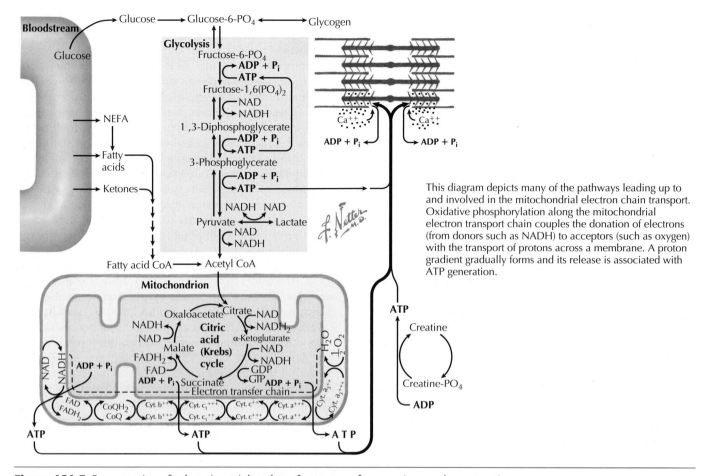

Figure 121-7 *Regeneration of adenosine triphosphate for source of energy in muscle contraction.*

clinical presentations, including vomiting, lethargy, and seizures. Whereas defects in ketone catabolism are associated with persistent ketosis and acidosis, defects in ketone synthesis present with hypoketotic hypoglycemia and acidosis. Metabolites of isoleucine and leucine metabolism are often found in certain enzyme deficiencies caused by defects along the corresponding catabolic pathways. Thus, treatment efforts for these disorders include avoidance of fasting and may include protein restriction. Urgent management to reduce catabolism should be instituted during acute episodes.

Disorders of Complex Molecules

This section includes several disorders with defects in the synthesis or catabolism of complex molecules and includes several diseases of cellular organelles, including lysosomal storage and peroxisomal disorders, disorders of intracellular trafficking and processing, such as AAT deficiency, congenital disorders of glycosylation (CDGs), and defects of cholesterol synthesis. Each tends to have a progressive degenerative course.

LYSOSOMAL DISORDERS

Lysosomes are cellular organelles that are important in the degradation of complex molecules. Various acid hydrolases within the lysosome may be deficient, leading to accumulation

of enzyme substrates in various tissues. The particular storage material that accumulates defines the type of lysosomal storage disorder (LSDs), such as mucopolysaccharidoses, sphingolipidoses, and mucolipidoses. Lysosomal protein transport out of the lysosome may also be defective. Most but not all LSDs are autosomal recessive (i.e., Hunter and Fabry syndromes are X-linked). The clinical presentation and age of onset vary by disease. LSDs, particularly the mucopolysaccharidoses, are often associated with characteristic physical examination findings, including corneal clouding, coarse facies, organomegaly with liver disease, and skeletal abnormalities (Figure 121-8). Urine screening tests and enzyme assays are commonly used for diagnosis. Treatment is generally supportive in nature, but enzyme replacement and bone marrow transplantation have been effective in several disorders.

PEROXISOMAL DISORDERS

Peroxisomes are cellular organelles with various functions, including β-oxidation of very-long-chain fatty acids (VLCFAs), α-oxidation of branched fatty acids, bile acid synthesis, glyoxylate metabolism, and plasmalogen synthesis. Most disorders are autosomal recessive except X-linked adrenoleukodystrophy. Zellweger-spectrum disorders and rhizomelic chondrodysplasia punctata type 1 are defects of peroxisomal biogenesis and result from multiple enzymatic defects. Zellweger syndrome is the

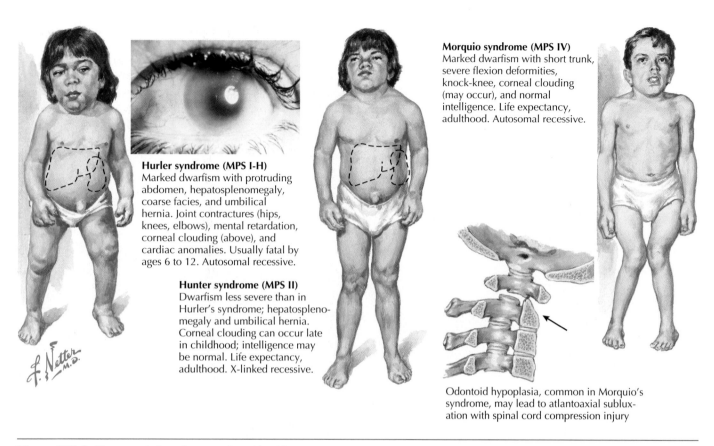

Hurler syndrome (MPS I-H)
Marked dwarfism with protruding abdomen, hepatosplenomegaly, coarse facies, and umbilical hernia. Joint contractures (hips, knees, elbows), mental retardation, corneal clouding (above), and cardiac anomalies. Usually fatal by ages 6 to 12. Autosomal recessive.

Hunter syndrome (MPS II)
Dwarfism less severe than in Hurler's syndrome; hepatospleno-megaly and umbilical hernia. Corneal clouding can occur late in childhood; intelligence may be normal. Life expectancy, adulthood. X-linked recessive.

Morquio syndrome (MPS IV)
Marked dwarfism with short trunk, severe flexion deformities, knock-knee, corneal clouding (may occur), and normal intelligence. Life expectancy, adulthood. Autosomal recessive.

Odontoid hypoplasia, common in Morquio's syndrome, may lead to atlantoaxial subluxation with spinal cord compression injury

Figure 121-8 *Characteristics of mucopolysaccharidoses.*

most severe, with seizures, hepatomegaly, and dysmorphic features in infancy. Primary hyperoxaluria, X-linked adrenoleukodystrophy, and adult Refsum disease are examples of peroxisomal disorders with single enzyme deficiencies. X-linked adrenoleukodystrophy classically presents in young boys with developmental regression, seizures, and adrenal insufficiency but also has a later-onset form. Dietary management and bone marrow transplantation are in investigative phases. Classic biochemical findings associated with each disorder assist with diagnosis. For example, serum VLCFAs are elevated in peroxisomal β-oxidation disorders. Enzyme assays and molecular testing are available for most.

Congenital Disorders of Glycosylation

CDGs are caused by defects in glycosylation, an important processing step in the intracellular function of many proteins. CDGs, also referred to as carbohydrate-deficient glycoprotein syndromes, may have defects in either N- or O-linked glycosylation. Type 1a (phosphomannomutase deficiency) is the most common N-linked disorder and classically presents with failure to thrive, developmental delay, abnormal subcutaneous fat, cerebellar hypoplasia, liver disease, and facial dysmorphia. Treatment options are limited to supportive care. Type 1b (mannosephosphate isomerase deficiency), which presents with failure to thrive, hypoglycemia, chronic diarrhea, and liver disease, may benefit from mannose supplementation.

Laboratory evaluation for N-linked disorders involves isoelectric focusing of transferrin (although other proteins may analyzed), in which there are characteristic protein migration patterns. Examples of O-linked disorders include multiple hereditary exostoses and muscle-eye-brain disease.

FUTURE DIRECTIONS

IEM form a large group of diseases that many physicians are likely to encounter during their careers. A wide range of phenotypes in all age groups exist, although most IEM present in infancy or childhood. Although infants and intellectually impaired individuals may present with non-specific symptoms and signs, biochemical disease should be on the differential diagnosis of critically ill patients or those with presentations characteristic of IEM in whom an alternative diagnosis has not been ascertained. Treatment options are growing, and NBS is allowing earlier diagnosis and improved outcomes. These disorders comprise a dynamic field in which researchers are progressively defining the pathophysiology, improving diagnostic methods, and expanding therapies.

SUGGESTED READINGS

Berry GT: Inborn errors of carbohydrate, ammonia, amino acid, and organic acid metabolism. In Taeusch HW, Ballard RA, Gleason CA, editors: *Avery's Diseases of the Newborn*, ed 8, Philadelphia, 2005, Elsevier Saunders, pp 227-257.

Berry GT: Introduction to the metabolic and biochemical genetic diseases. In Taeusch HW, Ballard RA, Gleason CA, editors: *Avery's Diseases of the Newborn*, ed 8, Philadelphia, 2005, Elsevier Saunders, pp 271-326.

Blau N, Hoffmann GF, Leonard J, Clarke JTR, editors: *Physician's Guide to the Treatment and Follow-up of Metabolic Diseases*, ed 1, Heidelberg, Germany, Springer Verlag, 2006.

Burton B: Inborn errors of metabolism in infancy: a guide to diagnosis, *Pediatrics* 102(6):E69, 1998.

Clarke JTR, editor: *A Clinical Guide to Inherited Metabolic Diseases*, ed 3, Cambridge, UK, Cambridge University Press, 2005.

Fernandes J, Saudubray JM, van den Berghe G, Walter JH: Inborn Metabolic Diseases: Diagnosis and Treatment, ed 4, Heidelberg, Germany, Springer Verlag, 2006.

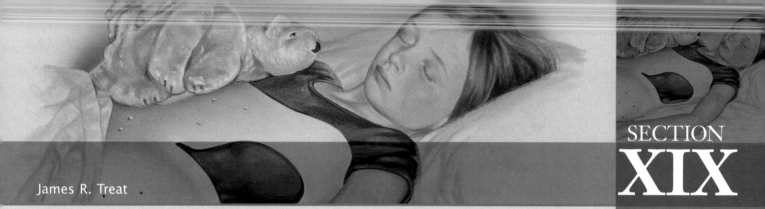

SECTION

XIX

James R. Treat

Dermatologic Disorders

Dermatologic Morphology

122

Lara Wine Lee

BASIC STRUCTURE OF THE SKIN

The skin has three basic layers: the epidermis, dermis, and subcutaneous tissue (Figure 122-1). Throughout these layers are additional structures and appendages that contribute to the skin's functionality.

Epidermis

The outermost layer of the skin, the epidermis, is composed primarily of keratinocytes to form a stratified epithelial tissue that functions primarily to protect against the external environment and prevent water loss. The innermost layer of the epidermis consists of the basal cells at the dermal–epidermal junction. Basal cells divide to form keratinocytes, which undergo an evolution by initially flattening out to form the stratum granulosum. The keratinocytes eventually die and form the outermost barrier, the stratum corneum, which is continually replenished. The epidermis also has melanocytes, the melanin-producing cells of the skin, Langerhans' cells, which are dendritic cells derived from macrophages and perform immune surveillance, as well as Merkel's cells, which are mechanosensory touch receptors.

Dermis

The dermis is composed primarily of a matrix of fibroblasts that produce the support structure of the skin by synthesizing collagen and elastic fibers. The part of the dermis closest to the epidermis is the more cellular layer, the papillary layer. The papillary dermis supports unmyelinated nerve endings that transmit sensations of pain, itch, and temperature. Deep to this is the reticular layer, which is dense in collagen and elastic fibers. Both layers contain blood and lymphatic vessels. In addition, the dermis supports most of the skin's appendages, including the hair follicle, apocrine and eccrine sweat glands, and sebaceous glands.

Subcutaneous Tissue

The subcutaneous tissue of the skin serves to conserve body heat and as a protective cushion. The subcutaneous tissue is composed primarily of adipocytes, which play important roles in glucose and fat metabolism. In addition, factors released by adipocytes contribute to wound healing, vascular remodeling, and the inflammatory and immune responses. A fibrous network anchors the adipocytes to deeper structures, such as muscular fascia and periosteum.

APPROACH TO DERMATOLOGIC MORPHOLOGY AND DISEASE

Recognition of cutaneous lesions begins with basic understanding of dermatologic terminology and morphology. As with any other disease process, diagnosis of cutaneous disease begins with a thorough history and physical examination. A thorough examination includes careful inspection of the body surface, including the mucous membranes, nails, and hair. The differential diagnosis is guided by the distribution and configuration of lesions. More careful examination of individual lesions, including inspection and palpation, helps identify the primary lesion. The primary lesion is defined as the basic, most representative lesion. Lesions often undergo secondary changes as a result of scratching, infection, or treatment. Identification of the primary lesions allows accurate description and aids in generation of a differential diagnosis.

Primary Lesions

Primary lesions (Figure 122-2) are characterized by their diameter and depth. A *macule* is a flat lesion that can be seen by changes in skin color but cannot be felt. The border may be well circumscribed or may gradually blend into the surrounding skin. It may be of any size, but the term is generally used to describe lesions smaller than 1 cm. Flat lesions larger than 1 cm are termed *patches*. Similar to macules, *papules* are small (<1 cm) lesions but are palpable with the greatest mass above the surface of surrounding skin. Larger elevated skin lesions are termed *plaques*. Plaques may be formed by a confluence of papules or can be the primary lesion. Palpable, solitary lesions whose mass is primarily below the surface, in the dermis and subcutaneous tissue, are termed either *nodules* (0.5-2 cm) or *tumors*. Tumors may be benign or malignant.

Primary lesions are also characterized by the presence of fluid or debris-filled cavities. For example, a small (<1cm) fluid-filled lesion is termed a *vesicle*. Larger fluid-filled lesions are *bullae*. Discrete, elevated lesions that contain purulent debris are *pustules*. The contents may be infectious or reactive. A larger purulent collection that is palpable but may contain deeper components is an *abscess*.

Other primary lesions include a *wheal* (*hive*), which is a firm, elevated lesion that is secondary to dermal edema. Wheals vary in size and shape, are usually pink to red, and may be transient. A *cyst* is a well-circumscribed, deep lesion that is covered by normal epidermis. It may contain fluid or semisolid debris.

Secondary Lesions

Primary lesions may undergo changes caused by evolution, irritation, infection, or application of treatments. Although it is important to recognize the secondary lesions, these changes often have less diagnostic utility than the primary lesion. *Scales* are layers of the stratum corneum that have desquamated but still remain attached to the skin surface. *Crusts* are thick accumulations of cellular debris, blood, pus, or serum. *Erosions* are superficial (involving only the epidermis) losses of tissue, resulting in depression of the surface. They generally heal without

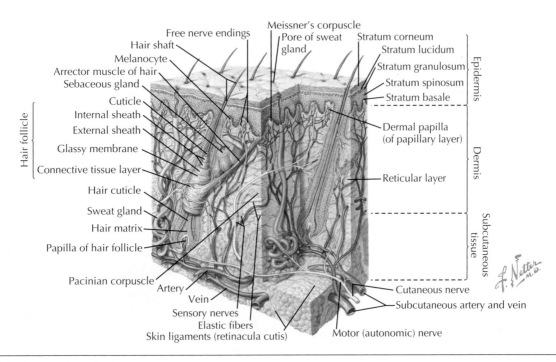

Figure 122-1 *Cross-section of skin.*

scar formation. In contrast, deeper tissue loss that extends into the dermis and even subcutaneous tissue is called an *ulcer*. Ulcers often heal with scarring. Ulceration or erosions that are linear and result from scratching are termed *excoriations*. *Fissures* form at sites of chronic inflammation. They are sharply demarcated, linear disruptions in the epidermis with extension into the dermis. *Lichenification* is a marked thickening of the epidermis that results in exaggeration of skin markings (Figure 122-3). Lichenification is a result of chronic irritation caused by inflammation, rubbing, or scratching.

Healing of lesions may result in secondary changes as well. For example, atrophic changes of the epidermis or dermis result in depressions in the skin surface. *Epidermal atrophy* is demonstrated by very thin, nearly translucent skin with loss of markings. Such areas are susceptible to mechanical damage. *Dermal atrophy* manifests as depressions with overlying normal skin color and markings. Scars may form at the sites of injury. A *scar* is a permanent change in the skin after an injury that results in fibrosis. Scars may be hypertrophic, which is an exaggerated response to skin damage that remains within the boundaries of the original injury. Hypertrophic scars are differentiated from *keloids*, which continue to grow long after the injury and can grow well outside the boundary of the initial insult.

Color of Lesions

Another important characteristic of lesions is how they compare with the patient's normal skin color. Lesions that are darker than the surrounding skin may be hyperpigmented. Inflammation can lead to hyperpigmentation. Other examples of hyperpigmentation include nevi, transient pustular melanosis of the newborn, and café-au-lait spots (see Chapters 124 and 126). Increased dermal pigmentation often results in a bluish

discoloration of lesions, such as seen in dermal melanocytosis (colloquially termed *Mongolian spots*). Lesions may also be hypopigmented, such as postinflammatory hypopigmentation, tinea versicolor, or ash leaf spots of tuberous sclerosis. Depigmented lesions have lost all pigment and can be differentiated from hypopigmented lesions by Wood's lamp examination. An example of depigmented disorders is vitiligo. Whereas lesions that are pink to red may be inflammatory in origin, more intense red to purple lesions are often vascular.

Configuration of Lesions

Additional diagnostic information can be gained from correct identification of the configuration or shape of individual or grouped lesions. Helpful terminology not only provides a specific description of the lesions' shape but also helps indicate the underlying process. Whereas *discrete* lesions describe those that remain as distinct and separated from surrounding areas of disease, *confluent* describes lesions that have coalesced or merged. *Clustered* lesions are grouped on one area. *Linear* lesions occur in a band or line and suggest a reactive dermatitis, such as poison ivy, or may follow developmental lines, such as an epidermal nevus.

Specific description of the shape of lesions provides further information. To label a lesion round gives little specific information, but describing it as *annular* (Figure 122-4) specifies a ring-shaped lesion with a raised or erythematous border and central clearing. Common examples of annular lesions include tinea infections, erythema migrans, and granuloma annulare. *Discoid* lesions are also round but tend to be more solid in nature. Other round lesions include *nummular* (Figure 122-5), *targetoid* (containing-concentric rings), and *guttate* (droplike) lesions; the latter is commonly used to describe a form of psoriasis

Type of primary lesion	Appearance	Description	Example	Type of primary lesion	Appearance	Description	Example
Macules	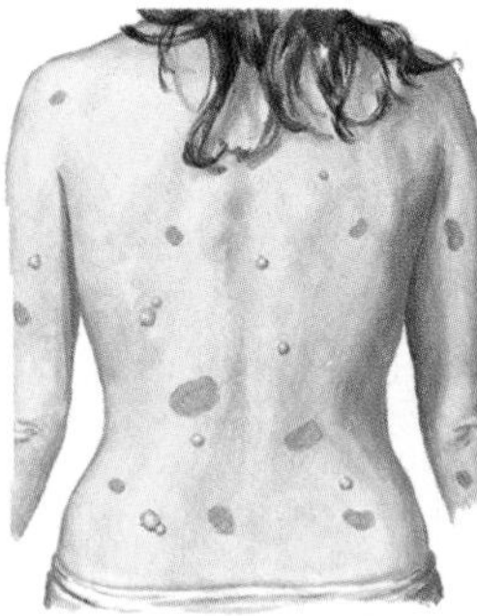	Flat changes in skin color of any size though generally less than 1 cm, may be rounded, irregular or fade into surrounding skin.	Café au lait macules, freckles, capillary malformations	Vesicle	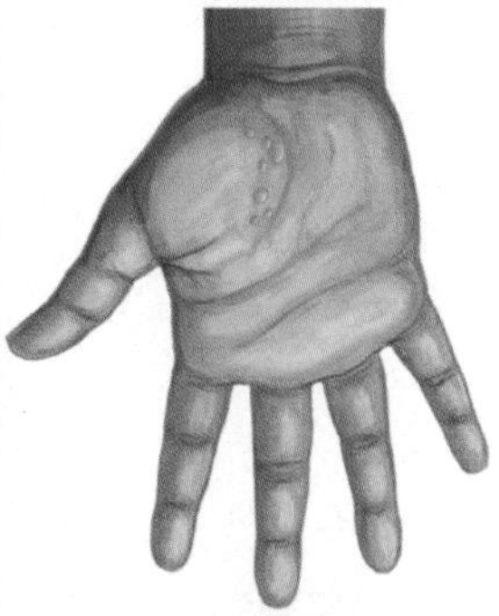	Circumscribed, fluid filled elevation up to 1 cm in diameter	Coxsackie virus, Herpes simplex virus, varicella, miliaria crystallina
Patches	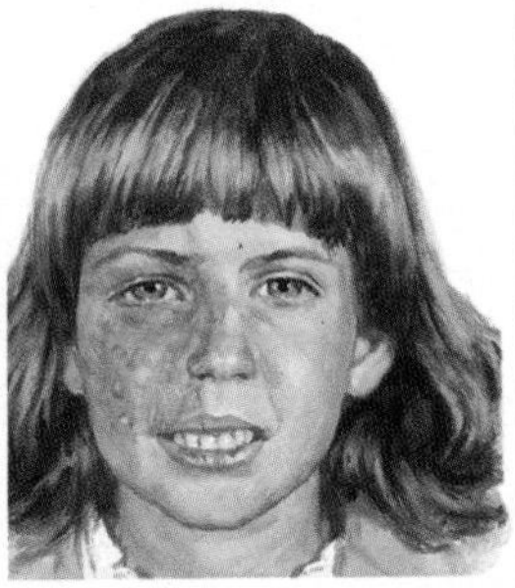	Greater than 1 cm flat lesion with color change, common colors include red (vascular lesion) darker (hyperpigmented) or lighter (hypopigmented or depigmented) than surrounding skin	Port wine stain, Mongolian spot, vitiligo	Bullae	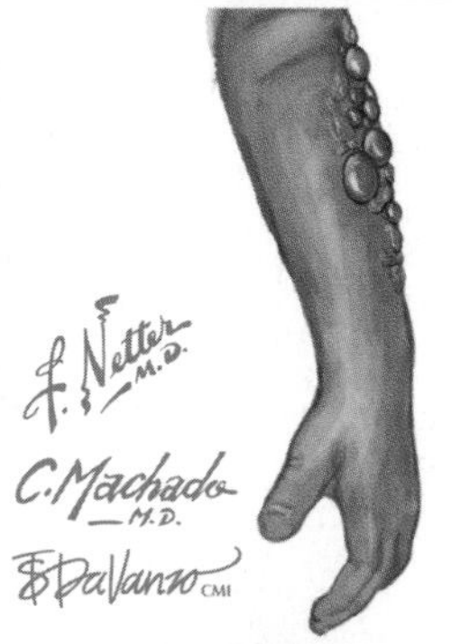	Circumscribed, fluid-filled elevation greater than 1 cm in diameter. Flaccid bullae (superficial, involving the epidermis) rupture easily and intact lesions may not be evident. Tense bullae (subepidermal) remain intact.	Bullous impetigo, sucking blisters, Epidermolysis bullosa, blistering distal dactylitis, insect bite reaction
Papules	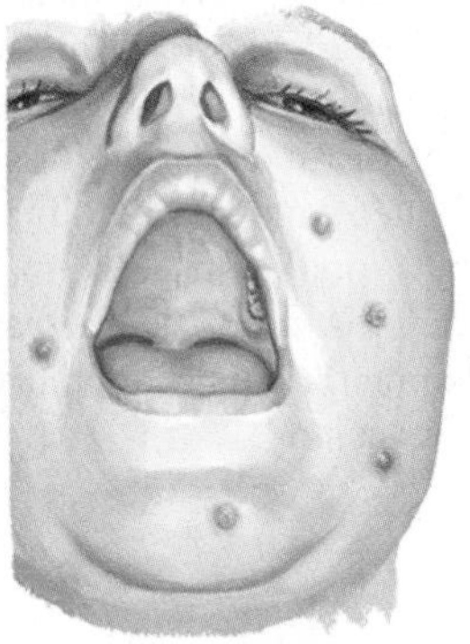	Solid elevations less than 1 cm, may have overlying color change or blend with surrounding skin	Molluscum contagiosum, dermal nevus, verruca/wart milia	Pustule	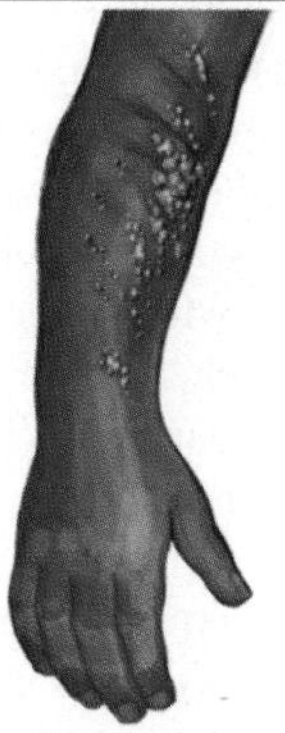	Less than 1 cm, circumscribed elevaton of the skin containing purulent material.	Folliculitis, transient pustular melanosis, infantile acropustulosis
Plaques	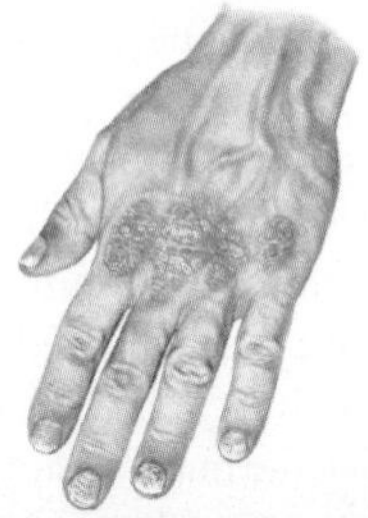	Elevated, flat-topped circumscribed lesion greater than 1 cm in diameter. May be formed by the confluence of papules.	Psoriasis, nevus sebaceous, lichen planus	Abscess	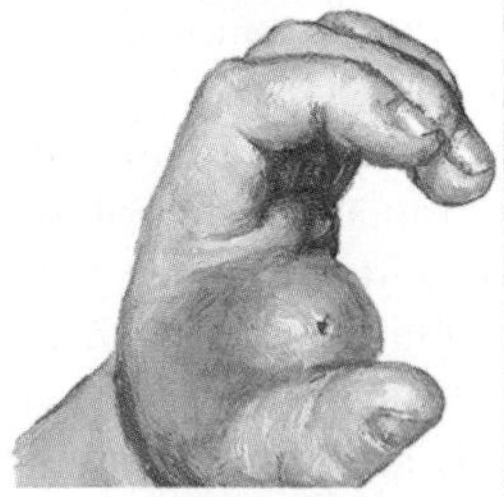	Circumscribed, elevated lesion greater than 1 cm containing purulent fluid.	Staphylococcal abscess, hidradenitis suppurativa, acne conglobata
Nodules or tumors	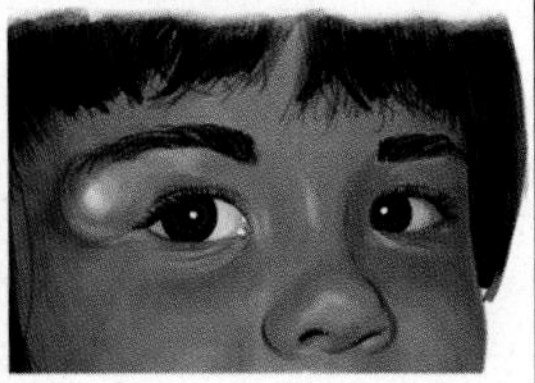	Circumscribed solid lesion less than 2 cm that involves the dermis and may include the subcutaneous tissue. Tumors are greater than 2 cm.	Dermoid cyst, Juvenile xanthogranuloma, neurofibroma, hemangiomas, lipoma	Wheal	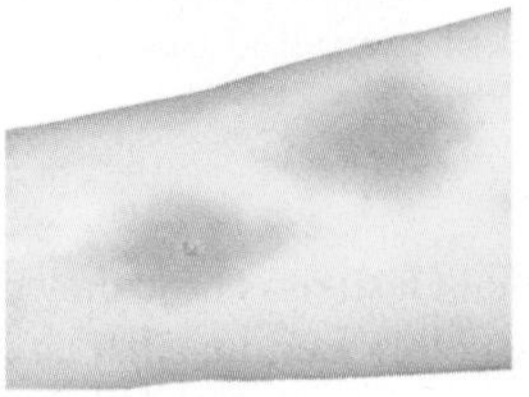	An evanescent, elevated lesion that represents dermal edema. Lesions may vary in size and shape and are often surrounded by macular erythema.	Urticaria (hives), bug bite reaction (papular urticaria), urticarial vasculitis

Figure 122-2 *Primary lesions.*

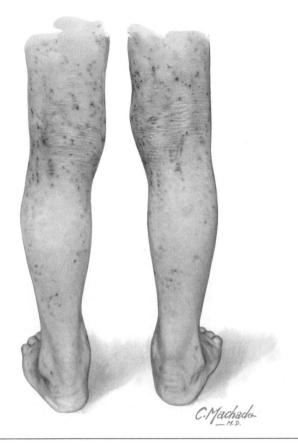

Figure 122-3 *Flexural lichenification.*

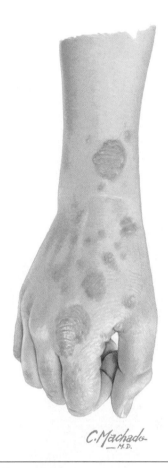

Figure 122-5 *Nummular eczema.*

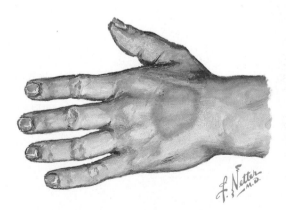

Figure 122-4 *Annular lesion.*

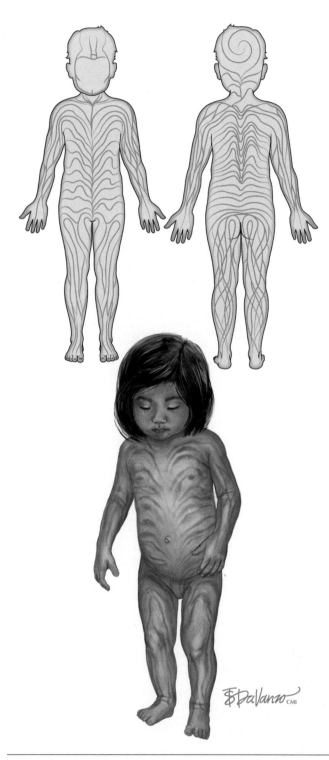

in children that occurs after acute streptococcal infection. *Umbilicated* lesions have a central depression; common examples include molluscum contagiosum and varicella.

Serpiginous describes lesions that have linear and curving elements as though following the track of a snake. *Reticulated* lesions have a netlike or lacy configuration, such as cutis marmorata or livedo reticularis. *Morbilliform* is a term that refers to a measles-like eruption. It consists of red macules and papules that may be discrete or confluent on large areas of the body surface. Common examples of morbilliform eruptions include Kawasaki's disease and drug eruptions. Lesions that have a variety of shapes are described as *multiform*.

Distribution of Lesions

Many cutaneous lesions have predilections for specific areas. Although these are discussed in more detail with specific disease processes, some generalizations about lesion distribution may be helpful in initial diagnosis. Linear eruptions may follow a *dermatomal* pattern, thus affecting the skin supplied by a single spinal nerve. Linear lesions may also follow *lines of Blaschko*, lines of embryologic development of the skin (Figure 122-6). These cutaneous lesions represent a form of genetic mosaicism; examples include epidermal nevi, lichen striatus, and some congenital disorders. Lesions that arise only in sun-exposed areas may represent a disorder of photosensitization or one precipitated by sun exposure.

SUGGESTED READINGS

Bolognia JL, Orlow SJ, Glick SA: Lines of Blaschko, *J Am Acad Dermatol* 31(2 pt 1):157-190, 1994.

Proksch E, Brandner JM, Jensen JM: The skin: an indispensable barrier, *Exp Dermatol* 17(12):1063-1072, 2008.

Figure 122-6 *Linear lesions.*

123

Vascular Disorders

Lara Wine Lee

Vascular lesions of the skin are a common pediatric problem with a wide range of clinical presentations. In 1996, the International Society for the Study of Vascular Anomalies adopted Mulliken and Glowacki's classification (Table 123-1). There are two categories based on biologic and clinical characteristics: vascular tumors and vascular malformations. Vascular tumors are neoplasms of vascular structures that grow by hyperplasia. Vascular malformations are local anomalies in vascular development that do not demonstrate proliferation.

VASCULAR TUMORS

Recent classification distinguishes three major types of vascular tumors, hemangiomas, tufted angiomas, and hemangioendotheliomas. Although these vascular tumors are generally benign, they have significant associated clinical consequences.

Infantile Hemangiomas

ETIOLOGY AND PATHOGENESIS

Hemangiomas of infancy are the most common infantile tumors, occurring in up to 1% to 2% of all infants and up to 10% in whites. These benign proliferations of endothelial cells affect females four times more often than males. The growing incidence of hemangiomas has been attributed to an association between hemangiomas and premature birth. Other factors that are associated with an increased incidence of hemangiomas include multiple gestations, assisted reproduction, chorionic villus sampling, increased maternal age, and preeclampsia. However, many of these factors may not be independent. Although most hemangiomas are sporadic occurrences, a positive family history does increase the incidence, and both autosomal dominant inheritance and syndromic associations are reported.

CLINICAL MANIFESTATIONS

Hemangiomas are classified as superficial, deep, or mixed lesions. Superficial hemangiomas, involving the papillary dermis, are red and protuberant. Superficial hemangiomas have well-defined borders. Deep lesions invade the reticular dermis and superficial fat. They tend to have a blue-purple discoloration with normal skin texture. The margins of deep lesions may be ill defined. Most lesions have both superficial and deep components (Figure 123-1). A mature hemangioma contains characteristics of capillaries, venules, and arterioles.

Although subtle skin changes may be present at birth, most hemangiomas do not become evident until the first few weeks of life when they undergo a period of rapid growth that may last 6 to 9 months. Growth then slows, and most cease growing by 10 to 12 months of age. Spontaneous involution and regression occurs after the cessation of growth. The first sign of regression is the appearance of grayish changes on the surface of the hemangioma. Although the vascular elements of the tumor may completely regress, they are often replaced by fibrofatty tissue that results in permanent skin changes (30%), including scarring, atrophy, telangiectasias, or permanent discoloration. Although some lesions will not fully regress, more than 60% of lesions have completed their regression by age 5 years, with almost all lesions completed by age 9 years.

MANAGEMENT

Most infantile hemangiomas are of little clinical significance and require no therapy. Treatment is based primarily on the location, size, and potential for complications. Lesions that affect vision, breathing, eating, or bowel habits or those that ulcerate or are large and likely to lead to significant cosmetic abnormalities may necessitate therapy. The mainstays of treatment include pulsed-dye laser therapy and corticosteroids. Pulsed-dye laser results in a high response rate for superficial hemangiomas but is typically reserved for ulcerated lesions because superficial hemangiomas will likely regress fully anyway. Steroid-resistant, life-threatening lesions may require treatment with chemotherapeutic agents such as vincristine or interferon-α (INF-α). Recent data suggest the efficacy of oral propranolol in shortening the course of infantile hemangiomas. Although propranolol therapy is well tolerated, care should be taken in children with abnormal vasculature, reactive airway disease, or underlying cardiac conditions.

The most common complication of rapidly proliferating hemangiomas is ulceration. Ulceration is most common in perineal and perioral hemangiomas and can be quite painful. Ulcerated hemangiomas are also at risk for superinfection. Hemangiomas in select locations may have unique complications. Nasal tip hemangiomas cause significant disfigurement. Periocular hemangiomas disrupt visual development, and early referral to an ophthalmologist is prudent. Hemangiomas along the jaw line or neck (beard distribution) of the head and neck (see Figure 123-1) have a high association with airway lesions that may cause life-threatening airway obstruction. Spinal dysraphism is associated with midline lumbosacral lesions, and magnetic resonance imaging (MRI) is indicated. Infants with multiple cutaneous hemangiomas warrant evaluation for visceral hemangiomas.

Congenital Hemangiomas

Congenital hemangiomas are fully formed at birth. Although they may follow a growth pattern consistent with infantile hemangiomas, a subset has distinctive growth patterns and characteristics. Noninvoluting congenital hemangiomas (NICHs) do not have a proliferative phase and grow only in proportion to the child's growth. NICHs are usually round, deep tumors with surface telangiectasias and a purplish coloration. The lesions usually have a rim of pallor. Rapidly involuting congenital

Table 123-1 International Society for the Study of Vascular Anomalies Classification of Vascular Anomalies

Vascular Tumors	Vascular Malformations

• Infantile hemangiomas
• Congenital hemangiomas
  • Rapidly involuting
  • Noninvoluting
• Tufted angiomas
• Kaposiform hemangioendothelioma
• Other hemangioendotheliomas
• Acquired vascular tumors
  • Pyogenic granuloma
  • Targetoid hemangioma
  • Glomeruloid hemangioma
  • Microvenular hemangioma
	• Slow-flow vascular malformations
	  • Capillary malformations
	    • Port-wine stain
	    • Telangiectasia
	    • Angiokeratoma
	  • Venous malformation
	    • Common sporadic VM
	    • Glomuvenous malformation
	  • Lymphatic malformation
	• Fast-flow vascular malformations
	  • Arterial malformation
	  • Arteriovenous malformation
	  • Arteriovenous fistula
	• Complex-combined vascular malformations

VM, venous malformation.
Adapted from ISSVA classification as reported in Color Atlas of Vascular Tumors & Vascular Malformations.

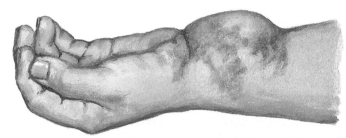

Hemangioma in wrist of young child

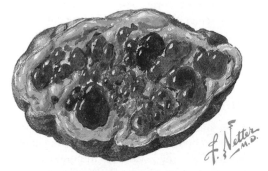

Sectioned hemangioma

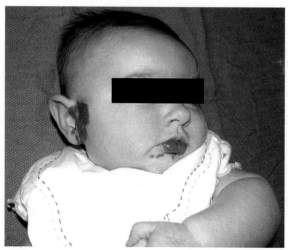

Hemangioma in a beard distribution. *Reprinted with permission for Zaoutis LB, Chiang VW. Comprehensive Pediatric Hospital Medicine. Figure 153-3. Mosby, Elsevier. 2007.*

Figure 123-1 *Hemangioma.*

hemangiomas (RICHs) have accelerated regression and may even show signs of involution at birth. They may appear similar to NICH or infantile hemangiomas and have generally involuted within the first year of life.

PHACES Syndrome

Large, segmental facial hemangiomas may be associated with PHACES (posterior fossa malformations, hemangiomas, arterial anomalies, cardiac anomalies, eye abnormalities, sternal cleft or supraumbilical raphe) syndrome (Figure 123-2). The most common associated feature of PHACES syndrome is posterior fossa malformations, particularly Dandy-Walker type and cerebellar hypoplasia. Arterial anomalies and stenosis affecting arteries of the head and neck are found in one-third of patients. Cardiac anomalies such as coarctation are also common and can be in atypical locations along the course of the aorta. Less common associations include eye anomalies and sternal clefting or supraumbilical raphe. PHACES should be considered in any child presenting with a large, segmental facial hemangioma. Suspected patients should be referred to a neurologist for complete neurologic evaluation, including MRI or magnetic resonance angiography of the brain and neck as well as cardiac evaluation. Ophthalmologic evaluation should also be considered.

Tufted Angiomas

Tufted angiomas are uncommon benign vascular tumors that develop within the first year of life. Located most commonly on the thorax, tufted angiomas are red to blue subcutaneous nodules

and plaques. Tufted angiomas grow slowly with lateral extension, and regression is uncommon.

Kaposiform Hemangioendothelioma

Kaposiform hemangioendothelioma (KHE) is a locally aggressive vascular tumor. KHE may initially present with a similar appearance to infantile hemangiomas, but the lesions become nodular and violaceous. KHE may be present at birth and commonly affects children younger than 2 years of age. Boys and girls are equally affected. KHE may invade local soft tissue and bone.

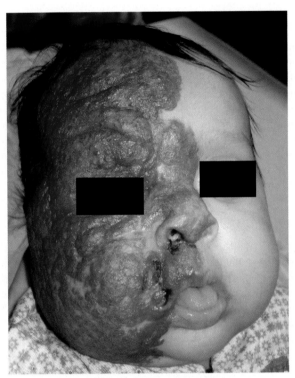

Large segmental facial hemangioma of PHACES syndrome.

Figure 123-2 *PHACES syndrome.*

Kasabach-Merritt Phenomenon

Rapidly expanding vascular tumors are associated with Kasabach-Merritt phenomenon, a consumptive coagulopathy of thrombocytopenia, coagulopathy, and microangiopathic hemolytic anemia. Unfortunately, the original description of this phenomenon was attributed to hemangiomas, but it was later found that the Kasabach-Merritt phenomenon happens exclusively with tufted angiomas, KHEs, and hemangiopericytomas. In Kasabach-Merritt phenomenon, infants present with acute enlargement of the vascular lesions and bleeding complications. Kasabach-Merritt phenomenon requires immediate medical attention because the mortality rate can be as high as 30%. Smaller lesions may be amenable to surgical excision with or without embolization. Lesions that cannot be resected present somewhat of a therapeutic challenge. Systemic corticosteroids are often used, but resistant lesions may require treatment with chemotherapeutic agents such as INF-α and vincristine.

Pyogenic Granuloma

Pyogenic granulomas are acquired vascular tumors that present as red to brown papules. Usually solitary, pyogenic granulomas can occur anywhere on the skin and mucous membranes but frequently are at sites of trauma. Lesions are benign but frequently bleed with slight trauma. Shave excision with electrodessication at the base is often adequate for resolution of these lesions.

VASCULAR MALFORMATIONS: SLOW-FLOW LESIONS

Capillary Malformations

NEVUS FLAMMEUS

Capillary malformations (CMs) are the most common vascular malformation of infancy, occurring in 0.3% of live births. *Port-wine stain* and *nevus flammeus* are other terms for congenital CMs. They are present at birth, appearing as a flat vascular "stain." CMs may appear to change color with the Valsalva maneuver caused by increased flow or may slightly darken with rises in hemoglobin, but they remain flat. CMs are composed of an increased number of ectatic dermal capillary-like vessels. They are hypothesized to arise embryologically from errors of vascular development. The incidence is equivalent in boys and girls.

Sporadic CMs may be associated with other congenital anomalies. Underlying spinal dysraphism has been reported with midline lumbosacral lesions, especially if there is a secondary lesion such as a dimple, nodule, or tuft of hair. Progressive hypertrophy of underlying tissue can also be seen, and this can lead to hemihypertrophy of the affected area. Although CMs are generally sporadic, familial and syndromic associations are well reported.

STURGE-WEBER SYNDROME

Sturge-Weber syndrome is a neurocutaneous disorder of facial port-wine stains and vascular malformation of the leptomeninges and eye. First described by Sturge in 1879, the syndrome has now been defined as the following triad: (1) port-wine stain involving at least the V1 (ophthalmic) branch of the trigeminal nerve, (2) ipsilateral leptomeningeal angiomatosis, and (3) ipsilateral vascular malformation of the choroidal vasculature of the eye. Children with Sturge-Weber syndrome have complications from leptomeningeal involvement, most commonly seizures within the first year of life (>50%). Transient or residual impairment, such as hemiplegia, is reported in up to 30% of patients. Glaucoma is the most common manifestation of the vascular anomaly of the eye.

The decision to treat a patient with CMs is based on the cosmetic impact of a lesion. Pulsed-dye laser therapy achieves significant lightening and may prevent the hypertrophy or vascular nodules, which can develop later on in life. Laser therapy, with a wavelength of 585 to 600 nm, targets oxyhemoglobin, leading to destruction of ectatic vessels without significant damage to surrounding skin structures.

NEVUS SIMPLEX

A subset of CMs called nevus simplex or "Salmon patches," are better known by colloquial names based on the location of the lesion. "Angel's kisses" occur on the glabella and eyelids, and "stork bite" describes those on the back of the neck. Nevus simplex is a common newborn birthmark, occurring in approximately 30% of all newborns. These lesions should be differentiated from true CMs because of their transient nature and thus require no treatment. Lesions that persist may not be evident unless the child is crying or straining, and parents should be counseled about this "recurrence."

TELANGIECTASIAS

Telangiectasias are permanent dilatations of small vessels of the skin. They generally blanch with direct pressure. Telangiectasias may be primary disorders of blood vessel development or secondary to any process that damages blood vessel endothelium, including sun damage, aging, or systemic disease. Although most telangiectasias are sporadic, they may be associated with hereditary syndromes such as ataxia-telangiectasia, generalized essential telangiectasia, or hereditary hemorrhagic telangiectasia. Pulsed-dye laser may be used to treat cosmetically unfavorable telangiectasias.

ANGIOKERATOMA

Angiokeratomas are collections of dilated superficial dermal vessels with overlying epidermal hyperkeratosis. They present as dark red to purple papules or plaques. Clustered plaques of angiokeratomas may be present at birth. Acquired angiokeratomas can be isolated or found at sites of trauma. Multiple, diffuse angiokeratomas on the abdomen, buttocks, and thighs, or angiokeratoma corporis diffusum, are most commonly associated with X-linked recessive deficiency of α-galactosidase (Fabry's disease). Other metabolic conditions, particularly lysosomal storage diseases, are associated with diffuse angiokeratomas. The diagnosis is made by urine oligosaccharide analysis.

Venous Malformations

Venous malformations (VMs) most commonly affect cutaneous and mucosal structures but can involve internal structures as well. VMs are often isolated bluish lesions with cutaneous and mucosal involvement. Although most VMs are present at birth, they do become more prominent as the patient ages. VMs should not have an associated warmth or palpable flow such as a thrill. VMs are composed of collections of ectatic thin-walled vessels that are deficient in smooth muscles. Significant bony abnormalities may result from deeper involvement. Although VMs are common sporadic lesions, rare familial and syndromic associations are found. There are no histologic differences between inherited and sporadic VMs. Blue rubber bleb syndrome is a rare condition of the skin, gastrointestinal, and other internal organ VMs. Maffucci's syndrome is a rare disorder of VM and benign cartilage enlargement (endochondromas) that may be associated with chondrosarcoma.

Recommended diagnostic imaging of choice in VMs is MRI, which can define the extent of the lesion and involvement of underlying structures. Head and neck VMs are associated with vascular anomalies of the brain. Sclerotherapy is effective in providing symptomatic relief and shrinking lesions or as an adjuvant therapy to surgical excision. Lesions, particularly on the extremities, respond well to compression and support devices. Lesions prone to thrombotic events can be treated with low-dose aspirin, and systemic coagulopathy often responds to low-molecular-weight heparin.

Glomuvenous Malformations

Some venous malformations have an additional cell type, the peripheral chemoreceptor, the glomus cell. Approximately 5% of all VMs contain glomus cells, so they are more appropriately named glomuvenous malformations (GVMs) or glomangiomas. These lesions are important to distinguish from the more common VM because therapy differs. GVMs are bluish-purple and raised and have a cobblestone surface. GVMs are often painful with compression. GVMs may be sporadic or familial but do have a high rate of familial inheritance (38%-63%). GVMs are often amenable to excision.

Lymphatic Malformations

Lymphatic malformations are aberrantly connected collections of lymphatic channels and lymphatic cysts. Diffuse lymphatic malformation is termed *lymphedema*. Primary lymphedema is characterized by the age of presentation; congenital lymphedema (type I or Nonne-Milroy disease), ages 1 to 35 years (type II or lymphedema praecox), or older than 35 years of age (lymphedema tarda).

Localized lymphatic malformations are characterized as either deep "macrocystic" lesions" or superficial "microcystic" lesions. Most lesions present by 2 years of age, with approximately 70% noted at birth. Continual expansion of lesions may be caused by progressive dilatation of the abnormal channels.

Clinical sequelae of lymphatic malformations largely depend on their location. Congenital malformations often lead to structural abnormalities. Lesions of the extremities can lead to impairment and overgrowth. Large lesions may present with consumptive sequelae such as hypoproteinemia and hypogammaglobulinemia. Lymphocytes can sequester in lymphatic malformations, leading to lymphopenia and susceptibility to infection. Leakage of lymph fluid may affect local structures, resulting in chylous effusions or ascites. Surgical resection, when possible, is the recommended therapy for lymphatic malformations.

Lymphatic malformations and lymphedema are associated with a number of genetic syndromes, including Turner, Noonan, and Down syndromes. Prenatally diagnosed cystic hygromas are associated with chromosomal abnormalities in 62% of cases, most commonly Turner's syndrome (33%).

VASCULAR MALFORMATIONS: FAST-FLOW LESIONS

Arteriovenous Malformations

Arteriovenous malformations (AVMs) are uncommon vascular malformations that represent a connection of arterial and venous channels without a capillary bed. They are found equally in males and females, and most are present at birth. Their clinical appearance may vary from erythematous macules and plaques to larger nodules. Unlike other vascular lesions, they are associated with increased warmth, pulsation, or audible flow, such as a bruit or thrill. Imaging, such as ultrasonography with Doppler flow, computed tomography, or MRI, confirms diagnosis of an AVM. AVMs may stay fairly quiescent or enter a period of growth. Locally aggressive lesions can cause deeper invasion, including bone involvement, ulceration, or hemorrhage. Treatment of AVMs is most successful when undertaken early and involves embolization with resection when anatomically feasible.

SUGGESTED READINGS

Boon LM, Mulliken JB, Enjolras O, Vikkula M: Glomuvenous malformation (glomangioma) and venous malformation: distinct clinicopathologic and genetic entities, *Arch Dermatol* 140(8):971-976, 2004.

Bruckner AL, Frieden IJ: Infantile hemangiomas, *J Am Acad Dermatol* 55(4):671-682, 2006.

Drolet BA, Swanson EA, Frieden IJ, et al: Infantile hemangiomas: an emerging health issue linked to an increased rate of low birth weight infants, *J Pediatr* 153(5):712-715, 5.e1, 2008.

Enjolras O, Wassef M, Chapot R: Introduction: ISSVA Classification. *Color atlas of vascular tumors and vascular malformations.* Cambridge, UK, 2007, Cambridge University Press, pp 3-11.

Garzon MC, Huang JT, Enjolras O, et al: Vascular malformations. Part II: associated syndromes, *J Am Acad Dermatol* 56(4):541-564, 2007.

Guggisberg D, Hadj-Rabia S, Viney C, et al: Skin markers of occult spinal dysraphism in children: a review of 54 cases, *Arch Dermatol* 140(9):1109-1115, 2004.

Maguiness S, Guenther L: Kasabach-Merritt syndrome, *J Cutan Med Surg* 6(4):335-339, 2002.

Sans V, Dumas de la Roque E, Berge J, et al: Propranolol for severe infantile hemangiomas: follow-up report, *Pediatrics* 124:e423-e431, 2009.

Stier M, Glick S, Hirsch R: Laser treatment of pediatric vascular lesions: port wine stains and hemangiomas, *J Am Acad Dermatol* 58(2):261-285, 2008.

Hyperpigmented Skin Disorders

124

Vikash S. Oza

From the newborn period through young adulthood, hyper-pigmented skin lesions are one of the most common findings on physical examination. Although often of cosmetic concern, the true importance of appropriate diagnosis lies in the fact that certain hyperpigmented skin conditions may serve as the first clinical indicator of an underlying genetic disorder, neurocutaneous syndrome, metabolic condition, or endocrinopathy. The goals of this chapter are to introduce clinicians to the characteristic features of common hyperpigmented skin lesions, associated diagnoses that should be considered, and the management of certain skin conditions.

ETIOLOGY AND PATHOGENESIS

Disorders of skin pigmentation reflect disturbances in the complex homeostasis of melanin production. Neural crest cell-derived melanocytes lie at the basal layer of the epidermis and produce melanin in lysosomal-like structures termed *melanosomes*. Melanosomes are transported from melanocytes to surrounding keratinocytes via dendritic extensions, and most melanin is found within the keratinocyte. Differences in skin pigmentation reflect not a difference in the number of melanocytes, which remains relatively constant, but a difference in the size, distribution, and number of melanosomes within keratinocytes.

Hyperpigmented skin lesions can be described as being either circumscribed or diffuse in nature. Focal areas of hyperpigmentation reflect local influences ranging from the degree of ultraviolet radiation to biochemical signaling from neighboring keratinocytes to inflammatory mediators such as prostaglandins and leukotrienes. Disorders with diffuse hyperpigmentation may in part be caused by increased production of melanocyte-stimulating hormone (MSH) as exemplified in conditions such as Addison's disease. MSH is a byproduct of adrenocorticotropic hormone (ACTH), secretion from the pituitary and stimulates the melanocytes' melanin production. Disruption of the production, maturation, or transportation of melanosomes results in many of the conditions discussed within this chapter. A discussion of nevi and disorders of melanocyte overgrowth is provided in Chapter 126.

CIRCUMSCRIBED HYPERPIGMENTED SKIN LESIONS

Freckles (Ephelides)

Freckles are the most common hyperpigmented macules seen in childhood. They are light to dark brown in color, smaller than 3 mm in diameter, irregular in contour, and found on sun-exposed areas such as the face, upper back and chest, and dorsal surface of the arms. They are not present at birth and develop over childhood. They are found most often in individuals with red hair and fair skin. The typical pattern is for freckles to increase in number and prominence in the summer and fade in the winter. The development of excessive freckling may suggest an underlying photosensitivity, as seen in xeroderma pigmentosum. Although benign in nature, individuals with lighter pigmented skin who are predisposed to the development of freckles are at higher risk of developing malignant melanoma.

Lentigines

Lentigines are round, brown to black macules, 4 to 10 mm in diameter that increase in number during adolescence and, at times, can be almost indistinguishable from ephelides. Clinically, lentigines occur anywhere on the body, not just in sun-exposed areas, and do not fade in the winter. Lentigines are quite common and benign when few in number. However, when multiple, lentigines constitute the primary clinical feature of a number of syndromes. The most important syndromes with lentigines as a defining feature are LEOPARD (lentigines, electrocardiogram abnormalities, ocular hypertelorism, pulmonary stenosis, abnormal genitalia, retardation of growth, and deafness) syndrome, also known as multiple lentiginous syndrome, Peutz-Jeghers syndrome, and Carney's complex (Figure 124-1 and Table 124-1). The clinician evaluating a patient with innumerable lentigines on examination should keep the above diagnoses in mind, especially if lentigines are noted on mucosal surfaces or cross the vermillion border because these are not features of benign lentiginosis.

Café-au-Lait Spots

Café-au-lait spots (CALS) are one of the most common hyperpigmented lesions, with one or two CALS present in approximately 25% of school-age children. Although CALS may be noted at birth, many CALS develop in early infancy and may increase in size and number throughout childhood. They are sharply defined, round to oval in shape, and light brown and homogenous in color and can range from 2 mm to more than 20 cm in diameter. CALS occur anywhere on the body but are generally located on the trunk and lower extremities, sparing the face and upper extremities. Similar to lentigines, CALS are benign in nature but may signal an underlying systemic disease.

The two most common disorders in which CALS are the principal cutaneous feature and may be the primary clinical finding at the time of diagnosis are neurofibromatosis type I (NF1) and McCune-Albright syndrome. The CALS seen in NF1 are multiple and have a smooth circumference often compared to the "coast of California" (Figure 124-2). The number or distribution of CALS is not associated with the severity of disease in NF1. Other principal cutaneous findings in NF1 are described in Table 124-2. Although one or two CALS are quite common, fewer than 1% of children younger than 5 years of age have more than five CALS without having NF1 or the newly described Legius' syndrome. Recent literature suggests that

LEOPARD Syndrome

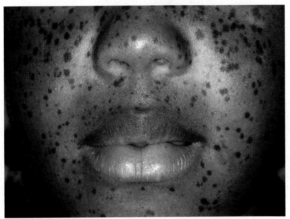

This patient has multiple lentigines with relative sparing of mucous membranes. (*Reprinted with permission from Cohen BA. Pediatric Dermatology. Mosby, Elsevier. Philadelphia, 2005.*)

Peutz-Jeghers Syndrome

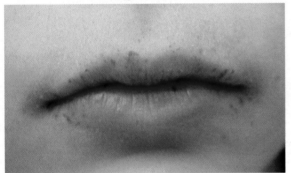

Note patient's characteristic mucocutaneous lentigines.

Figure 124-1 *Lentigines.*

many patients previously labeled as having mild NF-1 in fact have an "NF-like syndrome" termed *Legius' syndrome*, resulting from the autosomal dominant inheritance of a mutation in the *SPRED-1* gene. Legius' syndrome is characterized by multiple CALS, skin fold freckling, and an increased risk of macrocephaly and learning disabilities but without the other distinguishing features of NF-1 (see Chapter 76 for diagnostic criteria for NF-1). The CAL of McCune-Albright syndrome tends to be unilateral and large, stops abruptly at the midline, creating a segmental appearance, and has a jagged border likened to the "coast of Maine" (see Figure 124-2). Other associated features of McCune-Albright syndrome include precocious puberty and polyostotic fibrous dysplasia, although many children with large segmental café-au-lait macules have no associated syndrome. The clinician should consider the number and size of CALS along with other salient features by examination and history to guide their workup.

Mastocytosis

Cutaneous mastocytosis is defined by the collection of mast cells within the skin. Lesions of mastocytosis typically develop before the age of 2 years, but new lesions may be normal up to age 5 years. If mastocytosis develops after this age or if there are prominent symptoms of too much systemic histamine (watery diarrhea, consistent dermal flushing), a workup for systemic mastocytosis or mast cell leukemia should be considered. The time course for typical childhood-onset disease is self-limited, with 50% of cases resolving by puberty and the other 50% showing a significant reduction in symptoms. Cutaneous mastocytosis can be grouped into three forms: mastocytoma, urticaria pigmentosa, and diffuse cutaneous mastocytosis.

The term *mastocytoma* is used if only a few isolated lesions are present, but urticaria pigmentosa is defined by the presence of multiple smaller lesions. Mastocytomas typically develop in

Table 124-1 Major Lentiginous Syndromes

	Lentigines Distribution	Defining Features
LEOPARD syndrome	Neck and upper trunk (less often face, arms, palms, soles, and genitalia)	• Lentigines • Electrocardiograph abnormalities • Ocular hypertelorism • Pulmonary stenosis • Abnormal genitalia • Retardation of growth • Deafness (sensorineural)
Peutz-Jeghers syndrome	Mucocutaneous (lips and buccal mucosa; rarely, gums, palate, and tongue); elbows; palms; soles; and the nasal, periorbital, periumbilical, perianal, and labial regions	• Mucocutaneous lentigines • Gastrointestinal hamartomous polyps • Increased risk of early-onset adenocarcinomas affecting the GI tract, pancreas, breast, thyroid, and reproductive organs
Carney complex	Face, vermillion border of lips (not on buccal mucosa), conjunctiva, vaginal or penile mucosa	• Hyperpigmented cutaneous lesions (lentigines, CALS, and blue nevi) • Myxomas of heart, skin, and breast • Endocrine hyperactivity consistent with multiple endocrine neoplasia syndrome

CALS, café-au-lait spots; GI, gastrointestinal.

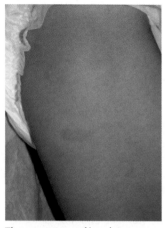

Three separate café-au-lait spots on the lower extremity of an infant.

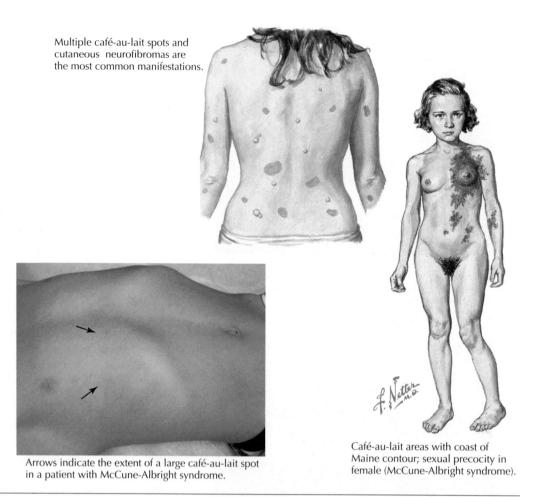

Multiple café-au-lait spots and cutaneous neurofibromas are the most common manifestations.

Arrows indicate the extent of a large café-au-lait spot in a patient with McCune-Albright syndrome.

Café-au-lait areas with coast of Maine contour; sexual precocity in female (McCune-Albright syndrome).

Figure 124-2 *Café-au-lait spots.*

Table 124-2 Cutaneous Findings in Neurofibromatosis Type I

	Age of Onset	Clinical Findings
Freckling	3-5 years old	Located in the skin folds of the axilla and inguinal area
Neurofibromas	Develop after puberty	Fleshy subcutaneous nodules with a violaceous hue occurring anywhere on the body
Plexiform neurofibromas	Present at birth or shortly thereafter	Soft tissue swelling often underlying a large, irregular CALS with overlying hypertrichosis; can grow rapidly, resembling a "bag of worms"

CALS, café-au-lait spots.

infancy manifesting as isolated flesh-colored to yellow-orange papules or plaques with a classic "peau d'orange" (orange peel) surface (Figure 124-3). Urticaria pigmentosa presents as multiple, tens to hundreds, of papules and plaques found throughout the skin, typically sparing the palms and soles. Urticaria pigmentosa is the most common form of mastocytosis and clinically can be mistaken for other hyperpigmented lesions ranging from CALS to purpura. Last, diffuse cutaneous mastocytosis is not as common as the two previous forms and reflects diffuse infiltration of the skin with mast cells, giving the skin a thickened and doughy texture with a yellow discoloration.

Symptoms from cutaneous mastocytosis result from mast cell release of proinflammatory mediators such as histamine and prostaglandins. Local release produces edema, surrounding erythema, and even the formation of vesicles or bullae that may mimic cutaneous herpes or a bullous disorder of childhood. Systemic release can manifest as a range of symptoms, including flushing, colicky abdominal pain, nausea, diarrhea, hypotension, and rarely wheezing and respiratory distress. Beyond recognizing its typical appearance, the diagnosis of mastocytosis can be made by eliciting a positive Darier's sign. The Darier's sign involves stroking a solitary lesion to trigger mast cell degranulation, leading to the appearance of edema, erythema, and

Mastocytoma

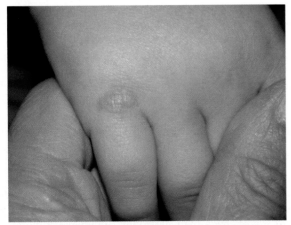

Flesh colored mastocytoma on dorsum of the hand.

Darier's sign

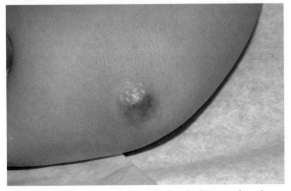

Stroking a mastocytoma leads to localized edema and erythema.

Figure 124-3 *Mastocytosis.*

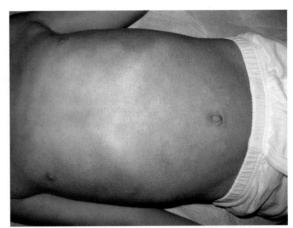

Widespread tan patches illustrating post-inflammatory changes in a patient with eczema.

Figure 124-4 *Postinflammatory hyperpigmentation.*

occasionally vesiculation at the site (see Figure 124-3). The mainstay of management of children with mastocytosis involves avoidance of the triggers of mast cell degranulation, including physical triggers (friction, pressure, or extremes in temperature), certain medications (aspirin, nonsteroidal antiinflammatory drugs [NSAID], opiates, amphotericin, topical polymyxin B), systemic anesthetics (pancuronium, decamethonium), alcohol, and iodine contrast media. Symptoms can be controlled with nonsedating histamine type 1 antagonists such as loratadine or cetirizine, and only rarely is an epinephrine pen needed for a history of severe reactions.

Acanthosis Nigricans

Acanthosis nigricans presents as dark brown, velvety thickening of skin folds classically involving the axilla and the posterior and lateral neck folds. Verrucous hyperpigmented thickening may also involve the knuckles, flexor regions of the elbows and knees, and the perineum. Acanthosis nigricans is strongly associated with obesity and insulin resistance and should raise the suspicion for type II diabetes and polycystic ovarian syndrome. Excess circulating insulin is believed to bind to insulin and insulinlike growth factor receptors on keratinocytes and dermal fibroblasts,

leading to the hyperkeratosis seen histologically in acanthosis. In large sample studies, approximately 90% of patients with type II diabetes have acanthosis nigricans on examination. Furthermore, the presence of acanthosis nigricans in obese individuals with fairer complexion is essentially predictive of insulin resistance. All obese individuals with acanthosis nigricans should be evaluated for underlying insulin resistance.

Dermal Melanosis

Dermal melanosis, more commonly known as a mongolian spot, is one of the most common hyperpigmented lesions seen in the newborn period. They are poorly circumscribed patches that are slate-gray to blue-green in color. The prevalence of mongolian spots varies greatly by ethnicity, with up to 90% of black infants, 80% of Asian infants, and 10% of white infants affected. These lesions are typically found on the buttocks or lumbar sacral area or less commonly on the back, flanks, shoulder, or lower extremities and generally fade by 2 years of age. Mongolian spots are benign in nature; however, the presence of extensive atypical mongolian spots has very rarely been associated with Hunter's syndrome or GM1 gangliosidosis.

Postinflammatory Hyperpigmentation

Postinflammatory hyperpigmentation is commonly seen throughout childhood. Local inflammatory mediators stimulate melanin production by melanocytes, leaving areas of hyperpigmentation in a distribution pattern consistent with the prior inflammatory insult (Figure 124-4). Common causes in childhood include eczematous eruptions, acne, mechanical trauma, and skin infections. Individuals with darker complexions are most often affected. Management involves treating any ongoing inflammation, particularly important in cases of atopic dermatitis and acne vulgaris, and appropriate sunscreen to avoid further hyperpigmentation, and the pigmentation will fade over months to years.

LINEAR CIRCUMSCRIBED HYPERPIGMENTED LESIONS

In the evaluation of a child with linear hyperpigmentation, the clinician should note whether the pattern of hypermelanosis follows the lines of Blaschko. The lines of Blaschko represent embryologic lines of ectodermal development that have a V or "fountain" shape on the back, an S or "whorl" pattern on the flanks, and a linear pattern on the extremities.

Incontinentia Pigmenti

The most important diagnosis to consider in cases of hyper-pigmentation following the lines of Blaschko is incontinentia pigmenti (IP; Bloch-Sulzberger syndrome). IP is an X-linked dominant disorder affecting largely girls because boys typically die in utero, and has been attributed to a mutation in nuclear factor-κB essential modulator (NEMO). The cutaneous component of the syndrome has four distinct phases: vesicular, verrucous, hyperpigmented, and hypopigmented. The vesicular phase is noted in the first 2 weeks of life with vesicles on an inflammatory base following a linear pattern on the trunk and extremities (Figure 124-5). With any blistering in the neonatal period, herpetic or bacterial infections should always be considered. In the vesicular stage, leukocytosis and peripheral eosinophilia are typically present. The vesicular phase typically fades by 4 months and is followed by the eruption of verrucous papules and plaques in a linear distribution on the extremities that fade by 6 months of age. The third stage, noted between 12 and 26 weeks and lasting up until young adulthood, is characterized by whorls of hyperpigmentation on the torso and extremities following the lines of Blaschko, which do not occur in the same areas affected in stages 1 and 2 (see Figure 124-5). Stage IV develops in adulthood and involves streaks of hypopigmentation and alopecia most commonly affecting the extremities. The importance of making of a diagnosis of IP is that this syndrome is associated with multiple noncutaneous findings involving the following: teeth (absence of teeth, conical or peg-shaped teeth), nails (nail dystrophy, subungual tumors), hair (alopecia), eyes (strabismus, optic atrophy, retinal neovascularization, placing infants at risk for retinal detachment), and the central nervous system (infantile spasms and seizures, spastic paralysis, and mental retardation). Children with IP should be followed by a pediatric ophthalmologist or retinal specialist, especially during the first year of life, and be monitored for seizures.

DIFFUSE HYPERPIGMENTATION

Generalized hyperpigmentation may indicate an underlying endocrinopathy or be a side effect of certain medications. Common disorders leading to hyperpigmentation are Addison's disease, hyperthyroidism, Cushing's disease, acromegaly, hemochromatosis, and chronic renal and hepatic disease. In the case of Addison's disease, Cushing's disease, and acromegaly, an increased production of ACTH and its byproduct melanotropin-stimulating syndrome stimulates melanocytes to produce melanin. Hyperpigmentation is seen most notably in sun-exposed areas, skin creases on the palms and soles, and mucous membranes. Medications known to cause variable degrees of hyperpigmentation include NSAIDs, minocycline, antimalarials, amiodarone, psychotropic drugs (phenothiazine, imipramine), clofazimine, azidothymidine, chemotherapeutics (5-fluorouracil, bleomycin, cyclophosphamide, daunorubicin, doxorubicin), and heavy metals (gold, silver, bismuth, mercury). The hyperpigmentation associated with medications will fade with discontinuation but is often a process that takes months to years.

Incontinentia Pigmenti Stage 1

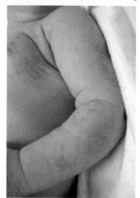

Highlighting the linear vesicles with erythematous base.

Incontinentia Pigmenti Stage 3

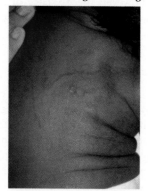

Hyperpigmentation in whorled pattern.

Figure 124-5 *Incontentia pigmenti.*

SUGGESTED READINGS

Bauer AJ, Statakis CA: The lentiginoses: cutaneous markers of systemic disease and a window to new aspects of tumourigenesis, *J Med Genet* 42:801-810, 2005.

Berlin AL, Paller AS, Chan LS: Incontinentia pigmenti: a review and update on the molecular basis of pathophysiology, *J Am Acad Dermatol* 47:169-187, 2002.

Boyd KP, Korf BR, Theos A: Neurofibromatosis type 1, *J Am Acad Dermatol* 61:1-14, 2009.

Briley LD, Phillips CM: Cutaneous mastocytosis: a review focusing on the pediatric population, *Clin Pediatr (Phila)* 47:757-761, 2008.

Lacz NL, Vafaie J, Kihiczak NI, et al: Postinflammatory hyperpigmentation: a common but troubling condition, *Int J Dermatol* 43:362-365, 2004.

Sinha S, Shwartz RA: Juvenile acanthosis nigricans, *J Am Acad Dermatol* 57:502-508, 2007.

Spurlock G, Bennett E, Chuzhanova N, et al: *SPRED1* mutations (Legius syndrome): another clinically useful genotype for dissecting the neurofibromatosis type 1 phenotype, *J Med Genet* 46:431-437, 2009.

Acne

Erin Pete Devon

125

*A*cne vulgaris is the most common skin condition of teenagers, affecting up to 85% of adolescents and frequently continuing into adulthood. Increases in circulating hormones during puberty stimulate acne formation, which often occurs at a time of emotional insecurity. In addition to physical scarring, patients with severe acne can experience significant psychological morbidity. Pediatricians are often the first health care providers to care for patients with acne and have the opportunity to make a positive impact.

ETIOLOGY AND PATHOGENESIS

An appreciation of the pathogenesis of acne facilitates a better understanding of targeted treatments. Acne develops in the pilosebaceous unit (Figure 125-1). There are four primary factors involved: abnormal keratinization, increased sebum production, proliferation of *Propionibacterium acnes* bacteria, and inflammation. With the onset of adrenarche, there is an increase in androgen production and a resultant increase in sebum secretion. Each sebaceous gland has a different threshold of androgen sensitivity, effecting an individually unique response to puberty. Simultaneously, there is increased proliferation of keratinocytes and decreased desquamation. The accumulation of sebum and keratinocytes leads to the formation of the microcomedo, the precursor to acne lesions. *P. acnes*, a normal skin inhabitant, thrives in this lipid-rich environment. The organisms release chemotactic factors, setting up an inflammatory response. Depending on the contribution of each primary factor, a microcomedo can evolve into a closed comedo (whitehead), open comedo (blackhead) (Figure 125-2), or an inflammatory pustule, papule, or nodule if the sebum, keratin, and microorganisms, with the accumulation of inflammatory cells, rupture into the dermis.

Extrinsic factors can exacerbate acne. Although many patients erroneously believe that acne is caused by not keeping the skin clean, cleansing the face helps clear the skin of surface lipids but does not help prevent acne. Furthermore, aggressive cleansing with washcloths or loofahs as well as manipulation and squeezing of lesions can aggravate them by provoking an inflammatory response and can also lead to scarring. Additionally, cosmetics, hair preparations, and occlusive clothing can all worsen facial and body acne. Stress can also lead to an increase in androgenic hormones and thus exacerbate acne.

There is little evidence to show that particular foods worsen acne. One study has shown an increased self-reported rate of acne during adolescence with consumption of milk. However, this relationship was thought to be secondary to acnegenic hormones and bioactive molecules in milk. Further study is needed in this area to prove or disprove any possible association.

Climate also seems to affect acne, with summer attenuating symptoms, yet this correlation is confounded by the fact that summertime generally harbors less stress, which has been associated with acne flares.

CLINICAL PRESENTATION

Acne is a disease that can be seen in the first year of life, early childhood, the prepubertal period, and puberty. Neonatal cephalic pustulosis, formerly referred to as neonatal acne, appears in the first 3 months after birth and usually resolves in 1 to 3 months. In neonates, it is extremely important to exclude other bacterial, viral, or fungal causes, but a physician should also consider milia, erythema toxicum neonatorum, transient neonatal pustulosis, and sebaceous gland hyperplasia. Infantile or toddler acne is less common and usually presents between 3 and 6 months of life and can last 1 to 2 years. This is not typically associated with precocious puberty or a hormonal imbalance but needs to be considered in conjunction with a thorough history and physical examination. See Table 125-1 for a comparison of acne seen in neonates and toddlers. Acne can present in any location where there are sebaceous glands. In addition to the face, it is frequently found on the neck, upper chest, shoulders, and back (see Figure 125-2). There are multiple classification systems used to talk about acne, but a description of the lesions and their locations is most helpful. The resolution of acne may leave postinflammatory changes that usually resolve themselves but may take weeks to months, especially in darker pigmented patients. Moderate and severe acne can leave permanent scars.

The diagnosis of acne is relatively straightforward. Typical acne includes comedones, papules, pustules, and nodules in the distribution of the face, upper back, and chest. Acne that begins at an abnormal age, particularly severe acne, acne accompanied by an abnormal growth history or virilization, or acne that is recalcitrant to treatment, should be further evaluated. The physician may want to consider an underlying disorder, such as premature adrenarche, precocious puberty, Cushing's syndrome, congenital adrenal hyperplasia, and gonadal or adrenal tumors, or an alternative diagnosis if the lesions are not typical (Box 125-1). Perioral dermatitis and facial angiofibromas are shown in Figure 125-3.

MANAGEMENT

The initial evaluation of a patient with acne begins with a complete history. Most patients have no relevant history of systemic disease, but particular attention must be paid to a history or physical examination that is consistent with signs of endocrine dysfunction in patients with an atypical age of presentation and lesion morphology. Hyperandrogenism can cause abnormal weight gain, menstrual irregularities, hirsutism, and signs of insulin resistance such as acanthosis nigricans. Elevated cortisol levels can cause hypertension, striae, or a buffalo hump. Signs of virilization such as decreased breast size, alopecia, and clitoromegaly can be attributable to an underlying adrenal or ovarian tumor. In addition, acne-associated spondyloarthropathies have been associated with severe acne, including acne fulminans,

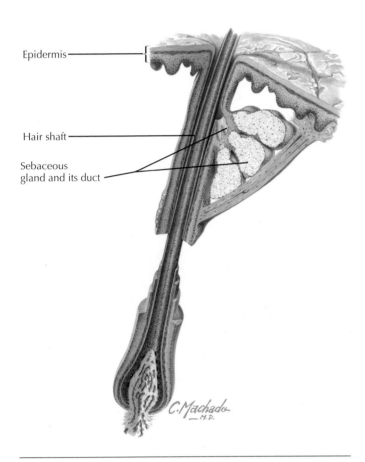

Figure 125-1 *Pilosebaceous unit.*

PAPA (pyogenic arthritis, pyoderma gangrenosum, and acne), and SAPHO (synovitis, acne, pustulosis, hyperostosis, osteomyelitis) syndrome. A complete medication history must also be taken. The physical examination should focus on the type and location of the lesions, postinflammatory changes, and scarring. In cases with red flags for an underlying systemic disease, laboratory evaluation may include measuring levels of free and total testosterone, DHEA-S (dehydroepiandrosterone sulfate), follicle-stimulating hormone, luteinizing hormone, 17 α-hydroxyprogesterone, and prolactin. Some experts also recommend an adrenocorticotropic hormone (ACTH) stimulation test. Bone age is a useful radiologic study for hyperandrogenism. A referral to an endocrinologist is also appropriate.

Treatment of acne should begin with good skin hygiene. Patients should be instructed to use nonirritating, noncomedogenic cleansers, which should be applied gently without scrubbing or using any harsh washing materials, as well as noncomedogenic moisturizers and sunscreen. Patients should be counseled that acne takes weeks to clear, and close follow-up should be arranged to assess the efficacy of treatment, side effects, and barriers to compliance. Often, teenagers will give up too early on therapy that would have been successful if they had been counseled that it will take weeks for full effect.

In general, when choosing a topical treatment, the vehicle should complement the patient's skin type and be realistic for its distribution of placement. For example, whereas gels may provide some drying action, creams are less likely to dry but more likely to leave a white film in dark-skinned patients.

See Figure 125-4 for an acne treatment algorithm for the initial management strategies for the treatment of acne.

Topical Retinoids

Topical retinoids are considered the foundation of maintenance and treatment therapy of both comedonal and inflammatory acne. They help regulate keratinocyte desquamation and have a direct antiinflammatory effect, preventing microcomedone formation and allowing greater access for topical antibiotic treatment, if being used.

This treatment should be used at the onset of therapy and applied to all affected areas. Topical retinoids can cause irritation, erythema, burning, and pruritus, so it is recommended to start with reduced frequency of application for improved compliance. A pea-sized amount allocated into four equal parts is sufficient to cover the entire face.

Caution should be taken when adding multiple therapies at the same time because they can all be drying. It is generally better to start with a lower strength formulation and increase it as needed. Cream formulations of retinoids are less potent but also less irritating than their gel counterparts. See Table 125-2 for examples of topical retinoids available in the United States.

Topical Benzoyl Peroxide

The key to acne treatment is targeting the different etiologies in the pathogenesis of acne development. Multiple studies have shown that patients treated with a combination of therapies have better results than those treated with monotherapy.

Benzoyl peroxide is a well-known topical bactericidal antimicrobial. It has excellent efficacy on its own and is the mainstay of most over-the-counter acne therapies. It is an excellent first-line medication and is available as a cleanser, gel, cream, and lotions in concentrations ranging from 2.5% to 10%. Another benefit of benzoyl peroxide is that resistance to *P. acnes* is not seen, and it decreases the development of antibiotic resistance when used concomitantly with topical antibiotics. Skin irritation is the most common side effect, which improves with usage. As with topical retinoid therapy, a common practice to decrease the irritation is to start use either every other day and slowly build up or short contact therapy for 1 hour at a time and then slowly increase the length of therapy. Patients should be advised that benzoyl peroxide can bleach materials and fabrics it touches.

Topical Antibiotics and Combination Products

Topical antibiotics should be used for mild inflammatory acne. This treatment works by decreasing the residing *P. acnes* and its resultant proinflammatory cytokines that transform comedones into papules, pustules, and nodules, as well as possessing antiinflammatory effects. Available topical antibiotics are erythromycin (solution, gel, ointment) and clindamycin (solution, gel, lotion). These products are generally well tolerated, but their drawback is the rapid development of *P. acne* resistance. The resistance can be decreased when used together with benzoyl

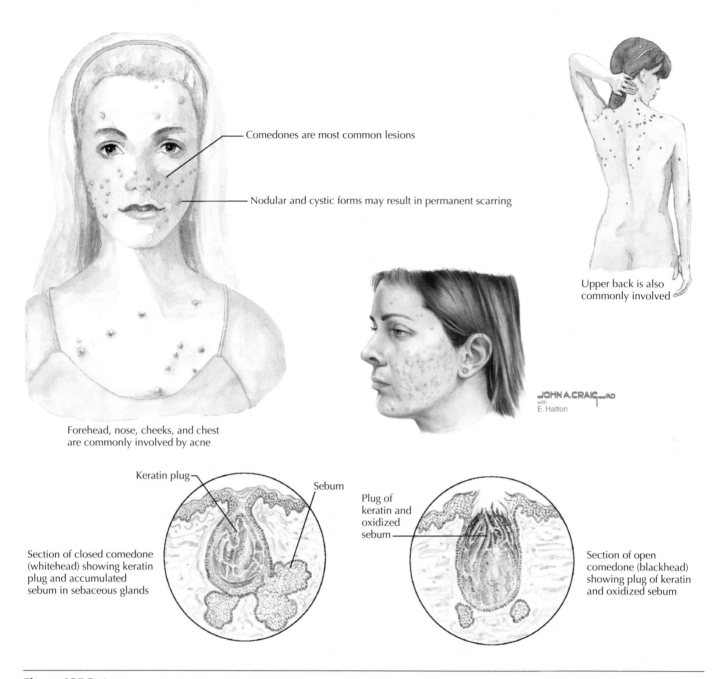

Comedones are most common lesions

Nodular and cystic forms may result in permanent scarring

Upper back is also commonly involved

JOHN A. CRAIG AD
with
E. Hatton

Forehead, nose, cheeks, and chest are commonly involved by acne

Keratin plug

Sebum

Plug of keratin and oxidized sebum

Section of closed comedone (whitehead) showing keratin plug and accumulated sebum in sebaceous glands

Section of open comedone (blackhead) showing plug of keratin and oxidized sebum

Figure 125-2 *Acne.*

Table 125-1 Acne in Neonates and Early Childhood

	Causes	Clinical Appearance	Expected Course
Neonatal cephalic pustulosis	Stimulation of sebaceous glands by maternal hormones Inflammatory reaction to the colonization of *Malassezia* spp.	Papules and pustules to the forehead, cheeks, chin, chest, and back	Nonscarring and self-limited No treatment needed but may be treated with topical antifungal for faster resolution
Toddler acne or aseptic facial granulomas	Hyperplasia of sebaceous glands secondary to androgenic stimulation	Comedones, papules, pustules, nodules Boys are more commonly affected	Risk of scarring with inflammatory lesions Treatment with topical therapy or systemic therapy as needed Has been associated with earlier and more severe adolescent acne

Box 125-1 Differential Diagnosis of Acne Vulgaris

- Keratosis pilaris
- Perioral dermatitis
- Facial angiofibromas
- Miliaria
- Drug history (i.e., corticosteroid-induced acne)
- Folliculitis
- Verruca vulgaris
- Pseudofolliculitis barbae

Table 125-2 Topical Retinoids

Retinoids	Comments	Side Effects
Tretinoin (available in cream, gel, solution, microsphere gel)	Tretinoin is affected by light and degrades to a greater extent when used together with benzoyl peroxide.	Irritation, erythema, burning, pruritus
Adapalene (available in gel or cream)	Well tolerated at its lowest concentration but can be less effective. May be used concomitantly with benzoyl peroxide	
Tazarotene (available in gel or cream)	More irritating but effective at comedolysis. Tazarotene is contraindicated during pregnancy.	

peroxide. Topical combination products that contain benzoyl peroxide along with erythromycin or clindamycin may be more effective but are more expensive.

Systemic Antibiotics and Other Systemic Therapies

Oral antibiotics should be used for the treatment of moderate to severe acne or widespread involvement of the trunk. Although

maintaining retinoid therapy is important for the prevention of acne, as already mentioned, treatment with oral antibiotics should be discontinued after a taper with the resolution of inflammatory lesions (Table 125-3).

Oral contraceptives containing estrogen, spironolactone, an androgen antagonist, and isotretinoin are therapies for patients

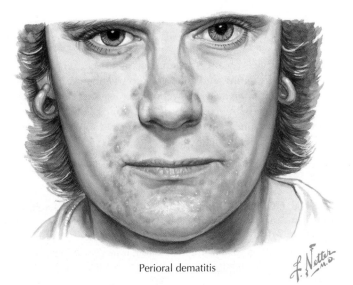

Perioral dematitis

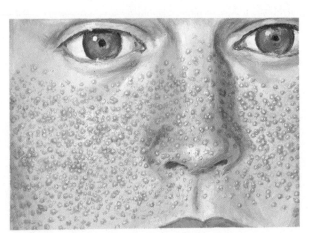

Facial angiofibromas

Figure 125-3 *Perioral dermatitis and facial angiofibromas.*

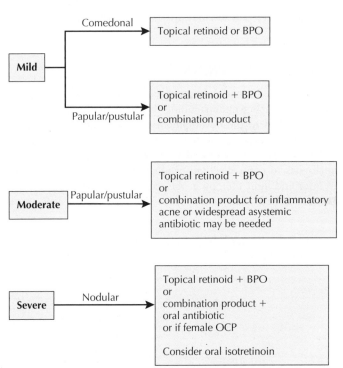

BPO = benzoyl peroxide, OCP = oral contraceptive
Adapted from Yan AC, Treat JR, *Beyond First-Line Treatment: Mangement Strategies for Maintaining Acne Improvement and Compliance.* Cutis 82; 18-25, 2008.

Figure 125-4 *Acne treatment algorithm.*

Table 125-3 Systemic Therapies for Acne

Medication	Comments	Some Notable Side Effects
Erythromycin	Useful in younger patients who have contraindications to tetracycline use	GI upset, drug interactions
Tetracycline	Avoid in children younger than 8 years of age and pregnant women because of permanent discoloration of the teeth and abnormal skeletal development Should not be taken with calcium-based foods or medications because they will decrease absorption	GI upset, photosensitivity, tooth discoloration
Doxycycline		Phototoxicity, GI upset
Minocycline		Pseudotumor cerebri, vertigo, SLE-like reaction, systemic hypersensitivity and Stevens-Johnson syndrome, and autoimmune hepatitis
Oral contraceptives containing estrogen	Ortho Tri-Cyclen, Estrostep, and Yaz are approved by the FDA for acne	Increased risk of thromboembolism, weight changes, mood changes
Spironolactone		Menstrual irregularities
Isotretinoin	Possible correlation with isotretinoin and depression has been made; the FDA has implemented iPLEDGE, a program that monitors all patients who are prescribed isotretinoin	Teratogenicity, hypertriglyceridemia, leukopenia, and elevated liver function test results; more commonly, patients develop dry skin, eyes, and mucosa

FDA, Food and Drug Administration; GI, gastrointestinal SLE, systemic lupus erythematous.

who have severe acne and have not responded to first-line therapy. Of note, certain forms of contraception, such as Depo-Provera shots, have been shown to worsen acne. Isotretinoin, a vitamin A derivative, is best suited for nodulocystic acne. It is extremely successful and may provide more long-lasting benefits than other acne therapies.

FUTURE DIRECTIONS

Determining the pathophysiology of acne has led to targeted therapies. Further understanding the molecular mechanisms of acne can lead to the development of new treatments, such as medication targeting toll-like receptors on the membranes of inflammatory cells, activated by *P. acnes*, and using vitamin D analogues to control sebum production. Additionally, the role of laser and light therapy in the treatment of acne is currently being studied. However, successful application of these technologies relies on a therapeutic doctor-patient relationship, individualized therapy, and adherence to treatment. Promoting adherence with medication reminders via text messages, self-monitoring with diaries, support groups, and telephone follow-up is another aspect being investigated to contribute to the successful management of acne.

SUGGESTED READINGS

Thiboutot D, Gollnick H, Bettoli V, et al: New insights into the management of acne: an update from the Global Alliance to Improve Outcomes in Acne group, *J Am Acad Dermatol* 60(5 suppl):S1-S50, 2009.

Yan AC, Treat JR: Beyond first-line treatment: management strategies for maintaining acne improvement and compliance, *Cutis* 82(2 suppl 1):18-25, 2008.

Zaenglein AL: Expert recommendations for acne management, *Pediatrics* 118:1188-1199, 2006.

Nevi

Leslie Castelo-Soccio and James R. Treat

126

ETIOLOGY AND PATHOGENESIS

Common moles, or melanocytic nevi, are benign proliferations of melanocytes called nevus cells. They can appear tan, light brown, brown, or black in color. Nevi can be congenital or acquired. They can be typical or atypical (dysplastic). There are also other varieties of nevi such as blue nevi, halo nevi, and Spitz nevi that have some special clinical and histologic features that distinguish them from common moles.

Melanocytic nevi are extremely common in children, with almost 100% of white children developing at least one nevus by early childhood. Although most nevi are benign, trying to differentiate nevi from melanoma or nevi that have developed melanoma within them can be challenging. Melanoma is uncommon in children, with an incidence of one per million children per year. However, there has been an increase in their incidence. The Surveillance, Epidemiology and End Results (SEER) database confirms an increased incidence of approximately 2.9% per year in children from 1973 to 2001. In this database analysis, cutaneous melanoma was more common in girls (55%) and in patients older than 10 years of age (90.5%). Younger children with melanoma were more likely to be nonwhite and male. They typically presented with a primary tumor of the head and neck with regional or distant metastases. It is important to recognize and appropriately manage various types of nevi and to reduce the risk of malignant transformation.

CLINICAL MANIFESTATION AND MANAGEMENT

Common Acquired Melanocytic Nevi

Common nevi typically begin to develop in early childhood, and new nevi may continue to arise into the third decade (Figure 126-1). These lesions have a variety of presentations depending on where the nests of nevus cells reside, and they are named accordingly. Those with nevus cells at the dermal-epidermal junction are known as junctional nevi, and those with nevus cells in the dermis are intradermal nevi. Those with cells in both compartments are called compound. The shapes and sizes vary, but most are smaller than 6 mm in size. They are more common in sun-exposed areas, where increased sun exposure leads to more moles in these areas. In general, children with lighter pigmented skin have more nevi than those with darkly pigmented skin. Children with families with increased nevi also have more moles, suggesting a genetic component to the total number of lifetime moles acquired. Studies in first-degree relatives and twins suggest that genetic factors have a significant impact on the number of moles independent of skin color or sun exposure.

The distribution of nevi can vary with skin pigmentation. Those with darker pigment have more nevi on acral locations, including the palms, soles, and nail beds. Nevi in acral sites are usually dark in color and have streaks of pigment that follow the dermatoglyphs.

Dysplastic or Atypical Nevi

These are atypical nevi that have some asymmetry, size larger than 6 mm, variable color, and irregular borders (Figure 126-2). They frequently contain both a macular and papular component and variegated color (pink, brown, tan). They show architectural disorder histologically and are categorized by many pathologists as mildly, moderately, or severely atypical. Atypical moles typically begin to develop around puberty. The tendency to develop these nevi is genetic, with some families having multiple atypical nevi but no family history of melanoma but other families having both an increased risk of atypical moles and melanoma (familial atypical mole and melanoma syndrome [FAMM]).

Nevi that change in size, shape, color, or surface (bleeding, crusting, ulceration, thickening) or show signs of inflammation deserve evaluation and consideration for biopsy. Additionally, pain, itch, or tenderness also suggest that the nevus should be evaluated. With this said, however, symmetrical enlargement can be a normal finding in younger patients because the nevus grows with the patient. Uniform darkening after sun exposure can also occur. Chronic rubbing can also make nevi change color. Acquired nevi should be excised if they show signs of malignant transformation. They can also be removed surgically if they are in a location that is not practical for observation or if they are persistently irritated because of location such as at the waistline or neckline. All other nevi can be serially followed for change by skin examination, photography, or both.

When children have multiple moles, it is helpful to look at the clinical appearance of all of the nevi. Nevi are often very similar. This has been called the "signature" of the nevi and again highlights that nevi are programmed by genetics. A nevus that looks different from this signature should be looked at with suspicion. A new nevus is usually not concerning in a child or adolescent if it fits the signature. It is critical to perform a complete skin examination, including the scalp. Some evidence suggests that children who develop scalp nevi are at increased risk for acquiring a large number of nevi. Prophylactic removal of all nevi is not recommended because many melanomas develop de novo not from a preexisting nevus, and there is no evidence that removing all nevi decreases the risk of melanoma.

Congenital Nevi

Congenital melanocytic nevi (CMN) are characterized by being present at birth or within a few months of birth. Rarely, they do not become visible until up to 2 years of age. Congenital nevi are divided into giant (>20 cm), medium (1.5-2 0cm), and small (<1.5 cm). The colors of CMNs are variable with a range from tan to black. CMNs change over time. At birth and during early infancy, they may appear more uniform in color and flat. With

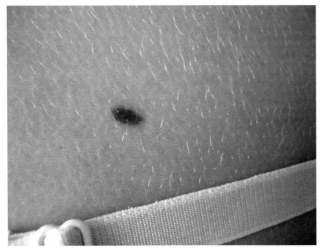

Common nevus on the trunk of a 10-year-old child.

Figure 126-1 *Common nevus.*

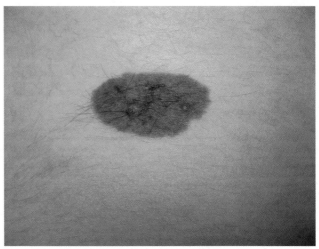

An intermediate sized nevus with terminal hairs.

Figure 126-3 *Medium-sized congenital nevus.*

time, they can become elevated and developed variegated pigmentation and a rough surface. Nodules and papules can develop within the lesion, and although most of these are benign, they need to be evaluated for malignant transformation. Over time, they can also develop dark terminal hairs (Figure 126-3).

Giant congenital nevi show the highest risk for neurocutaneous melanosis (melanocytes in the central nervous system [CNS]) and melanoma. The lifetime risk of melanoma in giant congenital nevi is 5% to 10%, but the peak risk is before puberty. This is in contrast to smaller congenital nevi, in which the risk for developing melanoma is highest after puberty. Neurocutaneous melanoma (NCM) occurs more commonly in patients with posterior axial giant congenital nevi and more than 20 satellite lesions. NCM is best detected by magnetic resonance imaging (MRI). There is some debate about screening MRIs to look for NCM because most patients with NCM are asymptomatic. If screening MRI is to occur, there is some evidence to suggest it should occur before the brain has myelinized (age 4 to 6 months).

It is thought that myelin protein can obscure subtle deposits of melanocytes. Patients with lumbosacral lesions should have MRI to look for tethered cord or other abnormalities of the spine. NCM has been divided into symptomatic and asymptomatic forms. The prognosis for symptomatic NCM is poor even when patients do not develop melanoma. Neurologic manifestations typically occur before the age of 2 years but can present into the second and third decades of life. The clinical signs of NCM are most often related to the space-occupying effects of growing melanocytes in the CNS. These include but are not limited to headaches, vomiting, generalized seizures, cranial nerve palsies, and developmental delay. Structural CNS anomalies such as Dandy-Walker malformations have also been reported in patients with symptomatic NCM. NCM without symptoms is more common. It is still unclear whether these patients are at an increased lifetime risk of CNS melanoma or future neurologic symptoms.

Management of giant CMNs is difficult. Surgical excision (typically in stages and sometimes only partial) does decrease the incidence of melanoma. Prophylactic excisions should occur between 6 and 9 months of age because the risk of melanoma is high in infancy, but the anesthesia risk is lower after 6 months of age. However, it should be noted that even total resection does not eliminate the risk of melanoma because it is impossible to excise all nevus cells because these nevus cells often track deep, and there may be other sites in CNS. Additionally, many giant CMNs are not operable. There must always be a risk:benefit analysis before surgery. The low incidence of melanoma overall may be a reason to follow patients clinically rather than perform large surgeries that can have cosmetic and long-term consequences (including other cancers such as squamous cell carcinoma occurring in the scar). Treatment decisions are tailored for each patient. All CMN patients and their parents need proper instruction in self-skin examinations, which should be performed each month. They need education about atypical changes they should be looking for in the lesions, including changes in size, shape, or color as well as development of papules, nodules, bleeding, or ulceration.

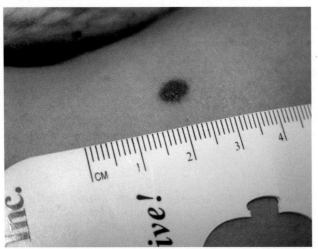

Slightly atypical nevus on the arm of a child.

Figure 126-2 *Dysplastic nevus.*

Cutaneous photography can be helpful to follow lesions. Physical examinations should be scheduled regularly with total skin exams, including palpation of the nevus and any scars, examination of lymph nodes, and a complete review of systems. Biopsy of suspicious lesions should not be delayed.

The management of small and medium melanocytic nevi is controversial. The lifetime risk of developing melanoma is somewhere between 0% and 5%, and it is rare to undergo malignant transformation in childhood. Lesions can be followed and surgically removed in later childhood when the child can participate in the decision. The risk for melanoma increases in puberty. If it is decided not to remove the lesion, serial examinations and photographs should be used for evaluation. Surgery should be considered sooner if it is burdensome to follow the lesion for the patient and family or anxiety is high. If a change is noted, the lesion should be biopsied. Patients and their families should be aware of CMN support groups such as Nevus Network (www.nevusnetwork.org).

Special Nevi

NEVUS SPILUS OR SPECKLED LENTIGINOUS NEVUS

Nevus spilus is a speckled nevus that typically occurs at birth or during early infancy. They present as lightly colored tan patches at birth commonly on the trunk. They later develop darker macules, papules, and hyperpigmentation within this tan background. The prevalence depends on age, with 0.2% reported for newborns and 2.3% for adults. This is likely because they can be mistaken for café-au-lait macules early. It is believed that these nevi may be a variant of CMN. They have a similar risk for melanoma as similarly sized CMN and should be followed clinically for change by inspection and palpation.

BLUE NEVUS

These are blue papules or nodules that typically begin in adolescence and grow slowly (Figure 126-4). They are composed of dermal melanocytes and melanophages, and the depth of the melanocytes in the dermis accounts for their blue color. There are three variants: common, cellular, and epitheloid. The common type is usually solitary on the dorsal hands and feet and occasionally the face. The cellular type has a predilection for the buttock and sacral region and occasionally is present at birth. Epithelioid blue nevi can be numerous and can be seen in Carney's complex (a disorder of myxomas, lentigines, endocrine abnormalities or neoplasms, and schwannomas). Melanomas can rarely arise in blue nevi. Clinically, the dark blue color may resemble a nodular melanoma. Usually, the clinical history of slow growth is what distinguishes the two. Small blue nevi can be followed clinically. Those in difficult locations to follow such as the scalp or sacrococcygeal area can be surgically removed.

SPITZ NEVI

Spitz nevi are acquired nevi that are usually benign but have some overlap features with melanoma histologically. They appear very rapidly anywhere on the body but with a predilection for the face or extremities and can be red, red-brown, and sometimes black in color. They are usually very symmetrical. Grouped or agminated Spitz nevi can occur. Clinically, they can look like common acquired nevi, pyogenic granulomas if red in color, or verruca vulgaris if the surface is more verrucous or melanomas. Suspected Spitz nevi should be biopsied and evaluated histopathologically to rule out atypical features. There is a lot of debate about what margins to take around a Spitz nevus. Atypical Spitz nevi and those that cannot be distinguished from a melanoma are treated like melanomas of the same depth and characteristics.

HALO NEVI

These are lesions that are characterized by a central pigmented nevus surrounded by an area of depigmentation (Figure 126-5). These occur most commonly in adolescents on the back. They occur in 5% of white children 6 to 15 years of age. The central

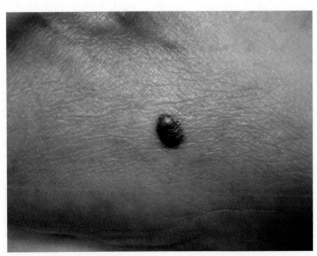

Blue nevus on dorsal foot of adolescent.

Figure 126-4 *Blue nevus.*

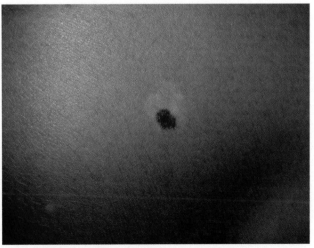

Halo nevus on the trunk of a child.

Figure 126-5 *Halo nevus.*

area may darken but more commonly lightens or regresses over time. There are many lymphocytes surrounding the melanocytes on histology, suggesting an immunologic response to the nevus cells. Halo nevi may herald the onset of vitiligo. Regressing melanoma may also have an associated leukoderma, but typically it is not a symmetrical process as in the halo nevus. Full examination is indicated to rule out a concurrent melanoma. The decision to biopsy the central nevus is based on the same criteria as for other acquired nevi.

SUGGESTED READINGS

Bolognia JL: Too many moles, *Arch Dermatol* 142:508, 2006.

DeDavid M, Orlow S, Provost N, et al: Neurocutaneous melanosis: clinical features of large congenital melanocytic nevi in patients with manifest central nervous system melanosis, *J Am Acad Dermatol* 35:529-538, 1996.

Dennis LK, Vanbeek MJ, Beane Freeman LE, et al: Sunburns and the risk of cutaneous melanoma: does age matter? A comprehensive meta-analysis, *Ann Epidemiol* 18(8):614-627, 2008.

Frieden I, William M, Barkovich A: Giant congenital melanocytic nevi: brain magnetic resonance findings in neurologically asymptomatic children, *J Am Acad Dermatol* 31:423-429, 1994.

Friedman RJ, Farber MJ, Warycha MA, et al: The "dysplastic" nevus, *Clin Dermatol* 27(1):103-115, 2009.

Gelbarb SN, Tripp JM, Marghoob AA: Management of Spitz nevi: a survey of dermatologists in the United States, *J Am Acad Dermatol* 47:224-230, 2002.

Goodson AG, Grossman D: Strategies for early melanoma detection: approaches to the patient with nevi, *J Am Acad Dermatol* 60(5):719-735, 2009.

Huynh PM, Grant-Kels JM, Grin CM: Childhood melanoma: update and treatment, *Int J Dermatol* 44:715-723, 2005.

Marghoob AA, Borrego JP, Halpern AC: Congenital melanocytic nevi: treatment modalities and management options, *Semin Cutan Med Surg* 26:231-240, 2007.

Mateus C, Palangie A, Franck N, et al: Heterogeneity of skin manifestations in patients with Carney complex, *J Am Acad Dermatol* 59(5):801-810, 2008.

Morgan CJ, Nyak N, Cooper A: Multiple Spitz naevi: a report of both variants with clinical and histopathological correlation, *Clin Exp Dermatol* 31:368-371, 2006.

Prok LD, Arbuckle HA: Nevi in children: a practical approach to evaluation, *Pediatr Ann* 36:39-45, 2007.

Schaffer JV: Pigmented lesions in children: when to worry, *Current Opin Pediatr* 19(4):430-440, 2007.

Schaffer JV, Orlow SJ, Lazova R, et al: Speckled lentiginous nevus: within the spectrum of congenital melanocytic nevi, *Arch Derm* 137:172-178, 2001.

Tripp JM, Kopf AW, Marghoob AA, et al: Management of dysplastic nevi: a survey of fellows of the American academy of dermatology, *J Am Acad Dermatol* 46:674-682, 2002.

Michael D. Gober and James R. Treat

*A*ppropriate nutritional intake is an important aspect in children's overall health. Although health care workers in developing countries are confronted daily with patients with various forms of nutritional deficiencies, these important health issues can also manifest in affluent countries with abundant food supplies. Infants and children require sufficient calories and nutrients for normal growth and development. Malnutrition in general is considered by the World Health Organization to be one of the most important risk factors for illness and premature death.

ETIOLOGY AND PATHOGENESIS

In the developing world, the most common form of malnutrition is protein-energy malnutrition caused by local food supply shortages or inappropriate use of foods not meant to replace infant formula. In developed countries, malnutrition is primarily related to chronic illness, malabsorption associated with gastrointestinal (GI) disease, or restrictive dietary habits. These conditions may be attributable to psychiatric or behavioral conditions such as anorexia nervosa, fad diets, inappropriate diet supplementation in the context of suspected food allergy, an impoverished living environment, or neglect or abuse. Recognition of the cutaneous findings associated with nutritional abnormalities is vital because these deficiencies may be easily corrected.

CLINICAL PRESENTATION

Protein-Energy Malnutrition

The majority of nutritional deficiency is associated with either poor dietary intake or GI malabsorption. Protein-energy malnutrition is divided into two major categories, marasmus and kwashiorkor. Marasmus is caused by insufficient total caloric intake and classically is seen in the context of food deprivation. Conversely, kwashiorkor is associated with inadequate protein intake in the setting of normal caloric intake. Indeed, kwashiorkor was initially described in children whose caloric intake was almost entirely derived from corn. Protein-losing enteropathies or diets consisting entirely of rice, milk because of concerns for milk intolerance are known causes of kwashiorkor in developed countries.

A child with marasmus is defined as having less than 60% of expected body weight for age in the absence of edema or hypoproteinemia. This form of malnutrition presents with loss of subcutaneous fat and muscle wasting, leading to an overall emaciated appearance. The skin is typically dry, thin, and wrinkled. Hyperpigmentation, fine scale, increased lanugo hair, nail fissures, and purpura are other cutaneous findings associated with marasmus.

Children with kwashiorkor also exhibit a lower body weight than expected for age, ranging from 60% to 80% of expected body weight. However, unlike in marasmus, these children also exhibit edema and hypoproteinemia stemming from insufficient dietary protein or the underlying medical condition leading to intestinal protein loss. Overall, the presence of mild hypoproteinemic edema in early disease gives the appearance of a well-fed, overweight child. However, recognition of the cutaneous findings help establish the diagnosis. Pigment alterations are the most common skin finding in patients with kwashiorkor, presenting as hypo- or hyperpigmentation after minor injury. In mild cases, superficial desquamation occurs that has the clinical appearance of enamel paint, which can progress in more severe cases to large areas of erosions, particularly on the extremities and buttocks, with an appearance similar to flaking paint. These areas are commonly secondarily infected with bacteria or colonized with *Candida* spp. Children also can present with skin atrophy, redness, and purpura. The hair is often dry, sparse, and lighter in color. Under conditions of repeated episodes of protein malnutrition followed by periods of adequate protein intake, the hair may have alternating light and dark bands, termed the flag sign, which correspond to the different episodes of protein nutritional status. Other important findings helpful in establishing the diagnosis of kwashiorkor include edema, irritability, anorexia, apathy, hepatomegaly from fatty infiltration of the liver, and failure to thrive.

Zinc Deficiency

Zinc is an element that is a required component of many enzymes involved in the synthesis and degradation of lipids, protein, and nucleic acid. Classic skin findings of zinc deficiency include erythematous and slightly eroded plaques involving the extremities, diaper area, and periorificial area. The facial involvement often involves the lower cheeks and chin but spares the skin above the upper lip, giving a "U" appearance. The rash can present with exudate, crust, vesicles, and bullae (Figure 127-1). Chronic zinc deficiency often manifests with lichenified plaques. *Candida* spp. and *Staphylococcus aureus* superinfections are common in this disorder. Other cutaneous findings of zinc deficiency include stomatitis, angular chelitis, blepharitis, nail-fold inflammation with possible nail dystrophy, and hair thinning with areas of complete alopecia. In addition to dermatitis, diarrhea is a commonly associated symptom. The severity is highly variable and does not correlate with the development of cutaneous findings. Children with zinc deficiency also characteristically are irritable, have problems eating and sleeping, and are growth impaired.

Acquired zinc deficiency is associated with poor dietary intake or underlying GI disease, leading to malabsorption. In addition to acquired zinc deficiency, an inherited cause of zinc deficiency has been identified. This disorder, termed *acrodermatitis enteropathica*, is caused by an autosomal recessive mutation in the zinc transporter gene *SLC39A4*. Because human breast milk (but not formula or cow's milk) contains zinc-binding proteins that aid in zinc absorption, these patients typically present

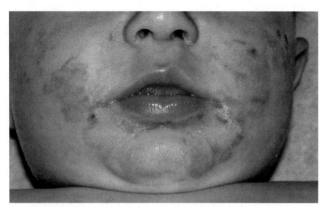

Clinical photograph of zinc deficiency. *Photograph courtesy of Albert Yan, MD.*

Figure 127-1 *Zinc deficiency.*

1 to 2 weeks after weaning from breast milk. Interestingly, various case reports of exclusively breastfed infants with zinc deficiency demonstrated decreased zinc levels in breast milk despite normal maternal serum zinc. These infants do not exhibit a defect with intestinal zinc absorption, classifying this disorder, termed *transient neonatal zinc deficiency*, as an acquired zinc deficiency unlike acrodermatitis enteropathica. Transient neonatal zinc deficiency has been linked with maternal mutations in the zinc transporter gene *SLC30A2*, which is responsible for transport of zinc into breast milk. Understanding the genetic cause of zinc deficiency is important because the levels of zinc supplementation for acquired zinc deficiency and acrodermatitis enteropathica differ, and zinc oversupplementation can potentially result in immune dysfunction. The diagnosis of other specific nutritional deficiencies, including essential fatty acid (EFA) deficiency and biotin deficiency, should be considered when suspecting zinc deficiency because of the similarity in cutaneous manifestations of these three disorders (see below).

Essential Fatty Acid Deficiency

The EFAs are long-chain polyunsaturated fatty acids that must be obtained through the diet. The clinically most important EFAs include linoleic acid and linolenic acid, which are components of the cell membrane and aid normal barrier function of the stratum corneum by contributing to lamellar granule formation. Furthermore, linoleic acid can be metabolized to arachidonic acid, an important molecule that can ultimately be converted into prostaglandins, leukotrienes, and thromboxane.

EFA deficiency is usually seen in the context of other deficiencies; however, children receiving parenteral nutrition without proper lipid supplementation can present with isolated EFA deficiency. In addition, children with fat malabsorption disorders such as biliary atresia, cystic fibrosis, or short bowel syndrome are at risk of developing EFA deficiency, particularly if they are supplemented primarily with medium-chain triglycerides. The cutaneous findings of EFA deficiency resemble those seen in zinc deficiency, including dry, scaling, erythematous skin that has a periorificial predilection. The hair often

becomes lighter in color or may be lost entirely. Children can also present with poor wound healing as well as growth problems and increased susceptibility to infections.

Biotin Deficiency

Biotin, which is also known as vitamin H or vitamin B7, is a water-soluble vitamin B complex nutrient that functions as a cofactor for carboxylases, which are enzymes involved in gluconeogenesis and the metabolism of amino acids and fatty acids. Biotin deficiency occurs in children receiving total parenteral nutrition without biotin supplementation. Unusual diets consisting of many raw eggs can lead to biotin deficiency because of high levels of the protein avidin in raw egg whites that binds and inactivates biotin. Biotin is also produced by bacteria in the large intestines, so broad-spectrum antibiotics may trigger a biotin deficiency because of altered intestinal flora. Other drugs, particularly anticonvulsants such as phenytoin, phenobarbital, and carbamazepine, have the potential to cause biotin deficiency because of their impairment of biotin absorption.

The inherited form of biotin deficiency is called *multiple carboxylase deficiency*. Two distinct genes have been associated with this disorder, holocarboxylase synthetase and biotinidase, two enzymes required for utilization of biotin. Holocarboxylase synthetase deficiency typically presents during infancy, and biotinidase deficiency presents in children between 3 months of age and 2 years of age. Recently, a case report of a child with multiple carboxylase deficiency despite normal dietary biotin intake and normal holocarboxylase synthetase and biotinidase suggests that a biotin transport protein deficiency can also cause biotin deficiency.

Cutaneous findings of biotin deficiency include a periorificial dermatitis resembling zinc deficiency, alopecia, blepharitis, and conjunctivitis. Organic aciduria; developmental delay; and neurologic findings such as seizures, ataxia, and hypotonia are also seen in children with biotin deficiency. Children also are at increased risk of fungal infections because of decreased immune function. In neonates, holocarboxylase synthetase deficiency often initially presents with metabolic acidosis, and without prompt recognition of the diagnosis and appropriate supplementation, it can lead to death. Although the cutaneous findings associated with all types of biotin deficiency can be reversed with supplementation, the neurologic impairment related to biotin deficiency may be permanent, further supporting the need for recognition of this deficiency.

Niacin Deficiency

Niacin is a water-soluble nutrient that is part of the vitamin B complex. Deficiency of niacin, also known as vitamin B3, leads to pellagra. The classic skin manifestations of pellagra are symmetric erythema typically occurring on sun-exposed sites associated with itching and burning that can form blisters and crusts after sunlight exposure. The lesions later become coarse, dry, and hyperpigmented. On the upper chest, keratotic hyperpigmented plaques associated with pellagra are commonly known as Casal's necklace. Oral findings include edema, atrophic glossitis, and stomatitis (Figure 127-2). Patients with niacin deficiency also develop GI symptoms, such as abdominal pain, vomiting,

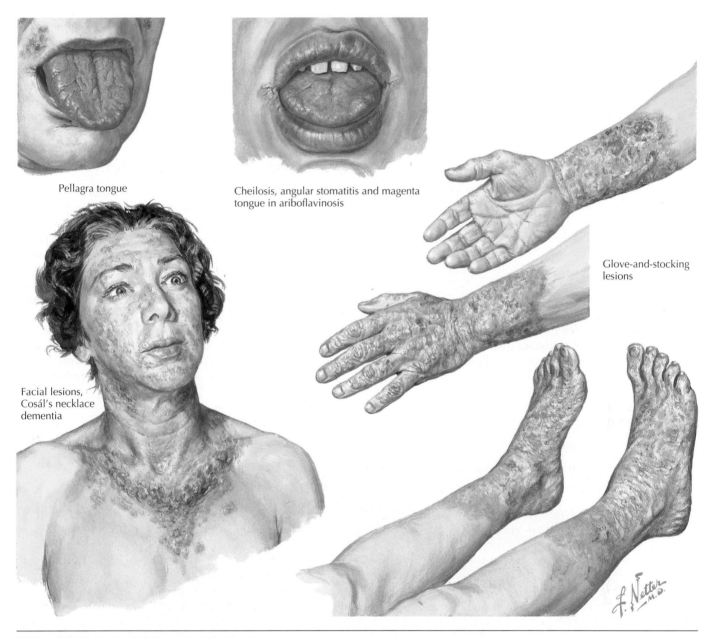

Pellagra tongue

Cheilosis, angular stomatitis and magenta tongue in ariboflavinosis

Glove-and-stocking lesions

Facial lesions, Cosál's necklace dementia

Figure 127-2 *Niacin deficiency (pellagra).*

and diarrhea, and neurologic complaints, such as vertigo. Although the symptoms of pellagra are often summarized into the three Ds—dermatitis, diarrhea, and dementia—the full spectrum of the disease is not usually seen during the early stages and is rare in pediatric patients. Although niacin is found in most foods, it is not absorbed well from corn, and thus children whose diet is almost entirely corn are at high risk of developing pellagra. Tryptophan can be converted to niacin in the body; therefore, conditions associated with tryptophan malabsorption increase the risk of developing pellagra-like symptoms. Hartnup's disease is a genetic condition in which patients have a genetic mutation in the neutral amino acid transporter gene (*SLC6A19*), resulting in poor intestinal tryptophan absorption and the potential for developing symptoms of pellagra. Drugs such as isoniazid and 5-fluorouracil that inhibit the conversion

of tryptophan to vitamin B3 or phenytoin that can decrease total serum tryptophan also increase susceptibility to development of pellagra.

Other Vitamin B Complex Deficiencies

Vitamin B6 is also known as pyridoxine, which is converted in the body into pyridoxal-5-phosphate, a coenzyme important in amino acid metabolism. Deficiency of vitamin B6 manifests with oral changes typical of all vitamin B complex deficiency, including glossitis and stomatitis. A dermatitis similar to pellagra can also be observed, likely because vitamin B6 is a cofactor in the enzyme important for the conversion of tryptophan to niacin. Vitamin B6 deficiency can manifest as a periorificial, scaly rash that resembles seborrheic dermatitis.

Deficiency of vitamin B12 (cyanocobalamin) and folic acid (vitamin B9) have similar clinical findings, and the most common is megaloblastic anemia. Cutaneous findings include painful atrophic glossitis and angular chelitis similar to many other vitamin B complex deficiencies. Dark-skinned patients may also present with hyperpigmentation with a predilection for the flexural areas, creases of the palms and soles, and nails. Many foods are fortified with folic acid, making isolated deficiency rare. Vitamin B12 is important in DNA synthesis, so children with various chronic anemias such as sickle cell disease have increased folic acid requirements. Vitamin B12 deficiency is rare in infants because the maternally derived stores last approximately 1 year. A strict vegetarian diet (veganism) is associated with vitamin B12 deficiency as well as decreased intestinal absorption caused by gastric intrinsic factor deficiency (pernicious anemia).

Vitamin C Deficiency

Vitamin C, also known as ascorbic acid, is commonly found in fresh fruit and vegetables. Scurvy, a deficiency in vitamin C, occurs in children almost exclusively because of poor dietary habits or if parenteral nutrition is exposed to light for too long because ascorbic acid is broken down by light. Follicular hyperkeratosis and abnormally curly hairs known as corkscrew hairs typically on the forearms, legs, and abdomen are observed in patients with scurvy. Other characteristic skin findings are perifollicular hemorrhage, ecchymoses, loosening of teeth, gingival hyperplasia, and bleeding gums (Figure 127-3). Subperiosteal bleeding can cause epiphyseal separation, resulting in a paucity of spontaneous limb movements (pseudoparalysis). Vitamin C is important in collagen biosynthesis; however, the mechanism of bleeding susceptibility in scurvy is not entirely known.

EVALUATION AND MANAGEMENT

When evaluating a patient with a suspected nutritional deficiency, a thorough history is of primary importance. Obtaining a complete diet history helps identify any potential deficiencies. Parental concerns about food allergy occasionally lead to severe dietary restrictions and present with a nutritional deficiency. Cultural dietary restrictions may not be readily apparent without careful investigation. Systemic illnesses that cause intestinal malabsorption should also be considered in the differential diagnosis. Laboratory testing for levels of the various nutrients will help confirm the diagnosis. If proper supplementation does not result in resolution of the symptoms, genetic testing for mutations in the various transport proteins associated with a given deficiency can be helpful as in the case of *SLC39A4* for zinc.

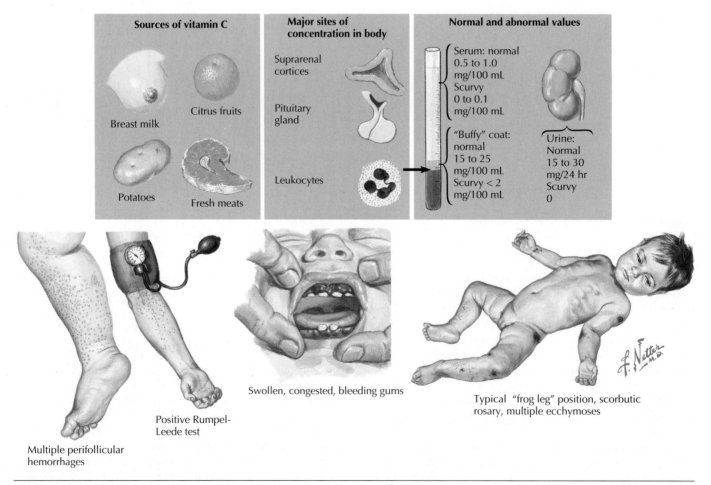

Figure 127-3 *Vitamin C deficiency (scurvy).*

FUTURE DIRECTIONS

Studies are ongoing to further identify any genetic abnormalities that may predispose individuals to nutritional deficiencies. Proper labeling of food products to help educate the public on proper dietary habits, particularly for infants to prevent inadvertent nutritional deficiency, is also an area of active work.

SUGGESTED READINGS

Heath ML, Sidbury, R: Cutaneous manifestations of nutritional deficiency, *Curr Opin Pediatr* 18:417-422, 2006.

Maverakis E, Fung MA, Lynch PJ, et al: Acrodermatitis enteropathica and an overview of zinc metabolism, *J Am Acad Dermatol* 56:116-124, 2007.

Ruiz-Maldonado R, Orozco-Covarrubias L: Nutritional diseases. In Bolognia JL, Jorizzo JL, Rapini RP, editors: *Dermatology*, ed 2, St. Louis, 2008, Elsevier.

Index

Page numbers followed by "f" indicate figures, "t" indicate tables, and "b" indicate boxes.

Eczema herpeticum, 115
Edema
  with burn injury, 39-40
  cerebral, associated with diabetic ketoacidosis, 27
  in nephrotic syndrome, 385
  in primary herpes, 559f
Edrophonium (Tensilon) test, 511-512
Edwards syndrome, 745
Elbow
  injuries, 151-153
    dislocation, 152, 153f
    overuse injuries, 152-153
  supracondylar fractures, 135-136
Electrical burns, 40
Electrocardiography, for ARF and RHD, 302
Electroencephalogram (EEG), 468
  for neurologic assessment in neonate, 644
Electrolyte loss, in diabetic ketoacidosis, 26-27
Electrolyte transport, abnormal, in CF, 247f
Electrolytes
  changes, with severe acute malnutrition, 90t
  requirements for, 82
Electron microscope findings, nephrotic syndrome, 387f
Electron transport chain, 777
Elliptocytosis, hereditary, 308
Emergencies
  anaphylactic reaction, 110-111
  hypertensive, 291-293
  neurologic
    altered level of consciousness, 63-65
    increased intracranial pressure, 65-66
    status epilepticus, 62-63
Emphysema, congenital lobar (CLE), 234
Empyema, 239
Encephalopathy, hypoxic-ischemic, 640, 644
Endocardial cushion development, 252-253
Endocarditis, infective
  clinical presentation, 590
  evaluation and management, 590-592
  pathogenesis, 590
Endocrine dysfunction
  in CKD, 402
  in trisomy 21, 743
Endocrine-mediated diarrhea, 710
End-organ dysfunction, hypertensive, 291-292
Endoscopy
  GI, 696
  for GI bleeding, 688t, 689
  for hepatobiliary disease, 727
  wireless capsule, 701
Endotheliopathy, from HUS, 394-395
Endotracheal tube (ETT), 4-5
Energy metabolism disorders
  defects in ketone metabolism, 777-778
  fatty acid oxidation disorders, 772-773, 777
  primary lactic acidosis, 777
Enfuvirtide, 600t
Entamoeba histolytica, 623
Enterobius vermicularis, 623
Enterocolitis, necrotizing, 652-653
Enterovirus infections
  nonpolio, 615-616
  of oral soft tissues, 206
Enthesitis-related arthritis, 160
Eosinophilia, 316-318
Eosinophilic gastroenteritis, 706-707, 709f
Eosinophils, 315f
Ependymomas, 354t
Ephelides, 792
Epicanthal folds, 741f
Epidermis, 782

Epididymitis, 554t, 556t
Epidural abscess, 579f
  etiology and pathogenesis, 580-581
  management and therapy, 581-582
Epidural hematoma, 48f
Epigastric hernias, 714, 717f
Epiglottitis, 212-213, 214t
Epilepsy syndromes, 466-467, 469f
  genetic, 641t
Epinephrine
  in resuscitation, 8-9
    of neonate, 670
  for shock, 15t
  treatment for anaphylaxis, 110
EpiPen, 112
Epiphyseal extrusion index, 145f
Epiphyseal lesions, differential diagnosis, 76t
Epiphysis
  complete separation from shaft, 134f
  slipped, 144f
Epstein-Barr virus (EBV), 609
  diagnosis of, 210-211
  link with Hodgkin lymphoma, 346
Ergocalciferol (vitamin D₂), 100
Erosion
  of cartilage, in psoriatic JIA, 161f
  mucosal, GI tract, 683-685
  secondary skin lesion, 782-783
Erysipelas, 563, 565f
Erythema, in JDMS, 164f
Erythema infectiosum, 615
Erythema nodosum, 700f
Erythrasma, interdigital, 621f
Erythroblastosis fetalis, 659f
Erythrocytapheresis, 330
Erythrocyte features, in Wright-stained blood smears, 315f
Escherichia coli, enterohemorrhagic (EHEC), 390
Esophageal atresia, 653-655
Esophageal varices, 725f
Esophagitis, 680
Esophagus
  developmental anomalies, 676
  gastroesophageal reflux, 678
  motility disorders, 676-680
  traumatic injuries to, 680-682
Essential fatty acid deficiency, 808
Essential hypertension, 290f
Essential thrombocytosis, 322
Ethanol, toxic ingestion, antidote, 60t
Ethylene glycol, toxic ingestion, 57t
  antidote, 60t
Ewing's sarcoma family of tumors (ESFT), 367-369
EWS rearrangements, 368
Excessive and inappropriate insulin, hypoglycemia secondary to, 450-454
Exchange transfusion
  complications of, 658
  for hyperbilirubinemia, 636, 638f
Excision, surgical, for burns, 44f
Exercise, for children with diabetes, 447
Exophthalmos, 426
Exposure assessment
  for injury and trauma, 47
  in resuscitation, 9-10
External acoustic meatus, 188f
External genitalia, differentiation, 754f
External hernias
  abdominal wall, 714
  inguinal, 714
  umbilical, 714
Extracorporeal membrane oxygenation (ECMO), 36, 286

Extrahepatic bile ducts, 724f
Extraintestinal manifestations, of IBD, 698-699, 700f
Extraintestinal parasites, 626-629
  clinical presentation, 628t
Extrinsic compression, of bowel, 690
Exudative pleural effusions, 239
Eye disorders
  abnormal red light reflex, 192
  of adnexal structures, 194-195
  associated with
    cerebral palsy, 488t
    cystic renal disease, 410t
  of eye movement, 192
  in neurofibromatosis, 483f
  red eye, 193-194
Eye(s)
  evaluation for dysmorphic disorders, 738t
  in Glasgow Coma Scale, 9f
  injury to, 50
  intracerebral hemorrhage effects, 498f
  ocular trauma, 195-196
  orbital spread of sinus infection, 544f

F
Face
  burns to, 40f
  injury to, 50
  and limb, genetic syndromes, 763
Facial angiofibromas, 801f
Facial features
  in Cornelia de Lange syndrome, 760f
  in Smith-Magenis syndrome, 750
Facial nevus, in tuberous sclerosis, 480f
Facial pain, headache attributed to, 473t-476t
Factitious hyperinsulinism, 452
Factor VIII, 333-334
Failure to thrive, 77
  clinical presentation, 102-103
  differential diagnosis, 76t
  etiology and pathogenesis, 102
  organic causes, 104-105
  psychosocial factors contributing to, 103-104
  social services, 105-106
  supplemental feeds, 105
Familial hemiplegia, 473t-476t
Familial hyperbilirubinemia, 636f
Familial juvenile systemic granulomatosis, 183
Familial short stature, 458, 464
Family history, for glomerulonephritis, 383
Fanconi anemia, 318t
Fanconi syndrome, 434
Fast-flow lesions, arteriovenous malformations, 790-791
Fat malabsorption
  in CF, 248
  resulting in diarrhea, 706, 709-710
Fats, dietary requirements, 82
Fatty acid oxidation disorders, 453, 772-773, 777
Febrile seizures, 466
Fecal impaction, 713
Fecal osmolar gap, 704
Feeding
  difficulties with, treatment of, 105
  evaluation, for failure to thrive, 103
  history, in evaluation of wheezing, 221
Femoral anteversion, 141-142
Femoral neck stress fractures, 153
Femur fractures, 138
Fetal circulation, 256
Fever
  acute complication of sickle cell disease, 326
  rheumatic. See Rheumatic fever
  in roseola, 614